midwifery

Preparation for Practice 5e

BOOK 2

midwifery
Preparation for Practice 5e

Sally Pairman, Sally K Tracy, Hannah G Dahlen, Lesley Dixon

ELSEVIER

ELSEVIER

Elsevier Australia. ACN 001 002 357
(a division of Reed International Books Australia Pty Ltd)
Tower 1, 475 Victoria Avenue, Chatswood, NSW 2067

ISBN (Two-Book set): 978-0-7295-4381-1
ISBN (Book 2): 978-0-7295-4383-5

National Library of Australia Cataloguing-in-Publication Data

NATIONAL LIBRARY OF AUSTRALIA

A catalogue record for this book is available from the National Library of Australia

Content Strategist: Libby Houston
Content Project Manager: Shruti Raj
Edited by Laura Davies
Proofread by Melissa Faulkner
Copyrights Coordinator: Saravanan Murugan
Cover and internal design by Georgette Hall
Index by Innodata Indexing

Typeset by GW Tech

Printed in India by Multivista Global Pvt. Ltd, Chennai.

Contents

Detailed contents

BOOK 2: Midwifery practice

BOOK 2

Midwifery practice

SECTION 1

Autonomous practice

CHAPTER 20

Overview of reproductive physiology

Sally Baddock

LEARNING OUTCOMES

Learning outcomes for this chapter are:

1. To describe the key structures in the female and male reproductive systems and relate these to the processes of reproduction
2. To outline the physiological changes and hormonal control of the ovarian and uterine cycles
3. To describe the process of fertilisation and implantation
4. To list key events in the continuum of development from zygote to embryo to mature fetus
5. To describe the development and functioning of fetal, uteroplacental and feto-placental circulation
6. To describe maternal anatomical and physiological changes associated with pregnancy, and the role of hormones in the maintenance of pregnancy.

CHAPTER OVERVIEW

This chapter focuses on the physiological processes associated with conception and pregnancy. This begins with the formation of the gametes in the female and male reproductive systems, and continues with an overview of embryology from fertilisation until birth. It includes the simultaneous development of the placenta to support the embryo, and the physiological changes associated with pregnancy occurring in the woman. A good understanding of these physiological processes is essential if a midwife is to make informed decisions with regard to monitoring the woman and fetus and interpretation of test results. It also enables informed discussion with the woman regarding the changes occurring to her body as the fetus develops, and an understanding of the factors that contribute to a healthy environment for normal embryological and fetal development.

For ease of study, the development of the embryo and placenta and the changes in the woman through pregnancy are presented as separate topics, but the processes are interwoven and simultaneous. The scope of this chapter is limited, but further reading is provided at the end of the chapter for a more in-depth exploration of specific topics. Some of the online resources listed provide animations that can help with the understanding of complex anatomical changes.

KEY TERMS

blastocyst
conception
embryology
gonadotrophins
hypothalamic–pituitary
implantation
morula
oogenesis
spermatogenesis
uteroplacental circulation

INTRODUCTION

A good understanding of the physiological processes underpinning conception and pregnancy is essential if a midwife is to make informed decisions with regard to monitoring the woman and fetus and to interpretation of test results. It also enables informed discussion with the woman regarding the changes occurring to her body as the fetus develops, and an understanding of the factors that contribute to a healthy environment for normal embryological and fetal development. This chapter explores the physiological processes in the male and female that enable conception and then follows the development of the embryo / fetus, the placenta and the physiological changes in the woman that support pregnancy. A significant focus is on the hormonal changes that drive these processes. Readers are advised to use this chapter as an adjunct to texts such as that by Blackburn (2017) or Rankin (2017).

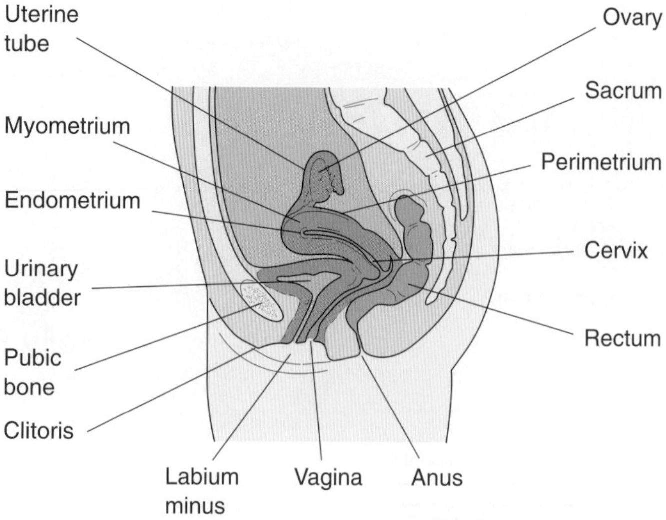

FIGURE 20.1 The female pelvic region: schematic sagittal section (Based on Moore & Persaud, 1998)

FEMALE AND MALE REPRODUCTIVE SYSTEMS

The physiological roles of the female and male reproductive systems are to produce and maintain sex cells (gametes), to transport the gametes to the site of fertilisation and to produce and secrete sex hormones, which control the reproductive process. The female reproductive system has the additional role of supporting the developing fetus. The structures of the female and male reproductive systems underpin these roles.

Anatomy of the female reproductive system

The female reproductive system consists of a pair of female gonads, commonly referred to as the ovaries, as well as a number of accessory ducts—specifically the uterine or fallopian tubes, the uterus and the vagina. The ovaries and the accessory ducts make up the internal female genitalia. The external female genitalia are referred to as the vulva and consist of the mons pubis, labia majora, labia minora, clitoris and vestibule. The mammary glands of the female are also important in the reproductive system following reproduction.

Female internal genitalia

The structures of the female internal genitalia are depicted in Fig. 20.1.

The ovaries have two important roles in the reproductive system: to produce female sex cells (oocytes) through the process of **oogenesis**, and to produce the female sex hormones—the oestrogens (oestradiol, oestrone and oestriol) and progesterone.

The uterine tubes link the ovaries and the uterus, although there is no anatomical connection. The distal ends of the uterine tubes end in fimbriae (fingerlike projections), which waft the ovulated ovum in the peritoneum towards the opening of the fallopian tube. Contractions of smooth muscle in the walls of the uterine tubes and the wafting action of cilia lining the walls aid oocyte movement (fertilised or not) to the uterus.

The uterus is a hollow cavity consisting of three regions: the fundus, the body and the cervix. The fundus is the region superior to the uterine tubes. The body is the major portion of the uterus and is the site where **implantation** occurs. The cervix is the region that connects the uterus with the vagina and consists of the cervical canal, the internal os and external os. The uterus is a thick-walled organ with three layers: the perimetrium (outer layer), the myometrium (thick muscle layer) and the endometrium (the inner mucosal lining). The perimetrium is a thin serous layer composed of epithelial cells derived from the visceral peritoneum. The myometrium is the thickest layer of the uterus. It is comprised of smooth muscle that is responsible for uterine contractions. The endometrium consists of two layers: the stratum basalis, which lies next to the myometrium, and the stratum functionalis—the outer mucosa that is shed during menstruation (Fig. 20.2).

The vagina is often referred to as the 'birth canal', and is the region of the internal female genitalia that connects to the external female genitalia. The vagina is a passage for semen during intercourse and for menstrual blood during menstruation. The epithelial cells that line the vagina produce glycogen, which is metabolised to lactic acid by the vaginal microflora. This results in the vagina having an acidic pH, which protects against foreign microorganisms as well as destroying many sperm cells that enter the vagina.

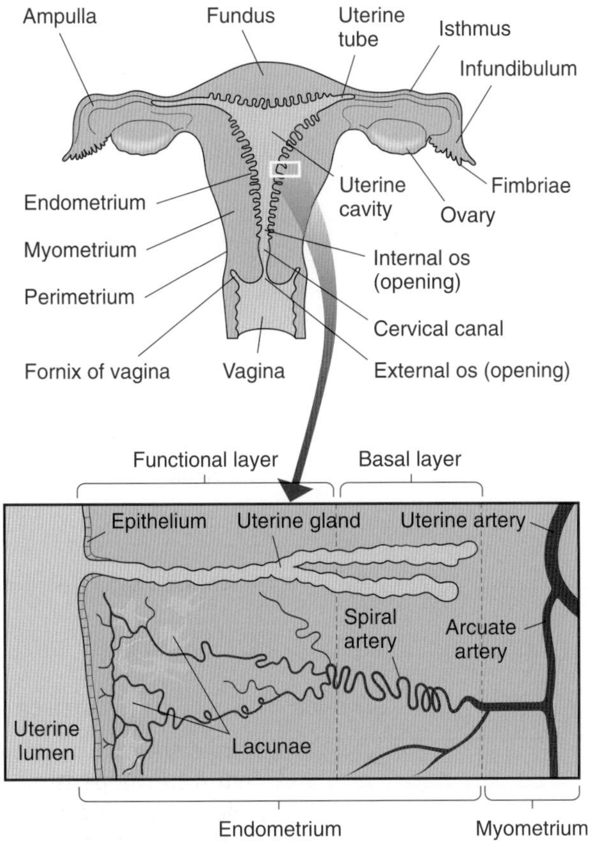

FIGURE 20.2 Female reproductive organs
(Based on Moore & Persaud, 1998)

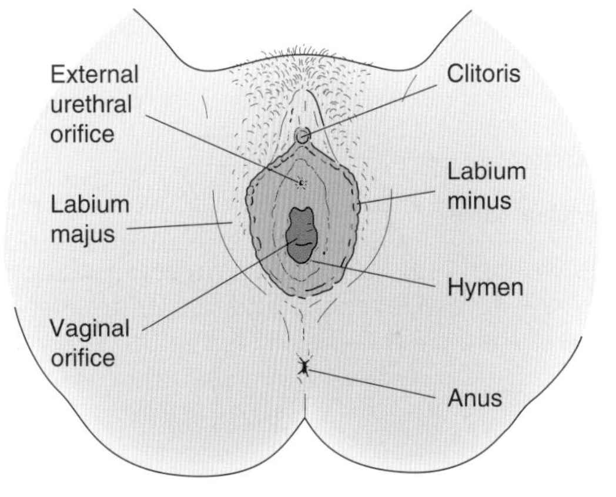

FIGURE 20.3 External female genitalia: the labia are spread apart to show the external urethral and vaginal orifices within the vestibule area
(Based on Moore & Persaud, 1998)

CRITICAL THINKING EXERCISE

Discuss the physiological and anatomical aspects of the uterus that make it a suitable organ for supporting and nurturing an embryo/fetus.

Female external genitalia

The female external genitalia or vulva—mons pubis, labia majora, labia minora, clitoris and hymen—are shown in Fig. 20.3.

Mammary glands

The mammary glands or breasts are also present in the male but produce milk only in the female. The breasts are a type of sweat gland (sudiferous gland), positioned over the pectoralis major and serratus anterior muscles and attached by connective tissue. Suspensory ligaments support the breasts and are present between the skin and the deep fascia of the muscle. The areola is the region surrounding the nipple and contains modified sebaceous (oil) glands, known as Montgomery's tubercles, which help to keep the tissue protected and supple by secreting a lubricant. Each breast contains adipose tissue, which determines the size of the breast but not the capacity or function of the breast. Within the breast clusters of alveoli, milk-secreting glands are connected to fine ducts that merge into ever larger ducts until these merge into a primary milk duct that leads to the nipple. Each breast contains 4–18 primary milk ducts. The milk is produced in the alveoli and passes into the branching duct system. Previously it was thought that small ducts from each lobule drained into a lactiferous sinus that opened onto the nipple surface, but ultrasound has demonstrated that these sinuses do not exist. This suggests that ducts transport breast milk, rather than store it. There is sometimes dilation of the ducts following milk ejection but this resolves as milk flows (Ramsay et al., 2005). The two hormones important in lactation are prolactin, secreted by the anterior pituitary, and oxytocin, secreted by the posterior pituitary. Prolactin is important for milk production and oxytocin is important in the let-down or milk-release reflex.

The female pelvis

The pelvic bones provide points of attachment for the lower limbs and transmit the weight of the trunk to these limbs, and provide support to the pelvic organs. The size and shape of the female pelvis in relation to the fetal skull is an important determinant of successful childbirth.

The pelvic (hip) girdle

The pelvic girdle consists of a pair of hip (innominate) bones. They join anteriorly at the symphysis pubis and meet posteriorly with the sacrum to form the sacroiliac joint. Together, the innominate bones, sacrum and coccyx form the deep basin-like structure known as the bony pelvis. Each innominate bone actually consists of three separate bones: the ilium, the ischium and the pubis (Figs. 20.4 and 20.5). In infancy these three bones are

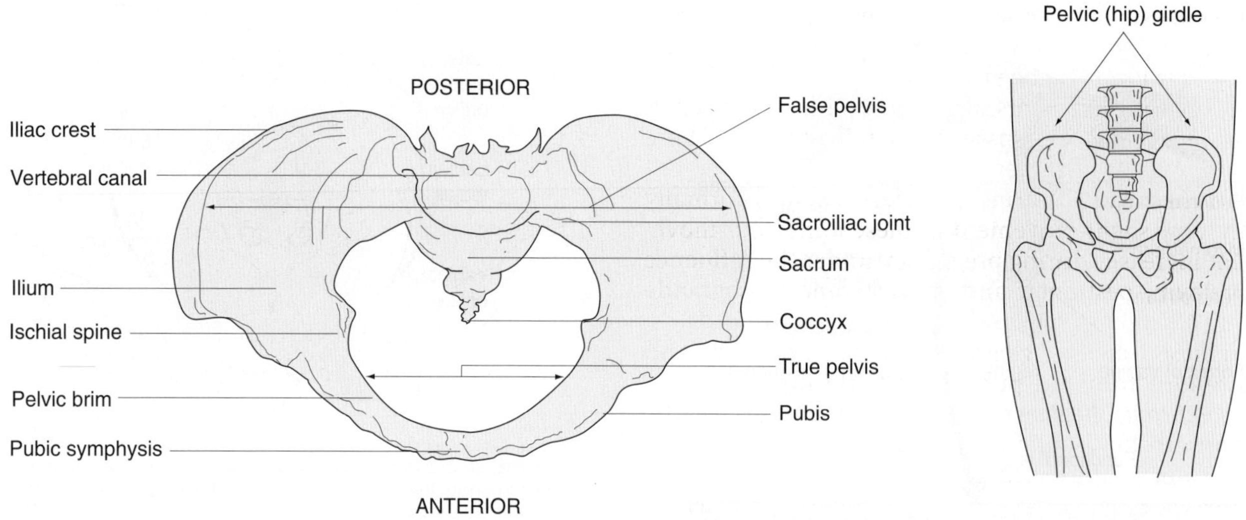

FIGURE 20.4 Female pelvis: superior view
(Based on Tortora, 2006)

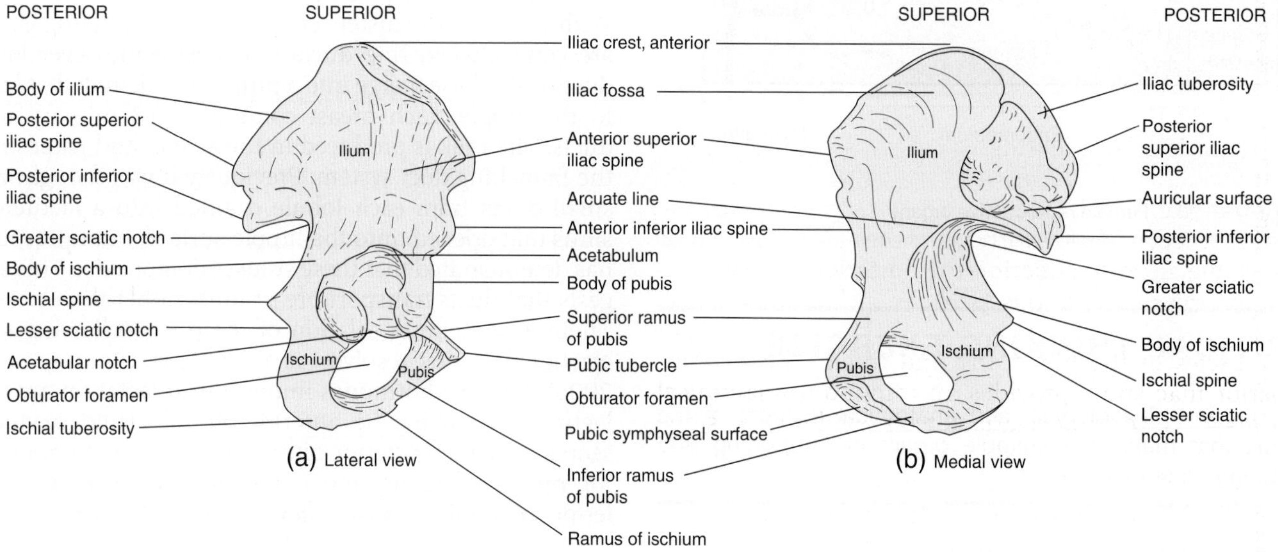

FIGURE 20.5 The right hip bone: (a) lateral view; (b) medial view
(Based on Tortora, 2006)

separate. By puberty most growth is completed, and the three bones fuse at the acetabulum (cup-shaped hollow in the bone). Growth continues in other areas of the pelvis (i.e. the iliac crests, the ischial tuberosities—bumps or protuberances on the ischium) until the early twenties (Huseynov et al., 2016) or even early thirties (Sharma et al., 2016).

Joints of the pelvic girdle

The pelvic bones are characterised by three joints (see Fig. 20.4):

- sacroiliac—between sacrum and ilium
- pubic symphysis—unites the two pubic bones anteriorly
- hip (coxal)—between coxal (innominate) bones and femur.

Ligaments associated with the pelvic girdle

Ligaments are dense bands of fibrous tissue that serve to reinforce joints and to maintain bones in their correct anatomical arrangement. They contain collagen and elastic fibres. The elastic fibres enable ligaments to stretch, and this assists in the softening of the pubic symphysis and sacroiliac joints during pregnancy. This softening is stimulated by hormones such as relaxin, oestrogen and progesterone. Joint laxity may lead to backache and joint instability (Casagrande et al., 2015) although a systematic review suggests that the level of evidence for an association between levels of relaxin and pelvic pain during pregnancy is low (Aldabe et al., 2012).

The following ligaments support the joints of the pelvis.

- *Sacroiliac ligaments*—span the sacroiliac joints. These are very strong ligaments that transmit the weight of the trunk, head and arms to the legs. There is normally only very slight movement at these joints, but movement increases during pregnancy under the influence of relaxin, oestrogen and progesterone (Casagrande et al., 2015).
- *Symphysis pubis ligaments*—bridge anteriorly and posteriorly from one pubic bone to the other.
- *Sacrotuberous ligaments*—run from the sides of the sacrum to the ischial tuberosities (across the greater and lesser sciatic notches).
- *Sacrospinous ligaments*—run from the sides of the sacrum to the ischial spines (across the greater sciatic notch).
- *Sacrococcygeal ligaments*—run from the sacrum to the coccyx.
- *Inguinal ligaments*—run from the anterior superior iliac spine to the lateral edge of the pubic bone, forming the groin.

Bones of the pelvic girdle

Ilium

The ilium is a large flaring bone that forms the major part of the hip bone. It consists of a body and ala (wings). Important landmarks include the iliac crests, which are the thickened, superior portions of the alae, and the iliac spines: the anterior superior, the posterior superior, the anterior inferior and the posterior inferior. The iliac spines provide important points of muscle attachment for muscles of the hip, trunk and thigh. The anterior superior iliac spine provides an important anatomical landmark. The greater sciatic notch provides for passage of the sciatic nerve and the iliac fossa is found on the medial surface of iliac alae. The auricular surface is the point of articulation between the ilium and the sacrum, and the ileopectineal line runs anteriorly and inferiorly from the auricular surface. Together with the sacral promontory, the ileopectineal line defines the pelvic brim—that is, the superior margin of the true pelvis (Rankin, 2017) (Fig. 20.6).

Ischium

The ischium forms the posterior inferior part of the hip bone and appears L or arc shaped. It is composed of a superior portion, the body, and an inferior portion, the ramus (or the branch). Important landmarks include the ischial spines, which project medially into the pelvic cavity and are the points of attachment for the sacrospinous ligament. The lesser sciatic notch allows nerves and blood vessels to pass through on their way from the pelvis to the thigh. The ischial tuberosities bear our upper body weight when we sit. They also provide attachments for hamstring muscles and the sacrotuberous ligament (Rankin, 2017).

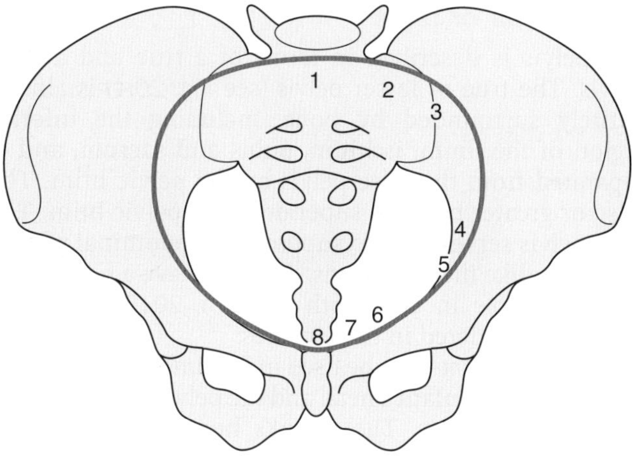

FIGURE 20.6 The pelvic brim: 1 = sacral promontory; 2 = sacral ala; 3 = sacroiliac joint; 4 = ileopectineal line; 5 = ileopectineal eminence; 6 = superior pubis ramis; 7 = body of pubic bone; 8 = symphysis pubis
(From Stables & Rankin, 2005)

Pubic bones

The pubic bones form the anterior part of the innominate bone and are V-shaped. Important landmarks include the pubic crests, which are formed by the anterior border of the pubic bones, and the pubic tubercle, which provides attachment for the inguinal ligament. The obturator foramen is an opening covered by a membrane through which the obturator nerve and blood vessels pass. The pubic arch is formed from inferior borders of pubic rami. This structure is wider in females, serving to increase the anteroposterior diameter of the pelvic outlet (Rankin, 2017).

Sacrum

The sacrum is formed by five fused sacral vertebrae, attached superiorly to the fifth lumbar vertebrae and inferiorly to the coccyx. Its two alae articulate with the ilium at the sacroiliac joint. The ventral and dorsal sacral foramina are openings situated laterally on the sacrum through which nerves and blood vessels pass.

Sacral promontory

The first sacral vertebra has a distinct anterosuperior bulge: the sacral promontory. The degree to which this structure projects into the pelvic cavity has clinical implications for labour and childbirth.

Coccyx

The coccyx, a small triangular-shaped bone, is formed from three to five fused vertebrae. The coccyx articulates with the inferior border of the sacrum via the sacrococcygeal ligament. The coccyx is seen to project less into the pelvic outlet in the female and is slightly more able to move posteriorly than seen in the male pelvis. This positioning and mobility of the coccyx assist the descent of the infant head during childbirth.

Pelvis, true or false

The pelvis is described in terms of a true and a false pelvis. The true or lesser pelvis (see Fig. 20.4) is almost entirely surrounded by bone, including the inferior region of the ilium, ischium, pubis and sacrum, and is separated from the false pelvis by the pelvic brim. The false or greater pelvis is superior to the pelvic brim. The false pelvis serves only to support the abdominal viscera and so, unlike the true pelvis, does not have a potentially restrictive role in childbirth (Rankin, 2017). The true pelvis is considered in three planes:

- The *pelvic brim*—can be used in pelvimetry to establish whether the infant's head and the pelvis share compatible dimensions. The infant's head passes through the pelvic brim when it engages in late pregnancy or during the onset of labour.
- The *pelvic cavity*—the dimensions of this area are normally enhanced by the curvature of the sacrum. The rounded shape of the cavity encourages rotation of the baby's head; the ischial spines can reduce the dimensions of the pelvic cavity. The infant's head is considered engaged when it has reached the level of the ischial spines as well as when the fetal head is flexed and the widest diameter of the fetal head (suboccipitobregmatic of 9.5 cm and biparietal diameter of 9.5 cm) have passed into the brim of the pelvis (Rankin, 2017).
- The *pelvic outlet*—can be described as the anatomical or the obstetric outlet. The anatomical outlet refers to the lower border of the pelvis and is not significant in terms of birth; but the obstetric outlet, the constricted lower portion of the pelvis, is more relevant. It is bounded by the subpubic arch, the ischial spines, the sacrospinous ligaments and the lower border of the sacrum (Rankin, 2017). The sacrococcygeal joint is flexible to a degree, which allows the coccyx to move posteriorly out of the way during childbirth.

The maximum diameter of the pelvis through which the infant's head can pass differs for all three planes. Initially the largest diameter is in the transverse plane (pelvic brim), but the anteroposterior diameter becomes the largest at the pelvic outlet, particularly in females who possess a classical gynaecoid pelvis where the angle of the subpubic arch is equal to or greater than 90° (Rankin, 2017). Measurements of the diameter of the pelvis at the brim, cavity and outlet are presented in Table 20.1.

The shape of the pelvis can vary between individuals. Although the gynaecoid shape is most common in women, three other types have been described: the android, anthropoid and platypelloid pelvis. These are illustrated in Fig. 20.7.

- The android pelvis has male-type features. It is characterised by a small inlet that is somewhat heart shaped. The side walls converge, causing the pelvis to narrow as the fetus descends. The ischial spines are prominent and the angle of the subpubic arch is less than 90°. This type of pelvis is least suited to childbearing.

Table 20.1 Pelvic measurements

	Anteroposterior (cm)	Oblique (cm)	Transverse (cm)
Brim	11	12	13
Cavity	12	12	12
Outlet	13	12	11

(Source: Stables & Rankin, 2010)

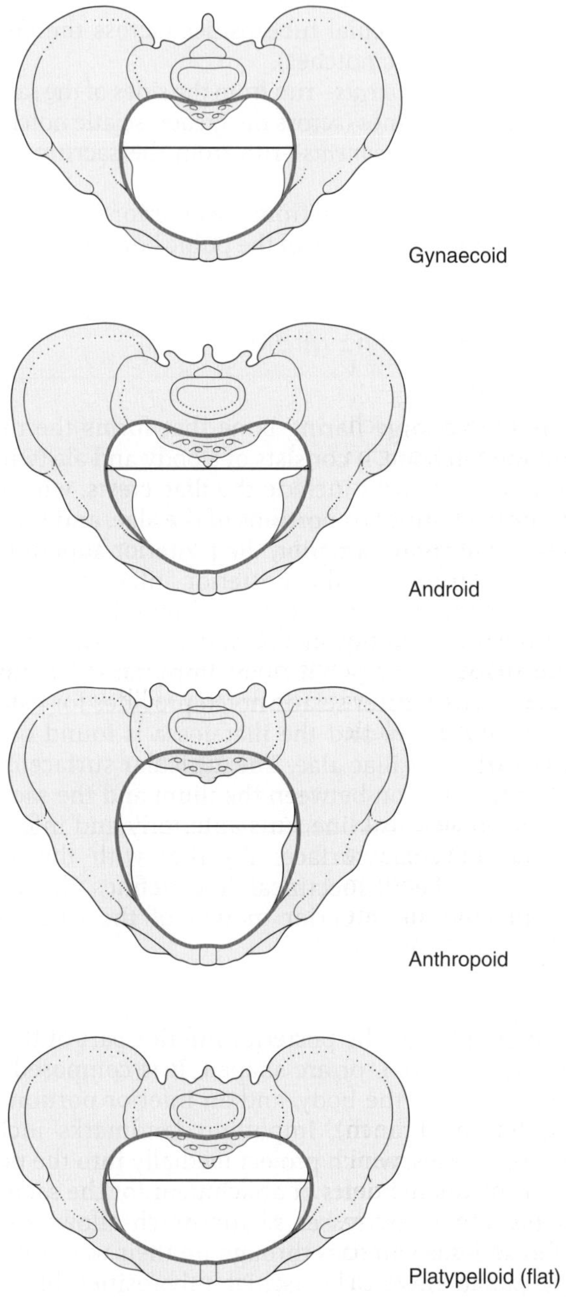

FIGURE 20.7 Shapes of the pelvic brim
(From Coad & Dunstall, 2005)

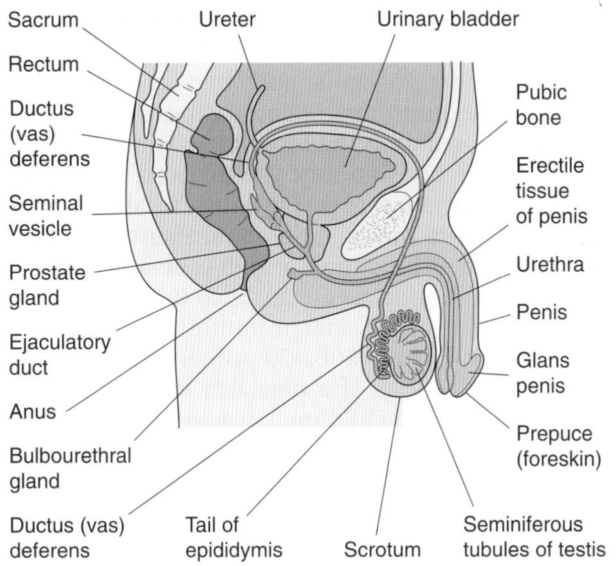

FIGURE 20.8 The male pelvic region: schematic sagittal section
(Based on Moore & Persaud, 1998)

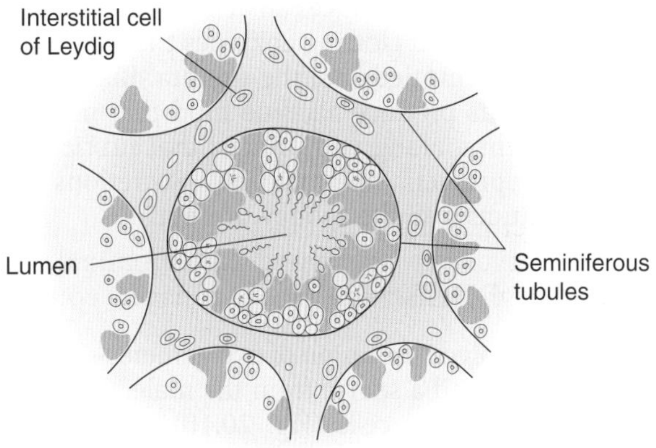

FIGURE 20.9 The testis in cross-section: illustrating the seminiferous tubules and interstitial cells of Leydig
(Based on Bray et al. 1994)

- In the anthropoid pelvis the anteroposterior diameter is greater than the transverse diameter, but the pelvis is generally large all over. The side walls are parallel or flare outwards, ischial spines are not prominent and the subpubic angle may be normal or wide. The pelvis is so large that delivery may occur without rotation.
- In the platypelloid pelvis there is a reduced anteroposterior diameter. The side walls diverge, the cavity is shallow and the ischial spines are blunt with a wide subpubic angle. The fetus may have difficulties entering the brim, but not after this.

The shape of the pelvis does not necessarily predict whether a successful vaginal delivery is likely; the size of the fetal head in relation to the pelvis is more important (Rankin, 2017).

Childbirth is dependent on the ability of the baby to move, to ensure that the maximum diameter of the baby's skull moves to align with the maximum diameter of the pelvis. These manoeuvres are called the mechanism of labour and are outlined in the later chapters on this topic.

Anatomy of the male reproductive system

The structures of the male reproductive system (Fig. 20.8) include the testes, penis, accessory ducts (epididymis, vas deferens or ductus deferens, ejaculatory ducts and urethra) and the accessory glands (prostate gland, seminal vesicles and bulbourethral glands).

The paired testes each contain coiled seminiferous tubules, which are the site of sperm production (Fig. 20.9). The sperm are moved from the seminiferous tubules to the coils of the epididymis by peristalsis. Secretions from the adjacent Sertoli cells in the seminiferous tubules build up pressure and contribute to the movement of sperm.

In the epididymis, sperm mature and become motile after approximately 14–21 days. During ejaculation, peristaltic contractions move spermatozoa from the epididymis to the vas deferens, through the ejaculatory duct and into the urethra. The urethra runs from the urinary bladder to the outside of the body, with part of the urethra (spongy urethra) running through the penis. The urethra has the dual role of transporting urine and sperm to exit the body.

During sexual excitement, the three columns of erectile tissue surrounding the urethra become engorged with blood, resulting in erection. This enables the penis to enter the vagina during sexual intercourse. Further stimulation leads to ejaculation of semen (sperm and secretions).

Accessory sex glands and semen

Semen is the alkaline fluid that protects, nourishes and transports sperm during ejaculation. Two to five millilitres are ejaculated during orgasm, containing 50–100 million sperm / mL. At least 20 million sperm / mL are necessary for fertility. However, 90% of the fluid is made up of secretions from the seminal vesicles, prostate gland and bulbourethral glands.

Seminal vesicles release alkaline secretions into the ejaculatory duct that contain several chemicals, including fibrinogen, fructose and prostaglandins. Fibrinogen helps to coagulate semen just after ejaculation, and this contributes to retention of semen in the region of the uterine cervix until the sperm become motile. Fructose nourishes the sperm, and prostaglandins aid fertilisation by making the cervical mucus more receptive. Prostaglandins also stimulate uterine contractions, which suck semen into the uterus and fallopian tubes, enabling them to reach the ampulla as soon as 5 minutes after ejaculation, to up to 6 hours later. These secretions also dilute epididymal inhibitory factor, which is thought to suppress the motility of spermatozoa.

The prostate gland produces an acidic, milky fluid containing citric acid and clotting enzymes that aid coagulation, and this is emptied into the urethra. Bulbourethral (Cowper's) glands produce alkaline fluid that neutralises the acidic urethra, along with mucus that lubricates the urethra and protects spermatozoa. Secretions travel through the ducts into the spongy urethra.

Gametogenesis

Fertilisation involves the union of two gametes—an oocyte from the female and a sperm from the male. Gametes are highly specialised sex cells (Fig. 20.10). Gametogenesis (formation of the sex cells) necessarily involves halving the number of chromosomes in each cell, by a type of cell division called meiosis, and by altering the shape of the cells. In females this process is termed oogenesis and in males it is called **spermatogenesis**. When the two gametes join at fertilisation, the full number of chromosomes is restored.

Oogenesis

Oogenesis is the process by which mature female sex cells are formed. Much of this process occurs in the fetus prior to birth. Oogonia in the fetus multiply by mitotic division and develop into primary oocytes (containing 46 chromosomes). The first meiotic division also begins before birth, but is arrested until after puberty. Completion of the first meiotic division is linked to the ovarian cycle. Each month, following puberty, several primary oocytes begin to develop but only one matures to complete the first meiotic division 36–48 hours before ovulation (Moore et al., 2013). This division results in a large secondary oocyte containing most of the cytoplasm, and a smaller non-functional polar body that soon degenerates. Each has 23 chromosomes (22 autosomes and 1 sex chromosome). At ovulation the secondary oocyte begins the second meiotic division, but the division is completed only if fertilisation occurs. Once again, almost all the cytoplasm goes to one cell, the mature oocyte; a second polar body is non-functional and degenerates. The cellular divisions of oogenesis are outlined in Fig. 20.11.

The mature oocyte is a large, immotile cell, just visible to the naked eye. Up to 800,000 primary oocytes may be present in the ovaries of a newborn female infant, but many regress during childhood, leaving about 40,000 at puberty. During the reproductive life of a female, about 400 oocytes mature and are released during ovulation (Moore et al., 2013).

Spermatogenesis

Spermatogenesis describes the development of spermatogonia (primitive germ cells) into spermatozoa. This process begins at puberty and continues through adult life. At puberty, the spermatogonia increase in number by mitotic division and grow and change to form primary spermatocytes ($2n$ chromosomes). Each primary spermatocyte undergoes the first meiotic division to form two secondary spermatocytes (n chromosomes) and the second meiotic division to result in four spermatids (n chromosomes).

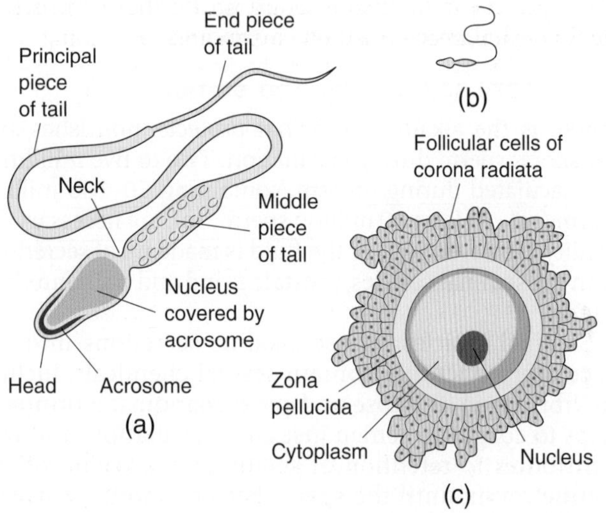

FIGURE 20.10 Male and female gametes. (a) Parts of the human sperm (×1250). The head, composed mostly of the nucleus, is partly covered by the acrosome, an organelle containing enzymes. The tail consists of three regions: middle piece, principal piece and end piece. (b) Sperm drawn to about the same scale as the oocyte. (c) Human secondary oocyte or ovum (×200) surrounded by the zona pellucida and corona radiata
(Based on Moore & Persaud, 1998)

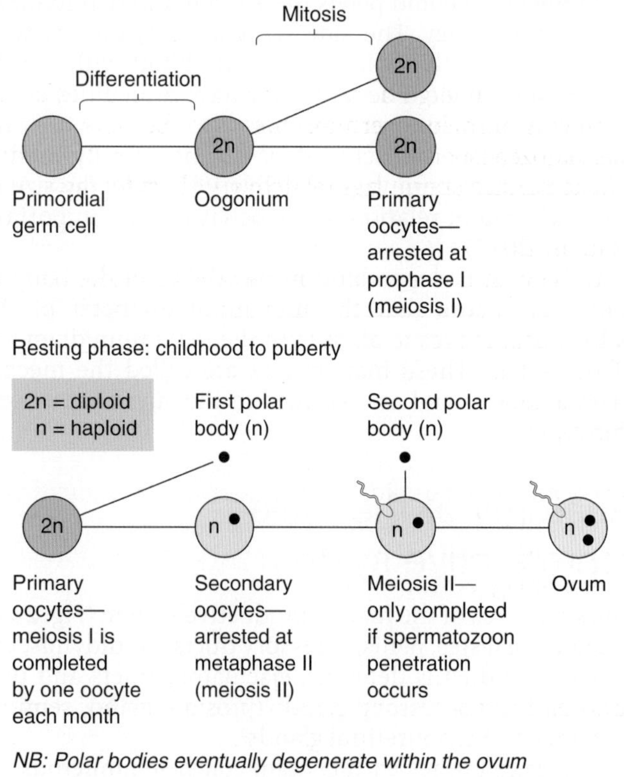

FIGURE 20.11 Arrest of oocyte meiosis
(Based on Coad & Dunstall, 2001)

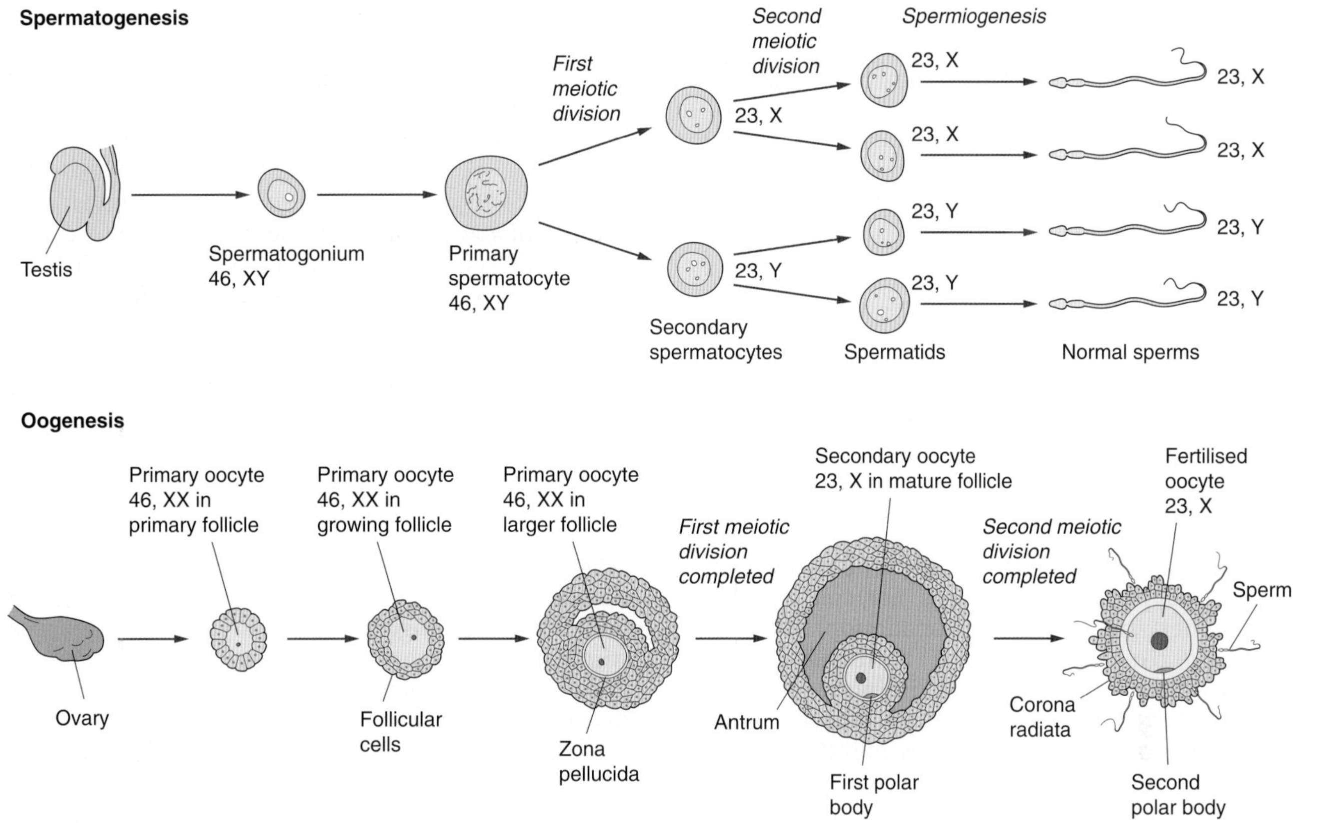

FIGURE 20.12 Comparison of oogenesis and spermatogenesis
(Based on Moore & Persaud, 1998)

Spermatids undergo a considerable change in shape, in a process termed spermiogenesis, to become mature spermatozoa (sperm).

The mature sperm has relatively little cytoplasm. It is divided into a head, midpiece and tail, and is motile. The head is the largest structure. It contains the nucleus with the chromosomes and is covered anteriorly by the acrosome—a structure containing enzymes that facilitate penetration of the ovum at fertilisation. The midpiece is rich in energy-producing mitochondria, which fuel the lashing movements of the tail. Spermatogenesis takes about 2 months to complete and continues throughout the reproductive life of a male (Moore et al., 2013). The sperm move to the epididymis, where they are stored and become functionally mature.

A comparison of oogenesis and spermatogenesis is shown in Fig. 20.12.

Female reproductive cycles

Females undergo monthly reproductive cycles starting at puberty and continuing through the reproductive years. These cycles are controlled by the hypothalamic–pituitary–ovarian hormones and result in changes in the ovary that lead to release of one secondary oocyte per month, and in changes in the uterus in preparation for implantation of the fertilised ovum. If fertilisation does not occur, the cycle begins again under the influence of the **hypothalamic–pituitary** hormones. For simplicity, the reproductive cycle is described as an average 28-day cycle. There is considerable individual variation, but the cycle length is most commonly between 26 and 34 days (Blackburn, 2017).

Ovarian cycle

The ovarian cycle (Fig. 20.13) includes three phases: the follicular or preovulatory phase, the ovulatory phase or ovulation, and the postovulatory or luteal phase.

Follicular phase

In the follicular phase the ovarian follicles, containing an oocyte, mature. Ovarian follicles are found in the cortex of the ovary and contain a variety of cells including primary or secondary oocytes, granulosa cells and theca cells. Oocytes are surrounded by a thick membrane, the zona pelucida, and in mature follicles there is a large fluid-filled cavity, the antrum.

Follicles are present in several forms: primordial (the most undeveloped), primary, secondary and Graafian or vesicular (the most mature).

- Primordial follicles contain primary oocytes and are the type of follicle present at birth. The first meiotic

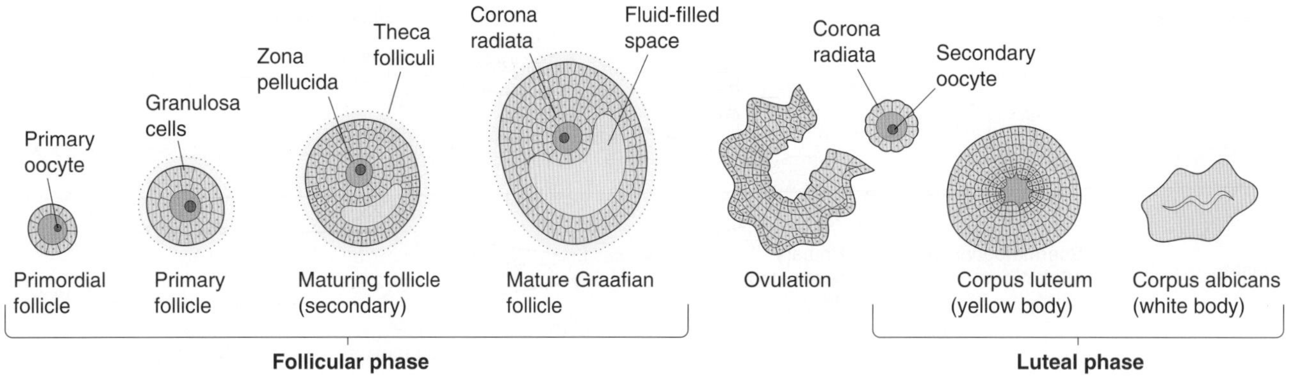

FIGURE 20.13 The ovarian cycle
(Based on Coad & Dunstall, 2001)

division has already begun in utero, but the process is arrested part way and does not continue again until puberty, when levels of gonadotrophin-releasing hormone (GnRH), luteinising hormone (LH) and follicle-stimulating hormone (FSH) increase.
- The primary follicle is formed in response to the increased level of the hormones mentioned above. The hormones signal the cells surrounding the oocyte to proliferate and form a layer of granulosa cells. These cells allow nutrients and signalling molecules to reach the oocyte.
- The secondary follicle is formed when a layer of connective tissue, called the theca folliculi, develops around the follicle and an antrum begins to develop with it. The thecal cells, together with the granulosa cells, produce steroid hormones (mainly oestrogens with small quantities of progesterone). The secondary follicle is also characterised by the zona pellucida, which surrounds the oocyte and is released along with the oocyte at ovulation.
- Graafian or vesicular follicles are the final and most mature form of ovarian follicle. This stage of follicular development is characterised by a large antrum and a follicular size of approximately 2.5 cm diameter. Due to its size it bulges from the ovary midway through the ovarian cycle.

The completion of meiosis I, in which a secondary oocyte and the first polar body are formed, occurs about 36 hours before ovulation (Blackburn, 2017). Meiosis II continues but is not completed until fertilisation occurs. The process of meiosis results in the genetic material in each oocyte being halved from 46 chromosomes ($2n$) to 23 chromosomes (n).

Ovulation

The ovulatory phase begins when oestrogen levels peak and ends when the vesicular follicle ruptures, releasing the secondary oocyte surrounded by the zona pellucida and corona radiata (the crown of granulosa cells around the zona pellucida). Ovulation is under hormonal control, as follows: LH interacts with LH receptors on the granulosa cells, increasing the production of oestrogen by the dominant follicle. A rise in oestrogen levels 48 hours before ovulation triggers the LH surge. The high level of LH stimulates production of prostaglandins ($PGF_{2\alpha}$ and PGE_2), and allows the primary oocyte to complete the first meiotic division and become a secondary oocyte. Simultaneously, levels of oestrogen drop and proteolytic enzymes are synthesised, which break down the thecal cells and assist rupture of the vesicular follicle (Blackburn, 2017).

Luteal phase

This is the final stage of the ovarian cycle. The ruptured follicle remains in the ovary and the antrum begins to fill with clotted blood. The granulosa and some thecal cells form a structure called the corpus luteum (yellow body). This is an endocrine structure capable of producing progesterone and smaller amounts of oestrogen. The purpose of the corpus luteum is to provide progesterone until the placenta is adequately formed. If fertilisation does not occur, the corpus luteum degenerates into a corpus albicans (white body) and is degraded through lysosomal activity.

Uterine cycle

The uterine cycle occurs in the same time frame as the ovarian cycle and is similarly controlled by changes in hormonal levels (Fig. 20.14). It consists of three stages: the menstrual phase (days 1–5), the proliferative phase (days 6–14) and the secretory phase (days 15–28). The following is a review of each stage.

Menstrual phase

Menstruation is triggered by several factors. The first is a drop in levels of progesterone and oestradiol (one form of oestrogen). The second is a change in the ratio of prostaglandins and prostacyclins (hormone-like compounds) that cause vasoconstriction and increased coiling of the spiral arterioles, leading to a decrease in blood flow to the stratum functionalis of the uterus. The cells in the stratum functionalis become ischaemic and necrosed, and slough away from the stratum basalis.

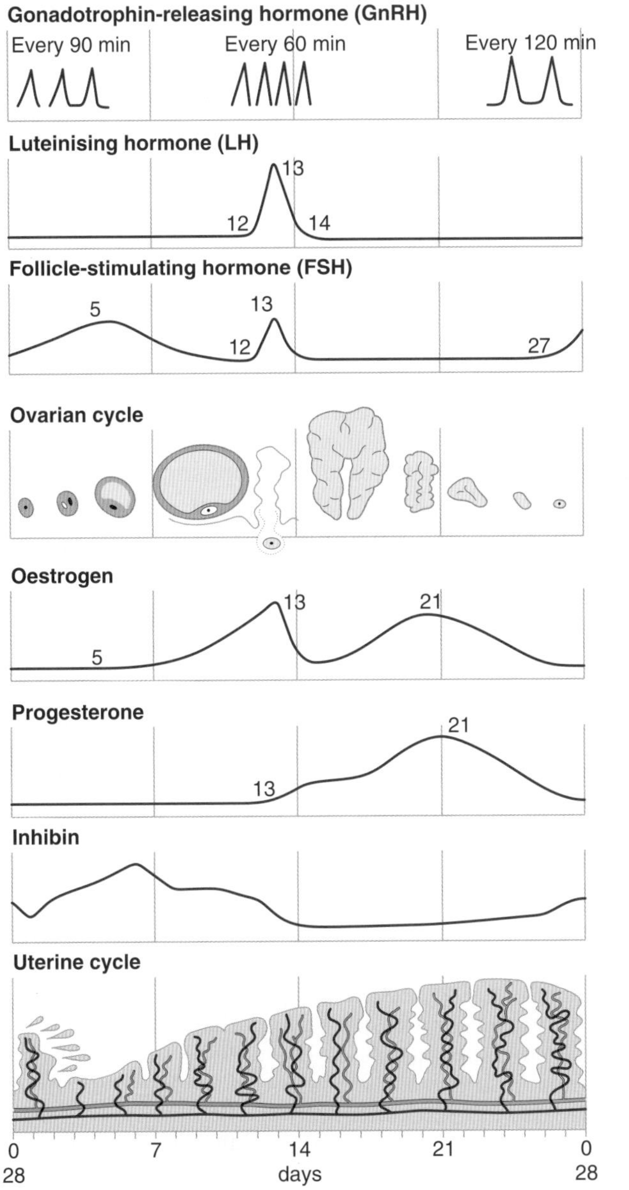

FIGURE 20.14 Uterine cycle and hormone levels
(Based on Coad & Dunstall, 2001)

The straight arterioles dilate, contributing to menstrual flow (Blackburn, 2017).

Proliferative phase

In the proliferative phase, the stratum functionalis of the endometrium begins to thicken as endometrial cells proliferate. Arterioles regenerate and endometrial glands develop. These changes occur in response to increased levels of oestradiol. The mucus produced by the cervix also responds to these hormones. Its consistency becomes less viscous and less stretchy, showing little or no ferning (spinnbarkeit test), thus becoming more receptive to sperm. Variation in the length of the proliferative phase accounts for most of the variation in uterine cycles (Blackburn, 2017).

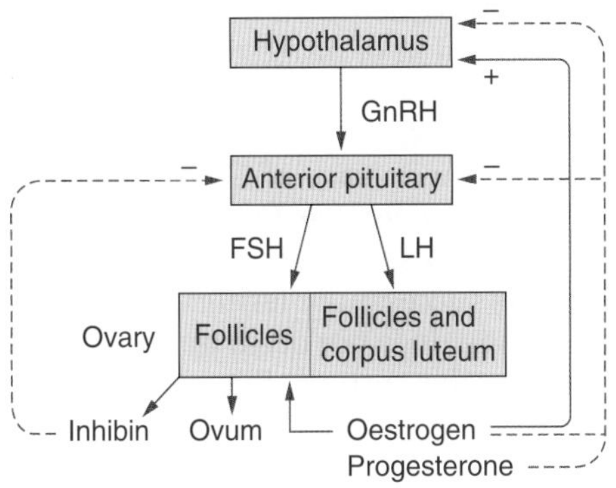

FIGURE 20.15 Control of follicular development and oestrogen secretion
(Based on Bray et al., 1994)

Secretory phase

The secretory phase occurs following ovulation, when levels of progesterone are high. The influence of progesterone results in further thickening of the stratum functionalis, an increase in the number of blood vessels and increased coiling and dilation of blood vessels. Finally, the endometrial glands begin secreting glycogen.

Hypothalamic–pituitary–ovarian (HPO) axis

The female reproductive system is regulated by a variety of hormones produced by the brain (the hypothalamus and the pituitary gland) and the ovaries (Fig. 20.15).

Hypothalamus

The hypothalamus produces a peptide hormone called gonadotrophin-releasing hormone (GnRH) within its neurons. This hormone stimulates the release of several hormones from the anterior pituitary gland, specifically FSH and LH.

Pituitary gland

The anterior pituitary gland produces and secretes many hormones, including FSH, LH and prolactin. LH and FSH are glycoproteins that enhance each other's actions (act synergistically) in regulating the ovarian cycle.

FSH, along with oestrogen produced by the ovaries, acts on the granulosa cells of the follicles to stimulate growth and produce FSH receptors and LH receptors. The granulosa cells of a primordial follicle undergo limited growth without FSH (Blackburn, 2017).

LH acts on the thecal cells, instigating the production of androgens that are converted to oestrogens by the granulosa cells. This increases the oestrogen level and inhibits the development of other follicles by inhibiting FSH (negative feedback). At the same time, one follicle becomes dominant and secretes high levels of oestradiol, allowing granulosa cell development in that follicle. As levels of oestradiol increase, the release of GnRH is triggered by positive feedback, allowing increased levels of LH and FSH to complete the maturation of follicles, and an LH surge triggers ovulation within 12–24 hours. The

LH surge is accompanied by a drop in oestrogen and an increase in production of progesterone from the follicle.

Following ovulation, increasing levels of oestrogen and progesterone exert a powerful negative-feedback effect, inhibiting the release of GnRH and subsequently LH and FSH. This negative feedback prevents further maturation of follicles—important if the oocyte released at ovulation was successfully fertilised. However, in most cycles, fertilisation does not occur and the corpus luteum degenerates into the corpus albicans, resulting in a decreased level of progesterone. The low progesterone levels cease to inhibit GnRH, which begins to rise, followed by an increase in LH and FSH and the beginning of the follicular phase.

Prolactin is a protein hormone that stimulates milk production. Levels of prolactin rise during pregnancy, but human placental lactogen (hPL) and progesterone prevent the binding of prolactin to receptors in the breast. After birth, prolactin stimulates milk production.

RESEARCH ACTIVITY

A recent New Zealand longitudinal study looked at almost 1400 couples who had been trying to conceive for more than 12 months. All couples initially assessed by a fertility service between 1998 and 2005 were followed for birth outcomes to the end of 2014. More than 60% gave birth in the study period and just under 50% did not require treatment to conceive successfully. However, the study confirmed the importance of early referral for older women while providing evidence that younger women without severe diagnosis or lengthy infertility could be provided more opportunity to conceive spontaneously (Righarts et al., 2017).

However, some couples who have experienced difficulty in conceiving may require fertility treatment. Pharmacological treatment has the aim of retrieving multiple oocytes to increase the chance of pregnancy. GnRH agonists are widely used to stimulate ovarian cycles (Kasum et al., 2014). High-order multiple pregnancies are also identified as being commonly associated with the use of fertility drugs—because of multiple ovulations or more than one embryo replacement.

Identify the physiological mechanism that explains the way in which GnRH agonists can assist fertility.

Ovaries

The ovaries produce the oestrogens (oestradiol, oestrone and oestriol), progesterone and inhibin.

Oestrogens are produced in the ovaries by granulosa cells within the follicles and the corpus luteum. During a woman's reproductive years the main oestrogen is oestradiol. Although the concentration of this is less than that of oestrone, it has a greater oestrogenic potency and is responsible for most of the effects of oestrogen in the female reproductive system. However, during pregnancy oestriol becomes the main oestrogen secreted (Blackburn, 2017). The stimulus for oestrogen release is primarily FSH and, to a lesser extent, LH. Oestrogens are responsible for various functions, including:

- developing and maintaining the female reproductive structures such as the endometrial lining of the uterus, and secondary sexual characteristics such as fat content of the breasts, abdomen, mons pubis and hips, voice pitch, broadness of the pelvis, distribution of underarm and pubic hair, and the development of breasts
- maintaining fluid and electrolyte balance—by influencing the action of aldosterone, sodium reabsorption in the renal tubules is stimulated leading to increased reabsorption of water; diuresis is also reduced through the action of antidiuretic hormone (ADH)
- increasing the rate at which amino acids enter cells—thereby altering protein metabolism, allowing cells to grow and multiply; this action is supported by the influence of growth hormone
- regulating oxytocic receptors
- stimulating uterine tube contractility to assist sperm motility and to retain the ovum (Blackburn, 2017).

Progesterone is produced in the ovaries by granulosa cells, primarily of the corpus luteum. Therefore, progesterone levels peak in the postovulatory phase when the corpus luteum is active, and fall if pregnancy does not occur and the corpus luteum degenerates. LH is the stimulus for progesterone release. Progesterone has various functions, including:

- preparing the endometrium of the uterus to receive a fertilised ovum
- preventing sperm entry into the uterus by promoting changes in the cervical mucus
- increasing basal body temperature by influencing the thermostat located in the hypothalamus
- relaxing the muscle of the uterine tubes during the luteal phase to assist passage of the fertilised ovum to the uterus (Blackburn, 2017).

Inhibin is produced in the ovaries by granulosa cells of the follicles and corpus luteum. It exerts negative-feedback controls on FSH release during the growth of the dominant follicle and the corpus luteum.

CLINICAL POINT

1. Body temperature rises after ovulation, in response to progesterone, and is used in natural family planning to indicate the fertile phases of the reproductive cycle.
2. Hormonal contraceptives contain levels of oestrogen and/or progesterone that cause feedback control on the HPO axis to prevent follicle development and ovulation. Some contraceptives use the cervical mucus-changing properties of progesterone (e.g. the minipill).

Summary: homeostatic control of the reproductive cycle

Whereas the follicular phase of the cycle is characterised by the positive feedback of oestrogen prompting an LH surge, the luteal phase is characterised by negative feedback. GnRH, LH and FSH production is controlled by negative-feedback mechanisms linked to the ovarian hormones in the HPO axis (oestrogens, progesterone and inhibin). If the secondary oocyte is not fertilised, the ovum dies within 24 hours and the corpus luteum deteriorates. The levels of oestrogens and progesterone therefore drop, triggering the production of GnRH, LH and FSH, which begins the reproductive cycle (ovarian and uterine cycles) again. If fertilisation and implantation occur (pregnancy), levels of oestrogen and progesterone remain elevated because the **blastocyst** secretes the hormone human chorionic gonadotrophin (hCG), which maintains the corpus luteum and its hormone production (see the following Clinical Point). The placenta then takes over producing oestradiol and progesterone by 6–10 weeks of gestation.

CLINICAL POINT

Pregnancy test

The developing syncytiotrophoblast secretes hCG into the maternal circulation to maintain the pregnancy by stimulating the corpus luteum to continue producing oestrogens and progesterone. This hormone is the basis of the pregnancy test, as hCG increases rapidly over the first 9 weeks, then more slowly until 10–12 weeks and finally declines. An antibody test can detect hCG in the blood approximately 9 days after fertilisation and in the urine 10–12 days after fertilisation. This is usually well before the woman is aware that she is pregnant (Rankin, 2017).

RESEARCH ACTIVITY

Hormone replacement therapy (HRT) has previously been suggested to reduce the risk of cardiovascular disease. However, a study, the Women's Health Initiative (WHI) trial published in the *Journal of the American Medical Association* in 2002, in fact identified that HRT increased the risk of cardiovascular disease in healthy postmenopausal women. The study was halted early because it was decided that these results presented an unacceptable risk for the participating women (Rossouw et al., 2002). HRT had also been used to treat the symptoms of menopause, but following the trial this usage was brought into question because of the published risk. Subsequent analysis (Stefanick et al., 2006) highlighted the complexity of the different hormone replacement regimens and the impact of age and time since the last physiological exposure to hormones. Langer (2017) and Thorley (2016) each report in commentaries that, whereas not all women have indications for HRT, those who do and who initiate them within 10 years of menopause experience benefits—both short term (vasomotor, dyspareunia) and long term (bone health, coronary risk reduction).

1. Explain why HRT may reduce these symptoms.
2. What is the concern about the use of HRT?

Hypothalamic–pituitary–testicular control in the male

Hypothalamic–pituitary–testicular (HPT) control in the male is not cyclical like HPO control in the female. The HPT axis regulates physiological changes in the testes from puberty onwards. GnRH is secreted by the hypothalamus every 70–90 minutes, which triggers the anterior pituitary to secrete LH and FSH.

LH directly stimulates both the production of testosterone from cholesterol and the process of spermatogenesis, whereas FSH primarily facilitates spermatogenesis.

Testosterone is produced by the Leydig (interstitial) cells adjacent to the seminiferous tubules (see Fig. 20.9) and diffuses across the basal membrane to influence the spermatogonia and Sertoli cells directly. Testosterone levels are maintained by negative feedback to the hypothalamus and anterior pituitary, via the HPT axis.

Summary points

- The structures of the female and male reproductive systems are designed to produce and transport gametes: ova and sperm.
- Gametogenesis involves meiotic cell divisions that halve the chromosome number: oogenesis produces ova in the ovaries, and spermatogenesis produces sperm in the testes.
- Following puberty, a single oocyte is released from the ovary each month under the control of the hormones of the HPO axis.
- Ovarian hormones stimulate monthly vascular and glandular development of the uterus in preparation for pregnancy.
- Hormones of the HPT axis stimulate sperm production from puberty onwards.
- Sperm are produced in the seminiferous tubules and are stored in the epididymis until ejaculation.
- Semen released at ejaculation includes an average 300 million sperm and 2–5 mL of secretions from the accessory glands to aid nourishment and support of the sperm.

EMBRYOLOGY

Embryology is described as the study of 'the origin and development of a human being from a zygote to the birth' (Moore et al., 2008, p. 2) and it is suggested that development is a continuum that starts at fertilisation, includes birth and continues after birth, with development of teeth, bones, reproductive structures and so on. The process finishes by about the age of 25 years. This section is limited to antenatal development, which begins with **conception**. Conception refers to fertilisation that results in pregnancy; the probability of a viable conception has been calculated at less than 40%–50% per menstrual cycle (Blackburn, 2017). The processes needed to produce a viable oocyte and a viable sperm have been described earlier in this chapter. This section examines fertilisation and the factors that contribute to successful fertilisation, implantation, development of the embryo and fetus, and development of the placenta.

Fertilisation

Fertilisation normally occurs in the ampulla of the fallopian tube. The beginning of fertilisation occurs when the sperm passes through the zona pellucida and makes contact with the secondary oocyte. This is most likely to occur if sperm enter the vagina just prior to or during ovulation, because sperm must undergo capacitation and the acrosomal reaction (see below) prior to fertilisation, and these processes require several hours.

Sperm transport

During sexual intercourse, approximately 300 million sperm are released into the vagina in about 3 mL of semen. Chemicals present in the semen cause coagulation of the sperm (see Accessory sex glands, above). This may help retain sperm in the vagina and protect against the acidic environment of the vagina. The coagulum is then dissolved in 20–60 minutes by activation of a further enzyme (fibrinolysis) in the semen. The alkaline pH of the semen facilitates sperm motility. Within a minute of sperm deposition, sperm can be detected in the cervix and uterus. However, most sperm are lost through vaginal leakage and never enter the cervix. Those that do survive may survive in the cervix for hours and be nourished by the cervical mucus. Further progress towards the uterus is dependent on the consistency of the mucus, which is determined by oestrogen and progesterone (see Uterine cycle, above). Sperm most probably move both by their own propulsion and by the action of uterine cilia, causing semen to flow through the uterus to the fallopian tubes (Johnson, 2013).

Capacitation and the acrosomal reaction

Capacitation is stimulated by secretions in the oestrogen-dominated uterus and fallopian tubes. As the sperm move through the fallopian tubes, glycoproteins and seminal plasma proteins are removed from the plasma membrane over the acrosome (head of spermatozoa), leading to activation. The capacitated sperm contacts the corona radiata around the secondary oocyte. Enzymes are released from the acrosome (acrosome reaction) and are able to digest a tunnel through the corona radiata and zona pellucida (Johnson, 2013).

> **CLINICAL POINT**
>
> When sperm are recovered following ejaculation and placed with ova in vitro, fertilisation takes several hours to occur. In contrast, sperm recovered from the uterus or fallopian tube are capable of immediate fertilisation. This suggests that sperm attain a fertilising capacity (capacitate) during their journey through the female reproductive tract (Johnson, 2013).

Sperm need 4–10 hours in the female reproductive tract before they can fertilise an ovum. Sperm remain activated for only a short time, but a supply of sperm persists for some time as sperm stored in the folds of the mucosa of the cervix trickle gradually through the capacitating uterus to the fallopian tube, where they become activated. This allows a greater time following intercourse in which activated sperm are available to fertilise the ovum (Johnson, 2013).

The sperm 'bind' with specific receptors (glycoproteins) on the surface of the zona pellucida. Once the spermatozoon penetrates the zona pellucida (between 5 and 20 minutes), it is in the cytoplasm of the ovum. Several hundred sperm can bind on the zona pellucida but only one sperm can penetrate this layer, owing to an event called *syngamy*. This causes changes in the electrical potential and chemical composition of the zona pellucida that prevent other sperm from penetrating once one has done so (Johnson, 2013).

The cell membranes of the oocyte and sperm fuse, and the head and tail of the sperm enter the oocyte, leaving the sperm's plasma membrane behind (Fig. 20.16). The oocyte completes the second meiotic division, forming a mature oocyte and a second polar body. The nucleus of the mature ovum becomes a female pronucleus and the polar body disintegrates. Within the oocyte, the nucleus of the sperm enlarges to become the male pronucleus and the tail disintegrates. The two pronuclei can no longer be distinguished from one another. The membranes of the pronuclei fuse, and a *zygote* is formed (Moore et al., 2013). The zygote has 46 chromosomes: 22 autosomes and 1 sex chromosome from each gamete. The zygote is genetically unique, containing a new combination of chromosomes that is different from that of either of the parents. Fertilisation is completed within 24 hours of ovulation (Moore et al., 2013).

Factors that facilitate fertilisation

The ovum survives for only 12–24 hours after ovulation. Similarly sperm probably survive only up to 24 hours in the female reproductive tract (Moore et al., 2013). They require at least 4–6 hours, sometimes 10 hours, in the female reproductive tract to become activated. Sexual intercourse up to 24 hours before and approximately 12 hours after ovulation may result in fertilisation.

Changes in the female reproductive tract mean the female is most receptive to sperm at around the time of ovulation. Increased oestrogen levels at this time have many effects, such as:

- increasing the contractility of the fallopian tube, which assists sperm transport
- decreasing the viscosity of the cervical mucus
- altering the molecular structure of the mucus to form small channels that allow sperm through.

Sperm are attracted to the oocyte by chemotaxis (Sun et al., 2005) and thermotaxis (Boryshpolets et al., 2015). Progesterone released after ovulation stimulates the acrosomal reaction (Shah et al., 2003) and also increases the viscosity of the cervical mucus during the luteal phase, preventing further sperm access.

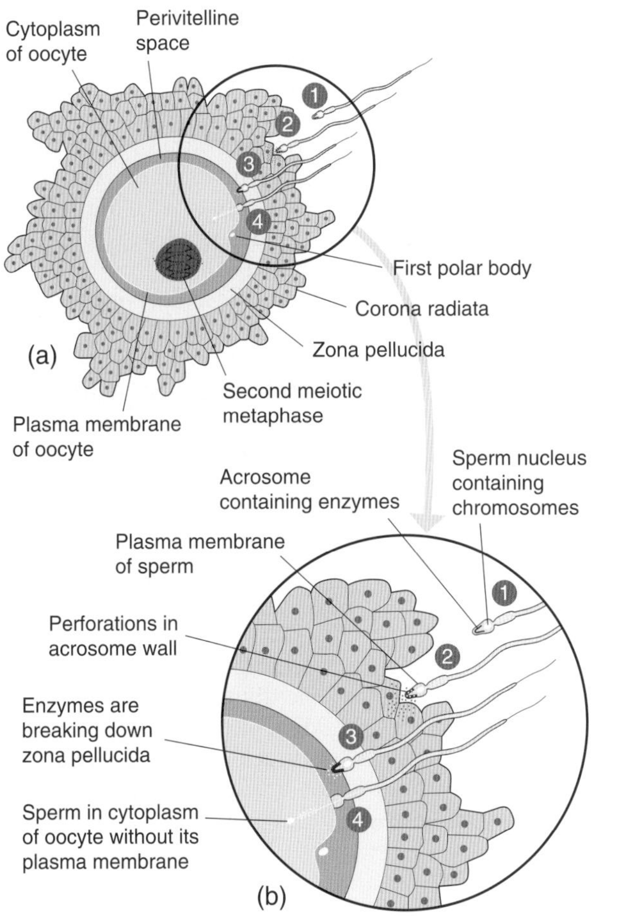

FIGURE 20.16 Acrosome reaction and sperm penetrating an oocyte. The details of the area outlined in (a) are shown in (b): 1 = sperm during capacitation; 2 = sperm undergoing the acrosome reaction; 3 = sperm digesting a path through the zona pellucida; 4 = sperm after entering the cytoplasm of the oocyte (Based on Moore & Persaud, 1998)

Cleavage and formation of blastomeres

The zygote remains in the ampulla of the fallopian tube for about the first 24 hours and then is swept towards the uterus by ciliary action over the next 3–4 days (Moore et al., 2013). The zygote undergoes repeated mitotic divisions, called cleavage, as it moves towards the uterus. Cleavage increases the number of cells—blastomeres—but not their size, and they are still contained within the zona pellucida. The cytoplasm of the ovum provides the energy and nutrients for the mitotic divisions. The first division into the two-cell stage occurs about 30 hours after fertilisation (Moore et al., 2013). Further divisions occur about every 12–24 hours. By 3 days, there are 12–15 blastomeres, which now change shape, forming a solid cluster within the zona pellucida, called a *morula*.

The **morula** enters the uterine cavity at day 4–5, and as uterine secretions pass through the zona pellucida into the morula, a fluid-filled space, the blastocyst cavity, is formed (Moore et al., 2013). As the cavity forms, the surrounding blastomeres separate into two areas:

- the *trophoblast*—the thin layer of cells around the outside that give rise to the fetal part of the placenta, the chorion
- the *inner cell mass*—the inner group of blastomeres that give rise to the embryo, yolk sac and amnion.

The conceptus is now called a *blastocyst*. The blastocyst floats in the uterine cavity for about 2 days as the zona pellucida disintegrates. This allows more-rapid growth of the blastocyst. Uterine secretions containing nutrients, glycogen, mucopolysaccharides and lipids maintain the blastocyst. Approximately 6 days after fertilisation, the blastocyst attaches to the endometrium and begins to implant (Moore et al., 2013).

Fig. 20.17 summarises the processes of cleavage and implantation during the first week. The technique of assisted reproduction may involve transfer of cultured blastomeres into the uterus.

Steps of implantation

Implantation of the blastocyst normally occurs in the posterior or anterior wall of the uterine body, with the inner cell mass oriented towards the epithelium of the endometrium. Implantation is essential to maintain nourishment of the blastocyst. The following points detail the steps involved in implantation, also illustrated in Fig. 20.18.

1. The trophoblast differentiates into two layers: the outer syncytiotrophoblast (maternal side of the placenta) and the inner cytotrophoblast (fetal side of the placenta).
2. The cytotrophoblast forms new syncytial cells, the chorionic villi and the amnion.
3. The syncytiotrophoblast is diffuse tissue with no cell membranes. Projections of the syncytiotrophoblast extend through the endometrial epithelium and connective tissue (stroma), releasing proteolytic enzymes, which break down the maternal tissues. This allows the blastocyst to burrow into the endometrium. The syncytiotrophoblast is not rejected by the mother, possibly because it does not have transplantation antigens (Blackburn, 2017). Slight bleeding may occur during this time, and can be mistaken for light menstrual bleeding (Blackburn, 2017).
4. The blastocyst is nourished by glycogen and lipids that diffuse from the stromal cells and glands of the eroded tissue.
5. By day 9, degradation by the proteolytic enzymes causes spaces (lacunae) to appear in the syncytiotrophoblast. Individual lacunae fuse to form lacunal networks and these fill with fluid from the endometrial glands (Blackburn, 2017). Nutrients diffuse from the lacunae to the embryo.
6. Concurrent development of the inner cell mass occurs. At about day 7, a layer of cells, called the hypoblast, forms on the side of the inner cell mass adjacent to the blastocyst cavity (Moore et al., 2013). Formation of a *bilaminar disc* (a two-layered embryo) with a layer of epiblast and hypoblast is complete by day 8. This embryonic disc

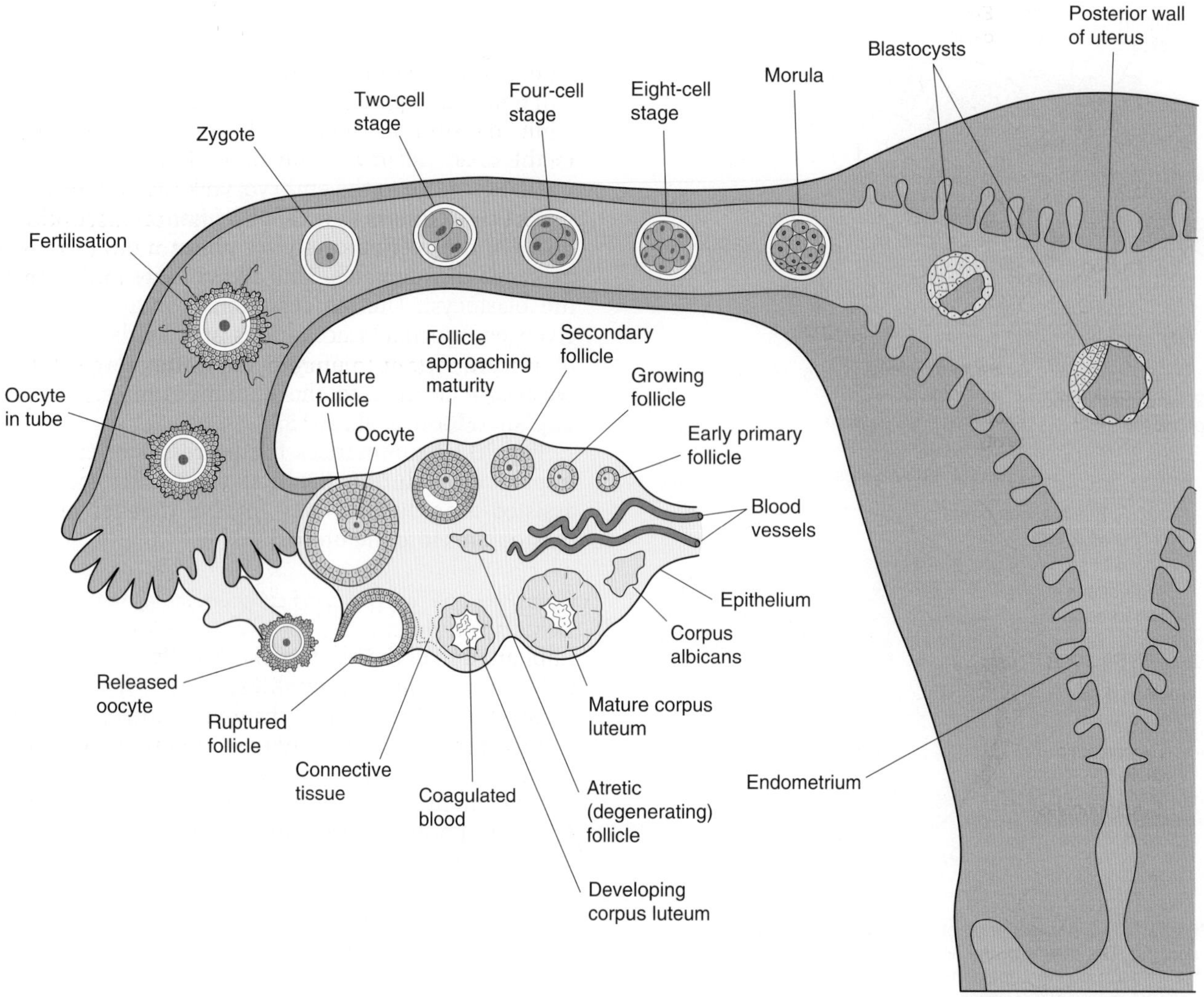

FIGURE 20.17 Summary of the ovarian cycle, showing cleavage and implantation
(Based on Moore & Persaud, 1998)

forms the germ cells that will produce all the tissues and organs of the embryo (described in the next section).

7. By day 10 the conceptus is completely implanted in the endometrium, covered by a closing plug, and by day 12 it is covered by regenerated endometrial epithelium (Moore et al., 2013).

Changes in the endometrium

The uterine endometrium is in the secretory phase during implantation. During this phase there is proliferation of endometrial glands, providing a source of nutrition for the blastocyst. The spiral arterioles form a prolific network of blood vessels supplying the dense capillary bed beneath the epithelial layer of the endometrium.

Following implantation, the endometrium changes in structure and is known as the decidua. Increasing progesterone facilitates enlargement of the decidual cells and accumulation of glycogen and lipids. These cellular changes, in combination with the vascular changes of the endometrium, are known as the decidual reaction.

Three areas of the decidua are defined by their location relative to the implantation site:

- The *decidua basalis* is the region beneath the site of implantation. This develops into the maternal part of the placenta.
- The *decidua capsularis* is the area covering the implantation site. This disappears as the chorion is formed.
- The *decidua parietalis* (vera) is the remainder of the uterine lining. The chorion and decidua parietalis eventually fuse, obliterating the uterine cavity.

Although the posterior wall of the body of the uterus is the most common site for implantation, the blastocyst may implant over the internal os of the cervix or cervical canal, resulting in placenta praevia. Extrauterine implantation results in an ectopic pregnancy. The most common site is the ampulla or infundibulum of the fallopian tube.

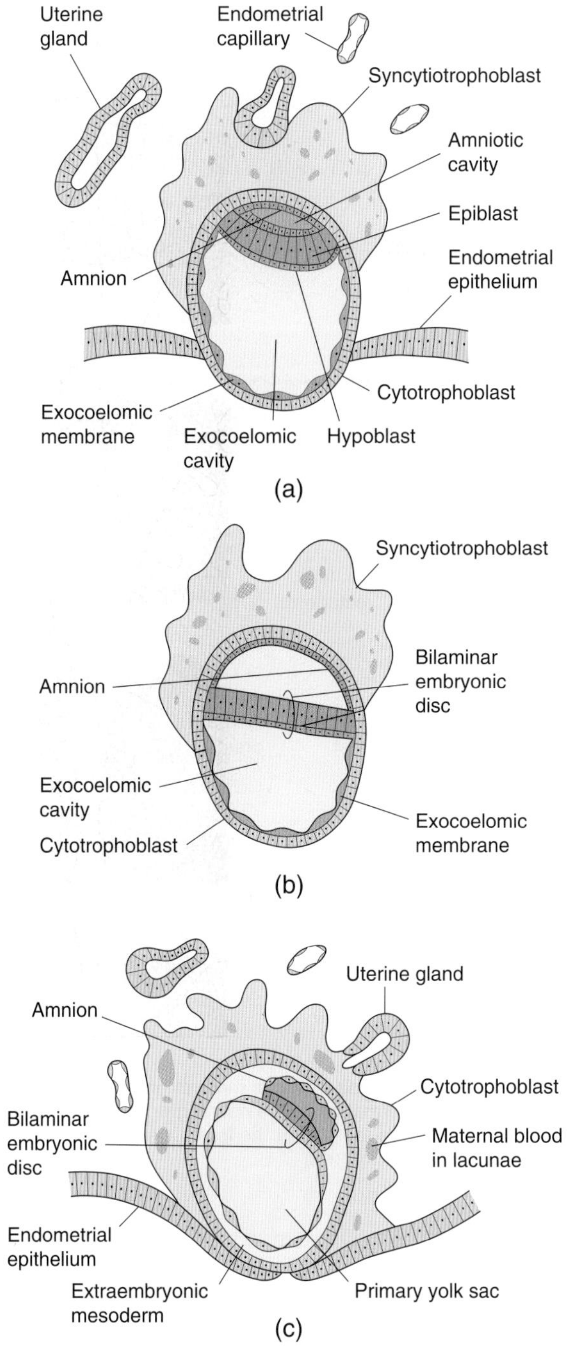

FIGURE 20.18 Implantation of a blastocyst into the endometrium: (a) section through a blastocyst partially implanted in the endometrium; (b) slightly older blastocyst after removal from the endometrium; (c) section through a blastocyst of about 9 days implanted in the endometrium
(Based on Moore & Persaud, 1998)

By the time implantation is complete, at 10–12 days, the inner cell mass has differentiated into a bilaminar disc and the trophoblast has developed into the syncytiotrophoblast and the cytotrophoblast. The syncytiotrophoblast has formed maternal lacunae and the cytotrophoblast has formed chorionic villi. Further development of the embryo, placenta and fetal membranes occurs simultaneously.

Development of the embryo

The embryonic period refers to the period from the third to the eighth week after fertilisation. During this time the embryo develops from a bilaminar flat disc (see Fig. 20.18) to an embryo with all the major organ systems and a functioning cardiovascular system. The embryo is vulnerable to developmental disruption from a wide range of teratogens—environmental agents such as infections, hyperthermia, drugs and radiation exposure, and nicotine and narcotics exposure—leading to major congenital abnormalities.

It is important to understand embryological development. It explains why a healthy lifestyle prior to conception and during early pregnancy is important in order to provide the best possible environment for normal development of the embryo, and why women of reproductive age should avoid potential teratogens at all times. This vulnerable phase of embryological development often occurs before a woman is aware that she is pregnant. Understanding normal embryological development also helps to understand abnormal development (e.g. cleft palate) and has led to the development of processes that can correct some abnormalities.

In considering embryological development, this section reviews changes in the third week and then focuses on the principles that govern development, rather than the detailed development of organ systems, which is beyond the scope of this text. (See the Further reading and Online resources lists at the end of this chapter for more detailed accounts.)

The embryo in week 3

Development during the embryonic period is very rapid and this makes it a vulnerable time. Gastrulation is the reorganisation of cells of the bilaminar disc (week 2) to form the trilaminar disc (Moore et al., 2013). The notochord and somites also form in week 3, and neurulation begins.

Gastrulation

A line of epiblast cells undergoes very rapid division to form the primitive streak along the midline. Cells from the primitive streak migrate down to form a layer of mesoderm between the epiblast and hypoblast (Fig. 20.19), resulting in the trilaminar disc. The primitive streak continues to form mesoderm through the fourth week and then degenerates (Moore et al., 2013). All body organs and structures are derived from these three germ layers (ectoderm, mesoderm and endoderm).

Notochord and somite formation

A chord of mesodermal cells migrates to form the notochord, a rigid tube that defines the head–tail axis of the embryo and plays a key role in signalling the development of unspecialised embryonic cells into specialised adult tissues and organs (Moore et al., 2013). The notochord forms the framework for the development of the axial skeleton (bones of head and spinal cord) and the neural plate, which develops into the primitive nervous system. Paired segments of mesoderm also form on either side of the

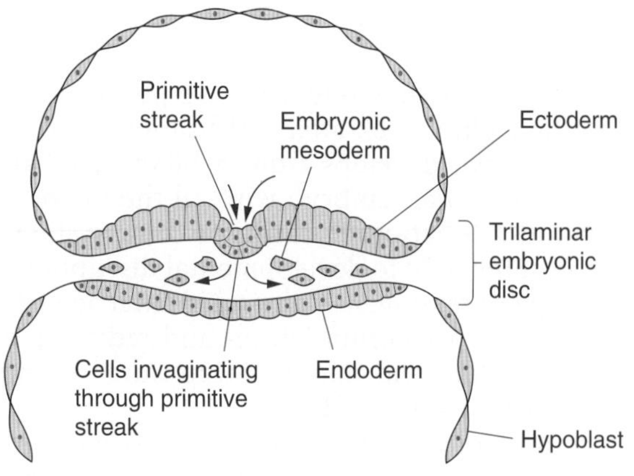

FIGURE 20.19 Invagination of the cells of the primitive streak to form a trilaminar disc
(Based on Coad & Dunstall, 2001)

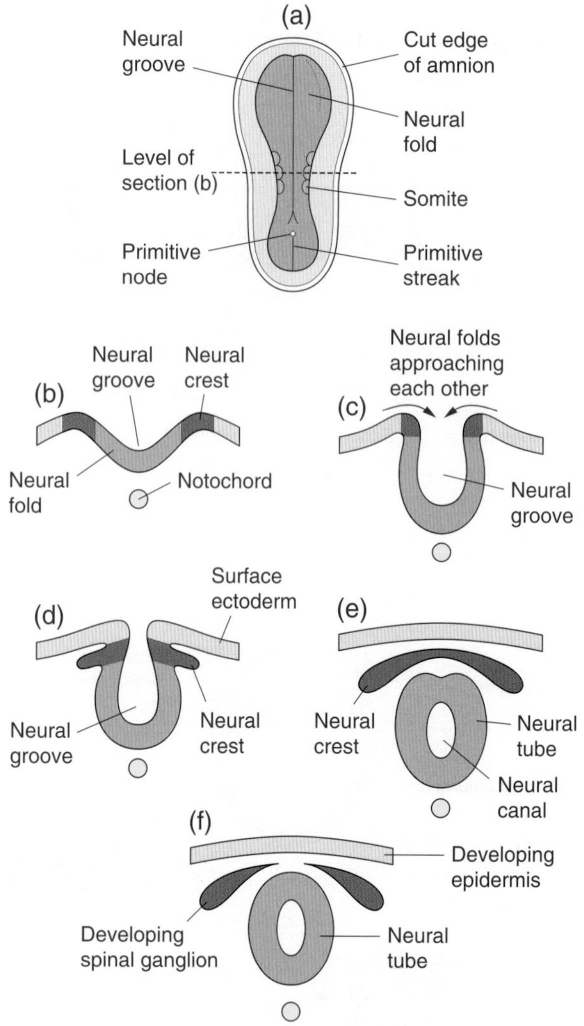

FIGURE 20.20 Transverse sections through progressively older embryos, showing formation of the neural groove, neural tube and neural crest up to the end of the fourth week
(Based on Moore & Persaud, 1998)

notochord. These are somites, which eventually give rise to the axial skeleton and associated musculature as well as the overlying dermis of the skin. About 38 pairs of somites appear between days 20 and 30, and 42 to 44 pairs are present by the fifth week. They form prominent elevations and can be used to determine an embryo's age at this time (Moore et al., 2013).

Neurulation

The notochord induces thickening of the embryonic ectoderm to form the neural plate. A longitudinal groove develops in the plate and neural folds form above this. The folds fuse to form the neural tube—the primordium of the central nervous system (Fig. 20.20). Incomplete fusion of the tube results in congenital defects of the central nervous system (e.g. spina bifida).

Other changes during the third week include blood vessel formation. By the end of the week, nutrition is delivered by a primitive **uteroplacental circulation**, the framework for development of the nervous system is present, and the embryo begins organogenesis. A number of fundamental processes guide organogenesis and development of the embryo.

Cellular processes that control embryological development

Embryological development involves growth, differentiation and organisation. Growth involves an increase in cell number and cell size, while differentiation involves the creation of new types of cells and tissues. Organisation describes how the new units become coordinated into functional units (Blackburn, 2017). Gene families within the embryo are known to control development. By the two- to four-cell stage, activated genes produce intercellular signalling proteins, which regulate cellular activity and development. Environmental factors can interact with groups of genes to turn them on and off at precise intervals.

The mechanisms controlling these processes are complex, but a number of processes have been described that contribute to development. These include: cell differentiation, induction, differential cell proliferation, programmed cell death, changes in cell size, cell migration, cell recognition and adhesion, folding and differential maturity. The following description of these processes has been adapted from Blackburn (2017).

Cell differentiation

The zygote contains one set of chromosomes, with the blueprint for the development of at least 350 different cell types that make up the body. Initially, cell division produces cells that are identical, but differentiation begins at the end of the first week, when the blastomeres of the morula develop into either cells of the inner cell mass or cells of the trophoblast. Remembering that all cells have the same genetic code, the process of differentiation involves restricting some areas of development while enabling others. This is regulated by gene families, which are switched on to produce specific proteins in a particular order (Blackburn, 2017).

Induction

Cells can influence cells in another part of the embryo by induction. Once again this process relies on signalling proteins (from inductors) and the ability of some cells to bind these proteins and respond (inducers). Development of many parts of the embryo is by secondary induction, where one change induces the next and so forth. For example, formation of the structures of the eye involves a series of inductions: the forebrain is induced to form the optic cup, which then induces adjacent tissue to form the lens of the eye, which then induces the surrounding tissue to form the cornea. Interfering with a step in the induction process may prevent the later stages occurring (Blackburn, 2017).

Differential cell proliferation

Differential cell proliferation is the process whereby groups of cells grow at different rates. This can give the impression of cells sinking into tissues if adjacent cells proliferate rapidly and build up in one area. This can be seen in the development of the neural groove. Rapid cell proliferation often precedes a period of differentiation. Congenital defects can result if proliferation is inhibited—by teratogenic agents, for example. Proliferation can also be inhibited through lack of space—for example, with a diaphragmatic hernia, the intestinal contents are pushed into the thoracic cavity, where they can inhibit lung growth (Blackburn, 2017).

Programmed cell death

Programmed cell death, where cells are destroyed by lysosomal enzymes, is a normal part of embryological development. This is the process whereby hollow tubes are formed (e.g. the trachea and parts of the gut). It also accounts for the disappearance of the webbing between fingers and toes. If the enzyme release is inhibited, congenital malformations such as syndactyly, bowel atresia or imperforate anus may result. Overactive enzymes can produce micromelia (shortened limbs) (Blackburn, 2017).

Cell size and shape change

Chemical changes in cell microtubules, the skeleton within the cell, are responsible for changing cell shape (e.g. elongation of the cell). The process can be inhibited (e.g. by toxins from microorganisms). Other changes in cell shape (e.g. swelling or shrinking) can be induced by changes in osmotic balance (Blackburn, 2017).

Cell migration

Development of structures often involves migration of cells to different areas. This is a controlled process whereby the leading edge of the cell elongates (due to microtubule elongation) and adheres to a new contact point. Contraction of the cell towards the contact point completes the migration. Again, interference with the microtubule enzymes may impede migration—for example, Hirschsprung's disease (a lack of intestinal ganglion cells) results from failure of neural crest cells to migrate. In the central nervous system, at 3–6 months gestation, there is migration of millions of neurons from their original site in the periventricular area to their eventual location in the cerebrum and cerebellum. Interference with this migration can result in defects in central nervous system function and organisation (Blackburn, 2017).

Cell recognition and adhesion

Recognition and adhesion involves interaction of specific substances, such as cell surface enzymes, on one cell with complementary substances or adhesion molecules on another cell. An example of this is when the neural folds meet and fuse to form the neural tube. Adhesion may be prevented if there is interference with cell membrane substrates. This may be the mechanism for cleft palate or neural tube defects (Blackburn, 2017).

Folding of the embryo

The embryo starts as a straight line of cells but undergoes folding to adapt to the available space as it grows. Transverse folding results in a cylindrical shape, whereas longitudinal folding results in the head and tail folds (Blackburn, 2017).

Differential maturity

This process refers to the fact that different organ systems mature at different rates; for example, the gut is structurally complete at birth whereas the alveoli of the lungs and the long bones continue maturation after birth. This explains why different organ systems are vulnerable to damage by toxins at different stages of development.

Any malfunction of these fundamental processes results in impaired development. Understanding the basic principles may help to see why seemingly unconnected pathologies occur as congenital defects. The above processes are responsible for the cascade of changes resulting in organogenesis (development of the organ systems) (Blackburn, 2017).

Organogenesis: highlights of weeks 4 to 8

All the major organ systems and structures of the body form from the three germ layers of the trilaminar disc. Table 20.2 lists visual highlights of the changes seen in the embryo (adapted from Moore & Persaud, 2008). This is a critical period in human development, as it is a time of most-rapid cell division and the time of greatest vulnerability to teratogens. Different organ systems undergo rapid change at different times, and this leads to the variable impact of teratogens on different structures. Critical periods for the different organ systems are illustrated in Fig. 20.21.

CRITICAL THINKING EXERCISE

1. Identify three potential teratogens.
2. Identify the stage of pregnancy at which exposure to these teratogens would be most damaging.
3. Describe the likely congenital abnormalities that would result from this exposure.

Table 20.2 Overview of embryonic development from 4 to 8 weeks

Week of gestation	Visual highlight
4	• Embryo straight, C-shape developing • Somites form • Neural tube fusing, but open at rostral and caudal ends • Branchial arches present (develop into primitive face, jaws and neck) • Forebrain prominent • Upper limb buds appear, then lower limb buds • Otic pits present (internal ears) • Tapered tail obvious • Beating heart prominent
5	• Rapid development of brain and head enlargement • Face touches heart prominence • Hand plates develop in upper limbs
6	• Limb buds (especially upper) more differentiated into elbow and wrist • Ridges (digital rays) in hand plates obvious (forerunners of digits) • External ear canal and auricle (pinna) formed • Pigmented eye obvious • Head disproportionately large and bent over • Some straightening of neck and thorax
7	• Umbilical herniation (intestines enter extraembryonic coelom in umbilical cord) • Notches appear between digital rays of hand plates • Liver is prominent
8	• Short, webbed digits of hands gradually lengthen • Notches appear between digital rays of the feet • Stubby tail disappears • Head disproportionately large • Neck apparent • Eyelids more obvious and eyes open • Auricles of external ears are low set • Sexuality of external genitalia not easily determined

(Adapted from Moore & Persaud, 2008)

The fetus: from 9 weeks to birth

The fetal period is mainly a time of growth and functional maturation. There is rapid body growth, while head growth slows. A fetus is capable of surviving independently at 32–4 weeks gestation. Data from Australia (Sharp et al., 2018) and from a meta-analysis including 65 studies from high-income countries (Myrhaug et al., 2019) report survival in a neonatal intensive care unit may be possible from 22 to 26 weeks, although survival for babies under 24 weeks gestation is commonly associated with neurological impairment (Myrhaug et al., 2019; Sharp et al., 2018). A survey in Australia of 133 neonatologists and registered nurses suggested that they would 'almost always' resuscitate an infant of 24 weeks gestation (Oei et al., 2000). Similar results were identified from a survey of obstetricians at non-tertiary facilities; however, healthcare professionals at these non-specialist facilities were shown to often underestimate survival of extremely premature infants (Gooi et al., 2003).

RESEARCH ACTIVITY

There is strong evidence to support increased folic acid intake prior to pregnancy to reduce neural tube defects (NTDs). There remains a debate over mandatory fortification of foods with folic acid. In 2006 Bower et al. used a published model to estimate the number of neural tube defects that could be prevented in Australia and New Zealand by increasing levels of folic acid intake. The model estimated that an increase from 0.1 mg to 0.2 mg folic acid per day would result in the prevention of 49 (95% confidence interval (CI) 27–84) NTDs per year in Australia in total, 7 (95% CI 4–11) NTDs in Australian Aboriginal infants and 11 (95% CI 6–18) NTDs in New Zealand. Following mandatory fortification of wheat flour for bread making, an increase in red cell folate concentration and a reduction in NTD in the Australian Aboriginal population was reported (Bower et al., 2016) However such improvements are not consistently reported. Analysis of a large data set in the USA following mandatory fortification of cereal grains with folic acid in 1998 did not find fortification with folic acid was associated with a significant

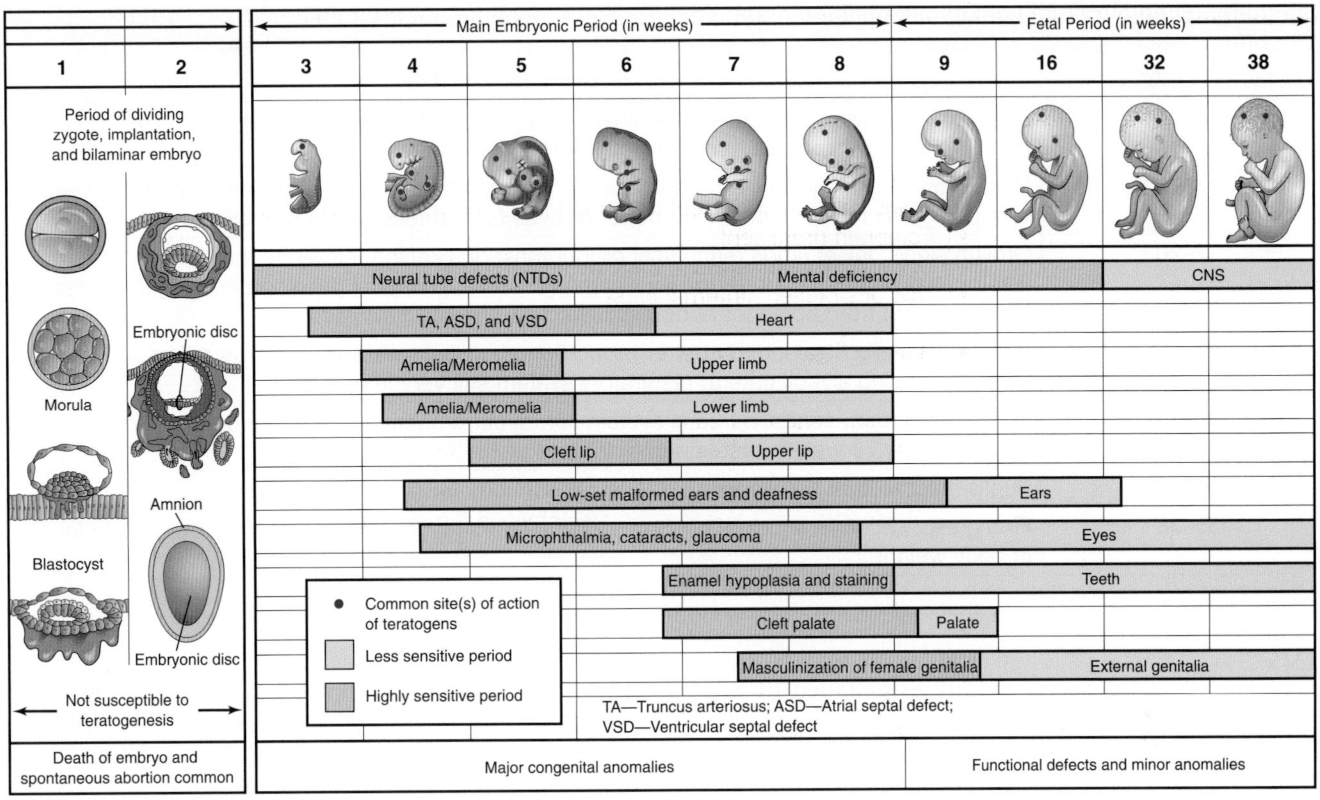

FIGURE 20.21 Critical periods for the different organ systems
(Based on Moore & Persaud, 1998)

decrease in the prevalence of NTDs at the population level (Murphy & Westmark, 2020). A Cochrane review reported that fortification of wheat flour with folic acid may reduce the risk of neural tube defects but due to the small number of studies and limitations in study design this was described as low-certainty evidence (Tablante et al., 2019).

In 2009 in New Zealand the recommendation was to increase voluntary fortification of bread. Subsequent mathematical modelling indicated the increased number of breads with fortification resulted in a marginal increase in folate intakes. This was calculated to be inferior to the impact of mandatory fortification (Evans et al., 2014).

Folate in the diet and the synthetic supplement, folic acid, are metabolised through a complex series of reactions. There is evidence that a mutation in one of the enzymes in this pathway, methylene-tetrahydrofolate reductase (MTHFR), may impact on levels of folate and unmetabolised folic acid. This is a growth area of research and more needs to be understood about the impact of mutations in MTHFR on a range of health issues (Boas et al., 2015; Plumptre et al., 2015).

1. What is the role of folic acid in preventing neural tube defects?
2. Does folic acid cross the placenta?
3. A review of supplementation in 39 countries identified that the majority (69.4%) recommend a healthy diet plus a folic acid supplement of 400 μg/d from pre-conception (4–12 weeks) until the end of the first trimester of pregnancy (8–12 weeks), consistent with the WHO recommendation (Gomes et al., 2016). What is the recommended level of supplementation in New Zealand and Australia? Is fortification of foods mandatory in Australia and New Zealand? Food Standards Australia New Zealand (FSANZ) develops food standards for both New Zealand and Australia. Information can be found at: https://www.foodstandards.gov.au/consumer/nutrition/folicmandatory/Pages/default.aspx

The developmental level at birth may affect adult health. Several studies support a link between low birth weight and increased risk of coronary heart disease, stroke, hypertension and non-insulin-dependent diabetes in adults (Barker, 2004; Kajantie et al., 2005).

Table 20.3 outlines some visual highlights of fetal development. The developing embryo and fetus is supported by the development of extraembryonic structures.

Development of the placenta and fetal membranes

The placenta is a fetomaternal organ—that is, it has fetal and maternal regions that develop from the trophoblast region in the blastocyst. Development begins in the second

Table 20.3 Overview of fetal development

Week of gestation	Visual highlight
9–12	Eyes can close; sex distinguishable externally by 12 weeks; red blood cells produced in liver at first, then mainly in spleen; urine excreted into amniotic fluid
13–16	Head proportionately smaller; ossification of skeleton begins; ovaries differentiated (16 weeks) with primordial follicles containing oogonia; eyes face anteriorly, not laterally now
17–20	Growth slows; lower limbs reach final proportions; quickening felt by mother, brown fat forms (site of heat production); uterus fully formed (18 weeks); vaginal development begun, testes begin descent from posterior abdominal wall (20 weeks)
21–25	Substantial weight gain; body better proportioned; cells in walls of lungs secreting surfactant to keep developing alveoli patent; respiratory system still very immature
26–29	Lungs developed; central nervous system can direct breathing, bone marrow produces red blood cells by 28 weeks; testes begin descent at 28–32 weeks
30–34	Pupils react to light (31 weeks); white fat 8% of body weight
35–38	Firm grasp; circumferences of head and abdomen equal (36 weeks); growth slows; white fat 16% of body weight

(Adapted from Moore & Persaud, 1998)

week. The placenta becomes fully established by 8–10 weeks, and full size by the fourth month. The placenta separates the maternal and fetal circulatory systems, yet allows ready exchange of many substances such as respiratory gases and nutrients between the mother and fetus. The placenta is the main site for the production of hormones that maintain the pregnancy, although initially hormones are supplied from the corpus luteum in the ovary. Secretion of hCG by the trophoblast maintains the corpus luteum until the placenta is able to take over hormone production by 8–10 weeks. The chorioamniotic membrane develops around the fetus and contains the amniotic fluid. It is metabolically active tissue that produces hormones.

Uteroplacental and fetoplacental circulation

Development of the fetal membranes and the placenta, along with development of embryonic blood vessels for transport, enables a more efficient exchange mechanism for the developing embryo than the cell-to-cell diffusion during early development.

Maternal lacunae

Primitive circulation develops as the syncytiotrophoblast erodes the glands and blood vessels of the endometrial tissue to form lacunae (spaces). Evidence indicates that, during the first trimester, trophoblastic plugs prevent blood flow from the spiral arterioles into the lacunae (Johnson, 2013; Khong, 2004). This means that embryonic development is in a relatively hypoxic environment (James et al., 2006; Johnson, 2013). Secretions from the endometrial glands initially fill the lacunae, allowing nutrients and oxygen to diffuse to the embryonic disc, and wastes and carbon dioxide to diffuse from the embryonic disc into maternal circulation. This primitive uteroplacental circulation is present by day 13. Towards the end of the first trimester, the lacunar networks develop into the intervillous spaces of the placenta, which fill with blood, providing fluid with a higher oxygen content for fetal exchange. By this time the fetus has developed blood vessels in the villi and mechanisms to cope with the higher levels of oxygen available from the maternal blood (Blackburn, 2017; James et al., 2006; Johnson, 2013).

Chorionic villi

During the second week, the cytotrophoblast invades the areas of syncytiotrophoblast between the lacunae and forms fingerlike projections called the chorionic villi. Further chorionic villi develop as the syncytiotrophoblast continues to invade the decidua. Villus development is stimulated by growth factors and the relatively hypoxic environment (Johnson, 2013). Blood vessels develop within the villi by 18–21 days, and a primitive fetoplacental circulation operates between embryonic blood in the villi, embryonic vessels and the primitive heart by 20–21 days. Villi can be two types, anchoring or branch villi, with similar numbers of both. Branch villi facilitate maternal–fetal exchange via diffusion, whereas anchoring villi attach the placenta to the decidua (Blackburn, 2017).

Formation of the smooth chorion and amnion

The chorionic villi initially cover the entire surface of the chorionic sac, but during the eighth week they disintegrate in some areas, forming the smooth chorion, and develop in other areas, forming the villous chorion. Degeneration occurs in areas compressed against the decidua capsularis as they lose their blood supply and become the smooth chorion and thus the chorionic membrane. In the area of membrane against the decidua basalis, the villi growing into the endometrium proliferate, and these become the chorionic villi of the fetal placenta (Moore et al., 2013).

The amnion is formed from embryonic ectoderm (see Embryology section earlier in the chapter). Initially the amnion encloses a small cavity, the amniotic cavity, situated above the embryonic disc, but the membrane and cavity enlarge to surround the embryo (Fig. 20.22). The amniotic membrane is pushed against the chorion and they form the chorioamniotic membrane, a double membrane sac surrounding the fetus. The membranes do not fuse, but rather are separated by 200 mL of amniotic fluid and mucus produced in the amnion. The chorion contains blood vessels that atrophy as pregnancy progresses; the amnion does not have a blood supply, but nutrients pass to it from the chorionic blood vessels. The amnion attachment to the fetus is reduced to the site of the umbilical cord. The membranes continue to grow until the 28th week, after which stretching accommodates the increased fetal size (Blackburn, 2017). Connective tissue is heavily interwoven with collagen, allowing stretching and providing strength.

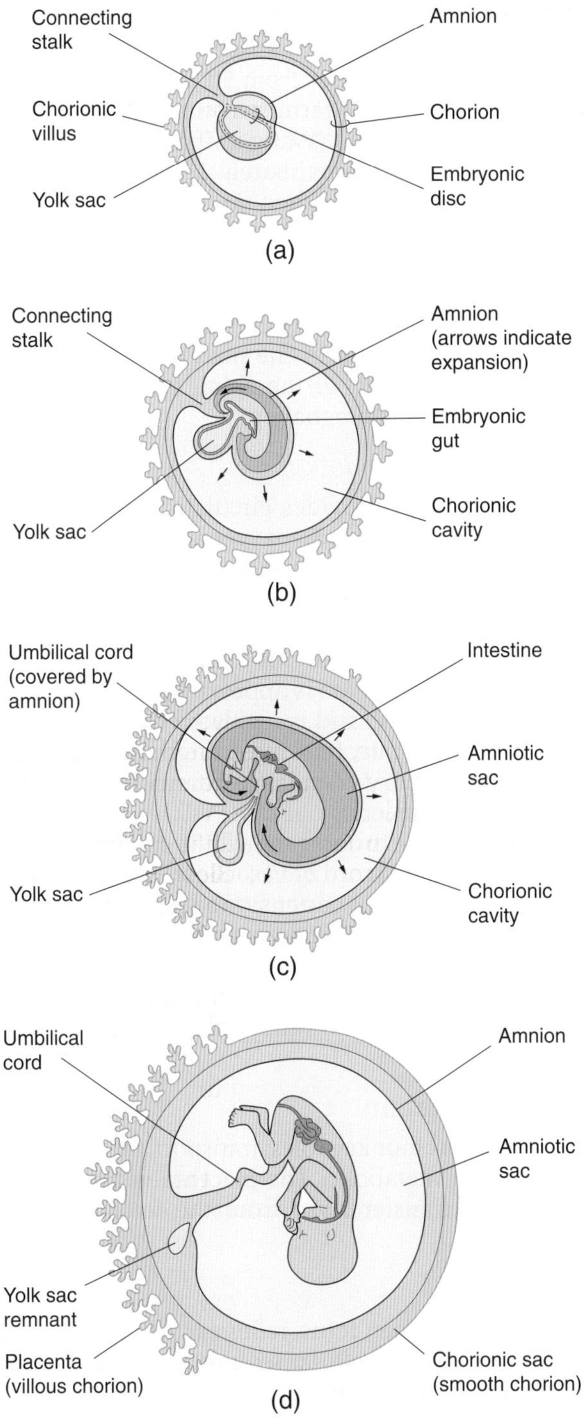

FIGURE 20.22 Steps showing how the amnion enlarges, fills the chorionic sac and envelops the umbilical cord: (a) 3 weeks; (b) 4 weeks; (c) 10 weeks; (d) 20 weeks
(Based on Moore & Persaud, 1998)

The amnion can rupture independently of the chorion and form amniotic bands of tissue. These bands can constrict and reduce blood supply to fetal parts, sometimes causing amputation (Guzman-Huerta et al., 2013).

The fetal membranes have a high metabolic rate, similar to that of the liver. They are active in synthesising many chemicals such as amniotic fluid, nutrients, renin and prostaglandins. The enzyme phospholipase A_2, necessary for prostaglandin synthesis, is found in the membranes and decidua, and the prostaglandin precursor arachidonic acid is also found in the membranes. The chorion stores hormones such as progesterone.

Amniotic fluid

Amniotic fluid is contained in the membranes and has several functions. It allows fetal movement and protects the fetus from changes in pressure and temperature. Protection from infection comes from antibacterial factors, such as transferrin (which binds iron needed by bacteria), fatty acids (which interfere with bacterial membranes), immunoglobulins and lysozymes (which destroy bacteria) (Blackburn, 2017).

The formation of amniotic fluid relies on diffusion of water and solutes from several sources. Initially there is some secretion by amniotic cells; however, most of the fluid diffuses from the interstitial fluid of the decidua parietalis and from blood in the intervillous spaces of the placenta across the amniochorionic membrane to the amniotic cavity. Exchange also occurs between the fetus and the amniotic cavity. The fetus swallows amniotic fluid, which is excreted by the fetal respiratory tract and fetal renal system (urine present in bladder by 11 weeks). Prior to keratinisation of the skin, which occurs by about 24 weeks, the skin is a major pathway for exchange of amniotic fluid (Blackburn, 2017; Modena & Fieni, 2004). Maternal hydration can alter amniotic fluid volume and there is some evidence that maternal resting in the left lateral recumbent position increases the production of fetal urine and amniotic fluid (Kahrama et al., 2011).

Amniotic fluid is composed of 98%–99% water, with the remaining 1%–2% comprising electrolytes, creatinine, urea, bile, renin, glucose, hormones, fetal cells, lanugo and vernix. The composition and volume change with the age of gestation of the fetus. If the volume of amniotic fluid is above or below the expected level for the gestational age of the fetus, conditions such as polyhydramnios or oligohydramnios can occur, with both maternal and fetal consequences.

Formation of the yolk sac (umbilical vesicle)

As the epiblast migrates to form the amnion, cells from the hypoblast migrate around the blastocyst cavity to form the extracoelomic cavity, which is modified to become the primary yolk sac, also termed the umbilical vesicle as the sac does not contain yolk (Moore et al., 2013). The embryonic disc is situated between the amniotic cavity and the yolk sac. The yolk sac is important for nutrient transfer in the second and third weeks. Early blood cell formation occurs in the wall of the yolk sac from the third to the sixth week, when the liver takes over this role. During the fourth week, part of the yolk sac is incorporated into the embryo as the primitive gut, and its endoderm develops into the epithelium of the respiratory and digestive tracts. The remainder degenerates to a small 5-mm structure by 10 weeks and disappears by 20 weeks (see Fig. 20.22) (Moore et al., 2013).

Placental circulation in the mature placenta

Once embryonic circulation is established, oxygen and nutrients diffuse from the secretions or blood entering the maternal intervillous spaces, through the walls of the branch villi, and then enter the embryonic capillaries in the chorionic villi. Carbon dioxide and waste products are exchanged in the opposite direction. Maternal and fetal blood do not mix unless the placenta tears away from the decidua (Fig. 20.23).

The placenta acts as a barrier to very few substances. Some large molecules with a particular shape and charge cannot pass—for example, heparin cannot cross but warfarin can. The placenta becomes thinner as pregnancy advances, and many drugs given to the mother are detected in fetal plasma.

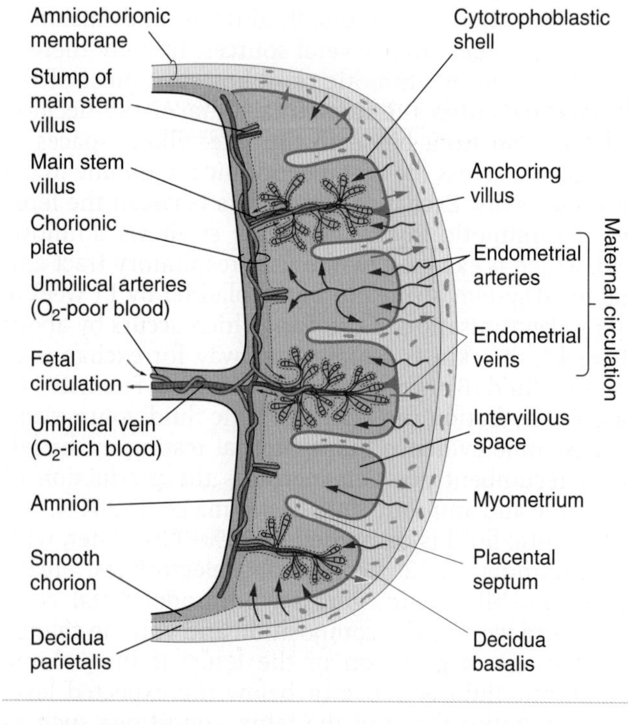

FIGURE 20.23 A full-term placenta: transverse section showing the relation of the fetal part to the maternal part
(Based on Moore & Persaud, 1998)

Maternal placental circulation

Maternal blood enters the intervillous space from the spiral arteries in the endometrium. Blood spurts towards the roof of the intervillous space and then flows around the villi, allowing exchange of gases and nutrients. Blood then leaves the intervillous spaces via the endometrial veins. Blood flow increases from 50 mL / min at 10 weeks to 600–800 mL / min at term, accounting for 20% of the increased cardiac output (Wang & Zhao, 2010). The intervillous spaces hold approximately 150 mL of blood, and this is continually replenished (Moore et al., 2013). During labour, uterine contractions prevent blood entering the intervillous spaces, but sufficient blood is retained there (150 mL) for fetal exchange of oxygen, nutrients and so on (see Fig. 20.23). It is hypothesised that a dysfunctional implantation of the placenta associated with impaired development of the spiral arteries may cause hypertension during pregnancy.

Fetal placental circulation

The umbilical cord provides circulatory connection between mother and fetus. Deoxygenated blood leaves the fetus via two umbilical arteries to the placenta, and oxygenated blood comes from the placenta via the umbilical vein. Wharton's jelly, consisting of collagen, muscle and mucopolysaccharide, cushions the blood vessels. Fetal blood flow in the placenta is approximately 500 mL / min (Wang & Zhao, 2010), and is regulated by several factors, such as fetal heart rate, fetal left-to-right shunts, and systemic and pulmonary vascular resistance (see the section Fetal circulation, below).

If the blood flow around the villi is compromised (e.g. prolapse of umbilical cord or vasoconstriction of maternal blood vessels due to hypertension), fetal hypoxia occurs. This may be indicated by decelerations in fetal heart rate and can lead to fetal death. A chronic reduction in uteroplacental circulation can result in intrauterine growth restriction owing to reduced supply of nutrients and oxygen to the fetus.

Placental function

The placenta has four key roles: transport, immunological, endocrine and metabolic. The placenta is also the main route of heat transfer away from the fetus (Blackburn, 2017).

Transport role

The embryo, and then fetus, relies exclusively on the placenta for transport of cellular requirements. This includes the transport of the following substances:

- Respiratory gases, oxygen and carbon dioxide—the rate of delivery is dependent on maternal and fetal blood flow. Any factors that impede uterine or fetal blood flow can lead to fetal hypoxia. Inhaled anaesthetics readily cross the placenta to the fetus, as does carbon monoxide produced from the incomplete combustion of cigarette smoke.

- Nutrients—these constitute the bulk of substances transferred. Glucose, water and all vitamins cross rapidly. Small amounts of free fatty acids are transferred, whereas there is little or no transfer of maternal cholesterol, phospholipids or triglycerides. Transferrin, an iron-transport protein, crosses the placenta and delivers iron to the fetus (Moore et al., 2013).
- Hormones—steroid hormones cross freely; protein hormones are generally not transported to the fetus, but small amounts of thyroid hormones do cross slowly (Moore et al., 2013).
- Waste products—carbon dioxide, urea, uric acid and conjugated bilirubin are all transported quickly across the placenta (Moore et al., 2013).
- Electrolytes—are freely exchanged. This includes any intravenous fluids given to the mother, which can interfere with fetal fluid balance (Moore et al., 2013).
- Normal cellular transport mechanisms—of simple and facilitated diffusion, active transport and pinocytosis—allow movement of these substances between the maternal and fetal circulation. However, many harmful substances can also pass freely by the same mechanisms. These include the following:
- Drugs—almost all drugs can pass freely and many result in compromise for the fetus; for example, alcohol can cause fetal alcohol syndrome, narcotics may result in heroin addiction in the newborn, and sedatives and analgesics such as pethidine used in labour can cause respiratory depression in the newborn. Antibiotics cross the placenta and this may be beneficial.
- Infectious agents—several viruses can cross the placenta and cause fetal infection—for example, rubella, poliomyelitis, measles and HIV. In some cases (e.g. rubella), severe congenital malformations may result.

Fig. 20.24 summarises the range of substances that are transported across the placenta.

Increased transport of substances occurs as pregnancy progresses. This is due to a decrease in the distance between maternal and fetal blood as placental development occurs, an increased volume of blood transported and greater fetal demands. Many factors can influence placental transport, such as maternal nutritional status or exercise. Disease states that influence maternal nutrient level, such as diabetes mellitus, or influence blood flow, such as hypertension, also affect placental transfer.

Immunological role

The placenta provides an effective barrier against most large bacterial microorganisms; however, most viruses and some smaller bacteria can pass to the fetus. Protection is afforded by maternal antibodies, particularly immunoglobulin G (IgG) antibodies, which cross the placenta and provide passive immunity against some diseases such as measles, diphtheria and smallpox. Maternal antibodies do not protect against chickenpox or pertussis (whooping cough) (Moore et al., 2013). Transfer of antibodies can be disadvantageous—an example is transfer of rhesus (Rh) antibodies to a fetus following antibody production by a mother with Rh− blood who has been exposed to Rh+ blood. If the fetus is Rh+ this can lead to haemolytic disease of the newborn (erythroblastic fetalis). Despite having a different genetic composition from that of the mother, the trophoblast is protected from generating an immune response in the mother (Gaunt & Ramin, 2001; Rankin, 2017).

Endocrine role

Several hormones that maintain pregnancy are synthesised in the placenta: oestrogens, progesterone, hCG and hPL. These hormones are discussed later in the section on pregnancy.

Metabolic role

The placenta synthesises glycogen, cholesterol, fatty acids and enzymes, which are used by the embryo/fetus and

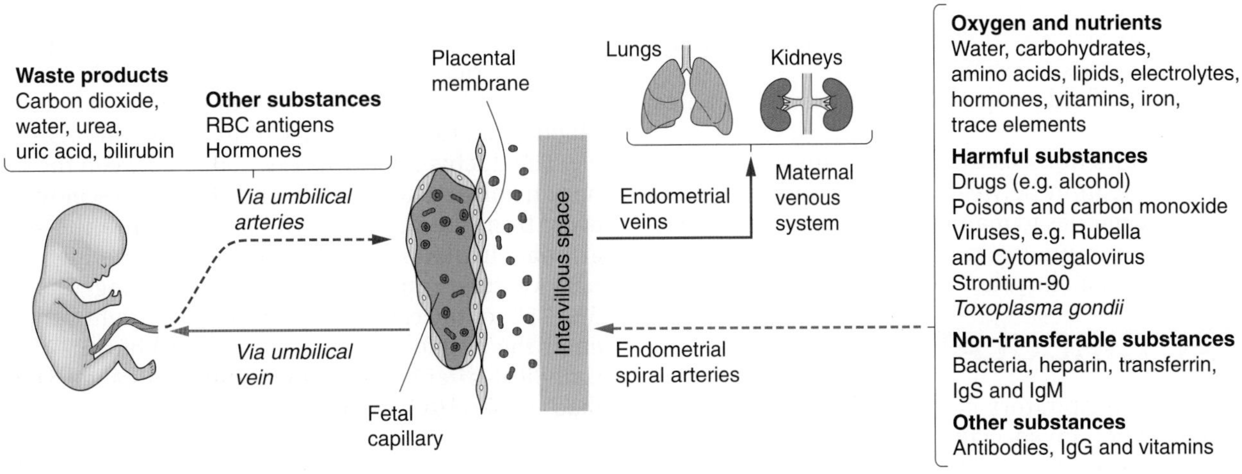

FIGURE 20.24 Substances transported across the placenta. RBC = red blood cell; Ig = immunoglobulin
(Based on Moore & Persaud, 1998)

the placenta. This is particularly important in early pregnancy (Moore et al., 2013).

CRITICAL THINKING EXERCISE

Explain the advantages to the embryo of the placental circulation. How is nutrition provided prior to this (e.g. during the blastocyst stage)?

Summary of placental and fetal membrane development

- The placenta begins to form as the syncytiotrophoblast invades the endometrium.
- Maternal blood vessels and glands are eroded to form lacunae, and these link over time to form the blood-filled maternal intervillous spaces.
- The cytotrophoblast invades the areas between the lacunae to form the fetal chorionic villi, which are invaded by fetal blood vessels.
- Exchange of nutrients and wastes occurs via cell transport mechanisms such as diffusion and active transport between the blood in the fetal vessels and the secretions or blood in the intervillous spaces. Transport involves crossing the membrane of the chorionic villus and the endothelium of the fetal capillary.
- Maternal blood arrives at the intervillous spaces from the uterine arteries and leaves in the uterine veins. On the fetal side, blood arrives at the placenta from the umbilical arteries and leaves in the single umbilical vein.
- A double membrane develops around the embryo. The outer chorion is formed from the cytotrophoblast, while the inner amnion is formed from migrating ectoderm from the embryonic disc.
- The fetal membranes are metabolically active, producing amniotic fluid and hormones involved in pregnancy.
- The amniotic fluid circulates through the fetus in the digestive, respiratory and renal systems, and is also exchanged across the skin.
- The amniotic fluid protects the fetus from mechanical stress.
- The main functions of the placenta are to provide a transport medium between the fetus and mother, to produce hormones to maintain pregnancy, and to provide some immunological protection to the fetus. It also has a metabolic role.

FETAL CIRCULATION

The fetal cardiorespiratory systems have several physiological and structural specialisations that allow survival in a fluid environment. The fetal circulatory system delivers oxygen and nutrients to the fetal tissues and removes metabolic waste products, but the fetus relies on the placenta for oxygenation of the blood, and not its own lungs, which remain dormant and fluid filled until birth. Fetal breathing movements can be detected on ultrasound by week 10 (Blackburn, 2017); however, the lungs and associated pulmonary blood vessels do not reach adequate maturity until 28 weeks gestation. Premature delivery with associated immaturity of the lungs and pulmonary vasculature can result in respiratory distress syndrome (RDS).

In the fetus, several structures (see below) are present to divert blood from the immature lungs to the placenta for gas exchange. This leads to the mixing of oxygenated and deoxygenated blood in the atria, aorta and vena cava, which lowers levels of oxygen saturation.

Characteristics

Fetal circulation is characterised by fast flow, low vascular resistance (due to the low-resistance umbilical and placental circulations) and high pulmonary vascular resistance. The oxygen content of fetal blood is lower than that of the neonate, but fetal haemoglobin (HbF) has a higher affinity for oxygen to manage this hypoxic state.

Structures

The fetal structures—umbilical vein, umbilical arteries, ductus venosus, foramen ovale and ductus arteriosus—ensure that the fetal circulation is routed to the placenta for oxygenation and that most of the blood bypasses the lungs, which are non-functional (Fig. 20.25). The placenta is a low-resistance pathway, taking 40% of the fetal cardiac output. The umbilical vein carries oxygenated blood from the placenta to the inferior vena cava (IVC), either indirectly via the hepatic portal system or directly via the ductus venosus. The ductus venosus is a low-resistance pathway that bypasses the liver and takes 40%–60% of blood flow, thereby enabling a large amount of the oxygenated blood to reach the heart directly. Deoxygenated blood from the lower part of the fetal body mixes in the IVC with oxygenated blood from the ductus venosus just before the IVC enters the right atrium.

The foramen ovale is an opening in the septum between the right and left atria that allows 50%–60% of the blood to shunt directly to the left atrium. The rest of the blood flows to the ductus arteriosus via the right ventricle. The ductus arteriosus is situated between the pulmonary trunk and aortic arch, and shunts 60% of the blood away from the pulmonary circulation into the systemic arterial circulation via the aortic arch. The high pulmonary vascular resistance of the deflated lungs allows only 5%–15% of the cardiac output from the right ventricle to enter the pulmonary circulation (Blackburn, 2017). The umbilical arteries carry deoxygenated blood from the iliac arteries back to the placenta.

Oxygen saturation of fetal blood

The fetus has high oxygen demands for its metabolic needs and this is reflected in the high cardiac output,

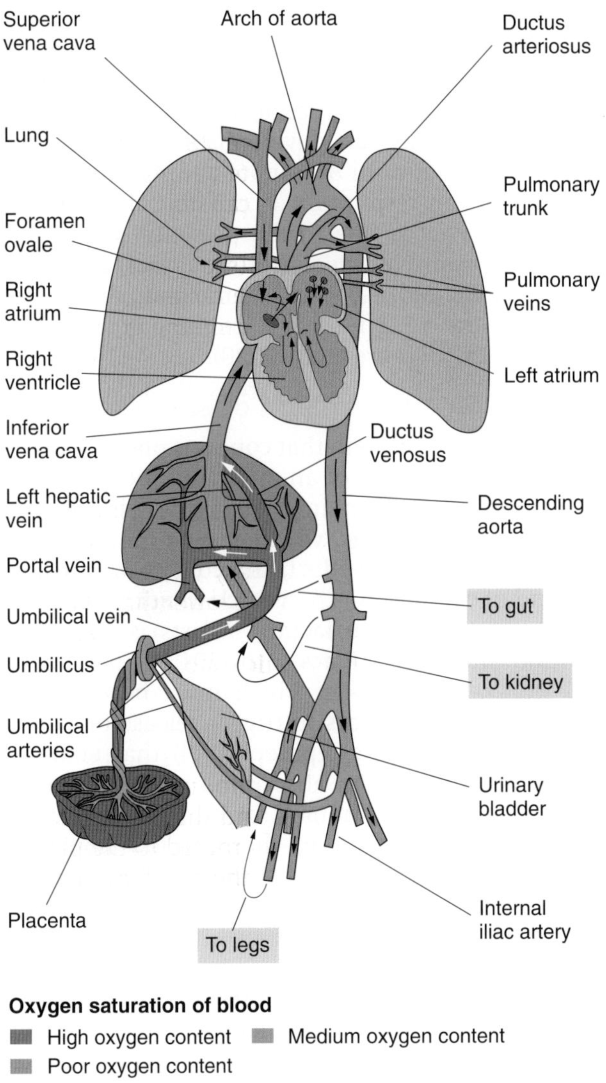

FIGURE 20.25 Schematic illustration of the fetal circulation
(Based on Moore & Persaud, 1998)

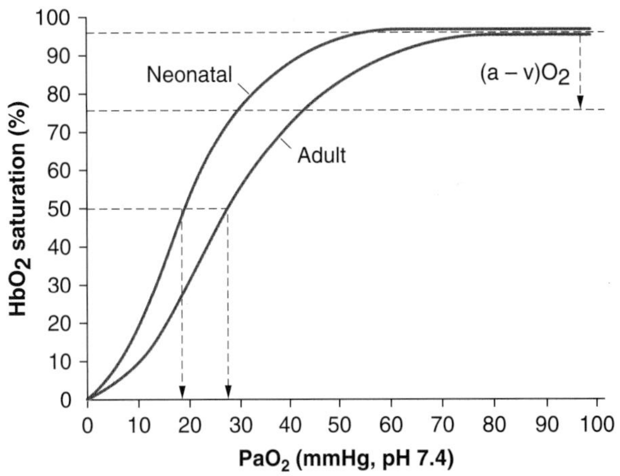

FIGURE 20.26 Oxyhaemoglobin curves of blood: from term infants at birth and from adults
(Based on Blackburn, 2003)

which is 250 mL / min per kg compared with the adult value of 85 mL / min per kg. Fetal heart rate is also high at 155 b.p.m. at 20 weeks and 140 b.p.m. at 40 weeks (Blackburn, 2017).

The highest oxygen saturation occurs in the umbilical vein at 70% (32–5 mmHg), falling to 65% (26–8 mmHg) in the left atrium and ascending aorta. This blood, at 65% saturation, also perfuses the fetal brain and coronary arteries. Blood returning from the lower limbs to the hepatic circulation and from the superior vena cava to the right atrium is very desaturated, at 25% (16–17 mmHg) even less than the 50% (18–19 mmHg) saturated blood returning to the placenta via the umbilical arteries (see Fig. 20.25).

There is a maternal–fetal oxygen gradient at the placenta (maternal partial arterial oxygen pressure P_aO_2 is 33 mmHg, fetal P_aO_2 is 28 mmHg), which facilitates oxygen diffusion into the umbilical vein. Fetal blood is uniquely able to maintain oxygen saturation at a higher level for a given P_aO_2 than adult blood. This is due to the increased affinity that HbF has for oxygen, which improves saturation and allows more oxygen to reach the tissues (Blackburn, 2017).

The fetal oxyhaemoglobin dissociation curve is shifted to the left of the maternal oxyhaemoglobin (HbO_2) dissociation curve, and illustrates that HbF binds more oxygen at lower saturations, and equally that very low saturations must be reached before significant oxygen will be released from the HbF (Fig. 20.26).

Development of fetal circulation and lungs

The cardiovascular system is the first embryonic system to start functioning. This facilitates more efficient distribution of oxygen and nutrients around the growing mass of the embryo. An indication of the level of development at various gestational ages follows. (More detail is available from the Further reading list at the end of the chapter.)

By 3–4 weeks the heart tube, containing one atrium and one ventricle, is beating. Development of the lungs is paralleled by development of the pulmonary circulation, but lungs do not take on a gas-exchange function until birth. By 3–4 weeks a lung bud has appeared at the caudal end of the laryngotracheal tube, and blood vessels, which will be the future pulmonary arteries, have formed branches to the lung bud. By 8–10 weeks the heart has four chambers with mitral and tricuspid valves, and bronchi and bronchioles have formed in the lungs (Fig. 20.27). Development of pulmonary blood vessels is concurrent with development of the bronchi.

By 20 weeks, pulmonary vascularisation is prominent and development of pulmonary terminal sacs from the respiratory bronchioles is ongoing. Lung fluid secretion begins from the terminal sacs and pulmonary capillaries.

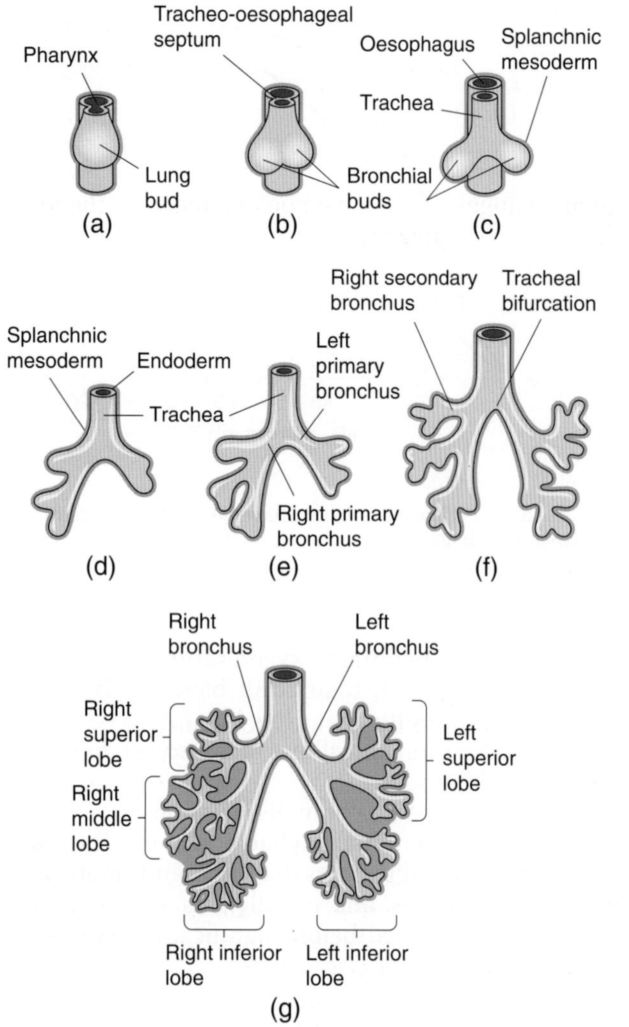

FIGURE 20.27 Successive stages in the development of the bronchi and lungs: (a) to (c) 4 weeks; (d) to (e) 5 weeks; (f) 6 weeks; (g) 8 weeks
(Based on Blackburn, 2003)

Fetal breathing movements are well established. They occur 40%–80% of the time, and at a rate of 30–70 breaths/minute (Blackburn, 2017; Bolt et al., 2001).

Fetal breathing movements

Fetal breathing movements cause movement of amniotic fluid and are important for their role in stimulating development of the lungs. The diaphragm appears to play a more significant role than the thorax in fetal breathing movements (Blackburn, 2017). Lung development is dependent on sufficient thoracic space for lung development, sufficient amniotic fluid and fetal breathing movements. These breathing movements increase closer to term (Moore et al., 2013).

At 25 weeks, respiration is possible because some primitive alveoli have developed, but severe respiratory insufficiency is likely if the baby is born prematurely. At this time the terminal sacs are sparse, and lined with thick cuboidal epithelial cells; pulmonary capillaries are still developing and there is insufficient surfactant in the alveoli. From 26 to 28 weeks, terminal air sacs develop and form clusters in conjunction with extensive capillary networks. Terminal sac development continues until birth and beyond, until 8 years of age. At 28 weeks, gas exchange during respiration is possible if birth occurs prematurely. This is due to the presence of clusters of thin-walled primitive alveoli (terminal sacs) and pulmonary capillaries. At 32–6 weeks, surfactant production by cells within the alveoli—type II pneumatocytes—begins (Bolt et al., 2001; Moore et al., 2020).

Composition and function of surfactant

Surfactant is a lipoprotein that contains phospholipids. It prevents the formation of an air/water interface, which reduces surface tension in the alveoli. This increases compliance of the lungs, which means they can be inflated for relatively less effort, and collapse of the alveoli at the end of expiration is prevented (Blackburn, 2017).

The presence of surfactant assists absorption of lung fluid after birth (Blackburn, 2017). This amounts to 25 mL/kg body mass, which must be excreted or absorbed. Labour appears to trigger release of catecholamines (e.g. adrenaline (epinephrine)) that enable the switch from secretion to absorption of lung fluid. The sudden change in pulmonary blood flow at birth also helps remove lung fluid in the first few hours. This change from secretion to absorption of lung fluid is critical for survival of the baby and the process is mediated through the activation of airway epithelial sodium channels (Helve et al., 2009).

Glucocorticoid and thyroid hormones enhance surfactant synthesis, the former by increasing glycogen depletion as well as by increasing phospholipid synthesis. Glycogen depletion leads to changes in the alveoli, such as thinning and increased size of the alveoli, along with increasing the numbers of type II pneumatocytes. If insufficient surfactant is present at birth, ventilation is impaired resulting in infant respiratory distress syndrome (IRDS). Thyroid hormones increase the rate of phospholipid synthesis (Blackburn, 2017; Bolt et al., 2001).

Clinical applications

Conditions that inhibit glycogen depletion in the lungs, such as insulin-dependent diabetes, may inhibit surfactant synthesis if the condition is not well controlled. Insulin inhibits glycogen breakdown, effectively decreasing the substrate needed for phospholipid synthesis, and the structural changes associated with glycogen depletion are inhibited (Blackburn, 2017).

Some conditions accelerate lung maturity by inducing stress in the fetus, therefore increasing secretion of glucocorticoids and catecholamines (e.g. preeclampsia, intrauterine growth restriction (IUGR), premature rupture of the membranes) (Blackburn, 2017). Several studies have shown that antenatal administration of glucocorticoids to women increases fetal surfactant production and reduces the occurrence of IRDS. A systematic review and meta-analysis of six trials which analysed 5698 singleton pregnancies provided further evidence that administration of antenatal steroids at ≥ 34 weeks gestation reduced neonatal respiratory morbidity (Saccone & Berghella, 2016). Neonates requiring ventilation may be given surfactant via an endotrachial tube.

CRITICAL THINKING EXERCISE

Explain how the anatomical features specific to the fetal circulation contribute to effective gas exchange in utero. Compare the mechanisms required for gas exchange in utero and following birth.

Summary of fetal circulation

- Fetal circulation is characterised by fast flow, low vascular resistance and high pulmonary vascular resistance.
- Fetal structures divert blood from the lungs to the placenta. These are the umbilical vein, umbilical arteries, ductus venosus, foramen ovale and ductus arteriosus.
- The high oxygen needs of the fetus are met by a high cardiac output. HbF enhances oxygen transfer from maternal blood. This is reflected in a shift to the left of the HbO_2 dissociation curve of the fetus.
- Oxygenated blood from the umbilical vein mixes with deoxygenated blood returning in the vena cava, producing 'mixed blood' with reduced oxygen saturation. This returns to the heart and circulates to the tissues via branches of the aorta. Branches from the internal iliac arteries flow into the umbilical arteries to return to the placenta.
- At 25 weeks gestation, respiration is possible as some primitive alveoli have developed, but the epithelial lining is thick, pulmonary capillaries are sparse and insufficient surfactant is produced.
- At 28 weeks, further development of the terminal air sacs, capillaries and surfactant makes gas exchange possible.
- Fetal breathing movements facilitate development of the lungs.
- Surfactant increases the compliance of the lungs and facilitates fluid reabsorption after birth.

MATERNAL CHANGES ASSOCIATED WITH PREGNANCY

Pregnancy is associated with major physiological changes that enable the woman to support the in utero growth and development of the baby, from the beginnings as a one-celled organism until reaching term as a complex human being. This process takes an average of 266 days (38 weeks) from the time of fertilisation, or 280 days if the time is taken from the first day of the last menstrual bleeding. The maternal physiological changes associated with the growing fetus and with the changes to the body systems are predominantly controlled by hormones, in some instances facilitated by the increase in size of the fetus. The function of these hormones and the subsequent changes to maternal body systems are the focus of this section on pregnancy.

Hormones of pregnancy

There are a vast number of hormones and neurohormones, growth factors and proteins produced by the placenta during pregnancy. The maternal physiological and anatomical changes during pregnancy are largely controlled by the following hormones:

- human chorionic gonadotrophin (hCG)
- human placental lactogen (hPL)
- oestrogens
- progesterone.

Human chorionic gonadotrophin

Human chorionic gonadotrophin is a glycoprotein, similar in structure to luteinising hormone, secreted by the trophoblast. It can be detected in the blood 9 days after fertilisation and in the urine 10–12 days after fertilisation (Rankin, 2017).

It is linked to many maternal changes in the first trimester. Probably most importantly, it prevents the degeneration of the corpus luteum and stimulates it to continue secreting oestrogens and progesterone until the placenta takes over this role. Changes in smell, taste and saliva seem to be correlated with the level of hCG, which has been linked to feelings of nausea in the first trimester. It may also have an immunosuppressant role that reduces maternal rejection of the placenta (Blackburn, 2017).

Human placental lactogen

Human placental lactogen is a polypeptide, similar to growth hormone, secreted by the syncytiotrophoblast. Synthesis begins 5–10 days after implantation and levels increase to a peak just before term (Blackburn, 2017). It facilitates growth, changing maternal metabolism to maximise the nutrients available to the fetus in utero. Three key metabolic changes facilitated by hPL are as follows:

- It reduces maternal utilisation of glucose by reducing the response of maternal cells to insulin—it is an insulin antagonist. This raises the maternal blood glucose level and makes more glucose available to the fetus.
- It mobilises maternal lipid stores, releasing fatty acids as the maternal energy source, leaving glucose for fetal uptake.
- It accelerates amino acid transfer to the fetus.

Steroid hormones

The steroid hormones oestrogen and progesterone, responsible for the maintenance of pregnancy, are initially

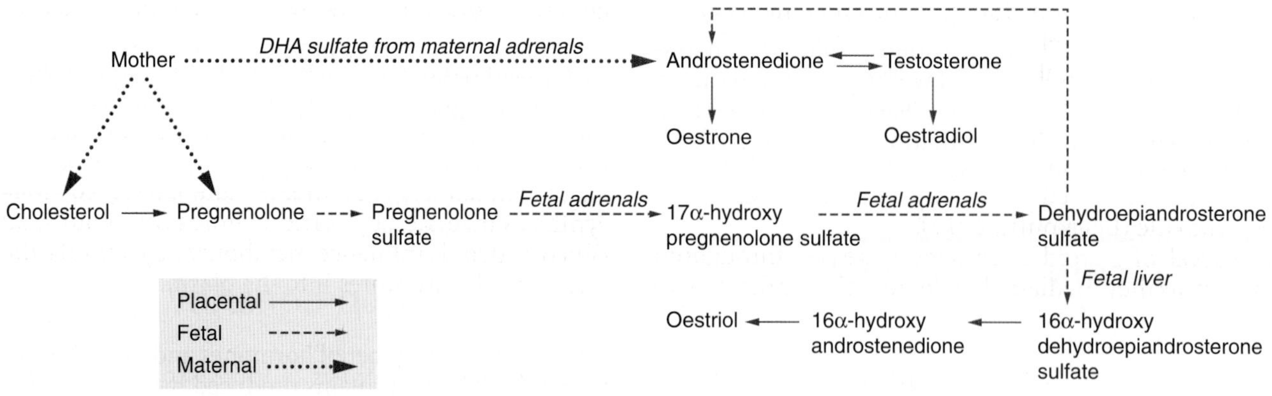

FIGURE 20.28 Summary of the principal routes by which the human fetoplacental unit synthesises oestrogens
(Based on Johnson & Everitt, 2000)

released from the corpus luteum in the ovaries. The placenta takes over this role at about 7 weeks gestation. The synthesis is complex, involving the mother, placenta and fetus, as each lacks the enzymes necessary for independent synthesis. Fig. 20.28 illustrates the interconnections in the pathways for synthesis. The common precursor for steroid synthesis is cholesterol; the synthesis of cholesterol is increased in pregnancy to meet the demand for steroid synthesis.

Oestrogens

Three types of oestrogens are synthesised in the ovaries and placenta: oestriol, beta oestradiol and oestrone. Oestriol, the weaker form, is the most common oestrogen; it increases most significantly during pregnancy. In a non-pregnant woman, oestriol is synthesised from beta oestradiol and oestrone in the ovaries; however, during pregnancy oestriol synthesis relies on enzymes in the fetal liver and on dehydroepiandrosterone sulfate (DHEAS) from the fetal adrenals for synthesis. There is a rapid increase early in pregnancy, which slows between 24 and 32 weeks, and then there is a surge in oestriol at 34–6 weeks. Measurement of oestriol levels was one of the earliest methods of monitoring fetal wellbeing, but this technique is no longer used (Blackburn, 2017).

Oestrogens stimulate growth of tissues by increasing protein synthesis. They cause the hyperplasia and hypertrophy of the uterus, the increased vascularisation of the uterus and the development of the mammary ducts and alveolar tissue in the breasts. Oestrogens also cause swelling and softening of connective tissues (e.g. cervix, nipples and ligaments) by increasing the water content in the extracellular matrix and reducing the adhesion of the collagen fibres in connective tissues. Angiotensin and aldosterone levels increase under the influence of oestrogens, leading to fluid retention. Oestrogens increase the sensitivity of the uterus to progesterone and, along with progesterone, increase the sensitivity of the maternal respiratory centre to carbon dioxide.

These functions of oestrogens contribute to some of the minor discomforts of pregnancy. Water retention mediated by oestrogen can lead to oedema. Pelvic discomfort can result from relaxation of the pelvic ligaments, stretching of the sacroiliac and sacrococcygeal joints, and the increasing elasticity of the symphysis pubis.

Progesterone

Progesterone is secreted by the corpus luteum initially, and then by the placental syncytiotrophoblast. The fetus is not essential for progesterone synthesis, and therefore levels are not indicative of fetal wellbeing. Placental progesterone enters both the maternal and fetal circulation and is broken down and excreted in the urine as pregnanediol.

Progesterone increases the secretory activity of the decidual cells of the uterus, which supply nourishment for the embryo (as discussed in the section on the placenta, earlier in the chapter). Along with other uterotonic inhibitors, progesterone lowers smooth muscle excitability, particularly in the myometrium, to prevent uterine contraction, but also in the ureters, stomach and intestines. It increases the sensitivity of the maternal chemoreceptors to carbon dioxide, thus stimulating ventilation at lower partial arterial carbon dioxide pressure (P_aCO_2) values than before pregnancy. Progesterone also has a role in implantation, and in helping to suppress the maternal immunological response (Blackburn, 2017). Fetal adrenal hormone production relies on progesterone as an essential precursor.

Progesterone-induced relaxation of smooth muscle results in many of the minor discomforts of pregnancy, such as:

- oesophageal reflux (heartburn), due to relaxation of the oesophageal sphincter
- nausea and vomiting, which may be potentiated by reduced peristalsis
- urinary tract infections, which increase in pregnancy owing to stasis of urine caused by relaxation of the smooth muscle in the ureters and bladder
- varicose veins and haemorrhoids, due to dilation of the veins in the legs and rectal region

- postural hypotension, due to venous pooling resulting from reduced peripheral resistance in the blood vessels in the lower limbs (Rankin, 2017).

As well as the smooth muscle relaxation effect, progesterone has a thermogenic effect, increasing body temperature by 0.5–1.0°C, and it stimulates hyperventilation owing to the increased sensitivity of chemoreceptors to carbon dioxide (Blackburn, 2017).

The level of steroid hormones increases throughout pregnancy, as they mediate changes to facilitate the growth and nourishment of the fetus.

CRITICAL THINKING EXERCISE

Knowing the impact that hPL has on metabolism during pregnancy, explain how this hormone facilitates fetal growth.

Endocrine glands

The placenta secretes both hormones and neurohormones throughout pregnancy that have wide ranging effects on maternal and fetal physiology in pregnancy and have a role in initiation of labour. The role of the placenta in synthesising hormones such as hCG, hPL, oestrogens and progesterones has already been discussed. It has a further role in producing neurohormones such as corticotrophic-releasing hormone (CRH), thyrotrophin-releasing hormone (TRH), adrenocorticotrophic hormone (ACTH) and beta endorphin (Voltolini & Petraglia, 2014). As such, the placenta has a significant impact on all aspects of pregnancy and birth.

Pregnancy is also associated with an increase in size of the anterior pituitary gland and increases in secretion of adrenocorticotrophic hormone (ACTH). This is probably the result of placental corticotrophic-releasing hormone (CRH) stimulation rather than of hypothalamic CRH stimulation. Placental CRH is present in low levels during pregnancy, increases throughout pregnancy and has a role in the initiation of labour (Voltolini & Petraglia, 2014). Increases in prolactin, thyrotrophin and melanocyte-stimulating hormone occur and in the third trimester an increase in pituitary beta endorphin and spinal endorphins is detected. Endorphin increase is linked to the increase in pain threshold in the latter part of pregnancy. The posterior pituitary increases secretion of oxytocin but ADH levels are similar to non-pregnant levels (Voltolini and Petraglia, 2014). However, the osmoreceptors in the hypothalamus are adjusted to the lower osmotic pressure of pregnancy (Blackburn, 2017).

Not all hormones are increased. Levels of **gonadotrophins** (FSH and LH) are depressed via negative feedback owing to the increasing levels of steroid hormones (oestrogen and progesterone). This prevents further ovulation during pregnancy.

The adrenal gland increases corticosteroid (glucocorticoid and aldosterone) production. Cortisol, the main glucocorticoid, increases two- to threefold by term, and the diurnal rhythm of release continues, higher levels being secreted in the morning than in the evening.

Increases in corticosteroids have been linked to the formation of striae gravidarum or 'stretch marks'. The cause is unclear but may be related to reduced adhesiveness between collagen fibres and decreased collagen synthesis mediated by corticosteroids (Blackburn, 2017). Glucocorticoids influence metabolism by stimulating the release of glucose stores into the plasma.

The thyroid gland increases in size in response to low levels of iodine in the blood. During pregnancy, iodine clearance by the kidneys is increased. As iodine is an essential component of the thyroid hormones (thyroxine, T_4 and tri-iodothyronine, T_3), this stimulates hypertrophy of the thyroid and an associated increase in release of T_3 and T_4. However, there is also increased circulating thyroxine-binding globulin during pregnancy, and therefore there is no actual increase in thyroid hormone activity (Blackburn, 2017). There is evidence linking increased levels of T_4 to nausea and vomiting in pregnancy (Forbes, 2014). In fact, women with pre-existing hyperthyroidism may experience some relief of symptoms during pregnancy owing to the increased level of thyroxine-binding globulin (Blackburn, 2017). Increased release of parathyroid hormone facilitates increased calcium absorption from the gut and decreased excretion by the kidneys, and therefore increased calcium is available to the fetus.

REFLECTIVE THINKING EXERCISE

Hormones initiate widespread physiological changes during pregnancy. Reflect on the diversity of these changes and consider how you would explain these to a pregnant woman to aid her understanding of her changing physiology.

Changes to the reproductive system

The reproductive system probably undergoes the most obvious changes associated with pregnancy. There is considerable enlargement of the uterus, softening of the cervix, engorgement of the vulva, and growth and development of the breasts. These changes are to accommodate the growing fetus and to prepare for birth and nutrition of the baby.

Uterus

Under the influence of oestrogen, the uterine muscle fibres undergo hypertrophy and hyperplasia, resulting in a spherical, thick-walled (25 mm) uterus by 20 weeks (Blackburn, 2017). Following this, the uterus grows by distension as the growing fetus stretches the muscle fibres. During the third trimester, this results in a thinner-walled (5–10 mm) cylindrical-shaped uterus that is easily indented, the fetus being easily palpated and fetal movements visible. The uterine mass increases from 50 grams pre-conception to approximately 1100–1200 grams at term, and the uterine cavity changes from a capacity of 10 mL to one of 5 L (Blackburn, 2017).

The uterine muscle supports and protects the fetus. It has both contractile and elastic properties, which equip the uterus to accommodate growth during pregnancy and to generate tension during labour. The myometrium comprises four layers, which have different roles in preparing for birth:

- The inner, circular layer runs in a spiral around the cornua, lower uterine segment and cervix and stretches during labour.
- The middle, oblique layer contracts to expel the fetus and constrict blood vessels after the placenta is birthed—commonly referred to as the 'living ligatures'.
- The two outer, longitudinal layers contract and shorten during labour to cause thickening of the upper segment, which maximises the expulsive force exerted on the baby during labour.

The different layers of muscle have different embryonic origins and may respond differently to uterotonic agonists and antagonists (Blackburn, 2017). Uterine muscle is sparsely innervated by adrenergic neurons, which disappear from the myometrium at term.

The lower uterine segment muscles are replaced by connective tissue, and this enables stretching in late pregnancy. Uterine blood vessels hypertrophy and become more coiled up until 20 weeks, and then uncoiling occurs as the uterus distends. Stretching of the broad ligament may cause painful sensations during the second and third trimesters. Whereas the myometrium is capable of spontaneous activity, progesterone, relaxin, nitric oxide and prostacyclin exert an inhibitory effect (Blackburn, 2017). However, as pregnancy progresses there is an increase in frequency of contractions, about a 5% increase per week. These contractions are commonly referred to as 'Braxton Hicks' contractions. Contractions are more common at night and least common in the early afternoon. Contractions in the second trimester are irregular and painless but may become uncomfortable during the third trimester. The changes in character of the contractions are due to structural and functional changes in the myometrium mediated by changing oestrogen and progesterone (Blackburn, 2017).

Table 20.4 lists some of the key changes that occur as the uterus enlarges.

Table 20.4 Stages of uterine development

Week of gestation	Characteristic uterine changes
12	• Uterus rises out of the pelvis in an upright position, often to the right • Cervical isthmus stretches • Fundus can be palpated abdominally above symphysis pubis
20	• Uterus becomes thicker and rounded • Fallopian tubes become more vertically positioned
30	• Lower uterine segment can be identified
36	• Uterus reaches the xiphisternum • Fetus moves down into the lower region of the uterus

(Adapted from Rankin, 2017)

Cervix

The cervix is primarily composed of connective tissue covered in a thin layer of smooth muscle. Changes occur throughout pregnancy, and by the second trimester the cervix becomes swollen as it softens and widens owing to the effect of oestrogens, prostaglandins, progesterone, relaxin and nitric oxide on the collagen fibres and water content. These changes culminate in cervical ripening, in preparation for labour. A plug of thick mucus, or operculum, resulting from proliferation of the cervical mucosa and glands, protects the cervix from ascending infection (Blackburn, 2017).

Vagina

Several changes to the vagina occur owing to the effects of oestrogens, but primarily there is increased blood flow, leading to venous engorgement. The vagina contains no glands and relies on the cervix to produce mucus (Rankin, 2017). The increased blood supply to the vagina and cervix areas produce a bluish-purplish colour known as Jacquemier's sign. The uterine arteries pulsate and this can be palpated in the lateral fornices of the vagina, known as Osiander's sign (Rankin, 2017). There is marked shedding of superficial mucosal cells, which leads to increased vaginal discharge (leucorrhoea), and normal bacteria of the vagina (Döderlein's bacilli) interact with increased glycogen in the mucosal cells, increasing the acidity of the vagina. This provides protection against some pathogens but provides an environment conducive to the growth of *Candida albicans* and *Trichomonas vaginalis* (Rankin, 2017).

Haematological changes

Major alterations to the composition of blood occur during pregnancy. Changes protect against the normal blood loss of around 500 mL that occurs at birth, maintain cardiac output despite widespread vasodilation, promote rapid haemostasis during placental separation and increase protection against bacterial infection. These normal changes are reflected in blood screening results.

Haemodilution

Blood volume increases by 30%–40% (approximately 1500 mL) between about 7 and 34 weeks gestation, but there can be considerable individual variation, ranging from a minimal increase up to a twofold increase (Blackburn, 2017). The additional blood volume is accommodated in the uterus, breasts, muscles, kidneys and skin. It is important to note that the plasma increases at a faster rate than the cellular components. This leads to haemodilution, which is reflected in decreased concentration of many elements, such as haemoglobin, immunoglobulins, platelets and plasma proteins.

Plasma volume begins to increase at around 7 weeks and increases very rapidly during the second trimester, reaching a 40%–50% increase by weeks 28 to 32 (Blackburn, 2017). Increasing oxygen demand due to the growing tissues and increased metabolism stimulates erythropoiesis. This increases more slowly and reaches only about a 2%–30% increase in red cell volume (250–450 mL), thus remaining less than the total plasma increase (Fig. 20.29). The resulting haemodilution decreases the blood viscosity by 20%, which has the advantage of decreasing the workload of the heart (Blackburn, 2017).

Haemoglobin concentration falls as a result of haemodilution, from a range of 120–58 g/L in a non-pregnant woman to 116–39 g/L in the first trimester of pregnancy, to 97–148 g/L in the second trimester and to 95–150 g/L in the third trimester (Abbassi-Ghanavati et al., 2009).

Although a decrease in haemoglobin concentration is a normal consequence of haemodilution, there are also increased requirements for iron during pregnancy, to meet the demands of increased erythropoiesis (iron is an essential component of haemoglobin) and the needs of the growing fetus. Plasma iron can be increased by dietary intake, mobilisation of iron stores and increased maternal absorption of iron in the intestines, particularly in the latter stages. This mirrors the increased transfer to the fetus at this time. Serum ferritin levels also fall as stored iron is released from the liver, spleen and bone marrow to boost haemoglobin levels. If a woman's iron stores are not adequate at the start of pregnancy, a deficiency may lead to decreased erythropoiesis, as fetal needs are met at the expense of maternal needs for iron and supplementation may be required (Lowensohn et al., 2016). There is considerable controversy as to whether iron supplements are required to meet the normal increased demands of pregnancy (Brion et al., 2008; Ziaei et al., 2008). A literature review of routine iron supplementation of women did not show benefit (Lowensohn et al., 2016).

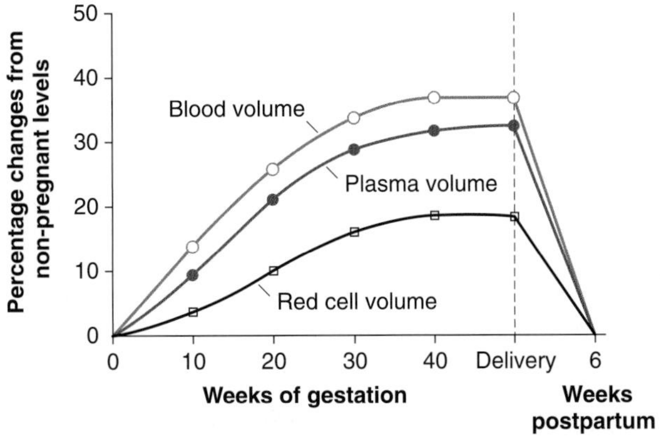

FIGURE 20.29 Changes in blood volume, plasma volume and red blood cell volume during pregnancy and postpartum
(Based on Blackburn, 2003)

White cell count, particularly the neutrophil count, increases during pregnancy to give more protection against bacterial infections. However, the concentration of immunoglobulins (IgA, IgG, IgM) decreases owing to haemodilution and suppression of the immune system.

Plasma proteins also increase but haemodilution lowers the concentration, particularly of albumin, which lowers the osmotic pressure of the plasma. This means there is a greater tendency for fluid movement to the interstitial compartment, and this coupled with the increased water retention mediated by oestrogen leads to an increased possibility of oedema (Blackburn, 2017).

Changes to blood coagulability

Clotting factors such as fibrinogen and factors VII, VIII, IX, X and XII increase, and this leads to hypercoagulability of the blood, despite a decrease in platelet count (due to haemodilution). Although the hypercoagulable state promotes clot formation, this is partially balanced by the increase in fibrinolytic activity (due to increased plasminogen) leading to a balance between clot formation and clot lysis. Bleeding times tend not to change (Blackburn, 2017).

The haematological changes of pregnancy result in an increase in blood volume, and in erythrocytes, leucocytes and coagulation factors, although the greater increase in plasma leads to decreased concentration of many components. Abnormalities in the increases of plasma or cellular constituents may flag underlying pathology; for example, preeclampsia is associated with smaller-than-usual increases in plasma volume (Blackburn, 2017).

Cardiovascular system

Plasma volume increases as a result of increased activity of the renin–angiotensin system and of oestrogens, which increase fluid retention by the kidneys. Cardiac output increases by 30%–50% owing to this increased blood volume (Blackburn, 2017)—an increase from an average of 5 L/min at 10 weeks to approximately 6.5 L/min at 25 weeks. Increased cardiac output is largely determined by increases in stroke volume (30% increase), but the heart rate also increases by 15% (Blackburn, 2017). Despite these changes in cardiac output, blood pressure remains the same or drops slightly. This is due to the decrease in total peripheral resistance (TPR) facilitated by the actions of progesterone. Progesterone causes the smooth muscle in the arterial walls to relax, thus enabling vasodilation. Mean arterial pressure is determined by the cardiac output and the total peripheral resistance, and therefore an increase in cardiac output accompanied by a decrease in TPR results in reasonably constant blood pressure. Smooth muscle in the walls of the veins similarly relaxes, increasing the venous capacity.

Blood flow distribution

As the blood volume increases during pregnancy, it is distributed such that the uterus receives the greatest amount, with an increase from 50 mL / min at 10 weeks to 500 mL / min at term (Blackburn, 2017). Eighty percent of the uterine blood supply is directed to the intervillous spaces of the placenta to meet fetal requirements (see section on placental function, earlier in the chapter).

Early in pregnancy there is a significant decrease in the resistance of renal blood vessels, leading to the kidneys' early ability to accommodate increased cardiac output. This decrease in resistance reaches a maximum by 8 weeks, and may be under the influence of nitric oxide, prostacyclin and atrial natriuretic factor (Blackburn, 2017). Skin and mucous membranes receive up to a 70% increase in blood flow by week 36. This can contribute to heat intolerance, sweating and nasal congestion. Nasal congestion and changes in upper airway patency may lead to increased snoring during pregnancy (Sarberg et al., 2014).

The supine position has a marked effect on cardiac output, especially in later pregnancy when the weight of the uterus is greater. By the third trimester, the supine position results in compression of the vena cava by the uterus, leading to decreased venous return and hence cardiac output (Fig. 20.30). A change from lying on the left side to lying supine can result in a 25%–30% decrease in cardiac output (Blackburn, 2017).

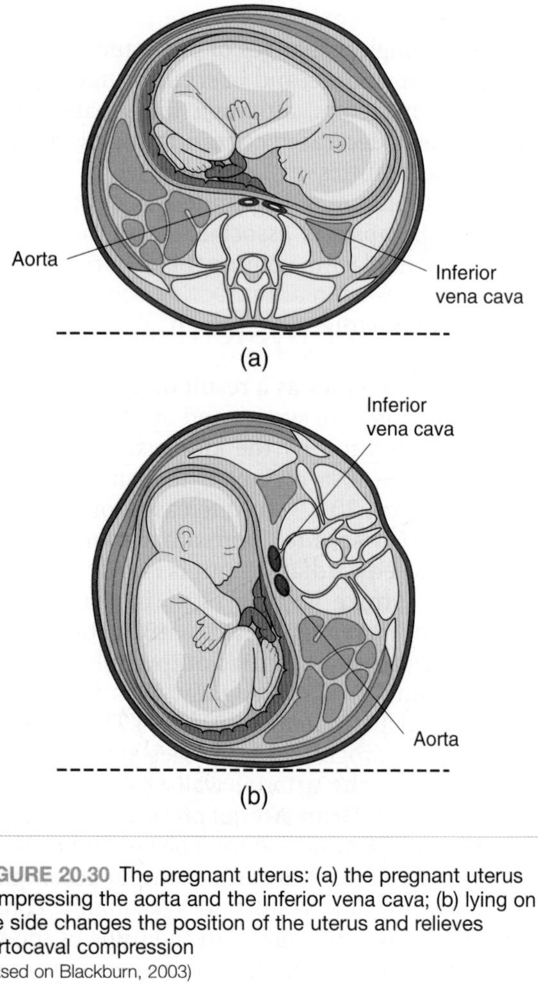

FIGURE 20.30 The pregnant uterus: (a) the pregnant uterus compressing the aorta and the inferior vena cava; (b) lying on the side changes the position of the uterus and relieves aortocaval compression
(Based on Blackburn, 2003)

CRITICAL THINKING EXERCISE

- Why is an increased blood volume during pregnancy likely to be an advantage?
- What compensatory mechanisms occur to maintain blood pressure during pregnancy?

Respiratory system

Several factors influence ventilation during pregnancy. These include an increase in the basal metabolic rate, leading to increased oxygen consumption (20%) and carbon dioxide production, and increased sensitivity of the chemoreceptors to P_aCO_2, an effect caused by progesterone. The result is an increase in ventilation of 40% from 7 L / min to 10 L / min, contributed mainly by an increase in tidal volume of 25%–40%. The increased ventilatory drive from increased chemoreceptor sensitivity leads to hyperventilation—that is, ventilation greater than metabolic need—and this may also account for the sensation of dyspnoea sometimes encountered during pregnancy (Blackburn, 2017). Anatomical changes include flaring of the ribs and a raised position of the diaphragm (4 cm) due to uterine enlargement. Functional residual capacity (volume of air left in the lungs at the end of expiration) and residual volume (volume remaining in the lungs at the end of a forced expiration) are both decreased. During sleep, changes in ventilatory drive and metabolic rate, reduced residual volume and changes in upper airway patency may increase the risk of snoring and of sleep-disordered breathing.

RESEARCH ACTIVITY

There is currently considerable research interest in Australasia and internationally in the link between sleep-disordered breathing (which can be indicated by snoring) and preeclampsia, diabetes and other health conditions (Guilleminault et al., 2000; Laposky & Pemberton, 2021). A greater frequency of snoring has been found among women with preeclampsia (controls 32%, pregnant women 55%, women with preeclampsia 85%) ($p < 0.001$) (Izci et al., 2005) and a greater frequency of witnessed sleep apnoeas has also been associated with pregnancy-induced hypertensive disease (Perez-Chada et al., 2007). Hypertensive pregnant women who reported habitual snoring had twice the risk of obstructive sleep apnoea than hypertensive women who did not (relative risk 2.0 (95% CI 1.4–2.8)), suggesting that pregnant women with hypertension should be investigated for obstructive sleep apnoea (O'Brien et al., 2014). Sleep-disordered breathing is two to three times higher during pregnancy and, while treatments to protect breathing during sleep are available, more research is needed to assess their effectiveness in reducing cardiorespiratory complications in pregnancy (Laposky & Pemberton, 2021).

1. What is the clinical treatment for sleep-disordered breathing?
2. What could be the physiological mechanism linking sleep-disordered breathing with preeclampsia?

Renal system

The renal system must handle the increased metabolic wastes of the mother and the wastes from fetal metabolism. Renal function involves the processes of filtration, reabsorption and secretion, all of which are altered to some extent during pregnancy. Glomerular filtration rate (GFR) increases by up to 40%–50% in the first trimester, and falls significantly in the last 3–4 weeks (Blackburn, 2017). The increase is a result of increased renal blood flow, facilitated by decreased renal vascular resistance. Reabsorption of electrolytes is increased as activity of the renin–angiotensin–aldosterone system increases, owing to oestrogen and progesterone stimulation. This prevents excessive loss of sodium and other solutes and may balance the faster excretion rate.

Glycosuria is common. Glucose reabsorption depends on a carrier mechanism in the renal tubules. At high GFRs this mechanism can become saturated, leaving glucose in the filtrate to be excreted from the body. Proteinuria at levels of 0.3 g/day is also common, probably linked with increased leakiness of the glomerulus. Renal clearance of many substances (e.g. creatinine and iodine) increases, partly because of the increased GFR (Blackburn, 2017).

Progesterone is responsible for dilation and possible kinking of the ureters from 10 weeks. Dilation of the ureters and partial obstruction due to ureteral compression at the pelvic brim, along with relaxation of the smooth muscle in the bladder, can lead to urinary stasis and greater risk of infection during pregnancy. The risk of infection in the static urine is also increased as the urine may contain glucose, protein and amino acids, which support bacterial growth. The reduced movement of urine also facilitates upward movement of bacteria increasing the susceptibility to pyelonephritis (Blackburn, 2017).

Increased frequency of micturition is normal in early pregnancy owing to the increased renal plasma flow and increased excretion by the kidneys. It is also normal later in pregnancy due to the pressure of the fetus and uterus on the bladder.

The renin–angiotensin–aldosterone system continues to have a role in the regulation of blood pressure during pregnancy.

Musculoskeletal system

Hormonal changes during pregnancy lead to increased laxity of joints with maximum effect in the last weeks when the pelvic capacity increases. In particular, the symphysis pubis, sacroiliac and sacrococcygeal joints soften and facilitate widening of the pelvis. The increased mobility of the joints also allows the coccyx to be pushed out of the way during labour.

Relaxation of the ligaments is related to relaxin and oestrogen. Animal studies indicate relaxin remodels collagen fibres to reduce their diameter. Relaxin contributes to symphysis widening, which begins around 10–12 weeks gestation. This normally does not exceed 10 mm (Borg-Stein & Dugan, 2007). A correlation has been identified between relaxin levels and lower back pain or symphysial pain (Casagrande et al., 2015), although a systematic review of six studies suggested there is minimal evidence for this association (Aldabe et al., 2012).

Other physiological changes such as weight gain, cardiovascular changes, pulmonary changes and oedema can also contribute to musculoskeletal complaints (Ireland & Ott, 2000). There is evidence for increased bone remodelling during pregnancy but not for changes in overall bone mass (Borg-Stein & Dugan, 2007).

Integumentary system

Melanocyte-stimulating hormone increases during pregnancy and causes deeper pigmentation of the skin. This can lead to a patchy mask on the face, called chloasma, or a pigmented line on the abdomen from the pubis to the umbilicus, called linea nigra. The areola darkens and toughens, as does the perineum, which can also stretch more. In many areas of the body, stretching occurs in the collagen layer of the skin where adipose tissue is most concentrated (e.g. breasts, abdomen and thighs). Stretch marks—striae gravidarum—occur as red stripes and may result from the increased corticosteroids (see earlier section on the endocrine glands).

Gastrointestinal system

Pregnancy can result in a number of minor discomforts associated with the digestive system. These are mainly a result of the effect of progesterone and include oesophageal reflux, heartburn and constipation.

Effect of progesterone on smooth muscle

Oesophageal sphincter malfunction allows oesophageal reflux of stomach contents, resulting in heartburn. This is exacerbated by higher intra-abdominal pressure in later pregnancy (Rankin, 2017).

Lowered stomach tone and motility (peristalsis) and reduced gastric secretion mean food stays in the stomach longer (up to 48 hours during labour). This may be worsened by narcotics. It should be noted that drugs given orally (e.g. anticonvulsants) may not be absorbed adequately.

Nausea and vomiting may result from a combination of effects, such as decreased peristalsis and increased intra-abdominal pressure. High levels of hCG and sex steroids may also play a role by stimulating the vomiting centre receptors in the medulla (Rankin, 2017).

A lower rate of peristalsis in the intestines facilitates increased absorption of nutrients, but the increased transit time and subsequent increased water reabsorption in the large intestine may lead to constipation. Compression and displacement of the bowel by the enlarging uterus may aggravate the situation (Rankin, 2017).

Sleep in pregnancy

Among the many physiological changes that occur during pregnancy are changes to sleep. Some changes to sleep are a result of physiological changes of pregnancy and it is not clear what the role of disturbed sleep in late pregnancy might have. There is evidence that poor sleep quality and duration in late pregnancy may impact on maternal and fetal health including an association with postnatal depression (Okun et al., 2009) and some evidence for an association with length of labour and mode of delivery (Lee & Gay 2004).

Sleep disruption measures include delayed sleep onset time (sleep latency), increased waking after sleep onset (WASO), deceased sleep efficiency (time asleep / time in bed) and increased daytime sleepiness and daytime napping. Women also report restless sleep, low back pain, leg cramps and frightening dreams (Hertz et al., 1992). An increase in snoring (Hutchison et al., 2012) is well documented, as well as sleep-disordered breathing and obstructive sleep apnea during pregnancy, which can be linked to hypertension in pregnancy (Dominguez et al., 2018). The biological mechanism for these adverse outcomes may be related to disturbances in the immune and hormonal systems (Okun, 2019). Some measures of sleep such as longer sleep duration (> 9 hours) and daily daytime naps have shown an association with late stillbirth (≥ 28 weeks gestation), however restless sleep is shown to be protective of late stillbirth (Cronin et al., 2020). Sleep education (Ladyman et al., 2020) and cognitive behaviour therapy (Bei et al., 2019) are non-pharmacological interventions with the potential to improve sleep.

Dental health

Fluid retention in the connective tissue of the gums can lead to a 'spongy' feeling and increased vascularity can result in increased bleeding of the gums during pregnancy. Hormonal changes also impact on dental health during pregnancy making the woman more vulnerable to dental problems—highlighting the need for good dental hygiene and for antenatal dental assessment (George et al., 2016).

Summary of maternal changes in pregnancy

- Maternal changes associated with pregnancy are largely mediated by the steroid hormones, initially from the corpus luteum maintained by hCG, and later from the placenta.
- Other hormones such as hPL, cortisol and aldosterone mediate many changes.
- Under the influence of oestrogen and progesterone the uterus increases in size, with increased glandular secretions and increased vascularisation. Spontaneous myometrial contractions are largely suppressed by progesterone and other uterotonic inhibitors. The cervix softens as adhesion between collagen bundles is reduced and it is infiltrated by water.
- Oestrogen and the renin–angiotensin system increase sodium and water retention throughout pregnancy, increasing the blood volume by 40%. Plasma volume increases more than the red cell volume, resulting in haemodilution.
- Despite increases in haemoglobin, albumin and immunoglobulins, etc., there is a decrease in the concentration of these blood components. Decreased albumin concentration results in decreased colloid osmotic pressure and possible oedema. A state of hypercoagulability exists owing to increased coagulation factors.
- Progesterone-mediated vasodilation leads to reduced total peripheral resistance and this more than compensates for the effects of increased blood volume. Blood pressure does not normally increase. The increase in cardiac output is due to an increase in both stroke volume and heart rate. A redistribution of blood flow sends approximately 20% of the cardiac output to the uterus, with 80% of this serving the placenta.
- Changes to the ribcage facilitate ventilation. Progesterone and oestrogen increase sensitivity of the respiratory centre to carbon dioxide, resulting in mild hyperventilation. Tidal volume increases to supply increased oxygen to meet increased metabolic needs, and residual volume is reduced.
- Increased GFR leads to increased micturition early in pregnancy. Renin–angiotensin leads to retention of sodium and water. Mild glycosuria, proteinuria and increased clearance of creatinine result from normal changes in renal function. Smooth muscle relaxation, mediated by progesterone, can lead to stasis of urine and increased risk of urinary tract infection.
- Progesterone-mediated smooth muscle relaxation leads to many of the minor discomforts of pregnancy (e.g. oesophageal reflux, constipation, backache); hCG may be linked to feelings of nausea.
- Modifications of the woman's physiology during pregnancy allow her to meet the many needs of the fetus (including cardiorespiratory, nutritional, metabolic and renal) without compromise to her own wellbeing, and to prepare for birth.

REFLECTIVE THINKING EXERCISE

During pregnancy there are major changes to physiology. Consider your discussions with pregnant women and reflect on how you could introduce more focus on the underlying physiology to build greater understanding of these changes.

Conclusion

Adaptations by the woman's physiology during pregnancy allow her to support the developing fetus to grow into a healthy baby while maintaining her own wellbeing. Near term especially, there are considerable challenges in meeting, in particular, the respiratory, nutritional, metabolic and renal needs of the fetus without compromise to the woman. Pregnancy also prepares the woman and the fetus for birth.

Review questions

1. Outline the action of the combined oestrogen/progesterone contraceptive pill with reference to the hypothalamic–pituitary–ovarian axis.
2. List three physiological factors that promote successful fertilisation.
3. Explain why teratogens tend to cause more severe developmental problems when exposure occurs in the first 8 weeks of pregnancy.
4. Describe the process of gastrulation, name the layers of germ cells present in the trilaminar disc, and name one function of the notochord.
5. Outline the barriers a molecule of oxygen (O_2) must pass as it diffuses from the maternal lacuna to the fetal chorionic villus, and describe the factors that facilitate this movement.
6. Name each vessel that transports blood from the fetus to the placental circulation and back.
7. Outline the mechanism that maintains normal blood pressure during pregnancy despite an increase in blood volume.
8. Describe the process of haemodilution that occurs during pregnancy.
9. Explain why oedema may occur in pregnancy.
10. Provide a physiological explanation for each of mild glycosuria, mild proteinuria and oedema that are common in pregnancy.

Online resources

Animation of fetal circulation: Fetal circulation right before birth | Circulatory system physiology | NCLEX-RN | Khan Academy: https://www.youtube.com/watch?v=-IRkisEtzsk.

Baby circulation right after birth | Circulatory system physiology | NCLEX-RN | Khan Academy: https://www.youtube.com/watch?v=jFn0dyU5wUw.

Food Standards Australia New Zealand (FSANZ) develops food standards for both New Zealand and Australia. Their fact sheet on folic acid fortification can be found here: https://www.foodstandards.gov.au/consumer/nutrition/folicmandatory/Pages/default.aspx.

NICE guidelines on antenatal care (updated 2019): http://www.nice.org.uk/CG62.

NZ Ministry of Health information on folate and folic acid: http://www.health.govt.nz/our-work/preventative-health-wellness/nutrition/folate-folic-acid#current_policy.

Online textbooks which provide excellent diagrams and descriptions of embryological development (check your library for access):

Johnson MH. *Essential Reproduction.* 7th ed. Chichester. West Sussex: Wiley-Blackwell; 2013.

Moore KL, Persaud TVN, Torchia MG. *Before We Are Born: Essentials of Embryology and Birth Defects (electronic resource).* Philadelphia, PA: Saunders/Elsevier; 2013.

References

Abbassi-Ghanavati M, Greer LG, Cunningham FG. Pregnancy and laboratory studies: a reference table for clinicians. Obstet Gynecol. 2009;114(6):1326–1331.

Aldabe D, Ribeiro DC, Milosavljevic S, et al. Pregnancy-related pelvic girdle pain and its relationship with relaxin levels during pregnancy: a systematic review. *Eur Spine J.* 2012;21(9):1769–1776.

Barker DJ. The developmental origins of chronic adult disease. *Acta Paediatr Suppl.* 2004;93(446):26–33.

Bei B, Pinnington DM, Shen L, Blumfield M, et al. A scalable cognitive behavioural program to promote healthy sleep during pregnancy and postpartum periods: protocol of a randomised controlled trial (the SEED project). 2019; *BMC Pregnancy Childbirth,* 19(1), 254. doi:10.1186/s12884-019-2390-8.

Blackburn S. *Maternal, Fetal and Neonatal Physiology: A Clinical Perspective.* 2nd ed. St Louis, MO: WB Saunders; 2003.

Blackburn S. *Maternal, Fetal and Neonatal Physiology: A Clinical Perspective.* 5th ed. Saunders/Elsevier; 2017.

Boas WV, Goncalves RO, Costa OL, et al. Metabolism and gene polymorphisms of the folate pathway in Brazilian women with history of recurrent abortion. *Rev Bras Ginecol Obstet.* 2015; 37(2):71–76.

Bolt RJ, van Weissenbruch MM, Lafeber HN, et al. Glucocorticoids and lung development in the fetus and preterm infant. *Pediatr Pulmonol.* 2001;32(1):76–91.

Borg-Stein J, Dugan SA. Musculoskeletal disorders of pregnancy, delivery and postpartum. *Phys Med Rehabil Clin N Am.* 2007; 18(3):459–476.

Boryshpolets S, Perez-Cerezales S, Eisenbach M. Behavioral mechanism of human sperm in thermotaxis: a role for hyperactivation. *Hum Reprod.* 2015;30(4):884–892.

Bower C, de Klerk N, Hickling S, et al. Assessment of the potential effect of incremental increases in folic acid intake on neural tube defects in Australia and New Zealand. *Aust N Z J Public Health.* 2006;30(4):369–374.

Bower C, Maxwell S, Hickling S, et al. Folate status in Aboriginal people before and after mandatory fortification of flour for bread-making in Australia. *Aust N Z J Obstet Gynaecol.* 2016; 56(3):233–237.
Bray JJ, Cragg PA, Macknight AD, et al. *Lecture Notes on Human Physiology.* 3rd ed. Oxford: Blackwell Scientific; 1994.
Brion MJ, Leary SD, Smith GD, et al. Maternal anemia, iron intake in pregnancy, and offspring blood pressure in the Avon Longitudinal Study of Parents and Children. *Am J Clin Nutr.* 2008; 88(4):1126–1133.
Casagrande D, Gugala Z, Clark SM, et al. Low back pain and pelvic girdle pain in pregnancy. *J Am Acad Orthop Surg.* 2015;23(9): 539–549.
Coad J, Dunstall M. *Anatomy and Physiology for Midwives.* Edinburgh: Elsevier; 2001.
Coad J, Dunstall M. *Anatomy and Physiology for Midwives.* 2nd ed. Edinburgh: Elsevier; 2005.
Cronin RS, Wilson J, Gordon A, et al. Associations between symptoms of sleep-disordered breathing and maternal sleep patterns with late stillbirth: Findings from an individual participant data meta-analysis. *PLoS One.* 2020; 15(3), e0230861. doi:10.1371/journal.pone.0230861.
Dominguez JE, Habib AS, Krystal AD. A review of the associations between obstructive sleep apnea and hypertensive disorders of pregnancy and possible mechanisms of disease. *Sleep Med Rev.* 2018;42:37–46.
Evans SE, Mygind VL, Peddie MC, et al. Effect of increasing voluntary folic acid food fortification on dietary folate intakes and adequacy of reproductive-age women in New Zealand. *Public Health Nutr.* 2014;17(7):1447–1453.
Forbes S. Pregnancy sickness and parent-offspring conflict over thyroid function. *J Theor Biol.* 2014;355:61–67.
Gaunt G, Ramin K. Immunological tolerance of the human fetus. *Am J Perinatol.* 2001;18(6):299–312.
George A, Lang G, Johnson M, et al. The evaluation of an oral health education program for midwives in Australia. *Women Birth.* 2016;29(3):208–213.
Gomes S, Lopes C, Pinto E. Folate and folic acid in the periconceptional period: recommendations from official health organizations in thirty-six countries worldwide and WHO. *Public Health Nutr.* 2016;19(1):176–189.
Gooi A, Oei J, Lui K. Attitudes of Level II obstetricians towards the care of the extremely premature infant: a national survey. *J Paediatr Child Health.* 2003;39(6):451–455.
Guilleminault C, Querra-Salva MSC, Poyares D. Normal pregnancy, daytime sleeping, snoring and blood pressure. *Sleep Med.* 2000; 1(14):289–297.
Guzman-Huerta ME, Muro-Barragan SA, Acevedo-Gallegos S, et al. Amniotic band sequence: prenatal diagnosis, phenotype descriptions, and a proposal of a new classification based on morphologic findings. *Rev Invest Clin.* 2013;65(4):300–306.
Helve O, Pitkänen O, Janér C, et al. Pulmonary fluid balance in the human newborn infant. *Neonatology.* 2009;95(4), 347–352. doi:10.1159/000209300
Hertz G, Fast A, Feinsilver H, et al. Sleep in normal late pregnancy. *Sleep.* 1992;15(3):246–51.
Huseynov A, Zollikofer CP, Coudyzer W, et al. Developmental evidence for obstetric adaptation of the human female pelvis. *Proc Natl Acad Sci USA.* 2016;113(19):5227–5232.
Hutchison BL, Stone PR, McCowan LM, et al. A postal survey of maternal sleep in late pregnancy. *BMC Pregnancy & Childbirth.* 2012;12:144.
Ireland ML, Ott SM. The effects of pregnancy on the musculoskeletal system. *Clin Orthop Relat Res.* 2000;372:169–179.
Izci B, Martin SE, Dundas KC, et al. Sleep complaints: snoring and daytime sleepiness in pregnant and pre-eclamptic women. *Sleep Med.* 2005;6(2):163–169.
James JL, Stone PR, Chamley LW. The regulation of trophoblast differentiation by oxygen in the first trimester of pregnancy. *Hum Reprod Update.* 2006;12(2):137–144.
Johnson MH. *Essential Reproduction.* 7th ed. Chichester. West Sussex: Wiley-Blackwell; 2013.
Johnson MH, Everitt BJ. *Essential Reproduction.* 5th ed. Oxford: Blackwell Science; 2000.
Kahrama O, Çeçen K, Temur I, et al. Effects of the maternal position and rest on the fetal urine production rate: a prospective study conducted by 3-dimensional sonography using the rotational technique (Virtual Organ Computer-Aided Analysis). *J Ultrasound Med.* 2011;30:481–486.
Kajantie E, Osmond C, Barker DJ, et al. Size at birth as a predictor of mortality in adulthood: a follow-up of 350 000 person-years. *Int J Epidemiol.* 2005;34(3):655–663.
Kasum M, Simunic V, Vrcic H, et al. Follicular progesterone elevations with ovulation induction for IVF. *Gynecol Endocrinol.* 2014;30(8): 537–541.
Khong TY. Placental vascular development and neonatal outcome. *Semin Neonatol.* 2004;9(4):255–263.
Ladyman C, Gander P, Huthwaite M, et al. Sleep HAPi: A Feasibility and Descriptive Analysis of an Early and Longitudinal Sleep Education Intervention for Pregnant Women. *Behav Sleep Med.* 2020; 1–18. doi:10.1080/15402002.2020.1772265.
Langer RD. The evidence base for HRT: what can we believe? *Climacteric.* 2017;20(2):91–96.
Laposky AD, Pemberton VL. Sleep-Disordered Breathing and Pregnancy-Related Cardiovascular Disease. *J Womens Health (Larchmt)* 2021; 30(2), 194–198. doi:10.1089/jwh.2020.8869.
Lee KA, Gay CL. Sleep in late pregnancy predicts length of labor and type of delivery. *American Journal of Obstetrics and Gynecology.* 2004;191(6):2041–6.
Lowensohn RI, Stadler DD, Naze C. Current concepts of maternal nutrition. *Obstet Gynecol Surv.* 2016;71(7):413–426.
Modena AB, Fieni S. Amniotic fluid dynamics. *Acta Biomed Ateneo Parmense.* 2004;75(suppl 1):11–13.
Moore KL, Persaud TVN. *Before We Are Born: Essentials of Embryology and Birth Defects.* 5th ed. London: WB Saunders; 1998.
Moore KL, Persaud TVN., Torchia MG. *Before We Are Born: Essentials of Embryology and Birth Defects.* 7th ed. Philadelphia: WB Saunders; 2008.
Moore KL, Persaud TVN, Torchia MG. *Before We Are Born: Essentials of Embryology and Birth Defects (electronic resource).* Philadelphia: PA Saunders / Elsevier; 2013.
Moore KL, Persaud TVN, Torchia MG. *Before We Are Born: Essentials of Embryology and Birth Defects.* 10th ed. Edinburgh: Philadelphia : Elsevier 2020
Murphy ME, Westmark CJ. Folic Acid Fortification and Neural Tube Defect Risk: Analysis of the Food Fortification Initiative Dataset. *Nutrients.* 2020;12(1):247. doi: 10.3390/nu12010247. PMID: 31963665; PMCID: PMC7019961.
Myrhaug HT, Brurberg KG, Hov L, et al. Survival and Impairment of Extremely Premature Infants: A Meta-analysis. *Pediatrics.* 2019; 143(2). doi:10.1542/peds.2018-0933.
O'Brien LM, Bullough AS, Chames MC, et al. Hypertension, snoring, and obstructive sleep apnoea during pregnancy: a cohort study. *BJOG.* 2014;121(13):1685–1693.
Oei J, Askie LM, Tobiansky R, et al. Attitudes of neonatal clinicians towards resuscitation of the extremely premature infant: an exploratory survey. *J Paediatr Child Health.* 2000;36(4):357–362.
Okun ML, Hanusa BH, Hall M, et al. Sleep complaints in late pregnancy and the recurrence of postpartum depression. *Behav Sleep Med.* 2009;7(2):106–17.
Okun ML. Sleep disturbances and modulations in inflammation: Implications for pregnancy health. *Social and Personality Psychology Compass.* 2019.

Perez-Chada D, Videla AJ, O'Flaherty ME, et al. Snoring, witnessed sleep apnoeas and pregnancy-induced hypertension. *Acta Obstet Gynecol Scand.* 2007;86(7):788–792.
Plumptre L, Masih SP, Ly A, et al. High concentrations of folate and unmetabolized folic acid in a cohort of pregnant Canadian women and umbilical cord blood. *Am J Clin Nutr.* 2015;102(4): 848–857.
Ramsay DT, Kent JC, Hartmann RA, et al. Anatomy of the lactating human breast redefined with ultrasound imaging. *J Anat.* 2005; 206(6):525–534.
Rankin J. *Physiology in Childbearing With Anatomy and Related Biosciences.* 4th ed. Edinburgh: Elsevier; 2017.
Righarts AA, Gray A, Dickson NP, et al. Resolution of infertility and number of children: 1386 couples followed for a median of 13 years. *Hum Reprod.* 2017;32(10):2042–2048.
Rossouw JE, Anderson GL, Prentice RL, et al. Writing Group for the Women's Health Initiative Investigators. Risks and benefits of estrogen plus progestin in healthy postmenopausal women: principal results from the Women's Health Initiative randomized controlled trial. *JAMA.* 2002;288(3):321–333.
Saccone, G., & Berghella, V. Antenatal corticosteroids for maturity of term or near term fetuses: systematic review and meta-analysis of randomized controlled trials. *BMJ.* 2016: 355, i5044. doi:10.1136/bmj.i5044
Sarberg M, Svanborg E, Wirehn AB, et al. Snoring during pregnancy and its relation to sleepiness and pregnancy outcome – a prospective study. *BMC Pregnancy Childbirth.* 2014;14:15.
Shah C, Modi D, Gadkar S, et al. Progesterone receptors on human spermatozoa. *Indian J Exp Biol.* 2003;41(7):773–780.
Sharma K, Gupta P, Shandilya S. Age related changes in pelvis size among adolescent and adult females with reference to parturition from Naraingarh, Haryana (India). *Homo.* 2016; 67(4):273–293.
Sharp M, French N, McMichael J, et al. Survival and neurodevelopmental outcomes in extremely preterm infants 22–24 weeks of gestation born in Western Australia. *J Paediatr Child Health.* 2018;54(2), 188–193. doi:10.1111/jpc.13678.
Stables D, Rankin J. *Physiology in Childbearing With Anatomy and Related Biosciences.* 2nd ed. Edinburgh: Elsevier; 2005.
Stables D, Rankin J. *Physiology in Childbearing With Anatomy and Related Biosciences.* 3rd ed. Edinburgh: Elsevier; 2010.
Stefanick ML, Anderson GL, Margolis KL, et al. Effects of conjugated equine estrogens on breast cancer and mammography screening in postmenopausal women with hysterectomy. *JAMA.* 2006;295(14):1647–1657.
Sun F, Bahat A, Gakamsky A, et al. Human sperm chemotaxis: both the oocyte and its surrounding cumulus cells secrete sperm chemoattractants. *Hum Reprod.* 2005;20(3):761–767.
Tablante EC, Pachón H, Guetterman HM, et al. Fortification of wheat and maize flour with folic acid for population health outcomes. *Cochrane Database Syst Rev,* 2019;7(7):CD012150. doi:10.1002/14651858.CD012150.pub2.
Thorley J. HRT for menopause: a delicate balance. *Lancet Diabetes Endocrinol.* 2016;4(1):25.
Tortora G. *Brief Atlas of the Skeleton, Surface Anatomy and Selected Medical Images.* Hoboken, NJ: John Wiley & Sons; 2006.
Voltolini C, Petraglia F. Neuroendocrinology of pregnancy and parturition. *Handb Clin Neurol.* 2014;124:17–36.
Wang Y, Zhao S. Placental blood circulation. In: Wang Y, Zhao S, eds. *Vascular Biology of the Placenta. Ch. 2.* San Rafael, CA: Morgan & Claypool Life Sciences; 2010:3–12.
Ziaei S, Mehrnia M, Faghihzadeh S. Iron status markers in nonanemic pregnant women with and without iron supplementation. *Int J Gynaecol Obstet.* 2008;100(2):130–132.

Further reading

Blackburn S. Maternal, *Fetal and Neonatal Physiology: A Clinical Perspective.* 5th ed. Saunders / Elsevier; 2017.
Lowensohn RI, Stadler DD, Naze C. Current concepts of maternal nutrition. *Obstet Gynecol Surv.* 2016;71(7):413–426.
Moore KL, Persaud TVN, Torchia MG. *Before We Are Born: Essentials of Embryology and Birth Defects (electronic resource).* Philadelphia, PA: Saunders / Elsevier; 2013.
Ramsay DT, Kent JC, Hartmann RA, et al. Anatomy of the lactating human breast redefined with ultrasound imaging. *J Anat.* 2005;206(6):525–534.
Rankin J. *Physiology in Childbearing With Anatomy and Related Biosciences.* 4th ed. Edinburgh: Elsevier; 2017.
Voltolini C, Petraglia F. Neuroendocrinology of pregnancy and parturition. *Handb Clin Neurol.* 2014;124:17–36.

CHAPTER 21

Nutrition and physical activity foundations for pregnancy, childbirth and lactation

Emma Le Lievre and Jade Wratten

LEARNING OUTCOMES

Learning outcomes for this chapter are:

1. To discuss the role and dietary sources of macronutrients and key micronutrients in pregnancy and lactation and identify when supplementation may be warranted
2. To discuss what food to avoid in pregnancy to prevent food-borne illnesses, such as listeria
3. To examine appropriate gestational weight gain and the impact of obesity during the childbirth period
4. To consider nutrition during labour and during lactation
5. To discuss appropriate physical activity during pregnancy and postpartum.

CHAPTER OVERVIEW

This chapter outlines the foundational knowledge required for a midwife when working with women during the childbearing period in regards to nutrition and physical activity. The importance of adequate nutrition cannot be understated. It is required to support healthy progression of the pregnancy and to maintain the health of the mother and growing fetus. Inadequate nutrition has been found to lead to poor outcomes during the childbearing period, and is also linked to later-life disease. A fundamental knowledge and understanding of macronutrients and micronutrients in pregnancy is vital for midwives to optimise information sharing with women regarding nutrition. Specific nutritional information shown in this chapter can be shared by midwives and utilised by women to assist in promoting health, positive pregnancy outcomes in regards to appropriate gestational weight gain and food safety in pregnancy. Increased gestational weight gain and obesity in pregnancy presents a challenge to midwives and is associated with many risks; this chapter will outline these with specific midwifery practice points highlighted to ensure that balanced and evidence-based information is shared appropriately with women who are obese, keeping them at the centre and focus of their care. Intrapartum nutrition considerations will be explored. Dietary information remains of high importance in the postnatal period with energy requirements during lactation actually exceeding those of pregnancy. Adequate intake is important and is required to maintain the health of the mother, with deficiencies in the newborn usually being indicative of deficiencies in the mother. Finally, this chapter will cover the importance of physical activity in a healthy pregnancy and the benefits and safety considerations that should be applied to physical activity during this time. Specific recommendations for exercise prescription during pregnancy and the return to physical activity following the birth are also covered.

KEY TERMS

dietary supplements
exercise
food safety
gestational weight gain
macronutrients
micronutrients
nutritional foundation for lactation
nutrition in labour
maternal obesity
physical activity

INTRODUCTION

Food is primarily consumed to sustain our appetite and to provide our bodies with the energy and nutrients required to function; food is also used in celebration and bringing people together, therefore often has a strong cultural significance.

The importance of a balanced diet and engaging in regular physical activity during pregnancy cannot be understated. These have an impact on maternal and fetal wellbeing, pregnancy outcomes and later-life diseases in both the infant and the mother. Midwives work in partnership with women and their family/whānau and are perfectly positioned to share nutritional and activity guidance with women at a time when many are open to receiving messages regarding health. Embracing these messages could have a positive impact not only on the woman and her current pregnancy but also on her and her family's long-term health.

REFLECTIVE THINKING EXERCISE

Consider what factors influence how and what a woman eats. How might this be different between individual women or between women from different locations and socioeconomic backgrounds? How might politics and other social factors influence one's nutrition?

Dietary recommendations

There are many messages in society surrounding food, nutrition and health, many of which are led by advertising and marketing from food companies seeking to increase their share of the market. This information can be misleading and does little to support clear or sustainable healthy-eating habits. Both the Australian Government National Health and Medical Research Council (NHMRC) (2013) and the New Zealand Ministry of Health (MOH) (2020) have published dietary and activity guidelines which include information for pregnant and lactating women. Many of the recommendations are consistent between countries with only subtle differences present. Summaries of the guidelines are outlined in Box 21.1 and Box 21.2. It is important that midwives are familiar with key public health messages unique to their country of practice. Table 21.1 outlines the number of servings from each food group that are recommended during pregnancy and lactation, compared to the non-pregnant person. Table 21.2 gives examples of servings for each food group. Some women will be familiar with the concept of serving sizes and food groups; others will be discovering this for the first time. Working with women and their families taking into account their existing knowledge is crucial in delivering health messages.

Box 21.1 Australian Dietary Guidelines

Guideline 1
To achieve and maintain healthy weight, be physically active and choose amounts of nutritious food and drink to meet your daily needs.

Guideline 2
Enjoy a wide variety of foods from the five groups every day and drink plenty of water.

Guideline 3
Limit intake of foods containing saturated fat, added salt, added sugars and alcohol.

For women who are pregnant, planning a pregnancy or breastfeeding, not drinking alcohol is the safest option.

Guideline 4
Encourage, support and promote breastfeeding.

Guideline 5
Care for your food, prepare and store it safely.

Box 21.2 New Zealand Eating Statements for New Zealand Adults

Eating statement 1
Enjoy a variety of nutritious foods every day.

Eating statement 2
Choose and/or prepare foods and drinks with unsaturated fats, with little to no added sugar, that are low in salt, that are mostly 'whole' and less processed.

Eating statement 3
Make plain water your first choice over other drinks.

Eating statement 4
If you drink alcohol keep your intake low.

Pregnancy: Stop drinking alcohol if you could be pregnant, are pregnant or are trying to get pregnant.

Breastfeeding: when breastfeeding, it is best to be alcohol-free.

Eating statement 5
Buy or gather, prepare, cook and store food in ways that keep it safe to eat.

Pregnancy: Take extra care to protect yourself from foodborne illness if you are pregnant.

Eating statement 6
Encourage, support and promote breastfeeding.

(Source: Ministry of Health, 2020a)

Table 21.1 Recommended minimum servings per food group Australia and New Zealand

	Vegetables	Fruit	Grain foods	Legumes, nuts, seeds, fish and other seafood, eggs, poultry or red meat with fat removed	Milk and milk products	Approximate number of additional servings from the five food groups*
Women						
19–50	5	2	6	2.5	2.5	0–2.5
Pregnant 19+	5	2	8.5	3.5	2.5	0–2.5
Lactating 19+	7.5	2	9	2.5	2.5	0–2.5
Men						
19–50	6	2	6	3	2.5	0–3

*Additional servings may be needed for taller or more active adults (NHMRC, 2013 as cited in Ministry of Health, 2020a)

Table 21.2 Serving size examples for each food group

Vegetables	A standard serving of vegetables is about 75 g (100–350 kJ), which is about the same as: • ½ cup cooked vegetables • ½ cup canned vegetables • 1 cup green leafy or raw salad vegetables • ½ medium potato or similar sized piece of kūmara, taewa, taro, cassava • 1 medium tomato.
Grain foods, mostly wholegrain and those naturally high in fibre. Wholegrain options should be chosen where possible	A standard serve (500 kJ) is about the same as: • 1 slice (40 g) wholegrain bread • ½ medium (40 g) wholegrain roll or flat bread • ½ cup (75–120 g) cooked rice, pasta, noodles, wheat • ½ cup (120 g) cooked porridge • ¼ cup (30 g) muesli • 2 breakfast wheat biscuits • ⅔ cup cereal flakes • 3 (35 g) crispbreads or crackers.
Fruit	A standard serve of fruit is about 150 g (350 kJ), which is about the same as: • 1 medium apple, banana, orange or pear • 2 small apricots, kiwifruit or plums • 1 cup diced or canned fruit (drained and with no added sugar) • 1 cup frozen fruit, e.g. mango, berries.
Milk and milk products, mostly low and reduced fat	A standard serve (500–600 kJ) is about the same as: • 1 cup (250 ml) low or reduced fat fresh, UHT long-life, reconstituted powdered milk or buttermilk • 2 slices (40 g) or a 4 × 3 × 2 cm piece of cheese such as Edam • ¾ cup (200 g) low- or reduced-fat yoghurt • 1 cup (250 ml) calcium-fortified plant-based milk alternatives (with at least 100 g of added calcium per 100 mL).
Legumes, nuts, seeds, fish and other seafood, eggs, poultry and/or red meat with fat removed	A standard serve (500–600 kJ) is about the same as: • 1 cup (150 g) cooked or canned beans, lentils, chickpeas, or split peas (preferably with no added salt) • 170 g tofu • 30 g nuts, seeds, peanut or almond butter, tahini or other nut or seed paste (no added salt) • 100 g cooked fish fillet (about 115 g raw) or one small can of fish • 2 large (2 × 60 g = 120 g) eggs • 80 g cooked lean chicken (100 g raw) • 65 g cooked lean meat such as beef, lamb, pork, veal (90–100 g raw)—no more than 500 g cooked (700–750 g) red meat each week

(Source: Ministry of Health, 2020a)

Dietary energy

Energy is required in the body for metabolic processes, physiological functions, muscular activity, heat production, growth and synthesis of new tissue. It is released from food components by oxidation. Dietary energy is found in macronutrients (carbohydrates, proteins, fats) and to a lesser degree alcohol (Table 21.3).

Energy is used by the body for basal metabolism, which includes a number of functions necessary for life. The amount of energy used for these functions is called the basal metabolic rate (BMR) and represents 45–70% of daily energy expenditure. BMR is significantly influenced by age, gender, body size and composition, and varies significantly person to person. Physical activity—both the activities of daily living (occupational, schoolwork, housework) and discretionary activity (activity done as part of exercise, sport, social and cultural interactions)—is the most modifiable determinant of energy need and is second largest after the BMR. Finally, energy is also expended through processing food into nutrients. This process results in heat production and oxygen consumption and can result in an approximately 10% increase in the BMR. Pregnancy and lactation further increase energy requirements to accommodate the needs of the growing fetus, placenta, expanding maternal tissue, additional maternal effort (both at rest and when engaging in physical activity) and through lactogenesis.

Recommended energy intake is therefore dynamic and highly individualised. A joint publication by the NHMRC, Australian Government Department of Health and Ageing and New Zealand Ministry of Health has produced Estimated Energy Requirements for various populations. Table 21.4 outlines the recommended increased energy requirements for pregnancy and lactation. These recommendations do not take into account individual circumstance and should only be used as a guide to support discussions with women.

Table 21.3 Energy density of micronutrients

Micronutrient	Energy (kj)
Fats	37
Carbohydrates	17
Protein	17
Alcohol	29

Table 21.4 Estimated additional energy requirements: pregnancy and lactation

Pregnancy 1st trimester	No additional requirement
Pregnancy 2nd trimester	Addition 1.4 MJ / day
Pregnancy 3rd trimester	Additional 1.9 MJ / day
Lactation	Additional 2.0–2.1 MJ / day

NUTRITION IN PREGNANCY

Women are often unaware of the differences between micronutrients and macronutrients or what constitutes a healthy diet, therefore, the midwife needs to identify and build the woman's understanding and knowledge of what is healthy whilst incorporating a holistic, individualised approach

MACRONUTRIENTS

Macronutrients include fats (lipids), carbohydrates and proteins, which provide the body with the energy required for basic life functions and all cell processes in the body. Each macronutrient renders different amounts of energy and different pathways for their utilisation. An understanding of macronutrients is important; however, many factors contribute to one's nutrition and a holistic approach is always required.

Fats

There are three main types of naturally occurring fatty acids that comprise dietary fats: saturated, monounsaturated and polyunsaturated. Saturated fats occur mainly in animal-based foods; polyunsaturated and monounsaturated fats occur mainly in plant-based foods.

Fat plays an important role as a potent energy source, insulator and protector of the body's organs; fat can also be stored and used for energy long after it has been consumed. Some fats are essential, such as linoleic acid, an omega-6 fat, and alpha-linolenic acid, an omega-3 fat, which are essential fats required for growth and development. These fats cannot be synthesised by the body and therefore must be consumed in our diet from foods, hence making them 'essential'. One of the primary functions of these fats is to produce long-chain polyunsaturated fatty acids (LCPs), which are found in particularly high concentrations in the central nervous system and retina. LCPs are also consumed in our diet, particularly in nuts, seeds, meat, dairy and fatty fish.

Prescribing recommended daily intake of fats is complex and requires an understanding of these different types of fat, and which are most important to elicit positive health outcomes and avoid negative health outcomes associated with dietary fat intake.

Carbohydrates

Carbohydrates are a major nutritional energy source providing energy to cells, particularly the brain, which requires glucose for its metabolism. Carbohydrate intake is necessary to avoid ketoacidosis. Carbohydrates are particularly significant during pregnancy due to increased energy demands to accommodate fetal growth, maternal and fetal metabolism and lactogenesis.

Carbohydrates are further divided into simple sugars and complex carbohydrates. Simple sugars are present in fruit (fructose), milk (lactose) and table sugar (sucrose).

The body's major energy source comes from glucose, another simple sugar, which is the most abundant carbohydrate. Glucose is the building block for complex carbohydrates or, more specifically, the starches. Starches are a storage form of carbohydrate present in plants such as grains, legumes and root vegetables.

Carbohydrates should account for the majority of energy intake during pregnancy, however, the type of carbohydrate consumed is important to prevent large fluctuations in blood glucose levels. The rate at which dietary carbohydrate, specifically glucose, is absorbed into the bloodstream can be measured, and is referred to as the glycaemic index (GI). Some carbohydrates present in food are rapidly digested in the digestive tract, thereby entering circulation quickly. This can result in a large increase in blood glucose followed by a sudden drop in blood glucose. Foods containing these types of carbohydrates are referred to as having a high GI value. In contrast, some carbohydrates are digested more slowly, allowing for a slow and steady rise in blood glucose that is not followed by a sudden drop in blood glucose levels. Foods containing these types of carbohydrates are referred to as having a low GI value. For sustained energy, foods with a low GI value are recommended.

Dietary fibre

In addition to simple and complex carbohydrates, dietary fibre may also be considered a type of carbohydrate. Unlike simple sugars and starches, the human body lacks the enzymes required to break down dietary fibre. Dietary fibre is classified as either soluble or insoluble. Foods rich in soluble fibre include fruits and vegetables, oats, barley and legumes, whereas foods rich in insoluble fibre include wheat, whole grains and most vegetables. The benefits of dietary fibre include increased satiety, regular bowel movements, a reduction in blood cholesterol levels and modulation of blood glucose levels.

Protein

Protein occurs in all living cells (plant and animal). Amino acids, assembled in long chains are the building blocks of protein. The body stores protein in order to utilise it for its many other roles such as providing a structural component to muscles, connective tissue and bone, repair of tissues, maintaining fluid balance, blood pressure and enzymatic activity, transporting substances throughout the body and the formation of hormones and antibodies. Dietary intake of protein is important to ensure that the body has the correct mix of amino acids, the building blocks of protein. There are 20 amino acids, of which nine are considered essential. The body is unable to produce essential amino acids in adequate amounts and therefore they must be obtained from dietary sources. Animal proteins contain all nine essential amino acids, whereas plant proteins are limited in at least one.

During pregnancy the requirement for dietary protein is slightly higher than in prepregnancy, to account for the development of maternal and fetal tissues. The protein requirements are based on body weight: for every kilogram of body weight a non-pregnant woman should consume between 0.8 and 1.0 g of protein, approximately 60 g per day increasing by another 0.48 g/kg for pregnancy (NHMRC, 2013). This is reflected in recommendations to increase servings during pregnancy and lactation (Table 21.1) (MOH 2020a; NHMRC, 2013). Examples of protein servings are outlined in Table 21.2.

Historically, there have been concerns about the safety of high-protein diets in pregnancy. While more recent studies have not substantiated these concerns, they have also not found any benefits associated with protein intake over and above the recommended dietary intake (Halldorsson, et al. 2021).

CRITICAL THINKING EXERCISE

A woman you are providing midwifery care for has indicated to you that she is vegetarian. She consumes dairy products, but no other animal foods. She has followed this diet for 6 years and is keen to continue the diet during pregnancy.

1. What questions about her diet might you ask her, and why?
2. What nutrients might you be concerned about with her diet, and why?
3. What plan of care would you develop with her to ensure that she meets the energy and nutrient requirements of pregnancy?

MICRONUTRIENTS

Micronutrients are vitamins and minerals small in size, but vital to health and optimal functioning of the body during pregnancy. They do not produce energy, but they are required in assisting and releasing energy yielded from macronutrients. Micronutrients have many specific targeted functions during pregnancy such as DNA synthesis and cell division. Deficiencies may lead to an array of conditions affecting not just the mother, but also the pregnancy, fetus and breastfed infant. While nutritional requirements often increase in pregnancy, the body undergoes specific physiological adaptations (usually increased absorption) that assist in securing or attempting to secure any additional requirement for micronutrients. Furthermore, some micronutrients are susceptible to destruction by cooking, and therefore short cooking times are preferable to long ones.

Supplementation in pregnancy

Iodine and folic acid are the only routinely recommended **dietary supplements** during pregnancy and breastfeeding. Instead, eating a wide range of foods from all food groups along with getting sufficient safe sun exposure will usually provide the micronutrients required by the pregnant or breastfeeding body. In the event of deficiency, or for those at increased risk of deficiency, supplementation can be considered.

Minerals

Iron

Iron is a trace mineral utilised as a component of a number of proteins including haemoglobin, myoglobin, cytochromes and enzymes. Haemoglobin is important for transport of oxygen to tissues throughout the body. Almost two-thirds of the body's iron is found in haemoglobin. A further one-quarter of the body's iron is found in readily metabolised stores such as ferritin or haemosiderin in the liver and reticulo-endothelial system. The remaining iron is utilised by a variety of body functions.

A 2014–15 survey showed that nearly 8.7% of women over the age of 15 in New Zealand were anaemic (MOH, 2020b). The prevalence of anaemia varies by age and ethnic group, with women experiencing higher rates than the general population (Table 21.5). In Australia, Aboriginal and Torres Strait Islander women and teenage mothers have been shown to be at higher risk of anaemia during pregnancy (Government of South Australia, 2016).

Table 21.5 Prevalence of iron deficiency anaemia in New Zealand

Population group	Rate of anaemia (%)	
	General population (15 yrs +)	Women (15 yrs +)
Total	6.9	8.7
Age group (years)		
15–24	3.7	5.2
25–34	4.5	8.6
35–44	9.1	15.6
Ethnic group		
Māori	6.5	8.5
Pacific	10.9	16.6
Asian	7.9	1.5
European/other	6.4	7.8

(Adapted from Ministry of Health, 2020b)

Iron in pregnancy

It is challenging for many women to achieve and maintain optimal levels of iron during pregnancy. The body's need for iron increases as pregnancy progresses from the second trimester onwards to meet the demands of the growing fetus. The ability to absorb iron also increases during pregnancy but requirements are up to six times higher than that of a non-pregnant woman. Iron is important for brain function and brain development, with deficiencies being associated with premature birth, small-for-gestational-age (SGA) infants, general weariness, fatigue, having an increased susceptibility to infections and depression in the postnatal period (Milman et al., 2016). Dietary sources of iron and other minerals are given in Table 21.6.

Table 21.6 Dietary sources of minerals

Mineral	Animal sources	Plant sources
Iron	• Red meat (beef, venison) • Poultry • Fish and seafood • Eggs	• Legumes (kidney beans, chickpeas, lentils, green peas, soy beans) • Wholegrain or fortified breads and breakfast cereals • Green leafy vegetables (silverbeet, spinach) • Dried fruits • Nuts (cashews, walnuts, peanuts) • Seeds (sunflower and sesame) • Blackstrap molasses • Marmite and Vegemite
Calcium	• Milk • Cheese • Yogurt • Tinned fish with bones (salmon, sardines)	• Green leafy vegetables (spinach, cabbage, leeks, broccoli, bok choy, kale) • Peanuts, almonds and sesame seeds
Zinc	• Red meat • Seafood	• Whole grains • Legumes • Nuts • Seeds • Wheatgerm
Iodine	• Fish • Seafood	• Seaweed

Haem iron, found in animal sources, is more bioavailable than non-haem iron and, being protected by the haem molecule, is less likely to be affected by inhibitors. Non-haem iron is found in both animal and plant sources; however, it is heavily influenced by promoters and inhibitors of iron, with most likely only 10% of the iron being available to be absorbed (Milman, 2012). Women who rely on non-animal or plant-based sources of iron should be encouraged to take steps to optimise iron absorption through promoters and avoid inhibitors of iron absorption.

Iron optimisation and absorption

Obtaining optimal iron even when dietary intake is good can be challenging because dietary iron is poorly absorbed, with only 30% of the total iron available to use within the body.

Promoters include meat and vitamin C. Therefore, having a meal with vitamin-C-rich foods such as broccoli, tomatoes, capsicums, kiwifruit or citrus fruits will assist in optimal absorption. Cigarette smoke will inhibit iron absorption, as will tannins present in black teas and red wines, which are polyphenols and act as inhibitors reducing iron absorption by up to 40%. It is recommended that alcohol is avoided, and black tea is consumed 2–3 hours before or after a meal. Phytates are another inhibitor of iron absorption; these are phosphate-containing molecules present in legumes, nuts, and whole grains that bind iron, rendering it unavailable for absorption. Soaking legumes, roasting nuts and fermenting whole grains decreases the phytate content of these foods, thereby decreasing their effect on iron absorption (Bechoff & Dhuique-Mayer, 2017). Finally, high doses of calcium and zinc, such as the level present in supplements, when consumed with iron-rich foods or iron supplements have been reported to inhibit iron absorption (Milman, 2011)—highlighting one concern with multivitamin use in pregnancy.

When using supplementation to treat iron deficiency, there is evidence to suggest that traditional dosing regimes prescribed may not be optimising iron absorption. A small 2017 study found that iron supplementation was optimised when higher doses were prescribed on alternate days (120 mg iron every second day versus 60 mg iron daily) (Stoffel et al., 2017).

Calcium

Calcium is essential for development and maintenance of the skeleton and involved in blood pressure control, nerve impulses, muscle contraction and secretion of some hormones. It is stored in teeth and bones where it provides structure and strength. Deficiencies in infants can cause growth delays and bone malformations also known as rickets; and low bone density or osteoporosis which is common in western cultures. Osteoporosis is a leading cause of morbidity amongst older populations in Australia and New Zealand, particularly postmenopausal women. During pregnancy, low calcium is associated with preeclampsia (Adams et al., 2021).

Calcium levels fall during pregnancy, thus sufficient intake through diet is important to meet the maternal and fetal needs. Physiological adaptions during pregnancy result in increased absorption of calcium meaning that the recommended daily intake for calcium does not increase during pregnancy (MOH, 2020), however, women need to be aware of existing recommendations and how to achieve them as a part of a well-balanced diet.

Calcium is present in many animal and plant foods and, like iron, the bioavailability of calcium is much higher in animal foods than in plant foods (see Table 21.6). Some plant foods do have well-absorbed calcium, however, the calcium present in plant foods may interact with various inhibitors, including phytates, and be inhibited by high doses of minerals, such as iron, and oxalates (Sivakumaran et al., 2014). Oxalates are compounds present in foods such as spinach, rhubarb and chocolate. Like phytates, they bind calcium, rendering it unavailable for absorption in the intestinal tract.

For women at high risk of preeclampsia, calcium supplementation is recommended—particularly for women who have low dietary intake of calcium with 1.5–2.0g oral elemental calcium recommended (MOH, 2022).

Zinc

Zinc is an important component of over 80 enzymes that are involved in many reactions including cell replication and growth, regulation and gene expression, optimal immune function and hormone activity. Zinc is required in greater amounts during pregnancy and lactation and has a role in embryogenesis, fetal growth and milk production. Findings from several observational studies suggest that zinc deficiency during pregnancy increases the incidence of neural tube defects (NTDs), fetal death and malformations, low birth weight, premature rupture of membranes and increased antenatal and intrapartum complications. However, a 2021 review and meta-analysis of 15 studies found a relationship between maternal zinc status and preterm birth, but no statistically significant relationship with other adverse feto-maternal outcomes (Iqbal & Ali, 2021).

Iodine

Iodine is an essential component for the thyroid hormones, responsible for regulating body temperature and involved with processes surrounding metabolism, reproduction and growth. Iodine deficiency during pregnancy can cause an enlargement of the thyroid gland known as goitre and in infants can lead to neonatal cretinism, stunted growth, cognitive deficiencies, deafness, motor rigidity and hypothyroidism (Toloza et al., 2020). Iodine is present in only a limited number of foods, with fish, seafood and seaweed being the richest natural sources in Australia and New Zealand (Table 21.6). In Tasmania and inland regions of New Zealand the iodine content of the soil is very low, resulting in the plants grown in these areas being poor sources for dietary intake of iodine. The increasing prevalence of iodine deficiencies (including goitre) in the populations of Australia and New Zealand triggered their governments to enforce the mandatory use of iodised salt in the manufacturing of bread in 2009, with the exception of organic breads; however, despite fortification the populations of these two countries remain 'mildly' iodine deficient (Australian Institute of Health and Welfare (AIHW), 2016). This poses an extra concern for pregnancy due to an increased iodine requirement, making achieving adequate iodine levels in pregnancy more of a challenge. In 2010, routine supplementation for all pregnant women of 150 μg of iodine was introduced and was recommended to be offered (Table 21.7). It is also advised that breastfeeding mothers continue to take this supplement because breastfed infants gain iodine via the breast milk. Even with compensatory mechanisms, adequate intake of iodine via breast milk is difficult to gain in even mildly iodine-deficient areas when mothers are not supplemented. A recent study found that breastfed infants of mothers who were supplemented with iodine remained deficient, which poses the question of whether the current 150 μg tablet is sufficient (Andersen & Laurberg, 2016).

Mercury

Mercury is a contaminant that can be toxic if consumed in large quantities. It occurs naturally in seawater, rivers and lakes and can be present in fish as a result. Quantities of mercury in fish vary between species, location and diet. It is advised that pregnant women become familiar with the amount and types of fish that are safest to consume. High levels of mercury have been linked with adverse outcomes in the infant. Australia and New Zealand have different recommendations regarding the amount of fish it is safe to consume based on the species of fish available in each country. Information about mercury content in fish can be found at the Food Standards Australia New Zealand website and the Ministry for Primary Industries website (see Online resources).

Vitamins

Folate/folic acid

Folate (vitamin B_9) is required for the body to make DNA and RNA and metabolise amino acids necessary for cell division. Humans cannot make folate, making it an essential nutrient. Folate can be obtained through the diet, however, only 50%–70% of dietary folate consumed is absorbed leaving many individuals with low levels.

Folate in pregnancy

As folate is required for cell replication and division it is particularly significant for pregnancy and fetal development. Folate deficiencies are associated with cleft lip, cleft palate, placental abruption, low birth weight, miscarriage and most commonly neural tube defects such as spina bifida, anencephalus and encephaloceles (Haider & Bhutta, 2012). Folic acid is the synthetic form of folate, with its supplementation known to reduce the incidence of NTDs (De-Regil et al., 2015). Women are encouraged to supplement with folic acid from 4 weeks prior to conception through to 12 weeks gestation (MOH, 2020). The recommended dose of folic acid varies between Australia and New Zealand and depending on risk assessment (Table 21.7) with higher doses recommended for at-risk women.

Folic acid fortification

The difference in recommended dosage of folic acid supplementation between Australia and New Zealand is

Table 21.7 Folic acid and iodine supplementation recommended in Australia and New Zealand

	Dose	Population	Duration
Folic acid	**Australia** 400–500 μg daily New Zealand 800 μg daily	All pregnant women not included below	At least four weeks before pregnancy (or as soon as pregnancy is discovered) until the end of the first 12 weeks of pregnancy)
	Australia and New Zealand 5 mg daily	• Maternal NTD • Previous pregnancy affected by an NTD or a child or close family member with an NTD • Paternal NTD or paternal family history of NTD • Receiving insulin treatment for diabetes • Taking medication known to affect folate metabolism such as anti-epileptics • Prepregnancy BMI > 35 (RANZCOG)	
Iodine	**Australia and New Zealand** 150 μg daily	All pregnant and lactating women	Throughout pregnancy and lactation

a result of folic acid fortification of food that occurs in Australia but not New Zealand.

Over 60 countries fortify a food source, commonly wheat and bread, with folic acid—with Australia commencing mandatory fortification in 2009.

In New Zealand only 16.2% of women are folate sufficient, with lower rates in women aged 15–24 compared to those aged 25–44 (Gluckman & Beaglehole, 2018). Folate insufficiency was found to be more prevalent in Asian populations compared to non-Asian and in women residing in more deprived neighbourhoods. In July 2021 the New Zealand Government announced that it will be making fortification of bread-making wheat flour with folic acid mandatory. There will be a two-year transition period (ending in 2023) to allow industry to make the necessary adjustments (Ministry for Primary Industries/Manatū Ahu Matua, 2021). Therefore, the recommended supplementations in pregnancy in New Zealand may change to align with Australian recommendations in the future.

Vitamin B_{12}

Vitamin B_{12}, unlike other water-soluble vitamins, can be stored within the liver; it is involved in folate and fatty acid metabolism, DNA synthesis, red blood cell production in bone marrow and the production of myelin (Pawlak et al., 2013). During pregnancy, vitamin B_{12} is stored in the placenta and is transferred to the fetus with a newborn having approximately double the vitamin B_{12} concentration of the mother (Rashid, et al., 2021). Vitamin B_{12} deficiency, in pregnancy, can lead to developmental, cognitive and neurological impairments (Wang et al., 2012) and results in high levels of homocysteine, which is associated with cardiovascular disease and is termed megaloblastic anaemia. Food sources of vitamin B_{12} are outlined in Table 21.8. There are no reliable plant-based food sources for vitamin B_{12}. While serum vitamin B_{12} levels fall during pregnancy, women who consume a mixed diet usually have sufficient stores of vitamin B_{12} to meet the demands of the growing fetus.

Table 21.8 Dietary sources of vitamins

Vitamin	Animal sources	Plant sources
Folate/folic acid		• Spinach • Silverbeet • Broccoli • Cabbage • Yeast extracts • Whole grains • Kidneys • Asparagus • Legumes • Wheatgerm
Vitamin B_{12}	• Meats • Poultry • Fish • Seafood • Dairy products • Eggs	Vitamin B_{12} fortified forms of: • Soy milk • Yeast extracts • Spreads (margarine)
Vitamin A	Preformed vitamin A • Liver (recommended to avoid in pregnancy) • Eel • Eggs • Butter	Provitamin A (carotenoids) Plants of dark green and orange colour: • Carrots • Apricots • Mangoes • Pumpkin • Silverbeet • Spinach
Vitamin D	• Fatty fish 1.4–9.9 µg per 100 g (56–396 IU) • Salmon fillet (farmed) 22.9–30.6 µg per 100g (916–1224 IU) • Cows' milk (standard, 3.3% fat) 0.3–0.6 µg per 100g (12–24 IU) • Eggs (equiv. 2 large eggs) 1.5 µg (60 IU)	

B_{12} and plant-based diets

A deficiency of vitamin B_{12} is more common in those who consume a vegetarian, vegan or 'plant-based' diet because B_{12} is not found in plant sources. A plant-based diet describes a wide range of dietary patterns that contain none or lower amounts of animal products and increased amounts of vegetables, fruit, cereals and nuts. An increasing proportion of the population are embracing plant-based diets due to the lowered environmental impact of this diet; it is therefore important for midwives to be aware of the relationship between plant-based diets and vitamin B_{12} deficiency (Rashid et al., 2021).

The Ministry of Health recommend that pregnant women who follow a vegan diet receive B_{12} supplementation even if they are showing no signs of deficiency (Ministry of Health, 2020). Internationally, there have been calls for neonatal screening programs to identify vitamin B_{12} deficiency in the neonate, especially in populations where plant-based diets are common (Rashid et al., 2021). A 2021 study in Southern India ($n=1169$) found the presence of maternal vitamin B_{12} deficiency in early pregnancy predicted vitamin B_{12} deficiency in the neonate (Finkelstein, et al., 2021).

Vitamin A

Vitamin A is a fat-soluble vitamin essential for cellular differentiation, vision, growth and immune function, with a deficiency leading to night blindness and vision impairment. Vitamin A is complex and is present in two forms: preformed vitamin A and pro-vitamin A (Table 21.8). Although excess consumption of carotenoids can result in a staining and orange pigment seen in the skin, this is not associated with toxicity. High intakes, however, of preformed vitamin A from supplements and consumption of liver during pregnancy have been known to have a teratogenic effect (Maia et al., 2019). It is generally recommended that pregnant women therefore avoid liver and liver products and any supplements that contain more than the recommended dietary intake of vitamin A of 800 µg/day.

Vitamin D

Vitamin D is responsible for increasing intestinal absorption of calcium. The most important compounds in humans are vitamin D_3 (colecalciferol) and D_2 (ergocalciferol). The primary natural source of vitamin D is synthesis of cholecalciferol in the lower layers of the skin epidermis, this process is dependent on sun exposure (specifically exposure of UVB rays). Both cholecalciferol and ergocalciferol can be ingested in the diet, however, dietary sources in Australia and New Zealand account for less than 10% of total vitamin D requirements because few foods contain vitamin D or are fortified with vitamin D (MOH, 2020).

Vitamin D and pregnancy

Vitamin D aids absorption of calcium during pregnancy, which assists with muscle function, bone health, the absorption of calcium and the formation of the fetal skeleton (Wagner et al., 2012). Symptomatic deficiencies in pregnancy are rare; however, mothers who have low levels may give birth to infants with an increased risk of becoming deficient. Deficiencies in children are serious and can lead to seizures and softening of the bones as seen in rickets. While dietary sources of vitamin D should be encouraged (Table 21.8) it is found in only small amounts within foods and most of the vitamin D we need can be achieved from skin exposure to sunlight. With high rates of skin cancer, Australians and New Zealanders are encouraged to follow sun-safe messages, which are critical in the prevention of skin cancer, but coupled with current lifestyle factors these may also be hindering women from achieving optimal vitamin D status (MOH, 2020). In Australia and New Zealand, the current recommended adequate intake for pregnancy and lactating women is 5 µg/day or 10 µg/day for women at risk of vitamin D deficiency (Box 21.3) (NHMRC, 2006, cited in MOH 2020a, 2020d).

CRITICAL THINKING EXERCISE

Explain the difference between soluble and insoluble vitamins. How are they transported and used differently within the body? How may this knowledge assist your understanding of the potential food sources for each group of vitamins and of their required frequency of consumption?

REFLECTIVE THINKING EXERCISE

How will you respond to a woman you meet in early pregnancy who asks you which supplements she should take now that she is pregnant?

Box 21.3 Risk factors for vitamin D deficiency

Women are at risk of vitamin D deficiency if they (MOH, 2020d):

- have darker skin
- completely avoid sun exposure for religious, personal or medical reasons, including by applying sunscreen to exposed skin every day
- have liver or kidney disease, or are on certain medications (e.g. some anticonvulsants) that affect vitamin D levels
- live in an area south of Nelson-Marlborough in winter.

FOOD SAFETY DURING PREGNANCY

Food safety is important during pregnancy. As a result of suppressed immunity during pregnancy, women are more susceptible to foodborne illness. *Listeria monocytogenes, Toxoplasma gondii,* some strains of *Salmonella* and occasionally *Campylobacter* can cause a number of adverse maternal and fetal outcomes if exposure occurs during pregnancy. Box 21.4 outlines food safety techniques that should be used every day but especially when pregnant.

Challenges occur when women restrict their food intake based on fear of infection, hence unfortunately not meeting their increased nutrient requirements in pregnancy; these women would benefit from the guidance of a midwife in highlighting plenty of low-risk alternative food options and ensuring women understand the principles of safe food storage as well as the importance of consuming a well-balanced diet.

Box 21.4 Food safety tips

When buying food:

- always check the use-by date of each food before buying it
- avoid foods with damaged packaging—for example, dented or swollen tins, ripped packaging, broken seals
- choose undamaged and unripe (or just-ripe) fresh vegetables and fruit.

If gathering food:

- always wash food like pūhā and watercress thoroughly after gathering or buying from others who have gathered it.

When storing food:

- keep the fridge at or below 4 degrees Celsius
- store raw meat away from other food, for example, on the bottom shelf of the fridge so the raw meat juices do not drip on to other food
- follow storage advice on labels
- cover leftovers and store them in the fridge (within two hours of cooking) and use within two days of cooking.

When preparing and cooking food:

- always thoroughly wash hands with soap and water, and dry them, before handling food or between handling raw meat and other food
- always prepare food on clean surfaces and with utensils that have been cleaned with hot, soapy water
- reheat any leftovers until they are steaming hot before eating them
- be aware of food that is at higher risk of being contaminated by pathogens—for example, raw meat (including chicken), milk products, fish or shellfish, and sprouts. For these foods:
  - store and cook them safely
  - if in doubt about the safety of the food, throw it out.

Food safety while breastfeeding

- Food safety advice for women who are breastfeeding is the same as for non-pregnant adults.

Listeria

Listeria monocytogenes is a Gram-positive bacterium found naturally in soil and vegetation. An infection with *L. monocytogenes* results in non-specific symptoms similar to a mild flu with fever, diarrhoea and sore throat; however, listeria can be passed to the fetus through the placenta or through the vagina during birth. Listeria infection during pregnancy can result in miscarriage, premature pre-term rupture of membranes, fetal distress, premature labour, chorioamnionitis, placental abruption and fetal demise; furthermore neonatal risks include meningitis and sepsis (Craig et al., 2019).

Despite the low incidence of listeriosis, general **food safety** principles should be promoted particularly during pregnancy to reduce a woman's risk further (Box 21.4). Both raw and processed foods are a potential source of listeria. Foods that have been cooked and then chilled are ideal breeding grounds for listeria; therefore foods stored in the refrigerator longer than 12 hours may contain it. Fortunately, high heat destroys this pathogen; therefore reheating foods can significantly reduce the risk of contracting listeriosis.

Toxoplasmosis

Toxoplasmosis is caused by a single-cell parasite called *Toxoplasma gondii* and is a significant infection during pregnancy. Congenital toxoplasmosis occurs in infants following maternal transmission. It can result in miscarriage, fetal death, and syndromes including neurologic and neurocognitive deficits that result in a significant burden of disease globally (Torgerson & Mastroiacovo, 2013). Human infection can result from the ingestion or handling of undercooked or raw meat containing tissue cysts, or from direct contact with cats, or ingesting food or water contaminated by oocytes excreted in the faeces of cats.

Women should be aware of food safety strategies (Box 21.4) and those specific to reducing the risk of contracting toxoplasmosis, in particular the cross-contamination of hands after gardening in areas where there could be cat faeces, or cleaning up after animals.

Pica

Most women report some dietary aversions or dietary cravings during pregnancy that disappear following birth. For the most part, these do not have a great impact on nutrient intake. The consumption of non-food items such as dirt, starch, chalk, clay, paint or rubber is cause for concern due to potential toxic levels of lead, or consumption of parasites. This practice is referred to as pica. Some view pica as an eating and mental health disorder, whereas others have theorised that pica is a biological response to the consequence of nutrient deficiencies; women with pica more often have deficiencies in iron and calcium (Cardwell, 2013). Pica has been associated with lead poisoning, hypokalaemia and lower maternal haemoglobin levels at birth. Although the true prevalence of pica in pregnancy is unknown and may be difficult to ascertain, it is important to be aware of the potential consequences of pica as it relates to pregnancy (Cardwell, 2013).

GESTATIONAL WEIGHT GAIN

Achieving a healthy **gestational weight gain** is important to maternal, fetal and infant health, irrespective of maternal prepregnancy body mass index (BMI) and is a message that all women should receive as early as possible during pregnancy. The general consensus for recommended gestational weight gain (GWG) is shown in Table 21.9. Ethnicity and age are not differentiated in this table. Despite some support for modification in relation to these factors, the evidence is currently not clear enough to support specific recommendations (Siega-Riz et al., 2009, 2010).

What is known is that low GWG is associated with preterm birth and low-birth-weight infants, and that high GWG is associated with preeclampsia, gestational diabetes, large-for-dates infants, depression, caesarean section and postpartum weight retention (Alavi et al., 2013; Johnson et al., 2013).

Women with excessive weight gain during pregnancy are less likely to lose the excess weight after the birth. Cumulative excessive weight gain over the childbearing years negatively impacts on women's health and increases the likelihood of subsequent child and adolescent overweight and obesity (Martin et al., 2014). Achieving an appropriate gestational weight gain is therefore an important consideration not only for optimal pregnancy outcomes in a current pregnancy, but also for the health of future pregnancies.

Nutritional information and interventions provided to women during pregnancy can optimise appropriate GWGs (Oteng-Ntim et al., 2012). Continuity models of midwifery care, for example, which provide individualised ongoing care in a trusting and supportive relationship, have the potential to support optimal weight gain.

Dieting or restricting food is not recommended in pregnancy, with studies showing that the offspring of women who are not meeting their nutritional requirements such as those dieting or in periods of famine are at increased risk of later-life diseases such as cardiovascular disease and diabetes (Barker, 1994; Lillycrop & Burdge, 2015). This is thought to be due to fetal programming, a concept in which gene expression is changed during pregnancy in response to environmental influences. These changes or 'resetting' of physiological parameters can emerge in adult life and result in a range of long-term consequences. Women who have a high BMI may inadvertently lose weight during pregnancy owing to a healthier lifestyle and diet interventions in pregnancy, which is favourable; however, they should refrain from reducing their intake below that recommended.

At the first pregnancy visit midwives should identify and record the woman's height and weight, which can then be used to identify the woman's BMI and optimal weight gain. Where prepregnancy BMI is not known, a weight gain of 0.5–2 kg in the first trimester may be assumed (Institute of Medicine (IOM) & National Research Council (NRC), 2009). The NZ guideline for healthy weight gain during pregnancy (2014) also identifies that:

- BMI should be calculated from measured height and measured weight at booking/first visit (ideally before 10 weeks gestation). If the woman presents after 10 weeks gestation, the BMI can still be calculated from measured height and weight, and weight gain can still be advised based on best estimate of prepregnancy BMI.
- Women should be encouraged, where appropriate, to monitor (using the same scales each time) and record

Table 21.9 Recommended weight gain during pregnancy based on prepregnancy BMI

Prepregnancy BMI (kg/m²)	Recommended weight gain (kg)	Rates of weight gain in 2nd and 3rd trimester (kg)
Underweight: <18.5	12.5–18	0.51 (0.44–0.58)
Normal: 18.5–24.9	11.5–16	0.42 (0.35–0.50)
Overweight: 25–29.9	7.0–11.5	0.28 (0.23–0.33)
Obese: ≥30.0	5–9	0.22 (0.17–0.27)

[a] Calculations assume a 0.5–2 kg weight gain in the first trimester.
BMI (body mass index) is calculated as weight (kg) divided by height squared (m^2).
(Source: Ministry of Health, 2020a)

their own weight regularly (for example, monthly) during pregnancy and in the postpartum period and bring a copy of this information to antenatal visits for discussion as part of their care plan. If it is not possible for a woman to record their own weight, they can ask to be weighed at antenatal visits.

A discussion on weight gain during pregnancy is important as is informing women that weight gain is unnecessary in the first trimester and should follow a linear pattern from late into the second trimester. Self-reported weight and height measurements do show a tendency for larger weights to be underreported, which can have significant implications for maternal serum screening (MSS) results and customised growth charts, highlighting a challenge for midwives to gain accurate information whilst continuing to work in a woman-centred way (Fuber & McGowan, 2011; Hildingsson & Thomas, 2012).

REFLECTIVE THINKING EXERCISE

Recording an accurate prepregnancy BMI (or early pregnancy if not possible) is important for establishing accurate GWG recommendations and also in receiving accurate MSS results and when using customised growth charts. Tracking gestational weight gain through pregnancy also may identify risk and highlight opportunities for midwives to discuss diet and nutrition. However, weighing women at each visit is still under debate, with some women finding the focus on weight unpleasant, embarrassing and stigmatising. How do you think midwives can tackle this issue and continue to provide quality woman-centred care with regards to recording BMI and tracking GWG?

MATERNAL OBESITY

Jane Raymond

Maternal obesity presents one of the most serious challenges to face midwifery practice this century, with significant impacts on the health of pregnant women, their babies and their families.

Defining obesity

The term 'obese' is defined by the World Health Organization (WHO, 2000) as a body mass index greater than 30 kg/m^2. Some classify the term more specifically, referring to a BMI between 30–39.9 as class I obesity, with morbid obesity (class II) being 40–49.9 and maternal super obesity (class III) being >50 kg/m^2 (Cunningham & Teale, 2013; Marshall et al., 2012). Although some may find these terms useful in classifying the extent or severity of obesity, women may find such a label derogatory and therefore actual BMI numbers would appear to be a sufficient objective reference (Table 21.10).

Prevalence of obesity in Australasia

Obesity rates continue to rise within both the general and pregnant populations worldwide. A significant toll in relation to obesity is being taken on specific populations. In New Zealand in 2019–20, 30.9% of all adults over 15 were reported as being obese. This was higher in Māori and Pacific populations where the rate of obesity was 47.9% and 63.4% respectively (MOH, 2020c)

In Australia, Indigenous populations are 1.2 times as likely to be overweight compared to non-Indigenous populations (77% compared with 66%) and 1.5 times as likely to be obese (47% compared with 31%) (Australian Bureau of Statistics (ABS), 2019).

Perinatal complications associated with obesity

Pregnant women who are obese are at risk of a multitude of complications (Catalano & Shankar, 2017). These include fetal anomaly, gestational diabetes, hypertensive

Table 21.10 Classifications of obesity by body mass index

New Zealand classification	BMI value (kg/m^2)	Risk of health conditions
Underweight	<18.5	Not applicable
Healthy weight	18.5–24.9	Average
Overweight	25.0–29.9	Increased
Obese	≥30.0	Substantially increased
Obese (class I)	30.0–34.9	Moderate
Obese (class II)	35.0–39.9	Severe
Obese (class III): 'extreme obesity'	≥40.0	Very severe

(Source: Ministry of Health, 2015)

disorders including preeclampsia, large-for-dates and macrosomic infants and stillbirth (Liu et al., 2016; Magann et al., 2013). During birth women who are obese are more likely to be in labour longer and/or more likely to have induction of labour, premature labour, postpartum haemorrhage and require more internal fetal surveillance when compared to women in the healthy BMI weight category (Chin et al., 2012; Cunningham & Teale, 2013; Fyfe et al., 2011, 2012). Additionally, obese women are up to five times more likely to give birth by caesarean section (Chin et al., 2012; Dennedy et al., 2012; Marshall et al., 2012), and experience difficult anaesthetic procedures and reduced success of vaginal birth after caesarean section (Ehrenberg & Wissler, 2010; Mace et al., 2011; Tipton et al., 2011).

In the postnatal period, obesity is associated with longer hospital stays, thromboembolism, wound infections and lower rates of breastfeeding. Infants born to women who are obese are more likely to experience respiratory distress, hypoglycaemia and jaundice, and need intensive care treatment more often than infants born to non-obese mothers (McIntyre et al., 2012).

The experience of women who are obese

Women's experience of their maternity care when obese can provide insights for all health professionals to consider. Women who are obese report a much less positive experience of their maternity care. They describe a heavy focus on risk, less continuity of care, more fear of childbirth and unpleasant ultrasound experiences, and feel humiliated and under scrutiny (Heslehurst et al., 2015; Hildingsson & Thomas, 2012).

The significant risks associated with obesity have led to a term 'the medicalisation of obesity' where women who are obese are considered high risk and managed and treated accordingly. Although risk identification is aimed at keeping women and babies safe, the weighting and focus on risk has the potential to disempower women who are obese and depersonalise their care (McGlone & Davies, 2012). Women who are obese may be considered a vulnerable group; evidence suggests that they are less likely to attend for 'routine' healthcare than women of normal weight owing to negative attitudes of caregivers (Brownell et al., 2005), and therefore may be reluctant to engage in antenatal care. Given these vulnerabilities, women who are obese need the opportunity to build trusting relationships with a limited number of caregivers. Many, however, experience complicated pregnancies and consequently meet a greater number of carers, making it challenging to obtain consistent support (Hildingsson & Thomas, 2012; Mills et al., 2013).

Care of women who are obese

It is recommended that women who are obese are informed at their first antenatal visit of how their weight, and their GWG, may impact on their health and their pregnancy in a respectful and supportive manner (Department of Health, 2020). It is further recommended that obese women are monitored more closely during pregnancy than women of normal weight (Department of Health, 2020; Royal Australian and New Zealand College of Obstetricians and Gynaecologists (RANZCOG), 2013). Local guidelines are likely to include some or all of the following: higher doses of folic acid in early pregnancy, a wide range of surveillance methods for congenital abnormalities, regular ultrasound growth scans with customised growth charts because accurate growth assessment by palpation is often difficult, early glucose tolerance testing for gestational diabetes and increased number of visits to monitor blood pressure, and attend anaesthetic and obstetric referrals.

Adverse outcomes increase proportionally with increased BMI; therefore women with a BMI >50 kg/m^2 have higher risk for complications compared with a woman with a BMI of 30 (Marshall et al., 2012). Many obese women will experience a healthy pregnancy and a normal birth, but midwives should be alert to the need to act promptly when changes occur. Referrals at the outset of pregnancy, or as complications arise, should be made in line with appropriate guidelines, as for all women. Within Australia and New Zealand the National Midwifery Guidelines for Consultation and Referral specify that midwives should seek consultation with a medical practitioner regarding the plan for care of women with a BMI above 35 kg/m^2 (level B/consultation category) (Australian College of Midwives, 2014; MOH, 2022). Women with a BMI above 40 kg/m^2 should be referred for medical care at a secondary or tertiary level but, where appropriate, the midwife may continue to provide midwifery care throughout the pregnancy.

Care of obese women in labour is often a fine balancing act for midwives—managing actual and potential complications whilst striving to prevent a cascade of intervention. For example, guidelines suggest early epidurals in labour with continuous fetal surveillance, but these also result in restricted maternal movement (Ehrenberg & Wissler, 2010; Mace et al., 2011). This can be a challenging situation for midwives who promote the value of upright positions and remaining active during labour to increase the likelihood of normal birth. It is acknowledged that insertion of an epidural may be difficult in obese women, causing anxieties for anaesthetic staff who will not wish to be caught unprepared (Bell & Cronje, 2010). Early anaesthetic consultation, preferably during pregnancy, and a clear management plan in line with the woman's wishes documented in her medical record, will assist decision making during labour.

The reason why obese women are more likely to have longer labours, caesarean section and postpartum haemorrhage is thought to be due to the myometrium of the uterus not contracting efficiently. In situations where there is no fetal compromise, women who are obese may be offered longer times for labour progress than women who are not obese. Allowing more time may help to promote vaginal birth as opposed to a caesarean section, with its associated complications (Chin et al., 2012). Postnatally, additional support will be required for breastfeeding, owing to the earlier cessation often associated with maternal obesity (Molinaro & Fan, 2015).

Maternal obesity presents significant challenges to midwifery practice. It is essential that women are provided with options for models of maternity care that provide midwifery continuity of carer, albeit within a collaborative framework for consultation and referral. Midwives are in a position to offer a stronger focus on factors that support health rather than a focus on what causes disease during pregnancy, and are encouraged to work alongside women who are obese in a positive manner (McGlone & Davies, 2012). Midwives need to maintain their knowledge base around maternal obesity and related issues, and continue to share information, collaborate with other maternity care providers, and assess risk appropriately while supporting women's autonomy and choice.

REFLECTIVE THINKING EXERCISE

It has been suggested that women who are obese should be offered an epidural early in labour. The rationale for this is to prevent difficulties with insertion in advanced labour, due to the higher likelihood of caesarean section in labours where women are obese. What implications may this have for the woman and her labour? What advantages and disadvantages are there with an early epidural? What information is required to be shared with the woman to ensure her decision is fully informed?

NUTRITION IN LABOUR

Childbirth is an energy-demanding process that requires adequate energy and hydration. Without adequate energy intake, body stores of glycogen and adipose tissue will be used to sustain energy requirements. As the period of fasting increases, ketones begin to appear in the blood. It is largely accepted that some amount of ketosis during childbirth is normal. However, as ketones begin to spill into the urine, the body becomes depleted of sodium and potassium, resulting in dehydration, which may lead to maternal or fetal acidosis. It is important, therefore, to ensure adequate nutrition and hydration to prevent such large aberrations in acid–base balance.

Since the mid 1900s and following the move to hospital birth, many hospitals worldwide implemented policies on restricting oral intake during childbirth. The primary rationale for this restriction was to lower the risk of Mendelson's syndrome, now termed pulmonary aspiration syndrome, in which stomach acids and food could be aspirated into the lungs during general anaesthesia. Eating in labour increases gastric volume theoretically, increasing the risk of pulmonary aspiration. A 2013 Cochrane review, however, found fasting in labour does not guarantee decreased gastric contents or less acidity (Singata et al., 2010, 2013). Fortunately, regional anaesthetics are now a common practice for operative births and pulmonary aspiration is extremely rare (Singata et al., 2013). In their review, Singata et al. (2013) conclude that there is no justification for restricting food and drink during labour and women should be free to eat and drink (or not) as they wish.

NUTRITIONAL FOUNDATION FOR LACTATION

Dietary recommendations for lactating women often focus on the increased energy demand of lactation (Tables 21.1 and 21.4) Ford et al. (2020) call for an increased focus on the consequences of an unbalanced diet on the breastfeeding dyad. They also call for a larger public health focus specifically on the breastfeeding dyad rather than seeing breastfeeding as a continuum of pregnancy or an extension of healthy adult eating (Ford et al., 2020).

The nutritional quality of breast milk is fairly constant regardless of maternal diet; however, although diet does not affect actual lactogenesis, concentrations of micronutrients in breast milk are influenced by the mother's dietary intake with deficiencies in the mother often translating to deficiencies in the infant. This is especially true regarding certain nutrients such as vitamin D, A, B_2, B_6, B_{12}, iron, iodine and also fatty acids (Valentine & Wagner, 2013). Whilst supplementation of the infant is recommended only with respect to vitamin K for prevention of haemorrhagic disease in the newborn and vitamin D for at-risk infants, infants may not reach their full health potential if the maternal diet is poor.

As B vitamins are predominantly sourced in grains, meats and fortified foods, women who consume restrictive diets such as vegetarian, vegan or gluten-free diets and who live in areas where no fortification exists run the risk of not having adequate concentrations in their breast milk (Valentine & Wagner, 2013).

Concentrations of vitamin A in breast milk are higher in women who consume a diet rich in vitamin A, which is important for optimal vision and eye function. Likewise, the content of fatty acids in breast milk is influenced by dietary factors and increased amounts are associated with improved cognition and attention scores of children; hence lactating women should be encouraged to consume two to three servings of fish per week (Valentine & Wagner, 2013).

Iodine is important for infants with regards to their neurodevelopment, with low levels in breast milk being indicative of low maternal dietary intake—hence the recommendation for women in Australia and New Zealand (low-iodine locations) to supplement through pregnancy and breastfeeding (FSANZ, 2016, 2019; MOH, 2020).

Breast milk is not a good source of vitamin D and prolonged exclusive breastfeeding (over six months) may increase the risk of vitamin D deficiency. While studies have found that maternal supplementation is associated with increased vitamin D concentrations in breast milk, routine supplementation is not recommended in New Zealand (MOH, 2020c). Lactating women should be encouraged to consume foods high in vitamin D while breastfeeding.

PHYSICAL ACTIVITY DURING PREGNANCY

Internationally, **physical inactivity** is a primary risk factor for non-communicable diseases and was estimated to cost INT$54 billion in direct healthcare in 2013 (WHO, 2018). The World Health Organization (WHO) estimates that 23% of adults and 80% of adolescents (aged 11–17) do not meet the WHO global recommendations of physical activity for health (WHO, 2018). In Australia and New Zealand, physical activity guidelines for pregnant women without serious pre-existing health conditions are the same as for the general population.

Benefits of physical activity during pregnancy

Regular physical activity during pregnancy benefits both the woman and her baby. Maternal benefits include: reduced likelihood of developing gestational diabetes mellitus, pre-eclampsia (Mottola et al., 2018) and gestational hypertension; prevention of excessive gestational weight gain; reduced symptoms of depression (RANZCOG, 2020); improved cardiovascular function; and improved strength and lean muscle mass. Improved sense of wellbeing and enhanced sleep are also associated with regular physical activity during pregnancy (Prather et al., 2012). Some of these factors work together; for example, body image satisfaction during pregnancy is an important determinant of psychological wellbeing (Rauff & Downs, 2011), and regular physical activity contributes to both.

Benefits to the fetus are often a motivating factor for women when considering physical activity during pregnancy. These include lower (healthy) birth weights and increased gestational ages (Prather et al., 2012).

Safety considerations relating to physical activity during pregnancy

There are some risks associated with any physical activity, in pregnant and non-pregnant populations, and there are some safety considerations which are unique to pregnancy. Risks of physical activity are relatively small but include concerns related to maternal hypoglycaemia, dizziness and fainting, strains and sprains and a reduced blood supply to the placenta, risk of fetal hyperthermia and premature labour (Ministry of Health, 2020). Absolute and relative contraindications to physical activity during pregnancy should be considered when you are providing advice to women about physical activity (Box 21.5).

Box 21.5 Absolute and relative contraindications to aerobic exercise during pregnancy

Absolute contraindications

- Haemodynamically significant heart disease
- Intrauterine growth restriction in current pregnancy
- Poorly controlled hypertension
- Restrictive lung disease
- Incompetent cervix/cerclage
- Multiple gestation at risk for premature labour
- Persistent second- or third-trimester bleeding
- Placenta praevia after 26 weeks gestation
- Premature labour during the current pregnancy
- Ruptured membranes
- Pregnancy-induced hypertension
- Severe anaemia
- Unexplained persistent vaginal bleeding
- Cervical insufficiency/cerclage
- Pre-eclampsia/pregnancy-induced hypertension
- Uncontrolled hypertension
- Multiple pregnancy at risk of preterm labour

Relative contraindications

- Unevaluated maternal cardiac arrhythmia
- Chronic bronchitis or other respiratory disorder
- Poorly controlled type 1 diabetes
- Extreme morbid obesity
- Extreme underweight
- Eating disorder
- History of extremely sedentary lifestyle
- Intrauterine growth restriction in current pregnancy
- Poorly controlled hypertension/preeclampsia
- Orthopaedic limitations
- Poorly controlled seizure disorder
- Poorly controlled thyroid disease

(Reproduced from RANZCOG, 2016)

Australian and New Zealand recommendations for physical activity during pregnancy

New Zealand and Australia have similar guidelines for physical activity during pregnancy (Box 21.6 and Box 21.7). Pregnant women should be advised to stop exercising and seek advice from their care provider if they experience any of the warning signs to terminate physical activity (Box 21.8).

Physical activity during pregnancy—women who are currently active

Women engaging in regular physical activity should be encouraged to continue doing so while being guided by the physical activity guidelines for their country. Information sharing should include the benefits and safety precautions during pregnancy as well as the warning signs to terminate physical activity and when to contact their care provider (Box 21.8). Women should also be aware that increased recovery time between periods of physical activity may be warranted when pregnant.

Physical activity during pregnancy—previously sedentary women

Pregnant women who have been sedentary will benefit from engaging in physical activity during pregnancy. These women will require different support and guidance to those who have been physically active before pregnancy. Discussion about the national physical

Box 21.6 Ministry of Health Activity Statements for New Zealand Adults

Activity Statement One

Sit less, move more!

Break up long periods of sitting

Activity Statement Two

Do at least two and a half hours (150 minutes) of moderate or one and a quarter hours (75 minutes) of vigorous physical activity spread throughout the week

Pregnancy: Pregnant woman should aim to do two and a half hours of moderate-intensity physical activity spread over at least three days per week (preferably some activity every day)

Activity Statement Three

For extra health benefits aim for five hours of moderate or two and a half hours of vigorous physical activity spread throughout the week

Pregnancy: Pregnant women should seek advice from a health care professional with specialist knowledge about the impact of vigorous-intensity activity if competing in events or significantly more active than Activity Statement Two

Activity Statement Four

Do muscle strengthening activities at least two days each week

Pregnancy: Pregnant women may also benefit from doing stretching and pelvic floor muscle training daily

Activity Statement Five

Doing some physical activity is better than doing none

Pregnancy: All pregnant women without serious health conditions should be regularly physically active through a variety of aerobic and resistance activities

(Reproduced from Ministry of Health, 2020a)

Box 21.7 Australian Government Department of Health Guidelines for Physical Activity During Pregnancy

Amount of physical activity

During pregnancy aim to:

- Be active on most, if not all days of the week
- Do moderate intensity activities for two and a half to five hours each week or vigorous intensity activities for one and a quarter to two and a half hours each week
- 30–60 minutes moderate or 15–30 minutes vigorous activity most days
- Muscle strengthening activities at least twice weekly
- Break up long periods of inactivity
- Pelvic floor exercises—daily during pregnancy and start again as soon as possible after birth

(Reproduced from Department of Health, 2021)

Box 21.8 Warning signs to terminate physical activity while pregnant

- Vaginal bleeding
- Dyspnoea before exertion
- Dizziness or feeling faint that does not resolve with rest
- Headache
- Muscle weakness
- Sudden swelling of the ankles, hands or face
- Calf pain or swelling (need to rule out thrombophlebitis)
- Uterine contractions or pain in the lower back, pelvic area or abdomen (potentially indicating pre-term labour)
- Decreased fetal movement
- Amniotic fluid leakage

(Adapted from ACSM, 2014 and RANZCOG, 2016)

activity recommendations is important, however, the focus should be on the message that any amount of physical activity is beneficial. Gradual increases in physical activity may result in these women meeting the physical activity guidelines, but this should be a goal secondary to the introduction of any amount of physical activity. Sufficient recovery between periods of physical activity is critical during pregnancy, particularly in previously sedentary women.

Exercise prescription and exercise response in pregnancy

Pregnancy is a time when a woman's body undergoes significant anatomic and physiologic changes caused by gestational hormones to support the growing fetus. These changes in the anatomy and physiology of pregnant women lead to differing exercise responses compared to the non-pregnant woman. Box 21.9 outlines some of these changes and exercise prescription considerations that should be applied to physical activity.

CRITICAL THINKING EXERCISE

What are some of the benefits of physical activity during pregnancy? How would you encourage someone to start physical activity if they come into pregnancy inactive? What strategies would you use to moderate physical activity levels in someone who believes more is better?

Midwifery Practice Scenario

You have just met a woman for her booking visit and she reports being highly active. On further questioning you find out she regularly exercises five to six times a week for an hour or more; most of her exercise is cardiovascular based but she also has one netball training session and game. What advice would you give her with regard to her exercise as her pregnancy progresses?

Box 21.9 Pregnancy adaptations and exercise prescription considerations

Increase in body weight The increase in body weight as pregnancy increases is associated with increased pressure on joints. Weight-supported activities such as water-based exercise or stationary cycling may be more tolerable to a pregnant woman compared to weight-bearing exercises such as walking.

Changes in weight distribution The altered centre of gravity that occurs with the change in weight distribution as the pregnancy progresses may influence balance. Exercise prescription should include activities that avoid sudden or frequent changes in direction, particularly for women beginning an exercise program for the first time.

Increase in ligament laxity The increase in ligament laxity that occurs in pregnancy should be considered when recommending exercise. In the absence of robust research RANZCOG recommend women take care when engaging in weight-bearing exercise and activities involving frequent and rapid changes in direction and avoid activities involving jumping. Stretching activities should be slow and controlled, not ballistic.

Decrease in blood pressure Women should avoid rapid changes in posture (i.e. from lying or sitting to standing) to minimise the risk of dizziness or fainting. Exercise should be completed with a slow and sustained cool down.

Enlarged uterus As the uterus grows with advancing pregnancy the weight of the gravid uterus may obstruct venous return. Women after the end of the first trimester are advised to avoid exercises in a supine position for prolonged periods of time. Such exercises should be modified to be conducted in a sitting or standing posture.

Avoiding trauma For women who wish to continue with activities that involve a risk of falling or receiving abdominal trauma (e.g. horseriding, team sports), the midwife should discuss the potential risks to support informed decision making.

(Adapted from RANZCOG, 2016)

POSTPARTUM PHYSICAL ACTIVITY

Benefits of postpartum exercise include reduced depressive symptoms (Pritchett et al., 2017) and overall improved psychological wellbeing, improved cardiovascular fitness, decreased urinary stress and incontinence, decreased lactation-induced bone loss, reduced gestational weight retention and reduced postpartum weight gain.

Not returning to physical activity after childbirth for previously active women is associated with prolonged periods of inactivity (Brown et al., 2009). Therefore, counselling women postpartum or ideally during pregnancy about the benefits of physical activity postpartum is important and can have an impact on lifelong health behaviours.

One difficulty in counselling women around postpartum exercise is that there are very few clear guidelines, as the recommendations need to be individualised to the woman's pregnancy, labour and birth history as well as her exercise history and goals. Evenson et al. (2015) discuss this in their review of international guidelines for postpartum exercise. In general, they recommend a delay to regular physical activity until there is some resolution of the hormonal and physical effects of pregnancy (normally about 6 weeks postpartum).

Exercise guidelines for the general population (Australia and New Zealand) also apply to women postpartum but women should be advised that fatigue should guide their physical activity. Achieving the level of exercise recommended should be considered the eventual goal. Box 21.10 outlines guidelines for beginning exercise following a normal vaginal birth. Returning to physical activity following an instrumental birth or caesarean section should be delayed, and follow the post-procedural advice given to the woman.

Box 21.10 General guidelines for exercise during the postpartum period after a normal birth

- Stretching, pelvic floor exercises, and relaxation and breathing exercises are safe to perform in the immediate postpartum period.
- Begin gentle walking as early in the immediate postpartum period as is comfortable for the mother.
- Do not rush getting back 'into shape'.
- Do not get overly fatigued; rest intervals during exercise may be helpful.
- Fatigue should be used to guide participation.
- Abdominal exercises should start slowly and torque exercises should be avoided.
- Maintain proper nutrition and hydration.
- Beginning a moderate intensity aerobic exercise program should be delayed until after six weeks postpartum.

Postpartum exercise and breastfeeding

Concerns about the impact of breastfeeding are often cited as a barrier to engaging in postpartum exercise. Women should be reassured that during this time mild to moderate exercise is safe to engage in, although strenuous and exhaustive exercise should be avoided. Ensuring adequate hydration before, during and after exercise is important, as too is ensuring adequate caloric intake. Exercising after feeding baby or when breasts are empty can reduce discomfort (Mottola, 2003).

Midwifery Practice Scenario

You are caring for a woman who has given birth 6 weeks ago and is ready to start gentle exercise again. What advice would you give her to help her get back into exercise? Her partner is concerned that exercising will reduce her milk supply and she won't be able to breastfeed their baby. Think about the information and education you will need to provide for her to minimise this risk and allow her to allay the fears of her partner.

Pelvic floor exercises

Urinary incontinence (UI) has an impact on exercise participation in the years following pregnancy, and pelvic floor exercises should be discussed during both pregnancy and postpartum. A systematic review of the effect of pelvic floor exercises demonstrated that pelvic floor muscle training is effective if a supervised training protocol is used, follows strength-training principles that emphasise close to maximum contractions and lasts at least 8 weeks (Mørkved & Bø, 2014). Women should be advised to start pelvic floor exercises from as early in pregnancy as possible, and to continue them until at least 6 months postpartum.

REFLECTIVE THINKING EXERCISE

UI impacts on a woman's ability to partake in physical activity following the birth of her child. It can also impact on movement in late-stage pregnancy. This is a condition that a number of women associate with age and not pregnancy. Think about the advice you would give as a midwife to minimise the risk and/or impact of UI in a first-time mum.

Conclusion

Nutrition, diet and physical activity during pregnancy, childbirth and lactation are vitally important and can lead to improved outcomes in mothers and their infants in both the short and the long term. For optimal maternal and fetal health, adequate intakes of macro- and micronutrients are required. This chapter has focused on many nutrients including fatty acids, iron, zinc, iodine, vitamin D, vitamin B_{12} and folate. Women will benefit from the knowledge that midwives share with regards to these nutrients, their role in health and hence the importance of the foods that are good sources. Midwives can also use their knowledge to share what supplements may be recommended acknowledging both general and individualised supplementation philosophies.

Optimal nutrition will also support the lactating infant and, although lactation and energy will not be influenced by the maternal diet, deficiencies in mothers are associated with deficiencies in breastfed infants.

Excess gestational weight gain and maternal obesity is a common occurrence today and is associated with significant adverse outcomes, presenting a challenge to midwives who provide individualised care and promote and support normal birth amongst an ever-increasing environment of medicalised risk management of these women. Nutrition and physical exercise can assist in preventing and reducing these risks.

Review questions

1. How does the body mass index assist midwives in providing midwifery care? How can it be used appropriately?
2. Name food sources of each macronutrient and state their role and importance in pregnancy.
3. What impact do iron, iodine and vitamin D deficiency have in pregnancy and lactation?
4. What are the risks associated with excess gestational weight gain and/or maternal obesity?
5. What are the advantages and disadvantages of supplements? What supplements might you recommend to all women during pregnancy and which supplements might you recommend only for certain situations?
6. Why is food safety important during pregnancy?
7. Why are energy intake and hydration important during labour?
8. What are the contraindications to physical activity during pregnancy?
9. How does physical activity help to alleviate some of the discomforts of pregnancy?
10. What are some of the special considerations unique to pregnancy that should be considered when planning or undertaking physical activity?
11. What are some general guidelines to consider when discussing postpartum physical activity with women?

Acknowledgements

The authors would like to acknowledge the work of Megan Gibbons, who contributed to the previous edition of this text.

Online resources

Activity and Nutrition Aotearoa: http://www.ana.org.nz/.
American College of Sports Medicine: http://www.acsm.org.
Australia and New Zealand Food Standards Authority: http://www.foodstandards.gov.au/Pages/default.aspx.
Australian Dietary Guideline: https://www.eatforhealth.gov.au/guidelines.
Australian Government Department of Health: http://www.health.gov.au/.
Australian Sports Commission: http://www.ausport.gov.au/.
Dietitians Association of Australia: http://www.daa.asn.au.
Five Plus a Day: http://www.5aday.co.nz/.
Food Standards Australia New Zealand: https://www.foodstandards.gov.au/.
Food Standards Australia New Zealand—Mercury in fish: http://www.foodstandards.gov.au/consumer/chemicals/mercury/Pages/default.aspx.
New Zealand Dietitians Association: http://www.dietitians.org.nz.
New Zealand Food Safety in Pregnancy: https://www.mpi.govt.nz/dmsdocument/3675-Food-Safety-in-Pregnancy.
New Zealand Ministry for Primary Industries—Food Safety: http://mpi.govt.nz/food-safety.
New Zealand Ministry for Primary Industries—Mercury: https://www.mpi.govt.nz/food-safety-home/safe-levels-of-chemicals-in-food/mercury-levels-fish/.
New Zealand Ministry of Health: http://www.health.govt.nz/.
New Zealand Nutrition Foundation: http://www.nutritionfoundation.org.nz/.
Sport New Zealand: http://www.sportnz.org.nz/.
Sports Medicine Australia: http://sma.org.au/.
Vegetarian Resource Group: http://www.vrg.org/nutrition/veganpregnancy.php.
World Health Organization (Obesity): http://www.who.int/nutrition/topics/obesity/en/.

References

Adams J, Sorenson J, Pollard E, et al. Evidence-based recommendations for an optimal prenatal supplement for women in the U.S., Part Two: Minerals. *Nutrients*. 2021;13(6) doi: https://doi.org/10.3390/nu13061849.

Alavi N, Haley S, Chow K, et al. Comparison of national gestational weight gain guidelines and energy intake recommendations. *Obes Rev*. 2013;14(1):68–85.

American College of Sports Medicine (ACSM). *Resource Manual for Guidelines for Exercise Testing and Prescription*. 7th ed. Baltimore: Lippincott Williams & Wilkins; 2014.

Andersen S, Laurberg P. Iodine supplementation in pregnancy and the dilemma of ambiguous recommendations. *Eur Thyroid J*. 2016;5(1):35–43. doi:10.1159/000444254.

Australian Bureau of Statistics. *Health risk factors – diet body mass, blood pressure, physical activity [Data cube]. National Aboriginal and Torres Strait Islander Health Survey 2018–19*. 2019 Online: https://www.abs.gov.au/statistics/people/aboriginal-and-torres-strait-islander-peoples/national-aboriginal-and-torres-strait-islander-health-survey/2018–19 accessed 29 June 2021.

Australian College of Midwives (ACM). *National Midwifery Guidelines for Consultation and Referral*. Vol. 3, no. 2. 2014. Online: http://www.midwives.org.au/shop/new-national-midwifery-guidelines-consultation-and-referral.

Australian Institute of Health and Welfare (AIHW). *Monitoring the Health Impacts of Mandatory Folic Acid and Iodine Fortification*. Cat. no. PHE 208. Canberra: AIHW; 2016.

Barker DJP. *Mothers, Babies and Disease in Later Life*. London: BMJ Publishing Group; 1994.

Bechoff A, Dhuique-Mayer C. Factors influencing micronutrient bioavailability in biofortified crops. *Ann N Y Acad Sci*. 2017; 1390(1):74–87.

Bell R, Cronje J. Anaesthetic management of the obese parturient. In: Richens Y, Lavender T, eds. *Care for Pregnant Women who are Obese*. London, UK: Quay Books; 2010:133–139.

Brownell K, Puhl R, Schwartz M, et al. *Weight Bias*. New York: Guildford Press; 2005.

Brown W, Heesch K, Miller Y. Life Events and Changing Physical Activity Patterns in Women at Different Life Stages. *Annals of Behavioural Medicine*. 2009;37:294–305. doi:10.1007/s12160-009-9099-2.

Cardwell MS. Eating disorders during pregnancy. *Obstet Gynecol Surv*. 2013;68(4):312–323.

Catalano P, Shankar K. Obesity and pregnancy: mechanisms of short term and long term adverse consequences for mother and child. *BMJ*. 2017;356. doi: 10.1136/bmj.j1.

Chin JR, Henry E, Holmgren CM, et al. Maternal obesity and contraction strength in the first stage of labour. *Am J Obstet Gynecol*. 2012;207(2):129.e1–129.e6.

Craig A, Dotters-Katz S, Kuller J, et al. Listeriosis in Pregnancy: A Review. *Obstet Gynecol Surv*. 2019;74(6):362–368.

Cunningham CE, Teale GR. A profile of body mass index in a large rural Victorian obstetric cohort. *Med J Aust*. 2013;198(1): 39–42.

Dennedy MC, Avalos G, O'Reilly MW, et al. The impact of maternal obesity on gestational outcomes. *Ir Med J*. 2012;105(Suppl 5): 23–25.

Department of Health, Australian Government, 2021, Guidelines for Physical Activity During Pregnancy, online: https://www.health.gov.au/resources/publications/physical-activity-and-exercise-during-pregnancy-guidelines-brochure

Department of Health Clinical Practice Guidelines: *Pregnancy Care 2020* Online: http://www.health.gov.au/antenatal.

De-Regil LM, Peña-Rosas JP, Fernández-Gaxiola AC, et al. Effects and safety of periconceptional folate supplementation for preventing birth defects. *Cochrane Database Syst Rev*. 2015;(12): CD007950, doi:10.1002/14651858.CD007950.pub3.

Ehrenberg HM, Wissler RN. Special concerns for the obese patient. In: Powrie RO, Greene MF, Camann W, eds. *de Swiet's Medical Disorders in Obstetric Practice*. 5th ed. Oxford, UK: Wiley-Blackwell; 2010:615–620 (Ch. 27). doi:10.1002/9781444323016.

Evenson R, Mottola M, Owe K, Rousham E, Brown W. Summary of International Guidelines for Physical Activity Following Pregnancy. *Obstet Gynaecol Surv*. 2015;69(7):407–414. doi:10.1097/OGX.0000000000000077.

Finkelstein J, Fothergill A, Krisher J, et al. Maternal vitamin B12 deficiency and perinatal outcomes in southern India 2021. *PLoS ONE*. doi:10.1371/journal.pone.0248145.

Food Standards Australia New Zealand (FSANZ). *Iodine and pregnancy*. 2016. Online: http://www.foodstandards.govt.nz/consumer/generalissues/pregnancy/Pages/iodineand pregnancy.aspx.

Food Standards Australia New Zealand (FSANZ). *Iodine fortification*. 2019. Online: http://www.foodstandards.govt.nz/consumer/nutrition/iodinefort/Pages/default.aspx.

Ford E, Underwood M, German J. Helping Mom Help Baby: Nutrition-Based Support for the Mother-Infant Dyad During Lactation. *Frontiers in Nutrition*. 2020;7(54) https://dx.doi.org/10.3389%2Ffnut.2020.00054.

Fuber C, McGowan L. A qualitative study of the experiences of women who are obese and pregnant in the UK. *Midwifery*. 2011;27(4):437–444.

Fyfe EM, Anderson NH, North RA, et al. Risk of first-stage and second-stage caesarean delivery by maternal body mass index among nulliparous women in labour at term. *Obstet Gynecol*. 2011;117(6):1315–1322.

Fyfe EM, Thompson JMD, Anderson NH, et al. Maternal obesity and postpartum haemorrhage after vaginal and caesarean delivery among nulliparous women at term: a retrospective cohort study. *BMC Pregnancy Childbirth*. 2012;12:112.

Gluckman P, Beaglehole R. *The health benefits and risks of folic acid fortification of food*. 2018. Online: https://www.pmcsa.org.nz/wp-content/uploads/The-health-benefits-and-risks-of-folic-acid-fortification-of-food.pdf.

Government of South Australia, Department of Health. *Clinical Guideline: Anaemia in Pregnancy. South Australian Perinatal Practice Guidelines*. 2016. Online: http://www.sahealth.sa.gov.au/wps/wcm/connect/33aa3b804ee1d163abb0afd150ce4f37/Anaemia-pregnancy-WCHN-PPG-12052012.pdf?MOD=AJPERES.

Haider BA, Bhutta ZA. Multiple-micronutrient supplementation for women during pregnancy. *Cochrane Database Syst Rev*. 2012;(11):CD004905, doi:10.1002/14651858.CD004905.pub3.

Halldorsson T, Birgisdottir B Brantsaeter A, et al. Old Question Revisited: Are High-Protein Diets Safe in Pregnancy? *Nutrients*. 2021;(13):440. https://www.mdpi.com/2072-6643/13/2/440#.

Heslehurst N, Russell S, Brandon H, et al. Women's perspectives are required to inform the development of maternal obesity services: a qualitative study of obese pregnant women's experiences. *Health Expect*. 2015;18(5):969–981.

Hildingsson I, Thomas J. Perinatal outcomes and satisfaction with care in women with high body mass index. *J Midwifery Womens Health*. 2012;57(4):336–344. doi:10.1111/j.1542-2011.2011.00141.x.

Institute of Medicine (IOM), National Research Council (NRC). *Weight Gain During Pregnancy: Reexamining the Guidelines*. Washington, DC: National Academies Press; 2009.

Iqbal S, Ali I. *Effect of maternal zinc supplementation or zinc status of pregnancy complications and perinatal outcomes: An umbrella review of meta-analyses 2021*. doi.org/10.1016/j.heliyon.2021.e07540.

Johnson J, Clifton RG, Roberts JM, et al. Pregnancy outcomes with weight gain above or below the 2009 Institute of Medicine guidelines. *Obstet Gynecol*. 2013;121(5):969–975.

Lillycrop K, Burdge G. Maternal diet as a modifier of offspring epigenetics. *J Dev Orig Health Dis*. 2015;6(2):88–95. doi:10.1017/S2040174415000124.

Liu P, Xu L, Wang Y, et al. Association between perinatal outcomes and maternal pre-pregnancy body mass index. *Obes Rev*. 2016; 17(11):1091–1102.
Mace HS, Paech MJ, McDonell NJ. Obesity and obstetric anaesthesia. *Anaesth Intensive Care*. 2011;39(4):559–570.
Maia S, Souza A, Caminha M, et al. Vitamin A and Pregnancy: a Narrative Review. *Nutrients*. 2019;11(3):681. doi:10.3390/nu11030681.
McGlone A, Davies S. Perspectives on risk and obesity: towards a 'tolerable risk' approach? *Br J Midwifery*. 2012;20(1):13–17.
McIntyre DH, Gibbons KS, Flenady VJ, et al. Overweight and obesity in Australian mothers: epidemic or endemic? *Med J Aust*. 2012;196(3):184–188.
Magann EF, Doherty DA, Sandlin AT, et al. The effects of an increasing gradient of maternal obesity on pregnancy outcomes. *Aust N Z J Obstet Gynaecol*. 2013;53:250–257.
Marshall NE, Guild C, Cheng YW, et al. Maternal superobesity and perinatal outcomes. *Am J Obstet Gynecol*. 2012;206(5):417.e1–417.e6.
Martin JE, Hure AJ, Macdonald-Wicks L, et al. Predictors of postpartum weight retention in a prospective longitudinal study. *Matern Child Nutr*. 2014;10(4):496–509.
Mills AE, Schmied VA, Dahlen HG. 'Get alongside us', women's experiences of being overweight and pregnant in Sydney, Australia. *Matern Child Nutr*. 2013;9:309–321.
Milman N. Iron in pregnancy—how do we secure an appropriate iron status in the mother and child? *Ann Nutr Metab*. 2011; 59(1):50–54.
Milman N. Oral iron prophylaxis in pregnancy: not too little and not too much! *J Pregnancy*. 2012;2012:514345. doi:10.1155/2012/514345.
Milman N, Paszkowski T, Cetin I, et al. Supplementation during pregnancy: beliefs and science. *Gynecol Endocrinol*. 2016; 32(7):509–516.
Ministry for Primary Industries/*Manatū Ahu Matua. Fortification of flour with the B vitamin folic acid*. 2021 Online: https://www.mpi.govt.nz/food-business/bakery-and-grain-based-products/folic-acid-fortification-of-bread/.
Ministry of Health (MOH). *Section 88 Primary Maternity Services Notice 2007*. 2007, updated 2015, 2017 2019, 2020. Online: http://www.health.govt.nz/publication/section-88-primary-maternity-services-notice-2007.
Ministry of Health (MOH). *Supplement (Tablet) to Take When Pregnant and Breastfeeding*. 2010. Online: http://www.health.govt.nz/our-work/life-stages/maternity-services/supplement-tablet-take-when-pregnant-or-breastfeeding.
Ministry of Health (MOH). *Understanding Excess Body Weight: New Zealand Health Survey*. 2015. Online: http://www.health.govt.nz/publication/understanding-excess-body-weight-new-zealand-health-survey.
Ministry of Health (MOH). *Guidance for Healthy Weight Gain in Pregnancy*. 2014, updated 2016. Online: http://www.health.govt.nz/publication/guidance-healthy-weight-gain-pregnancy.
Ministry of Health (MOH). *Eating and Activity Guidelines for New Zealand Adults: Updated 2020*. 2020a. Wellington: Ministry of Health. Online: https://www.health.govt.nz/system/files/documents/publications/eating-activity-guidelines-new-zealand-adults-updated-2020-jul21.pdf.
Ministry of Health (MOH). *Biomedical Data Explorer 2014/15: New Zealand Health Survey [Data File]*. 2020b. Online: https://minhealthnz.shinyapps.io/nz-health-survey-2014-15-biomedical/.
Ministry of Health (MOH). *Annual data explorer 2019/20: New Zealand Health Survey [Data File]*. 2020c. Online: https://minhealthnz.shinyapps.io/nz-health-survey-2019-20-annual-data-explorer/.
Ministry of Health (MOH) *Companion Statement on Vitamin D and Sun Exposure in Pregnancy and Infancy in New Zealand: A supplement to the Consensus Statement on Vitamin D and Sun Exposure in New Zealand*. 2020d. Online: https://www.health.govt.nz/system/files/documents/publications/companion-statement-vitamin-d-sun-exposure-pregnancy-infancy-nz-dec20.pdf.
Ministry of Health (MOH). *Diagnosis and Treatment of Hypertension and Pre-eclampsia in Pregnancy in New Zealand: A clinical practice guideline*. 2022.
Ministry of Health (MOH). *Guidelines for Consultation With Obstetric and Related Medical Services (Referral Guidelines)*. 2022.
Molinaro A, Fan WQ. Does an elevated BMI in breastfeeding mothers influence the success of breastfeeding at 8 weeks of age compared to non-obese mothers? *J Paediatr Child Health*. 2015;51(S1):139–148.
Mørkved S, Bø K. Effect of pelvic floor muscle training during pregnancy and after childbirth on prevention and treatment of urinary incontinence: a systematic review. *Br J Sports Med*. 2014;48(4):299–310. doi:10.1136/bjsports-2012-091758.
Mottola M, Exercise in the postpartum period: Practical Applications. *Current Sports Medicine Reports*. 2003:362–368. doi:10.1007/s11932-002-0049-
Mottola M, Davenport M, Ruchat S, et al. Canadian guideline for physical activity throughout pregnancy. *Br J Sports Med*. 2018;52:1339–1346. doi:10.1136bjsports-2018-100056.
National Health and Medical Research Council of Australia (NHMRC). *Australian Dietary Guidelines*. Canberra: NHMRC; 2013.
Oteng-Ntim E, Varma R, Croker H, et al. Lifestyle interventions for overweight and obese pregnant women to improve pregnancy outcome: systematic review and meta-analysis. *BMC Med*. 2012;10(1):47.
Pawlak R, Parrott SJ, Raj S, et al. How prevalent is vitamin B12 deficiency among vegetarians? *Nutr Rev*. 2013;71(2):110–117.
Prather H, Spitznagle T, Hunt D. Benefits of exercise during pregnancy. *PM R*. 2012;4(11):845–850.
Pritchett R, Daley A, Jolly K. Does aerobic exercise reduce postpartum depressive symptoms? A systematic review and meta-analysis. *British Journal of General Practice*. 2017;67(663):e684–e691.
Rashid S, Meier V, Patrick H. Review of Vitamin B_{12} deficiency in pregnancy: a diagnosis not to miss as veganism and vegetarianism become more prevalent. *Eur J Haematol*. 2021;106: 450–455. doi:10.1111/ejh.13571.
Rauff EL, Downs DS. Mediating effects of body image satisfaction on exercise behaviour, depressive symptoms, and gestational weight gain in pregnancy. *Ann Behav Med*. 2011;42(3):381–390.
Royal Australian and New Zealand College of Obstetricians and Gynaecologists (RANZCOG). *Management of Obesity During Pregnancy: College Statement*. C-Obs 49. 2013, reviewed 2017. Online: https://www.ranzcog.edu.au/RANZCOG_SITE/media/RANZCOG-MEDIA/Women%27s%20Health/Statement%20and%20guidelines/Clinical-Obstetrics/Management-of-obesity-(C-Obs-49)-Review-March-2017.pdf?ext=.pdf.
Royal Australian and New Zealand College of Obstetricians and Gynaecologists (RANZCOG). *Exercise during pregnancy*. 2016. Online: https://ranzcog.edu.au/RANZCOG_SITE/media/RANZCOG-MEDIA/Women%27s%20Health/Statement%20and%20guidelines/Clinical-Obstetrics/Exercise-during-pregnancy-(C-Obs-62).pdf?ext=.pdf.
Royal Australian and New Zealand College of Obstetricians and Gynaecologists (RANZCOG). *Exercise during pregnancy guidance*. C-Obs 62. 2020. Online: https://ranzcog.edu.au/statements-guidelines2020.
Siega-Riz AM, Viswanathan M, Moos MK, et al. A systematic review of outcomes of maternal weight gain according to

the Institute of Medicine recommendations: birthweight, fetal growth, and postpartum weight retention. *Am J Obstet Gynecol.* 2009;201(4):339.e1–14, doi: 10.1016/j.ajog.2009.07.002.

Siega-Riz AM, Deierlein A, Stuebe A. Implementation of the new Institute of Medicine gestational weight gain guidelines. *J Midwifery Womens Health.* 2010;55(6):512–519.

Singata M, Tranmer J, Gyte GML. Restricting oral fluid and food intake during labour. *Cochrane Database Syst Rev.* 2010;(1): CD003930, doi:10.1002/14651858.CD003930.pub2.

Singata M, Tranmer J, Gyte GML. Restricting oral fluid and food intake during labour. *Cochrane Database Syst Rev.* 2013;(8): CD003930, doi:10.1002/14651858.CD003930.pub3.

Sivakumaran L, Huffman S, Sivakumaran S. *The Concise New Zealand Food Composition Tables.* 11th ed. Palmerston North, NZ: New Zealand Institute for Plant and Food Research Limited and Ministry of Health; 2014.

Stoffel N, Cercamondi C, Brittenhan G, et al. Iron Absorption from oral iron supplements given on consecutive versus alternate days and as single morning doses versus twice-daily split dosing in iron depleted women: two open-label, randomized controlled trials. *The Lancet Haematology.* 2017. doi:10.1016/S2352-3026(17)30182-5.

Tipton AM, Cohen SA, Chelmow D. Wound infection in the obese pregnant woman. *Semin Perinatol.* 2011;35(6):345–349. doi:10.1053/j.semperi.2011.05.020.

Toloza F, Motahari H, Maraka S, Consequences of severe iodine deficiency in pregnancy: evidence in humans. *Frontiers in Endocrinology.* 2020;11:409 doi:10.3389/fendo.2020.00409.

Torgerson P, Mastroiacovo P. The global burden of congenital toxoplasmosis: a systematic review. *Bulletin of the World Health Organization.* 2013;91:501–508.

Valentine CJ, Wagner CL. Nutritional management of the breast-feeding dyad. *Pediatr Clin North Am.* 2013;60(1):261–274.

Wagner CL, Taylor SN, Dawodu A, et al. Vitamin D and its role during pregnancy in attaining optimal health of mother and fetus. *Nutrients.* 2012;4(3):208–230.

Wang ZP, Shang XX, Zhao ZT. Low maternal vitamin B(12) is a risk factor for neural tube defects: a meta-analysis. *J Matern Fetal Neonatal Med.* 2012;25(4):389–394.

World Health Organization (WHO). *Guideline Obesity: Preventing and Managing the Global Epidemic. Report of a WHO Consultation. WHO Technical Report Series 894.* Geneva: WHO; 2000. Online: http://www.who.int/nutrition/publications/obesity/WHO_TRS_894/en/.

World Health Organization (WHO). *Global action plan on physical activity 2018–2030: more active people for a healthier world.* 2018. Online: https://apps.who.int/iris/bitstream/handle/10665/272722/9789241514187-eng.pdf?sequence=1&isAllowed=y.

Further reading

Goonewardene M, Shehata M, Hamad A. Anaemia in pregnancy. *Best Pract Res Clin Obstet Gynaecol.* 2012;26(1):3–24.

Grant CC, Wall CR, Yates R, et al. Nutrition and Indigenous health in New Zealand. *J Paediatr Child Health.* 2010;46(9): 479–482.

Hilliard AM, Chauhan SP, Zhao Y, et al. Effect of obesity on length of labour in nulliparous women. *Am J Perinatol.* 2012;29(2): 127–132.

Maile MD, Blum JM. The search for an evidence-based method of reducing aspiration anaesthesia and analgesia. *Anesth Analg.* 2012;115(1):5–6, doi:10.1213/ANE.0b013e31824cb90e.

CHAPTER 22

Screening and assessment

Caroline Homer

LEARNING OUTCOMES

Learning outcomes for this chapter are:

1. To explain the concept of screening during pregnancy
2. To discuss the known benefits and disadvantages of screening procedures
3. To describe the common tests, examinations and other procedures offered or recommended to women
4. To discuss the ethical, legal and social dilemmas accompanying the use of innovative medical technologies in antenatal screening
5. To evaluate critically the current screening tests offered to pregnant women and to understand the limitations of current methods as well as the emerging technologies that may change screening in the future
6. To demonstrate an awareness of some of the more contentious areas for screening in pregnancy.

CHAPTER OVERVIEW

Screening is a way of detecting a predisposition for a condition or a disease in people who are considered otherwise healthy and without any signs of the condition that is screened for. It can involve specific tests, or simple questions. A screening test is not a diagnosis or a diagnostic test. It merely brings to our attention someone or a group of women who may be at higher risk of having a disorder or disease. The next step, once a screening test has shown positive results, is for the woman to undertake further tests, which may be more expensive, invasive and time consuming. Screening usually begins early in pregnancy to check whether a woman has any conditions or infections that could affect her or her baby's health but it will also occur at different time points through the pregnancy. There are also screening tests recommended for the baby and these will be discussed later in this text.

It is important always to explain the purpose of any test that is offered or recommended, and women need to decide whether they wish to have any particular test. The information that tests provide may help you and the woman to consider certain pathways or treatments during the antenatal period. The test results will also invariably affect the way women make choices during their pregnancy. If women decline tests that are recommended in evidence-based guidelines, it is important to document this and to ensure that the woman understands any ramifications.

This chapter discusses the screening and assessment techniques currently undertaken in New Zealand and Australia, which form the basis of the assessments made during the antenatal visits as discussed in Chapter 23. The chapter is not intended as a 'cookbook' guide on when and how to advise women about screening. You will be aware of the different screening policies at the national and area healthcare service levels. This chapter is intended to introduce the reader to current debates and information appropriate to practice.

The author of this chapter is Australian and so much of the chapter is from this perspective, recognising that at times the recommendations between Australia and New Zealand differ. Where there is a difference, the New Zealand recommendations are highlighted. In addition, clinical practice recommendations in all countries alter from time to time as new evidence becomes available and as guidelines are updated. It is always important to clarify the current recommendations for your country through your Ministry of Health or professional college.

KEY TERMS

asymptomatic bacterial vaginosis
asymptomatic bacteriuria
blood group
Chlamydia trachomatis
diabetes
group B *Streptococcus*
hepatitis B virus (HBV)
hepatitis C virus (HCV)
human immunodeficiency virus (HIV)
preeclampsia

INTRODUCTION: SCREENING GUIDELINES

In Australia and New Zealand there are various sets of evidence-based guidelines prepared and published to guide women and maternity care providers through the maze of screening options available for women during pregnancy.

In Australia, National Clinical Practice Guidelines for Pregnancy Care have been developed by the Australian Government in collaboration with state and territory governments (Australian Government Department of Health, 2020). The guidelines are designed to support Australian maternity services to provide high-quality, evidence-based antenatal care to healthy pregnant women. The recommendations cover a wide range of care including routine physical examinations, screening tests and social and lifestyle advice for women with an uncomplicated pregnancy. The full guidelines can be accessed on the Australian Government Department of Health website at http://www.health.gov.au/.

In New Zealand, the Ministry of Health has developed national clinical guidance for the maternity sector. The guidance has targeted specific topics that have been identified as areas of variability within the sector. The topic relevant to this chapter is related to the screening for gestational diabetes (Ministry of Health, 2014a).

The National Screening Unit provides another source of screening guidance for women in New Zealand. In relation to pregnancy there is guidance on screening for HIV in pregnancy and antenatal screening for Down syndrome and other conditions (Ministry of Health, 2014b). The guidance is mainly targeted for women and families but also provides useful ways of explaining tests for providers. More details are on their website: https://www.nsu.govt.nz/pregnancy-newborn-screening.

In many countries like Australia and New Zealand, guidance from the National Institute for Health and Care Excellence (NICE) in the United Kingdom is often used as a basis for care. The 2021 update of the 2008 guidelines (NICE, 2008) is available on their website—see: https://www.nice.org.uk/guidance/ng201.

The World Health Organization (WHO) has also released their recommendations on antenatal care for a positive pregnancy experience (WHO, 2016). These include a section on screening and assessment including on HIV, anaemia, domestic violence and ultrasound scans. Some of the recommendations are more targeted to low–middle income countries but many have resonance for countries such as Australia and New Zealand.

In all the guidelines, it is recommended that women seek care early in pregnancy to ensure a comprehensive assessment is made according to the best available evidence. With the new tests available for screening for chromosomal abnormalities, having the first antenatal visit before 10 weeks is advisable (NICE, 2008). This means that women have time to receive information on their options and make decisions about screening tests.

SCREENING TESTS

A good screening test should be able to discriminate clearly between those who are at high risk and those who are not. It should be safe, have a reasonably defined cut-off level, and be both valid and reliable. Although these latter two terms are often used interchangeably, they are distinct. *Validity* is the ability of a test to measure what it sets out to measure, usually differentiating between those with and those without the disease. In contrast, *reliability* indicates repeatability (Grimes & Schulz, 2002, p. 882); it refers to a method of measurement that consistently gives the same results (NICE, 2008).

However, being labelled as at 'high risk' is useful only if something can be done to alter or decrease the risk. In addition, risk factors are not things that cause an outcome—they are only markers of a particular situation, and serve to alert the midwife to the fact that diagnostic tests might be required to ascertain whether or not the woman has a certain condition. This leads us to our first ethical dilemma.

Screening differs from the traditional clinical use of tests in several important ways. When we believe there is something wrong with us, it prompts us to consult an expert (perhaps a doctor) about the complaint or problem, and this in turn prompts testing to confirm or exclude a diagnosis. By contrast, screening engages apparently healthy women who are not seeking medical help (and might prefer to be left alone). In addition, the occurrence of false-positive results and true-positive results may lead to unnecessary interventions. Although the anxiety induced by a correct diagnosis may be overwhelming, those incorrectly thought to have a problem suffer as well. For example, although failing to diagnose sexually transmitted diseases can have important health implications, incorrectly labelling people as infected can affect relationships and damage lives (Grimes & Schulz, 2002).

Assessing the effectiveness of a test

There are four indices of the validity of a test: sensitivity, specificity, and predictive values of positive and negative.

Sensitivity

Sensitivity is sometimes termed the 'detection rate'. It describes the ability of a test to find those with the disease (Grimes & Schulz, 2002). In diagnostic testing, sensitivity refers to the chance of having a positive test result given that you have the disease. A 100% sensitivity means that all those with the disease will test positive, but this is not the same the other way around. A woman could have a positive test result but not have the disease—this is called a 'false positive'. The sensitivity of a test is also related to its 'negative predictive value' (true negatives); a test with a sensitivity of 100% means that all those who get a negative test result do not have the disease. To judge fully the accuracy of a test, its specificity must also be considered (NICE, 2008).

Specificity

Specificity denotes the ability of a test to identify those without the condition (Grimes & Schulz, 2002). In diagnostic testing, this refers to the chance of having a negative test result given that you do not have the disease. A 100% specificity means that all those without the disease will test negative, but this is not the same the other way around. A woman could have a negative test result yet still have the disease—this is called a 'false negative'. The specificity of a test is also related to its 'positive predictive value' (true positives); a test with a specificity of 100% means that all those who get a positive test result definitely have the disease. To judge fully the accuracy of a test, its sensitivity must also be considered (NICE, 2008).

For the purposes of this chapter, it is important to understand the concepts of sensitivity and specificity broadly so that you understand how screening works in real life. For example, for any continuous outcome measurement (e.g. blood glucose level), the sensitivity and specificity of a test will be inversely related. If we place the cut-off for abnormal blood glucose level at a very low point, thereby producing perfect sensitivity (i.e. we manage to identify all those women with **diabetes**), the low cut-off identifies all those with diabetes. However, the trade-off is poor specificity—that is, those women who also have blood glucose at the level specified but are part of the 'healthy distribution' (i.e. at one end of 'normal') are incorrectly identified as having abnormal values. Placing the cut-off higher yields the opposite result: all those who are healthy are correctly identified (perfect specificity), but the cost here is missing a proportion of women who do have diabetes. Selecting a cut-off point is a compromise, mislabelling some healthy people and some people with diabetes. Where the cut-off should be depends on the implications of the test.

As in other areas of maternity care, there is debate about what constitutes evidence-based screening and what does not. The evidence for screening is not always collected before a test is introduced into practice and this often creates difficulties in undertaking research to build up the evidence base. In addition, there are some healthcare providers and some in the general community who feel that just because a test exists it should be used. This can mean that many women can be subjected to a test that does not have a sufficient evidence base and this can have unintended consequences in terms of overtreatment or unnecessary intervention.

CRITICAL THINKING EXERCISE

Review the recommendations in the Australian National Antenatal Guidelines (Australian Government Department of Health, 2020). Each recommendation is classified as an 'evidence-based recommendation', a 'consensus-based recommendation' or a 'practice point'. The different classifications are because of the strength of evidence behind each one. Find out the definition of each of these different classifications and find an example of a recommendation under each one.

- Why do you think some topics have higher-level evidence than others?
- What does this say about the challenges of obtaining the evidence?

THE FIRST STEP IN EFFECTIVE SCREENING

The first step in screening is to engage the women in a comprehensive first antenatal visit, to talk with her about the pregnancy and what she wants, and her general health, and to identify any factors that may need further consideration. This will involve discussion of previous experiences of labour, birth and the postpartum period. It is also important to ascertain the support network available and the priorities for medical consultation, if this is recommended.

Review of current and past maternity history

At the first visit, talk with the woman about her pregnancy and what she wants in terms of care. At this time you will ascertain the number of pregnancies she has had (gravida) and the number of births (parity). Understanding her past history, including whether she has had miscarriages or abortions, pre-term labour and birth, or has had a stillbirth or a neonatal death, will help guide your discussion about screening.

As in all aspects of midwifery care, ask open-ended questions and provide her with an opportunity to discuss issues and ask questions; discuss the involvement of her partner/family in antenatal care and offer verbal information supported by written or other appropriate form of information (e.g. on topics such as diet and lifestyle, available pregnancy care services, maternity benefits, screening tests, breastfeeding) (Australian Government Department of Health, 2020).

POINTS IN PREGNANCY FOR ASSESSMENT AND TO RECOMMEND OR OFFER SCREENING

For most women in Australia and New Zealand, a schedule of 7–10 antenatal visits will be usual. The World Health Organization recommends that a minimum of eight contacts is recommended to reduce perinatal mortality and improve women's experience of care (WHO, 2016).

First antenatal visit

At the first antenatal visit a number of activities should take place including providing woman-centred and respectful care, undertaking a comprehensive history, doing a general health assessment and providing information and support. Screening is only one component of care. For more detailed description of the holistic approach to care, see the Australian antenatal clinical practice guidelines (Australian Government Department of Health, 2020).

General assessment

At the first antenatal visit it is important to undertake a comprehensive history including discussion around the:

- current pregnancy (planned, unplanned, woman wishes to proceed with/terminate pregnancy)
- medical (past history, medicines, family history, cervical smears, immunisation)
- obstetric (previous experience of pregnancy and birth)
- smoking, nutrition, alcohol, physical activity and drug use
- expectations, partner/family involvement, cultural and spiritual issues, concerns, knowledge, pregnancy, birth, breastfeeding and infant feeding options
- concerns about family violence and other issues at home.

A clinical assessment at this point will:

- discuss the date of last menstrual period and offer ultrasound scan for gestational age assessment to be carried out between 8 and 14 weeks of pregnancy; the practice in New Zealand is to combine this early ultrasound for dating purposes with the nuchal transparency (NT) screening
- measure height and weight and calculate body mass index (BMI)
- measure blood pressure
- test for proteinuria
- ask questions about previous mental health disorders and psychosocial factors that affect mental health
- administer the Edinburgh Postnatal Depression Scale (EPDS) at this visit or as early as practical in pregnancy.

New Zealand practice: mental health screening

In New Zealand, midwives ask about the woman's mental health history and feelings about the pregnancy at the booking visit, as well as reviewing the woman's emotional and social situation during the pregnancy (New Zealand College of Midwives (NZCOM), 2015). The Edinburgh Postnatal Depression Scale was designed as a postnatal assessment tool, and in New Zealand it is not recommended for use as a routine mental health screening tool during pregnancy. Continuity of care under the New Zealand midwifery partnership model supports the development of relationships that provide the forum for discussions about mental health and enables the midwife to identify mental health changes that may occur during pregnancy.

Screening tests recommended and/or offered

The following tests are recommended at the first antenatal visit (Australian Government Department of Health, 2020):

- blood group and antibodies, full blood count and haemoglobin
- HIV, hepatitis B virus and hepatitis C virus, rubella non-immunity, syphilis and asymptomatic bacteriuria (midstream urine (MSU) sample)
- *Chlamydia* testing for women younger than 30
- *Chlamydia* and gonorrhoea testing should be considered for women in areas with a high prevalence of sexually transmitted infections.

Routine testing for vitamin D status is not recommended unless there are specific concerns about the local geographical issues or ethnicity in relation to access to sunlight.

The possibility of chromosomal abnormalities is a concern for many women. Therefore, in the first trimester, all women/couples should be given information about the purpose and implications of testing for chromosomal anomalies to enable them to make informed choices about whether to have any tests. The recommendations from the Australian national antenatal guidelines are to offer screening for chromosomal abnormalities to be carried out between 9 and 14 weeks of pregnancy (Australian Government Department of Health, 2020, p. 54). Women also need to be supported to access testing for chromosomal anomalies in a timely manner, especially those who live in non-metropolitan areas.

Ongoing assessment and screening in antenatal care

Most women in Australia and New Zealand will have 7–10 antenatal visits. The content of each visit will vary slightly depending on the context and individual needs, any concerns raised or identified at the first antenatal visit and local policies.

Although screening and assessments are important at each visit, time should also be made to enable the woman to discuss her expectations and experiences as well as raise any issues and/or concerns that may have arisen since her last visit. The provision of psychosocial support is essential at every antenatal visit. Information should be provided to women on general health issues including nutrition, alcohol, smoking, symptom relief if conditions common in pregnancy are being experienced, breastfeeding and reducing the risk of sudden unexpected death in infancy (SUDI). The role of antenatal care is also to build the woman's confidence in her ability to give birth and look after her new baby. Engaging with the woman's partner and support network is important, especially if they will be with her during her labour and birth and the early weeks after the baby is born.

Information sharing should be tailored for her needs. Many women like written information but other forms such as internet resources or videos may be more appropriate. Time should be made for the woman to direct the type of issues and questions she wants discussed.

Box 22.1 is adapted from NICE (2008) and the Australian Antenatal Clinical Practice Guidelines (Australian Government Department of Health, 2020) and provides an overview of the typical trajectory of assessment and screening.

Box 22.1 Additional specific activities at subsequent antenatal visits

16–19 weeks

- Review, discuss and record the results of all tests undertaken.
- Reassess planned pattern of care for the pregnancy and identify whether additional care or referral is needed.
- Assess fetal growth.
- Offer fetal anatomy scan to be carried out at 18–20 weeks gestation.
- Offer women the opportunity to be weighed, encourage self-monitoring of weight gain and discuss weight change, diet and level of physical activity.

20–27 weeks

- Assess fetal growth.
- Discuss fetal movements, including the need for prompt contact with a health professional if there are any concerns about reduced or absent movements.
- Measure blood pressure.
- Test for proteinuria in women who have clinical indications of preeclampsia (e.g. high blood pressure). In New Zealand, the practice is to test for proteinuria with a dipstick, and send sample for protein:creatinine ratio (PCR) if 1+ protein or more.
- Offer women the opportunity to be weighed, encourage self-monitoring of weight gain and discuss weight change, diet and level of physical activity.
- Test for hyperglycaemia between 24 and 28 weeks gestation.
- Repeat ferritin testing if levels were identified as low in the first trimester.

28 weeks

- Assess fetal growth.
- Discuss fetal movements, including the need for prompt contact with a health professional if there are any concerns about reduced or absent movements.
- Test for anaemia, blood group and antibodies.
- Recommend anti-D to Rhesus-negative non-isoimmunised women (Australia only).
- Measure blood pressure.
- Test for proteinuria in women who have clinical indications of preeclampsia (e.g. high blood pressure). In New Zealand, the practice is to test for proteinuria with a dipstick, and send sample for protein:creatinine ratio (PCR) if 1+ protein or more.
- Offer women the opportunity to be weighed, encourage self-monitoring of weight gain and discuss weight change, diet and level of physical activity.
- Test for hyperglycaemia if this has not already been tested.
- Enquire about mental health and administer the EPDS.

29–34 weeks

- Assess fetal growth.
- Discuss fetal movements, including the need for prompt contact with a health professional if there are any concerns about reduced or absent movements.
- Review, discuss and record the results of tests undertaken at 28 weeks.
- Reassess planned pattern of care for the pregnancy and identify women who need additional care, arranging referral if required.
- Give information, with an opportunity to discuss issues and ask questions on preparation for labour and birth, including the birth plan, recognising active labour and positively managing the pain of normal labour (this may need to take place earlier in remote areas).
- Discuss breastfeeding (e.g. skin-to-skin contact at birth, early feeding, rooming-in, attachment, exclusive breastfeeding, feeding on demand, partner support); discuss safe infant formula feeding if a woman chooses to formula feed.
- Measure blood pressure.
- Test for proteinuria in women who have clinical indications of preeclampsia (e.g. high blood pressure). In New Zealand, the practice is to test for proteinuria with a dipstick, and send sample for protein:creatinine ratio (PCR) if 1+ protein or more.
- Offer women the opportunity to be weighed, encourage self-monitoring of weight gain and discuss weight change, diet and level of physical activity.
- Offer repeat ultrasound at 32 weeks to women whose placenta extended over the internal cervical os (the opening of the cervix into the vagina) in the 18–20-week scan.
- Recommend a second dose of anti-D to Rhesus-negative non-isoimmunised women at 34 weeks (Australia only).

35–7 weeks

- Assess fetal growth.
- Discuss fetal movements, including the need for prompt contact with a health professional if there are any concerns about reduced or absent movements.
- Give information, including care of the new baby, reducing risk of sudden and unexpected death in infancy (SUDI), newborn screening tests and vitamin K prophylaxis, psychosocial support available in the postnatal period including maternal and child health services and psychosocial supports, with an opportunity to discuss issues and ask questions.
- Assess fetal presentation by abdominal palpation from 36 weeks and confirm suspected malpresentation by ultrasound.
- For women whose babies are not a cephalic presentation, discuss a range of options, including external cephalic version for breech presentation.

Box 22.1 Additional specific activities at subsequent antenatal visits—cont'd

- Offer testing for group B *Streptococcus* if organisational policy is to test all women routinely.
- Measure blood pressure.
- Test for proteinuria in women who have clinical indications of or risk factors for preeclampsia (e.g. high blood pressure). In New Zealand, the practice is to test for proteinuria with a dipstick, and send sample for protein:creatinine ratio (PCR) if 1+ protein or more.
- Offer women the opportunity to be weighed, encourage self-monitoring of weight gain and discuss weight change, diet and level of physical activity.

38–40 weeks

- Assess fetal growth.
- Give information, including normal length of pregnancy, onset of labour, with an opportunity to discuss any fears and worries and ask questions.
- Discuss fetal movements, including the need for prompt contact with a health professional if there are any concerns about reduced or absent movements.
- Measure blood pressure.
- Test for proteinuria in women who have clinical indications of preeclampsia (e.g. high blood pressure). In New Zealand, the practice is to test for proteinuria with a dipstick, and send sample for protein:creatinine ratio (PCR) if 1+ protein or more.
- Offer women the opportunity to be weighed, encourage self-monitoring of weight gain and discuss weight change, diet and level of physical activity.

Women who have not given birth by 41 weeks

- Give information, including discussion about options for prolonged pregnancy (e.g. membrane sweeping), with an opportunity to discuss issues and ask questions.
- Discuss fetal movements, including the need for prompt contact with a health professional if there are any concerns about reduced or absent movements.
- Measure blood pressure.
- Test for proteinuria in women who have clinical indications of preeclampsia (e.g. high blood pressure). In New Zealand, the practice is to test for proteinuria with a dipstick, and send sample for protein:creatinine ratio (PCR) if 1+ protein or more.
- Offer women the opportunity to be weighed, encourage self-monitoring of weight gain and discuss weight change, diet and level of physical activity.

(Source: Australian Government Department of Health (2020) Clinical Practice Guidelines: Pregnancy Care. Canberra: Department of Health.)

COMMON SCREENING TESTS OFFERED TO WOMEN DURING PREGNANCY

Assessing gestational age

Accurate knowledge of gestational age is valuable for pregnancy care. Pregnancies can be dated based on last menstrual period (LMP) or ultrasound, with evidence demonstrating that ultrasound is superior. Over the years there have been concerns raised about the side effects of ultrasound especially as they become more common and frequent. The most recent study specifically examining this issue found no clear association between ultrasound scanning and intellectual performance (Kieler et al., 2005). Nevertheless, ultrasound is a technology and carries costs and so should be used only when clinically indicated. In Australia, it is recommended that women should be offered an early ultrasound scan to determine gestational age, detect multiple pregnancies and accurately time fetal anomaly screening. This will ensure consistency of gestational age assessments and reduce the need for induction of labour after 41 weeks (Australian Government Department of Health, 2020). Ideally, this early scan should be performed between 8 weeks 0 days and 13 weeks 6 days.

New Zealand practice: ultrasound for gestational age

In New Zealand, a routine first-trimester scan is not justified if dating is the sole (or major) reason for the scan, as an NT scan (undertaken between 11 weeks and 13+6 for first-trimester fetal anomaly screening) can give reliable dating information. For women who decline screening for chromosomal anomalies, a dating scan would be appropriate in place of the NT scan. If a woman declines all pregnancy ultrasounds, estimation of gestational age is calculated by LMP and clinical assessments.

Screening for chromosomal anomalies

There is an increasing number of biochemical tests and ultrasound techniques that are now able to identify those pregnant women who have a higher chance of chromosomal anomalies such as trisomy 21 (Down syndrome), trisomy 18 (Edwards syndrome) and trisomy 13 (Patau syndrome). Some of these conditions are not compatible with live birth; some are associated with long-term and serious morbidity (Australian Government Department of Health, 2020).

In the first trimester, all women should receive appropriate written information concerning screening including the purpose and implications of testing for chromosomal anomalies so as to enable them to make informed choices about whether to have the tests (Australian Government Department of Health, 2020).

In Australia and New Zealand, many women choose to have the combined test, which includes:

- maternal serum testing of pregnancy-associated placental protein-A (PAPP-A) and free beta human chorionic gonadotrophin (β-hCG)
- ultrasound measurement of fetal nuchal translucency thickness.

The blood for biochemical analysis should be collected between 9 weeks and 13 weeks 6 days gestation, and ultrasound assessment should take place between 11 weeks and 13 weeks 6 days gestation.

Women should be notified of their screening result, irrespective of the risk, in a format that they understand. Those women with an increased risk of chromosomal anomaly should be offered further counselling and diagnostic testing within 72 hours or as soon as possible.

For women who are greater than 14 weeks gestation, second-trimester maternal serum screening may be offered, which involves a blood test taken between 14 and 20 weeks.

The New Zealand National Screening Unit has some excellent resources and frequency asked questions for women that will be useful for midwives (https://www.nsu.govt.nz/).

New non-invasive screening tests

As a replacement for the combined first-trimester testing, a new test known as cfDNA testing or non-invasive prenatal testing (NIPT) is starting to be offered in Australia and New Zealand although it is not covered under public or private health insurance. The test involves sequencing DNA fragments in the women's serum, mapping each DNA sequence to a reference genome to determine its chromosome of origin, and counting the number of fragments arising from each chromosome. If the fetus is affected by trisomy, a greater than expected number of the relevant chromosome will be present in maternal serum (Australian Government Department of Health, 2020). The test can be conducted from 10 weeks gestation onwards.

The test is a screening not a diagnostic test. Women also need to be informed that, although it may have a higher detection rate for common chromosomal abnormalities than the combined tests described above, it may not detect other, less common chromosomal abnormalities.

Diagnosis of chromosomal anomalies

Screening tests provide women with the estimated probability of having a baby with a chromosomal abnormality. For those who have an increased chance, ongoing diagnostic testing is offered. Diagnostic tests are based on chromosomal analysis of cells collected using:

- chorionic villus sampling (CVS) (tissue from the villi of the chorion [part of the placenta])—testing takes place any time after 11 weeks pregnancy, or
- amniocentesis (to sample fetal skin cells in the amniotic fluid)—testing takes place after 15 weeks pregnancy.

The results of the test are not immediate as the cells need to be cultured. The results can sometimes be available in 3 days but in some cases can take up to 3 weeks.

How to discuss testing with women

Undertaking a diagnostic test for a chromosomal abnormality can be a very stressful time for a woman and her partner. It is therefore important to explain (Australian Government Department of Health, 2020):

- the anomalies that may be diagnosed
- the available tests, the gestational stage at which they should be undertaken, the process of the procedure and the risks involved
- the possibility that the procedure may not be successful or the result may not accurately reflect the fetal status
- the possibility of other fetal anomalies that are not identified by the test
- the time frame for receiving results and making further decisions if necessary
- options to consider if a chromosomal anomaly is identified (e.g. continuation of the pregnancy or termination where this is permitted under jurisdictional legislation) and the need for additional care if the pregnancy continues (e.g. specialist management of the pregnancy and the baby)
- long-term implications for the woman and her family of having an affected baby and the health and development issues for children with the condition
- the impact on a woman and her family of a false-negative or false-positive result (e.g. anxiety among women receiving false positives may remain)
- costs involved and how they are to be met.

REFLECTIVE THINKING EXERCISE

Considering the words we use

Consider the antenatal care you have provided recently to a woman. This care may have been in a community-based clinic setting, a hospital clinic or at home. Reflect upon the information you provided to the woman, particularly in relation to your explanation of risks and benefits of different screening tests and especially the words and terminology you used. Reflect upon these questions:

- How effective do you feel you were in explaining the issue?
- How did she respond to your information?
- Did you use any words that could have been more carefully chosen if you could press a rewind button?

Read the article by Nicky Leap (2012) and reflect upon the words we use in antenatal care to convey risks. Are there any other words or expressions you could use in the future?

Write these down and try them out in your next occasion of providing antenatal care.

Indications for genetic counselling

Indications vary for referral to a genetic counsellor, and may include a known or suspected hereditary disease within the family, mother's maternal age more than 35 years for a first baby, paternal age more than 40 years, previous recurrent pregnancy loss (three or more) or an unexplained stillbirth or neonatal death. Consanguinity or a specific ethnic group (e.g. Ashkenazi Jewish for Tay–Sachs disease) requires genetic counselling. Maternal metabolic disorders such as thyroid disease, phenylketonuria or maternal type 1 diabetes may also require referral. Certain ethnic/geographical populations such as African, Southeast Asian and Mediterranean groups have significantly higher rates of haemoglobinopathies and require antepartum screening. Further testing may involve maternal blood tests, ultrasound or invasive sampling (e.g. genetic amniocentesis or CVS) for genetic assays.

SCREENING FOR INFECTIONS

Bacterial

The most common bacterial infections that will be addressed in this section include asymptomatic bacteriuria, asymptomatic bacterial vaginosis, chlamydia, syphilis and group B *Streptococcus*.

Asymptomatic bacteriuria

Asymptomatic bacteriuria is the persistent bacterial colonisation of the urinary tract (usually by *Escherichia coli*) without symptoms. It is common in pregnancy (Australian Government Department of Health, 2020). Detection of all women with asymptomatic bacteriuria is important, as 25%–30% will develop symptomatic urinary tract infection while pregnant and the infection increases the risk of pyelonephritis, premature labour and pre-term rupture of the membranes.

Women should be offered routine screening for asymptomatic bacteriuria by MSU culture early in pregnancy.

Asymptomatic bacterial vaginosis

Asymptomatic bacterial vaginosis results from the relative deficiency of normal *Lactobacillus* species in the vagina and relative overgrowth of anaerobic bacteria. Bacterial vaginosis is asymptomatic for 50% of women in pregnancy (Joesoef & Schmid, 2002) but may result in a vaginal discharge that can be grey in colour with a characteristic 'fishy' odour (Brocklehurst et al., 2013). The condition is associated with an increased risk of pre-term birth. Despite this, routine screening of all pregnant women for bacterial vaginosis is not currently recommended (Australian Government Department of Health, 2020).

Women who report symptoms that are suggestive of bacterial vaginosis should be offered antibiotic treatment. Interestingly however, although antibiotics are effective in eradicating bacterial vaginosis, treatment does not change the risk of pre-term birth, low birth weight or premature rupture of the membranes in women at low risk of pre-term birth (Brocklehurst et al., 2013). For women with a previous pre-term birth, treatment of bacterial vaginosis may reduce the risk of pre-term prelabour rupture of membranes and low birth weight (Brocklehurst et al., 2013; Kieler et al., 2005).

Chlamydia trachomatis

Chlamydia trachomatis is a sexually transmitted infection. It is usually spread by vaginal or anal sex without a condom. The infection has long-term implications for women including chronic pelvic pain, pelvic inflammatory disease, infertility and ectopic pregnancy. There are also implications in pregnancy including pre-term birth and intrauterine growth restriction.

The infection is asymptomatic in at least 70% of women and the majority of infections clear spontaneously without morbidity (Geisler et al., 2008; Rogers et al., 2008). *Chlamydia* is the most common bacterial sexually transmitted infection in Australia and New Zealand. In Australia, the notification rate was relatively stable between 2011 and 2015 but increased by 13% between 2015 and 2017. It is highly prevalent among younger people, with around 80% of all diagnoses being in young people. In Australia, the rates of infection are highest in remote areas (Kirby Institute, 2018).

It is recommended therefore that *Chlamydia* testing should be offered at the first antenatal visit to pregnant women younger than 30 years and to all pregnant women in areas of high prevalence (Australian Government Department of Health, 2020).

Midwifery Practice Scenario

Amira is a midwife working in a midwifery continuity of care program. She is seeing Li, who is pregnant with her first baby. Li is 26 years old and this was a planned pregnancy. She is now 24 weeks pregnant and Amira has seen Li for all her antenatal visits so far. Today Amira needs to discuss the results of her *Chlamydia* screen that was undertaken at the last antenatal visit. Li was screened as the guidelines recommend offering *Chlamydia* testing at the first antenatal visit to pregnant women younger than 30 years. The screening test was positive for *Chlamydia*. Li is shocked as she has not had any symptoms. Amira explains that genital chlamydial infection is asymptomatic in at least 70% of women so it is not surprising that she has not had symptoms.

Amira finds *Chlamydia* to be a difficult issue to discuss as it is a sexually transmitted infection and it means that she needs to discuss possible infection of her current and past sexual partners. Can you reflect upon ways that you as a midwife can discuss sexual partners and behaviours with women?

Li asks whether *Chlamydia* infection during pregnancy is a risk to herself or her baby. If you were Amira, how would you explain the risks during pregnancy? Can you explain the treatment? What further information could you provide for her to take home to talk with her partner about?

Syphilis

Syphilis is a sexually acquired infection caused by *Treponema pallidum*. Syphilis may be asymptomatic and remain latent for many years. The availability of penicillin reduced the prevalence of syphilis significantly, and the disease is not common in most parts of New Zealand or Australia.

Infectious syphilis has significant overwhelming health effects if not treated in pregnancy. These include adverse pregnancy outcomes such as stillbirth and congenital syphilis. In pregnant women with early, untreated syphilis, 70%–100% of infants will be infected and one-third will be stillborn. Congenital syphilis can be fatal at a young age and can also cause permanent impairment, debilitation and disfigurement (Chakraborty & Luck, 2008; Richens & Mabey, 2013).

In Australia, there has been a considerable increase in the notification rate of infectious syphilis from 7.8 per 100,000 in 2013 to 18.3 per 100,000 in 2017 with this increase in both men (119%) and significantly in women (309%) (Kirby Institute, 2018).

It is recommended that all women should be offered testing at the first antenatal visit as treating syphilis benefits both mother and baby (Australian Government Department of Health, 2020). In addition, in Australia repeat testing is recommended early in the third trimester (28–32 weeks) and at the time of birth for women at high risk of infection or reinfection.

Group B Streptococcus

Group B *Streptococcus* (*S. agalactiae*; GBS or GBBS) is a beta-haemolytic, Gram-positive aerobic coccobacillus. It is a common bacterium that can colonise people of all ages without symptoms. It is generally found in the gastrointestinal tract, vagina and urethra. The bacteria can be passed from mother to baby during labour and lead to infection in the first week of life (early onset infection). Late-onset infection can develop up to 3 months of age (Phares et al., 2008). Prevention focuses on addressing early-onset disease in newborns, which is the most common cause of serious infection in newborn babies (Centers for Disease Control and Prevention, 2010).

Early-onset GBS infection (EOGBS) in neonates usually occurs within the first 24 hours after birth, although it is defined as that occurring within the first 7 days. Late-onset GBS infection occurs from 7 days until 3 months of age, and is less aggressive.

EOGBS infection is acquired by vertical transmission from mother to baby (Clifford et al., 2011). In colonised women, the intensity of colonisation is directly related to the risk of transmission to the neonate (Gilbert, 2003). GBS bacteriuria reflects heavy colonisation (Heath, 2007) and increases the risk of GBS disease in the neonate (Oddie & Embleton, on behalf of the Northern Neonatal Network, 2002). Early neonatal colonisation risk is increased if there has been prolonged rupture of membranes (>18 hours), maternal intrapartum pyrexia, chorioamnionitis or a previous infant with GBS infection, low birth weight or prematurity (<37 weeks) (Oddie & Embleton, on behalf of the Northern Neonatal Network, 2002). Although approximately 70% of cases of EOGBSD are in term babies (≥37 weeks gestation), mortality case-fatality rates of approximately 20% have been documented in pre-term infants, compared with 2%–3% in term infants (Phares et al., 2008; Schrag et al., 2000). In a population-based study in the United States, the mortality rate for pre-term infants with EOGBSD was 23%, highlighting the risks for this group (Centers for Disease Control and Prevention (CDC), 2005).

The highest incidence of the disease is in young infants and it is a significant cause of morbidity and mortality in newborns (CDC, 2010). About 1%–2% of infants born to GBS-colonised mothers will develop early-onset infection. In this group there is a 6% fatal outcome, which is higher in pre-term infants.

Screening options

There are two approaches to screening to reduce the incidence of GBS infection in neonates: (1) a risk factor-based approach, and (2) a routine antenatal culture-based approach. The approach varies across Australia and New Zealand and both approaches have benefits and risks. Each organisation should decide on one approach and high rates of adherence to the chosen approach (Australian Government Department of Health, 2020; Homer et al., 2014).

A risk factor-based approach. Women are assessed for risk factors which increase the risk of neonatal EOGBS sepsis. The risk factors include:

- previous GBS-affected infant
- GBS bacteriuria at any time during the current pregnancy
- pre-term (<37+0 weeks) in established labour
- maternal intrapartum pyrexia ≥38°C
- signs and symptoms of suspected chorioamnionitis
- rupture of membranes ≥18 hours.

If any of these risk factors are present, intravenous antibiotics are recommended in labour.

Routine antenatal culture-based approach. All pregnant women between 35+0 and 37+0 weeks gestation are recommended to self-collect either a combined low vaginal–perianal or a combined vaginal–rectal swab.

If a woman has had a previous baby diagnosed with GBS sepsis or she has been confirmed as having GBS bacteriuria in her current pregnancy, further antenatal screening is not required, but intravenous antibiotics are indicated. Women booked for an elective caesarean section still require routine antenatal GBS screening. Women who have a history of GBS colonisation in a previous pregnancy should not be assumed to be positive in the current pregnancy and should be tested in the current pregnancy.

Women who are positive in the routine antenatal screen for GBS colonisation (within 3–5 weeks prior to birth) should be informed of their status and receive the recommended intravenous antibiotics to minimise the risk of sepsis in their neonates.

Women who are negative in the routine antenatal screen for GBS colonisation in their current pregnancy do not require intravenous antibiotics for GBS.

CRITICAL THINKING EXERCISE

1. Find out the GBS screening approach used in your country/context/health area.
2. What can you see are the benefits and risks of the approach selected in your area?
3. Write down three things that you will say to women about GBS infection, screening and the benefits and risks.
4. Practise this with a colleague and try to improve the 'script' you provide to women.

Viral infections

The most common viral infections that will be addressed in this section include cytomegalovirus, hepatitis B and C, HIV, herpes, toxoplasmosis and rubella. Table 22.1 gives an overview of the common infections and the mode and rate of transmission.

Cytomegalovirus (CMV)

Cytomegalovirus (CMV) is a member of the herpes virus family. Most people who acquire the virus after birth experience few or no symptoms. CMV remains latent in the host after primary infection and may become active again, particularly during times of compromised immunity including pregnancy (Australian Government Department of Health, 2020).

Table 22.1 Intrauterine viral transmission

Virus	Mode/rate of transmission
Cytomegalovirus (CMV)—a member of the herpes virus family.	Prenatal infection affects 1%–2% of live births. Virus replicates in the uterus, infects the placenta, and then is transmitted to the fetus. Transmission rate is approx. 50% in women with primary infection. It remains latent in the host after primary infection and may become active again, particularly during times of immune compromise.
Herpes simplex virus (HSV-2)—a virus causing painful sores of the anus or genitals that may lie dormant in nerve tissue. Not to be confused with HSV-1, a virus that causes cold sores.	Infrequent prenatal infection. Transmission occurs primarily at the time of birth (80%) and also possibly through an ascending infection after the membranes rupture.
Human immunodeficiency virus (HIV)—infection with HIV begins with an asymptomatic stage with gradual compromise of immune function, eventually leading to acquired immunodeficiency syndrome (AIDS).	Transmission primarily at the time of birth. Isolated cytotrophoblasts infected in vitro. (The most common way to diagnose HIV infection is by a test for antibodies against HIV-1 and HIV-2. HIV antibodies are detectable in at least 95% of patients within 3 months of infection.)
Hepatitis B virus (HBV)—a virus that affects the liver. It has an incubation period of 6 weeks to 6 months, and is excreted in various bodily fluids including blood, saliva, vaginal fluid and breast milk; these fluids may be highly infectious.	Transmission primarily perinatal. Some intrauterine infection from maternal blood (5%).
Hepatitis C virus (HCV)—a virus known to be one of the major causes of liver cirrhosis, hepatocellular carcinoma and liver failure; HCV is a major public health concern.	Intrauterine infection and at birth (2%–12%).
Human parvovirus B19—a viral infection transmitted from animals. Infection during pregnancy can result in fetal hydrops and death.	Placental infection associated with inflammatory cytokines. Complications in early gestation.
Rubella virus—the pathogenic agent of the disease rubella and the cause of congenital rubella syndrome when infection occurs during the first weeks of pregnancy. Humans are the only known host of this virus.	Placental infection during primary maternal infection. Transmission in first trimester (80%) and second trimester (25%).
Human papillomavirus (HPV)—a viral infection spread through skin-to-skin contact. HPV is a group of more than 100 different viruses. It causes genital warts and plays a causative role in cervical dysplasia and cervical cancer.	Infection via maternal genital secretions at birth.
Varicella zoster virus—a virus in the herpes family that causes chickenpox during childhood and may reactivate later in life to cause shingles in immunosuppressed individuals.	Congenital infection low (2%). Transmission during primary infection in late gestation (25–50%).

(Source: Pereira et al., 2005)

The available evidence does not support routine antenatal CMV screening for all women. The Australian guidelines do recommend testing for cytomegalovirus to women who come into frequent contact with large numbers of very young children (e.g. child care workers), using serology (cytomegalovirus-specific IgG only) and also offering testing for cytomegalovirus to pregnant women if they have symptoms suggestive of cytomegalovirus that are not attributable to another specific infection or when imaging findings suggest fetal infection (Australian Government Department of Health, 2020).

It is important that all pregnant women are given advice about the basic hygiene measures to help reduce the risk of cytomegalovirus infection, including avoiding contact with a child's saliva or urine and hand washing after such exposure.

Hepatitis B virus (HBV)

Hepatitis B virus is an acute and chronic communicable disease that causes major liver disease (Australian Government Department of Health, 2020). Infection can be prevented through vaccination. The virus has an incubation period of 6 weeks to 6 months and is excreted in various body fluids including blood, saliva, vaginal fluid and breast milk, which may be highly infectious. Adults who have hepatitis B may have no symptoms. After infection, some people do not clear the virus; they become carriers and may pass on the infection to other people including an unborn baby (Australian Government Department of Health, 2020). The transfer of hepatitis B from mother to child can be prevented by prompt immunoprophylaxis at birth.

It is recommended therefore that all women undergo hepatitis B virus testing at their first antenatal visit as effective postnatal intervention can reduce the risk of mother-to-child transmission (Australian Government Department of Health, 2020).

Hepatitis C virus (HCV)

Hepatitis C virus is a blood-borne virus that is one of the major causes of liver cirrhosis, hepatocellular carcinoma and liver failure (Webster et al., 2015). Perinatal transmission is the main source of hepatitis C in Australian children (Raynes-Greenow et al., 2015). Currently, there is no effective means to prevent the transfer of hepatitis C from mother to child (Dunkelberg et al., 2014).

Recently, new treatments have emerged for hepatitis C (known as direct-acting antiviral agents) that can clear the infection and essentially cure the disease. These have not been tested in pregnancy as yet, or in breastfeeding (Aebi-Popp et al., 2016; Rac & Sheffield, 2014), however, women who are diagnosed with hepatitis C in pregnancy may choose to start such treatments soon after the birth of the baby. Therefore, it is now recommended that all women be offered testing for hepatitis C at the first antenatal visit (Australian Government Department of Health, 2020). Hepatitis C screening is not undertaken as part of routine pregnancy blood tests in New Zealand. A risk-based approach to hepatitis C screening is taken.

Human immunodeficiency virus (HIV)

Human immunodeficiency virus (HIV) is a blood-borne infection that is initially asymptomatic but involves gradual compromise of immune function, eventually leading to acquired immunodeficiency syndrome (AIDS). Undiagnosed HIV infection during pregnancy has serious implications for the health of both the woman and her child. Early HIV diagnosis can reduce the risk of mother-to-child transmission and the rate of disease progression in the mother (Siegfried et al., 2011).

There are a number of interventions that can prevent or reduce mother-to-child transmission of HIV (Siegfried et al., 2011). These interventions may also address immediate and ongoing health issues for the mother. Therefore, it is recommended that all women should be offered HIV testing at the first antenatal visit (Australian Government Department of Health, 2020; Ministry of Health, 2014b).

Rubella

Rubella, also known as German measles, is an infection caused by the rubella virus. It is usually a mild self-limiting disease with few complications. If pregnant women contract rubella during the first trimester, however, it can affect the pregnancy and lead to congenital rubella syndrome at birth. There is no treatment to prevent or reduce mother-to-child transmission of rubella once infection has been detected in pregnancy. Vaccination during pregnancy is contraindicated because of fears that the vaccine could be teratogenic (Australian Government Department of Health, 2020).

There are a number of recommendations in relation to rubella in pregnancy (Australian Government Department of Health, 2020). These are:

- Testing for rubella immunity is recommended at the first antenatal visit to identify women at risk of contracting rubella and enable postnatal vaccination to protect future pregnancies.
- Inform women who have been vaccinated against rubella before they were aware of the pregnancy that the baby is highly unlikely to have been affected by the vaccine.

In addition, women identified as non-immune to rubella antenatally should be advised to avoid contact with people experiencing possible symptoms of rubella.

Herpes simplex virus

Both herpes simplex virus (HSV) type 1 and HSV type 2 can cause genital herpes. Because the infection is chronic, genital herpes has become the most common STI among women. The prevalence of the genital HSV infection can cause a wide spectrum of disease. First-episode infections, which represent new acquisition of HSV, usually are most severe and recurrent infections may be milder. However, many primary infections are unrecognised by either patient or care provider. Recurrences are usually limited to the genital area. Most women with HSV-2 do not know they have genital herpes because their recurrences are mild and infrequent. Such women may have non-specific genital conditions and may have been receiving treatment for other genital conditions, such as recurrent yeast infections, urinary tract infections or allergic rashes in the genital area. An important feature of HSV infection is intermittent reactivation, with or without accompanying symptoms, and resultant shedding of the virus in the genital tract.

Routine herpes testing for people without symptoms is not recommended (CDC, 2017). Herpes simplex is most often spread to an infant during birth if the mother has HSV in her vagina at the time of the birth. Babies are most at risk from neonatal herpes if the mother contracts genital HSV late in pregnancy. Women with visible genital herpes lesions or prodromal symptoms at the time of labour therefore need careful assessment to advise about the best mode of birth as a caesarean section may be recommended. Women without visible lesions or prodromal symptoms will usually be able to labour because they have a low risk of neonatal HSV transmission.

It is difficult to make the diagnosis of genital herpes on clinical grounds alone. The classic presentation of a painful cluster of vesicles and ulcers occurs in a small proportion of women, and most women will have atypical lesions such as abrasions, fissures or itching without obvious lesions. Conversely, even in at-risk women with a presentation compatible with genital herpes, up to 20% of women will not have genital herpes. Thus, a definitive diagnosis should be confirmed by a laboratory test even if the infection was established in the past on clinical grounds.

Toxoplasmosis

Caused by the protozoan parasite *Toxoplasma gondii*, primary toxoplasmosis infection is usually asymptomatic in healthy women. Once infected, a lifelong antibody response provides immunity from further infection.

Routine antenatal serological screening for toxoplasmosis should not be offered because the harms of screening may outweigh the potential benefits. Pregnant women should be advised of primary prevention measures to avoid toxoplasmosis infection (Australian Government Department of Health, 2020) such as:

- washing hands before handling food
- thoroughly washing all fruit and vegetables, including ready-prepared salads, before eating
- thoroughly cooking raw meat and ready-prepared chilled meals
- wearing gloves and thoroughly washing hands after handling soil and gardening
- avoiding cat faeces in cat litter or in soil.

Coronavirus (COVID-19) testing

The announcement of the global COVID-19 pandemic by the World Health Organization (WHO) on 11 March 2020 has seen rapid and radical changes to the way healthcare is delivered around the world.

Serologic tests measure the antibody response in an individual. Antibodies to COVID-19 are produced over days to weeks after infection with the virus. The presence of antibodies indicates that a person was infected with the COVID-19 virus, irrespective of whether the individual had severe or mild disease, or even asymptomatic infection (WHO, 2021).

There are currently no evidence or recommendations to routinely screen pregnant women for coronavirus, the virus that causes COVID-19.

The evidence base on COVID-19 generally, as well as in pregnancy, is growing quickly and by the time this edition is published there are likely to be many thousands more papers and guidelines issued. It is recommended that readers should check the latest guidance in Australia and New Zealand to determine the most up-to-date screening approaches.

SCREENING FOR CLINICAL CONDITIONS

Blood group and Rhesus D status

Identifying the woman's **blood group** and Rhesus D (RhD) status is important to prevent haemolytic disease of the newborn (NICE, 2008). This should occur at the first antenatal visit. Rhesus-negative women should be advised to receive anti-D prophylaxis. In health services where routine anti-D prophylaxis is not offered, anti-D is recommended within 72 hours of a sensitising event.

The Royal Australian and New Zealand College of Obstetricians and Gynaecologists (RANZCOG) guidelines for the use of RhD immunoglobulin (anti-D) in obstetrics (RANZCOG, 2020) provide a clear plan of the timing and process for the use of RhD immunoglobulin (anti-D).

At this point in time, New Zealand has not adopted a policy of routine antenatal administration of anti-D for pregnant women with a Rhesus-negative blood group. Anti-D is recommended for women who experience sensitising events including amniocentesis, chorionic villus sampling, trauma to the abdomen, antepartum haemorrhage, external cephalic version (whether or not successful) and confirmed fetal–maternal haemorrhage.

Diabetes

Hyperglycaemia is raised blood glucose level in pregnancy and includes a range of conditions from impaired fasting glucose and impaired glucose tolerance (prediabetes), preexisting type 1 diabetes, preexisting type 2 diabetes (either previously diagnosed or diagnosed during pregnancy) and gestational diabetes (developing during pregnancy). Gestational diabetes can recur in later pregnancies. Women who develop gestational diabetes are at high risk of developing type 2 diabetes in later life (Australian Government Department of Health, 2020).

Diabetes identified during pregnancy is reasonably common in many high-income countries especially in certain populations (Moses et al., 2016). For example, Aboriginal and Torres Strait Islander women and women born in high-diabetes-risk regions (such as Polynesia, Asia and the Middle East) have higher rates of diabetes during pregnancy than other women (Australian Government Department of Health, 2020).

The prevalence of diabetes in pregnancy seems to have increased in Australia and New Zealand over the past decades. This may be due to increased rates of obesity and first-time mothers aged over 35 years as well as changed ethnic diversity as migration patterns alter in both countries.

Screening for diabetes in pregnancy

Screening for diabetes in pregnancy has gone through much iteration over the past 10 years. Assessing a woman's risk of diabetes, however, is important. It is recommended that at the first antenatal visit, healthcare providers assess a woman's risk of diabetes—including her age, BMI, previous gestational diabetes or high-birth-weight baby, family history of diabetes, presence of polycystic ovarian syndrome and whether she is from an ethnic group with high prevalence of diabetes (Australian Government Department of Health, 2020).

There is no universal agreement globally on the approach to screening for diabetes in pregnancy. However, the Australasian Diabetes in Pregnancy Society (ADIPS) (Nankervis et al., 2013), the American Diabetes Association (ADA, 2013), the Endocrine Society in the USA (Blumer et al., 2013), the International Association of Diabetes and Pregnancy Study Groups (IADPSG) (Metzger et al., 2010), the United States Preventive Services Task Force and the World Health Organization (WHO, 2013) all recommend universal screening. In New Zealand, early universal screening is recommended using glycated haemoglobin (HbA_{1c}) with later targeted screening (Ministry of Health, 2014a).

In Australia, the guidelines recommend a two-stage approach to screening with the recommendations stating (Australian Government Department of Health, 2020):

- Offer early testing for hyperglycaemia to women with risk factors for diabetes, including Aboriginal and Torres Strait Islander women.
- Between 24 and 28 weeks gestation, offer testing for diabetes to women who have not previously been tested in the current pregnancy. Offer repeat testing to women who were tested early in pregnancy owing to risk factors and had normal blood glucose on the initial test.

In New Zealand, the national guidelines make recommendations for the diagnosis of probable undiagnosed diabetes in early pregnancy and of gestational diabetes mid-trimester (Ministry of Health, 2014a):

- Universal screening using glycated haemoglobin (HbA_{1c}), as part of 'booking' antenatal blood tests (ideally before 20 weeks) will identify women with probable undiagnosed diabetes or prediabetes.
- Women who have a normal HbA1c at booking are recommended to have a 1-hour 50-g polycose screening test at 24–8 weeks, with follow-up diagnostic glucose tolerance test if the results are above the reference range.
- At 24–8 weeks gestation, all women not previously diagnosed with diabetes who are at high risk of gestational diabetes (HbA_{1c} of 41–9 mmol/mol) should be offered the diagnostic 2-hour, 75-g oral glucose tolerance test.

Diagnostic classifications

There is some controversy about the optimal diagnostic threshold for diabetes in pregnancy. There are concerns that if the blood sugar level criteria levels are too low then too many women will be diagnosed with diabetes in pregnancy, which could increase unnecessary surveillance and interventions. Alternatively, if the criteria levels are too high, women may not be diagnosed, which means they may be subject to the adverse effects and impacts of diabetes.

The WHO and IADPSG have developed criteria that are commonly used in many settings (Table 22.2). It is important that care providers are aware of which diagnostic criteria are used in their own setting and apply these consistently.

CRITICAL THINKING EXERCISE

1. Find out the screening for hyperglycaemia approach used in your country/context/health area.
2. What are the blood sugar levels used in your setting to diagnose diabetes in pregnancy?
3. What is your advice to women about a general healthy lifestyle to reduce the risk of diabetes? Consider issues such as a balanced diet, being physically active and avoiding excessive weight gain during their pregnancy.
4. Practise this discussion with a colleague and try and improve the 'script' you provide to women.

Screening for hypertension in pregnancy

Hypertensive disorders in pregnancy and **preeclampsia** remain major causes of maternal and perinatal mortality,

Table 22.2 WHO/IADPSG criteria for diagnosis of diabetes in pregnancy

Diabetes in pregnancy—one or more of the following criteria are met	
Fasting plasma glucose	≥7.0 mmol/L (126 mg/dL)
2-hour plasma glucose	≥11.1 mmol/L (200 mg/dL) following a 75-g oral glucose load
Random plasma glucose	≥11.1 mmol/L (200 mg/dL) in the presence of diabetes symptoms
Gestational diabetes—one or more of the following criteria are met at any time during pregnancy	
Fasting plasma glucose	5.1–6.9 mmol/L (92–125 mg/dL)
1-hour plasma glucose	≥10.0 mmol/L (180 mg/dL) following a 75-g oral glucose load
2-hour plasma glucose	8.5–11.0 mmol/L (153–199 mg/dL) following a 75-g oral glucose load
(Source: WHO, 2013)	

accounting for 15% of maternal deaths and 4% of perinatal deaths. A key aim of antenatal care is the timely detection and management of women with hypertension in pregnancy (Australian Government Department of Health, 2020; WHO, 2016).

Hypertensive disorders during pregnancy include (Lowe et al., 2014):

- *chronic hypertension*—blood pressure ≥140 mmHg systolic and/or ≥90 mmHg diastolic confirmed before pregnancy or before 20 completed weeks pregnancy, without a known cause (essential hypertension), associated with a secondary cause such as existing kidney disease (secondary hypertension) or associated with measurement in a healthcare setting ('white-coat hypertension')
- *gestational hypertension*—new-onset hypertension (defined as a blood pressure ≥140 mmHg systolic and/or ≥90 mmHg diastolic) after 20 weeks pregnancy with no maternal or fetal features of preeclampsia, followed by return of blood pressure to normal within 3 months after the birth
- *preeclampsia*—a multisystem disorder characterised by hypertension and involvement of one or more other organ systems and/or the fetus, with raised blood pressure after 20 weeks pregnancy commonly the first manifestation and proteinuria a common additional feature (although not required to make a clinical diagnosis)
- *superimposed preeclampsia*—development of one or more of the systemic features of preeclampsia after 20 weeks pregnancy in a woman with chronic hypertension.

In preeclampsia, hypertension is accompanied by one or more of the following features (Lowe et al., 2014):

- impaired kidney or liver function
- haematological involvement
- neurological symptoms (headache, visual disturbances, stroke, convulsions)
- pulmonary oedema
- fetal growth restriction
- placental abruption.

CLINICAL POINT

Measuring blood pressure in pregnancy

1. At the first antenatal visit, blood pressure should be recorded on both arms to exclude rare cardiac abnormalities. Variation between arms should be less than 10 mmHg.
2. The woman should sit down with her feet supported. In labour, if the woman is lying down use the left arm.
3. Take measurements after the woman has been resting in this position for 2–3 minutes.
4. Clothing should be removed from the arm (not rolled up tightly above the cuff).
5. Use a standard-sized cuff for women with an arm circumference of ≤33 cm, and a large cuff for arm circumference >33 cm.
6. The woman's arm should be supported at heart level. Palpate systolic blood pressure at the brachial artery and inflate the cuff to 20 mmHg above this level.
7. Deflate the cuff slowly, at approximately 2 mmHg per second.
8. Record diastolic blood pressure reading using the Korotkoff V sound. If phase V is not present, then record phase IV.

(Source: Lowe et al., 2014)

Urine testing in pregnancy

Testing for proteinuria after the initial antenatal visit should be undertaken if a woman has risk factors for, or clinical indications of, preeclampsia—in particular raised blood pressure.

When testing for proteinuria, an automated dipstick machine should be used as manually read urine dipstick tests have high false-positive/negative rates. An automated machine may not be available in community settings and therefore a manual dipstick should be used. A MSU sample should be collected for a spot urine protein creatinine ratio if proteinuria is detected by either method (Lowe et al., 2014).

RESEARCH ACTIVITY

A discussion of fetal movements is essential to have with all women all the way through pregnancy.

Watch this short animation about encouraging women to trust their instincts and speak up when it comes to health concerns in pregnancy:

https://www.tommys.org/pregnancy-information/symptom-checker/i-just-think-something-wrong/always-ask-safer-pregnancy.

The animation is based on research. This is one of the papers—search for this paper online (it is available on Open Access):

Rance S, McCourt C, Rayment J, et al. Women's safety alerts in maternity care: is speaking up enough? *BMJ Quality and Safety* 2013;22:348–355.

In the paper, identify one example of:

- women's safety alerts
- the supportive roles of partners and relatives
- the need for staff to listen and respond.

How can midwives use this evidence to ensure that they value women's concerns and support women to speak up?

RESEARCH FINDINGS

Vitamin D screening in pregnancy is now very common in many healthcare settings globally. This is despite a lack of quality evidence showing that screening and giving supplementation are of benefit.

The Australian pregnancy care guidelines highlighted that, while recent studies have explored possible associations between vitamin D status in pregnancy and subsequent outcomes, this evidence is generally of low quality and heterogeneous (i.e. in definition of optimal level, timing of serum testing) and the findings are inconsistent. In addition, the evidence on the harms and benefits of vitamin D supplementation remains unclear.

Find the policy on vitamin D screening from your health service and consider the following questions:

- Is the policy based on evidence?
- What are the strengths and limitations of the policy?
- How does it differ from the Australian guidelines mentioned above?
- Are there reasons for this based on the population in your area?
- How will you incorporate the evidence in your practice given the guidelines?

Conclusion

This chapter has highlighted some of the common screening and assessments that contribute to the provision of quality antenatal care. When undertaking screening and assessments, it is important to make a follow-up plan to ensure that the woman has the opportunity to discuss the results and plan further testing should that be indicated. The midwife should always be aware that screening has the potential to cause anxiety given the potential to uncover pre-existing conditions in an otherwise well population.

Review questions

1. Why is screening in pregnancy important?
2. What is the difference between a screening test and a diagnostic procedure?
3. What is the specificity of a screening test and how is this different from the sensitivity of a screening test?
4. Is it ethically justifiable to offer screening in utero for a potentially untreatable genetic disorder? Why, or why not?
5. What is the incidence of hepatitis B in your area? What do you tell families who want to weigh up the pros and cons of hepatitis B vaccination of their baby at the time of birth? What are the long-term effects of hepatitis B? Does hepatitis B affect different populations differently?
6. What are the benefits and possible unintended consequences of screening for blood-borne viruses (e.g. HIV, hepatitis B, hepatitis C)?
7. What are the risks and benefits of screening for diabetes in pregnancy?

Acknowledgements

Thank you to Sally K Tracy, Joyce Cowan and Celia Grigg for important contributions in the previous edition.

Online resources

Australian Government Department of Health. Clinical Practice Guideline: Pregnancy Care; 2020: https://www.health.gov.au/resources/collections/pregnancy-care-guidelines-and-related-documents.

Australian Government Department of Health. Coronavirus (COVID-19) pandemic: https://www.health.gov.au/news/health-alerts/novel-coronavirus-2019-ncov-health-alert.

Commonwealth Government of Australia. Health Insight: blood tests during pregnancy: https://www.pregnancybirthbaby.org.au/pregnancy-checkups-and-scans.

National Centre for Health and Clinical Excellence (NICE): http://www.nice.org.uk.

New Zealand Government Manatū Hauora Ministry of Health. COVID-19 (novel coronavirus): https://www.health.govt.nz/our-work/diseases-and-conditions/covid-19-novel-coronavirus.

New Zealand Government. Pregnancy and newborn screening: https://www.nsu.govt.nz/pregnancy-newborn-screening.

Raising Children Network. Pregnancy section: https://raisingchildren.net.au/pregnancy/health-wellbeing.

Royal Australian and New Zealand College of Obstetricians and Gynaecologists (RANZCOG). A message for pregnant women and their families (COVID-19 information): https://ranzcog.edu.au/statements-guidelines/covid-19-statement/information-for-pregnant-women.

References

Aebi-Popp K, Duppenthaler A, Rauch A, et al. Vertical transmission of hepatitis C: towards universal antenatal screening in the era of new direct acting antivirals (DAAs)? Short review and analysis of the situation in Switzerland. *J Virus Erad.* 2016;2(1):52–54.

American Diabetes Association (ADA). Standards of medical care in diabetes—2013. *Diabetes Care.* 2013;36(suppl 1):S11–S66.aq.

Australian Government Department of Health. *Clinical Practice Guidelines: Pregnancy Care.* Canberra: Australian Government Department of Health; 2020.

Blumer I, Hadar E, Hadden D, et al. Diabetes and pregnancy: an Endocrine Society clinical practice guideline. *J Clin Endocrinol Metab.* 2013;98(11):4227–4249.

Brocklehurst P, Gordon A, Heatley E, et al. Antibiotics for treating bacterial vaginosis in pregnancy. Update. *Cochrane Database Syst Rev.* 2013;(2):1–30.

Centers for Disease Control and Prevention (CDC). Early-onset and late-onset neonatal group B streptococcal disease – United States, 1996–2004. *MMWR Morb Mortal Wkly Rep.* 2005;54:1205–1208.

Centers for Disease Control and Prevention (CDC). Prevention of perinatal group B streptococcal disease. Revised guidelines from CDC, 2010. *MMWR Morb Mortal Wkly Rep.* 2010;59(RR–10):1–36.

Centers for Disease Control and Prevention (CDC). *Genital Herpes Screening FAQ*; 2017. Online: https://www.cdc.gov/std/herpes/screening.htm.

Chakraborty R, Luck S. Syphilis is on the increase: the implications for child health. *Arch Dis Child.* 2008;93(2):105–109.

Clifford V, Garland S, Grimwood K. Prevention of neonatal group B *Streptococcus* disease in the 21st century. *J Paediatr Child Health.* 2011;48:808–815.

Dunkelberg J, Berkley E, Thiel K, et al. Hepatitis B and C in pregnancy: a review and recommendations for care. *J Perinatol.* 2014;34(12):882–891.

Geisler W, Wang C, Morrison S, et al. The natural history of untreated *Chlamydia trachomatis* infection in the interval between screening and returning for treatment. *Sex Transm Dis.* 2008;35(2):119–123.

Gilbert R. Prenatal screening for group B streptococcal infection: gaps in the evidence. *Int J Epidemiol.* 2003;33:2–8.

Grimes D, Schulz K. Uses and abuses of screening tests. *Lancet.* 2002;359(9309):881--884.

Heath P. Perinatal group B streptococcal disease. *Best Pract Res Clin Obstet Gynaecol.* 2007;21:411–424.

Homer C, Scarf V, Catling C, et al. Culture-based versus risk-based screening for the prevention of group B streptococcal disease in newborns: a review of national guidelines. *Women Birth.* 2014;27:46–51.

Joesoef M, Schmid G. Bacterial vaginosis. *Clin Evid.* 2002;7:1400–1408.

Kieler H, Haglund B, Cnattingius S, et al. Does prenatal sonography affect intellectual performance? *Epidemiology.* 2005;3:304–310.

Kirby Institute. *HIV, viral hepatitis and sexually transmissible infections in Australia: Annual surveillance report 2018.* Sydney: Kirby Institute, UNSW. Online: https://kirby.unsw.edu.au/report/hiv-viral-hepatitis-and-sexually-transmissible-infections-australia-annual-surveillance.

Leap N. The power of words revisited. *Essentially MIDIRS.* 2012;3(1):17–21.

Lowe S, Bowyer L, Lust K, et al. *The management of hypertensive disorders of pregnancy. Society of Obstetric Medicine of Australia and New Zealand (SOMANZ).* 2014. Online: http://www.somanz.org/documents/HTguideline2014Consultation-Draft120214.pdf.

Metzger B, Gabbe S, Persson B, et al. International association of diabetes and pregnancy study groups recommendations on the diagnosis and classification of hyperglycemia in pregnancy. *Diabetes Care.* 2010;33(3):676–682.

Ministry of Health. *Screening, Diagnosis and Management of Gestational Diabetes in New Zealand: A clinical practice guideline.* Wellington, NZ: Ministry of Health; 2014a. Online: https://www.health.govt.nz/publication/screening-diagnosis-and-management-gestational-diabetes-new-zealand-clinical-practice-guideline

Ministry of Health. *Recommendations for HIV testing of adults in healthcare settings; 2014b.* Online: http://www.health.govt.nz/our-work/diseases-and-conditions/.

Moses R, Wong V, Lambert K, et al. The prevalence of hyperglycaemia in pregnancy in Australia. *Aust N Z J Obstet Gynaecol.* 2016;56(4):341–345. doi:10.1111/ajo.12447.

Nankervis A, McIntyre H, Moses R, et al. *ADIPS Consensus Guidelines for the Testing and Diagnosis of Gestational Diabetes Mellitus in Australia.* Sydney: Australian Diabetes in Pregnancy Society; 2013.

National Institute for Health and Care Excellence (NICE). *Antenatal Care: Routine Care for the Healthy Pregnant Woman.* London: National Collaborating Centre for Women's and Children's Health; 2008, updated 2017.

New Zealand College of Midwives. *Midwives Handbook for Practice.* Christchurch, NZ: New Zealand College of Midwives; 2015.

Oddie S, Embleton N, on behalf of the Northern Network. Risk factors for early onset neonatal group B streptococcal sepsis: case–control study. *BMJ.* 2002;325:308–312.

Pereira K, Maidji E, McDonagh S, et al. Insights into viral transmission at the uterine-placental interface. *Trends Microbiol.* 2005;13(4):164–174.

Phares C, Lynfield R, Farley M, et al; Active Bacterial Core Surveillance/Emerging Infections Program Network. Epidemiology of invasive group B streptococcal disease in the United States 1999–2005. *JAMA.* 2008;299:2056–2065.

Rac M, Sheffield J. Prevention and management of viral hepatitis in pregnancy. *Obstet Gynecol Clin North Am.* 2014;41(4):573–592.

Rance S, McCourt C, Rayment J, et al. Women's safety alerts in maternity care: is speaking up enough? *BMJ Qual Saf.* 2013;22: 348–355.

Raynes-Greenow C, Polis S, Elliott E, et al. Childhood hepatitis C virus infection: an Australian national surveillance study of incident cases over five years. *J Paediatr Child Health.* 2015; 51(11):1115–1120.

Richens J, Mabey C. Sexually transmitted infections (excluding HIV). In: Farrar J, Hotaz PJ, Junghanss T, et al, eds. *Manson's Tropical Diseases.* 23rd ed. London: Saunders Elsevier; 2013; Ch. 23.

Rogers S, Miller W, Turner C, et al. Concordance of *Chlamydia trachomatis* infections within sexual partnerships. *Sex Transm Infect.* 2008;84(1):23–28.

Royal Australian and New Zealand College of Obstetricians and Gynaecologists (RANZCOG). *Use of RhD Immunoglobulin (Anti-D Immunoglobulin) during pregnancy and the post partum period*; 2020. Online: http://www.ranzcog.edu.au/the-ranzcog/policies-and-guidelines/.

Schrag S, Zywicki S, Farley M, et al. Group B streptococcal disease in the era of intrapartum antibiotic prophylaxis. *N Engl J Med.* 2000;342:15–21.

Siegfried N, van der Merwe L, Brocklehurst P, et al. Antiretrovirals for reducing the risk of mother-to-child transmission of HIV infection. *Cochrane Database Syst Rev.* 2011;(7):CD003510, doi:10.1002/14651858.CD003510.pub3.

Webster D, Klenerman P, Dusheiko G. Hepatitis C. *Lancet.* 2015;385: 1124–1135.

World Health Organization (WHO). *Diagnostic Criteria and Classification of Hyperglycaemia First Detected in Pregnancy.* Geneva: WHO; 2013.

World Health Organization (WHO). *WHO Recommendations on Antenatal Care for a Positive Pregnancy Experience.* Geneva: WHO; 2016.

World Health Organization (WHO). *Serology and Early Investigation protocols.* Geneva: WHO; 2021. Online https://www.who.int/emergencies/diseases/novel-coronavirus-2019/serology-in-the-context-of-covid-19.

Further reading

Australian Government Department of Health. *Clinical Practice Guideline: Pregnancy Care.* Canberra: Australian Government Department of Health; 2020. Online: https://www.health.gov.au/sites/default/files/documents/2021/02/pregnancy-care-guidelines-pregnancy-care-guidelines.pdf

Choosing Wisely Australia is another useful website that provides information to clinicians and consumers about improving the quality of healthcare by eliminating unnecessary and sometimes harmful tests, treatments and procedures: http://www.choosingwisely.org.au/home.

There is a wealth of information for women, partners and families on the Raising Children website. This site provides facts sheets and short videos that may be useful: http://raisingchildren.net.au/pregnancy/pregnancy_and_birth.html.

World Health Organization (WHO). *Recommendations on Antenatal Care for a Positive Pregnancy Experience.* Geneva: World Health Organization; 2016.

World Health Organization (WHO). *Serology and Early Investigation protocols for COVID-19.* Geneva: World Health Organization; 2021. https://www.who.int/emergencies/diseases/novel-coronavirus-2019/serology-in-the- context-of-covid-19

CHAPTER 23

Working with women in pregnancy

Celia Grigg and Kelly Kara

LEARNING OUTCOMES

Learning outcomes for this chapter are:

1. To discuss the organisation and essential components of antenatal care within the context of the midwifery model
2. To describe and explain the concept of 'decision points' as a framework for organising care
3. To list and describe routinely offered antenatal blood screening, blood pressure and urine screening tests, and vaccinations
4. To explain the purpose and process of abdominal palpation of pregnant women
5. To describe the assessment and significance of fetal movements
6. To discuss some of the physiological changes of pregnancy, with specific reference to nausea and vomiting, constipation and heartburn.

CHAPTER OVERVIEW

This chapter discusses antenatal care within the context of autonomous midwifery practice. It provides a broad overview of the issues of antenatal care, and considers some of the core technical components of clinical practice. Where possible, this discussion is based on reviewed research, in order to promote *evidence-informed midwifery practice*. The dearth of published research that meaningfully addresses midwifery questions is an ongoing problem in this regard. The chapter establishes a framework for understanding the *way* of doing things, as much as it provides instruction on *what* to do. As such, it seeks to interpret routine care with reference to the following set of guiding principles, which are fundamental for midwives working within the midwifery model:

- partnerships with women—women-centred, negotiated relationships
- continuity of care in the holistic process of pregnancy, birth and early parenting
- support and empowerment of childbearing women
- promotion of holistic wellness
- assessment and screening, which includes risk identification, knowledge/understanding and choices
- information sharing as a two-way process
- promotion of active, informed decision making by women
- health promotion and education within an appropriate 'adult learning' approach.

In this chapter, antenatal care is discussed within a broad practice model of midwife-led continuity of care. While this model characterises Aotearoa New Zealand's midwifery and maternity services, it is also becoming increasingly available in Australia and is the model to which the Australian midwifery profession aspires. The key components of routine antenatal care are identified using the New Zealand College of Midwives (NZCOM) 'decision points' as a framework (NZCOM, 2015). Some of these components are further developed in the explanatory sections that follow. The decision points refer to relevant issues raised in other chapters of this book, and readers are also referred to other reading and research activity where appropriate. Notwithstanding the model of care in which a midwife may practise, the aspects of antenatal care described in this chapter are applicable to any setting.

Of necessity, this chapter discusses antenatal care as a discrete entity, and it may be tempting to consider it as such. However, antenatal care is but a small part of a woman's experience of the broader process of pregnancy, and cannot be separated from childbearing as a holistic process, which includes pregnancy, birth and the postnatal period. Further, the meaning and effect of antenatal care is totally dependent on the individual woman and her personal context.

KEY TERMS

antenatal care
antenatal education
assessment and screening
booking visit
decision points
estimated due date (EDD)
exercise or physical activity
palpation
physiological changes
routine screening

INTRODUCTION: ANTENATAL CARE—WHAT IS IT?

Defining **antenatal care** as a conceptual entity, or even in terms of a list of discrete clinical components, is difficult. Definitions of antenatal care can vary markedly, depending on one's beliefs or understanding of the childbearing process, be it from a midwifery or a medical perspective. It is important to recognise how the midwife's perspective will influence the aims, scope and content of the antenatal care she provides, and the way in which she provides this care.

From a midwifery perspective, antenatal care is not an independent entity—it is an integral part of the whole childbearing experience. It usually represents the beginning of the journey that midwives and women will make together, which includes the time before, during and after the birth of the baby. For midwives working from a midwifery model, it is a time of forming and building a relationship with each woman and those who are important to her. It is a time when a partnership is negotiated, roles and responsibilities are identified, information is shared, options are discussed and choices are made and supported. In order for an effective partnership to be established, midwives need to consider the cultural safety of their care and the traditional power imbalance between health professionals and childbearing women (see Department of Health (DOH), 2020, pp. 30—35, and Midwifery Council Statement on Cultural Competence, 2011). This is an ongoing issue for midwives as indigenous women in both Australia and New Zealand continue to have poorer outcomes (Australian Institute of Health and Welfare, 2021; Perinatal and Maternal Mortality Review Committee (PMMRC), 2021). The antenatal period is also a time when notions of wellness and normality within the context of pregnancy are supported and promoted (Browne et al., 2014; DOH, 2020; Sword et al., 2012).

Each woman and each midwife brings their respective knowledge and expertise together in this new relationship. A woman brings her knowledge of her past and present physical wellness (and that of her family), her personal, social, emotional and cultural realities, her experiences of pregnancy (present and sometimes previous) and her plans for her birth and mothering. A midwife brings her knowledge of the childbearing process, supports its normality, identifies risks and shares information that enables the woman to make informed decisions throughout.

However, much of what constitutes contemporary antenatal care throughout the world remains strongly rooted in the 'medical' model within which it developed. Widespread, institutionalised, routine antenatal care began less than 80 years ago, as a mass-screening program with the aim of reducing maternal and perinatal mortality, and brought 'pregnancy' under medical supervision and control for the first time in human history (Wagner, 1994). The history and politics of antenatal care will not be discussed here. They are well articulated by many authors, such as Oakley (1984), Strong (2000), Katz Rothman (1989), Donnison (1988) and, in New Zealand, Donley (1998). What is of significance in this context are the *beliefs* and *assumptions* that continue to underpin the structure and content of various aspects of antenatal care. Traditionally, and in many contemporary contexts, antenatal care consists of a prescribed set of acts based around the clinical monitoring and screening of all pregnant women, regardless of their health or risk status. This establishment of routine antenatal care was based on the notion that pregnancy is a state of pathology, rather than of normal physiology. Oakley (1984) argued that 'the most characteristic aspect of modern antenatal care is the clinical insistence on the probability of pathology in all childbearing' (p. 2). Over the past 80 years, technological advances have brought an ever-increasing array of screening tests, interventions and treatments. However, a recent Cochrane review states that 'few of the procedures commonly undertaken within antenatal care have been shown to have a major impact on maternal and perinatal morbidity or mortality, and some have no effect', although the findings from 'observational studies tend to show that women who receive antenatal care have lower maternal and perinatal mortality and better pregnancy outcomes' (Dowswell et al., 2015, p. 6). We do not know whether antenatal care is an effective intervention or just something those who are likely to have better outcomes receive. Further the review states that 'few of its common components have been formally evaluated, and there is little reliable evidence of the relative merits, hazards and costs of alternative packages of care'; despite this, the Cochrane reviewers suggest that 'it is reasonable to assume that antenatal care does confer some health benefits, although how it does so may be complex and multifactorial' (Dowswell et al., 2015, p. 6). It is extremely important that all those who provide care clearly articulate the scope and limitations of the screening and diagnostic tests used in antenatal care.

Some might argue that routine antenatal care fails to meet reasonable expectations of its relevance and effectiveness. If this is indeed the case, then it may be possible to mount a case to abandon it. However, such a proposition would be inappropriate from a midwifery point of view. Maternal and perinatal morbidity and mortality are not the only outcome measures of value. There has long been substantial evidence that midwifery-provided continuity of care has beneficial effects on other outcome measures, such as reduced anxiety and a greater sense of control (Oakley, 1992). While there may be different types of continuity (de Jonge et al., 2014) and continuity of care may be conceptualised differently by women (Jenkins et al., 2015), influenced by their knowledge and experience of it, it is relational continuity which is paramount and has been identified by others as 'everything' (Davison et al., 2015) or 'gold' (de Jonge et al., 2014).

Continuity of care is also associated with improved clinical outcomes, including reduced rates of intrapartum analgesia, amniotomy, instrument-assisted vaginal birth and episiotomy, and pre-term birth and fetal loss before 24 weeks gestation (Sandall et al., 2013, 2016). Further, there is evidence that women express higher levels of 'satisfaction', or have their expectations fulfilled (identified as a better measure in this context by Clark et al., 2015a, 2015b) with continuity of care (Forster et al., 2016). One mechanism by which it acts to improve clinical outcomes has been identified by Dove & Muir-Cochrane (2014), who found that midwives assumed a role as 'risk-negotiator' mediating relationships between women and other maternity care providers—a role which 'relied profoundly on the trust engendered in their relationships with women via continuity of care' (p. 1063).

An often-neglected aspect in discussions regarding antenatal care is what matters to women. A recent systematic review (Downe et al., 2015) provides an international perspective on this, and identifies a very generic concept of 'a positive pregnancy experience' as the composite outcome. The reviewers broke it down into four components:

> *maintaining physical and social normality;*
> *maintaining a healthy pregnancy for mother and baby (including preventing and treating risks, illness and death);*
> *effective transition to positive labour and birth; and*
> *achieving positive motherhood (including maternal self esteem, competence, autonomy.*
>
> (Downe et al., 2015, p. 532)

With these findings in mind, the authors recommended an antenatal care service which comprises three domains:

> *clinical care/therapeutic practices (biomedical interventions and tests, integrated with spiritual and religious practices, where appropriate);*
> *relevant and timely information (physiological, biomedical, as well as behavioural and sociocultural); and*
> *support (social, cultural, emotional and psychological).*
>
> (Downe et al., 2015, pp. 532–3)

The general framework of care set out in this chapter fits well into these domains. The key point is that antenatal care is a process that consists of more than just a series of medical tests and monitoring procedures. Although some of these tests may form part of the process, in the midwifery context they are not of themselves the essence of antenatal care—that is, they do not *define* it. Midwives need to claim and promote the potential of *holistic midwifery care,* and put this potential into practice in their work. For midwives, antenatal care is fundamentally about a relationship between two actively participating individuals (and the woman's support people) who bring their respective expertise together and work to maximise the health and wellbeing of the woman and her unborn child, and to prepare for labour, birth and parenting. From the midwifery perspective, the term 'routine antenatal care' is perhaps a misnomer, as there is no such thing as a 'routine' woman. Every woman is different, and each of her pregnancy experiences is unique.

Organisation of care

The provision of antenatal care in Australia and New Zealand has traditionally been based on a medically defined, controlled and provided system of assessment, screening and monitoring of pregnant women, which was initiated in Britain and established in the 1920s (Hall, 2001).

In *Australia* this remains largely unchanged, although there are increasing examples of alternative models (Brock et al., 2014), including Midwifery Group Practice (Haines et al., 2015; Maier, 2013), an Aboriginal Family Birthing Program (Brown et al., 2016; Middleton et al., 2017) and group antenatal care (Allen et al., 2015). In particular the legislation introduced into the Federal Parliament in 2009 extended access to the Pharmaceutical Benefits Scheme (PBS) and the Medicare Benefits Schedule (MBS), thereby enabling Endorsed midwives to provide antenatal care in the community under their own responsibility. The legislative changes opened up the possibility of midwifery models of care as alternatives to the mainstream maternity care systems. Under the new arrangements, Endorsed midwives wishing to provide care under Medicare and prescribe certain medicines under the PBS are required to demonstrate that they meet certain eligibility requirements and that they have collaborative arrangements in place, including appropriate referral pathways with hospitals and doctors, to ensure that women receive coordinated care and the appropriate expertise and treatment as the clinical need arises. Although controversial, it has been shown that these collaborative arrangements can work effectively for clinicians and women alike (see Ch. 18).

In *New Zealand,* legislation enabling an alternative organisation of care was introduced in 1990, which enabled women to choose, and midwives to provide, full and complete maternity care for well women without referral or deferral to doctors. The regulatory framework within which this occurs is currently referred to as 'Section 88' of the Primary Maternity Services Notice (Ministry of Health (MOH), 2007). Today, antenatal care in New Zealand is founded on the concept of a primary caregiver, known as a *lead maternity carer* (LMC), providing the majority of care and organising referral when care is outside the scope of practice of the LMC. Midwives are the LMC for 94.5% of the 92% of women who register with an LMC (MOH, 2020). (See Ch. 2 for a detailed discussion on the role and scope of LMCs in New Zealand.)

The antenatal visit

Antenatal visits are the main mechanism for the provision of antenatal care. They are negotiated and agreed upon between the woman and the midwife, and occur at prearranged times and locations at regular intervals throughout the woman's pregnancy. They are multidimensional and include several components, such as information sharing, **assessment and screening, active decision making** and **health promotion and education** (Fig. 23.1). Aspects of these dimensions will be illustrated and discussed throughout this chapter.

The number and timing of visits follow a pattern, which was established when the concept of antenatal care was introduced in the 1920s (Candy et al., 2003). This traditional pattern of antenatal visits—4-weekly from booking until

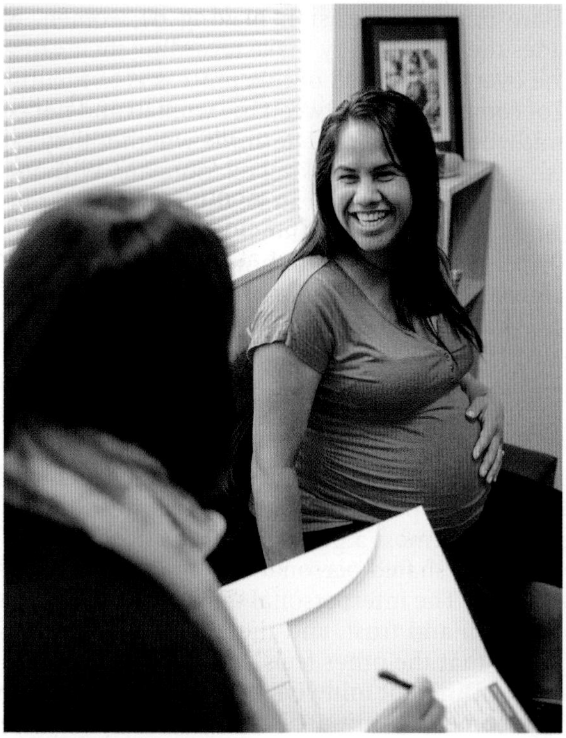

FIGURE 23.1 Antenatal visit
(Reproduced with the permission of the New Zealand College of Midwives)

28 weeks gestation, fortnightly until 36 weeks and weekly until birth—remains the standard of antenatal care today in Australia and New Zealand. (A large research survey undertaken by the International Confederation of Midwives in 2021 found that in many countries worldwide the nature of antenatal visits has been seriously disrupted due to the restrictions on face-to-face contact during COVID-19 (Tracy et al., in press).)

The 'routine' format has no particular scientific, medical, social or midwifery foundation, and has recently been the subject of debate and challenge. This challenge arose from the concept of 'evidence-based practice' and has led to the evaluation of this aspect of antenatal care (Enkin et al., 2000).

Determining the 'optimal' number of visits in routine antenatal care is extremely difficult. This is due to the complexity of the process of pregnancy itself, the diversity of childbearing women and the context-bound, multidimensional nature of antenatal care in general (Strong, 2000). Attempts to specify a particular number of visits have been based on research which measures only biomedical outcomes, such as incidence rates of preeclampsia, low birth weight, urinary tract infections, postpartum anaemia and perinatal mortality, although some studies have surveyed maternal satisfaction (Candy et al., 2003; Dowswell et al., 2015; Petrou et al., 2003). Current recommendations, based on these studies and other similar research, are for a schedule with a reduced number of antenatal visits. The British National Institute of Clinical Excellence (NICE) antenatal care guideline (2008, updated 2021) recommends, for well women, 10 visits for those having their first baby (primiparas) and seven for those having their second or subsequent baby (multiparas). The latest Australian pregnancy care clinical practice guidelines (DOH, 2020) precedes the same recommendation with the statement 'determine the schedule of antenatal visits based on the individual woman's needs' (p. 52). It is notable, however, that a reduction in women's satisfaction with fewer visits, as reported in research that studied this issue, has been minimised and largely ignored in these guidelines. Arguably, this illustrates the continuing dominance of the medical model as the foundation of contemporary antenatal care.

Issues concerning the length and location of antenatal visits are context bound in the same way as those associated with the number of visits, and the alternative options offered are equally constrained within sociopolitical limits. In the New Zealand model, the woman and midwife negotiate the length and location of visits, with each party making her respective personal and practice choices clear prior to any agreement to work together. Although there is no set optimal length for visits, enough time needs to be set aside to include discussion, assessment, decision making and documentation of the issues, such as those included in the 'decision point' framework set out later in this chapter. Visit times of less than 20 minutes are unlikely to be able to include all of the components in the decision-making framework. The time taken for visits will vary according to the practice styles of individual midwives, differences in the needs and personalities of women, the stage of the woman's pregnancy and her health status.

It is also important that the location of visits be one in which both the woman and the midwife feel relaxed and comfortable, and be available at the time most convenient to them. It needs to be safe, both personally and culturally, and afford appropriate privacy. The ideal location will be accessible and have appropriate facilities. If possible, it is valuable for the midwife to provide some of the antenatal care in the woman's home. This may help to alter the traditional power balance between care provider and receiver, and also provides valuable insight for the midwife into the woman's personal and social context.

A MIDWIFE'S STORY

When I arrived at the woman's home, I was surprised to find an ashtray in every room—including the toilet! She had told me previously that no one who lived in the house smoked. She hadn't mentioned that her grandmother, who lived close by, spent most of her time at her house, and smoked heavily. It was a delicate situation, with family relationships at stake, and required the full duration of the pregnancy to support the woman in negotiating smoke-free spaces in her own home. Visiting her at home and meeting her family gave me valuable insight into how to support the woman in making changes which would have a positive impact on her own health and that of her baby, without fracturing family relationships.

Summary points: the antenatal visit

- Negotiate frequency, location and length of visits.
- Visits should be multidimensional and include:
  - information sharing
  - assessment and screening
  - active decision making
  - health promotion
  - education.
- Antenatal visits are more than biomedical surveillance.

INITIAL CONTACT

Initial contact between a pregnant woman and a midwife is generally by phone. This call may simply be little more than an enquiry about the availability of the midwife. It may, however, evolve into a process of establishing more-substantial contact between the two, either as a continuation of the phone call or at a face-to-face meeting. This will represent the first meaningful exchange between the midwife and the pregnant woman. It is an opportunity for the woman to gain a first impression of the midwife—what she sounds like, her ways of practice and her availability. For the midwife, it is an opportunity to help the woman clarify what she is seeking, to share information about how she practises and to talk about the choices that are open to the woman.

There is no common understanding about the nature of this contact in terms of what it involves, or what its outcomes are expected to be. Women perceive its purpose in different ways. Some women are better informed about the process of arranging their care than others, and are very clear about what they want. Others have no clear understanding about the process or what will come out of it. It is the midwife's obligation to assist the woman through this initial contact by providing a framework for understanding the exchange, and a pathway through it.

Likewise, there is no standard terminology for, or description of, this initial contact. It may be referred to as the 'options' or 'check-out' visit or contact (to 'check out' meaning to gain a first impression or initial understanding of a person or a situation), and many midwives will have their own term for it. It is not the same thing as a 'booking' visit. The key feature differentiating this contact from a booking is that during the initial contact process the woman and midwife share information that will enable a decision to be made about whether they will work together. The booking visit, by contrast, occurs as a result of that decision having been made.

There is also no standard format for the process itself. While individual midwives will perceive and prioritise its various stages and content differently, it needs to include certain elements in order to be meaningful to childbearing women. For women having their first baby, the system and process are new and unknown. They will often require specific information from the midwife, and will frequently be dependent upon guidance from her; they often don't know what they need to know in order to make an informed decision. It is the midwife's role to facilitate informed decision making by women, which includes the choices they make regarding their caregiver.

The overall intention of this process is to identify the level of compatibility between the woman and her potential midwife, in order to determine whether they can establish a constructive working relationship. Without this, effective communication can be difficult, which can lead to a breakdown in the relationship between them, and in turn create the potential for a negative impact on social or clinical outcomes. Compatibility needs to occur at three levels—the interpersonal, the professional and the practical.

The interpersonal level

Each woman and midwife pair needs to feel that there is a comfortable personal connection between them. This is first and foremost a professional relationship, and not one based on shared personal experiences or a common background. The interpersonal dynamic is about a sense of relaxation and trust, and the ability to speak a social 'language' that the other feels comfortable with and understands. Different midwives will suit different women, and sometimes this initial discussion will result in a decision not to work together. This may be due to character and personality variables, about which we should not be surprised. The process is about establishing an effective human relationship (even if it is professional in nature) and so it should not be regarded as a sign of failure that a woman chooses not to work with a particular midwife.

Cultural factors are also key aspects of compatibility. It is important for women to have the opportunity to evaluate the cultural awareness and sensitivity of a midwife, and be confident that the midwife will be able to advocate for her culture-specific needs or desires.

The professional level

There is variation in the context and scope of practice among midwives. This variation is due in part to differences in belief and understanding of the nature of pregnancy, birth and parenting, and reflects the midwifery philosophy that underpins their practice. Midwives may also feel more or less comfortable in a range of settings. Some work comfortably with women in an obstetric setting, whereas others are most comfortable in the primary, community or home-birth context. The way in which midwives practise professionally will vary according to these beliefs as well as their levels of experience, personal confidence and comfort zones, and their skills or knowledge base.

There is also variation among women in their views, beliefs and understandings of the nature of pregnancy, birth and parenting. This will influence the expectations they have and the priorities they set for the type of care their midwife will provide. For example, before choosing a caregiver, a woman planning a home birth will want to know whether her choice will be genuinely supported by her midwife.

The practical level

There are a number of practical details of care that will need to be discussed. The first of these is the availability of the midwife to provide care for the woman's pregnancy, birth and postnatal period. This is focused on the estimated due date (EDD).

It is appropriate for midwives to inform women about arrangements for back-up when they are unavailable to provide care, such as during regular time off or illness, or when they are with another woman. In some practices, midwives work together in loose 'partnerships', and arrangements may or may not be made for women to meet their back-up midwives; in others, visits with the back-up midwife are an integral part of the care. There is also a moral obligation on midwives to inform women about their plans for holidays during the period of care.

A second major issue is the time and place of antenatal care. Women and midwives need to identify whether they can organise antenatal visits at a time and place that suits. This is affected by the context in which care is provided, and by the personal choices made by individual midwives. Some midwives provide clinic-based antenatal care on set days of the week. Others may negotiate with women to visit them in their homes for some or all of the antenatal care.

A MIDWIFE'S STORY

When Ana and I first met, she was 8 weeks pregnant with her first child. She told me of her plan to have an elective caesarean section; she came from a country that offered this option to all women. When asked why she feared vaginal birth so much, she recounted stories of traumatic vaginal births of women she knew. None of these were normal births. I informed her that one of my professional boundaries was to decline to work with women planning a caesarean section with no clinical indication. We talked through my reasoning. Our initial visit ended with the option of us working together on the basis of planning a normal birth, or her choosing to work with someone else. The following week she attended her prearranged appointment with an obstetrician and, after considering her options, called me to ask me to provide her maternity care. We began a journey together which eventually included a normal birth.

Summary points: initial contact

- The main purpose is to establish an equitable two-way partnership between the woman and the midwife:
  - both are active decision makers and negotiate their respective roles and responsibilities
  - both need the opportunity to make choices about whether or not they will work together.
- The midwife begins learning about:
  - the plans, beliefs and concerns the woman has about her pregnancy, childbirth and postnatal care
  - her social, cultural and physical history and context
  - issues that may make it inappropriate for her to provide care, such as when a woman has specific social or cultural needs, or an underlying medical condition that requires care and knowledge that is beyond the midwife's scope of practice.
- The woman learns about:
  - the midwife's personal beliefs regarding childbirth
  - her scope of practice
  - her professional boundaries
  - the practical arrangements that may affect the woman's choice of caregiver
  - the midwife's personality and practice, and whether she (the woman) can trust the midwife to provide the kind of care that she wants.
- This process should function as a positive screening process for both the woman and the midwife.
- Each has the right to choose to work with the other.
- Both woman and midwife share information, and actively participate and make decisions in a negotiated partnership.

THE BOOKING VISIT

The **booking visit** is, essentially, the beginning of the care relationship between the midwife and the woman and her family. It is an important part of the whole context of midwifery care, and of the antenatal care component in particular. It occurs early in the pregnancy and at the woman's home where possible, and includes the midwife, the woman and whomever else she chooses to have with her—partner, mother, sister or friend. The purpose of this visit is to formalise the arrangements for care, and to establish a foundation for the partnership. In other words, it is about defining the nature of the relationship between the woman and the midwife, and the context and meaning of antenatal care for both of them. It will:

- have a holistic focus
- be a two-way process of information sharing and decision making
- review the past, identify the present and plan the future
- include the identification of health, known ill-health, and risk markers for potential ill-health, for the woman or her baby
- include practical arrangements of care, in terms of frequency, time and place.

The booking visit happens as a result of a decision being made by the woman and midwife to work together. At this point, they will have already spoken by phone, and may have met, and will know a little about each other. If the initial contact or 'check-out' visit was not done face to face, it is preferable that the booking visit be held off until they have had an opportunity to meet. Alternatively, the visit could begin as a check-out opportunity for both, with a clearly identified endpoint for the meeting, in order to give some time and space for the woman to consider whether or not she would like to work with that midwife. If both are comfortable with each other, they may decide to formally begin the relationship at that point.

The booking visit represents the beginning of a shared journey. It is the beginning of a relationship that will last for at least 8 months (in the first instance), and encompass a special, powerful and life-changing period for the woman and her family. It is a time when many personal and private aspects of a woman's life will become shared with the midwife. As such, the booking is a great opportunity for the midwife to *get to know* the woman she will be working with. The woman's home is the ideal venue for this visit, as it is in her place and space, which can help to moderate the traditional hierarchical power dynamic between 'healthcare professional' and 'patient' to that of a more equitable partnership between midwife and woman.

Having the booking visit at the woman's home can also give the midwife important information about the woman's personal and social context. The midwife will be able to gain valuable insight into the woman's personality and outlook, her understanding of pregnancy and childbirth, and her life situation and lifestyle choices, when discussing her history and her present and future plans. There is as much to be learned from the *way* in which the woman talks about these things, and the way she responds to new information or options, as there is from *what* she says. During the discussion, the midwife can develop a sense of how the woman perceives her own role in the birth process—as an active 'doer' or a passive 'receiver' of care—as well as her understanding of health issues and the concept of risk in pregnancy.

Learning about *who* a woman is, in a holistic sense, is a central and integral component of the midwifery model. It is not an optional extra to the 'real' physical or clinical aspects, but an imperative for midwifery care, if an effective working relationship is to develop. Having this understanding helps the midwife to tailor the way she shares information with the woman, so that it may be meaningful for her. Midwives cannot identify what is appropriate for women if they know nothing of their personal, social or cultural 'self'. Sharing information or making recommendations that are irrelevant or inappropriate to their personal, social or cultural circumstances will be ineffectual, can be offensive, and may have a negative impact on the woman and the outcomes.

The booking visit and the process of establishing a partnership is not about 'becoming friends' or 'being nice'. It is about developing an effective working relationship at a professional level, between human beings.

REVIEWING THE PAST

The quality and quantity of information shared during the booking visit depends on a number of factors. The specific questions asked by the midwife, the way in which they are asked and the timing of them (in terms of when in the booking process they are asked) may influence a woman's responses, particularly when they relate to sensitive information such as that regarding sexually transmitted infections, abortions or abuse.

It is also important to recognise that a woman's knowledge of her family's health history and that of her own childhood illnesses or operations may be limited, perhaps because of poor access to those details, possibly as a result of family separation or dislocation. Some women may also have limited understanding of the details of treatments or the nature of medical procedures they have undergone. For example, the detail, meaning or significance of differing cervical treatments (such as loop surgery, cone biopsy, laser treatment and the associated terminology such as 'CIN I, II or III') are sometimes not known or understood by women. This means that women, understandably, are sometimes unable to provide the level of detail sought by midwives.

The midwife identifies risk markers from the woman's history, and discusses them with her. This discussion may include options for testing, screening, treatment, self-care, referral for consultation with situation-appropriate specialists, support and further information sharing.

CLINICAL POINT

Antenatal mental health—routinely review, screen, assess and act

Mental ill-health is an issue at any time, but the unique stresses, treatment limitations and life-changing experiences of pregnancy, birth and the postnatal period result in it being a time of particular risk with potentially serious consequences for both women and babies/children (Austin et al., 2011; Schmied et al., 2016). At its most serious it can result in the death of women or babies. For the period 2006–15 suicide was 'the leading "single" cause of maternal death in New Zealand' ... and 'almost seven times that reported for the UK for 2006–2014' (PMMRC, 2017, p. 128). At a lower level 'perinatal depression and anxiety are associated with poorer outcomes for women including risk of self-harm, poor physical health, breakdown in relationships, unhappiness in the maternal role and, for some, less capacity to nurture their infant' ... for children this can result in 'poorer cognitive functioning, impairments in language, physical, psychological, emotional and behavioural problems' (Schmied et al., 2016, p. 2). As the primary providers of maternity care, midwives are responsible for reviewing, screening, assessing and referring appropriately for mental health concerns—although not for treating mental ill-health.

The PMMRC report notes that 'repeat themes arising in recent maternal suicide reviews include lack of recognition of the risk for pregnant women presenting with suicidal ideation and failure to refer promptly for assessment and treatment, lack of information sharing between services, and discontinuation or changes of anti-depressant medication in pregnancy without full discussion of risks and/or clinical oversight' (PMMRC, 2017, p. 128).

During the booking visit, or at first contact, midwives need to ask women about past or present mental illness, past or present treatment by a specialist mental health service and family history of severe mental illness, including perinatal illness in a first-degree relative (PMMRC, 2017, p. 129). If a woman discloses a history of mental ill-health, it needs to be considered an important risk marker for both antenatal and postnatal ill-health and regular reviews need to be undertaken during pregnancy as part of their antenatal care. Any significant history or present ill-health requires both GP communication and specialist referral (with consent). While there are a number of screening tools available, the Australian clinical guidelines on pregnancy care recommend the use of the Edinburgh Postnatal Depression Scale (EPDS) for antenatal assessment, at least once early in pregnancy and preferably twice (DOH, 2018). (It is also recommended postnatally.) Women who score 10–12 need reviewing again at the next antenatal visit, those with a score of 13 referred, as they are likely to have depression and/or anxiety, and those with a score of ≥15 referral to a specialist (Austin et al., 2011; DOH, 2018).

There are a number of clinical guidelines for practice available (Austin et al., 2011; New Zealand Guidelines Group, 2008; NICE, 2021; Sanger et al., 2015). The Australian 'Clinical Practice Guidelines *Depression and Related Disorders–Anxiety, Bipolar Disorder and Puerperal Psychosis—the Perinatal Period*' are the most comprehensive, context relevant and holistic, although under update review (Austin et al., 2011, available online at http://resources.beyondblue.org.au/prism/file?token=BL/0891). A shorter summary article of these guidelines is also published (Austin et al., 2013). (Further reading from the New Zealand and Australian contexts: Ogbo et al., 2018; Schmied et al., 2013, 2016; Underwood et al., 2017; Waldie et al., 2015; Yelland & Brown, 2014.)

(See Ch. 22 for discussion on screening, assessment and consultation options, and Ch. 37 for discussion on risk markers and potential complications in pregnancy.)

Using a structured history incorporating a cue sheet (Box 23.1) is likely to get 'more and better information' than an unstructured format (Lilford et al., 1992). Documentation of shared information is very important for both the woman and the midwife. During the care, it is appropriate for the woman to carry her own maternity notes (DOH, 2020; NICE, 2019). Upon completion of care, the midwife also needs to keep either the original or a copy of these documents, in order to meet her respective professional and legal requirements.

Identifying the present

As part of the booking visit, the midwife also undertakes a 'current health review' (see Box 23.2) and an initial examination, in order to establish baseline information and facilitate the process of planning the care. All the issues identified in the 'current health review', and those raised in the aforementioned historical health review, have the potential to influence the process or outcome of pregnancy, although some are more significant than others. They should provide the midwife with cues as to the nature and detail of any physical examination that may be required.

Currently, there is no consensus as to the detail, make-up and content of a 'routine' initial physical

Box 23.1 Historical health review

Maternity: midwifery and obstetric

- Gravida—number of pregnancies (includes living children, miscarriage, termination of pregnancy, ectopic pregnancy, stillbirth, neonatal death)
- Parity—number of babies born at or beyond 20 weeks, pre-term (<37 weeks), post-term (>42 weeks)
- Contraceptive history
- Past pregnancy/pregnancies—date, place, pregnancy complications, labour spontaneous/induced, gestation, duration of complications, outcome, name, sex, weight, breast/artificial feeding, postnatal complications (PPH), social/economic/cultural issues
- Other

Risk markers

- Chronic hypertension—genetic hypertension or pre-eclampsia (degree), gestational diabetes
- Multiple pregnancy—congenital abnormalities, antenatal anaemia (Hb <105)
- Pre-term birth (<37 weeks)—small baby (IUGR/SGA), APH
- Post-term birth (>42 weeks)—large baby (>4500 g), shoulder dystocia
- Assisted birth (forceps/ventouse)—lower-segment caesarean section, vaginal birth after caesarean section, postpartum haemorrhage (>1000 mL or treated)
- Rh sensitisation/ABO incompatibility—perinatal infection
- Antenatal or perinatal depression/psychosis
- Other

Medical

- Essential hypertension, diabetes, heart disease
- Asthma, TB/pulmonary disease, thyroid disease
- Neurological disorder (epilepsy), musculoskeletal disease
- Renal/urinary tract disorder
- Haematology disorder, liver disease, digestive disorder
- STI, infertility, cervical abnormality/treatment
- Polycystic ovaries, fibroids, endometriosis
- Allergies, infections, vaginal/urinary tract abnormality/treatment
- HIV status risk (high/low; routine screening offer)
- MRSA risk (high/low)
- TB risk (high/low)
- Medical examination

Box 23.1 Historical health review—cont'd

- Surgery (what, when, complications)
- Blood transfusion
- Physical, sexual, psychological abuse
- Female genital mutilation/female circumcision
- Vitamin D deficiency
- Thromboembolism
- Haemoglobinopathies
- Other

Mental health

- Depression, anxiety, eating disorder, other: +/− treated (see Mental Health clinical point)

Family health

- Maternal—diabetes, hypertension/preeclampsia, multiple pregnancy, asthma, intellectual disability, haemoglobinopathy, allergies, mental ill-health, other
- Congenital abnormalities (maternal and/or paternal)—chromosomal, limb deformity, metabolic, neural tube defect, cardiac defect, cleft palate, dislocated hip(s), severe infant morbidity, SIDS/SUDI, other

ABO=ABO blood group; APH=antepartum haemorrhage; Hb=haemoglobin level; HIV=human immunodeficiency virus; IUGR=intrauterine growth restriction; MRSA=methicillin-resistant *Staphylococcus aureus*; PPH=postpartum haemorrhage; Rh=rhesus factor; SGA=small for gestational age; SIDS=sudden infant death syndrome; STI=sexually transmitted infection; SUDI=sudden unexpected death in infancy; TB=tuberculosis.

Box 23.2 Current health review

Physical

- General health
- Any underlying/ongoing health concerns
- Medical examination (as appropriate)
- Cervical smear screen—if/when (indicated now?)
- Any sign of current infection (review risk re STI)
- BP, pulse, MSU (for dipstick and culture if not NAD)
- Height (cm), weight (kg), calculate BMI
- Diet (details), exercise (details)
- Smoking (what, how much, readiness to reduce/stop)
- Alcohol, drugs (what, how much, readiness to reduce/stop)
- Safety from violence (if woman alone, or wait until the next visit or arrange another time; ask *all* women)
- Medications and supplements (details), folic acid
- COVID-19 vaccination status

Emotional/psychological

- General health, psychological/mental wellbeing (see Mental Health clinical point)
- Feelings about pregnancy and having a baby
- Planned/unplanned and welcome/unwelcome pregnancy

Social

- Autonomy, support, resources, employment, community 'belonging' or isolated
- Is there a current relationship—partner, husband? Is it stable and supportive?

Cultural

- Identity, integration/isolation, support, resources, needs
- Safety issues

Spiritual

- Any spiritual and/or religious beliefs that may influence needs, choices or care options
- Current pregnancy: establish EDD
- LMP (sure/unsure), known conception date
- EDD (consider 283-day option)
- Positive pregnancy test
- Menstrual cycle—regular/irregular/frequency, contraception, last cycle and menstruation normal (Y/N, details)

BMI=body mass index; BP=blood pressure; EDD=estimated due date; LMP=last menstrual period; MSU=midstream urine sample; STI=sexually transmitted infection.

examination of a well pregnant woman. Kean & Chan (2007) state that 'there is very little to be gained from a full formal physical examination' (p. 70). The Royal Australian and New Zealand College of Obstetricians and Gynaecologists (RANZCOG) guideline recommends 'a careful medical history and appropriate clinical examination should be undertaken' (RANZCOG, 2019a, p. 3), but gives no detail on what it should comprise, beyond body mass index (BMI). The Australian and WHO guidelines do not mention an initial physical examination (DOH, 2020; WHO, 2016). The current NICE (2019) guidelines recommend measurement of women's weight and height to identify their BMI, but not routine breast and pelvic examinations. In contrast, Frye (1998), in the context of midwifery care in the USA, recommends a full medical examination including the above checks and details such as assessment of lymph nodes, reflexes, mouth, eyes and lungs, in addition to the 'vital signs'. It is debatable whether such an examination is indicated, or within the scope of midwifery practice. Certainly, midwives generally work with well women, and should have sound knowledge of normal anatomy, physiology and organ and hormone function as well as being able to recognise signs of dysfunction, but a *routine* full examination may be both inappropriate and outside the midwifery scope of practice. To date, there is limited evidence available which addresses this issue to any significant degree.

It is important to distinguish between something that is offered routinely, and that which is offered in response to risk markers. For example, offering vaginal swabs as a screening test routinely is not currently recommended, but screening may well be indicated for a woman with a history of unsafe sex practice and/or *Chlamydia* infection. In such cases it is appropriate to discuss the option of carrying out a diagnostic test to identify whether there is a current infection, along with issues of self-care, and the potential risks from such an infection to the woman's health and wellbeing and that of her baby.

Planning the future

Working through the relevant aspects of the woman's past and present health status enables a foundation to be established, which facilitates effective planning for the future care of the woman. The midwife and the woman are now in a position to make decisions about the relevance or appropriateness of particular screening or diagnostic tests, and to determine whether there is a need for referral for specialist consultation. This may be to any one or a number of specialists and/or allied health providers, such as an obstetrician, dietitian, physiotherapist, psychiatrist, sexual health specialist or geneticist. They are also in a position to make decisions about those other matters that are outlined in decision point 1 (see Box 23.4).

CLINICAL POINT

Routine family/domestic violence screening

Domestic and family violence is recognised as a global health problem. It is recommended that all midwives routinely screening women for the risk of domestic and family violence (DFV). Awaiting self-identification from women, or screening based on 'perceived' signs or symptoms of risk, consistently misses up to 98% of women living with DFV. DFV is about power and control and includes behaviours causing physical, sexual or psychological harm including controlling behaviours, physical aggression, sexual coercion and psychological abuse (Baird et al., 2021). DFV is estimated to be experienced by approximately one in every three or four women, with one woman in six experiencing DFV during pregnancy (Auger et al., 2021). DFV is known to escalate during pregnancy, with the violence beginning during pregnancy for a quarter of women who experience DFV and worsening in frequency and severity where violence was previously occurring (Baird et al., 2021). Violence in pregnancy is associated with a number of additional and serious risks, which include: repeated miscarriage, antepartum haemorrhage (APH), premature rupture of membranes (PROM), premature labour, placental abruption and low-birth-weight babies. There is a definite correlation between DFV and concurrent child abuse.

DFV screening is a tool, which women accept and approve of, for exposing the hidden (Baird et al., 2021). Midwives are in a unique and privileged position, as they walk beside women at such a pinnacle transition in their lives. Remember that leaving a DFV relationship is a process, and you don't know which point a woman is at; but every single time you ask a woman directly, have a conversation about DFV, offer non-judgmental support and appropriate referral to specialist agencies, you are making a momentous difference to women suffering and surviving DFV.

Box 23.3 lists family/domestic violence resources in New Zealand and Australia.

Box 23.3 Additional resources—family/domestic violence

- Ministry of Health, New Zealand. *Family violence assessment and intervention guideline*. 2016: https://www.health.govt.nz/publication/family-violence-assessment-and-intervention-guideline-child-abuse-and-intimate-partner-violence
- Ministry of Health, Australia. *Pregnancy care guidelines: Part E: Social and emotional screening*. 2020: https://www.health.gov.au/resources/pregnancy-care-guidelines/part-e-social-and-emotional-screening/family-violence

A MIDWIFE'S STORY

'Maria', a woman from South America of strong religious faith, had unexpectedly become pregnant by 'Tom', a Kiwi man, which led to a rapid wedding. She worked part-time, had no family in New Zealand and did not drive. Tom shared care for his school-aged son from a previous relationship. He attended almost all antenatal visits, sitting in physical contact with Maria most of the time, overtly expressing his adoration of her. Family violence screening was carried out in the second trimester, at a rare visit when Maria was alone. No violence was disclosed.

Antenatally Maria often contacted the midwife with discomfort or pain. She experienced repeated thrush infections, some 'fainting episodes', significant pain from uterine fibroids, sacroiliac pain, headaches and constipation, suspected urinary tract infections and an episode of vaginal herpes lesions.

One afternoon, when Maria was at about 30 weeks gestation, Tom phoned the midwife asking if Maria had called, as she had 'stormed out of the house after an argument, in her *typical fiery South American manner*, saying she was bleeding and going to the hospital'. He told the midwife that she was not bleeding, just angry, and that there was nothing to be concerned about regarding the wellbeing of the woman or their baby. Maria didn't go to the hospital or call the midwife. The midwife accepted Tom's assurances and didn't follow up and check on the wellbeing of the woman. The incident was not mentioned at the next antenatal visit.

All of the family struggled to adjust postnatally, following a clinically necessary caesarean section birth. Tom reported that Maria was stressed and anxious, and struggling with caring for herself and their baby. At 3 weeks postpartum the midwife was called to see Maria on a Saturday evening, when Tom was out. Maria's left breast was reddened and very tender. After assessment, when it was clear that there was trauma to the breast which was not caused by a breast infection, the woman eventually disclosed that the redness, and developing bruising, had been caused by Tom's knee as he held her down during a fight 2 days earlier. Following the midwife's appropriate response to this injury, a further three episodes of physical violence during pregnancy were then disclosed, including Maria having had her head held under the water in a bath for a prolonged period as 'punishment' for a misdemeanour. Tom's son had also witnessed this violence.

The woman had not felt able to disclose the violence previously, partly because she accepted her husband's version of previous violence as being her own fault, and partly because she had defended herself and hit him back sometimes. She had not previously recognised Tom's refusal to shop for groceries and withholding of food money from her as family violence. The midwife was very pleased to have attended a workshop on family violence just the weekend prior to this incident. She felt equipped to use the phrases she had learned and provide appropriate information and support for the woman, in a way that she had not previously. Ongoing counselling and support was arranged for Maria from Women's Refuge, her GP and a home-help agency, and Tom and the family were to attend counselling. No further violence occurred prior to discharge from maternity care at 6 weeks postpartum. Maria chose to stay with Tom.

Questions

1. Describe the cues for potential family violence during the antenatal period. Consider:
   a. Tom's over-attentive behaviour and close physical contact during visits as potentially overprotective rather than adoring
   b. the frequent contact with the midwife reporting numerous types of physical pain and discomfort
   c. the episode when Maria left the house telling Tom she was bleeding and threatening to contact the hospital or midwife.
2. How might you, as Maria's midwife, have responded to those cues? Consider:
   a. arranging an antenatal visit alone with Maria for family violence screening (you might need to call her at work and generate a reason for the visit)
   b. discussing all types of family violence, including non-physical, and their unacceptability
   c. recording Maria's work hours and contact details, including an alternative postal address, and storing them separately from Maria's maternity notes
   d. providing written information for Maria (including a small card with emergency contact numbers which could be hidden in a shoe, possibly sent to her work address)
   e. reassuring Maria that she can call you at any time and you will help her get support from appropriate agencies, and that she is not to blame for the violence.

DECISION POINTS

Decision points are a significant new initiative in the organisation of antenatal care. They provide a systematic framework for organising care, and are articulated in the New Zealand College of Midwives' *Midwives' Handbook for Practice* (NZCOM, 2015). The Australian guidelines also list care recommendations for specific visits by gestation (DOH, 2020). A modified and expanded version of these decision points has been developed for this chapter, a key theme of which is a holistic midwifery approach to antenatal care.

The decision points are based on eight time frames, which are loosely tied to gestation periods through the course of pregnancy (Boxes 23.4–23.11). They consist of

Box 23.4 Decision point 1: the booking visit (before 12 weeks)

1 Information sharing

Choices for maternity care

Information on community groups and agencies

Woman's:

- plans regarding pregnancy, birth and early parenting (care plan)
- experience of pregnancy
- physiological changes (see explanatory sections)
- social, emotional, medical, physical, cultural situation

Midwife's practice—support, time off, how to contact, confidentiality

Communication needs assessment, e.g. interpreter

Folic acid supplementation, iodine supplementation (New Zealand)

Options for:

- antenatal education (see explanatory sections)
- place for birth
- midwifery student involvement, if relevant

2 Assessment and screening

Review history (see Box 23.1):

- maternity, medical, social, physical, psychological
- identify and discuss alerting factors or risk markers

Review current health status (see Box 21.2):

- physical, social, emotional/mental and cultural
- identify and discuss alerting factors or risk markers
- establish EDD (see explanatory sections)

Initial antenatal screening—routine (with informed consent)

- blood
  - routinely offered (see explanatory sections)
  - options from risk markers—STIs, TB, hepatitis C, vitamin D deficiency
- urine—MSU and dipstick urinalysis and/or microscopy and culture (see explanatory sections)

Screening options if risk markers from history or current health review:

- Down syndrome and other conditions—offer routine screening blood tests: MSS1 (combined with NT scan) or MSS2

3 Active decision making

LMC—decided prior to 'booking' process

Screening options—routinely offered and options due to 'risk markers'

Referral—if indicated and wanted—for 'specialist' input (e.g. obstetrician, dietitian, physiotherapist)

Meeting/involvement of midwifery student

Time, place, frequency of antenatal care

4 Health promotion and education

Lifestyle affirmation, or review 'readiness' for change

Diet, exercise, self-care, employment

Safety—physical, emotional, cultural

Avoiding infections—listeria, toxoplasmosis, STIs, etc

EDD=estimated due date; LMC=lead maternity carer; MSS1, MSS2=first- and second-trimester maternal serum screening; MSU=midstream urine sample; NT=nuchal translucency; STIs=sexually transmitted infections; TB=tuberculosis.

four categories of cues that provide a guiding form and structure for care. These cues alert the midwife to the components of what is currently considered appropriate and necessary in the provision of comprehensive antenatal care. The four categories include cues about information sharing, assessment and screening, active decision making, and health promotion and education. These categories are intended to assist the midwife to consider the various dimensions of care beyond the purely clinical aspects of it, and reflect a holistic understanding of the care process without being overly prescriptive. It is important that the midwife actively considers each aspect of care raised in the decision point framework with reference to the social, emotional, physical and cultural realities of each woman.

A range of components of routine antenatal care outlined in the decision points are described and discussed in detail in the explanatory sections which follow. These explanatory sections cover:

- estimated due date
- routine antenatal blood screening
- routine blood pressure screening
- routine urine screening
- physiological changes of pregnancy.

Details of the issues identified in the decision points but not covered in this chapter are covered in other chapters.

EXPLANATORY SECTIONS

Estimated due date (EDD)

While EDD has traditionally referred to the *expected* date for delivery, it does not here. *Estimated* due date is both more accurate a description and more midwifery friendly. Midwives do not *expect* women to give birth on this date, rightly so, with less than 5% of women doing so (Lynch & Zhang, 2007). The date is an estimate only.

Box 23.5 Decision point 2: 16 to 20 weeks

1 Information sharing

Decisions made since last visit—re screening, care plan, lifestyle changes

Results from screening or diagnostic tests, and implications discussed

Normal physiological changes (see explanatory sections)

Expectations re first fetal movements—timing range, initial irregularity

Options re employment and parental leave

2 Assessment and screening

Assess woman's physical and mental wellbeing—discuss options re physiological changes

Screen:

- urinalysis (see explanatory sections) blood pressure
- blood test: offer MSS2 for Down syndrome and other conditions, if screening not offered earlier (16 weeks optimal)
- discuss option of fetal anomaly scan (18–20 weeks), timing, expectations, limitations, information, diagnostic and decision options
- family violence (routine, see Ch. 9)

Assess baby's wellbeing:

- size (fundal height—see explanatory sections)
- growth, movements, heart rate (Doppler/Sonicaid)

3 Active decision making

Offer information on vaccination for coronavirus (COVID-19)

Scan (decision may be made after visit, form given if requested, self-booked)

Antenatal education decision made—classes booked if desired

Plans re infant feeding

4 Health promotion and education

Breastfeeding promoted—information, resources and support options

Self-care and lifestyle—diet, exercise, support re healthy changes, employment issues

Pelvic floor exercises

MSS2 = second-trimester maternal serum screening.

Box 23.6 Decision point 3: 20 to 24 weeks

1 Information sharing

Normal physiological changes (see explanatory sections)

Relationship issues—changes, support, involvement of partner/friends

Results from and experience of anomaly scan (if done)

2 Assessment and screening

Assess woman's physical and mental wellbeing—discuss options re physiological changes

Screen—urinalysis, blood pressure

Assess baby's wellbeing—size (fundal height), growth, movements, heart rate (Doppler/Sonicaid)

3 Active decision making

Place for the birth (if decided)—if hospital: booking forms and arrange visit

Any follow-up from anomaly scan indicated

4 Health promotion and education

Discussion re woman's own wellbeing and preparation for parenthood

Diet, exercise, support, stress minimisation, employment—as relevant/appropriate

Pizza is delivered—women give birth. Here EDD refers to an estimated due date.

Dating in history and Naegele's rule

Women have been calculating their menstrual cycles and pregnancies using lunar months for 'tens of thousands of years' (Frye, 1998). However, the method based on a set number of days following the last menstrual period (LMP) was proposed by Professor Boerhaave in 1709 and popularised by, and subsequently attributed to, Dr Naegele (Baskett & Naegele, 2000). Boerhaave proposed that gestation be calculated 'by counting one week after the last period and by reckoning the nine months of gestation from that time' (cited in Baskett & Naegele 2000, p. 1433). Neither man specified whether it is the first or last day of the LMP that is the start point.

The first day of LMP is currently taken as the starting point, to which nine months and seven days are added.

Box 23.7 Decision point 4: 24 to 28 weeks

1 Information sharing

Signs of premature labour and when to call midwife

Signs of baby's wellbeing—expectations re movements (see explanatory sections)

Normal physiological changes (see explanatory sections)

Discuss emotional and social situation—feelings re pregnancy, financial changes, career/employment implications and plans (timing of work reduction/finishing), support needs and options

2 Assessment and screening

Assess woman's wellbeing—discuss options re physiological changes

Screen:

- urinalysis, blood pressure
- routine blood screen offer—CBC, blood group and rhesus antibodies, gestational diabetes
- family violence (routine)

Assess baby's wellbeing—size (fundal height), growth, movements, heart rate (Pinard or Doppler/Sonicaid)

3 Active decision making

Routinely offer influenza and pertussis (Tdap) vaccination and discuss vaccination for COVID-19 (see Box 23.12)

Continue developing care plan—antenatal education start date, if appropriate, or alternative arrangements (books/videos, resources, support)

Preparations for change of life with new baby:

- emotional, social, practical
- car seat (bought or booked for hire), clothing and bedding

4 Health promotion and education

Postnatal sleeping arrangements—appropriate bed sharing, and risk markers re SIDS/SUDI

Self-care and support networks (check knowledge re community groups and agencies)

CBC=complete blood count; SIDS=sudden infant death syndrome; SUDI=sudden unexpected death in infancy; Tdap=tetanus, diphtheria, acellular pertussis.

Box 23.8 Decision point 5: 30 to 32 weeks

1 Information sharing

Check that the woman, and her family, are comfortable with planned place for birth and birth plan discussed, including expectations of midwifery care

Discuss options for working with pain in labour (see Chs 3 and 26)

Discuss signs of preeclampsia, and when to contact midwife

Discuss recommendation for woman going to sleep on her side for fetal wellbeing

Discuss family's expectations and preparations for life with a new baby

Discuss postnatal care plan—re vitamin K and newborn metabolic screen test

Discuss breastfeeding—'skin to skin', preparation, expectations and support

Discuss safe sleeping, normal newborn behaviour, newborn immunisations plan

2 Assessment and screening

Assess woman's wellbeing—discuss options re physiological changes (see explanatory sections)

Screen—urinalysis (glucose and protein), blood pressure

Assess baby's wellbeing—size (fundal height), growth, movements, heart rate

3 Active decision making

Postnatal care and support—community groups and agencies (well child services)

Plans for placenta

Plans for working with pain in labour

Plans for feeding baby—check knowledge, resources, support

4 Health promotion and education

Childcare arrangements (if applicable) for end of pregnancy, labour, early postnatal days

Support and resources for postnatal days

Self-care:

- review employment arrangements, emotional and social situation
- review woman's feelings about birth and parenting—support options

Box 23.9 Decision point 6: 34 to 36 weeks

1 Information sharing

Discuss signs of labour, expectations, support, beliefs and feelings about labour

If hospital birth planned:

- check that all know where it is, check cultural needs
- discuss policies which may affect the woman's choices

If home birth planned—discuss appropriate environment and gear needed

Reminder of recommendation for woman going to sleep on her side for fetal wellbeing

Physiological changes and expectations (see explanatory sections)

Discuss postnatal emotional and social changes and expectations—review mental health history and current wellbeing

2 Assessment and screening

Assess woman's wellbeing—discuss options re physiological changes

Screen:

- urinalysis (glucose and protein), blood pressure
- consider blood test of Hb (if woman taking iron or symptomatic) and Rh antibody (if woman Rh neg)

Assess baby's wellbeing:

- size (fundal height), growth, movements, heart rate
- presentation—if not cephalic, discuss referral options (36 weeks)

3 Active decision making

Birth plans identified

Preparation of other child(ren) for changes with new baby

Practical arrangements made for early postnatal days—meals in freezer or support as appropriate

Plans made for labour:

- support people, childcare, resources (food, comfort measures)
- home-birth gear together, or bag packed for hospital

4 Health promotion and education

Self-care—diet, exercise and lifestyle changes for this stage of pregnancy

Review emotional and social situation, review employment plans

Hb=haemoglobin level; Rh=rhesus factor.

The inherent variability in the length of different months has been negated with the conversion of the formula into pregnancy calculators as 'LMP plus 280 days' (Gestation Network, see Online resources). Naegele's rule relies on women's recall of their LMP, which is known to be variable (Wegienka & Baird, 2005). This rule has *all* women ovulating at the same time within a cycle, having a cycle of the same length (which is set at 28 days), and taking the same length of time to gestate. It uses the LMP as a proxy for conception date. A review of the literature reports that, due to variations in the timing of ovulation and conception, fertilisation can potentially occur over a broader time frame than previously defined, making Naegele's rule less reliable, even with a known LMP date (Hunter, 2009, p. 184). The British Confidential Enquiry into Stillbirths and Death in Infancy (CESDI) recommended that the formula be altered to account for variation in cycle length, proposing 'EDD=LMP+280 days+length of cycle–28 days' (cited in Stenhouse et al., 2003). While this might improve the accuracy of the date it is not commonly practised, with manual and online pregnancy calculators having no capacity for this adjustment. Arguably, Naegele's rule standardises pregnancy length as much as ultrasound does; both assume that human gestation is a set length from a particular marker point—Naegele from LMP and ultrasound from a fetal body part measurement at a particular gestation.

As humans do everything else at variable rates—begin to walk and talk, begin and end menstruating, etc.—we know that they will also gestate for varying lengths of time. Research has also variously identified maternal height, ethnicity, parity and age as potentially influential in the length of gestation, although not with predictive reliability (Rosser, 2000).

The EDD has taken on new significance in the contemporary context, with decisions regarding medical screening and interventions demanding standardised gestational age dating. Of significance here is the point that, when known, the LMP is still a worthwhile reference point, and where the planned EDD is postponed by more than 7 days then early fetal compromise could be present and this signals the need for midwives to pay particular attention to the growth and wellbeing of these babies. Using customised fetal growth charts is likely to provide a more accurate and useful monitoring tool than standardised measures for these women and their babies (see Online resources).

Box 23.10 Decision point 7: 38 to 40 weeks

1 Information sharing

Review signs of labour, expectations, support, beliefs and feelings about labour

Recognising labour, and when and how to contact midwife

Review woman's knowledge of risk markers:

- fresh vaginal blood loss
- reduced fetal movements
- signs of preeclampsia
- ruptured membranes (without contractions, meconium-stained liquor)

Physiological changes and expectations of timing of labour (discuss normal range)

Review blood results (if appropriate)

Discuss pregnancy over 40 weeks

Discuss postnatal care plan, support systems and visits by midwife and any well child caregiver (as applicable)

2 Assessment and screening

Assess woman's wellbeing—discuss options re physiological changes (see explanatory sections)

Screen:

- urinalysis (glucose and protein), blood pressure
- family violence, antenatal depression and/or anxiety (consider using cues or tools in Clinical Point sections)

Assess baby's wellbeing:

- size (fundal height), growth, movements, heart rate
- presentation, descent in the woman's pelvis, liquor volume

Review expected date of birth—check and confirm expected dates

3 Active decision making

Support networks arranged for labour, birth and postnatal

Confirm postnatal care plan re:

- vitamin K
- newborn metabolic screening test

4 Health promotion and education

Review self-care:

- adjustments to life without paid work (if relevant)
- support, opportunities
- diet, exercise, sleep, emotions, self-esteem

Review partner and/or family readiness, support, resources, arrangements for time off work

Discuss first breastfeed and importance of skin-to-skin contact

Box 23.11 Decision point 8: 41 to 42 weeks

1 Information sharing

Discuss wellbeing of woman and baby, family support

Discuss issues and options re 'post-dates' (see Ch. 38)

Discuss option of vaginal exam and membrane sweep/cervical massage

Discuss option of obstetric referral and timing and process of induction of labour, if no spontaneous onset of labour

2 Assessment and screening

Assess woman's wellbeing—discuss options re physiological changes (see explanatory sections)

Screen—urinalysis, blood pressure

Assess baby's wellbeing:

- size (fundal height), growth, movements, heart rate
- presentation, descent in the woman's pelvis, liquor volume
- screen—discuss option of cardiotocograph or scan, to assess baby's wellbeing if indicated
- discuss risk markers—reduced fetal movements, low liquor volume

3 Active decision making

Set plan re assessment of baby and woman's wellbeing—offer referral for consultation

4 Health promotion and education

Additional care and support options

Check support networks and resources

Ultrasound scan dating

Practice guideline recommendations

Currently, the available evidence and practice guidelines internationally state that ultrasound dating is more accurate than LMP-based dating (DOH 2020; NICE 2019). The Australian Government's *Clinical Practice Guidelines: Pregnancy Care* (2020) recommend offering women with an unsure conception date a scan between 8+0 and 13+6 weeks (p. 140), although noting the overlap in the timing of nuchal translucency screening scan between 11+0 and 13+6 weeks and raising the possibility of women having one scan for both measures (with informed consent).

Even with ultrasound gestational age dating, a known LMP remains an important reference point. For women who choose to have an ultrasound, the Australian *Clinical Practice Guidelines: Pregnancy Care* recommend the following (DOH, 2020, p. 140):

- *If the LMP was certain and menstruation regular, compare the LMP estimate to the ultrasound estimate:*
  - *ultrasound performed between 6 and 13 weeks pregnancy: if the two dates differ by 5 days or less, use the LMP estimate; if the dates differ by more than 5 days, use the ultrasound estimate*
  - *ultrasound performed between 13 and 24 weeks pregnancy: if the two dates differ by 10 days or less, use the LMP estimated; if the dates differ by more than 10 days, use the ultrasound estimate*
- *if the ultrasound was performed between 6 and 24 weeks pregnancy and the LMP was not certain or menstruation irregular, use the ultrasound estimate*
- *if the LMP was certain and menstruation regular and no ultrasound was performed between 6 and 24 weeks pregnancy (or none with a heartbeat), use the LMP estimate.*

Pregnancy calculators

Pregnancy or gestation calculators are the most common tool for midwives identifying women's EDD. They are subject to both intra- and inter-calculator variability (Ross, 2003), and so should be checked against each other and the most reliable chosen. The Gestation Network website (see Online resources) also has software which calculates EDD from the LMP—although, as with the cardboard calculators, it currently does not allow for variance in cycle length and works on the 280-day rule.

CRITICAL THINKING EXERCISE

Aroha is pregnant. She is not sure when her baby is due. The first day of her LMP was 15 February 2018. She has a regular cycle, which lasts 5 days, every 30 days.

1. Calculate the EDD using three different pregnancy calculators.
2. Calculate the EDD manually using Naegele's rule.
3. Calculate the EDD using the computer software mentioned in the text.
4. Compare the EDDs from each method, and consider the implications of any potential variation.
5. What information would you share with Aroha regarding her EDD?

Summary points: estimated due date

When working with women to identify their EDD, midwives should:

- identify the first day of LMP, if known
- ask whether it was a normal period in timing, length and volume
- ask about the normal cycle—length and regularity
- ask about contraceptive use prior to conception
- use Naegele's rule or the pregnancy calculator to get an EDD (consider using LMP plus 282 days for a 28-day cycle)
- discuss variability and expectations regarding the actual timing of the birth
- review pregnancy signs, symptoms and experiences and compare with estimated dating
- ask if they can palpate the woman's abdomen to compare uterine size with dates
- consider the option of a scan if the woman has no idea of LMP or timing of conception, and date-specific screening is to be undertaken, or if her uterine size is significantly mismatched with EDD on palpation.

Routine antenatal blood screening

The use of blood tests as a **routine screening** tool is routine in antenatal care, although there may be variation in the tests included or offered between states and countries (DOH, 2020; MOH, 2017; National Screening Unit (NSU), 2017). Currently, both Australia and New Zealand have the following tests offered routinely:

- blood group and rhesus factor
- rhesus, red cell and ABO antibodies
- full/complete blood count (FBC/CBC) in early pregnancy and 28 weeks
- syphilis
- hepatitis B
- rubella antibodies
- human immunodeficiency virus (HIV)
- Down syndrome and other conditions (first-trimester maternal serum screening in combination with nuchal translucency scan, or second-trimester maternal serum screening)
- diabetes (GDM, or undiagnosed type 1 or 2):
  - New Zealand also routinely offers screening for undiagnosed pre-existing diabetes (HbA_{1c}) with the first trimester antenatal blood test; and screening for gestational diabetes (GDM) at 24–8 weeks either polycose/oral glucose challenge test (OGCT), if no risk factors, or oral glucose tolerance test (OGTT), if risk factors (see guideline—MOH, 2014).
  - Australian guidelines recommend a two-stage approach, with the selective offer of first-trimester HbA_{1c} test for women with risk factors for diabetes, including

Aboriginal and Torres Strait Island women, and universal screening at 24–8 weeks (DOH, 2020, p. 206).

CLINICAL POINT

- In Australia, anti-D (Rh_0 (D) immunoglobulin) is offered prophylactically at 28 and 34 weeks gestation to women with Rhesus-negative blood groups, and also after any potentially sensitising events.
- In New Zealand, anti-D is offered only after any potentially sensitising events.

(For further discussion on anti-D and Rhesus sensitisation, see Ch. 22.)

CRITICAL THINKING EXERCISE

Mai is 14 weeks pregnant with her first child when she first seeks maternity care. She is 24 years old, and a recent immigrant of West African ethnic origin. She and her partner Ahut are well educated and have good English-language skills.

1. What tests would be carried out if you ordered 'routine' initial blood screening for Mai?
2. Describe what is being tested, and its potential significance.
3. What additional blood screening tests might you consider discussing with Mai and Ahut, and what information would inform this discussion?
4. What written information is available for them in your region, on either 'routine' or 'additional' blood tests?

For detailed discussion on the conditions being screened for, see Frye (1998). The issues of the nature of screening itself, informed choice and the politics regarding antenatal screening are also addressed in Ch. 22 and elsewhere, for example Grimes & Schulz (2002), Oats (2000), Searle (1997) and Strong (2000). Gates (2004) addresses some of the political issues involved, as do Parker et al. (2002) and Santalahti et al. (1998).

Debate continues over the appropriateness of universal versus risk-based screening, and opt-in versus opt-out screening, for the following conditions, with each currently offered to women considered to have risk factors in both New Zealand and Australia:

- hepatitis C (HCV)
- chlamydia
- gonorrhoea
- vitamin D deficiency
- haemoglobinopathies (e.g. sickle cell and thalassaemia)
- cytomegalovirus (CMV)
- tuberculosis (TB).

See Ch. 22 for discussion on these conditions and contemporary screening options offered. (See also Box 23.12 for additional resources for perinatal infections.)

Box 23.12 Additional resources—perinatal infections

The booklet 'Management of perinatal infections' (Palasanthiran et al., 2014), published by the Australasian Society for Infectious Diseases, has algorithms for the maternal and neonatal diagnosis and management of the following perinatal infections: cytomegalovirus, enterovirus, hepatitis B, hepatitis C, herpes simplex virus, human immunodeficiency virus, *Listeria,* tuberculosis, parvovirus, rubella, group B *Streptococcus,* toxoplasma, syphilis and varicella zoster virus. It is available free online at: http://www.asid.net.au/resources/clinical-guidelines.

Vaccinations for women during pregnancy

New Zealand

- Influenza recommended and government funded (available Mar–Dec) at any stage in pregnancy
- Pertussis (in combined tetanus, diphtheria, pertussis (Tdap) vaccine) recommended and government funded 28–38 weeks: (http://www.health.govt.nz/our-work/preventative-health-wellness/immunisation/new-zealand-immunisation-schedule)
- COVID-19 recommended and government funded (two vaccination course) appropriately spaced in pregnancy, as per current guidelines

Australia

- Influenza recommended and funded on national immunisation program (NIP) all year and any stage in pregnancy
- Pertussis (Tdap) recommended for third trimester, but not funded under NIP—contact state or territory health department for local funding details: http://www.immunise.health.gov.au/internet/immunise/publishing.nsf/Content/pregnant-women
- COVID-19 recommended and government funded (two vaccination course) appropriately spaced in pregnancy, as per current guidelines (see Commonwealth and state Health Department websites for all updates).

RESEARCH ACTIVITY

Syphilis

1. What is syphilis? How is it transmitted?
2. What are the stages, and what distinguishes them?
3. At which stage does it spread into the bloodstream?
4. How is it treated?
5. Why is it an issue for pregnant women?

Iron measures, levels and supplementation

In the context of routine antenatal care, the midwife uses the red cell results from the CBC primarily as part of the process of screening for iron deficiency anaemia (IDA). Potential signs and symptoms of anaemia include tiredness, dizziness, tinnitus, feeling cold, dry or itchy skin, infections, irritation or poor concentration, palpitations or breathlessness, tachycardia, headaches, pallor, glossitis and koilonychia (Coggins, 2001; Jordan, 2010). Anaemia is potentially a significant threat to the health and wellbeing of women and their babies. For example, for women it can result in lowered immunity, postnatal depression, difficulty with lactation; and for babies it can contribute to premature birth, low birth weight, reduced neonatal iron stores and impaired cognitive and psychomotor development (Crowther, 2010; Milman, 2012; Pavord et al., 2020; Ray et al., 2020). IDA is the most common cause of anaemia, with folate, vitamin $B_{12,}$ haemoglobinopathy and haemolytic anaemia as minor causes (Milman, 2008). Physiological changes induced by pregnancy may expose underlying anaemia, or it may develop during pregnancy.

Haemoglobin (Hb) levels have traditionally been used as a primary measure of anaemia, as 'about 70% of iron in the body is in haemoglobin' (Jordan, 2010, p. 250). There is ongoing debate over the appropriate reference ranges for Hb during pregnancy, the boundaries between physiological changes and pathological changes requiring intervention in the form of supplementation and whether routine supplementation is appropriate (Pasricha et al., 2018; Pavord et al., 2020; Peña-Rosas et al., 2015a). The Australian National Blood Authority (NBA, 2015) states that 'the optimal Hb level to be achieved through treatment during pregnancy has not been established' (p. 32). The current WHO Hb cut-off points for anaemia are <110 g/L in the first and third trimesters and <105 g/L in the second trimester (Pasricha et al., 2018). The Australian guidelines use the thresholds of 110 g/L until 20 weeks gestation and 105g/L for the rest of pregnancy (DOH, 2020, p. 196). The new UK guideline (British Society of Haematology) uses 110g/L for only the first trimester, 105g/L after 12 weeks and 100g/L postpartum (Pavord et al., 2020). Despite this debate, Hb remains the routine screening test recommended for IDA by the Australian and British guidelines (DOH, 2020; NICE, 2019; Pavord et al., 2020).

More recently there has been an increased focus on 'iron deficiency' (ID), where a woman has low iron stores but not anaemia. The measure used most commonly to detect this is serum ferritin (SF), which is being advocated as the best single marker of iron status in pregnancy, in the absence of inflammation (WHO, 2020). Its use in combination with Hb is advocated by some (Milman, 2006; Pasricha et al., 2010; Walsh et al., 2011). Parameters for pregnancy-specific reference ranges, normal physiological changes in SF and their clinical significance are not yet clearly established (Pavord et al., 2020). The WHO has set a cut off of <15mcg/L (WHO, 2020), which is the rate best supported by published evidence to date (Daru et al., 2017). (The only study which identified <30mcg/L has major limitations—see Daru et al., 2017). Also, SF can be raised in the presence of inflammation, so a high level is not necessarily indicative of high iron stores alone. The inclusion of SF in routine screening is not currently recommended; although the recently updated Australian guideline recommends the addition of SF to screening where there is high prevalence of IDA (DOH, 2020). The whole clinical picture needs consideration, and not any one measure in isolation.

There is no debate regarding the routine offer of screening of women for anaemia—it is recommended universally. Midwives may consider either routinely or selectively offering to check the SF level (along with the Hb) for women more likely to have ID or develop IDA—for example, those who have a history of anaemia, heavy menses or postpartum haemorrhage, recent blood donation, short time between pregnancies, multiple pregnancy, parity of ≥3, vegetarian/vegan or poor nutrition diet, low socioeconomic status, teenagers and indigenous women (Pasricha et al., 2010; Pavord et al, 2020).

The DOH, RANZCOG, NBA, British Society for Haematology and NICE guidelines recommend against routine iron supplementation (DOH, 2020; NBA, 2015; NICE, 2017; Pavord et al., 2020; RANZCOG, 2019b).This is supported by research indicating that iron supplementation for women with Hb levels >135 g/L may contribute to morbidity associated with high Hb levels (Dewey & Oaks, 2017). At issue here is the distinction between normal physiology and pathology. Supplementation with iron, or anything else, should be done with care and with cognisance of the indications for its use, and its potential effect on the physiology of pregnancy and on the sometimes-delicate balances which exist within the human body (Koleini et al., 2021). 'More is better' does not apply in this context (Dewey & Oaks, 2017).

All of the guidelines recommend that women with anaemia or ID be offered iron supplementation. Recent research has also identified alternate day oral supplementation is likely to be more effective than daily, due to it inducing a rise in serum hepcidin, and the reduction in gastric side effects (Stoffel et al., 2020; see also Roy & Pavord, 2018). (For further discussion on anaemia and related issues, see Ch. 21 for details of dietary options, and Ch. 33 for pharmacological options.)

The red cell values of a CBC may also signal haemoglobinopathies such as thalassaemia and sickle-cell anaemia, which require further testing and specialist care. Ethnicities with greater incidence of particular haemoglobinopathies are various, but include Māori and Pacific Islanders, as well as Asian, African, Mediterranean and Transcaucasian peoples (see Box 23.13 for additional information resources, and Ch. 32).

Routine blood pressure screening

Blood pressure measurement and monitoring is a core feature of routine antenatal care (Fig. 23.2). Blood pressure

Box 23.13 Additional resources—haemoglobinopathies

- Thalassaemia Australia: http://www.thalassaemia.org.au/
- UK Thalassaemia Society: http://www.ukts.org/

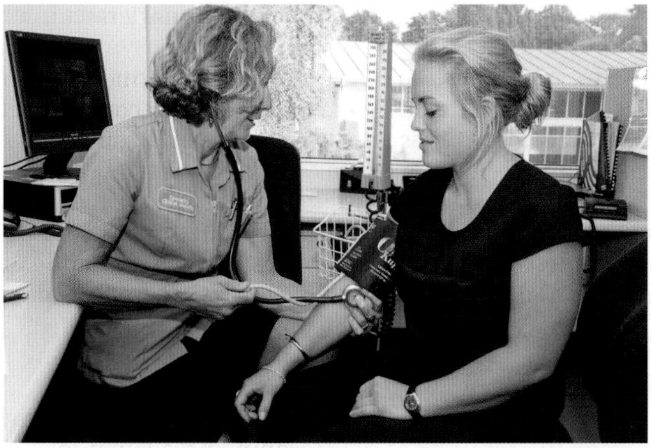

FIGURE 23.2 A midwife taking an antenatal blood pressure recording
(Reproduced with the permission of the New Zealand College of Midwives)

(BP) may be defined as 'the force exerted against the arterial walls when the heart pumps', and 'the blood pressure reading is a reflection of how hard the heart must work to adequately circulate the blood' (Frye, 1998, p. 420). Blood pressure changes in a healthy pregnancy are characterised by a fall in blood pressure, detectable in the first trimester, usually reaching its lowest point in the second trimester and rising to pre-conception levels towards the end of the third trimester (Lowe et al., 2014). Taking blood pressure is essentially a screening test for hypertension, and careful measurement is important as the technique used can significantly affect the accuracy of the reading.

CLINICAL POINT

How to measure blood pressure in pregnancy

1. Before you start, ensure the equipment is in good order (bladder has no leaks, slow deflation easy, calibrated yearly).
2. Use an appropriate cuff size—large if arm circumference >33 cm (bladder should encompass 80% of arm and secure snugly. BP will record higher if size or fit is inappropriate).
3. The woman should be sitting with feet and back supported and legs uncrossed, arm horizontal, supported and at heart level.
4. Take measurements after the woman has been seated in this position for at least 3 minutes.
5. If possible, palpate systolic BP at the brachial artery and inflate cuff to 20 mmHg above this level.
6. Deflate the cuff slowly, at approximately 2 mmHg per second.
7. Record systolic BP at Korotkoff I sound and diastolic BP at Korotkoff V (disappearance). Use phase IV only if phase V is not present.

(Sources: Brown et al., 2000; Taylor, 2004)

CRITICAL THINKING EXERCISE

Take the BP of a fellow student, using two different types of sphygmomanometer (and also trying different cuff sizes), and compare the readings. Using the same sphygmomanometer, compare the BP readings of the same woman, with her lying down and sitting up, and on different arms.

What are the implications of any differences found, for the accurate measurement of BP in the antenatal care of pregnant women?

RESEARCH ACTIVITY

Identifying blood pressure values

1. Who was Korotkoff?
2. What are Korotkoff sounds?
3. How many are there?
4. Which ones are used during pregnancy?

The Society of Obstetric Medicine of Australia and New Zealand (SOMANZ) recently updated (June 2015) its guideline for the management of hypertensive disorders of pregnancy, which are contemporary, comprehensive and well referenced; and very useful for midwives (available online) (Lowe et al., 2014).

Sustained elevated BP beyond normal values is referred to as hypertension, which presents some risk to the wellbeing of women and their babies (see Blackburn, 2007). SOMANZ (Lowe et al., 2014) defines hypertension in pregnancy as a systolic BP of ≥140 mmHg and/or a diastolic BP (Korotkoff V) of ≥90 mmHg (p. 3). The group identifies four classifications of hypertension, namely gestational hypertension (GH), preeclampsia (PE), chronic hypertension (CH) and PE superimposed on CH (Lowe et al., 2014). PE, if unrecognised, may develop into eclampsia, which is a major cause of maternal and perinatal morbidity and mortality NICE, 2021.

Preeclampsia

Preeclampsia is a multisystem disorder which is unique to pregnancy, and remains a condition that is difficult to predict, prevent or treat (see discussion in Ch. 37). The SOMANZ criteria for PE are as follows:

Hypertension arising after 20 weeks gestation and the new onset after 20 weeks gestation of one or more of (Lowe et al., 2014, p. 6):

- significant proteinuria—dipstick proteinuria subsequently confirmed by spot urine protein/creatinine ratio ≥30 mg/mmol
- renal insufficiency—serum/plasma creatinine (>90 μmol/L) or oliguria (<80 mL/4h)
- liver involvement—raised serum transaminases and/or severe epigastric/right upper quadrant pain
- neurological involvement—convulsions (eclampsia); hyperreflexia with sustained clonus; severe headache; persistent visual disturbances; stroke

- haematological disturbances—thrombocytopenia; disseminated intravascular coagulation (DIC); haemolysis
- pulmonary oedema
- fetal growth restriction.

Numerous risk markers have been identified over the years (see Ch. 37), although none reliably predict who will develop PE, or when or how unwell they will become.

The risk markers for PE (NICE, 2019) include women who:

- are having their first baby (or first baby with a different partner)
- are 40 years old or older
- last had a baby ≥10 years previously
- have a family history of PE (mother or sister)
- have a personal history of PE
- have a BMI of ≥35
- have a multiple pregnancy
- have pre-existing medical conditions (e.g. chronic hypertension, renal disease, diabetes, antiphospholipid antibodies)
- at booking, have a BP of ≥80.

In the contemporary Australasian context, this group of women may well represent the majority of the total childbearing population; yet only a fraction of the actual total will develop PE, and the majority of women in every one of the above groups will remain well and go on to give birth to a healthy baby. Although we cannot predict or prevent the development of PE, current routine antenatal BP screening does help identify some women who may be showing signs or experiencing symptoms that signal the need for closer monitoring or diagnostic testing; this may facilitate detection of PE prior to it causing morbidity or mortality (Enkin et al., 2000).

The distinction between isolated hypertension (be it chronic or gestational) and PE is an important one, with many more women having hypertension than those who go on to develop PE. Although it is important to recognise that chronic hypertension is a risk factor for the development of super-imposed PE and a range of other pregnancy complications (DOH, 2020).

Midwives have an important role in sharing information with women about the symptoms of PE, such as severe headaches, visual disturbances (not caused by postural hypotension), epigastric pain (not heartburn), or sudden marked swelling of the face, hands and feet. This information needs to be presented in a way that enables women to recognise and respond to symptoms appropriately, rather than frightening them into a hypersensitive state of anxiety. It is important that midwives and women maintain a sense of perspective regarding the actual incidence of this condition, as it is rare, affecting less than 5% of the childbearing population.

Routine urine screening

Urine screening has been considered a routine antenatal, although there is variation in both the method and the markers used, and no consensus about what constitutes best practice. The aim of urine screening is the detection of proteinuria (as a marker for PE and urinary tract infection) and bacteriuria (as a marker for an asymptomatic urinary tract infection). The dipstick urinalysis used routinely at every antenatal visit is easy to use, gives immediate results that are assessed by the midwife, and is markedly cheaper than laboratory microscopy and culture. Unfortunately, it has consistently been found to have poor sensitivity and predictive value for all of the variables it is used to test (DOH, 2020; National Collaborating Centre for Women's and Children's Health, 2008; Waugh et al., 2004).

Screening for proteinuria as a marker for preeclampsia

It is considered routine practice for midwives to ask women to pass urine at every antenatal visit, and to use a dipstick to assess the level of protein present, as part of the diagnosis of PE. The most recent SOMANZ guideline (2014) for the management of hypertensive disorders of pregnancy acknowledges issues with the sensitivity and specificity of dipstick testing, but states that '... in practice, dipstick testing is simple, cheap and an appropriate screening test', and that 'the presence of 2+ or 3+ proteinuria or repeated +1 dipstick testing increases both sensitivity and specificity and, therefore, should be assumed to represent significant proteinuria until proven otherwise by confirmatory tests' (Lowe et al., 2014, p. 7). This position is supported by other antenatal care guidelines (NICE, 2021, WHO, 2016) although the Australian Guidelines for Pregnancy Care (DOH, 2020) recommends testing at the first antenatal visit and states that repeated testing is of little benefit and should be confined to women with other risk factors such as new or pre-existing kidney disease or new or pre-existing hypertension.

Screening for asymptomatic bacteriuria

Routinely offering screening for asymptomatic bacteriuria early in pregnancy is now recommended in the Australian, Canadian, UK and WHO guidelines (DOH, 2020; Moore et al., 2018; NICE, 2021; WHO, 2016). Proteinuria on dipstick is also used to screen for asymptomatic bacteriuria in routine antenatal care, although some practitioners use dipsticks with additional measures for blood, leucocytes and nitrites for this purpose. The aim of screening is to identify those with asymptomatic bacteriuria and to offer (prophylactic) antibiotic treatment to reduce the incidence of pyelonephritis. Asymptomatic bacteriuria is defined as 'the persistent bacterial colonisation of the urinary tract (usually by *Escherichia coli*) without symptoms' (DOH, 2018, p. 252). Asymptomatic bacteriuria is reported to occur in between 2% and 10% of pregnant women, with significant variation between countries and communities, and greater incidence in women of low socioeconomic status (DOH, 2020; Smaill & Vazquez, 2019). Aboriginal Australian women have previously been found to have up to 16% rate of bacteriuria at the initial antenatal visit (Bookallil et al., 2005).

The physiological changes in the urinary tract make acute pyelonephritis much more likely during pregnancy. It is the risk of these women developing pyelonephritis, and its association with pre-term labour, that makes it of interest during pregnancy—although the association with pre-term labour is now less clear-cut than previously thought with conflicting findings from several large studies (Moore et al., 2018; Smaill & Vazquez, 2019). Asymptomatic urinary tract infection alone is not associated with pre-term birth (Chen et al., 2010; Smaill & Vazquez, 2019). If a woman develops pyelonephritis she may possibly have an increased risk of pre-term birth (most commonly at 33–6 weeks) along with other complications such as septicaemia, renal dysfunction and respiratory insufficiency (Smaill & Vazquez, 2019, p. 5). Women who present with clinical signs of pyelonephritis, which may include fever, chills, flank pain / costovertebral tenderness, dysuria and frequency, and possibly nausea and vomiting, need assessment and treatment.

The latest Cochrane review (Smaill & Vazquez, 2019) identified an overall incidence of pyelonephritis in the untreated group of women of 20%, but it ranged from 2.2% to 36% over 12 studies, only three of which have been published in the past 40 years, and vary in care, testing and treatment contexts. The review reported that treatment of asymptomatic bacteriuria will lead to approximately a 75% reduction in the incidence of pyelonephritis (Smaill & Vazquez, 2019). The review also assessed the evidence for the efficacy of antibiotic treatment of asymptomatic bacteriuria for pyelonephritis, pre-term birth and birthweight <2500 g as 'low' certainty evidence.

To date, only one of the studies identified has addressed any of the issues relating to antibiotics themselves, such as allergic reactions, yeast infections, gastrointestinal side effects, the impact on gut flora and the development of bacterial resistance. Bookallil et al. (2005) raised issues of potential exacerbation of *Candida* infection, 'adverse effects' and increased resistance to antibiotics. The Cochrane review does, however, note that the included research does not report on adverse or allergic reactions and that 'there are concerns about the effect of antibiotics on the human microbiome and the developing immune system' (Smaill & Vazquez, 2019, p. 17). The review also states that 'there is no evidence that non-pharmacological interventions, e.g. cranberry juice, are effective' (Smaill & Vazquez, 2019, p. 6). However, the pilot randomised control trial (RCT) cited to support this statement actually found that 'there may be a protective effect of cranberry ingestion against asymptomatic bacteriuria and symptomatic urinary tract infections in pregnancy' (Wing et al., 2008, p. 1367). Unfortunately, there has been no follow-up larger trial to test the robustness of these findings. Issues of the information and options given to, and choices made by, women have not been addressed in the research available on the topic.

The Australian guidelines (DOH, 2020) suggest two options for screening women for asymptomatic bacteriuria:

- midstream urine (MSU) and laboratory microscopy and culture
- MSU and dipstick test for blood, protein, nitrites and leucocytes, which is sent to the laboratory if there is a positive result in any of the four categories.

Women with asymptomatic bacteriuria have a potential risk of developing pyelonephritis and (prophylactic) antibiotics are generally effective, although they do not prevent recolonisation. Midwives need to consider their context of practice when deciding to offer women routine screening for asymptomatic bacteriuria. They need to provide information regarding the screening and treatment options available, including potential antibiotic risks and efficacy rates, in the context of the risks of women developing pyelonephritis, so as to facilitate active and informed decision making by women.

CLINICAL POINT

- In Australia—routine MSU sample taken at booking visit. In some remote areas it is sent only if dipstick is positive for leucocytes, nitrites, protein or blood.
- In New Zealand—MSU at booking is not routine; practice varies.

Screening for glycosuria as a marker for gestational diabetes mellitus

Screening for glycosuria on urinalysis is not considered to be the primary screening test for gestational diabetes mellitus (GDM). Its presence is interpreted as a potential sign of GDM, and blood glucose screening tests for GDM are offered to women (see Ch. 37). Glycosuria is not an independent or reliable marker of GDM; it can also reflect a lowered renal threshold, which is a normal physiological change of pregnancy. Although the NICE guidelines (2021) do note that significant glycosuria on urinalysis would be a reason to consider further testing to exclude gestational diabetes.

There is much ongoing debate regarding routine antenatal screening for GDM. This is reflected by three differing recommendations published:

- The New Zealand Guideline (MOH, 2014) recommends universal screening using HbA_{1c} as part of the 'booking' antenatal blood tests, and at 24–8 weeks the offer of diagnostic testing (75-g OGTT) for women at 'high risk' of GDM and screening (50-g OGCT) for all other women (MOH, 2014).
- The Australian Guideline (DOH, 2020) recommends first-trimester screening, using a fasting glucose or HbA_{1c}, for women with risk factors for gestational diabetes, including Aboriginal and Torres Strait Island women, and routine offer of screening for all women at 24–28 weeks gestation (except those diagnosed in the first trimester).
- The British NICE Guideline (2021) recommends risk-based screening for GDM.

These recommendations are generally referring to blood glucose screening tests. Urine screening, in the form of dipstick glycosuria, is a poor screening test and is no longer discussed as a screening test for gestational diabetes within the guidelines.

Summary: routine urine screening

Despite the questions raised over the sensitivity and predictive accuracy of dipstick screening for proteinuria, this is still generally considered a 'first-line' screening test for midwives to use at each antenatal visit. Given the potential impact of PE, and the fact that hypertension may not be present in over one-third of women who develop it, identifying proteinuria remains an important screening practice.

The usefulness of urine dipsticks for screening for GDM and asymptomatic bacteriuria is less clear. The offer of routine screening for asymptomatic bacteriuria is recommended in contemporary medical literature, using urine culture for reliable results. A routine screening offer by blood test for GDM has also become recommended practice, with some recommendations inclusive of a first-trimester screen and all inclusive of a second-trimester screening test.

It is important for midwives to be aware of the limitations of dipstick urine tests, and understand that they cannot be relied upon in themselves. The whole clinical and personal context of each woman needs to be considered when screening options are discussed and care choices are made. (See Chs 22 and 37 for fuller discussion on risk markers, screening and response to preeclampsia and gestational diabetes, and for details of the signs, symptoms and treatment options for urinary tract infection or pyelonephritis.)

Summary points

- Dipstick screening for proteinuria is an easily accessible first-line test.
- Dipstick screening for GDM or asymptomatic bacteriuria is less clearly useful.
- Consider the whole clinical and personal context of the woman.

CRITICAL THINKING EXERCISE

Marama is a well woman who is 32 years old. She is 10 weeks pregnant with her fifth pregnancy, and has two children.

1. What urine screening tests would you consider offering Marama?
2. Is there any further information you might seek from Marama that might influence the kinds of tests you discuss and offer her?
3. Could you discuss the purpose and reliability of urine screening tests and their results with Marama?

Palpation: hands-on learning, identification and assessment

Palpation, or examination by touch, is a process of the 'hands-on' identification and assessment of the position, growth and wellbeing of the baby (Fig. 23.3). It is an integral part of every antenatal visit, and is an acquired and highly valued midwifery skill. Each midwife has her own style, with the whole process being more than the sum of the parts described here. The process involves the gathering of small pieces of information, using the senses of hearing, seeing and touching, to put together an invisible four-dimensional 'puzzle'. It is also a significant time for two-way sharing of information. It is important for the midwife to discuss her plans with the woman, to explain the reasons for doing the examination, and to acknowledge the limitations of palpation (Enkin et al., 2000). She must seek the woman's consent, leaving open the option for her to decline, and check out any personal and cultural safety issues surrounding this intimate and exposing experience. The midwife asks about and listens to the woman's experience of her baby's growth and the nature and pattern of movements, and listens to the baby's heartbeat. She looks at the size and shape of the woman's abdomen, and notes her responses to palpation and to the baby's movements. The midwife uses touch to estimate the size and position of the baby, and its response to contact and voice. She also assesses the fluid volume and may identify other unexpected findings such as uterine fibroids. Observation and hands-on practice are the best way to learn the art and skill of effective palpation.

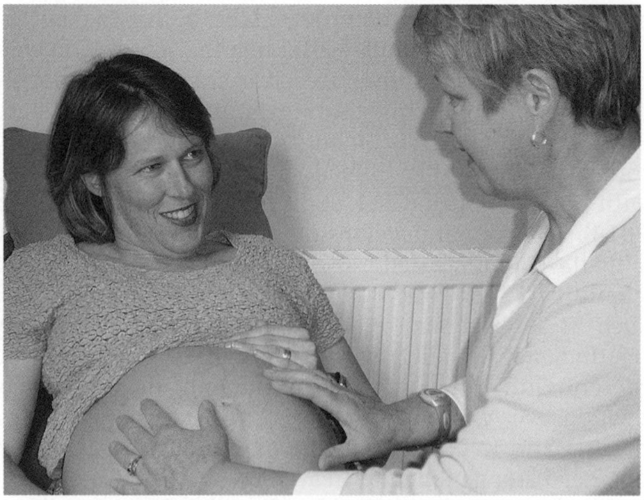

FIGURE 23.3 Abdominal palpation
(Reproduced with the permission of the New Zealand College of Midwives)

Context and preparation

The context within which the palpation occurs is a significant feature of the process. The comfort, privacy and safety of the physical environment are as important as meaningful communication between the midwife and the woman. The midwife should strive to ensure that the environment is appropriate, which will include a comfortable place on which the woman can lie down. This may be the floor (if in the woman's home), or a bed or sofa (couch), which is firm, wide and low enough to be used with comfort.

Equipment

The midwife should ensure that she has the necessary equipment for the palpation. This includes:

- Pinard stethoscope and (possibly) Doppler ultrasound, conductive gel, tissues
- watch with a second hand or counter

- privacy / modesty sheet
- tape measure (if appropriate).

Preparation

Prior to the palpation, the midwife should:

- have clean, warm hands (and short fingernails)
- affirm the woman's active role in the process
- caution her, if the palpation is occurring in later stages of pregnancy, about the possibility of hypotension while lying on her back
- ensure that the woman's privacy and modesty are protected and respected.

In preparation for the palpation, the woman should:

- be encouraged to empty her bladder
- lie down on her back, with her abdomen exposed or accessible for palpation
- be comfortable, with her head supported and perhaps her knees bent, with or without support under them.

During the palpation, the midwife should:

- take care not to focus exclusively on the woman's abdomen—maintain frequent verbal and eye contact
- tell the woman (and those with her) what she or he is doing / feeling for / finding
- encourage the woman to tell of any discomfort caused by palpating
- not palpate when the uterus is contracting—wait until it is relaxed
- guide the woman (include her partner, if she wishes) in palpating herself.

Techniques and methods

Palpation may be divided into five stages.

1. Initial visual assessment

Purpose. The purpose of this relatively brief stage in the process is to form an initial impression of the progress of the growing baby. It also provides an opportunity for discussion of the visible physiological changes; for example, she may have a linea nigra, increased hair growth or stretch marks.

Technique. Begin by establishing eye contact, once the woman is lying down. Ask her about her experiences of the baby's growth, movements and position as you look at her abdomen and begin the palpation. Check the size, shape and contours of the uterus, and consider these in relation to gestation, presentation and position. Match visible scars with your knowledge of her history. Note bruising or other signs of physical violence and, once she is upright again and if she is alone, ask about her experience and safety. Alternatively, follow up at another time, as appropriate.

2. Fundal assessment

Purpose. Fundal assessment identifies the uppermost part of the uterus and baby, from which the 'lie' and size of the baby are first distinguished, and initial information as to the 'presentation' is gained (see Box 23.14 for terminology). The 'lie' of the baby is the position of the baby's spine relative to the woman's spine, and is described as longitudinal, oblique or transverse (Fig. 23.4). The term 'presentation'

Box 23.14 Palpation terminology

- *Presentation*—refers to the part of the baby which lies at the woman's pelvic brim or in the pelvis. Options include: cephalic, breech, shoulder.
- *Presenting part*—refers to the part of the baby which lies closest to the cervix, i.e. the part which the fingers contact first during an internal examination. More specific than the presentation. Options include: vertex, face, brow; foot, sacrum; shoulder, elbow, hand, cord.
- *Lie*—is the relationship between the spine (long axis) of the baby and the spine (long axis) of the woman. Options include: longitudinal, oblique, transverse.
- *Attitude*—is the relationship of the baby's head and limbs to its trunk; usually expressed as a degree of flexion or extension. The degree to which the baby's head is flexed has real significance within the labour context, with a fully flexed head (chin on chest) having the smallest diameter to enable optimal descent through the woman's pelvis. It is generally assessed by vaginal examination rather than abdominal palpation.
- *Denominator*—is a landmark on the presentation which allows the degree of the rotation of the baby to be described. For each presentation one particular structure is nominated, the essential features being that it is a midline structure and that it is readily identifiable either by abdominal or vaginal examination. Options include:
  - the occiput—when the presenting part is vertex
  - the sacrum—when the presenting part is the buttock
  - the mentum or chin—when the presenting part is the face.

  A denominator is not usually used for the shoulder and brow presentations.
- *Position*—is the relationship between the denominator and eight points on the pelvic brim (left or right anterior, lateral or posterior; and direct anterior or posterior); for example, left occipitoanterior (LOA), right occipitolateral (ROL) or, less commonly, right sacroposterior (RSP). There are a multitude of options, although in reality the eight in Fig. 23.8 are the most common.
- *Engagement*—is when the widest presenting transverse diameter has passed through the brim of the pelvis.

(Sources: Bennett & Brown, 2003; Frye, 1998; Towler & Butler-Manuel, 1975)

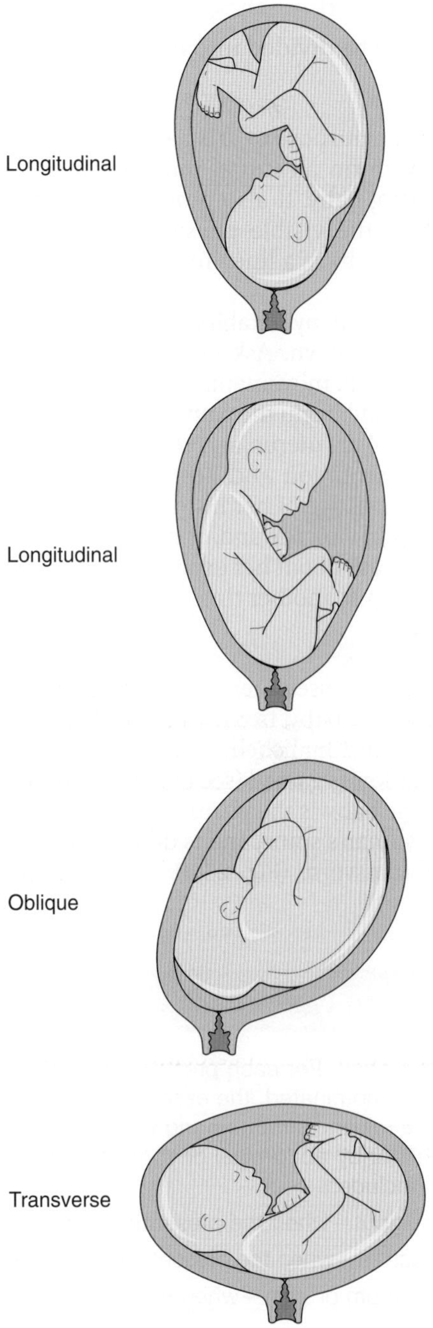

FIGURE 23.4 The lie of the baby
(Based on Henderson & Macdonald, 2004)

distinguishes the part of the baby that is lying lowest in the uterus, with cephalic, breech or shoulder the most common (Fig. 23.5). Cephalic presentations can be divided into vertex, brow or face; and breech presentations can be divided into frank, complete, footling or incomplete. In the first two trimesters, the fundal height is the primary palpation measure used to assess fetal growth, as the baby's small size makes it difficult to palpate, and its mobility makes identification of the lie or presentation irrelevant.

The second aspect of fundal assessment is the estimation of the size of the baby, which is compared with the expected size for the gestation. There are two methods used for comparing fundal height with gestation. Both have limitations, as fundal height varies with the position of the baby, the volume of liquor, and the size and shape of the woman. Assessing growth using fundal height, by landmark or measurement, is vulnerable to subjectivity and variability in technique between assessments and assessors. The record in detecting babies small for gestational age (SGA) or with fetal growth restriction/intrauterine growth restriction (FGR/IUGR) using abdominal palpation or measurement of fundal height (without customised charts, see below) is variable (Kesrouani et al., 2017; Morse et al., 2009). However, the currently available routine screening alternatives have not yet proved significantly better (Peter et al., 2015). For example, *routine* ultrasound assessing growth, amniotic fluid volume (AFV) or Doppler blood flow also have low predictive accuracy to date (Bricker et al., 2015; Haws et al., 2009). Babies that are SGA (IUGR or constitutionally small) are known to have high rates of morbidity and mortality after 24 weeks gestation (AIHW, 2021; PMMRC, 2021). In 2017–18 SGA (<10th centile) babies accounted for 27% of perinatal deaths of near-term normally formed babies in Australia (AIHW, 2021, p. 33). In New Zealand the perinatal related mortality rate by customised birthweight centile for SGA babies has improved, but the rate is still 8.72 compared with 1.87 for babies of appropriate size for their gestational age (PMMRC, 2021, p. 68). SGA is one factor amongst many that influence the wellbeing of women and babies, and therefore the growth and health of babies; indigeneity, ethnic minority, low socioeconomic status, age (teenagers), smoking, BMI and other health complications are all associated with higher rates of SGA and perinatal deaths (AIHW, 2021; PMMRC, 2021). Accurately assessing fetal size and growth is both important and an ongoing challenge for midwives.

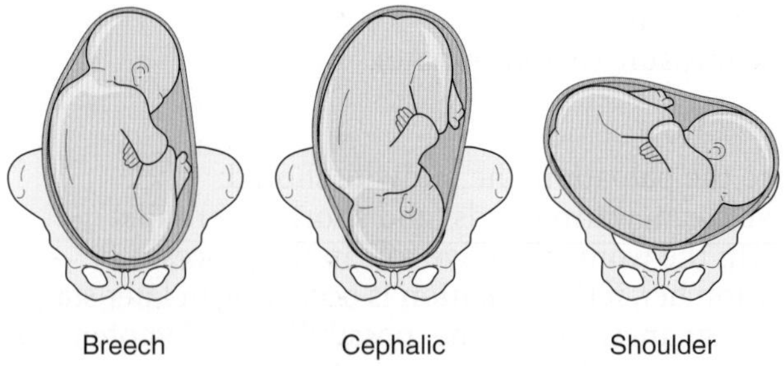

FIGURE 23.5 The presentation of the baby
(Based on Henderson & Macdonald, 2004)

The two methods of fundal assessment are described and discussed below.

'Landmark' guided fundal height assessment is a well-established practice, and is included in possibly every midwifery text. The 'landmarks' used are the symphysis pubis, umbilicus and xiphisternum (see Fig. 23.6). The growth of the fundus is expected to approximate this pattern, although there is variability between women and babies, as described above. McGeown (2001) notes that 'there is no scientific foundation for the use of the umbilicus

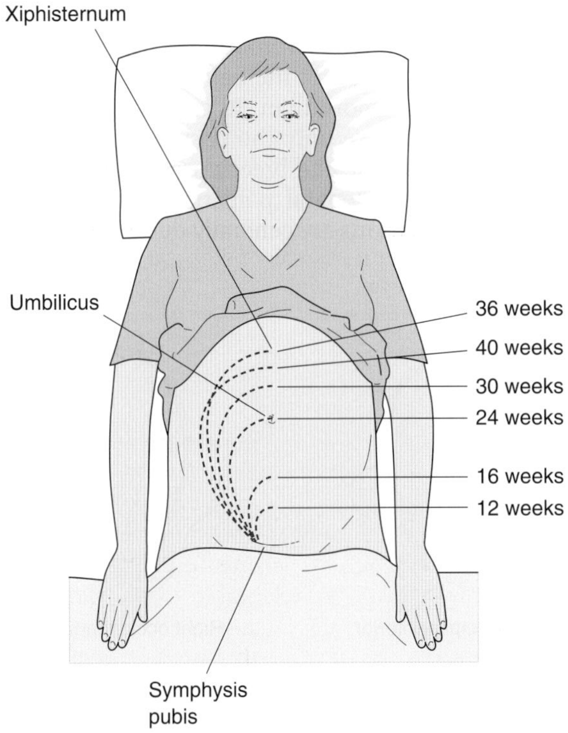

FIGURE 23.6 Landmarks of fundal height

as a landmark to indicate a specific gestational age, i.e. umbilicus=22/24/26 weeks gestation, dependent on which text one reads' (p. 191). Evidence regarding the reliability of fundal height assessment is mixed, with landmark assessments the least accurate (Morse et al., 2009). Despite the lack of supporting evidence, landmark assessment is used in practice as a guide for initial rough approximation; it should not be used in isolation.

Measurement of the fundal height is also common practice, and is recommended from 26 to 28 weeks gestation, at 2–3-weekly intervals (Morse et al., 2009). Fundal height (FH) measurement is taken using the uppermost part of the baby as the starting point and the top rim of the symphysis pubis as the end point. A flexible tape measure is held on the fundus, with the centimetre markers on the underside (to reduce bias), and laid on the skin along the longitudinal axis of the baby (Perinatal Institute, 2017). A new 'standardised' guide has been developed from a large international project (INTERGROWTH-21st Project, with website and resources), including the FH measurements for gestations 16–40 weeks and 3rd, 5th, 10th, 50th, 90th, 95th and 97th centiles for each gestation (Cheikh Ismail et al., 2016). The 50th centile is similar to the traditional FH measurement in centimetres (cm) to approximately equal the weeks of gestation up to 24 weeks, half a centimetre less than the gestation from 25 to 34 weeks, then gradually reducing until 40 weeks, when the 50th centile measurement is 38 cm (Cheikh Ismail et al., 2016, p. 6). For example, a woman who is 30 weeks would be expected to have an FH measurement of approximately 29.5 cm; a woman who is 36 weeks would have a 35-cm FH measurement if her baby was on the 50th centile (and she has a 'normal' BMI, and normal amniotic fluid volume, with her baby lying longitudinally). The actual measurements are inappropriate for large women, although after the first measurement is adjusted for a woman the relative growth of the baby should match the chart.

The 'customised growth charts' developed and commercialised in England by the West Midlands Perinatal Institute (Gardosi et al., 2000) calculate an optimal birthweight range adjusted for 'the physiological variables of maternal height, weight in early pregnancy, parity, ethnic group and by excluding known pathological variables such as smoking' (McGeown, 2001). The software is available from the Perinatal Institute website (http://www.gestation.net), and includes New Zealand and Australian versions. The charts facilitate better detection of SGA/IUGR babies (Cowan et al., 2021; McCowan et al., 2010; Roex et al., 2012) and large for gestational age (LGA) babies in Australasia (Pasupathy et al., 2012). The customised charts appear to be associated with improved outcomes; with a recent New Zealand study finding the use of the Growth Assessment Protocol, and its customised charts, associated with improved detection of SGA, without increasing obstetric intervention for SGA (Cowan et al., 2021). The charts are 'customised' to include four potentially influential factors, but cannot be 'individualised' to include many other influences found to be significant, such as obesity and maternal age (Anderson et al., 2013) and maternal birth weight, prepregnancy nutrition and exercise during pregnancy (McCowan et al., 2010). 'There is continued debate about the role of customisation of symphysis fundal height, estimated fetal weight and birthweight in screening for FGR' (O'Connor, 2016, p. 17). In addition to the chosen method of measuring fetal growth, conscientious midwifery care provided within the midwifery model and context of continuity arguably has the potential to improve outcomes, but it also lacks current data.

An ultrasound scan is recommended if the first fundal height measurement is <10th centile, or if consecutive measurements suggest no growth, slow growth or excessive growth when plotted on a customised growth chart. Fundal height measurement is not appropriate for some women—for example, those with a BMI of ≥35, having twins, with large fibroids or with polyhydramnios (Morse et al., 2009).

Summary. Measuring fundal height has been shown to be more accurate for detecting SGA babies than palpation alone. Recording of fundal height measurements on customised fetal growth charts is likely to improve detection rates for babies which are SGA or LGA.

Technique. First, find the fundus by working from the woman's chest towards her pelvis, using your finger pads (not tips) and pressing firmly enough to feel the increased resistance of the uterus relative to the other abdominal organs. The pressure required varies between women, with those having tight abdominal muscles or significant fat

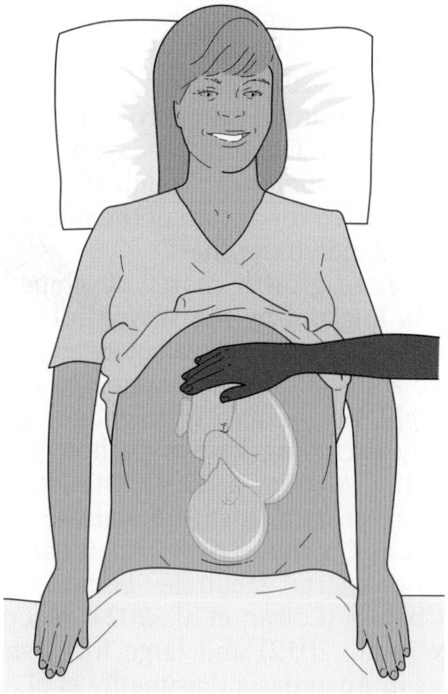

FIGURE 23.7 Identifying the fundal height

needing firmer pressure, but not so much as to cause pain (Fig. 23.7).

Once the fundus is found, cup your hand around it to define the shape and overall size of the uterus and the baby. The shape and height of the uterus help with identification of the lie of the baby. From approximately 28 weeks gestation, it is usually possible to identify the presentation of the baby by using the fingers, palm and heel of your cupped hand, or fingers and thumb extended, to identify which part of the baby is in the upper part of the uterus. You may use both hands, with one on either side of the part of the baby's body, to help with identification. The head feels hard and round, and is ballottable. The buttock may be firm in earlier gestations, but is never ballottable, as it is the extension of the torso / back.

Possible causes of discrepancies between the expected fundal height and gestation include:

- large or small baby
- multiple pregnancy
- molar pregnancy
- poly / oligohydramnios
- errors in gestational age estimation
- fibroids
- oblique or transverse lie.

3. Lateral assessment

Purpose. Lateral assessment involves palpation of the central part of the uterus. In the third trimester, it facilitates confirmation of the lie and presentation, and identifies the 'position' of the baby. The 'position' refers to the combination of the lie and presentation with the orientation of the baby—be it anterior, lateral or posterior. While the terminology used to define the baby's 'position' describes the position of the lowest part of the baby (the *denominator*) in relation to points on the woman's pelvis, it is primarily assessed by the location of the baby's back on palpation. Although there are more than 36 possible positions (see Frye, 1998), in practice only the positions relating to the most common cephalic and breech presentations are used in the context of antenatal palpation (Fig. 23.8). Other more unusual positions are generally described only by lie and presentation.

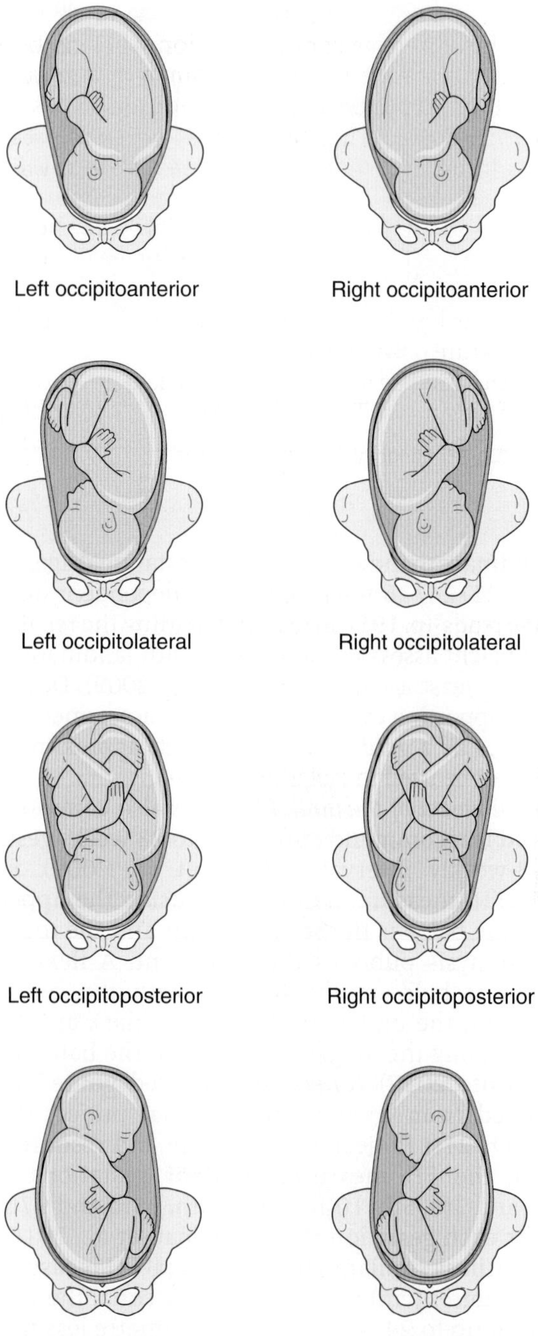

FIGURE 23.8 The most common positions of the baby
(Based on Fraser & Cooper, 2003)

Technique. There are two main techniques used for lateral palpation. The first involves 'walking' both hands across the woman's uterus and back again, using the pads of your fingers and keeping both hands close together, taking small 'steps' (Fig. 23.9). The second involves the use of one hand as an 'anchor' lying along the length of one side of the woman's uterus, while the other hand is used to examine the other side; then changing to use the other hand as 'anchor' (Fig. 23.10). Apply as much pressure as is needed to feel the baby, without causing discomfort to the woman—be aware of the possibility of causing discomfort and responsive to any signs of this. Effective communication will help both the woman and the midwife. Some women develop a sensitive spot or experience generalised tenderness. It is worthwhile considering how important it is to gather detailed information at any one antenatal visit. For example, at 32 weeks it is not important to identify more detail than the presentation and which side the back is on. If the baby wakes and moves prior to your finding the presentation or position, it can be helpful to spread both of your hands over the woman's uterus and feel the site and nature of the movements.

The back feels firm and can be 'tracked' for most of the length of the uterus. The limbs are small and knobbly and more likely to move during the palpation. If the baby is lying longitudinally and you cannot feel the back initially, broaden your search by bringing your hands to the woman's side closer to her back, as the baby's back may be tucked in closer to the woman's back, in a posterior position. If only the baby's limbs are palpable, the back will be in the opposite quadrant. For example, if limbs are felt in the right anterior area, the back will be in the left posterior position—check that area again to confirm this.

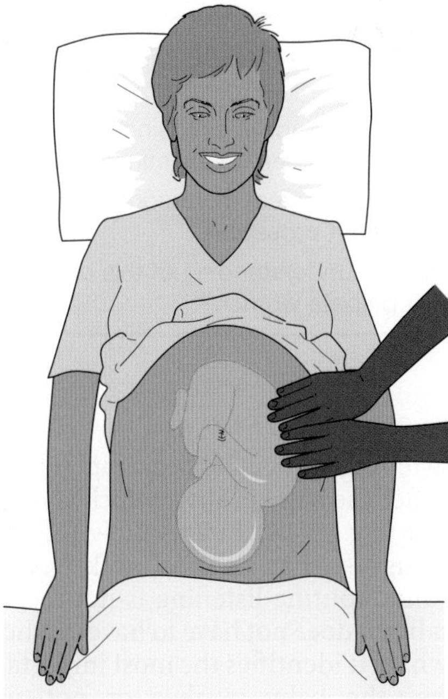

FIGURE 23.9 Lateral palpation: finding the back—'hand walking'

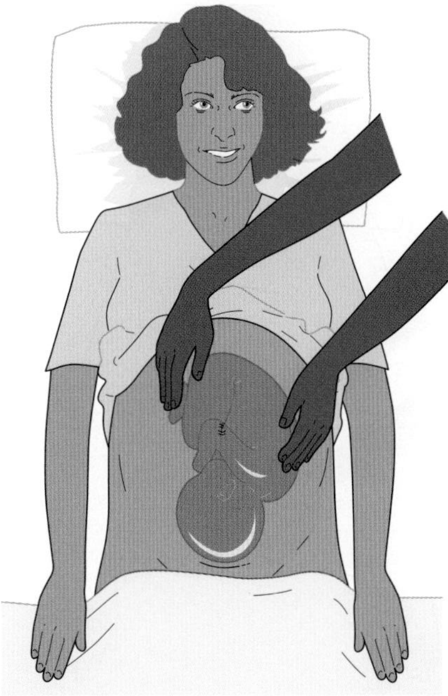

FIGURE 23.10 Lateral palpation: finding the back—'anchor hand'

Once the position of the back is identified, cup the fundus once more, to confirm the presentation by assessing the relationship between the top fetal pole (mostly the buttocks) and the back. Consider whether the top part moves when the back is pressed. It will move if it is the buttocks.

The amount of amniotic fluid or liquor can also be estimated during this part of the process. When palpating for the back, take note of how freely the baby is 'floating' in the uterine space. If there is reduced liquor (oligohydramnios), there will be minimal cushioning between the baby and the walls of the uterus. If there is excess liquor (polyhydramnios), the baby can be difficult to palpate, as it floats about (see Ch. 37 for discussion on the detail and significance of these conditions).

4. Pelvic palpation

Purpose. Palpating the lower part of the woman's uterus, just above the pelvic bones, is the final stage of the process. It serves to identify the part of the baby lying lowest (the 'presenting part') and should confirm your impressions from the fundal and lateral stages. It also enables the midwife to assess the descent of the presenting part into the pelvis. This may be more uncomfortable for the woman than the rest of the palpation, so use communication and sensitivity to manage this. If you work together, so that you press in with her out-breath, it may be less uncomfortable for her.

Technique. There are two techniques used for pelvic palpation. The first involves using both hands, initially placed midway between the woman's side and centre line, with fingertips touching the pubic bone (Fig. 23.10). Let the woman know when you are about to begin, then

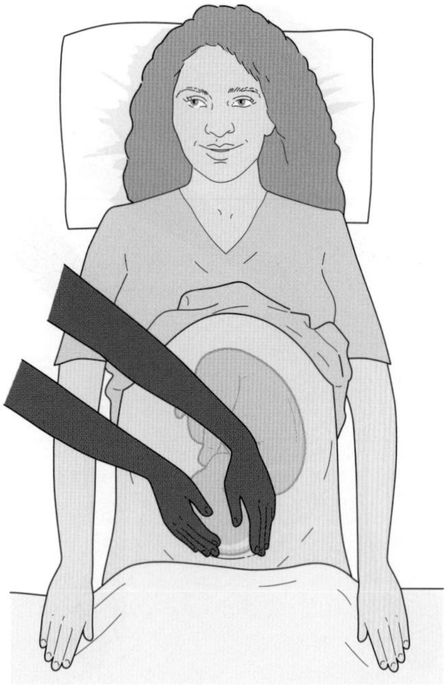

FIGURE 23.11 Pelvic palpation—feeling for the head using two hands

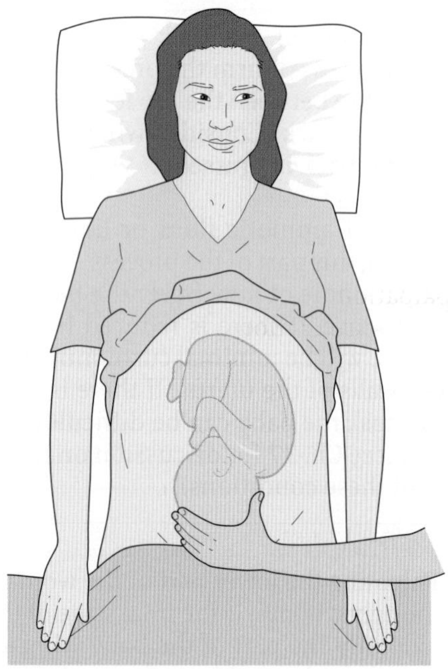

FIGURE 23.12 Pelvic palpation—ballotting the head with one hand

move the tips of your fingers towards the woman's back just above the pubic bone, feeling for the outer boundaries of the presenting part. The second technique (known as Pawlik's manoeuvre) uses one hand, with the heel of your hand beginning resting on the pubic bone and the thumb and fingers extended to reach either side of the presenting part (Fig. 23.12). The head feels hard on both sides, while the buttocks are irregular and soft on one or both sides. If the head is very well down in the pelvis, it may not be palpable, and the shoulder can feel like the buttocks, so it is worth rechecking the upper fetal pole.

Once the presenting part is identified, the next step is to assess its descent into the woman's pelvis. When palpating, you need also to assess the mobility of the presenting part (usually the head). If it is immobile, you need to assess the shape of the part that you can feel, considering whether it is broadening or narrowing from the top of the pubic bone. You are judging how much of the head has gone in, by how much of it is left above the pubic bone, and expressing it in fifths (Fig. 23.13). For example, if the head is immobile but broadening as you track its shape towards the torso, it may be one-fifth or two-fifths into the pelvis. It is defined as 'engaged' once the broadest part (the biparietal diameter) has descended below the pelvic rim. When documenting the descent, clearly note whether you are recording that which is palpable, or that which has descended (i.e. '2/5ths up/↑' or '3/5ths down/↓').

There are other measures of the baby's position which note the angle, 'flexion' or 'attitude' of the head, but they are not usually significant in the context of antenatal care (Frye, 1998). Of potential significance for a primiparous woman is whether the baby's head is engaged by 40 weeks. If it is not, the possibility of cephalopelvic disproportion (CPD) should be considered and discussed with the woman. Non-engagement for a primipara is not definitive of CPD and evidence shows that pelvic assessment or changed management, such as early induction of labour, does not improve outcomes (Enkin et al., 2000).

REFLECTIVE THINKING EXERCISE

1. How would you feel about exposing your abdomen for a healthcare professional to examine and touch?
2. What would help you feel more comfortable about undergoing such a procedure?
3. How might your understanding of this experience affect the way you palpate women?

5. Listening or auscultation

Purpose. Listening to the fetal heart rate (FHR) serves to identify whether the baby is alive, which is of great clinical significance (Fig. 23.14). Interestingly, the NICE guidelines (2017) suggest that, as it is unlikely to have any 'predictive value', routine listening is not recommended (p. 29). Arguably, it does not have to have predictive value to be worthwhile. It identifies the most important clinical state—whether the baby is alive or not—which has profound clinical and personal meaning and value for

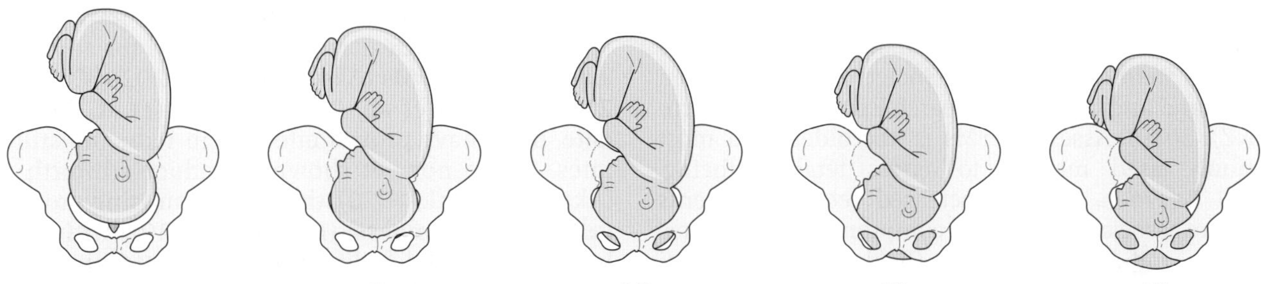

FIGURE 23.13 Assessing descent of the baby into the woman's pelvis

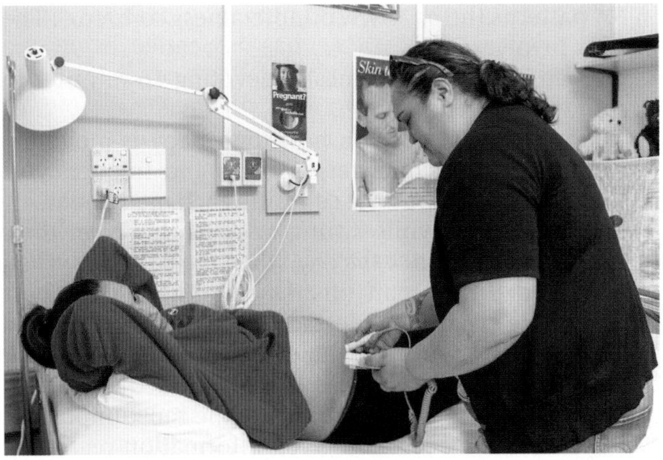

FIGURE 23.14 An antenatal Doppler assessment
(Reproduced with the permission of the New Zealand College of Midwives)

pregnant women and their families, particularly those who have miscarried previously. It is recommended here as an integral part of antenatal care, in contrast to the 2017 NICE guidelines. It appears that the option to use technology, in the form of portable Doppler ultrasound, has been taken up by the vast majority of pregnant women and midwives where it is available. Its ability to give instantaneous audible access to the baby's heartbeat from approximately 12 weeks gestation facilitates assessment of the wellbeing of babies before their movements can be felt, and before the HR can be heard via a Pinard stethoscope (24–8 weeks, in women with a normal body mass index).

Technique. Whether listening to the baby's heartbeat using a Pinard stethoscope or a Doppler, the basic technique is similar. Once the fundal height and/or position of the baby are identified, the instrument is placed on the woman's abdomen external to the baby's back. For example, if the baby is lying in a left occipitoanterior (LOA) position (see Fig. 23.8), the Pinard or Doppler should be placed in the lower left quadrant of the woman's abdomen. It is an acquired skill to hear the baby's heartbeat with a Pinard, as the experience is closer to feeling vibrations than hearing sound, and quite different from the sound that the Doppler produces. See Wickham (2002) for more detailed instructions on the use of the Pinard.

Summary points: palpation

Palpation:

- is a hands-on identification, assessment and information-sharing opportunity
- has limitations
- needs informed consent and personal/cultural sensitivity
- context and preparation are important.

There are five stages in palpation:

- initial visual assessment
- fundal assessment
- lateral assessment
- pelvic palpation
- listening or auscultation.

Fetal movements

Women who are having their first baby may feel its first movements from around 18 weeks gestation, although some may not feel them until as late as 21 weeks. Women having their second or subsequent baby may feel movements as early as 15 or 16 weeks. These movements are often referred to as 'flutters' or 'quickening', and are variously described as feeling like butterflies or bubbles. They are initially felt fleetingly, intermittently and irregularly. By 22 to 24 weeks, most women will be feeling many movements per day, and these will reflect a fairly regular sleep–wake pattern. Women may describe movements as kicks, flutters, swishes or rolls, which may change in nature during pregnancy; however, it is not normal for FMs to decrease at any gestation. 'As pregnancy advances it is normal to perceive increasingly strong movement, episodes of movements that are more vigorous than usual, fetal hiccups, and a diurnal pattern involving strong fetal movement in the evening' (Bradford et al., 2019, p. 2).

From about 28 weeks, fetal movements (FMs) may be regarded as a significant and reasonably reliable marker of a baby's wellbeing (Perinatal Society of Australia and New Zealand and Centre of Research Excellence Stillbirth (PSANZ), 2019). Assessing FMs is 'the oldest and most commonly used method to assess fetal wellbeing' (Heazell & Frøen, 2008). Decreased fetal movements (DFMs) are associated with fetal compromise and adverse pregnancy and birth outcomes (Bekiou & Gourrounti 2020; Turner et al., 2021; Warland et al., 2015). Using DFMs as the precursor measure for stillbirth is not clear cut, partly influenced by the frequency of DFM and the rarity of stillbirth (Bekiou & Gourrounti 2020; Turner et al., 2021). An international internet survey, of 1714 women who had experienced stillbirth after 28 weeks, found 30.5% reported significantly less fetal movement and 8.5% reported significantly more movement in the period prior to the baby's death; and no change in fetal movements was reported by 28% of respondents (Warland et al., 2015).

Unfortunately, no method of evaluating FMs has yet been found which reliably predicts fetal compromise in time to prevent stillbirth (Akselsson et al., 2020; Bekiou & Gourrounti 2020; Belussi et al., 2020; Flenady et al., 2021; Mangesi et al., 2015; Norman et al., 2018). This is further complicated by the lack of an internationally agreed definition of normal FMs or DFMs (PSANZ, 2019). FMs and maternal perceptions vary greatly. Some common associations have been found not to be robust, such as placental site, amniotic fluid index, BMI and parity (Bekiou & Gourrounti 2020; Bradford et al., 2018; Brown et al., 2016). A recent study in New Zealand of FM perception for women of normal and raised BMI found no difference in the perceived FM strength or frequency, with all women experiencing more FMs in the evening (Bradford et al., 2020). Further, cold drinks, loud noises, touching the abdomen or sitting in a cramped position did not stimulate FMs (Bradford et al., 2020).

While movement counting has been the most used means of identifying DFMs, women's perception of DFMs is now believed to be a better measure than a particular number of movements over any period of time (Bradford et al., 2019; Norman et al., 2018; PSANZ 2019). The comprehensive Australian and New Zealand clinical practice guideline for the care of women with DFMs recommends using maternal concern of DFM, which should override any definition of DFM based on numbers of fetal movements, and assessment of the woman and her baby as soon as possible after it's reported (PSANZ, 2019). It includes a recommended practice flow chart for practitioners to follow. It is of concern that the current evidence is that some midwives in Australia and New Zealand are giving poor or mixed information to women about fetal movements (Chan et al., 2021; McArdle et al., 2015; Peat et al., 2012; Pollock et al., 2020; Warland & Glover, 2017).

The focus of recent research has been on the efficacy of programs which raise the awareness of women, and often maternity care providers, of the importance of FMs, and give a clear response process for any woman experiencing DFMs (Akselsson et al., 2020; Chan et al., 2021; Flenady et al., 2021; Norman et al., 2018). To date, none have proved effective in reducing stillbirth rates. While not yet shown to reduce stillbirth rates (Akselsson et al., 2020), the most promising program is called 'mindfetalness' (Rådestad, 2012), with women both using it and feeling positive about it, reporting it as relaxing, decreasing worry, creating a relationship, and increasing their awareness of the unborn baby (Akselsson et al., 2017).

Mindfetalness—a mindful awareness of fetal movements and wellbeing—has the aim for the woman to consciously and restfully engage with her baby, and be aware of the FMs, so as to better recognise changes in FM patterns (http://www.mindfetalness.com/en/). The process involves:

- women in the third trimester devoting 15 minutes to mindfetalness daily
- asking them to focus on how their baby is moving—monitoring the character, strength and frequency of the movements, but not counting each movement.

It can be done while sitting or lying down on their (left) side, at any time of the day, when the baby is awake / moving and the woman unstressed, although the best time is in the evening (Rådestad, 2012).

The key message from the evidence is that *maternal awareness* of the significance of FMs, and their subsequent perception of a reduction, are the most important factors. Women need to be given information regarding expectations of FMs and what to do if these are not met. Healthcare professionals need to discuss FMs with women at each antenatal visit and respond to women's concerns and provide appropriate assessment and follow-up, as per the PSANZ guideline (https://stillbirthcre.org.au/wp-content/uploads/2021/03/Element-3_DFM-Clinical-Practice-Guideline-2.pdf). Women should contact their midwife on *the same day* if movements stop or reduce, and assessment is recommended as soon as possible and preferably within 2 hours, with CTG the first-line assessment along with a review of fetal growth and maternal wellbeing (PSANZ, 2019).

Clearly, the role of midwives as 'individualised information sharers' and listeners is critical in this context. Individualised care, planning and response are required, each woman's perception, personal and clinical situation, and past experience being important issues for inclusion. If women have good knowledge of appropriate expectations of FM, and they 'tune in' to their baby's movement pattern and routine, they are likely to be better able to identify and communicate marked changes in FM that may be significant to their baby's wellbeing. Midwives are able to affirm women's experience and knowledge of their baby's wellbeing, most of the time, but must also respond to any report of decreased fetal movements.

(See also Ch. 37.)

CRITICAL THINKING EXERCISE

Belinda is having her third baby and is 16 weeks pregnant. Liz is 26 weeks into her first pregnancy. Ella is 37 weeks pregnant with her first baby.

1. What would you ask each of these women about their baby's movements?
2. What differences would you expect in the frequency, pattern and nature of their babies' movements?
3. What factors might influence the women's understandings, expectations and experiences of the movements of their babies?

Antenatal education

Antenatal education is an integral part of the formal process of antenatal care in New Zealand, Australia and the rest of the Western world. Defining its aims, scope, role and efficacy, however, is not straightforward, as programs vary with the beliefs, expectations and frameworks of those who provide it (Brixval et al., 2015; DOH, 2018; Levett & Dahlen, 2019).

What is antenatal education?

The term 'antenatal education', when used generically, refers to information sharing between childbearing women (and their partners or friends) and caregivers or 'childbirth educators', which is intended to facilitate informed choices and decision making by the women about their pregnancy, childbirth and early postnatal period. It encompasses health promotion and preparation for childbirth and early parenting, and sometimes the development of social support networks, breastfeeding promotion / preparation and parental wellbeing. As such, it is integral to midwifery-provided antenatal care. It is not usually used to describe the active or passive learning that comes from books, the internet or other media, or which occurs between women and their friends or family.

During the past 50 years, however, 'antenatal education' (AE) has become the term used more specifically to describe face-to-face group sessions run by various providers which are additional to and separate from antenatal care per se. These courses are typically run for women in their third trimester, on the basis of weekly classes for approximately 2 hours, often over 5–8 weeks, or shorter more intensive sessions. Topics covered also vary considerably, but are likely to include at least some of the following aspects (Childbirth and Parenting Educators of Australia, 2018; MOH, 2015):

- *health promotion*—nutrition, exercise, relaxation and stress reduction; minimisation of alcohol, smoking and other 'hazardous substances'; 'pelvic awareness' and self-help for physiological changes of pregnancy
- *childbirth preparation*—signs and process of normal labour (expectations and coping skills); choices for labour and birth, such as place and pain management; unexpected outcomes, interventions (risks and appropriate use); role of support people and self-help strategies
- *parenting preparation*—establishing breastfeeding, care and safety of the newborn, appropriate clothing and equipment for babies, family and personal adjustments, support, expectations and coping strategies.

Who provides antenatal education and ho uses it?

At an organisational level, providers of AE can be divided into three broad groups:

- those associated with care provision, such as those run by hospitals or home-birth groups
- those run by community groups, such as Parents Centre or marae-based courses (New Zealand) or the Childbirth And Parenting Educators of Australia (Australia)
- those working as autonomous individuals offering private classes.

At the classroom level, the providers of AE vary greatly, with trained childbirth educators, health workers and midwives as the main leaders or facilitators. There is also considerable variation in the level and nature of training within and between these groups. Many classes have additional input from other healthcare professionals or special-interest user groups such as physiotherapists, lactation consultants or La Leche League leaders, doctors, psychologists, or those who have recently given birth. Traditionally, these classes have been used by white, middle- and upper-socioeconomic-status heterosexual couples having their first child, and not by indigenous peoples, teenagers, low-socioeconomic-status or gay couples, single women or those from ethnic minorities or other socially marginalised groups (Lumley, 1993; Redman et al., 1991).

What are the objectives of antenatal education, and how is it evaluated?

There is ongoing debate regarding the objectives, role, scope and potential impact of AE (Levett & Dahlen, 2019). A longstanding and still commonly expressed aim is to build women's confidence in their ability to give birth and care for their babies. It may also serve to build personal and social relationships, and develop shared experiences. These aims are not always realised, however, and research has identified numerous discrepancies between theory and practice in AE. These include differences between the experiences and perceptions of women and those of providers, in terms of needs, desired outcomes and the role and efficacy of AE overall (Barimani et al., 2018; Brady & Lalor, 2017; Cutajar & Cyna, 2018; Nolan, 2008a, 2008b, 2008c).

Addressing the potential impact of AE was a recent literature review and meta-analysis which included a range of study and AE types (1990–2018), and evaluated the effect of antenatal education on both physical and mental health outcomes (Hong et al., 2021). It reported physical outcomes, and found mixed results, with the AE programs associated with lower rates of epidural anaesthesia and caesarean section (Hong et al., 2021). AE programs were found to be associated with improved maternal self-efficacy and reduced stress, while they had no impact on anxiety, depression or satisfaction with the birthing experience (Hong et al., 2021). An earlier systematic review to assess the effects of AE on obstetric and psychosocial outcomes found insufficient evidence to draw conclusions (Brixval et al., 2015).

Evaluation of antenatal education beyond internal 'satisfaction' surveys or informal feedback is rare and potentially difficult (Gagnon & Sandall, 2007; MOH, 2015; Nolan, 2008a, 2008b, 2008c). 'Because of their complex, often disparate goals and ideologies, one cannot make general statements about the effects of antenatal classes as if they were a single entity' (Enkin et al., 2000, p. 24).

What is the role of the LMC midwife in antenatal education?

At the generic level, antenatal education is a core midwifery role. Throughout the antenatal period the midwife gets to know the woman and her supporters, and learns about her knowledge base and the beliefs, fears, plans and dreams she has about childbirth and caring for a baby. It is the midwife's role to share her belief in the woman's ability and in the process of childbirth. It is also her role to participate in health promotion and the preparation of the woman for birth and early parenting.

In relation to antenatal education classes, it is the midwife's role to inform women of the options available to them, and to discuss the various formats, content and underpinning philosophies of these. In order to do this, midwives should familiarise themselves with the local programs on offer. Midwives need to work with women for whom existing programs are inappropriate, to facilitate them accessing information and support which is more suited to their needs.

CRITICAL THINKING EXERCISE

Peter and Sue are in their mid thirties, Summer is 18 years old, and Aaliya and Hamsa are Somali refugees with fairly good English-language skills. All are having their first babies.

1. What antenatal education options are available in your region for these families?
2. What is the format, content and aim of the classes that are offered?
3. Who runs them, at both organisational and classroom levels?
4. How might you work with these families in order to see whether any of the classes available might meet their needs?

Exercise or physical activity in pregnancy

Exercise or physical activity in pregnancy has different meanings for different people. For some, it means gentle stretching exercises done as preparation for labour and birth, and is sometimes incorporated into group antenatal education (Brayshaw, 2003). For others, it means recreational sport or general physical fitness, in the form of aerobic exercise such as swimming, cycling, walking or team sports (Kramer & McDonald, 2006).

There is an increasing body of research which identifies exercise in pregnancy as improving or maintaining the health of women and their babies, benefiting physical, psychological, social and clinical health, and having more benefits and many fewer 'safety' issues and contraindications than previously thought (da Silva et al., 2017; Davenport et al., 2019; DOH, 2020; WHO, 2020). There is a building evidence base that regular physical activity in pregnancy can reduce the risk of many common pregnancy complications such as gestational diabetes and preeclampsia (WHO, 2020).

Historically, beliefs about exercise in pregnancy have varied with the social, cultural and political context of the time, with 'advice for physical activity reflect[ing] activities and behaviour deemed to be socially acceptable' (Rankin et al., 2000, p. 764). Arguably, this continues today, to some degree. Although there have been advice and guidelines provided regarding physical activity in pregnancy for centuries (Rankin et al., 2000) many pregnant women reduce their physical activity levels during pregnancy favouring a more sedentary lifestyle for a variety of reasons (Bauer et al., 2018).

Medical literature has focused, predominantly, on the physiological aspects of exercise, with some guidelines approaching exercise from a weight management perspective rather than a strategy for increasing wellbeing (NICE, 2010). Carrying out research on this issue is difficult, given the many confounding variables involved, which include underlying wellness and fitness levels, physiological and psychological changes induced by pregnancy, and the potential bias within any group of women who agree to participate in research on exercise.

Midwifery literature has explored some of the psychological and social aspects of exercise; for example, Coll et al. (2017), Connelly et al. (2015), Ekelin et al. (2018) and Findley et al. (2020) found that:

- many women discontinue regular prepregnancy exercise during pregnancy
- many women perceive that rest and relaxation are more important than exercise
- women are unaware of current exercise recommendations
- women believe they are being active although they are not meeting guidelines
- friends and family strongly influence exercising behaviour
- work- or time-related factors interfere with leisure-time physical activity

- the most common exercise belief was that exercise improves mood
- women lack motivation, support and/or resources to exercise
- physical limitations (e.g. nausea or fatigue) obstructed participation in exercise.

Recently, guidelines have become more consistent in the recommendation of regular, moderate-intensity physical activity throughout pregnancy being beneficial, except for a small number of women with contraindications. The 2020 WHO guidelines on physical activity and sedentary behaviour are clear that regular physical activity is recommended for all women, without contraindications, throughout pregnancy and postpartum. Many guidelines now specify aiming for at least 150 minutes of moderate-intensity activity each week (DOH, 2020; WHO, 2020). The comprehensive Australian guidelines recommendation is to advise women that low- to moderate-intensity physical activity during pregnancy is associated with a range of health benefits and is not associated with adverse outcomes. What is still unclear from the literature is which interventions by midwives are effective in changing the level of physical activity of pregnant women, in particular those who are not usually physically active. What is clear is that the attitudes, beliefs and behaviours that women (and midwives) have about exercise are rooted within their personal, social and cultural context, and cannot be addressed in isolation. Understanding more about the barriers and motivators for women is an important step for midwives (see Bauer et al., 2018; Coll et al., 2017; Connelly et al., 2015; Da Costa & Ireland, 2013; Ekelin et al., 2018; Findley et al., 2020). As with any other issue of health promotion, a complex process is involved, and it requires midwives to work in partnership with women and use effective communication, support and affirmation skills (Crafter, 1997).

REFLECTIVE THINKING EXERCISE

1. What are your personal beliefs about physical exercise?
2. How might these influence the way in which you discuss the role of exercise during pregnancy with pregnant women?
3. Consider potential barriers and motivators for women regarding exercise/physical activity.
4. Spend some time talking with pregnant women and practising midwives about their beliefs and behaviours with regard to the role of exercise during pregnancy.

Physiological changes of pregnancy

Pregnancy brings about many changes within a woman's body. Many of these **physiological changes** are experienced as unpleasant, and some are very distressing and debilitating (Box 23.15). They are commonly referred to as 'minor' discomforts or disturbances, which does not reflect the impact that some of these conditions have on many women and their families. The fact that they are common, natural and not 'pathological', and generally resolve as spontaneously as they arise, appears to contribute to the dismissal or minimisation of them by many caregivers.

There are marked differences in the incidence and severity of these changes, both between different women, and for the same woman during different pregnancies. There are also significant variations in the experiences, perceptions and responses of women to the changes caused by pregnancy. The sociocultural context within which women (and midwives) live also influences the way in which they respond. Arguably, in contemporary Western society, there is a lower tolerance for discomfort or pain among many, and an increased expectation that the negative aspects of physiological changes can be alleviated (without risk to the health of woman or baby), whether by the use of 'medicated' pharmacological remedies or by 'alternative' remedies. Further, contemporary lifestyles including diet, exercise and work patterns (paid and unpaid) may exacerbate these changes, and changing these factors can be difficult during pregnancy. Unfortunately, the very nature of physiological changes, as expressions of the normal physiology of pregnancy, makes them difficult to resolve with 'treatment' of any type. The focus is therefore on understanding the physiology and minimising the discomfort of these changes.

Responses to physiological changes vary widely, and a vast array of 'therapies' are used by women today. They include herbal medicine, homeopathy, acupuncture/acupressure, osteopathy, aromatherapy, reflexology, massage, reiki, hypnotherapy, Bach flower remedies, shiatsu and 'conventional' Western medicine. Additionally, there are numerous dietary and exercise approaches advocated by various healthcare professionals and lay people. Among them are those who advocate strongly for their particular therapies (both conventional and alternative), but evidence to date is very limited as to the efficacy and safety of many interventions for the alleviation of pain or discomfort caused by these changes. It is beyond the scope of this chapter to include a description or an evaluation of the range of therapeutic options for the physiological changes to be discussed, beyond the brief exemplar given on nausea and vomiting.

All interventions, including 'conventional' and 'alternative' medicines or remedies, should be treated with due respect and caution when being considered as treatments for physiological changes. (See the section on nausea and vomiting, below.) It should not be assumed that because something is 'natural' or 'alternative' that it is therefore any safer, of lower risk or more effective than 'conventional' or 'medical' options. It is important for midwives to carefully review the available evidence regarding the safety and efficacy of any intervention option they offer or recommend to women. Midwives should recognise the limits of their knowledge and training, and

Box 23.15 Physiological changes of pregnancy

Circulatory related to changes in blood vessels or lymph system:
- oedema
- carpal tunnel
- fainting and dizziness
- palpitations
- varicose veins—leg, vulval or anal (haemorrhoids)
- bleeding gums or nose

Muscle and ligament:
- leg cramps
- 'ligament' pain (abdominal)
- back pain
- sciatica
- symphysis pubis dysfunction
- incontinence
- uterine cramps—'irritable' uterus, Braxton Hicks contractions

Digestive:
- nausea and vomiting
- constipation
- heartburn and indigestion
- ptyalism
- bloating and excessive 'wind'
- diarrhoea

Breast—tenderness, growth, colour and size of areola, 'leaking'

Vagina—increased discharge, pH (thrush susceptibility)

Urinary—frequency, urinary tract dilation, shortening (UTI susceptibility)

Sleep—pattern, nature, insomnia, dreams

Nose—congestion, bleeds, hay fever

Hair—growth on skin (abdomen, face), loss from head

Skin—itching, pregnancy rash (PUPPP), acne, chloasma, linea nigra, stretch marks

Dietary—hypersensitivity to taste and/or smell, pica, appetite and metabolism changes

Sexuality—libido changes

Emotional—volatility and mood swings

Headaches and/or migraines

Tiredness/fatigue increased (1st and 3rd trimesters)

PUPPP=pruritic urticarial papules and plaques of pregnancy; UTI=urinary tract infection.

when discussing options and alternatives be able to refer on to those who are trained, accredited and accountable within their own profession when these therapies are outside their scope of practice.

When women describe discomfort or pain they are experiencing, midwives must take care to differentiate between physiological and pathological symptoms. For example:
- vomiting may be physiological or pathological, and caused either by bacterial or viral infection, or by hyperemesis
- indigestion needs to be distinguished from epigastric or chest (cardiac) pains
- normal physiological increase in vaginal discharge needs to be differentiated from infections, such as *Chlamydia* or thrush.

The physiological changes listed in Box 23.15 are the most common, and three of these will be discussed briefly here, as limited space does not permit a discussion of each and every one. Box 23.16 lists additional resources for managing physiological changes in pregnancy.

Box 23.16 Additional resources—physiological changes in pregnancy

- Balaskas (1998)
- Blackburn (2018)
- Jamil & Evennett (2000)
- Tiran (2018)

Nausea and vomiting in pregnancy (NVP or 'morning sickness')

Nausea and vomiting (NVP) is a common, very unpleasant, yet not well-understood condition of pregnancy. 'Nausea is the conscious recognition of subconscious excitation of the vomiting centre or an area close to it in the medulla. Vomiting is a complex series of movements which rids the gut of its contents when any part of it is irritated or distended' (Jordan, 2010, p. 131). While it is associated with raised levels of human chorionic gonadotrophin (hCG) hormone and changes in blood sugar levels, variability in incidence, severity and response to treatments are indicative of a multifactorial state. The mechanism causing it remains unknown (Matthews et al., 2015). Box 23.17 is a summary of a range of statistics on the occurrence and severity of NVP. These statistics have been sourced from Chandra et al. (2003), Einarson et al. (2013), Frye (1998), Gadsby et al., 2021, Matthews et al. (2015), and Wood et al. (2013).

NVP occurs predominantly in the first trimester. It is notoriously difficult to treat, in part because of the potentially greater harm that treatment poses to the baby during this critical developmental time, compared with other

> **Box 23.17 Incidence and severity of nausea and vomiting**
>
> Incidence
> - 69% of pregnant women experience it (range internationally 35–91%); 67% of these vomit
>
> Severity
> - Varies greatly—most women have symptoms by 8 weeks (94%)
> - One-third have symptoms by 5 weeks gestation
> - Resolves by 12–14 weeks for the majority of women
> - Resolves by 16–20 weeks for most (90%)
> - Not confined to the morning for most (80%–90%)
> - Causes lost work time (at least 25% in paid and unpaid work time)
> - Causes increased weight gain for some (frequent snacking to feel better) and weight loss for others (decreased appetite with moderate vomiting)
> - Emotional, social and psychological impact can be marked
> - Rated mild for 40%, moderate for 46% and severe for 14% of women
> - 1% of women with nausea and vomiting will develop the pathological condition of hyperemesis gravidarum (range internationally 0.3%–3.6%)
>
> (Sources: Chandra et al. (2003), Einarson et al. (2013), Frye (1998), Gadsby et al., 2021, Matthews et al. (2015), and Wood et al. (2013))

periods of pregnancy. Many treatments have been tried, including pharmaceuticals, herbal and homeopathic preparations as well as dietary, lifestyle and non-medicinal options such as acupuncture and acupressure. Unfortunately, the latest Cochrane review found a lack of high-quality evidence to back up any advice on evaluated treatments—both pharmaceutical and non-pharmaceutical (Matthews et al., 2015). Despite this, a wide variety of drugs are prescribed as antiemetics, the current most commonly used being dopamine antagonists, antihistamines, serotonin antagonists and vitamin supplements (O'Donnell et al., 2016). The history of conventional pharmaceutical medications for nausea and vomiting is notably marked by the tragic consequences of the use of the sedative and immunomodulatory drug thalidomide, which caused severe limb defects in babies. This situation illustrates the point that the widespread use of medications (pharmaceutical or herbal) should not be interpreted as proof of sound evidence of safety or efficacy. Recently, three systematic reviews into NVP have been published (Bustos et al., 2017; Matthews et al., 2015; O'Donnell et al., 2016). The most comprehensive of these is a 300-page Health Technology Assessment (HTA) report, which includes a range of study designs and provides readable summaries of each treatment (O'Donnell et al., 2016, available online; and its shorter published article by McParlin et al., 2016). The review by Bustos et al. (2017) includes comprehensive consideration of NVP pathogenesis. The HTA report concludes that, for mild symptoms of NVP, ginger, pyridoxine (vitamin B_6), antihistamines and metoclopromide, and for moderate symptoms pyridoxine-doxylamine, promethazine and metocloprimade, are 'associated with greater benefit than placebo'; ondansetron is associated with improvement for a range of symptom severity (McParlin et al., 2016, p. 1392). All pharmaceutical treatments require care with prescribing and midwives need to ensure that they have sound knowledge of their mechanism of action, potential interactions and contraindications before including them in their scope of practice.

It is also appropriate to be cautious about the use of alternative herbal medications. An example of these is ginger (*Zingiber officinale*). Despite its long tradition as a remedy for sickness, including NVP, ginger's pharmacological action is not yet fully understood (Bustos et al., 2017; Tiran, 2018). It has the potential to act as an anticoagulant, hypotensive, hypoglycaemic and a cholagoguic (stimulating bile secretion), and to interact with other medications such as sedatives, hypnotics, antacids and iron (Tiran, 2012). It is important that midwives treat this as a medication and treat it with due caution. As the maximal safe dose and length of treatment are not established, the use of ginger as a medication in capsule form should be approached with caution; it may cause unforeseen problems owing to the increased dosage that capsules facilitate above that which might have been ingested traditionally in its natural state as fresh root ginger, eaten or taken in a tea. Doses of between 450 and 2600 mg/day are used in the research (Hu et al., 2020, O'Donnell et al., 2016). It is generally suggested that a maximum daily dose of 1000 mg, divided into four doses of 250mg could be considered safe, although within the research there has been little consistency in dosage, form, treatment frequency or duration (DOH, 2020, Tiran, 2018). Ding et al. (2013, p. e29) identify the dosage of various forms of ginger, with the equivalent of 1000 mg:

- 1 teaspoon freshly grated root ginger
- 2 mL ginger liquid extract
- 4 cups prepackaged ginger tea
- 4 cups fresh ginger tea (1/2 tsp freshly grated ginger infused for 5–10 min)
- 2 pieces crystallised ginger.

Ginger biscuits, ale and syrups are not recommended because of their high sugar or alcohol content (Tiran, 2018). Further research is required on both conventional and herbal treatments for nausea and vomiting (Bustos et al., 2017; Fejzo et al., 2013; Matthews et al., 2015; O'Donnell et al., 2016; Tiran, 2018).

Alternative intervention for the treatment of nausea and vomiting, in the form of acupressure (Pericardium 6, Neiguan point) is showing promising results in most trials (Matthews et al., 2015; O'Donnell et al., 2016), and its 'chemical-free' nature arguably makes it a lower-risk option. Each of the alternative forms of therapy mentioned in the introduction earlier offers therapeutic options for nausea and vomiting which women may wish to consider, and midwives need to be able to make referrals as appropriate for the woman concerned.

Self-help responses to nausea and vomiting include lifestyle and dietary changes, which may provide some relief from this sometimes-debilitating condition that is recognised as having the potential to impact significantly on women's lives (Heitmann et al., 2017; Wood et al., 2013). Although the evidence base for many of these is limited or non-existent, they are the most widely accepted recommendations (Matthews et al., 2015; Wills & Forster, 2008). They include the following, sourced from the Auckland Home Birth Association (1993), Balaskas (1998), Chandra et al. (2003), Frye (1998), Jamil & Evennett (2000) and Wills & Forster (2008):

- increase rest periods
- minimise work and home stressors
- eat carbohydrate (and wait 20 minutes) before getting out of bed in the morning
- eat protein before going to bed, or if up during the night
- do low-energy / impact exercise, such as walking or yoga, after eating
- have regular small snacks of high protein and unprocessed carbohydrate (2–3 hourly)
- avoid refined, fried and spicy foods
- eat foods rich in B group vitamins
- eat five to six small 'meals' a day, rather than three large ones
- increase fluid (water, milk or juice) intake
- reduce coffee and tea intake if more than three cups per day.

Constipation

Constipation is difficult to define, but 'is present when a person strains to defecate and has infrequent bowel movements with no underlying cause' (Jordan, 2010, p. 271). Normal patterns for bowel movements vary significantly between women, and have been defined as anything from three per day to one every 3 days (Jordan, 2010). It is therefore not the frequency of bowel motion per se, but the discomfort and difficulty in passing one that is more significant in defining constipation. Constipation may also cause headaches, bloating, abdominal pain and impaired appetite (Jordan, 2010).

Constipation is caused by hormonal changes (which result in slowed bowel motility and changes in absorption patterns), by changes in food and fluid intake (volumes, times and types), and, for some, by reduced rates of exercise (Frye, 1998). Constipation is common during pregnancy, affecting up to 25% of women with the highest rates in the second trimester (DOH, 2020), although it is difficult to establish incidence rates owing to disclosure issues for women and other confounding variables, such as the effects of routine iron supplementation.

Dietary and lifestyle changes are the primary response to constipation during pregnancy (Rungsiprakarn et al., 2015). Both herbal and pharmaceutical laxatives should be used only as a short-term (1–2 weeks) last resort while dietary changes are made, as they can cause flora, fluid and electrolyte imbalances in the bowel and reduced gut motility and absorption of nutrients (Jordan, 2010).

Dietary changes include increased fibre intake, such as grains (whole or bran form), beans and lentils, brown rice, nuts, seeds and dried fruits. Fresh fruit and vegetables are an excellent source of fibre and have the advantage of providing both fibre and fluid together, as well as valuable nutrients. As most fibre absorbs fluid during digestion, it is important that women increase both fibre and fluid intake, as otherwise the increased intake of some types of fibre can aggravate rather than resolve constipation. Fluid intake is very important and water is optimal, with sugary drinks not recommended. There is no 'right' number of cups of fluid to have each day, but if a woman is constipated she is unlikely to be having enough fluid, either in foods or in liquid form. It is important that women drink plenty of fluid daily and not just when constipated. Prunes and kiwifruit, as fruit or juice, are excellent, but many women do not like or have access to them. Tea and coffee can worsen constipation by acting as diuretics so fluid is passed out as urine, not leaving enough in the intestine to keep the stool soft. The midwife should work individually with women, acknowledging their personal, social and cultural context, to find high-fibre foods and appropriate fluids that they might include in their diet. Regular consumption of these foods and fluids is important, rather than in response to constipation, as the bowel works best in a regular pattern or routine.

It is also worthwhile discussing issues of bowel motion pattern and technique with women. During pregnancy it may take longer to pass a motion because of slowed peristaltic action. It is important for a woman to take note of her body's natural urge to go to the toilet when it occurs and not put it off or hold on, as it may be some hours or the next day before another urge occurs, and by then more fluid has been absorbed from the faecal mass and greater compaction has occurred. If a woman has lost the natural regular urge to pass a bowel motion, she should be encouraged to make a regular time each day for trying—after meals being the best time, given the natural peristalsis that occurs with the intake of food. Positioning on the toilet and pushing technique can also affect ease or speed of passing a motion. Women should:

- sit on the toilet with knees higher than their hips (a footstool helps)
- have their legs hip-width apart
- lean forward with forearms resting on their knees (leaning back to push presses the stool against the posterior vaginal wall / pelvic floor and tenses the pelvic floor, when relaxation is needed)
- keep their back fairly straight, not rolled over
- let their tummy drop forward
- with the first push (using diaphragm), lift their heels and feel widening of the waist
- breathe out and push / grunt, relax, breathe deeply and try again
- try not to strain with prolonged pushes
- allow time for the peristaltic action, if it does not come

- try massaging their abdomen in a clockwise direction, starting at the right hip (possible until about 20 weeks gestation).

Heartburn

Heartburn (or gastro-oesophageal reflux) is a common experience for pregnant women, with different research citing incidence rates of between 30% and 80% (DOH, 2020; National Collaborating Centre for Women's and Children's Health, 2008). It is a very unpleasant condition in which stomach acid enters the lower oesophagus, causing a 'burning sensation' in the chest or back of the throat (Frye, 1998). It is caused by hormonal changes, which slow gastric motility and promote sphincter relaxation, and physical pressure from the growing uterus (Jordan, 2010). It tends to worsen as pregnancy progresses (Phupong & Hanprasertpong, 2015), and can cause major physical discomfort for women. It can interfere with content and pattern of eating, interrupt physical activity and sleeping, and result in considerable emotional and psychological distress for some women.

Numerous self-help measures for the relief of heartburn are listed below. Some will appeal to or work for one woman but not another, and some women find that something that helps initially may become ineffective as pregnancy progresses. Self-help measures for heartburn include the following:

- identifying foods which cause heartburn and avoiding them
- avoiding fried, fatty or spiced foods (for some women, bread causes heartburn)
- avoiding coffee, tea, alcohol and cigarettes, all of which worsen heartburn
- chewing food thoroughly and eating slowly
- eating apple, pineapple, papaya or kiwifruit with meals, as they have digestive enzymes which speed the breaking down and digestion of food
- eating four to six small meals a day, rather than three large ones (dividing the main meal onto two small plates and eating the second portion later or the next day reduces 'snack food' intake)
- eating the last meal of the day at least 2 hours before bedtime
- drinking plenty of fluid, but *not* with meals (they dilute digestive juices; wait 30 minutes)
- drinking milk or eating yoghurt
- chewing raw almonds or cashew nuts.

Other non-food-related strategies may include:

- checking posture, especially while sitting—slouching will worsen heartburn
- trying exercises that stretch the upper torso while sitting or standing (not lying)
- staying upright for 2 hours after eating—walking may help
- sleeping with upper body elevated, with bricks under the bed legs, or several pillows (Balaskas, 1998; Frye, 1998; Jamil & Evennett, 2000).

There are numerous herbal remedies available, in addition to the options from all the other therapies described earlier. There are also a number of medicated pharmaceutical options, which have varying levels of efficacy, and are variably supported by evidence (Jordan, 2010; Phupong & Hanprasertpong, 2015).

RESEARCH ACTIVITY

List 10 physiological changes associated with pregnancy, and identify the following:

- the nature of the condition
- the cause (if known)
- its incidence (frequency and timing during pregnancy)
- its natural course and resolution
- the potential for pathology
- relevant self-help measures.

REFLECTIVE THINKING EXERCISE

1. Consider the potential impact of physiological changes on the physical, psychological and social lives of pregnant women.
2. Identify your own scope of practice regarding interventions for treating or managing the physiological changes associated with pregnancy.
3. Identify referral options for 'out-of-scope' treatments.

Conclusion

This chapter has sought to provide an introduction to the care of pregnant women. It has presented an overview of the purpose and provision of antenatal care within the context of the midwifery model. A primary aim of the chapter has been to outline the key components of antenatal care, and describe a framework for organising these components in a relatively systematic and coherent way. These components include:

- the nature and process of establishing a relationship with a pregnant woman and her support people
- the principles involved in assisting or supporting a woman to make appropriate decisions regarding her pregnancy, and developing an individualised and effective care plan
- the assessment and monitoring of the health and wellbeing of a pregnant woman and her baby.

A framework of eight decision points has been presented, which comprise a set of four categories of cues, including information sharing, screening and assessment, decision making, and health promotion and information. They are intended to prompt the midwife to consider the holistic nature of antenatal care. While this framework strives to provide a clear structure to antenatal care, it is intended to act primarily as a set of cues for the midwife rather than a strict prescription. The partnership between a pregnant woman and her midwife is a unique one, and it is incumbent on the midwife to facilitate an effective process that meets the woman's individual needs and reflects her personal reality.

The chapter has also discussed some of the knowledge and skills a midwife might apply in the provision of antenatal care. These include:

- establishing an estimated due date
- abdominal palpation
- blood pressure measurement
- routine blood and urine screening options
- mental health
- describing the nature and significance of fetal movements
- antenatal education and exercise during pregnancy
- the concept of physiological changes associated with pregnancy, and issues related to the management of them.

A second objective of the chapter has been to argue for, and model the use of, reviewed research to promote evidence-informed midwifery in the provision of antenatal care. Much of what has traditionally been included in routine antenatal care has been based on anecdote and happenstance, rather than clear evidence that supports or refutes these practices. A good deal of the research reviewed to date either does not address issues of concern to midwives and childbearing women, is weak, or is primarily applicable to the type of antenatal care which is provided within the medical model. This has limited the extent to which the concept of evidence-based practice has been applied within this chapter. It is to be hoped that, in the future, midwives will be able to use evidence to inform their practice within the context of the midwifery model of care.

Review questions

1. What methods for establishing estimated due date are used in your region?
2. What antenatal blood tests are considered to be 'routine' in your region, and what are the 'normal' reference ranges for them?
3. Describe the physical, personal, social and emotional implications of positive blood screening tests for pregnant women and their families.
4. What are the contemporary diagnostic criteria for preeclampsia?
5. What are the essential components of measuring blood pressure?
6. What are the basic palpation techniques, and what information can be gained from abdominal palpation in antenatal care?
7. How might midwives help women to experience palpation positively?
8. What is the significance of fetal movements over the course of a woman's pregnancy, and how might a woman and her midwife monitor these?
9. What antenatal education and/or exercise classes are available in your region?
10. What place does exercise have in influencing the emotional and physical wellbeing of pregnant women, and what impact might social, personal or cultural factors have on exercise patterns?

Online resources

Department of Health (DOH). Clinical Practice Guidelines: Pregnancy Care. Canberra: Australian Government Department of Health; 2020: https://www.health.gov.au/resources/pregnancy-care-guidelines.

Gestation Network (gestation calculator, customised growth charts): http://www.gestation.net.

National Institute for Health and Clinical Excellence (NICE). Antenatal Care [update] 2021: https://www.nice.org.uk/guidance/ng201.

National Institute for Health and Clinical Excellence (NICE). Antenatal care for uncomplicated pregnancies. London: RCOG Press; 2008, 2019 update: https://www.nice.org.uk/Guidance/CG62.

Perinatal Institute (UK): http://www.perinatal.org.uk.

Palasanthiran P, Starr M, Jones C, et al, eds. Management of Perinatal Infections. 2nd ed. published by the Australasian Society for Infectious Diseases; 2014: https://www.asid.net.au/resources/clinical-guidelines.

References

Akselsson A, Georgsson S, Lindgren H et al. Women's attitudes, experiences and compliance concerning the use of Mindfetalness - a method for systematic observation of fetal movements in late pregnancy. *BMC Pregnancy & Childbirth.* 2017;17:359. Doi: 10.1186/s12884-017-1548-5.

Akselsson A, Lindgren H, Georgsson et al. Mindfetalness to increase women's awareness of fetal movements and pregnancy outcomes: a cluster-randomised controlled trial including 39,865 women. *BJOG* 2020;127:829-837.

Allen J, Kildea S, Stapleton H. How does group antenatal care function within a caseload midwifery model? A critical ethnographic analysis. *Midwifery.* 2015;31:489-497.

Anderson N, Sadler L, Stewart A, et al. Independent risk factors for infants who are small for gestational age by customised birthweight centiles in a multi-ethnic New Zealand population. *Aust N Z J Obstet Gynaecol.* 2013;53:136-142.

Auckland Home Birth Association. *A Guide to Healthy Pregnancy and Childbirth.* Auckland: Auckland Home Birth Association; 1993.

Auger N, Low N, Lee G, et al. Pregnancy outcomes of women hospitalized for physical assault, sexual assault, and intimate partner violence. *Journal of interpersonal violence.* 2021

Austin M-P, Highet N. *Guidelines Expert Advisory Committee. Clinical Practice Guidelines for Depression and Related Disorders—Anxiety, Bipolar Disorder and Puerperal Psychosis—in The Perinatal Period. A guideline for primary care health professionals.* Melbourne: beyondblue. 2011. Online: http://resources.beyondblue.org.au/prism/file?token=BL/0891.

Austin M-P, Middleton P, Reilly N. et al. Detection and management of mood disorders in the maternity setting: the Australian Clinical Practice Guidelines. *Women Birth.* 2013;26:2-9.

Australian Institute of Health and Welfare. *Australia's mothers and babies.* 2021. Cat. No. PER 101. Canberra: AIHW. https://www.aihw.gov.au/reports/mothers-babies/australias-mothers-babies

Baird K, Creedy D, Branjerdporn G, & Gillespie K. Red flags and gut feelings—Midwives' perceptions of domestic and family violence screening and detection in a maternity department. *Women and Birth.* 2021; 34(5): e468-e474.

Balaskas J. *New Natural Pregnancy.* 2nd ed. Sydney: Sandstone; 1998.

Barimani M, Forslund Frykedal K, Rosander M, & Berlin A. Childbirth and parenting preparation in antenatal classes. *Midwifery.* 2018;57:1-7.

Baskett T, Naegele F. Naegele's rule: a reappraisal. *BJOG.* 2000;107: 1433-1435.

Bauer C, Graf C, Platschek A, et al. Reasons, motivational factors, and perceived personal barriers to engagement in physical activity during pregnancy vary within the BMI classes: The Prenatal Prevention Project Germany. *Journal of Physical Activity and Health.* 2018;15(3), 204-211.

Bekiou A and Gourounti K. Reduced fetal movements and perinatal mortality. *Mater Sociomed.* 2020;32(3):227-234

Belussi F., Po G., Livi A, et al., Fetal Movement Counting and Perinatal Mortality. A systematic review and Meta-analysis. *Obstet Gynecol* 2020;135;453-62.

Bennett R, Brown L. *Myles' Textbook for Midwives.* 14th ed. London: Churchill Livingstone; 2003.

Blackburn S. Maternal, *Fetal and Neonatal Physiology a Clinical Perspective.* 3rd ed. Sydney: WB Saunders; 2007.

Blackburn S. *Maternal, Fetal and Neonatal Physiology a Clinical Perspective.* 5th ed. Philadelphia: WB Saunders; 2018.

Bookallil M, Chalmers E, Beel A. Challenges in preventing pyelonephritis in pregnant women in Indigenous communities. *Rural Remote Health.* 2005;5:395. Online: https://www.rrh.org.au/journal/article/395.

Bradford B, Cronin R, McKinlay C et al. A diurnal fetal movement pattern: Findings from a cross-sectional study of maternally perceived fetal movements in the third trimester of pregnancy. *PLoS ONE.* 2019; 14(6): e0217583.

Bradford B, Cronin R, McKinlay C, et al. Maternally perceived fetal movement patterns: the influence of body mass index. *Early Human Development.* 2020; 104922.

Bradford B, Thompson J, Heazell A et al. Understanding the associations and significance of fetal movements in overweight or obese pregnant women: a systematic review. *AOGC* 2018; 97, 13-24.

Brady V and Lalor J. Space for human connection in antenatal education: uncovering women's hopes using participatory action research. *Midwifery* 2017; 55:7-14

Brayshaw E. *Exercises in Pregnancy and Childbirth: A Practical Guide for Educators.* London: Books for Midwives; 2003.

Bricker L, Medley N, Pratt J.. Routine ultrasound in late pregnancy (after 24 weeks' gestation). *Cochrane Database Syst Rev.* 2015;(6):CD001451, doi:10.1002/14651858.CD001451.pub4.

Brixval C, Axelsen S, Lauemoller S, et al. The effect of antenatal education in small classes on obstetric and psycho-social outcomes—a systematic review. *Syst Rev.* 2015;4:20.

Brock E, Charlton K, Yeatman H. Identification and evaluation of models of antenatal care in Australia—a review of the evidence. *Aust N Z J Obstet Gynaecol.* 2014;54:300-311.

Brown M, Hague W, Higgins J, et al. Australasian Society for the Study of Hypertension in Pregnancy Consensus Statement: the detection, investigation and management of hypertension in pregnancy. *Aust N Z J Obstet Gynaecol.* 2000;40(2):139-155.

Brown S, Weetra D, Ah Kit J, et al. Improving access to antenatal care for Aboriginal women in South Australia: evidence from a population-based study. *Birth.* 2016;43(2):134-143.

Browne J, O'Brien M, Taylor J, et al. 'You've got it within you': the political act of keeping a wellness focus in the antenatal time. *Midwifery.* 2014;30:420-426.

Brown R, Higgins L, Johnstone E et al. Maternal perception of fetal movements in late pregnancy is affected by type and duration of fetal movement. *The Journal of Maternal-Fetal & Neonatal Medicine* 2016; 29(13):2145-2150. Doi: 10.3109/14767058.2015.1077509

Bustos M, Venkataramanan R, Caritis S. Nausea and vomiting of pregnancy—what's new? *Autonom Neurosci Basic Clin.* 2017; 202:62-72.

Candy B, Clement S, Sikorski J, et al. Antenatal visits. In: Wickham S, eds. *Midwifery Best Practice.* London: Books for Midwives; 2003:34-37.

Chan l, Gordon A, Warrilow K et al. Evaluation of Movements Matter: A social media and hospital-based campaign aimed at raising awareness of decreased fetal movements. *Aust NZ J Obstet Gynaecol* 2021; 1–9. Doi:10.1111/ajo.13360

Chandra K, Magee L, Einarson A, et al. Nausea and vomiting in pregnancy: results of a survey that identified interventions used by women to alleviate their symptoms. *J Psychosom Obstet Gynaecol.* 2003;24(2):71-75.

Cheikh Ismail L, Bishop D, Pang R, et al. Gestational weight gain standards based on women enrolled in the Fetal Growth Longitudinal Study of the INTERGROWTH-21st Project: a prospective longitudinal cohort study. *BMJ.* 2016;352:i555. doi:10.1136/bmj.i555.

Chen Y-K, Chen S-F, Li H-C, et al. No increased risk of adverse pregnancy outcomes in women with urinary tract infections: a nationwide population-based study. *Acta Obstet Gynecol Scand.* 2010;89:882-888.

Childbirth And Parenting Educators of Australia (CAPEA). *National competency standards for childbirth and early parenting educators.* 2018, 2nd edition. Online: https://capea.org.au/resources/competency-standards-for-childbirth-and-parenting-educators/

Clark K, Beatty S, Reibel T. Maternity care: a narrative review of what women expect across their care continuum. *Midwifery.* 2015a;31:432-437.

Clark K, Beatty S, Reibel T. 'What women want': using image theory to develop expectations of maternity care framework. *Midwifery.* 2015b;31:505-511.

Coggins J. Iron deficiency anaemia: a complication of pregnancy or a foregone conclusion? A midwife's view. *MIDIRS Midwifery Dig.* 2001;11(4):469-474.

Coll C, Domingues M, Goncalves H, et al. Perceived barriers to leisure-time physical activity during pregnancy: a literature review of quantitative and qualitative evidence. *J Sci Med Sport.* 2017;20:17-25.

Connelly M, Brown H, van der Pligt P, et al. Modifiable barriers to leisure-time physical activity during pregnancy: a qualitative study investigating first time mothers' views and experiences. *BMC Pregnancy Childbirth.* 2015;15:100.

Cowan J, McKinlay C, Taylor R, et al. Detection of small for gestational age babies and perinatal outcomes following implementation of the Growth Assessment Protocol at a New Zealand tertiary facility: An observational intervention study. *Aust NZ J Obstet Gynaecol.* 2021; 61: 339–346.

Crafter H. *Health Promotion in Midwifery: Principles and Practice.* London: Arnold; 1997.

Crowther S. Blood tests for investigating maternal wellbeing. *Pract Midwife.* 2010;13(10):48-52.

Cutajar L and Cyna A. Antenatal education for childbirth – epidural analgesia. *Midwifery* 2018; 64:48-52.

Da Costa D, Ireland K. Perceived benefits and barriers to leisure-time physical activity during pregnancy in previously inactive and active women. *Women Health.* 2013;53(2):185-202.

da Silva S, Ricardo L, Evenson K, et al. Leisure-time physical activity in pregnancy and maternal-child health: a systematic review and meta-analysis of randomized controlled trials and cohort studies. *Sports Med.* 2017;47:295-317.

Daru J, Colman K, Stanworth S et al., Serum ferritin as an indicator of iron status: what do we need to know? *Am J Clin Nutr* 2017;106(Suppl):1634S–9S; doi: 10.3945/ajcn.117.155960.

Davenport M, Ruchat S, Sobierajski F, et al. Impact of prenatal exercise on maternal harms, labour and delivery outcomes: a systematic review and meta-analysis. *British journal of sports medicine.* 2019; 53(2), 99-107.

Davison C, Hauck Y, Bayes S, et al. The relationship is everything: women's reasons for choosing a privately practising midwife in Western Australia. *Midwifery.* 2015;31:722-778.

de Jonge A, Stuijt R, Eijke I, et al. Continuity of care: what matters to women when they are referred from primary to secondary care during labour? A qualitative interview study in the Netherlands. *BMC Pregnancy Childbirth.* 2014;14:103.

Department of Health (DOH). *Clinical Practice Guidelines: Pregnancy Care.* Canberra: Australian Government Department of Health; 2018. Online: http://www.health.gov.au/internet/main/publishing.nsf/Content/4BC0E3DE489BE54DCA258231007CDD05/$File/Pregnancy%20care%20guidelines%206June18.pdf.

Department of Health (DOH). *Clinical Practice Guidelines: Pregnancy Care.* Canberra: Australian Government Department of Health; 2020. Online: https://www.health.gov.au/resources/pregnancy-care-guidelines.

Dewey K and Oaks B. U-shaped curve for risk associated with maternal hemoglobin, iron status, or iron supplementation. *Am J Clin Nutr* 2017;106(suppl):1694S–702S.

Ding M, Leach M, Bradley H. The effectiveness and safety of ginger for pregnancy-induced nausea and vomiting: a systematic review. *Women Birth.* 2013;26:e26–e30.

Donley J. *Birthrites: Natural Versus Unnatural Childbirth In New Zealand.* Auckland: Full Court Press; 1998.

Donnison J. *Midwives and Medical Men: A History of the Struggle for the Control of Childbirth.* London: Historical Publications; 1998.

Dove S, Muir-Cochrane E. Being safe practitioners and safe mothers: a critical ethnography of continuity of care midwifery in Australia. *Midwifery.* 2014;30(10):1063-1072. doi:10.1016/j.midw.2013.12.016.

Downe S, Finlayson K, Tuncalp O, et al. What matters to women: a systematic scoping review to identify the processes and outcomes of antenatal care provision that are important to healthy pregnant women. *BJOG.* 2015;123:529—539.

Dowswell T, Carroli G, Duley L, et al. Alternative versus standard packages of antenatal care for low-risk pregnancy. *Cochrane Database Syst Rev.* 2015;(7):CD000934, doi:10.1002/14651858.CD000934.pub3.

Einarson T, Piwko C, Koren G. Quantifying the global rates of nausea and vomiting of pregnancy: a meta-analysis. *J Popul Ther Clin Pharmacol.* 2013;20(2):e171–e183.

Ekelin M, Iversen M, Backhausen M, & Hegaard H. Not now but later–a qualitative study of non-exercising pregnant women's views and experiences of exercise. *BMC pregnancy and childbirth.* 2018; 18(1), 1-10.

Enkin M, Keirse M, Neilson J, et al. *A Guide to Effective Care in Pregnancy and Childbirth.* 3rd ed. Oxford: Oxford University Press; 2000. Online: http://2020ok.com/books/63/a-guide-to-effective-care-in-pregnancy-and-childbirth-19963.htm.

Fejzo M, Magtira A, Schoenberg F, et al. Antihistamines and other prognostic factors for adverse outcome in hyperemesis gravidarum. *Eur J Obstet Gynecol Reprod Biol.* 2013;170(1):71-76. doi:10.1016/j.ejogrb.2013.04.017.

Flenady V, Gardener G, Ellwood D et al. My Baby's Movements: a stepped-wedge cluster-randomised controlled trial of a fetal movement awareness intervention to reduce stillbirths. *BJOG.* 2021. Volume 129, Issue 1 p. 29–41: https://doi.org/10.1111/1471-0528.16944.

Findley A., Smith D, Hesketh K, & Keyworth C. Exploring womens' experiences and decision making about physical activity during pregnancy and following birth: A qualitative study. *BMC pregnancy and childbirth.* 2020; 20(1), 1-10.

Forster D, McLachlan H, Davey M-A, et al. Continuity of care by a primary midwife (caseload midwifery) increases women's satisfaction with antenatal, intrapartum and postpartum care: results from the COSMOS randomised controlled trial. *BMC Pregnancy Childbirth.* 2016;16:28.

Fraser D, Cooper M. *Myles Textbook for Midwives.* 14th ed. Edinburgh: Churchill Livingstone; 2003.

Frye A. *Holistic Midwifery. Vol. I. Care During Pregnancy.* Portland, OR: Labrys Press; 1998.

Gadsby R., Ivanova D., Trevelyan E., Hutton J, & Johnson S. The onset of nausea and vomiting of pregnancy: a prospective cohort study. *BMC Pregnancy and Childbirth.* 2021; 21(1), 1-7.

Gagnon AJ, Sandall J. Individual or group antenatal education for childbirth or parenthood, or both. *Cochrane Database Syst Rev.* 2007;(3):CD002869, doi:10.1002/14651858.CD002869.pub2.

Gardosi J, Mongelli M, Wilcox M, et al. *Gestation related optimal weight (GROW) program. Software version 3.* West Midlands Perinatal Institute, Birmingham. 2000. Online: www.gestation.net.

Gates E. Communicating risk in prenatal genetic testing. *J Midwifery Womens Health.* 2004;49(3):220-226.

Grimes D, Schulz K. Uses and abuses of screening tests. *Lancet.* 2002;359:881-884.

Haines HM, Baker J, Marshall D. Continuity of midwifery care for rural women through caseload group practice: delivering for almost 20 years. *Aust J Rural Health.* 2015;23(6):339-345. doi:10.1111/ajr.12232.

Hall M. Rationalisation of antenatal care. *Lancet.* 2001;357:1546.

Haws R, Yakoob M, Soomro T, et al. Reducing stillbirths: screening and monitoring during pregnancy and labour. *BMC Pregnancy Childbirth*. 2009;9(suppl 1):S5.
Heazell A, Frøen J. Methods of fetal movement counting and the detection of fetal compromise. *J Obstet Gynaecol*. 2008; 28(2):147-154.
Heitmann K, Nordeng H, Havnen G, et al. The burden of nausea and vomiting during pregnancy: severe impacts on quality of life, daily functioning and willingness to become pregnant again–results form a cross-sectional study. *BMC Pregnancy Childbirth*. 2017;17:75.
Henderson C, Macdonald S. *Mayes' Midwifery*. 13th ed. Edinburgh: Baillière Tindall; 2004.
Hong K, Hwang H, Han H et al. Perspectives on antenatal education associated with pregnancy outcomes: Systematic review and meta-analysis. *Women Birth*. 2021;34:219-230.
Hu Y, Amoah A, Zhang H. et al. Effect of ginger in the treatment of nausea and vomiting compared with vitamin B6 and placebo during pregnancy: a meta-analysis. *The Journal of Maternal-Fetal & Neonatal Medicine*. 2020; 1-10.
Hunter L. Issues in pregnancy dating: revisiting the evidence. *J Midwifery Womens Health*. 2009;54(3):184-190.
Jamil T, Evennett K. *The Alternative Pregnancy Handbook*. London: Judy Piathus; 2000.
Jenkins M, Ford J, Todd A, et al. Women's views about maternity care: how do women conceptualise the process of continuity? *Midwifery*. 2015;3:25-30.
Jordan S. *Pharmacology for Midwives, the Evidence Base for Safe Practice*. 2nd ed. Basingstoke: Palgrave Macmillan; 2010.
Katz Rothman B. *Recreating Motherhood: Ideology and Technology in a Patriarchal Society*. New York: Norton; 1989.
Kean L, Chan K. Routine antenatal management at booking clinic. *Obstet Gynaecol Reprod Med*. 2007;17(3):69-73.
Kesrouani A, Atallah C, AbouJaoude R, et al. Accuracy of clinical fetal weight estimation by midwives. *BMC Pregnancy Childbirth*. 2017;17:59. doi:10.1186/s12884-017-1242-7.
Koleini N, Shapiro J, Geier J & Ardehali H. Ironing out mechanisms of iron homeostasis and disorders of iron deficiency. *J Clin Invest*. 2021;131(11):e148671. Doi:10.1172/JCI148671.
Kramer M, McDonald S. Aerobic exercise for women during pregnancy. *Cochrane Database Syst Rev*. 2006;(3):CD000180, doi:10.1002/14651858.CD000180.pub2.
Levett K and Dahlen H. Perspective: Childbirth education in Australia: Have we lost our way? *Women Birth*. 2019;32:291-293.
Lilford J, Kelly M, Baines A et al. Effect of using protocols on medical care: randomised trial of three methods of taking an antenatal history. *BMJ* 1992; 305:1181-4.
Lowe S, Bowyer L, Lust K, et al. *Guideline for the Management of Hypertensive Disorders of Pregnancy*. Sydney: Society of Obstetric Medicine of Australia and New Zealand (SOMANZ); 2014 (updated June 2015). Online: http://somanz.org/downloads/HTguidelineupdatedJune2015.pdf.
Lumley J. Attenders and nonattenders at childbirth education classes in Australia: how do they and their births differ? *Birth*. 1993;2(3):123-130.
Lynch C, Zhang J. The research implications of the selection of a gestational age estimation method. *Paediatr Perinat Epidemiol*. 2007;21(suppl 2):86-96.
McArdle A, Flenady V, Toohill J, et al. How pregnant women learn about foetal movements: sources and preferences for information. *Women Birth*. 2015;28:54-59.
McCowan L, Roberts C, Dekker G, et al. on behalf of the SCOPE consortium. Risk factors for small-for-gestational-age infants by customised birthweight centiles: data from an international prospective cohort study. *BJOG*. 2010;117:1599-1607.
McGeown P. Detecting fetal growth abnormalities. *MIDIRS Midwifery Dig*. 2001;11(2):190-193.
McParlin C, O'Donnell A, Robson S, et al. Treatments for hyperemesis gravidarum and nausea and vomiting in pregnancy. *JAMA*. 2016;316(13):1392-1401.
Maier BJ. Antenatal group care in a midwifery group practice—a midwife's perspective. *Women Birth*. 2013;26(1):87-89. doi:10.1016/j.wombi.2012.02.002.
Mangesi L, Hofmeyr GJ, Smith V, et al. Fetal movement counting for assessment of fetal wellbeing. *Cochrane Database Syst Rev*. 2015;(10):CD004909, doi:10.1002/14651858.CD004909.pub3.
Matthews A, Haas D, O'Mathúna D, et al. Interventions for nausea and vomiting in early pregnancy. *Cochrane Database Syst Rev*. 2015;(9):CD007575. doi:10.1002/14651858.CD007575. pub4.
Middleton P, Bubner T, Glover K, et al. 'Partnerships are crucial': an evaluation of the Aboriginal Family Birthing Program in South Australia. *Aust N Z J Public Health*. 2017;41(1):21-26.
Midwifery Council of New Zealand. *Statement on cultural competence*. 2011. https://midwiferycouncil.health.nz/common/Uploaded%20files/About%20Us/Statement%20on%20cultural%20competence.pdf
Milman N. Iron and pregnancy—a delicate balance. *Ann Hematol*. 2006;85:559-565.
Milman N. Prepartum anaemia: prevention and treatment. *Ann Hematol*. 2008;87:949-959.
Milman N. Oral iron prophylaxis in pregnancy: not too little and not too much! *J Pregnancy*. 2012:514345. doi:10.1155/2012/514345.
Ministry of Health (MOH). *Section 88 Primary Maternity Services Notice*. Wellington, NZ: Ministry of Health; 2007. Online: http://www.health.govt.nz/our-work/life-stages/maternity-services/primary-maternity-services-notice-section-88.
Ministry of Health (MOH). *Screening, Diagnosis and Management of Gestational Diabetes in New Zealand: A Clinical Practice Guideline*. Wellington, NZ: Ministry of Health; 2014. Online: https://www.health.govt.nz/publication/screening-diagnosis-and-management-gestational-diabetes-new-zealand-clinical-practice-guideline.
Ministry of Health (MOH). *Maternity Consumer Surveys 2014*. Wellington, NZ: Ministry of Health; 2015a. Online: http://www.health.govt.nz/publication/maternity-consumer-survey-2014.
Ministry of Health (MOH). *Maternity Services - DHB Funded - Pregnancy and parenting information and education tier level two service specification*. 2015b. Online: https://nsfl.health.govt.nz/service-specifications/current-service-specifications/maternity-service-specifications.
Ministry of Health (MOH). *National Maternity Clinical Guidance*. Wellington, NZ: Ministry of Health; 2017. Online: https://www.health.govt.nz/our-work/life-stages/maternity-services/national-maternity-clinical-guidance.
Ministry of Health (MOH). *Report on Maternity. Primary Maternity Care, LMC type*. Web tool 2020. https://www.health.govt.nz/publication/report-maternity-web-tool
Moore, A., Doull, M., Grad, R., Groulx, S., Pottie, K., Tonelli, M., ... & Thombs, B. D. Recommendations on screening for asymptomatic bacteriuria in pregnancy. *CMAJ*. 2018;190(27), E823-E830.
Morse K, Williams A, Gardosi J. Fetal growth screening by fundal height measurement. *Best Pract Res Clin Obstet Gynaecol*. 2009; 23:809-813.
National Blood Authority (NBA). *Patient Blood Management Guidelines: Module 5 Obstetrics and Maternity*. Canberra: NBA; 2015. Online: https://www.blood.gov.au/pbm-module-5.
National Collaborating Centre for Women's and Children's Health (Commissioned by the National Institute for Health and Clinical Excellence). *Antenatal Care: Routine Care for the Healthy Pregnant Woman*. London: RCOG Press; 2008. https://www.nice.org.uk/guidance/cg62/evidence/full-guideline-corrected-june-2008-196748317.

National Institute for Health and Clinical Excellence (NICE). *Antenatal care for uncomplicated pregnancies*. London: RCOG Press; 2008, updated 2019. Online: https://www.nice.org.uk/Guidance/CG62.

National Institute for Health and Care Excellence (NICE). *Weight management before, during and after pregnancy*. Manchester: NICE Public Health Guidance. 2010. https://www.nice.org.uk/guidance/ph27.

National Institute for Health and Care Excellence (NICE). *Antenatal Care for Uncomplicated Pregnancies. Clinical Guideline.* London: NICE; 2017 (rev. ed.). Online: https://www.nice.org.uk/guidance/cg62.

National Institute for Health and Care Excellence (NICE). *Hypertension in pregnancy: diagnosis and management [NICE Guideline 133]*. London: RCOG Press, 2019. Online: https://www.nice.org.uk/guidance/ng133/resources/hypertension-in-pregnancy-diagnosis-and-management-pdf-66141717671365.

National Institute for Health and Clinical Excellence (NICE). *Antenatal care. NICE Guideline [NG201]*. London: RCOG Press; 2021. Online: https://www.nice.org.uk/Guidance/ng201.

National Screening Unit (NSU). *Antenatal Blood Test Fact Sheet.* New Zealand: Ministry of Health; 2017. Online: https://www.nsu.govt.nz/system/files/resources/antenatalbloodtests19jan16.pdf.

New Zealand College of Midwives (NZCOM). *Midwives Handbook for Practice*. 5th ed. Christchurch: NZCOM; 2015.

New Zealand Guidelines Group. *Identification of Common Mental Disorders and Management of Depression in Primary Care. An Evidence-based Best Practice Guideline*. Wellington: New Zealand Guidelines Group; 2008.

Nolan M. Antenatal survey (1) What do women want? *Pract Midwife*. 2008a;11(1):26–28.

Nolan M. Antenatal survey (2) What do women want? *Pract Midwife*. 2008b;11(2):32–35.

Nolan M. Antenatal survey (3) What do women want? *Pract Midwife*. 2008c;11(3):34–35.

Norman J, Heazell A, Rodriquez A et al Awareness of fetal movements and care package to reduce fetal mortality (AFFIRM): a stepped wedge, cluster- randomised trial. *Lancet* 2018; 392: 1629–38. Online: https://www.thelancet.com/journals/lancet/article/PIIS0140-6736(18)31543-5/fulltext.

Oakley A. *The Captured Womb.* Oxford: Blackwell; 1984.

Oakley A. *Social Support and Motherhood: The Natural History of a Research Project.* Oxford: Blackwell; 1992.

Oats J. Routine antenatal screening: a need to evaluate Australian practice [editorial]. *Med J Aust.* 2000;172:311–312. Online: www.mja.com.au/public/issues/172_07_030400/oats/oats.html.

O'Connor D. *Saving Babies' Lives, a Care Bundle for Reducing Stillbirth.* Leeds UK: NHS England; 2016. Online: https://www.england.nhs.uk/wp-content/uploads/2016/03/saving-babies-lives-car-bundl.pdf.

O'Donnell A, McParlin C, Robson SC, et al. Treatments for hyperemesis gravidarum and nausea and vomiting in pregnancy: a systematic review and economic assessment. *Health Technol Assess.* 2016;20(74):1–268. Online: https://www.ncbi.nlm.nih.gov/books/NBK390518/pdf/Bookshelf_NBK390518.pdf.

Ogbo F, Eastwood J, Hendry A, et al. Determinants of antenatal depression and postnatal depression in Australia. *BMC psychiatry*. 2018; 18(1):1-11.

Palasanthiran P, Starr M, Jones C, eds. *Management of Perinatal Infections.* 2nd ed. Sydney: Australasian Society for Infectious Diseases; 2014. Online: https://www.asid.net.au/resources/clinical-guidelines.

Parker M, Forbes K, Findlay I. Eugenics or empowered choice? Community issues arising from prenatal testing. *Aust N Z J Obstet Gynaecol.* 2002;42(1):10–14.

Pasricha S-R, Flecknoe-Brown S, Allen K, et al. Diagnosis and management of iron deficiency anaemia: a clinical update. *Med J Aust.* 2010;193(9):525–532.

Pasricha S-R, Colman K, Centeno-Tablante E et al. Revisiting WHO haemoglobin thresholds to define anaemia in clinical medicine and public health. *The Lancet Haematology*. 2018;(5):e60-e62.

Pasupathy D, McCowan L, Poston L, et al. on behalf of the SCOPE consortium. Perinatal outcomes of large infants using customised birthweight centiles and conventional measures of high birthweight. *Paediatr Perinat Epidemiol.* 2012;26:543–552.

Pavord S, Daru J, Prasannan N et al., UK guidelines on the management of iron deficiency on pregnancy. *British Journal of Haematology*. 2020;188:819-830.

Peat A, Stacey T, Cronin R, et al. Maternal knowledge of fetal movements in late pregnancy. *Aust N Z J Obstet Gynaecol.* 2012;52:445–449.

Peña-Rosas JP, De-Regil LM, Garcia-Casal MN, et al. Daily oral iron supplementation during pregnancy. *Cochrane Database Syst Rev.* 2015a;(7):CD004736, doi:10.1002/14651858.CD004736.pub5.

Perinatal and Maternal Mortality Review Committee (PMMRC). *Eleventh Annual Report of the Perinatal and Maternal Review Committee: Reporting Mortality 2015.* Wellington: Health Quality & Safety Commission; 2017. Online: https://www.hqsc.govt.nz/assets/PMMRC/Publications/2017_PMMRC_Eleventh_Annual_Report.pdf.

Perinatal and Maternal Mortality Review Committee (PMMRC). *Fourteenth Annual Report of the Perinatal and Maternal Review Committee: Reporting Mortality 2018.* Wellington: Health Quality & Safety Commission; 2021. Online: http://www.hqsc.govt.nz/our-programmes/mrc/pmmrc.

Perinatal Institute. *Customised growth charts*; 2017. Online: www.gestation.net.

Perinatal Society of Australia and New Zealand and Centre of Research Excellence Stillbirth (PSANZ). *Clinical practice guideline for the care of women with decreased fetal movements for women with a singleton pregnancy from 28 weeks' gestation.* Centre of Research Excellence in Stillbirth. Brisbane, Australia. 2019. Online: https://resources.stillbirthcre.org.au/elearn/resources/Element%203_DFM%20Clinical%20Practice%20Guideline.pdf

Peter V., Ho J, Vallipan J, et al. Symphysial fundal height (SFH) measurement in pregnancy for detecting abnormal fetal growth. *Cochrane Database Syst Rev.* 2015;(9):CD008136, doi:10.1002/14651858.CD008136.pub3.

Petrou S, Kupek E, Vause S, et al. Antenatal visits and adverse perinatal outcomes: results from a British population-based study. *Eur J Obstet Gynecol Reprod Biol.* 2003;106(1):40–49.

Phupong V, Hanprasertpong T. Interventions for heartburn in pregnancy. *Cochrane Database Syst Rev.* 2015;(9):CD011379, doi:10.1002/14651858.CD011379.pub2.

Pollock D, Ziaian T, Pearson E et al. Breaking through the silence in antenatal care: fetal movement and stillbirth education. *Women Birth.* 2020; 33:77-85.

Rådestad I. Strengthening mindfetalness. *Sexual & Reproductive Health.* 2012;3:59-60.

Rankin J, Hillan E, Mutrie N. An historical overview of physical activity and childbirth. *Br J Midwifery.* 2000;8(12):761–764.

Ray J, Davidson A, Berger H, et al Haemaglobin levels in early pregnancy and severe maternal morbidity: population-based cohort study. *BJOG.* 2020; 127:1154-1164, doi:10.1111/1471-0528.16216.

Redman S, Oak S, Booth P, et al. Evaluation of an antenatal education programme: characteristics of attenders, changes in knowledge and satisfaction of participants. *Aust NZ J Obstet Gynaecol.* 1991;31(4):310–316.

Roex A, Nikpoor P, Eerd E, et al. Serial plotting on customised fundal height charts results in doubling of antenatal detection of small for gestational age fetuses in nulliparous women. *Aust N Z J Obstet Gynaecol.* 2012;52:78–82.

Ross M. Circle of time: errors in the use of the pregnancy wheel. *J Matern Fetal Neonatal Med.* 2003;14(6):370–372.

Rosser J. Calculating the EDD: which is more accurate, scan or LMP? *Pract Midwife.* 2000;3(3):28–29.
Roy N., Pavord S., The management of anaemia and haematinic deficiencies in pregnancy and post-partum. *Transfusion Medicine* 2018; 28(2):107-116
Royal Australian and New Zealand College of Obstetricians and Gynaecologists (RANZCOG). *Routine Antenatal Assessment in the Absence of Pregnancy Complications. (Guideline C-Obs 3b).* Melbourne: RANZCOG; 2019a.
Royal Australian and New Zealand College of Obstetricians and Gynaecologists (RANZCOG). *Vitamin and mineral supplementation and pregnancy. Guideline C-Obs 25.* Melbourne: RANZCOG; 2019b.
Rungsiprakarn P, Laopaiboon M, Sangkomkamhang US, et al. Interventions for treating constipation in pregnancy. *Cochrane Database Syst Rev.* 2015;(9):CD011448, doi:10.1002/14651858.CD011448.pub2.
Sandall J, Soltani H, Gates S, et al. Midwife-led continuity models versus other models of care for childbearing women. *Cochrane Database Syst Rev.* 2013;(8):CD004667, doi:10.1002/14651858.CD004667.pub3.
Sandall J, Soltani H, Gates S, et al. Midwife-led continuity models versus other models of care for childbearing women. *Cochrane Database Syst Rev.* 2016;(4):CD004667, doi:10.1002/14651858.CD004667.pub5.
Sanger C, Haynes A, Mountain G, et al. Antenatal screening and early-intervention: a mental helath update from NSPCC. *Br J Midwifery.* 2015;23(6):388–390.
Santalahti P, Aro A, Hemminki E, et al. On what grounds do women participate in prenatal screening? *Prenat Diagn.* 1998;18:153–165.
Schmied V, Johnson M, Naidoo N, et al. Maternal mental health in Australia and New Zealand: a review of longitudinal studies. *Women Birth.* 2013;26:167–178.
Schmied V, Langdon R, Matthey S, et al. Antenatal psychosocial risk status and Australian women's use of primary care and specialist mental health services in the year after birth: a prospective study. *BMC Womens Health.* 2016;16:69. doi:10.1186/s12905-016-0344-0.
Searle J. Routine antenatal screening: not a case of informed choice. *Aust N Z J Public Health.* 1997;21(3):268–274.
Smaill FM, Vazquez JC. Antibiotics for asymptomatic bacteriuria in pregnancy. *Cochrane Database Syst Rev.* 2019;(11):CD000490, doi: 10.1002/14651858.CD000490.pub4.
Stenhouse E, Wright D, Hattersley A, et al. How well do midwives estimate the date of delivery? *Midwifery.* 2003;19:125–131.
Stoffel N, Zeder C, Brittenham G. et al. Iron absorption from supplements is greater with alternate day than with consecutive day dosing in iron-deficient anemic women. *Haematologica.* 2020;105(5):1232-1239.
Strong T. *Expecting Trouble: What Expectant Parents Should Know About Prenatal Care in America.* New York: New York University Press; 2000.
Sword W, Heaman M, Brooks S, et al. Women's and care providers' perspectives of quality prenatal care: a qualitative descriptive study. *BMC Pregnancy Childbirth.* 2012;12:29. doi:10.1186/1471-2393-12-29.
Taylor R. Correct technique for blood pressure measurement—why bother? *Midwifery News.* 2004;32:23.
Tiran D. Ginger to reduce nausea and vomiting during pregnancy: evidence of effectiveness is not the same as proof of safety. *Complement Ther Clin Pract.* 2012;18:22–25.
Tiran, D. Complementary therapies in maternity care: an evidence-based approach. *Singing Dragon.* 2018.
Towler J, Butler-Manuel R. *Modern Obstetrics for Student Midwives.* London: Lloyd-Luke Medical Books; 1975.
Tracy S.K., Pairman S., Kildea S., et al. Midwives Speaking Out on COVID-19: The International Confederation of Midwives (ICM) Global Survey. (In Press, under review PLOS 2022)
Turner J., Flenady V., et al Evaluation of Pregnancy Outcomes Among Women With Decreased Fetal Movements. *JAMA Netw Open.* 2021;4(4): e215071. doi:10.1001/jamanetworkopen.2021.5071
Underwood L, Waldie K, D'Souza S, et al. A longitudinal study of pre-pregnancy and pregnancy risk factors associated with antenatal and postnatal symptoms of depression: evidence from growing up in New Zealand. *Maternal and child health journal.* 2017; 21(4):915-931.
Wagner M. *Pursuing the Birth Machine: The Search for Appropriate Birth Technology.* Sydney: Ace Graphics; 1994.
Waldie K, Peterson E, D'Souza S, et al. Depression symptoms during pregnancy: evidence from Growing Up in New Zealand. *J Affect Disord.* 2015;186:66–73.
Walsh T, O'Broin S, Cooley S, et al. Laboratory assessment of iron status in pregnancy. *Clin Chem Lab Med.* 2011;49(7):1225–1230.
Warland J., Glover P., Talking to pregnant women about stillbirth. BMC Pregnancy and Childbirth 2015 Volume 15 Supplement 1 Proceedings of the Stillbirth Summit 2014
Warland J, Glover P. Fetal movements: what are we telling women? *Women Birth.* 2017;30:23–28.
Waugh J, Clark T, Divakaran T, et al. Accuracy of urinalysis dipstick techniques in predicting significant proteinuria in pregnancy. *Obstet Gynecol.* 2004;103(4):769–777.
Wegienka G, Baird D. A comparison of recalled date of last menstrual period with prospectively recorded dates. *J Womens Health.* 2005;14(3):248–253.
Wickham S. Pinard wisdom: tips and tricks from midwives (Part 1). *Pract Midwife.* 2002;5(9):21.
Wills G, Forster D. Nausea and vomiting in pregnancy: what advice do midwives give? *Midwifery.* 2008;24:390–398.
Wing D, Rumney P, Preslicka C, et al. Daily cranberry juice for the prevention of asymptomatic bacteriuria in pregnancy: a randomised, controlled pilot study. *J Urol.* 2008;180:1367–1372.
Wood H, McKellar L, Lightbody M. Nausea and vomiting in pregnancy: blooming or bloomin' awful? A review of the literature. *Women Birth.* 2013;26:100–104.
World Health Organization (WHO). *Global anaemia reduction efforts among women of reproductive age: impact, achievement of targets and the way forward for optimizing efforts.* Geneva: World Health Organization; 2020. Online: https://www.who.int/publications/i/item/9789240012202
World Health Organization (WHO). *WHO Recommendations on Antenatal Care for a Positive Pregnancy Experience.* Geneva: WHO; 2016. Online: http://www.who.int/reproductivehealth/publications/maternal_perinatal_health/anc-positive-pregnancy-experience/en.
World Health Organization (WHO). *WHO Recommendations on Antenatal Care for a Positive Pregnancy Experience: Ultrasound examination.* Geneva, Switzerland: WHO; 2018.
World Health Organisation (WHO). *WHO Guidelines on Physical Activity and Sedentary Behaviour.* Geneva: WHO. 2020. Online: https://www.who.int/publications/i/item/9789240015128.
Yelland J, Brown S. Asking women about mental health and social adversity in pregnancy: results of an Australian population-based survey. *Birth.* 2014;41(1):79–87.

Further reading

Balaskas J. *New Natural Pregnancy.* 2nd ed. Sydney: Sandstone; 1998.
Brayshaw E. *Exercises in Pregnancy and Childbirth: A Practical Guide for Educators.* London: Books for Midwives; 2003.
Department of Health (DOH). *Clinical Practice Guidelines: Pregnancy Care. Linking Evidence to Recommendations.* Canberra: Australian Government Department of Health; 2018.

Donley J. *Birthrites: Natural vs Unnatural Childbirth in New Zealand.* Auckland: Full Court Press; 1998.

Enkin M, Keirse M, Neilson J, et al. *A Guide to Effective Care in Pregnancy and Childbirth.* 3rd ed. Oxford: Oxford University Press; 2000. Online: http://2020ok.com/books/63/a-guide-to-effective-care-in-pregnancy-and-childbirth-19963.htm.

Fanslow JL, Kelly P, Ministry of Health. *Family Violence Assessment and Intervention Guideline: Child Abuse and Intimate Partner Violence.* 2nd ed. Wellington, NZ: Ministry of Health; 2016. Online: https://www.health.govt.nz/publication/family-violence-assessment-and-intervention-guideline-child-abuse-and-intimate-partner-violence.

Frye A. *Holistic Midwifery. Vol. I. Care During Pregnancy.* Portland, OR: Labrys Press; 1998.

Jamil T, Evennett K. *The Alternative Pregnancy Hand-Book.* London: Judy Piathus; 2000.

Jordan S. *Pharmacology for Midwives.* 2nd ed. Basingstoke, UK: Palgrave Macmillan; 2010.

Katz Rothman B. *Recreating Motherhood: Ideology and Technology in a Patriarchal Society.* New York: Norton; 1989.

Krishnaswamy S, Wallace E, Buttery J, et al. Antenatal pertussis vaccination: are we implementing best evidence into practice? *Aust N Z J Obstet Gynaecol.* 2016;56:552-555.

Milman N, Paszlowski T, Cetin I, et al. Supplementation during pregnancy: beliefs and science. *Gynecol Endocrinol.* 2016; 32(7):509-516. doi:10.3109/09513590.2016.1149161.

Ministry of Health (MOH). *Section 88 Primary Maternity Services Notice.* Wellington, NZ: MOH; 2007. Online: http://www.health.govt.nz/our-work/life-stages/maternity-services/primary-maternity-services-notice-section-88.

Ministry of Health (MOH). *Food and Nutrition Guidelines for Healthy Pregnant and Breastfeeding Women: A Back-Ground Paper.* Wellington, NZ: MOH; 2008. Online: https://www.health.govt.nz/system/files/documents/publications/food-and-nutrition-guidelines-preg-and-bfeed.pdf.

Ministry of Health (MOH). *Maternity Consumer Surveys 2014.* Wellington, NZ: MOH; 2015. Online: http://www.health.govt.nz/publication/maternity-consumer-survey-2014.

New Zealand College of Midwives (NZCOM). *Consensus Statement on Gestational Diabetes.* Christchurch: NZCOM; 2006.

New Zealand College of Midwives (NZCOM). *Midwives Handbook for Practice.* 5th ed. Christchurch, NZ: NZCOM; 2015.

Oakley A. *The Captured Womb.* Oxford: Blackwell; 1984.

Reiger K. *Our Bodies, Our Babies: The Forgotten Women's Movement.* Melbourne: Melbourne University Press; 2001.

Spangaro J, Koziol-McLain J, Zwi A, et al. Deciding to tell: qualitative configurational analysis of decisions to disclose experience of intimate partner violence in antenatal care. *Soc Sci Med.* 2016;154:45-53.

Strong T. *Expecting Trouble: What Expectant Parents Should Know About Prenatal Care in America.* New York: New York University Press; 2000.

Tiran D. *Natural Remedies for Morning Sickness and Other Pregnancy Problems.* London: Quadrille Publishing; 2001.

Yelland J, Brown S. Asking women about mental health and social adversity in pregnancy: results of an Australian population-based survey. *Birth.* 2014;41(1):79-87.

CHAPTER 24

Applied physiology for labour and birth

Sally Baddock

LEARNING OUTCOMES

Learning outcomes for this chapter are:

1. To outline the changes involved in myometrial activation and cervical ripening
2. To discuss the physiological factors that may be responsible for initiating labour
3. To outline the role of hormones in the maintenance of labour
4. To describe the physiology underlying the four stages of labour, including the physiology of effective uterine contractions, the mechanism of the second stage, the steps involved in placental separation in the third stage and the beginning of recovery from labour described as the fourth stage
5. To discuss physiological changes that occur to other systems to support labour
6. To describe fetal responses and identify measures of fetal wellbeing during labour.

CHAPTER OVERVIEW

This chapter focuses on the physiological processes associated with birth. This begins in the final weeks of pregnancy as changes occur to the uterus and cervix in preparation for birth and continues through the processes associated with the birth of the baby.

The physiology underlying labour includes many physical and chemical processes controlled by hormones. Before labour begins, hormones mediate the preparatory changes that occur in the uterus and cervix. The actual mechanisms that initiate labour are not clear, but they are associated with fetal, placental and maternal hormones. Progress in labour is largely mediated by hormones that govern **uterine contractions**. Effective contractions first lead to dilation of the cervix and then generate the pressure to birth the baby. The **mechanism of labour** describes the manipulations the baby must make to negotiate the pelvis and birth canal. Following the birth of the baby the placenta separates from the uterus and may be birthed without intervention, while continuing uterine contractions minimise blood loss from the placental site. Labour is a physically demanding time that is supported by changes to metabolism and probably changes to all body systems to facilitate the labour process. During labour the fetus is normally exposed to considerable stress.

These processes are the focus of this chapter. Additional readings are provided at the end of the chapter for a more in-depth exploration of specific topics.

KEY TERMS

cervical ripening
effacement
fetal responses
initiation of labour
mechanism of labour
myometrial activation
placental separation
stages of labour
uterine contractions
water and electrolyte balance

INTRODUCTION

Understanding the underlying physiology of labour is essential if a midwife is to make informed decisions about the progress of labour and if she is to be able to adequately assess the wellbeing of the woman and baby throughout labour. It also enables informed discussion with the woman throughout these times of major physiological change. This chapter explores the hormonal mechanisms that drive the physiological processes leading to the birth of the baby, birth of the placenta and also the initial recovery from labour.

PHYSIOLOGY OF LABOUR

Labour is a process where regular and coordinated muscular contractions of the uterus lead to gradual **effacement** and dilation of the cervix, followed by expulsive contractions, which result in the birth of the baby and placenta. For simplicity, the physiological changes that occur during this process can be divided into four **stages of labour**. Stage one describes the time when uterine contractions are of sufficient frequency, intensity and duration to cause effacement and dilation of the cervix. Stage two begins with the complete dilation of the cervix and ends with the birth of the baby, while stage three involves the birth of the placenta. The fourth stage refers to the first hour or two after birth when uterine tone is established and recovery from labour begins.

Physiologically there is no abrupt transition between the stages of labour or between the end of pregnancy and the onset of labour. The events leading to the onset of labour build gradually during the last weeks of the pregnancy, and there is overlap of physiological changes between the stages of labour.

The exact mechanisms that initiate and control labour are still not well understood. It is an extremely complex physiological process involving positive feedback and negative feedback loops and interconnections between maternal and fetal processes. Before exploring the physiology of labour, it is important to review the changes that occur in the uterus and cervix prior to active labour.

Uterine changes in preparation for labour

The myometrium consists of bundles of non-striated muscle fibres, intermixed with connective tissue, blood and lymph vessels and nerves. Throughout pregnancy the uterus is preparing for labour and there is an enormous increase in the bulk of the myometrium owing to hypertrophy and hyperplasia of the cells. Myometrial cells are smooth muscle cells and therefore are capable of spontaneous activity independent of external stimuli. Low-amplitude activity occurs even in a non-pregnant uterus. During pregnancy, however, contractions are largely prevented by uterotonic inhibitors, such as progesterone, relaxin, nitric oxide and prostacyclin, and those that do occur tend to be mild, irregular and non-synchronised (Di Renzo et al., 2016). Women are generally not aware of these contractions. As pregnancy progresses, contractions gradually increase in intensity and frequency until, in labour, strong, synchronous, effective contractions occur (Rabotti & Mischi, 2015).

Changes in the structure of myometrial cells enable them to contract more strongly and to maintain this through labour (Rabotti & Mischi, 2015). The initial changes are termed '**myometrial activation**'. Four main events occur during myometrial activation: the ratio of hormones changes, electrical activity increases, myometrial cells become more responsive, and there is an increase in numbers of ion channels. This occurs in the last few weeks of pregnancy as levels of uterotonic inhibitors decrease and those of oestrogen (estrogen) and contraction-associated proteins (CAPs) increase. CAPs include gap junction proteins, myometrial oxytocin receptors and prostaglandin receptors, and calcium and sodium channels (Blackburn, 2017). Increased gap junction formation facilitates the spread of electrical activity over the myometrium, and increased numbers of prostaglandin and oxytocin receptors enhance the responsiveness of target tissues to these uterotonins. Increased numbers of sodium ion channels facilitate sodium movement into the cells; this is required for electrical excitation. Increased numbers of calcium ion channels enable increased calcium movement into the cells; calcium is required for binding of myosin to actin during contraction (Rabotti & Mischi, 2015).

Cervical changes in preparation for labour

Another region of the uterus that undergoes changes is the cervix. During pregnancy, the cervix serves as a protective barrier from invading microorganisms and it is also important in retaining the fetus in the uterus (Word et al., 2007). Stretching of the cervix is resisted owing to its high content of connective tissue, which is made up of collagen fibre bundles embedded in a proteoglycan matrix.

Before effacement and dilation can occur, the cervix must change structure and soften or 'ripen', and this occurs towards the end of pregnancy. Results from studies using serial measurements of cervical length indicate that the process of **cervical ripening** precedes myometrial contractions of labour by several weeks (Word et al., 2007). The softening process is characterised by an infiltration of leucocytes, an increase in water and a decrease in collagen content of the cervix. Infiltration of the cervix by leucocytes and macrophages leads to the release of proteolytic enzymes that cause collagen degradation. Increases in hyaluronic acid levels and changes in blood vessel permeability increase the water content of the cervix. Increases in levels of glycoaminoglycans reduce the ability of collagen fibres to bind together (Johnson, 2013; Ravanos et al., 2015). The changes associated with cervical ripening are independent of myometrial contractions (Blackburn, 2017).

The process of cervical ripening is complex and depends on the hormones present at the end of pregnancy. Increases in oestrogen relative to progesterone and increases in relaxin levels promote collagen degradation. Nitric oxide levels in the cervix increase near term and may act with prostaglandin E_2 to induce vasodilation and facilitate neutrophil infiltration (Johnson, 2013). Stretching of the cervix results in the local release of prostaglandin $F_{2\alpha}$ ($PGF_{2\alpha}$) and the release of oxytocin from the posterior pituitary (the Ferguson reflex), which in turn increase uterine activity (Blackburn, 2017). In labour, cervical dilation is also enhanced by the use of upright positions—probably due to enhanced uterine contractions and greater movement of the fetus exerting forces on the cervix (Desseauve et al., 2017). Once the cervix is prepared physiologically and structurally, labour can begin.

WHAT INITIATES LABOUR?

In a number of mammalian species, the onset of labour is timed primarily by the fetus via secretions of the adrenal cortex, which increase oestrogen levels and subsequently $PGF_{2\alpha}$ in the uterus. $PGF_{2\alpha}$ activates myometrial contractions and cervical ripening (Johnson, 2013). In humans, it is likely that maternal as well as fetal mechanisms are involved, although the final pathway appears to involve activation of the fetal hypothalamic–pituitary–adrenal axis (Johnson, 2013; Ravanos et al., 2015).

CLINICAL POINT

Prostaglandin E_2 (PGE_2), administered vaginally, may be used to ripen the cervix or for induction of labour. Increased uterine electrical activity has been measured following PGE_2 application, with peak electrical activity measured 2–8 hours after PGE_2 application (Aviram et al., 2014).

PGE_2 is associated with lower rates of failed induction and higher rates of birth within a reasonable interval than amniotomy and/or oxytocin. There are a wide range of doses and formulations of vaginal PGE_2 with various gels, tablets, pessaries and slow-release inserts (Keirse, 2006). A meta-analysis of seven randomised controlled trials (RCTs) supported the effectiveness of vaginal inserts over repeated prostaglandin administration and indicated increased vaginal births, and less use of oxytocin but increased risk of hyperstimulation of the uterus in nulliparous women (Facchinetti et al., 2012). Further to this, a retrospective cohort study of >1000 women reported low-dose PGE_2 to be a safe method for induction of labour in grandmultiparous and great-grandmultiparous women (Haas et al., 2013). Obesity has been shown to reduce the effectiveness of PGE_2 in promoting cervical ripening (Gauthier et al., 2012) and underpins the suggestion that allowing more time for labour in overweight and obese women could result in increased vaginal deliveries (Carlson et al., 2015). Foley catheters are also used as a mechanical stimulus to dilate the cervix and are associated with a lower rate of uterine hyperstimulation than chemical induction methods (Chen et al., 2016).

CRITICAL THINKING EXERCISE

Why is it necessary for activation of myometrial cells and ripening/softening of the cervix to occur prior to labour?

Mechanisms leading to labour are mediated by changes in hormone levels. It is important to realise that hormone effectiveness is changed not only through increased synthesis and release of hormones, but also by reduction in the concentration of hormone-binding proteins or, alternatively, by increased number of receptors on target tissues. Thus the plasma concentration of a hormone may not reflect the degree of hormone binding at the local site.

It is known that increases in placental uterotonic hormones are linked to maturation of the fetal adrenal glands and the mechanical stretching of the uterus due to the growing fetus. Maternal adrenal glands and other endocrine or neural mechanisms may also play a role (Johnson, 2013).

A growing number of placental hormones have been identified, although their exact function in labour is not yet clear. The roles of some of the key hormones and chemical mediators that contribute to labour, such as corticotrophin-releasing hormone (CRH), prostaglandins (PGs), oxytocin, oestrogen, progesterone, relaxin and nitric oxide (NO), are outlined below.

Corticotrophin-releasing hormone

It is suggested that placental CRH plays an important role in the onset of labour (Grammatopoulos, 2008; Johnson, 2013), along with maturation of the fetal hypothalamic–pituitary–adrenal system (Ravanos et al., 2015). CRH is a neuropeptide produced by the hypothalamus, placenta, decidua, chorion and amnion. CRH receptors are found in the decidua and fetal membranes and in the myometrium. The complexity of control is highlighted by the fact that CRH appears to have a dual role: during pregnancy it promotes uterine quiescence; during labour, under the influence of oxytocin, it binds to different receptor types and promotes uterine contraction (Grammatopoulos, 2008; Ravanos et al., 2015).

There is strong evidence for the role of CRH in the **initiation of labour**. For example, placental CRH levels increase markedly after 35 weeks gestation, partly owing to a 60% decrease in protein binding of the hormone, and then CRH levels decrease by 50% within 20–30 minutes of birth. CRH levels are increased in pre-term labour (Ravanos et al., 2015) and in pregnancies complicated by pregnancy-induced hypertension and intrauterine growth restriction (Campbell et al., 1987; Petraglia et al., 1991), which may lead to pre-term labour.

Grammatopoulos & Hillhouse (1999) proposed that placental CRH initiates labour via mechanisms that increase production of placental oestriol (estriol, E_3, an active form of oestrogen) and fetal cortisol. The pathways for this are shown in Fig. 24.1. CRH stimulates the fetal adrenal gland

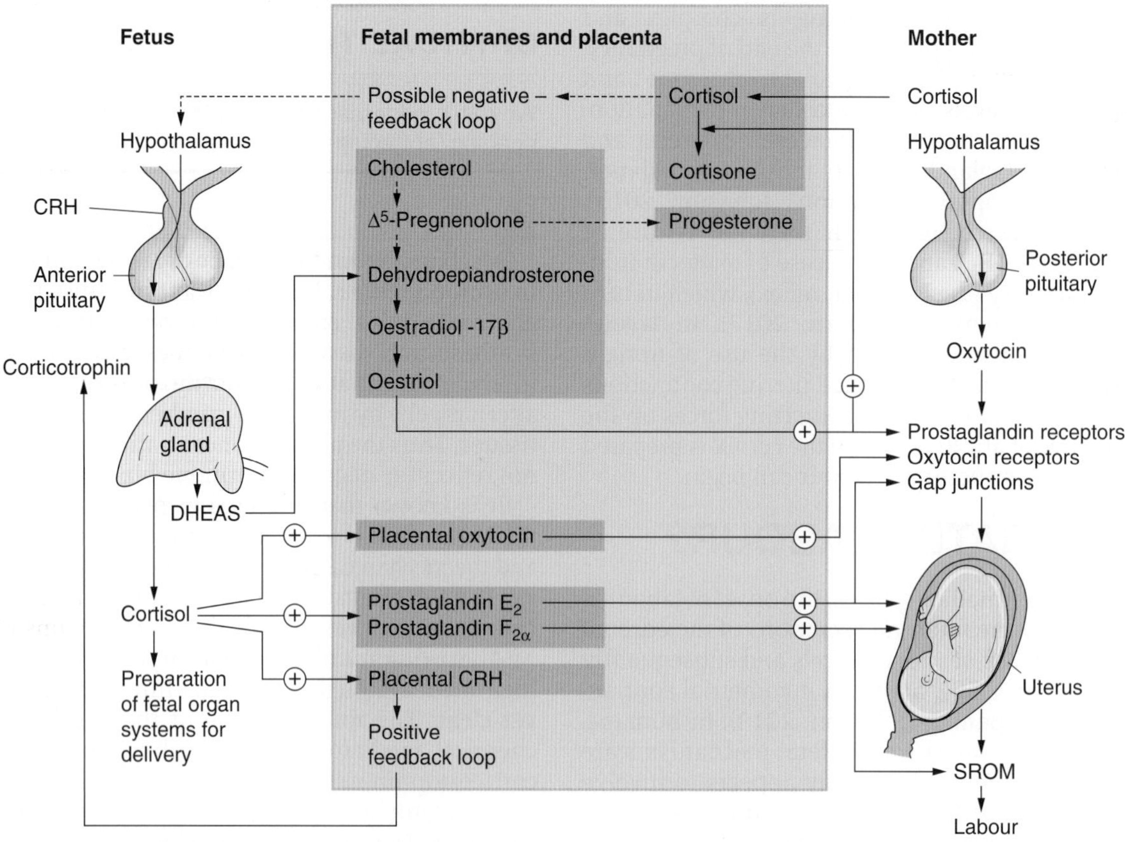

FIGURE 24.1 Proposed mechanism of labour induction at term. CRH = corticotrophin-releasing hormone; DHEAS = dehydroepiandrosterone sulfate; SROM = spontaneous rupture of the membranes
(Based on Blackburn, 2003)

to produce cortisol and the oestrogen precursor dehydroepiandrosterone sulfate (DHEAS). Fetal cortisol exerts positive feedback to increase placental CRH levels, and increases prostaglandin and oxytocin synthesis. DHEAS is an essential precursor to placental oestrogen synthesis, particularly oestriol, which drives other mechanisms associated with the initiation of labour. The specialised fetal adrenal cells responsible for DHEAS production atrophy after birth.

Although cortisol appears to have a role in the initiation of labour, some evidence suggests that labour may still progress when levels of fetal cortisol are low. For example, neither fetal anencephaly, where there is an absence of adrenocorticotrophic hormone (ACTH), nor adrenal hypoplasia, where cortisol production is reduced, necessarily result in prolonged labour but may be associated with post-term birth (Ravanos et al., 2015). Other clinical evidence indicates that, although maternal corticosteroid administration results in a decrease of fetoplacental oestrogen production, it does not delay the onset of labour (Johnson, 2013) as would be expected.

In summary, placental CRH behaves differently to hypothalamic CRH. Placental CRH may promote uterine quiescence during pregnancy and then enhance contractility during labour. It is suggested that, via the production of fetal cortisol and DHEAS, CRH leads to increased oestrogen production in the placenta, which drives the other mechanisms of labour such as an increase in numbers of oxytocin receptors and gap junctions and levels of prostaglandins.

Prostaglandins

Prostaglandins are lipids that are synthesised in tissues throughout the body. They are local hormones (paracrine hormones), which act at or near the place where they are synthesised. Prostaglandins are uterotonins directly responsible for uterine contraction. Two prostaglandins are particularly important in labour: PGE_2 and $PGF_{2\alpha}$. These prostaglandins stimulate smooth muscle fibres to contract, stimulate the formation of gap junctions in myometrial tissue, and increase calcium levels in myometrial cells. As mentioned previously, prostaglandins also have a role in softening the cervix, and enabling effacement and dilation (Arulkumaran et al., 2012; Johnson, 2013).

Levels of PGE_2 and $PGF_{2\alpha}$ in the amniotic fluid are known to increase before and during labour; however, evidence for an increase of these hormones in maternal plasma before labour begins is not conclusive (Johnson, 2013).

Prostaglandin synthesis has a complex pathway, outlined in Fig. 24.2. During labour, prostaglandins are synthesised by the decidua, cervix, placenta and fetal membranes. Arachidonic acid is the common precursor of both PGE_2 and $PGF_{2\alpha}$. It is produced by the action of phospholipase A_2

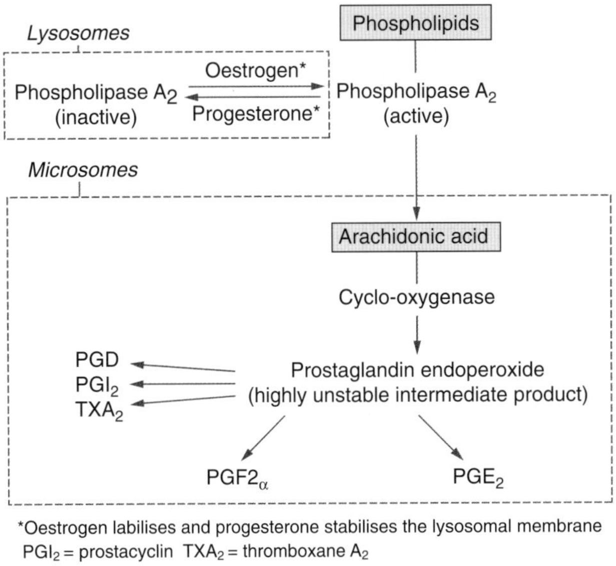

FIGURE 24.2 Biosynthesis of prostaglandins (PGs)
(Based on Johnson & Everitt, 1988)

on phospholipids in the fetal membranes and the decidua. Phospholipase A_2 is stored within lysosomes, which release the enzyme in the presence of oestrogen, and retain the enzyme in the presence of progesterone. Consequently, a rise in the oestrogen-to-progesterone ratio results in increased phospholipase A_2, leading to increased production of arachidonic acid and prostaglandin synthesis. Oxytocin also promotes prostaglandin release.

Other evidence that prostaglandins contribute to the initiation of labour comes from the finding that inhibitors of prostaglandin synthesis, such as the non-steroidal anti-inflammatory drug indomethacin, are effective at reducing pre-term labour (Arulkumaran et al., 2012).

Oxytocin

Another hormone essential for labour is oxytocin. Oxytocin is released into the systemic circulation from the posterior pituitary in response to tactile stimulation of the reproductive tract, particularly the cervix. This is known as the neuroendocrine reflex (Ferguson reflex) and is outlined in Fig. 24.3. There is also a local (paracrine) release of

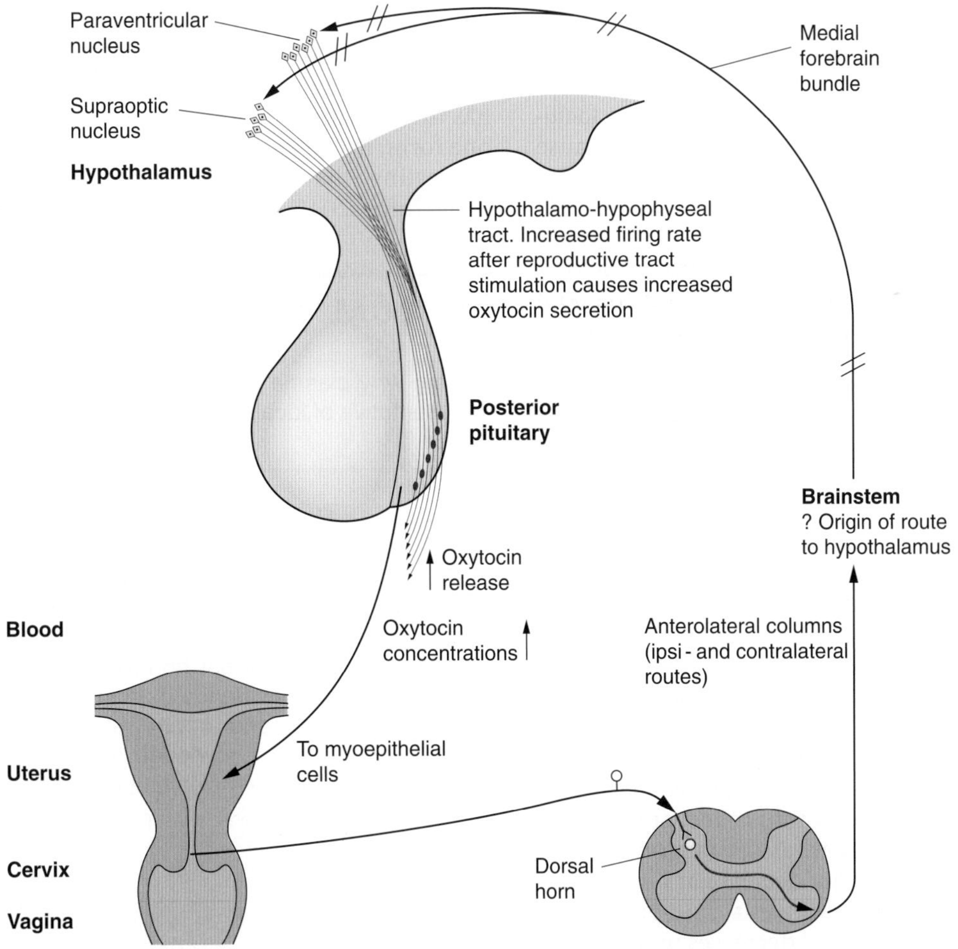

FIGURE 24.3 The neuroendocrine reflex (Ferguson reflex), showing underlying oxytocin synthesis and secretion
(Based on Johnson & Everitt, 1988)

oxytocin from the fetal membranes, decidua and placenta. There is little evidence that oxytocin initiates or is the primary uterotonin of labour, and it can be used clinically to induce labour only if the cervix is ripe. Plasma oxytocin levels do not increase physiologically until the second stage of labour, although local concentrations may increase before this. The importance of oxytocin for labour is demonstrated by the increase of oxytocin receptors in the decidua during pregnancy, reaching a 300-fold increase by term (Petraglia et al., 2010). Oxytocin binds to these decidual receptors, stimulates the release of prostaglandins from the decidua and stimulates uterine pacemakers.

There is considerable interest in the roles of oxytocin in addition to those of facilitating uterine contractions and breastfeeding. Research suggests oxytocin has a role in maternal care, parent–infant bonding and sex, as well as in relaxation and feelings of calm (Kosfeld et al., 2005; Mitre et al., 2016; Moberg, 2003; Uvnäs-Moberg et al., 2019). This perhaps has broader implications for factors impacting on the progress of labour, as well as mother–baby bonding.

Oestrogen (estrogen)

Oestrogen has a primary role in initiating many changes that are essential for labour, and levels begin to rise at about 34 weeks gestation (Blackburn, 2017). Oestrogen increases the sensitivity of the myometrial oxytocin receptors during pregnancy (Blackburn, 2017) and thus facilitates myometrial contractility but does not directly cause contractions (Ravanos et al., 2015). Oestrogen promotes the formation of CAPs and prostaglandin synthesis via increases in phospholipase A_2 release from lysosomes (Johnson, 2013). The synthesis of oestriol (the active oestrogen in pregnancy) by the placenta relies on the fetal adrenal precursor DHEAS, as outlined earlier (see Fig. 24.1). Therefore, maternal serum oestriol levels are an indicator of fetal hypothalamic–pituitary–adrenal maturity and elevated levels of oestriol are associated with the onset of labour (Blackburn, 2017; Norwitz et al., 1999).

Progesterone

Progesterone is also produced in the placenta. However, in contrast to oestrogen, it is not reliant on fetal precursors for synthesis and its role is in suppressing uterine excitement. Progesterone does this by promoting the uptake of intracellular calcium into the sarcoplasmic reticulum of the myometrium, and it works with nitric oxide to inhibit the production of CAPs. Progesterone also has a role in decreasing oxytocin binding during pregnancy, and it is suggested that removal of this effect at the onset of labour could facilitate myometrial contractions. Maternal plasma progesterone does not decrease at parturition, as it does in some animals (Norwitz et al., 1999; Ravanos et al., 2015), but there may be local decreases in progesterone activity through increased progesterone-binding protein. The decreased availability of progesterone and increased synthesis of oestrogen produce an increased oestrogen-to-progesterone ratio, allowing the uterotonic effects of oestrogen to dominate, enabling contraction of uterine muscle (Blackburn, 2017; Di Renzo et al., 2016).

Relaxin

Relaxin, like progesterone, supports quiescence of the uterus, and may inhibit oxytocin release (Blackburn, 2017). Relaxin is produced by the myometrium, decidua and placenta. Its levels are highest in the first trimester, but are measurable throughout pregnancy and fall rapidly after birth (Blackburn, 2017). Relaxin has a role in enhancing cervical ripening, and there is some evidence that exogenous application of relaxin promotes cervical ripening, with the advantage of not causing uterine hyperstimulation; however, the implications of clinical use of the hormone are not clear.

Nitric oxide

Nitric oxide (NO) is important in maintaining myometrial quiescence (Longo et al., 2003). It is produced by the decidua, fetal membranes, and fetal and placental vascular epithelium. NO is believed to interact with progesterone to inhibit the production of CAPs (Challis, 2001). Levels of NO in the myometrium decrease near term but increase in the cervix. NO production is dependent on the enzyme nitric oxide synthetase (NOS), which has three forms. There is an increase in the expression of one form, iNOS, in the cervix prior to the onset of labour, suggesting that NO contributes to cervical ripening (Blackburn, 2017; Ledingham et al., 2000).

CRITICAL THINKING EXERCISE

Explain why plasma levels of hormones are not necessarily representative of local changes that may initiate and maintain labour.

RESEARCH ACTIVITY

Sometimes we can gain an understanding of the normal function of hormones by seeing what happens when function is abnormal, as it can be easier to see the consequences of abnormal hormone function. Identify two examples where evidence from impaired function of fetal or maternal hormonal control at the initiation of labour has added to our knowledge of mechanisms that may contribute to the normal initiation of labour.

Summary: the hormonal contribution to labour

- Systemic plasma levels of hormones are not representative of local changes that may initiate and maintain labour.

- During pregnancy, hormones such as progesterone, relaxin and nitric oxide maintain the uterus in a quiescent state.
- Prior to labour, changes in the oestrogen-to-progesterone ratio facilitate activation of the uterine muscle, and ripening of the cervix occurs under the influence of prostaglandins, relaxin and nitric oxide.
- Following activation of myometrial cells and cervical ripening in the uterus, the myometrium responds to the uterotonins, oxytocin and prostaglandins.
- Initiation of labour probably involves both fetal and maternal influences.

FIRST STAGE OF LABOUR

During the first stage of labour, myometrial contractions lead to effacement and dilation of the cervix. The first stage is often divided into two phases: *latent* and *active*. In the latent phase, uterine contractions occur but cervical dilation is slow. The time frame for this phase varies considerably. In the active phase, strong, effective contractions lead to cervical dilation. While cervical dilation of 3 cm has been regarded as an indicator of active labour, there is considerable evidence that supports dilation of 6 cm as a more effective indicator (Hamilton et al., 2016; Oladapo et al., 2018; Zhang et al., 2010). Progress of labour has been shown to be slower than was originally described by Friedman, and current evidence suggests that labour dystocia should not be diagnosed before 6 cm dilation (Zhang et al., 2010).

Uterine contractions during the first stage

For contractions to be effective and result in effacement and dilation of the cervix, several processes must occur. The cervix must be softened, as described earlier; contractions must be coordinated so that all regions of the myometrium contract in unison under the influence of pacemaker cells, and there must be a descending gradient of uterine activity such that contractions are stronger at the uterine fundus and lessen towards the lower uterine segment. This gradient of activity allows retraction of the upper uterine segment to mediate the processes of effacement and dilation. Control of myometrial contractions is via the changing concentrations of placental hormones (prostaglandins, oxytocin, oestrogens, progesterone and relaxin), as described earlier.

Uterine muscle cells undergo some unique changes. For example, pacemakers located in each cornu of the uterus initiate contractions under the influence of local hormones. Gap junctions between the myometrial cells facilitate the rapid spread of electrical activity downwards over the muscle cells, facilitating almost-synchronous contraction of the myometrium so that maximum tension is generated in all myometrial cells at the same time. However, as expected, the strength of contraction is greater in the fundus and less in the lower uterine segment, owing to the relatively low muscle and high connective tissue content in the lower region of the uterus. Along with synchronous contraction, smooth muscle can also maintain tone between contractions, a characteristic called *retraction*. Due to retraction, the smooth muscle cells of the upper segment never fully relax and thus each contraction causes the muscle cells to become progressively shorter and fatter. Retraction of the upper segment enables shortening of the lower uterine segment so that the cervix becomes continuous with the lower uterine segment—that is, *effacement* (Rankin, 2017). The process is illustrated in Figs 24.4 and 24.5.

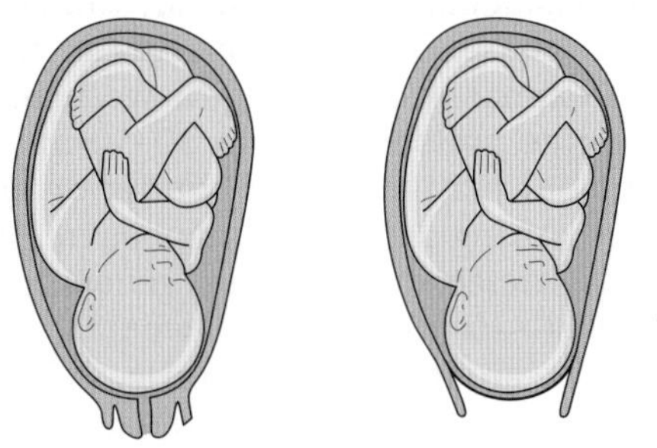

FIGURE 24.4 The uterus, showing dilation of the cervix and the formation of the lower uterine segment
(Based on Henderson & Macdonald, 2004)

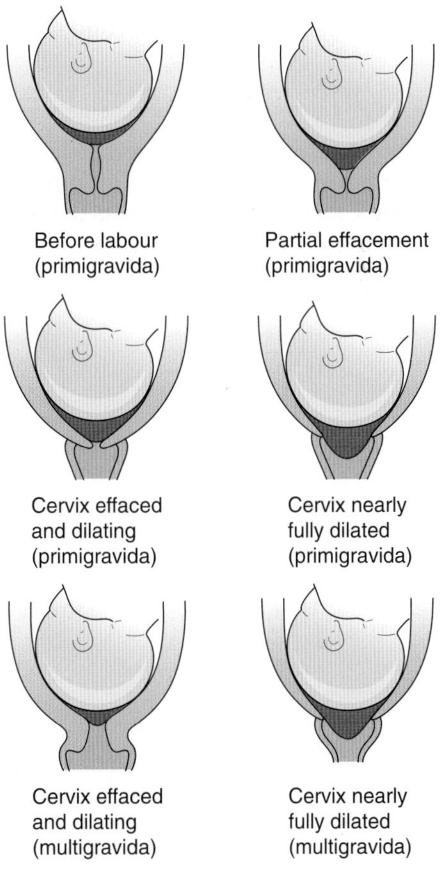

FIGURE 24.5 Effacement and dilation of the cervix
(Based on Henderson & Macdonald, 2004)

As contractions of the upper uterine segment of the uterus continue to pull on the lower segment, *dilation* of the external os is achieved. Full dilation of the cervix is measured at 10 cm. In the multiparous woman, effacement and dilation tend to occur as a single process. During the early stages of dilation, the operculum or mucous plug that was formed during pregnancy under the influence of progesterone is lost. This may appear as a blood-stained mucoid 'show'. The blood is due to the detachment of the chorion from the dilating cervix (Rankin, 2017).

There is a relationship between the pressure generated in the uterus during labour and the level of pain encountered at each phase. Generally, the uterus has a resting tone of approximately 10 mmHg between contractions, and intrauterine pressure rises to 30–50 mmHg during contractions but may reach 100 mmHg or more in the second stage during a Valsalva manoeuvre. Abdominal palpation can detect contractions generating pressure greater than 10–20 mmHg and a woman can perceive contractions at around 15–20 mmHg. Pain is usually felt when contractions generate pressures higher than 25 mmHg, but there is considerable variation among women (Blackburn, 2017). These intrauterine pressures are shown in Fig. 24.6. The pain may be due to ischaemia that occurs in muscle fibres during active contraction (visceral pain), and to stretching of the vaginal, perineal and pelvic tissues caused by the pressure of the presenting part (somatic pain) during the second stage.

Uterine contractions and the fetus

Effective myometrial contractions are needed to push the fetus downwards towards the vagina. This process induces a positive-feedback mechanism because as the upper uterine segment shortens and thickens, and the fetus is pushed downwards, the pressure on the cervix initiates the reflex release of oxytocin (neuroendocrine reflex). The more pressure, the greater is the release of oxytocin, which further facilitates uterine contractions.

There are other effects involving the fetus. For example, during contractions the force is transmitted along the length of the spine, forcing further flexion of the head, resulting in presentation of the smallest circumference to the cervical os (Rankin, 2017).

Also, as the fetal head is directed against the cervix, a small amount of amniotic fluid (the forewaters) is trapped in front of the head, separated from the remainder of the amniotic fluid (the hindwaters). This separation protects against ascending infection as long as the membranes are intact. There is another advantage to the fetus of intact membranes: the pressure of contractions is spread over the amniotic fluid, rather than being applied directly to the fetus. This avoids compression of the placenta between the fetus and wall of the uterus and thus facilitates fetal oxygen delivery during contractions (Rankin, 2017). Eventually, spontaneous rupture of the membranes (SROM) occurs under the force of the uterine contractions, though sometimes this is not until after the head / body is born.

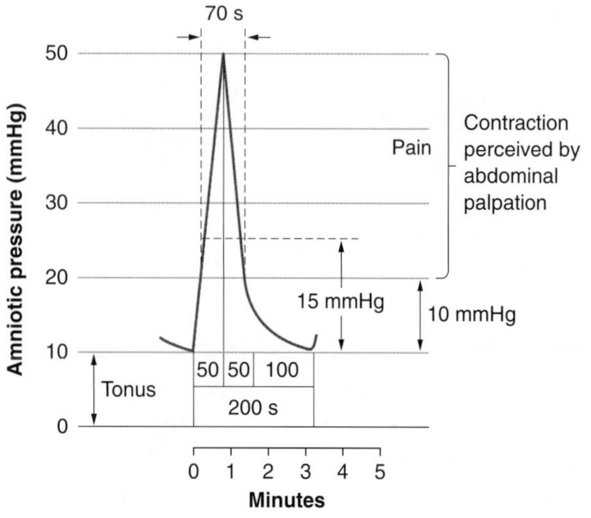

FIGURE 24.6 Correlation between abdominal palpation and intrauterine pressure tracing
(Based on Blackburn, *Maternal, Fetal and Neonatal Physiology: A Clinical Perspective*. 2nd ed. St Louis: WB Saunders Co, 2003)

RESEARCH ACTIVITY

Hiersch et al. (2015) developed a non-invasive way to measure uterine electrical activity while membranes were still intact and demonstrated that electrical activity increased throughout labour. Further, they found that electrical activity prior to rupture of the membranes was enhanced with greater cervical dilation, and was associated with lower maternal age and previous caesarean section. They identified that other studies have demonstrated that maternal age is associated with increase in operative vaginal deliveries, caesarean section and an increased need for oxytocin augmentation.

1. How might the study by Hiersch et al. (2015) lead to a possible explanation of increased intervention during labour in older women?
2. This was an observational study rather than an interventional one and lacked a control arm. How might this impact on the significance of the results?

Artificial rupture of the membranes (ARM) is sometimes performed with a view to increasing the progress of labour; however, this is not supported by the evidence and the procedure may expose the fetus to increased risk of infection and greater direct pressures during uterine contraction. Evidence from a Cochrane review of amniotomy for shortening spontaneous labour (Smyth et al., 2013), including 15 studies involving 5583 women, showed no shortening of the length of first or second stages of labour, no differences in maternal satisfaction of labour, no significant difference in maternal infection and a possible increase in caesarean section. There were some small differences in the length of second stage and in the chance of the newborn achieving an Apgar score of <7 at 5 minutes in the primiparous women only. All results need to be viewed with caution, however, because of the heterogeneity of the studies included in the analysis. The authors recommended that, on the basis of current evidence, amniotomy should not be introduced routinely as part of standard labour management and care (Smyth et al., 2013). In a more recent study of 15,000 women, early amniotomy was associated with increased odds of caesarean among obese women but was not associated with increased neonatal morbidity (Battarbee et al., 2020).

As the cervix nears full dilation, the first stage of labour merges into the transition phase and then into the second stage of labour. The transition phase is a poorly defined period and does not necessarily occur at full dilation. This phase is associated with very intense feelings, perhaps irritability and panic for the woman. On an emotional level this is regarded as the most difficult time for women and may lead to the expression of intense feelings of being unable to continue with the labour. The midwife has an important support role in reassuring the woman (Walsh & Downe, 2010).

THE SECOND STAGE OF LABOUR

The second stage of labour results in the birth of the baby. During the second stage of labour, uterine contractions are assisted by abdominal muscles and result in expulsive forces that move the baby through the pelvis and birth canal. There is a variable time until the presenting part of the fetus is visible (crowned) at the vulva. Crowning occurs once contractions force the fetus down and cause the presenting part to stretch the vagina and tissues of the pelvic floor. Crowning is generally associated with the urge to 'push', which may be overwhelming. The 'pushing urge' recruits the voluntary skeletal muscles of the abdominal wall and diaphragm. In this time, several changes occur. During each contraction, several bursts of spontaneous pushing of 5–6 seconds duration occur (Rankin, 2017), causing the presenting part of the fetus to be pushed against the perineum. The bladder is protected as it is pushed up into the abdominal cavity, and the rectum is flattened against the sacral curve, causing defecation of any contents. The effort of the second stage of labour causes sweating due to increased heat generated by muscle activity, and a rise in pulse rate in the woman. There are also pressure sensations on the rectum, and/or radiating pain in the thighs, due to pressure on the sacral plexus and the obturator nerve (Rankin, 2017).

Pushing during the second stage of labour

As well as the spontaneous desire to push that occurs during the second stage of labour, women are sometimes directed to push. However, evidence suggests that directed pushing may compromise fetal wellbeing by causing abnormalities in fetal heart rate (above 160 b.p.m. or below 110 b.p.m.) and reduced Apgar scores (Roberts, 2002; Yildirim & Beji, 2008). Also, mean umbilical arterial pH has been shown to be lower where women are subjected to sustained pushing (Yildirim & Beji, 2008). The reduction in pH may indicate fetal acidaemia caused by reduced blood flow to the placenta. (The physiology underlying fetal acidosis is described later, in the section on **fetal responses** during labour.) Therefore, due consideration should be given to abstaining from directed pushing when supporting a labouring woman. One RCT comparing spontaneous pushing with directed pushing did not show a significant difference in 5-minute Apgar scores less than 7 or admissions to neonatal intensive care, nor was there any significant difference in the duration of second stage, the risk of stage 3 or 4 perineal tears or spontaneous vaginal delivery. The level of evidence was moderate to very low quality (Lemos et al., 2017). Maternal satisfaction seems to be better after spontaneous pushing (de Tayrac & Letouzey 2016). More research is required in this area.

A study of antenatal education on the physiology of second stage of labour and how to push effectively, with complete relaxation of the pelvic floor muscles during spontaneous pushing, has not been shown to alter birth outcomes but women did state that they found the education helpful (Phipps et al., 2009). This was a small pilot RCT of 100 nulliparous women in Australia. Further research with a larger group has not been published but could be beneficial.

REFLECTIVE THINKING EXERCISE

Consider the following research study. One hundred low-risk primiparous women (38–42 weeks gestation), expecting a spontaneous vaginal delivery, were randomised to either a spontaneous pushing group (open-glottis pushing while breathing out) or a Valsalva-type pushing group (closed-glottis pushing while holding their breath) for the second stage of labour. Results indicated no significant differences in the incidence of episiotomy, perineal tears or postpartum haemorrhage between the two groups, but women in the spontaneous pushing group experienced a shorter second stage. The baby also fared better with spontaneous pushing, with higher 1- and 5-minute Apgar scores, and higher umbilical cord pH and P_aO_2 levels. After the birth, women expressed greater satisfaction with spontaneous pushing (Yildirim & Beji, 2008).

1. What would you consider to be the underlying physiological factors contributing to these results?
2. How do these results compare with the latest Cochrane review on the topic?
3. How would you interpret this for application to your practice?

Maternal position during the second stage of labour

Maternal position during labour has also received considerable research interest. Evidence suggests that maternal position influences the effectiveness of uterine contractions, fetal wellbeing, maternal comfort and the duration of labour (Blackburn, 2017). Magnetic resonance (MR) pelvimetry has identified that upright positions, compared with the supine position, can significantly increase female pelvic dimensions, suggesting that upright positions facilitate labour and birth (Michel et al., 2002). An RCT published in 2007 indicated that the squatting position may result in fewer instrumental deliveries, less extension of episiotomies and fewer perineal tears than the supine lithotomy position. This study reported no significant difference in the Apgar scores, fetal heart rate patterns or requirement for neonatal resuscitation (Nasir et al., 2007). A 2013 Cochrane systematic review (Lawrence et al., 2013) of 25 trials, including over 5000 women, reported many benefits of an upright posture in the first stage of labour, such as reduced duration of the first stage by one and a quarter hours for women randomised to upright as opposed to recumbent positions, and reduced likelihood of caesarean section and epidural. These benefits were not demonstrated for women with an epidural. In one trial, babies of mothers who were upright were less likely to be admitted to the neonatal intensive care unit. An upright position did not impact on the duration of the second stage or other measures of maternal or neonatal wellbeing (Lawrence et al., 2013). A more recent study confirmed that women in the sitting position at birth, compared with those in the horizontal/supine group, had a lower episiotomy rate (adjusted odds ratio (OR): 0.28; 95% confidence interval (CI): 0.14–0.56) and a non-significant higher intact perineum rate (adjusted OR: 1.40; 95% CI: 0.96–2.04) (Warmink-Perdijk et al., 2016). Upright positions also significantly reduced the rate of instrumental vaginal birth (Zang et al., 2021).

Increased blood loss (>500 mL) associated with an upright position in the second stage of labour has been demonstrated (Gupta et al., 2017; Zang et al., 2021), along with a small decrease in duration of second stage (Gupta et al., 2017). Increased blood loss with the upright position has been shown to be associated with perineal damage (de Jonge et al., 2007). More quality research is required.

If the second stage of labour is to be fully understood, not only the physiology but also the *mechanism* of labour needs to be explained.

CRITICAL THINKING EXERCISE

Identify situations or environments that tend to facilitate the progress of labour and provide physiological explanations as to the likely underlying mechanisms. Describe how you, as a midwife, could facilitate these types of situations.

REFLECTIVE THINKING EXERCISE

Thirty-five non-pregnant women were studied using MR pelvimetry in each of three positions: supine, hand-to-knee and squatting. Results identified that upright birthing positions expanded the female pelvic bone dimensions (Michel et al., 2002).

1. Why would the researchers have used non-pregnant women in this study?
2. Identify any advantages of MR pelvimetry compared with X-ray pelvimetry.
3. What differences might be expected in pregnant women (think of the impact of pregnancy hormones on joints during pregnancy)?
4. Is this study applicable to midwifery practice?

Mechanism of labour

Two issues complicate the birth of a human fetus: the curvature of the spine—a consequence of human upright posture—and the large size of the fetal head. In order to negotiate through the birth canal, the fetus must turn to take advantage of the widest diameter of each part of the pelvis. These movements are called the *mechanism of labour*. The pelvic inlet is widest in the transverse diameter, while the pelvic outlet is widest in the anteroposterior diameter. (Further information on the pelvis can be found in Ch. 20.)

It is useful for a midwife to visualise these unseen movements during the birth of the baby. The presentation and position of the fetus will determine the type of mechanism that occurs. According to Rankin (2017), all mechanisms of labour have the following principles in common: the fetus descends, the leading part of the fetus meets the resistance of the pelvic floor and rotates forwards to lie anteriorly under the symphysis pubis, and the emerging part of the fetus pivots around the pubic bone. The mechanism of labour for a normal presentation, where the head presents downwards, is outlined below and the stages are illustrated in Fig. 24.7. (Malpresentations of the fetus are discussed in Ch. 36.)

In a normal labour, the *lie* of the fetus (the long axis) is longitudinal, the fetal head is flexed (*attitude*), the *presentation* (part of the fetus which lies at the pelvic brim) is cephalic, the *position* (relative to points on the maternal pelvic brim) is right or left occipitoanterior, and the presenting part or *denominator* (part of the fetus which lies over the cervical os during labour) is the occiput (Rankin, 2017).

Descent

Descent of the fetal head may have occurred in the antenatal period so that labour begins with the head engaged (Rankin, 2017). However, a review of studies of non-engagement at the onset of labour by Dietze (2001) suggests that this may not be the norm, as non-engagement was reported in 50%–83% of nulliparous women assessed in early labour.

As the fetus descends through the pelvis, it changes position so that the fetal head can be accommodated by

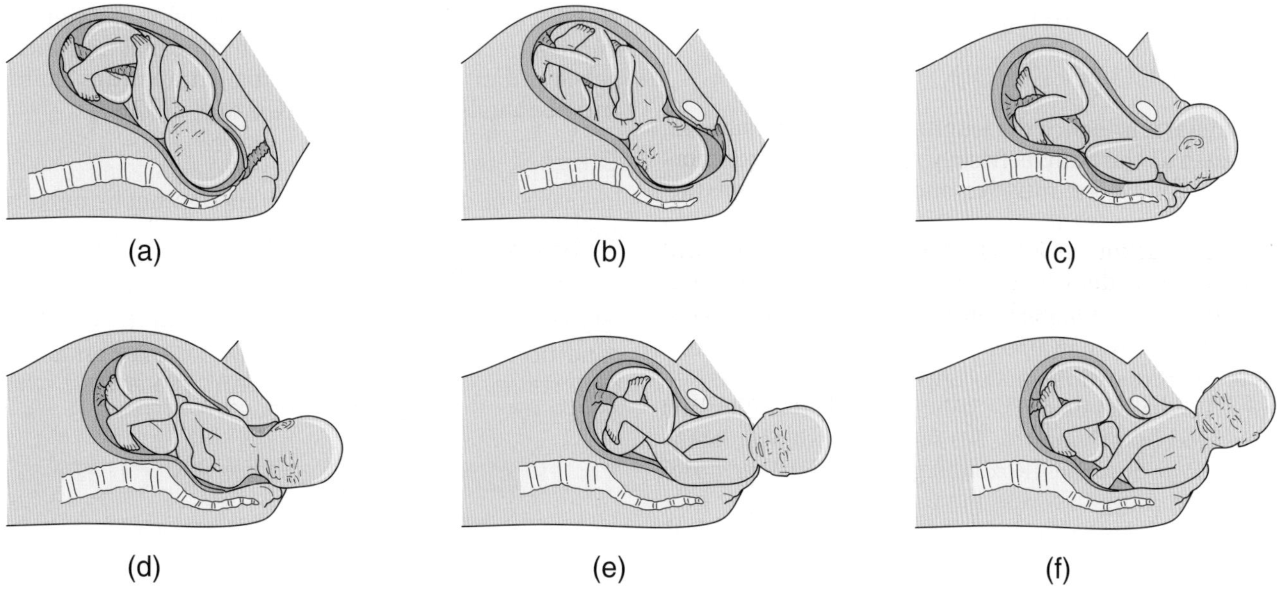

FIGURE 24.7 Normal labour showing: (a) engagement and flexion of the head, (b) internal rotation, (c) delivery by extension of the head after dilation of the cervix, and (d)–(f) sequential delivery of the shoulders

(Republished with permission from Johnson MH, Everitt BJ (1988) *Essential Reproduction*. 3rd ed. Blackwell Scientific, Oxford, permission conveyed through Copyright Clearance Center, Inc.)

the widest diameters of the woman's pelvis—the transverse diameter of the pelvic inlet, and the anteroposterior diameter of the pelvic outlet.

Flexion

Uterine contractions exert pressure down the fetal spine and lead to increased flexion of the fetal head because the head is attached to the spine nearer to the occiput than the sinciput. This increased flexion leads to presentation of the smallest diameter of the fetal head.

Internal rotation of the head

Following engagement, internal rotation of the fetal head aligns it with the anteroposterior diameter of the pelvic outlet and moves the occiput forwards to lie under the symphysis pubis. This occurs because of several influences: pressure exerted on the fetus by the uterine contractions, the shape of the pelvic floor and the presence of the ischial spines. This causes a slight twisting of the neck so that the head of the fetus is no longer in line with the shoulders (Rankin, 2017).

Extension of the head

The occiput now moves from beneath the pubic arch and pushes against the vaginal orifice. The head is born by extension (it is pushed upwards) and pivots on the suboccipital region around the pubic bone. The sinciput, face and chin sweep the perineum.

Restitution

Restitution occurs after the birth of the head, when the head returns to its original position in correct alignment with the shoulders.

Internal rotation of the shoulders and lateral flexion

Internal rotation occurs when the shoulders turn to fit the widest diameter of the pelvis (anteroposterior). The anterior shoulder reaches the pelvic floor and rotates forwards to lie under the symphysis pubis. This movement causes external rotation of the head so that the occiput lies laterally turned towards the woman's thigh. The anterior shoulder is usually born first as it moves under the pubic arch and the posterior shoulder passes over the perineum, although anecdotal reports suggest that in the upright position the impact of gravity often leads to release of the posterior shoulder first (Walsh, 2007). The spine undergoes lateral flexion to accommodate the curved birth canal and the rest of the body is born in that position (Rankin, 2017).

RESEARCH ACTIVITY

Dietze (2001) described the role of mobility of the sacroiliac joint during childbirth based on early X-ray evidence from Borell & Fernestrom (1957, cited in Dietze, 2001) and further interpretation by Ohlsen (1973, cited in Dietze 2001) that pressure from the fetal head during descent facilitated this movement at the sacroiliac joint. More recent computed tomography (CT) scans of women following birth support this finding of increased mobility of the sacroiliac joint associated with birth (Shibata et al., 2002).

1. What could be the advantages of increased mobility of the sacroiliac joint during the descent of the fetus?
2. What maternal position would facilitate this movement?

Factors that influence the progress of the second stage

Several factors influence the length of the second stage of labour, such as the bony pelvis, the fetal lie and presentation, the pelvic floor muscles and the position of the woman.

Bony pelvis

The relationship of the woman's bony pelvis to the size and lie of the fetus may affect progress. Very rarely, cephalopelvic disproportion may impede the progress of labour. The diameters of the pelvic brim and outlet can be measured by pelvimetry, but this does not accurately predict labour outcome (Rozenberg, 2007). Furthermore, studies attempting to assess the usefulness of X-ray pelvimetry have been criticised because of methodological weaknesses (Rozenberg, 2007). X-ray pelvimetry did not show any improved outcomes prior to a trial of labour in women with previous caesarean section or in those suspected of cephalopelvic disproportion, but one trial investigating the use of pelvimetry in breech presentation at term did indicate a significantly lower emergency caesarean section rate (Rozenberg, 2007).

The diameters of the woman's pelvis can be affected by the woman's position; for example, upright positions such as squatting can increase the size of the pelvic outlet (Michel et al., 2002; Nasir et al., 2007).

Various other unusual bony structures may slow the progress of labour (e.g. protruding sacral promontary, enlarged ischial spines).

Fetus

The lie and presentation of the fetus influence progress. A longitudinal lie with head presentation is most common, then longitudinal lie with breech. A transverse lie with shoulder presentation, however, cannot result in a vaginal birth. Passage through the vagina is facilitated by moulding of the fetal skull, which is made possible by the fontanelles (membrane-covered junctions between the cranial bones) and the unfused sutures of the fetal skull.

Pelvic floor muscles

The vagina passes through the muscles of the pelvic floor. As the fetus descends through the vagina, the levator ani muscles are pushed downwards and thin out, and the perineal body is stretched. In nulliparous women these muscles are being stretched for the first time, and this can lead to spasms and resistance against the descending fetus. Hence nulliparous women may have a longer second stage than multiparous women.

Position of the woman

The upright position maximises assistance from gravity, and has been shown to increase the effectiveness of uterine muscle contractions by potentially reducing aortocaval compression (Gizzo et al., 2014) and to decrease the length of the second stage of labour (Berghella et al., 2008; Lawrence et al., 2013). Upright positions also improve fetal alignment in the birth canal and increase pelvic outlet diameters reducing intrapartum maternal and neonatal complications (Gizzo et al., 2014).

Other

Increases in circulating adrenaline (epinephrine) associated with stress have been shown to decrease uterine contractions in the short term (Alehagen et al., 2005).

The duration of the second stage is more appropriately related to the progress of the labour and the satisfactory condition of woman and fetus, rather than an arbitrary time frame. Once the baby is born, the second stage is complete.

THIRD STAGE OF LABOUR

This is the stage when separation and birthing of the placenta and membranes occur, and mechanisms are initiated that minimise bleeding from the placental site. **Placental separation** usually starts with the contraction that births the baby (Rankin, 2017). This stage may be managed physiologically (no intervention) or actively (with intervention) (see Ch. 25). Physiological management (also known as 'expectant management') is a 'hands-off' approach, where the infant is encouraged to suckle to induce uterine contraction and the woman maintains an upright position to use the effect of gravity to deliver the placenta. Controlled cord traction is not used and the cord is clamped or tied and cut once it stops pulsating, or after the placenta is born. Active management involves the administration of a uterotonic, clamping of the cord and either controlled cord traction or maternal effort. Uterotonics (e.g. Syntocinon) induce uterine contraction.

The 2019 Cochrane review of maternal and infant outcomes of active compared to expectant management of third stage of labour reported on eight trials all conducted in the hospital setting (Begley et al., 2019). There was considerable clinical heterogeneity and low-quality evidence for the primary outcomes leading the authors to report findings conservatively, even though they were reported as statistically significant. They concluded that it is uncertain whether active management of the third stage reduces the risk of haemorrhage greater than 1000 mL at the time of birth in a population of women at mixed risk of excessive bleeding (Begley et al., 2019) but it probably decreases primary blood loss greater than 500 mL, and less use of therapeutic uterotonics. Adverse side effects likely included increases in maternal diastolic blood pressure, vomiting after birth, afterpains, use of analgesia after birth and more women returning to hospital with bleeding (outcome not prespecified). Infant birth weight was probably less with active management, likely due to the lower blood volume from early cord clamping. While the authors (Begley et al., 2019) suggest that women should be given information on the benefits and harms of both methods to support informed choice, the results should be treated with caution given the small number of trials, low level of evidence and lack of trials with women at low risk of bleeding. They also draw attention to the need for more research on early cord clamping and the potential adverse effects of some uterotonics. There is also a further question as to whether meta-analysis is the appropriate tool for a practice issue such as this given the impact of contexts such as birthing in hospital, primary birthing units or the home.

Retrospective analysis of data from low-risk cohorts of New Zealand women receiving continuity of care from a midwife lead maternity carer (LMC) identified that the majority of women had a postpartum blood loss of <500 mL and, of these women, more received physiological management of third stage (96%) than active management (93%) ($p < 0.05$) (Dixon et al., 2009). Further to this, the risk of blood loss >500 mL was more than twofold greater in the actively managed group compared with the physiologically managed group (relative risk (RR): 2.76; 95% CI: 2.44–3.12) (Dixon et al., 2013), as was the risk of blood loss >1000 mL (RR: 2.12; 95% CI: 1.39–3.22) (Davis et al., 2012). Women birthing in a primary maternity facility or at home were more likely to have physiological management and planned place of birth did not influence postpartum blood loss (Davis et al., 2012; Dixon et al., 2013). A further retrospective cohort study of 7548 women in Australia reported that skin-to-skin contact and breastfeeding within 30 minutes of birth was associated with an almost 50% reduction in postpartum haemorrhage (PPH) of >500 mL (Saxton et al., 2015).

Prospective research is required to clarify the risks and benefits associated with physiological and active management that take into account the model of midwifery care and the confidence of midwives/health professionals in providing physiological management.

Normally, the process of placental separation follows a particular pattern of events, outlined below.

Mechanism of placental separation

The placenta separates from the decidua basalis as a result of uterine contractions that cause retraction of the uterus and a 75% reduction in the area of the placental site (Fig. 24.8). Recordings of continuous ultrasound support the mechanism of separation as involving forceful uterine contractions that induce shear forces between the uterine wall and the stiffer tissue of the placenta, and cause the separation of the placenta (Fig. 24.8a). As the placenta separates a gradual thickening of the adjacent uterine wall is observed (Herman et al., 2002) (Fig. 24.8b). The weight of the placenta strips the membranes off the uterine wall and the placenta and membranes descend into the vagina and out of the body (Rankin, 2017) (Fig. 24.8c, d). The uterus retracts further and brings the walls of the uterus in apposition, which applies pressure to the placental site. The criss-cross arrangement of muscle fibres around the blood vessels (termed 'living ligatures') strangles the blood vessels, including the spiral arterioles supplying the placental site (Fig. 24.9). This prevents further blood loss. Fibrin plugs deposited in the torn ends of blood vessels further reduce blood loss. Uterine contractions are aided by putting the baby to the breast as stimulation of the nipples causes the reflex release of oxytocin from the posterior pituitary gland (Rankin, 2017).

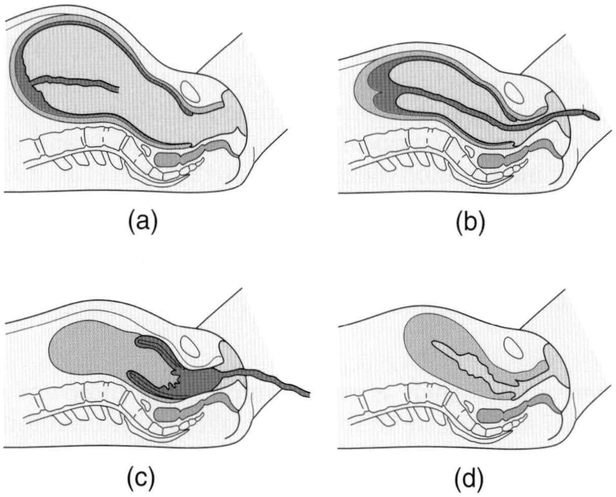

FIGURE 24.8 (a–d) The mechanism of placental separation
(Based on Henderson & Macdonald, 2004)

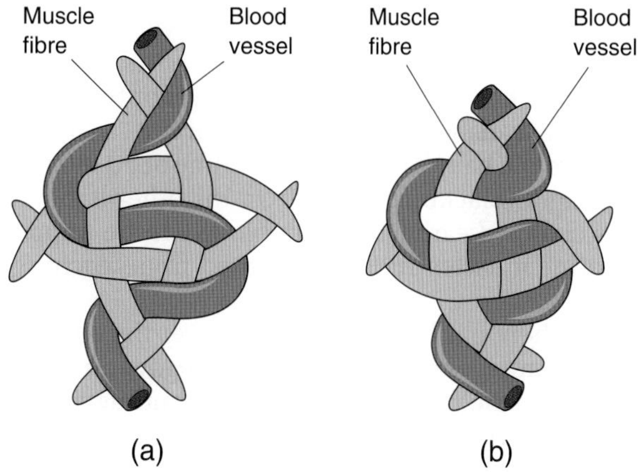

FIGURE 24.9 How the blood vessels run between the interlacing fibres of the uterus: (a) muscle fibres relaxed; (b) muscle fibres contracted
(Based on Henderson & Macdonald, 2004.)

It is normal to lose blood vaginally during the third stage with the separation of the placenta, but the impact of this blood loss depends not only on the volume lost but also on the general health of the woman. The World Health Organization defines a postpartum haemorrhage as a blood loss of equal to or more than 500 mL from the genital tract during the first 24 hours postpartum (Tunçalp et al., 2013). In low-income countries, where the prevalence of severe anaemia is high, a 500 mL blood loss can be life threatening for many women. While not underestimating the risk of PPH for any birth, it is also suggested that blood loss up to 1000 mL in healthy women may be considered physiological. The definition is further complicated by the difficulty of estimating blood loss, whether by measurement or by visual estimation. It has also been suggested that the 500 mL definition of PPH should be considered an alert level, and that PPH may be better defined as the volume of blood loss that is sufficient to cause deterioration in a woman's condition and thus require intervention (Begley et al., 2019; Sloan et al., 2010).

Complications associated with significant blood loss include cardiovascular shock, coagulation disorders, renal or liver failure and adult respiratory distress syndrome, and may result in death.

Cord clamping

Interventions such as cord clamping can interrupt the normal mechanism of the third stage, and if uterotonics are not administered then immediate cord clamping should not be necessary. If the mother suckles her baby, a reflex release of oxytocin occurs that stimulates uterine contractions. In the umbilical cord, vasoconstriction of the umbilical arteries occurs at birth in response to increasing partial pressure of oxygen (P_aO_2). This prevents blood flow from the baby to the placenta, but blood flow can occur from the placenta to the baby via the umbilical vein, which does not constrict. This occurs to a greater extent if the baby is held below the level of the placenta. A placental transfusion of 80 mL can occur—a significant increase to the baby's total blood volume of 70–80 mL / kg body weight (Blackburn, 2017). On the other hand, if the cord is clamped early, this extra blood can be trapped in the uterine muscles and be prevented from reaching the baby.

While there has been controversy over the advantages and disadvantages of early cord clamping (within the first minute after the birth of the placenta) and delayed cord clamping (more than 1 minute after the birth of the placenta or when the cord stops pulsating), there is considerable evidence identifying benefits to the infant and many clinical practice guidelines support delayed cord clamping. An observational study recording cord clamping time of 55 women birthing in a tertiary hospital in Aotearoa New Zealand reported that cord clamping of one minute or more occurred in almost all (93%) births and in over 60% deferred cord clamping of three minutes or more was used. The mean cord clamping time was 3.5 minutes (range 0.2–34 minutes) illustrating the widespread practice of delayed cord clamping in this sample of midwives (Hewitt, 2019). Results of a 2013 Cochrane review which included 15 RCTs supported delaying clamping of the umbilical cord in healthy term infants as this was shown to increase early haemoglobin concentrations and iron stores in infants at ages 3 and 6 months, although infants in the late-clamped group were also more likely to require phototherapy for jaundice (McDonald et al., 2013). These results have been supported by more recent RCTs (Ertekin et al., 2016; Kc et al., 2017). A further study reported that delayed cord clamping did not affect significantly the duration of the third stage of labour, nor measures of maternal haematology 48 hours after birth (De Paco et al., 2016). Ultrasound studies show blood may continue to move through the cord, both in arteries and the vein, up to and beyond five minutes post-birth (Boere et al., 2015).

A small RCT demonstrated improved brain myelination at 4 months of age for term babies that had over 5 minutes of placental transfusion (Mercer et al., 2018) and improved neurodevelopment in children at 4 years of age has been reported (Andersson et al., 2015).

Benefits of placental transfusion for non-breathing term infants have also been identified (Andersson et al., 2019). This is an important area for further research.

(Further information on this topic is included in Ch. 25.)

CRITICAL THINKING EXERCISE

A small group of physicians and midwives from a variety of birth settings including the home, birth centre and hospital were interviewed about their perceptions of when a change of practice was required to meet new evidence. Delayed cord clamping was selected as the exemplar practice for the study. The drivers of change identified were: (1) trusting colleagues, (2) believing the evidence, (3) honouring mothers and families, (4) knowing personal certainty and (5) protecting the integrity of the mother and the baby. The authors concluded that colleagues played a significant role in determining an individual's change in practice and that the evidence alone was never a sole driver of change (Leslie et al., 2015). Consider these findings in relation to your practice.

OTHER MATERNAL BODY SYSTEMS DURING LABOUR

Along with significant physiological changes that occur in the woman's reproductive system during labour, there are also changes to other body systems and processes. Metabolism alters to meet the increased energy demands of labour, along with changes to the respiratory and cardiovascular systems. Haematological changes maximise blood-clotting mechanisms and reduce the chances of haemorrhage. Water and electrolyte balance may be more difficult to maintain during labour.

Metabolism

Energy needs increase during labour, mainly because of the demands of both uterine and cardiac activity. Glucose is the prime energy source, but if the woman's intake is insufficient then oxidation of body fat (triglycerides) occurs to provide energy. Ketone bodies are produced through beta-oxidation of fats, and if excessive this can cause ketoacidosis, which may interfere with myometrial action (Rankin, 2017). Ketones can cross the placenta to the fetus and, because of their acidic nature, may depress fetal pH. It is normal for maternal blood pH to fall by 0.05 units, but it usually remains within the range 7.3–7.4 (Rankin, 2017).

Respiratory system

Normal breathing patterns are overridden by events in labour that prompt hyperventilation or hypoventilation, leading to changes in acid–base balance. This is at a time when increased oxygen is required to support strenuous myometrial contractions.

Mild respiratory alkalosis occurs as a result of hyperventilation during the late first stage of labour. Hyperventilation tends to increase if the woman is in pain or anxious. Excessive hyperventilation leading to a decreased partial pressure of carbon dioxide in the arterial circulation (P_aCO_2) and alkalosis can be potentially hazardous to both the mother and the fetus. Extremely low P_aCO_2 levels result in cerebral vasoconstriction and may reduce intervillous perfusion and blood flow (Blackburn, 2017). The resulting alkalosis shifts the oxygen–haemoglobin curve to the left and impairs the release of oxygen from the maternal blood to the fetus. This is during a time when oxygenation of the fetus may already be impaired during uterine contractions. Hyperventilation may also lead to dizziness and tingling in the mother owing to the low P_aCO_2 levels. Encouraging the woman to slow her respiration rate and promoting deep breathing between contractions can help reduce alkalosis (Blackburn, 2017).

Another factor to be aware of with respect to respiration during labour is the level of oxygen consumption, which increases with contractions. If there is insufficient time between contractions for replenishment of the blood supply, myometrial hypoxia may occur with associated increases in pain. With insufficient oxygen available, anaerobic metabolism is stimulated, which may lead to metabolic acidosis, most likely near the end of first-stage labour. Respiratory alkalosis, which normally occurs during labour, can compensate to some extent for mild metabolic acidosis. During second-stage labour, breath holding during pushing results in respiratory acidosis and increased P_aCO_2. This may reduce the uptake of CO_2 from the fetal circulation and result in fetal respiratory acidosis.

Cardiovascular system

Several changes occur in the cardiovascular system owing to the increased blood volume that is returned to the systemic circulation from the uterus with each contraction (300–500 mL). This increases cardiac output by about 30% during contractions in the first stage of labour and can increase cardiac output by up to 50% in the second stage. The increase is primarily due to increases in stroke volume (Ouzounian & Elkayam, 2012). Systolic blood pressure may rise by about 35 mmHg during contractions in the first stage and even more in the second stage (Blackburn, 2017). As there is little change in total peripheral resistance, the increase in blood pressure must be largely due to the increase in cardiac output. An increase in heart rate is usual, but a heart rate greater than 100 b.p.m. may indicate ketoacidosis. Cardiopulmonary blood volume also increases, but this increased load is not normally a problem unless a woman has cardiac complications.

Haematological changes

Birth of the baby is associated with blood loss (approximately 500 mL with a vaginal delivery) and rapid coagulation to compensate. The hypercoagulable state of pregnancy is increased in labour and this facilitates clot formation at the placenta. The release of thromboplastin during placental separation activates the extrinsic coagulation pathway. Immediately after birth there is an increased risk of coagulation disorders due to the hypercoagulable state. Other changes include an increase in haemoglobin concentration due in part to increases in erythropoiesis, but also to haemoconcentration associated with dehydration. There is an increase in numbers of leucocytes, particularly neutrophils, possibly due to stress (Blackburn, 2017).

CRITICAL THINKING EXERCISE

Is the hypercoagulable state of pregnancy always an advantage? What complications could be associated with this following birth? Identify some strategies for decreasing the risk of such complications.

Renal function

Maintaining **water and electrolyte balance** during labour is influenced by increased aldosterone secretion, which stimulates sodium retention, and by loss of water through sweating and increased respiration. A labouring woman can quickly become dehydrated, particularly if there is excessive blood loss. Fluid intake must be maintained to prevent dehydration. If administration of intravenous fluids is necessary, they must be monitored to avoid water intoxication. Oxytocin has an antidiuretic action and if added to the intravenous fluid it can increase the possibility of water intoxication. Careful monitoring is required.

FOURTH STAGE OF LABOUR

The fourth stage refers to the first hour or two after birth when uterine tone is established and recovery from labour begins. During this time, blood pressure reduces owing to redistribution of blood from the uterus and blood loss. Contractions of the uterus begin the process of involution and are the cause of afterpains. These pains may increase with the release of oxytocin associated with breastfeeding. Urine may have been retained owing to decreased bladder tone and possible trauma to the bladder, thus women should be encouraged to pass urine. Following the high energy requirement during the birth process, women may be hungry and in need of food and drink as this recovery phase progresses. (Further detail on the postpartum period is provided in Ch. 29.)

FETAL RESPONSES DURING LABOUR

While the woman is undergoing major changes associated with labour, the fetus is also experiencing major changes. The fetus is exposed to considerable stress during labour. Although this is necessary to provoke respiration and other processes, monitoring of fetal wellbeing is essential. Fetal heart rate monitoring provides a measure of fetal wellbeing during labour, with the goal of early detection of fetal hypoxia—although interpretation remains an inexact science. Monitoring can be via intermittent auscultation or continuous electronic monitoring, and there is evidence against routine use of continuous monitoring of low-risk women; a recent study has shown that continuous monitoring of low-risk women was associated with an approximately 20% increase in caesarean section rates, but the study was not powered sufficiently to detect possible important differences in perinatal mortality (Devane et al., 2017). A recent Cochrane review of RCTs included only three studies and reported that the quality of evidence was very low to moderate due to study design (Martis et al., 2017). The key reported findings were that caesarean sections due to fetal distress were associated with use of Doppler ultrasound or intermittent CTG compared with routine use of a Pinard stethoscope, but that there was no clear difference in neonatal outcomes of Apgar scores at 5 minutes after birth, neonatal seizures or perinatal mortality. Long-term outcomes for the baby such as neurodevelopmental disability or cerebral palsy were not reported. The study authors recommended that women, health practitioners and policy makers consider the lack of short- and long-term benefits for the mother or baby along with the increased caesarean section rate when making decisions about the type of monitoring.

The fetal heart rate is normally in the range of 110 to 160 b.p.m., with an average baseline of 140 b.p.m. (King & Parer, 2000). Factors that reduce oxygen delivery to the fetus, such as hyperactivity of the uterus, Valsalva pushes during the second stage and maternal supine position, may lead to fetal hypoxia and a drop in fetal heart rate.

Control of the fetal heart rate

An understanding of the control of fetal heart rate is important in interpreting fetal heart rate changes in labour. The fetal heart rate is controlled by the autonomic nervous system and the cardiovascular centre in the medulla oblongata of the brain. The medulla receives feedback from baroreceptors, chemoreceptors and inputs from higher cerebral centres. Efferent output to the heart is via the sympathetic and parasympathetic nerves. Heart rate variability (changes in timing from beat to beat) is the result of the multiple inputs and is an indicator of fetal wellbeing (King & Parer, 2000; Yli & Kjellmer, 2016). Fetal heart rate patterns and baseline readings are influenced by factors such as fetal blood supply and oxygen and carbon dioxide content of the blood, and therefore can also be used to indicate fetal wellbeing.

Baroreceptors in the aortic arch and the carotid arteries detect blood pressure. An increase in blood pressure will cause a rapid reflex drop in heart rate (mediated by parasympathetic nerves). This could occur during umbilical cord compression because as flow within the umbilical vein is slowed the pressure in the fetal arterial circulation increases (King & Parer, 2000; Yli & Kjellmer, 2016).

Chemoreceptors detect oxygen and carbon dioxide levels in the blood. Receptors are located in the aortic arch and central nervous system. Increases in carbon dioxide and decreases in oxygen levels in the fetus are mainly detected by the central receptors and cause a reflex decrease in heart rate, mediated by parasympathetic nerves. Decreased placental perfusion during uterine contractions may impair fetoplacental gas exchange and result in a gradual drop in arterial oxygen. Detection by the chemoreceptors results in a more gradual decrease in fetal heart rate—a late deceleration. In a well-oxygenated fetus, heart rate variability is maintained during the contraction; after the contraction, normal metabolism resumes and the bradycardia resolves (King & Parer, 2000; Yli & Kjellmer, 2016).

Non-asphyxial events can also influence heart rate variability and baseline levels (e.g. central nervous system depressants, beta-sympathomimetics, congenital neurological abnormalities and defective cardiac conduction).

Finally, it is important to note that bradycardic events in the fetus may cause hypoxia or be the result of hypoxia. Bradycardic events in the second stage occur secondary to fetal head compression and vagal (parasympathetic nerve) stimulation. The fetus can tolerate these bradycardic events as long as the heart rate remains above 80 b.p.m. and variability is maintained. If severe or prolonged, bradycardias resulting from impaired placental blood flow are likely to lead to fetal acidosis.

Fetal responses to hypoxia

During times of decreased placental blood flow, the fetus has mechanisms to maintain normal aerobic metabolism. First, blood flow can be redistributed to supply the vital organs (heart, brain and adrenals) at the expense of flow to the gut, kidneys and limbs; secondly, myocardial oxygen consumption can be reduced by reducing the heart rate (King & Parer, 2000; Yli & Kjellmer, 2016). If these mechanisms are not sufficient to meet metabolic needs, the fetus may change to anaerobic metabolism. Anaerobic metabolism produces energy, in the form of adenosine triphosphate (ATP), less efficiently than aerobic metabolism and it results in lactic acid production. Lactic acid is slow to cross the placenta, and may accumulate to cause metabolic acidosis in the fetus. Fetal heart rate patterns contribute to an assessment of fetal acid–base status (King & Parer, 2000; Yli & Kjellmer 2016).

CRITICAL THINKING EXERCISE

Suggest some physiological advantages and disadvantages of anaerobic metabolism in the fetus compared with aerobic metabolism.

RESEARCH ACTIVITY

Results from a study (Vogl et al., 2006) of 103 nulliparous women with uncomplicated singleton pregnancies indicated that the mode of delivery influenced both maternal and fetal stress hormone responses. Those undergoing elective caesarean section had significantly lower levels of cortisol, adrenaline and other stress hormones compared with vaginal birth, whether with no pain relief, epidural or use of ventouse.

1. What are the implications of this study?
2. Are there benefits for the neonate of increased stress at birth?

EPIGENETICS, LABOUR AND BIRTH

Epigenetics involves the study of behavioural and environmental factors which influence how genes work. Each cell in the human body has the same DNA and same genes, but epigenetics influences the expression of certain genes (turning them on) and the silencing of others (turning them off). Epigenetics influences the activity of genes but does not change the underlying DNA sequence.

Understanding of epigenetics is a rapidly developing field particularly significant in understanding long-term impacts on health and susceptibility to disease. This includes topics relevant to midwifery, such as the impact of stress, hypertension, preeclampsia, renal disease and impacts of pregnancy, labour and birth (Dahlen et al., 2016).

Studies have provided evidence for epigenetic effects during the antenatal and postnatal periods (Agarwal et al., 2018; Franzago et al., 2019) but little is known about the epigenetic influence of physiological birth or of medical interventions during labour and birth. An international, multidisciplinary research collaboration, EPIIC (Epigenetic Impact of Childbirth), has published hypotheses on epigenetic influences suggesting interventions such as the use of synthetic oxytocin, antibiotics, and caesarean section affect the epigenetic remodelling processes and subsequent health of the mother and baby (Dahlen et al., 2013). The hypotheses are underpinned by a review of current evidence and practice and suggest the epigenetic impact on genes could lead to long-term health issues related to immune responses, weight gain and metabolism.

To understand a possible mechanism for the long-term impacts of labour and birth on the baby, Uvnäs-Moberg et al. instigated a scoping review (Uvnäs-Moberg et al., 2020) of the literature. They focused on the possible role of epigenetic changes to oxytocin and oxytocin receptors in facilitating positive outcomes associated with vaginal birth and skin-to-skin contact of mother and baby. While evidence links endogenous oxytocin as the mediator of many of these positive health effects, they found no studies that reported epigenetic changes of oxytocin or oxytocin receptors in connection with physiological birth. This is a developing area of research and the authors noted that while there are no studies as yet affirming such epigenetic changes, further research is needed to explore this in more depth.

SUMMARY

- Before labour begins, *myometrial activation* occurs. This involves structural and chemical changes to the smooth muscle cells of the myometrium to enhance electrical transmission and contractility of the uterus. The process is controlled by hormones, particularly oestrogen.
- *Cervical ripening* must also occur before labour will proceed. This involves an inflammatory-like response that results in loss of collagen, increase in water content of the cervix and loss of collagen binding. This is mediated by oestrogen, relaxin, nitric oxide and prostaglandins. Stretching of the cervix leads to release of prostaglandins.
- The *physiological factors that may be responsible for initiating labour* include an increase in placental corticotrophin-releasing hormone, maturation of the fetal hypothalamic–pituitary–adrenal axis, an increase in levels of placental oestriol (synthesised from fetal precursors), an increase in levels of prostaglandins and a decrease in the effectiveness of the antiuterotonics progesterone, relaxin and nitric oxide. Pressure from the fetus against the uterus and cervix stimulates release of prostaglandins and oxytocin.
- *Maintenance of labour* depends on the presence of the uterotonic hormones, in part stimulated by the neuroendocrine reflex.
- The *first stage of labour* involves effacement and dilation of the cervix. This occurs only if myometrial contractions are effective. Contractions must be coordinated and show a decreasing gradient of activity with fundal dominance. They must generate sufficient pressure, last for sufficient time and be frequent enough to bring about dilation of the cervix until it is fully dilated at 10 cm.
- The *second stage of labour* begins at full dilation of the cervix and ends with the birth of the baby. The woman feels the urge to push, leading to contractions of the abdominal muscles for 5–6 seconds several times during each very strong, expulsive contraction of the uterus.
- The *mechanism of labour* describes the manipulations the baby must make to negotiate the narrow pelvis and birth canal. Progress during the second stage depends on effective expulsive contractions and is influenced by the shape of the bony pelvis, the lie and orientation of the fetus, the resistance of the pelvic floor and the position of the woman.
- Following the birth of the baby, uterine contractions separate the placenta from the uterus (the *third stage of*

labour). The placenta may be birthed without intervention or by active management, involving administration of an oxytocic drug, clamping of the cord and either controlled cord traction or maternal effort.

- During the *fourth stage of labour*, continuing uterine contractions minimise blood loss from the placental site and are facilitated by reflex oxytocin release, and enhanced by the suckling of the baby at the breast.
- Labour is a physically demanding time that is supported by *metabolic changes*. If glucose intake is insufficient, fatty acid oxidation provides energy. If excessive, this can result in ketone formation and ketoacidosis.
- Hyperventilation or hypoventilation during labour can lead to changes in *acid–base balance*. Hyperventilation with the resulting respiratory alkalosis can impair oxygen release from the maternal blood to the fetus. Maternal respiratory acidosis can reduce fetal transfer of CO_2 to the maternal circulation and lead to fetal respiratory acidosis.
- *Maternal cardiac output* increases with contractions as blood in uterine vessels is squeezed into the systemic circulation, and therefore during contractions the blood flow to the placenta is reduced.
- *Haematological changes* facilitate blood coagulation, but also increase the risk of coagulation disorders immediately after birth. Changes to aldosterone levels and increased water loss due to sweating may interfere with water and electrolyte balance during labour.
- During labour *the fetus is normally exposed to stress*. The heart rate is controlled by baroreceptor and chemoreceptor input and input from higher centres to the medulla oblongata. Asphyxial and non-asphyxial events can influence fetal heart rate and fetal heart rate variability.
- Monitoring of fetal heart rate and fetal heart rate variability provides *indicators of fetal wellbeing*. During times of decreased blood supply, the fetus can maintain energy requirements by redistribution of blood flow to vital areas, reduction of heart rate and oxygen needs, and if necessary switch to anaerobic metabolism, although this is less efficient and leads to lactic acid production.
- Epigenetics is a growing field of research including exploration into aspects of health such as stress, hypertension, preeclampsia, renal disease and impacts of pregnancy, labour and birth.

Conclusion

Labour is underpinned by many complex physiological processes driven by hormonal changes that are not fully understood. As pregnancy ends, labour begins with myometrial activation and cervical ripening and then a change in the balance of hormones drives the contractions that manipulate the fetus through the narrow pelvis and birth canal to be born. Contractions continue to facilitate the birth of the placenta. This is a physically demanding time for the woman and physiological changes to metabolic, cardiovascular, haematological and respiratory function facilitate the processes of labour and recovery. The fetus is well adapted to survive the stresses of normal birth, but if progress of labour is delayed this can lead to fetal compromise. After birth of the placenta the changes in hormone levels slowly return the woman's physiology to the non-pregnant state and the baby adapts to life in the extrauterine world.

Review questions

1. Describe four key changes to the structure of myometrial cells that occur during activation of the myometrium.
2. Outline the process contributing to softening/ripening of the cervix.
3. Identify at least one fetal and one maternal factor that probably contributes to the onset of labour. Include evidence for this.
4. Outline at least four roles of prostaglandin E_2 and prostaglandin $F_{2\alpha}$.
5. Describe the anatomical and physiological features of the upper uterine segment and the lower uterine segment that facilitate effacement of the cervix.
6. Explain why the birth of the baby (the mechanism of the second stage of labour) involves such a complex set of manoeuvres.
7. Describe two physiological or anatomical mechanisms that reduce the chance of haemorrhage at the placental site following birth of the placenta.
8. Describe the maternal breathing pattern that can bring about alkalosis and outline any impact this might have on fetal gas exchange.
9. Explain the mechanism underlying separation of the placenta in a normal birth.
10. Outline the reflex responses of the fetus to a decrease in P_aO_2.

Online resources

Te Ara Encyclopedia of New Zealand. Birth in Māori tradition: https://teara.govt.nz/en/te-whanau-tamariki-pregnancy-and-birth/page-1.
Centers for Disease Control and Prevention, 'What is epigenetics?': https://www.cdc.gov/genomics/disease/epigenetics.htm#:~:text=Epigenetics%20is%20the%20study%20of,body%20reads%20a%20DNA%20sequence.
Kahn Academy—videos on the basic physiology of labour: https://www.khanacademy.org/search?referer=%2F&page_search_query=physiology+of+labour.
National Institute for Health and Clinical Excellence (NICE). Intrapartum Care for Healthy Women and Babies. 2017 NICE guidelines and 2019 surveillance of intrapartum care for healthy women and babies (NICE guideline CG190): https://www.nice.org.uk/guidance/cg190.
New Zealand College of Midwives (NZCOM) Cochrane summaries for midwives: https://www.midwife.org.nz/research/cochrane-summaries-for-midwifery.
New Zealand College of Midwives (NZCOM) current consensus statements and guidelines: https://www.midwife.org.nz/quality-practice/practice-guidance/.
Smart Start New Zealand: https://smartstart.services.govt.nz.

References

Agarwal P, Morriseau TS, Kereliuk SM, et al. Maternal obesity, diabetes during pregnancy and epigenetic mechanisms that influence the developmental origins of cardiometabolic disease in the offspring. *Crit Rev Clin Lab Sci.* 2018;55(2), 71–101. doi:10.1080/10408363.2017.1422109.
Alehagen S, Wijma B, Lundberg U, et al. Fear, pain and stress hormones during childbirth. *J Psychosom Obstet Gynecol.* 2005; 26(3):153–165.
Andersson O, Lindquist B, Lindgren M, et al. Effect of delayed cord clamping on neurodevelopment at 4 years of age: a randomized clinical trial. *JAMA Pediatr.* 2015;169(7):631–638.
Andersson O, Rana N, Ewald U, et al. Intact cord resuscitation versus early cord clamping in the treatment of depressed newborn infants during the first 10 minutes of birth (Nepcord III) – a randomized clinical trial. *Maternal Health, Neonatology and Perinatology.* 2019;5(1):15. doi:10.1186/s40748-019-0110-z.
Arulkumaran S, Kandola MK, Hoffman B, et al. The roles of prostaglandin ep1 and 3 receptors in the control of human myometrial contractility. *J Clin Endocrinol Metab.* 2012;97(2):489–498.
Aviram A, Melamed N, Hadar E, et al. Effect of prostaglandin E2 on myometrial electrical activity in women undergoing induction of labor. *Am J Perinatol.* 2014;31(5):413–418.
Battarbee, A. N., Glover, A. V., & Stamilio, D. M. (2020). Association between early amniotomy in labour induction and severe maternal and neonatal morbidity. *Aust N Z J Obstet Gynaecol,* 60(1), 108–114. doi:10.1111/ajo.13031.
Begley, C. M., Gyte, G. M., Devane, D., McGuire, W., Weeks, A., & Biesty, L. M. (2019). Active versus expectant management for women in the third stage of labour. *Cochrane Database Syst Rev,* 2(2), Cd007412. doi:10.1002/14651858.CD007412.pub5.
Berghella V, Baxter JK, Chauhan SP. Evidence-based labor and delivery management. *Am J Obstet Gynecol.* 2008;199(5):445–454.
Blackburn S. *Maternal, Fetal and Neonatal Physiology: A Clinical Perspective.* 2nd ed. St Louis, MO: WB Saunders; 2003.
Blackburn S. *Maternal, Fetal and Neonatal Physiology: A Clinical Perspective.* 5th ed. Saunders / Elsevier; 2017.
Boere I, Roest AA, Wallace E, Ten Harkel AD, et al. Umbilical blood flow patterns directly after birth before delayed cord clamping. *Arch Dis Child Fetal Neonatal Ed.* 2015;100(2), F121–125. doi:10.1136/archdischild-2014-307144.
Campbell EA, Linton EA, Wolfe CD, et al. Plasma corticotropin-releasing hormone concentrations during pregnancy and parturition. *J Clin Endocrinol Metab.* 1987;64(5):1054–1059.
Carlson NS, Hernandez TL, et al. Parturition dysfunction in obesity: time to target the pathobiology. *Reprod Biol Endocrinol.* 2015;13:135. doi:10.1186/s12958-015-0129-6.
Challis JRG. Understanding pre-term birth. *Clin Invest Med.* 2001; 24(1):60.
Chen W, Xue J, Peprah MK, et al. A systematic review and network meta-analysis comparing the use of Foley catheters, misoprostol, and dinoprostone for cervical ripening in the induction of labour. *BJOG.* 2016;123(3):346–354.
Dahlen HG, Kennedy HP, Anderson CM, et al. The EPIIC hypothesis: intrapartum effects on the neonatal epigenome and consequent health outcomes. *Med Hypotheses.* 2013;80(5):656–662. doi:10.1016/j.mehy.2013.01.017.
Dahlen H, Downe S, Wright ML, et al. Childbirth and consequent atopic disease: emerging evidence on epigenetic effects based on the hygiene and EPIIC hypotheses. *BMC Pregnancy Childbirth.* 2016;16(1):4. doi:10.1186/s12884-015-0768-9.
Davis D, Baddock S, Pairman S, et al. Risk of severe postpartum hemorrhage in low-risk childbearing women in New Zealand: exploring the effect of place of birth and comparing third stage management of labor. *Birth.* 2012;39(2):98.
De Jonge A, Van Diem M, Scheepers P, et al. Increased blood loss in upright birthing positions originates from perineal damage. *BJOG: An International Journal of Obstetrics & Gynaecology.* 2007;114(3):349–355. doi:https://doi.org/10.1111/j.1471-0528.2006.01210.x.
De Paco C, Herrera J, Garcia C, et al. Effects of delayed cord clamping on the third stage of labour, maternal haematological parameters and acid–base status in fetuses at term. *Eur J Obstet Gynecol Reprod Biol.* 2016;207:153–156.
de Tayrac R, Letouzey V. Methods of pushing during vaginal delivery and pelvic floor and perineal outcomes: a review. *Curr Opin Obstet Gynecol.* 2016;28(6):470–476. doi:10.1097/gco.0000000000000325.
Desseauve D, Fradet L, Lacouture P, et al. Position for labor and birth: state of knowledge and biomechanical perspectives. *Eur J Obstet Gynecol Reprod Biol.* 2017;208:46–54.
Devane D, Lalor JG, Daly S, et al. Cardiotocography versus intermittent auscultation of fetal heart on admission to labour ward for assessment of fetal wellbeing. *Cochrane Database Syst Rev.* 2017;(1):CD005122.
Dietze M. A re-evaluation of the mechanism of labour for contemporary midwifery practice. *Midwifery Matters.* 2001;88:3–8.
Di Renzo GC, Giardina I, Clerici G, et al. Progesterone in normal and pathological pregnancy. *Horm Mol Biol Clin Investig.* 2016; 27(1):35–48.
Dixon L, Fletcher L, Tracy S, et al. Midwives' care during the third stage of labour. An analysis of the New Zealand College of Midwives Midwifery Database 2004–2008. *NZCOM J.* 2009;41: 20–25.
Dixon L, Tracy S, Guilliland K, et al. Outcomes of physiological and active third stage labour care amongst women in New Zealand. *Midwifery.* 2013;29:67–74.
Ertekin AA, Nihan Ozdemir N, Sahinoglu Z, et al. Term babies with delayed cord clamping: an approach in preventing anemia. *J Matern Fetal Neonatal Med.* 2016;29(17):2813–2816.
Facchinetti F, Fontanesi F, Del Giovane C. Pre-induction of labour: comparing dinoprostone vaginal insert to repeated prostaglandin administration: a systematic review and meta-analysis. *J Matern Fetal Neonatal Med.* 2012;25(10):1965–1969.
Franzago M, Fraticelli F, Stuppia L, et al. Nutrigenetics, epigenetics and gestational diabetes: consequences in mother and child. *Epigenetics.* 2019;14(3):215–235. doi:10.1080/15592294.2019.1582277.

Gauthier T, Mazeau S, Dalmay F, et al. Obesity and cervical ripening failure risk. *J Matern Fetal Neonatal Med.* 2012; 25(3):304–307.

Gizzo S, Di Gangi S, Noventa M, et al. Women's Choice of Positions during Labour: Return to the Past or a Modern Way to Give Birth? A Cohort Study in Italy. *BioMed Research International.* 2014;638093. doi:10.1155/2014/638093.

Grammatopoulos DK. Placental corticotrophin-releasing hormone and its receptors in human pregnancy and labour: still a scientific enigma. *J Neuroendocrinol.* 2008;20(4):432–438.

Grammatopoulos DK, Hillhouse EW. Role of corticotropin-releasing hormone in onset of labour. *Lancet.* 1999;354(9189): 1546–1549.

Gupta JK, Sood A, Hofmeyr GJ, et al. Position in the second stage of labour for women without epidural anaesthesia. *Cochrane Database Syst Rev.* 2017;(5):CD002006.

Haas J, Barzilay E, Chayen B, et al. Safety of labor induction with prostaglandin e2 in grandmultiparous women. *J Matern Fetal Neonatal Med.* 2013;26(1):49–51.

Hamilton EF, Warrick PA, Collins K, et al. Assessing first-stage labor progression and its relationship to complications. *Am J Obstet Gynecol.* 2016;214(3):358.e351–358. doi:10.1016/j.ajog.2015.10.016.

Henderson C, Macdonald S. *Mayes' Midwifery. A Textbook for Midwives.* 13th ed. Edinburgh: Baillière Tindall; 2004.

Herman A, Zimerman A, Arieli S, et al. Down-up sequential separation of the placenta. *Ultrasound Obstet Gynecol.* 2002;19(3): 278–281.

Hewitt, T. *Timing of cord clamping (TOCC): an observational study of cord clamping practice in a New Zealand maternity hospital. Unpublished master's thesis.* Otago Polytechnic. New Zealand.

Hiersch L, Salzer L, Aviram A, et al. Factors affecting uterine electrical activity during the active phase of labor prior to rupture of membranes. *J Matern Fetal Neonatal Med.* 2015; 28(14):1633–1636.

Johnson MH. *Essential Reproduction.* 7th ed. Chichester, UK: John Wiley; 2013.

Johnson MH, Everitt BJ. *Essential Reproduction.* 3rd ed. Oxford: Blackwell Scientific; 1988.

Kc A, Rana N, Malqvist M, et al. Effects of delayed umbilical cord clamping vs early clamping on anemia in infants at 8 and 12 months: a randomized clinical trial. *JAMA Pediatr.* 2017; 171(3):264–270.

Keirse MJ. Natural prostaglandins for induction of labor and pre-induction cervical ripening. *Clin Obstet Gynecol.* 2006;49(3): 609–626.

King T, Parer J. The physiology of fetal heart rate patterns and perinatal asphyxia. *J Perinat Neonatal Nurs.* 2000;14(3): 19–39.

Kosfeld M, Heinrichs M, Zak PJ, et al. Oxytocin increases trust in humans. *Nature.* 2005;435(7042):673–676.

Lawrence A, Lewis L, Hofmeyr GJ, et al. Maternal positions and mobility during first stage labour. *Cochrane Database Syst Rev.* 2013;(10):CD003934.

Ledingham M, Thomson A, Young A, et al. Changes in the expression of nitric oxide synthase in the human uterine cervix during pregnancy and parturition. *Mol Hum Reprod.* 2000;6(11):1041.

Lemos A, Amorim MM, Dornelas de Andrade A, et al. Pushing/bearing down methods for the second stage of labour. *Cochrane Database Syst Rev.* 2017;(3):CD009124.

Leslie MS, Erickson-Owens D, Cseh M. The evolution of individual maternity care providers to delayed cord clamping: is it the evidence? *J Midwifery Womens Health.* 2015;60(5): 561–569.

Longo M, Jain V, Vedernikov YP, et al. Effects of L-type Ca2+-channel blockade, K+ ATP-channel opening and nitric oxide on human uterine contractility in relation to gestational age and labour. *Mol Hum Reprod.* 2003;9(3):159.

McDonald SJ, Middleton P, Dowswell T, et al. Effect of timing of umbilical cord clamping of term infants on maternal and neonatal outcomes. *Cochrane Database Syst Rev.* 2013;(7):CD004074, doi:10.1002/14651858.CD004074.pub3.

Martis R, Emilia O, Nurdiati DS, et al. Intermittent auscultation (IA) of fetal heart rate in labour for fetal well-being. *Cochrane Database Syst Rev.* 2017;(2):CD008680.

Mercer JS, Erickson-Owens DA, Deoni, SCL, et al. Effects of Delayed Cord Clamping on 4-Month Ferritin Levels, Brain Myelin Content, and Neurodevelopment: A Randomized Controlled Trial. *The Journal of pediatrics.* 2018;203:266–272. e262. doi:10.1016/j.jpeds.2018.06.006.

Michel SCA, Rake A, Treiber K, et al. MR Obstetric pelvimetry: effect of birthing position on pelvic bony dimensions. *Am J Roentgenol.* 2002;179:1063–1067.

Mitre M, Marlin BJ, Schiavo JK, et al. A distributed network for social cognition enriched for oxytocin receptors. *J Neurosci.* 2016;36(8):2517–2535.

Moberg K. *The Oxytocin Factor: Tapping the Hormone of Calm, Love and Healing.* Cambridge: Da Capo Press, Pegasus Group; 2003.

Nasir A, Korejo R, Noorani KJ. Child birth in squatting position. *J Pak Med Assoc.* 2007;57(1):19–22.

Norwitz E, Robinson J, Challis J. The control of labor. *NEJM.* 1999; 341(9):660.

Oladapo OT, Diaz V, Bonet M, et al. Cervical dilatation patterns of 'low-risk' women with spontaneous labour and normal perinatal outcomes: a systematic review. *BJOG.* 125(8):944–954. doi:10.1111/1471-0528.14930.

Ouzounian JG, Elkayam U. Physiologic changes during normal pregnancy and delivery. *Cardiol Clin.* 2012;30(3):317–329.

Petraglia F, Coukos G, Volpe A, et al. Involvement of placental neurohormones in human parturition. *Ann N Y Acad Sci.* 1991; 622:331–340.

Petraglia F, Imperatore A, Challis JR. Neuroendocrine mechanisms in pregnancy and parturition. *Endocr Rev.* 2010;31(6): 783–816.

Phipps H, Charlton S, Dietz HP. Can antenatal education influence how women push in labour? *Aust N Z J Obstet Gynaecol.* 2009; 49(3):274–278.

Rabotti C, Mischi M. Propagation of electrical activity in uterine muscle during pregnancy: a review. *Acta Physiol.* 2015;213(2):406–416.

Rankin J. *Physiology in Childbearing With Anatomy and Related Biosciences.* 4th ed. Edinburgh: Elsevier; 2017.

Ravanos K, Dagklis T, Petousis S, et al. Factors implicated in the initiation of human parturition in term and preterm labor: a review. *Gynecol Endocrinol.* 2015;31(9):679–683.

Roberts JE. The 'push' for evidence: management of the second stage. *J Midwifery Womens Health.* 2002;47(1):2–15.

Rozenberg P. Is there a role for X-ray pelvimetry in the twenty-first century? *Gynécol Obstét Fertil.* 2007;35(5):491–492.

Saxton A, Fahy K, Rolfe M, et al. Does skin-to-skin contact and breast feeding at birth affect the rate of primary postpartum haemorrhage: results of a cohort study. *Midwifery.* 2015;31(11): 1110–1117.

Shibata Y, Shirai Y, Miyamoto M. The aging process in the sacroiliac joint: helical computed tomography analysis. *J Orthop Sci.* 2002;7(1):12–18.

Sloan NL, Durocher J, Aldrich T, et al. What measured blood loss tells us about postpartum bleeding: a systematic review. *BJOG.* 2010;117(7):788–800.

Smyth MDR, Alldred KS, Markham C. Amniotomy for shortening spontaneous labour. *Cochrane Database Syst Rev.* 2013;(1):

CD006167. Online: http://www.cochrane.org/CD006167/PREG_amniotomy-for-shortening-spontaneous-labour.
TunÇalp O, Souza JP, Gülmezoglu M, et al. New WHO recommendations on prevention and treatment of postpartum hemorrhage. *Int J Gynaecol Obstet.* 2013;123(3):254–256.
Uvnäs-Moberg K, Ekström-Bergström A, Berg M, et al. Maternal plasma levels of oxytocin during physiological childbirth - a systematic review with implications for uterine contractions and central actions of oxytocin. *BMC Pregnancy Childbirth.* 2019;19(1):285. doi:10.1186/s12884-019-2365-9.
Uvnäs-Moberg K, Gross MM, Agius A, et al. Are There Epigenetic Oxytocin-Mediated Effects on the Mother and Infant during Physiological Childbirth? *International journal of molecular sciences.* 2020;21(24):9503. doi:10.3390/ijms21249503.
Vogl SE, Worda C, Egarter C, et al. Mode of delivery is associated with maternal and fetal endocrine stress response. *BJOG.* 2006;113(4):441–445.
Walsh D. *Evidence-Based Care for Normal Labour and Birth.* New York: Routledge; 2007.
Walsh D, Downe S. *Essential Midwifery Practice: Intrapartum Care.* Chichester, UK/Ames, IA: Wiley-Blackwell; 2010.
Warmink-Perdijk WD, Koelewijn JM, de Jonge A, et al. Better perineal outcomes in sitting birthing position cannot be explained by changing from upright to supine position for performing an episiotomy. *Midwifery.* 2016;34:1–6.
Word RA, Li XH, Hnat M, et al. Dynamics of cervical remodeling during pregnancy and parturition: mechanisms and current concepts. *Semin Reprod Med.* 2007;25(1):69–79.
Yildirim G, Beji NK. Effects of pushing techniques in birth on mother and fetus: a randomized study. *Birth.* 2008;35(1):25–30.
Yli BM, Kjellmer I. Pathophysiology of foetal oxygenation and cell damage during labour. *Best Pract Res Clin Obstet Gynaecol.* 2016;30:9–21.
Zang Y, Lu H, Zhang H, Huang J, et al. Benefits and risks of upright positions during the second stage of labour: An overview of systematic reviews. *Int J Nurs Stud.* 2021;114:103812. doi:10.1016/j.ijnurstu.2020.103812.
Zhang J, Landy HJ, Branch DW, et al. Contemporary patterns of spontaneous labor with normal neonatal outcomes. *Obstet Gynecol.* 2010;116(6):1281–1287.

Further reading

American College of Obstetricians (ACOG). https://www.acog.org/Resources-And-Publications/Obstetric-Care-Consensus-Series/Safe-Prevention-of-the-Primary-Cesarean-Delivery. Identifies the need to revisit the definition of labour dystocia as a way of reducing the rate of primary caesarean deliveries.
Blackburn S. Parturition and uterine physiology. In: Blackburn S. *Maternal, Fetal and Neonatal Physiology: A Clinical Perspective.* 5th ed. Saunders/Elsevier; 2017:115–141.
Di Renzo GC, Giardina I, Clerici G, et al. Progesterone in normal and pathological pregnancy. *Horm Mol Biol Clin Investig.* 2016; 27(1):35–48.
Gupta JK, Sood A, Hofmeyr GJ, et al. Position in the second stage of labour for women without epidural anaesthesia. *Cochrane Database Syst Rev.* 2017;(5):CD002006.
Li X, Kruger JA, Nash MP, et al. Modeling childbirth: elucidating the mechanisms of labor. *WIREs Syst Biol Med.* 2010;2: 460–470. doi:10.1002/wsbm.65.
Martis R, Emilia O, Nurdiati DS, et al. Intermittent auscultation (IA) of fetal heart rate in labour for fetal well-being. *Cochrane Database Syst Rev.* 2017;(2):CD008680.
Rankin J. The onset of labour. In: Rankin J, eds. *Physiology in Childbearing With Anatomy and Related Biosciences.* 4th ed. Edinburgh: Elsevier; 2017:373–380.
Rankin J. The first stage of labour. In: Rankin J, eds. *Physiology in Childbearing With Anatomy and Related Biosciences.* 4th ed. Edinburgh: Elsevier; 2017:381–397.
Rankin J. The second stage of labour. In: Rankin J, eds. *Physiology in Childbearing With Anatomy and Related Biosciences.* 4th ed. Edinburgh: Elsevier; 2017:411–420.
Rankin J. The third stage of labour. In: Rankin J, eds. *Physiology in Childbearing With Anatomy and Related Biosciences.* 4th ed. Edinburgh: Elsevier; 2017:421–426.
Ravanos K, Dagklis T, Petousis S, et al. Factors implicated in the initiation of human parturition in term and preterm labor: a review. *Gynecol Endocrinol.* 2015;31(9):679–683.
Yli BM, Kjellmer I. Pathophysiology of foetal oxygenation and cell damage during labour. *Best Pract Res Clin Obstet Gynaecol.* 2016;30:9–21.

CHAPTER 25

Supporting women in labour and birth

Jacqui Anderson and Juliet Thorpe

LEARNING OUTCOMES

Learning outcomes for this chapter are:

1. To identify labour and birth as a continuum that integrates physical, psychological, emotional, social and spiritual processes
2. To demonstrate awareness of the effect of the labour, birthing environment and relationship with carers on each woman's experience
3. To explain the importance of woman-centred care based on the midwifery principles of partnership, continuity of carer, and holism
4. To perform evidence-informed care appropriate to the individual needs of each woman and her baby
5. To perform midwifery assessment skills to be able to monitor the woman and her baby's health, wellbeing and responses to the physiological changes during labour and birth and in the immediate postpartum period
6. To demonstrate how to facilitate and support the first few hours together for mother and baby.

CHAPTER OVERVIEW

This chapter takes a woman-centred approach to the midwifery care of women in physiological labour at term. Labour and birth are considered a single continuous process, from the beginning of labour until two hours following the birth, although the traditional divisions into stages of labour are discussed. Using the New Zealand College of Midwives' 'decision points midwifery care' as a framework, a midwife's work 'with woman' through labour and birth is examined (New Zealand College of Midwives (NZCOM), 2015). Underpinning this work is the midwife–woman relationship, **assessment skills**, decision making and the provision of supportive care that facilitates and enhances the normal physiological process of labour and birth no matter where the woman chooses to birth. Key midwifery principles of partnership, continuity of caregiver and the promotion of physiological birth also underpin this chapter.

KEY TERMS

active management
afterpains
assessment skills
baby's heart rate
continuity of carer
continuum of labour and birth
documentation
latent phase
lotus birth
non-directed pushing
normal physiological labour and birth
partnership
woman-centred care

INTRODUCTION

The ability to provide supportive midwifery care in labour is a multifaceted skill. A midwife's role in supporting women in labour begins in the antenatal period with the establishment of the relationship between each midwife and each woman (Guilliland & Pairman, 1995, 2010). For a midwife to be able to provide effective and individualised care, she must spend time with each woman, getting to know her and her desires and dreams for the birth of this baby. Spending time getting to know each other also enables trust to develop, and anxieties, fears and misconceptions to be acknowledged before labour starts (Bradfield et al., 2019; Fontein-Kuipers et al., 2018). Midwives have identified that developing a connection with the woman and providing woman-centred care are the essential elements of the midwifery model of care (ACM, 2019; Bradfield et al., 2019; Davis et al., 2021; NZCOM, 2015).

In this chapter we will explore the knowledge and skills needed by the midwife to be able to provide woman-centred care during labour and birth. Our discussion recognises that the midwifery definition of labour relies on each woman's perceptions, and is unique to the individual woman. It is therefore difficult to define in an exact way. However, within the midwifery model of care, the woman is the focus and therefore her perceptions are the governing factors when providing care in labour and birth (Perriman, et al., 2018).

Throughout this chapter the focus is on the importance of understanding what supports the physiological process of labour and birth. This then enables the midwife to assist in creating an environment that maximises the woman's potential for normal birth and a gentle transition for her newborn baby (Sandall et al., 2016).

DEVELOPING THE WOMAN–MIDWIFE RELATIONSHIP

The knowledge that a midwife gains through the partnership relationship established with each woman guides her ability to support the woman to use her own strength to labour and birth her baby. As the woman moves through the various stages of her labour, the midwife's role in facilitating and promoting **normal physiological labour and birth** relies on her ability to be 'with the woman' (Bradfield et al., 2019; Hildingsson et al., 2021). Research exploring women's views on the type of support they find valuable during labour and birth identifies that the quality of the support they receive may outweigh many other aspects of the birth experience (Downe et al., 2018; Olza et al., 2018). The parameters of normal labour and birth are individual to each woman. To be able to recognise what is 'normal' for each woman, a midwife needs to be available to her and alert to the ebbs and flows of that woman's experience. Unexplored fears and issues can exacerbate the challenges that occur in labour, and without this understanding a midwife will find it more difficult to provide **woman-centred care** (Leap & Hunter, 2016; Olza et al., 2020).

By truly being 'with' the woman, the midwife is able to recognise and acknowledge the complexity of a process that is at once emotional, spiritual and physical (Davis, 2019; Leap & Hunter, 2016). With this acknowledgement comes an understanding of the factors that may affect labour and birth both positively and negatively. Recent studies reinforce our understanding that women who receive care from a midwife they know are more likely to have a normal birth, fewer interventions during labour and birth and a more positive view of their childbirth experience (Hildingsson et al., 2021; McLachlan et al.; 2016; Sandall et al., 2016; WHO, 2018). Compassion and kindness are intrinsic to the role the midwife has in supporting a woman through labour and birth. The effect of our voice, our touch and our belief in the woman's strength and ability to birth her baby are as important (if not more important) than all the technology and tools at our disposal. The combination of the birth environment, relationships with partners and carers, the physiological processes of labour and birth, and psychological influences can have a profound effect on the progress of a woman's labour (Ayerle et al., 2018; Dahan, 2021; Dixon et al., 2013; Wrønding et al., 2019).

Decision points for midwifery care in labour and birth

Throughout this chapter, decision points are identified to provide a framework for provision of midwifery care. Developed by the New Zealand College of Midwives (NZCOM) in 1993 and revised in 2008 and 2015, the decision points identify those times when a midwife ought to make a midwifery assessment, although it is recognised that assessments are based on individual need (NZCOM, 2015). Relevant beyond Aotearoa New Zealand the decision points outline the information that needs to be shared between each woman and midwife at each assessment point, as well as the health information and midwifery care that should be provided. These decision points continue to be an important tool in supporting midwifery practice in any context.

THE CONTINUUM OF LABOUR AND BIRTH

Labour has traditionally been compartmentalised into arbitrary stages, unimaginatively labelled first, second, third and, more recently, fourth stages. For midwives and women, the reality is that labour and birth are a continuous process (Downe, 2000). Even so, as a woman

Box 25.1 Benefits of continuity of midwifery care for women in labour

- More women feeling in control during labour and childbirth
- More likely to have a spontaneous vaginal birth
- Reduced use of regional anaesthesia/analgesia
- Less episiotomy
- Less instrumental birth
- More likely to initiate breastfeeding

(Sources: Bradfield et al., 2019; Hildingsson et al., 2021; Sandall et al., 2016)

CLINICAL POINT

Common signs of labour

- Increasingly intense contractions, focused in the pelvis, that become painful
- Increasingly regular, longer and more-frequent contractions
- Vaginal discharge of blood-stained mucus (called a 'show'); may occur before contractions commence
- Vaginal discharge of clear fluid if membranes rupture spontaneously; can occur before contractions and is considered a sign of labour if accompanied by contractions and cervical dilation.
- Nausea and frequent bowel motions

moves into and through her labour process there are recognisable emotional and physical changes. It is important that midwives understand and recognise these changes, to support and identify normal progress. Reorienting thinking about labour to acknowledge the physiological process as experienced by women has led some researchers to define labour as consisting of:

- latent phase to the onset of active phase
- active phase to onset of transition
- transition to birth
- birth to skin to skin (Downe, 2000).

This chapter reflects this understanding of labour and birth as a *continuum,* and discusses midwifery care from the perspective of a midwife providing continuity of care (Box 25.1).

RECOGNISING LABOUR

Normal labour occurs between 37 and 42 weeks gestation. As a woman approaches the end of the pregnancy she will often experience an increase in the intensity of toning contractions (Braxton Hicks contractions) and commonly an increase in vaginal leucorrhoea/mucous. Other signals indicating that labour may be imminent include further descent of the baby into the pelvis and bouts of strengthening uterine activity. The advent of approaching labour can elicit intense emotional responses in some women, ranging from excited anticipation to acute apprehension. Midwives need to be sensitive to these feelings and changes, and be able to reassure women of the normality of these responses.

During the antenatal period, a midwife will have discussed with the woman the signs and symptoms to aid recognition of the beginnings of labour (see the following Clinical point). She will identify with the woman when to make contact and what information will be sought at this initial contact. It is helpful to summarise this discussion in the woman's notes so that she can remind herself of these points later as reassurance for her and her family.

Labour: latent phase to onset of active phase

The **latent phase** is recognised as a valid phase of labour, but is difficult to define and poorly understood (Hundley et al., 2017). It has been described as the start of uterine contractions until progressive dilation of the cervix commences. Confusing the latent phase with a poorly progressing active phase can lead to inappropriate and unnecessary interventions that may affect the outcomes for mother and baby (Kobayashi et al., 2017; Miller et al., 2020). This can occur because duration of the latent phase varies from woman to woman. There is no consensus in the literature on what constitutes the length of a normal latent phase. Definitions vary from 6–8 hours up to 24–36 hours (Hundley et al., 2017; NICE, 2014). Some women may not experience the latent phase of labour, but for those who do it can be a confusing and sometimes distressing time. It is common for women to need time, support and reassurance for labour to establish and become progressive (Beake et al., 2018; Rota et al., 2018). During the antenatal period, explanations of what women often experience in the latent phase may help prepare women and their families to understand what is happening. Being able to view labour and birth as a normal process enables a woman to find her way through her own unique experience. A woman may lose confidence, which may then slow the progress of her labour (Kobayashi et al., 2017). Encouraging her to listen to and trust her body, as well as being able to rest and fuel her body, enables the process of birth to happen at its own pace. Rest, food and fluids, supportive, professional midwifery care and the avoidance of unnecessary interventions will assist most women through this time (Beake et al., 2018). It is important to remember that slow progress in the first stage of labour does not necessarily mean the presence of a problem or abnormality (Simkin et al., 2017).

CRITICAL THINKING EXERCISE

Brigid is pregnant with her second baby. Three years ago Brigid gave birth to a daughter, Evie. The labour was unexpectedly fast and Brigid birthed Evie within 10 minutes of arriving at the hospital. Brigid has had many discussions during the pregnancy with her midwife Ruth about the trauma she felt after her last birth. The car ride was stressful and she felt overwhelmed in the hospital setting. As part of her current birth plan, Brigid and her partner Jonny are planning to birth at home and Brigid has been having regular mild–moderate contractions for the last 24 hours. The baby is deeply engaged in the pelvis and directly occipitoanterior, and Brigid's cervix is 2 cm dilated and softening. The fetal heart rate is normal and baby is moving well. Brigid feels that she is in early labour but not moving on to the active phase. Evie is awake and wanting attention from her Mum. Brigid is worried, tired and frustrated and wants to know what to do next as this experience feels so different to her labour with Evie.

- As Brigid's midwife what would be your advice having made your midwifery assessment?
- How would you address Brigid's physical and emotional needs at this time?
- How would you involve her support team in helping Brigid to cope with her latent labour?

FIRST DECISION POINT IN LABOUR

When the woman or her support person first informs the midwife that she is in labour

At this stage a woman begins to notice signs that she may be in labour, and makes contact with her midwife. The midwife will need to ask questions in order to assess whether the woman is in labour and whether she needs a physical assessment and attendance by the midwife. The midwife will gather information about the woman's wellbeing and how she is coping, and review the woman's history to this stage (Table 25.1). The following questions should be asked of the woman:

- Is she having discomfort / pain? When did this start? The midwife needs to ascertain whether the pain is caused by uterine activity / contractions.
- What are her contractions like? Where does she feel them? How often do they come? How long do they last?
- Can she talk through them? Does resting or being active change their pattern?
- How is she feeling? Who is there to support her?
- Has she had any vaginal discharge? If so, what does it look like (e.g. blood-stained, mucus or watery discharge)?
- Does she think her membranes have ruptured? If so, what colour is the liquor (e.g. clear, pink, green or brown / black)?
- Has her baby been moving in the last few hours?
- Does she want the midwife to attend?

On the basis of this assessment, the midwife will decide whether to visit the woman at home. Sometimes a woman can be reassured by phone that she is in the latent phase of labour and be asked to contact the midwife again when the contractions become more regular, frequent and painful, or if there are any other signs that labour is progressing. If the midwife is not certain of the progress of labour, then a home visit is advisable. Several studies have identified that women in the latent phase of labour who are planning to birth in a hospital or birthing unit should be encouraged to stay at home until labour establishes (Kobayashi et al., 2017; Miller et al., 2018; Rota et al., 2018). These studies show that women who are reviewed at home in early labour have shorter labours, fewer epidurals, less synthetic oxytocin augmentation and more positive birthing experiences. The key assessment is whether the woman is in latent or active labour.

Table 25.1 Factors that can affect the progress of labour

Supportive influences	Unsupportive influences
• Trust in the woman's body and the birthing process • Sensitive, nurturing, appropriate supporters • Comfortable environment—a feeling of safety, privacy, familiarity • Knowing that other children are well cared for • A known, trusted midwife who supports the birth plan • Opportunities for rest periods, able to eat and drink as she desires	• Unexplored fears and distrust of labour and birth • Inappropriate, insensitive supporters • Environment uncomfortable, noisy, distracting, lack of space and privacy • Woman's concern about her children or other family members • A midwife who is unfamiliar with and / or unsupportive of the birth plan • Tiredness and hunger

CLINICAL POINT

Characteristics of the latent phase

- The contractions are short, irregularly spaced and easily interrupted by inactivity and distractions (e.g. the woman's other children, unexpected visitors, loud noises, taking a bath).
- The woman may be able to sleep for short periods.
- The woman will often still feel hungry.
- The woman will still be connected to what is going on around her (e.g. she will join in on conversations and may be able to talk during a contraction).

If a visit is made, the midwife needs to carry out a full assessment of the woman and her baby and document this (see details of assessment later in the chapter). An abdominal examination to define the position and presentation of the baby and listen to the baby's heart rate gives the midwife and the woman information to reassure and guide further advice. If the baby isn't in an optimal position, recommendations can be made regarding strategies the woman can try to encourage optimal positioning (Simkin et al., 2017). Suggestions may include adopting forward-leaning positions, being on hands and knees, pelvic rocking and the avoidance of supine positions except when sleeping. Studies have indicated that these positions may encourage the baby into a more favourable occipitoanterior position and reduce back pain in labour (Guittier et al., 2016; Mylod, 2020). Vaginal examinations, while not generally warranted at this stage, may assist in the diagnosis of the latent phase, as minimal dilation will have occurred (Nash, 2020). This finding may provide some reassurance for the woman; however, observing her behaviour will also help the midwife differentiate between latent and active labour.

If the woman is in latent labour, understands what is happening in her body and is well supported at home by friends and family, it may then be appropriate to leave her. Her midwife may then return when she requires additional midwifery support and/or labour becomes active. The woman needs to know that the latent phase is normal and can be lengthy, and that it is not the time for clockwatching (Beake et al., 2018; Rota et al., 2018). The woman may be encouraged to continue with her usual activities, but to ensure that she continues to eat, rest and sleep so that she can find the focus and energy required when labour does establish.

At home, women can work with the latent phase by being able to rest in their own bed, walk in their garden, lean against their kitchen bench, kneel into a beanbag or take a warm bath. Women planning to birth in hospital should try to use all the resources available to them at home before going into the hospital environment, which does not favour the latent phase (Kobayashi et al., 2017; Rota et al., 2018). Being confined to one room and exposed to the sounds of other women in active labour does nothing to support the woman or give her confidence when she may have many hours of labour ahead of her.

Before leaving, the midwife needs to ensure that the woman knows how and when to make contact with her.

SECOND DECISION POINT IN LABOUR

When the woman wants intermittent support from the midwife

At this stage a woman contacts her midwife because she feels labour is progressing or changing and she wants more support. The midwife may have contacted the woman to ask about how she is feeling and how labour is progressing. As with the first decision point, a key assessment is to ascertain whether the woman is still in latent labour or if she is in established labour and, if the latter, how she is feeling in response to her labour. The woman should be visited at home and the assessments and discussions listed in Box 25.2 need to be considered.

If the woman is still in the latent phase, then midwifery care and advice will continue as before. If the woman has progressed into early labour, she may feel the need for intermittent support from the midwife. If the woman is well supported at home by friends and family, then the midwife may be able to leave for periods of time, always ensuring that she can be contacted if required and clearly stating when she will return for a further assessment (Carlsson, 2016). The woman is advised to eat and drink and move about as she wishes. Once labour establishes, the woman is likely to want continuous support from her midwife.

Box 25.2 What to consider for an early labour assessment

- Assess the woman's wellbeing, including her emotional and behavioural responses.
- Assess the adequacy of her food and fluid intake, and her ability to rest.
- Consider physical assessments including abdominal palpation, strength, length and frequency of contractions, blood pressure, maternal pulse and the baby's wellbeing including heart rate.
- If her membranes have ruptured, assess the colour of the liquor.
- Discuss the relevance of a vaginal examination at this point.
- Document findings, advice given and plan for ongoing care.

Labour: active phase to onset of transition

Active labour is characterised by contractions that increase in intensity, length and frequency. The pattern of contractions tends to be more regular and is less affected by external influences than contractions that characterise the latent phase. The active pattern of contractions causes effacement and dilation of the cervix and promotes the descent and rotation of the baby through the pelvis. The individuality of each woman's experience means that the frequency of contractions in active labour may vary, for example, from every 3 minutes for some women to every 10 minutes for others.

Traditionally, normal progress has been identified by a cervical dilation rate of 1 cm / hour in active labour. This definition was based on the work of Friedman in the 1950s and has been universally adopted to assess the parameters of 'normal' progress (Friedman, 1954). (For more detailed information on this aspect of labour progress, see Ch. 38.) However, in reality, many midwives and women know that what is slow progress for one woman may be acceptable for another. There is continuing debate about what actually constitutes a normal cervical dilation rate. Much of the research undertaken to identify 'normal' progress in labour has been undertaken in medicalised settings and has focused mainly on the rate of cervical dilation while ignoring other physiological changes and influences (Philpott & Castle, 1972; Seitchik, 1987; Studd, 1973). Later studies challenge the findings of this earlier research and instead use an holistic approach to labour assessment that centres on the woman and baby's wellbeing rather than on the length of labour alone (Abalos et al., 2020; Inde et al., 2018; Lundborg et al., 2020). One systematic review investigating the duration of labour in low-risk women found that normal labour for these women lasted longer than many clinicians expected (Oladapo et al., 2018). The authors found that an expectation of a minimum cervical dilation of 1 cm / hour was unrealistic for most healthy women (Ibid, 2017). Once again this challenges the traditional parameters identified by Friedman. These findings reiterate that the commonly used time frames associated with active labour criteria are overly stringent and warrant revision.

CLINICAL POINT

Characteristics of the active phase

- Contractions are of increasing regularity, strength, length and frequency.
- The woman needs to move about and cannot rest in one position for long.
- The woman will be less connected to what is going on around her and increasingly will not be able to talk through contractions: she will often go 'into herself' as the labour 'takes her over'.
- The woman may not feel like eating.
- On abdominal palpation, the presenting part is felt to have moved down further into the pelvis.
- On vaginal assessment of the cervix, increasing effacement, softening and dilation are felt, and the baby's head descends lower into the pelvis.

RESEARCH ACTIVITY

Familiarise yourself with the research on the duration of normal labour, for example Oladapo et al. (2018) and Abalos et al. (2020). What midwifery assessment skills will you use with women experiencing a labour that does not conform to the '1 cm cervical dilation per hour' paradigm?

CLINICAL POINT

When doing home visits to women in labour, bring a full birth kit in case of unexpected or unplanned home birth—see Table 25.2.

Note that it is advisable to keep a birth kit in your car when visiting women at home at any time, so that you are prepared for unexpected situations.

THIRD DECISION POINT IN LABOUR

When the woman wants continuous support from a midwife

As a woman becomes established in labour, she will usually want continuous support from her midwife. The active phase of labour requires complex midwifery care, as the midwife works in **partnership** with the woman. The midwife's role is to help the woman and her family and supporters to follow their birth plan, while at the same time making regular assessments of progress and determinations as to whether the progress is 'normal' for this woman and her baby. As labour advances, the woman will often require more support and encouragement to help her work through the challenges ahead.

Staying with the woman is an essential midwifery role. Continuous midwifery care during labour is recognised as benefiting both mother and baby (Bradfield et al., 2019; Olza et al., 2018; Perriman et al., 2018). Being 'with the woman' requires not only the physical presence of the midwife but also her focus and attention. Women identify that the quality of the 'presence' of the midwife is directly related to the midwife's energy and commitment to her (Hildingsson et al., 2021; Sandall et al., 2016). The midwife can also encourage the woman's support people to be as involved as the woman needs. It is not uncommon

Table 25.2 What to bring to a home birth

Preparation for home birth	Equipment for assessment and care of the woman and her baby	
	Woman	Baby
• A strong and well-founded belief in birth as a normal physiological process • An in-depth understanding of the physiology of normal birth • A continuous and unobtrusive presence that is eternally vigilant • A means of monitoring the wellbeing of the woman and her baby during labour, birth and the postbirth period • A copy of the woman's birth plan • A set of well-developed midwifery skills, including emergency skills • A list of telephone numbers for emergency assistance • A second midwife (present during late second stage and birth) • A set of clearly identified notes in which to record the details of events as they unfold • Birth notification documents • Prescription pad, referral pad	• Watch with a second hand • Stethoscope and sphygmomanometer • Thermometer, bath thermometer • Vaginal assessment swabs and solution (used if membranes have ruptured) • Sterile gloves for vaginal assessment/s and conduct of birth • Amnihook • Birth pack, large plastic sheet/incontinence sheets • Woman's own container for placenta or plastic bag • Container bags for soiled equipment/swabs • Torch with adequate light for suturing (a headlamp works well) • Suturing material: 20 mL syringe, 22-gauge needle, 1% plain lignocaine (20 mL ampoule) • Sterile vaginal swabs • Drugs: synthetic oxytocin (Syntocinon) 5- and 10-unit ampoules (keep refrigerated and use a cold storage container for transport) and synthetic oxytocin/ergometrine (Syntometrine) 1 mL syringes and needles • Oxygen available with Hudson mask • Cannulation equipment (16- and 14-gauge cannulae) and tourniquet • Normal saline and/or Ringer's lactate/Hartmann's and IV-giving set • Sharps disposal unit	• Pinard stethoscope and/or Doppler Sonicaid (one that is safe to use in water) • Suction equipment for the baby • Cord clamp (or traditional cord ties according to cultural practice) • Infant Laerdal bag and mask, and infant airways • Oxygen cylinder and gauge, tubing • Baby scales (weight conversion chart) • Tape measure • Vitamin K

For further information contact:
- Homebirth Aotearoa (New Zealand); New Zealand College of Midwives (http://www.midwife.org.nz)
- Australian College of Midwives (http://www.midwifes.org.au) for a copy of the application for accreditation as an independently practising midwife. This contains prompts for the midwife to consider skills in perineal repair, neonatal resuscitation and maternal resuscitation. In addition this asks the midwife to determine what she or he has available in terms of equipment for fetal monitoring and resuscitation, maternal assessment and care including resuscitation, drugs and communication equipment.

(Source: Table prepared by Maralyn Foureur, 2008)

for support people to have their own anxieties during the labour, which may impinge on their ability to support the woman. The midwife can guide support people to participate in nurturing the woman to maintain a positive environment.

If the woman is planning to have her baby in a maternity facility, she will need to transfer to the facility once she is in the active phase of labour and no longer wants to be at home. The midwife needs to be alert to the possible impact of this new environment on the woman and her support people. Some of these impacts have been identified in studies which found that even minimal physical and environmental interruptions to the birthing woman may interfere with her labour progress (Dahan, 2021; Olza et al., 2018;Wrønding et al., 2019). It is therefore important for women to encounter a welcoming birthing environment which enables her to be able to adjust to the change and develop a sense of being in a safe place to birth her baby.

CLINICAL POINT

What to consider when moving from home to hospital

- Visit at home to assess progress and discuss transfer to hospital with woman.
- Check the birth plan. Did the woman think she would feel more comfortable transferring in early or more established labour? How does she feel now?
- If unable to assess progress from observations and discussions with the woman, consider vaginal examination.
- Distance from the woman's home to the hospital—i.e. consider transfer time.
- Mode and availability of transport, comfort during transfer.
- Collect 'tools' to take into hospital—e.g. supporters, own pillow, wheat bag, food, drink, music, massage oils, car seat and clothes for baby, fresh clothes for the woman.
- Ensure equipment is available in case of unexpected, unplanned home birth.

Facilitating a supportive labour environment

Wherever a woman chooses to birth, it is important to assess the labour and birthing environment to take into account the wishes of the woman and the factors that will enhance and support her normal physiological labour (Dahan, 2021; Olza et al., 2018; Wrønding et al., 2019). These include, for example, ensuring adequate open spaces to move around, a nearby toilet, variety of comfortable furniture, low or adjustable lighting, support people and, for many women, privacy and quiet. Assisting the woman to make use of these 'tools' will help her to use her intuition and instinct to find the right place and positions for effective, active labour (Olza et al., 2018).

The birth space needs to feel safe for that woman. The concept of a 'safe place' incorporates both physical and psychosocial / spiritual safety that cannot be imposed on the woman (Carlsson, 2016; Dixon et al., 2013). Most women appear to labour most effectively when there is an atmosphere of calm and the focus is on her and her experience. Some women, however, feel self-conscious and prefer to be left alone or to have the distraction of their supporters' conversations, the television, their favourite music or even their children being busy around them. It is therefore important to talk to the woman to find out what she needs to feel safe. Being aware of the woman's cultural preferences is imperative for midwives when facilitating an appropriate environment for effective labour. For example, it may be inappropriate for there to be men (including the father of the baby) present, or it may be that the woman's entire family, including aunts, uncles and grandparents, are actively involved. There may be the need for prayers or incantations at specific times in labour and at the birth. Special foods and / or ceremonies may be important for some women and their families. The midwife's knowledge of these needs and preferences will help her to provide the woman with a safe space in which to labour and birth.

Most women who begin their labour spontaneously will do so at home (Table 25.3). It is well documented that women should be encouraged to stay at home when in early labour, and that women are more relaxed and have more options in their own environments (Kobayashi et al., 2017; Rota et al., 2018). For those women who choose not to birth at home, the timing for transfer to hospital is crucial. If too soon, it may disrupt the flow of labour and slow progress, thus risking unnecessary intervention. If too late, there is the risk of birthing somewhere unplanned, such as at home or—worse—in a car, where the environment may carry risks for the mother or baby.

A MIDWIFE'S STORY

Violet is a 30-year-old woman having her first baby. She has been well throughout the pregnancy and is now in active labour at 40 weeks. She went to the primary birthing unit 6 hours ago. She has her partner Chris and her good friend Helen with her for support. Her midwife Julie has just performed a vaginal examination and Violet's cervix is 6 cm dilated, the head is at the ischial spines and her membranes are intact. The fetal heart rate is within normal range and she has just passed some blood-stained mucus. Violet is having strong contractions every 2 minutes and has not wanted to move from lying on her side on the bed. She is saying that she wants an epidural and she can't do it any longer. She is pleading with Julie to 'do something'. Chris and Helen are also worried about Violet. The obstetric facility is a 45-minute car ride away.

- What midwifery assessments could assist Julie and Violet in developing a plan for this stage of the labour?
- What information could she be communicating to Violet and her family?
- What midwifery support would be helpful for Julie at this stage in Violet's labour?

Once the woman is admitted to hospital, creating a calm, positive, welcoming atmosphere will assist in reducing tension and anxiety and therefore be less likely to negatively affect the progress of labour (Dahan, 2021; Dixon et al., 2013; Olza et al., 2018). This can be a challenge when a woman is confined to one room. If the midwife arrives at the hospital before the woman, she can ensure that there is something available for the woman to drink, the lighting is dimmed and the room is warm. To make adequate space for the woman to be active in labour, consider placing the bed against the wall (or removing it from the room) and using beanbags, pillows and soft mats if available. This will signal to the woman

Table 25.3 Women's recognition of the spontaneous onset of labour

Reported signs and symptoms	Number (%)	
	Nulliparae	Multiparae
Recurrent pain	62 (32.8)	80 (44.4)
Non-recurrent pain	51 (27.0)	41 (22.8)
Watery loss	30 (15.9)	17 (9.4)
Blood-stained loss	17 (9.0)	16 (8.9)
Gastrointestinal symptoms	8 (4.2)	2 (1.1)
Emotional upheaval	8 (4.2)	14 (7.8)
Sleep disturbance	6 (3.2)	5 (2.8)
Other	7 (3.7)	5 (2.8)
Total	**189 (100)**	**180 (100)**

(Source: Adapted from Gross et al., 2003)

when she arrives that there is not an expectation that she lie on the bed.

A number of studies have shown that lying supine is not only uncomfortable for women but also does not aid the descent and rotation of the baby through the pelvis, and can contribute to fetal distress. Supine positions can compromise the uterine blood flow during labour and have been shown to decrease the intensity and frequency of contractions. The physical layout of the labour environment will have a significant influence on what positions a labouring woman adopts, and if a woman is given many options this will have a positive impact on the birth outcome (Dahan, 2021; Lawrence et al., 2013; Olza et al., 2018). There is clear evidence that when women are encouraged to take up whatever position they find most comfortable their labours progress effectively and, in some cases, may be slightly shorter (Ibrahim et al., 2020; Lawrence et al., 2013; NICE, 2014). The culture of the birthing facility will influence a woman's behaviour in labour, and if there is an expectation that the bed is to be used then she may feel pressured to do so.

Women who labour at home are rarely at a loss as to where to go or what to do next. Given the freedom of their own space, most women will adopt a variety of positions and use a number of rooms throughout their labour. If a woman is able to move freely at will and rest when her body tires, she will find the right places to labour in. The midwifery role is to be willing to support her wherever it is that she chooses to be, and to offer advice and suggestions when required.

Very few women at home will lie on their bed except when trying to rest or sleep, so when women move to the hospital environment from home the midwife needs to positively encourage and support women to continue moving freely and adopting different positions. By trying to make the labour room more home-like, midwives will assist in minimising disturbance to the flow of a woman's labour and this will be of significant benefit to a woman and her baby. This requires skill, effort and thought. As a woman's contractions increase in strength and intensity, the midwife needs to be constantly thinking ahead about what position changes, ideas and strategies she may need to suggest to support and encourage the woman through the challenges ahead.

CLINICAL POINT

Advantages of being upright in labour

- Increases uterine blood flow, which increases efficiency of uterine contractions and improves oxygen availability to the baby
- Assists rotation and descent of the baby through the pelvis
- Reduces the need for pharmacological analgesia
- Enables the woman to find the positions most comfortable for her and to be able to respond to her body's needs
- Has the potential to shorten the first stage of labour

A MIDWIFE'S STORY

Aroha is a 24-year-old woman who is in labour with her first baby. She and her partner Tipene have arrived at the Birthing Suite and Aroha really wants to birth in water but the room with the pool is not yet available. Her midwife Rosa arrives and establishes that Aroha is having contractions every 2–3 minutes and she is groaning with them. The midwifery coordinator of the Birthing Suite tells Rosa that the pool should be free soon and that Rosa will need to do a vaginal examination prior to Aroha being able to use the pool. Aroha says she is not sure if she can last that long and does not want a vaginal examination. As the midwife

- what strategies, tools and physical props would you have available to assist Aroha during this stage in her labour?
- how would you make an assessment of Aroha and her baby's wellbeing and how would your findings influence the plan you will make with Aroha and Tipene?

Eating and drinking in labour

Women experiencing normal labour should be free to eat and drink as their body demands (Ciardulli et al., 2017; Singata et al., 2013). The Cochrane Systematic Review of eating and drinking in labour found that there is no evidence identifying harms or benefits of restricting food and fluids in labour for women at low risk of complications (Singata et al., 2013). The reviewers concluded that women should be free to eat and drink in labour, or not, as they wish. However, caution is advised with food intake when women have been administered opioids, as these increase the potential for nausea and vomiting and cause slowing of digestive action (NICE, 2014). Labour is a physically challenging process and requires as much fuel as any other strenuous activity. Most women will still feel able to snack on light foods in early labour, but as the contractions intensify they may feel less inclined to eat. It is useful to talk with the woman prior to labour about what she thinks she may like to eat, and ensure that those foods are available to her. Most hospitals do not provide a particularly wide range of foods, so if the woman is planning to birth in hospital she may need to bring her own food with her. Some institutions have protocols that require labouring women to fast despite a lack of evidence supporting this practice. For many women this may not present a problem, as they are already unwilling to eat when in active labour. But for others, enforced hunger becomes an extremely unpleasant experience. Enforced hunger may also lead to acidosis, which contributes to poor progress in labour. Most of the research into nourishment during labour does not consider women's views or experiences. However a qualitative study undertaken in Turkey using a phenomenological methodology found that the participants indicated feelings of hunger, thirst and fatigue due to oral fluid and food intake restriction during labour and that this affected the natural course of labour (Ozkan et al., 2017). It appears that having the freedom to eat whenever and whatever she chooses enables a woman to be in control, and reinforces the concept that labouring women know what their bodies need (Ciardulli et al., 2017; Singata et al., 2013).

Women should be encouraged to drink according to their thirst, but may sometimes need prompting to drink when the labour becomes all-consuming. If a woman's fluid intake is inadequate or she is experiencing episodes of vomiting, she may become dehydrated, especially if the physical demands of her labour cause her to sweat excessively. This is particularly the case if the woman is labouring in a bath or birthing pool. One of the first symptoms of dehydration is fatigue, and this can disrupt the progress of labour and make it difficult for the woman to feel motivated and active. Decreased urine output may also be an indication for the need to increase fluid intake. If women are enabled to follow their inclinations about drinking, they are unlikely to become dehydrated (Ciardulli et al., 2017; Singata et al., 2013).

Working with contractions

When each woman experiences contractions, a midwife needs to observe their length, strength and frequency, the body language of the woman and the impact on the contractions of the positions she adopts. Many women who experience lower back and sacral pain will adopt a leaning-forward position or be on their hands and knees. Squatting or soaking in a warm bath may help those with intense suprapubic pain. Sitting on the toilet is an ideal place to be when the contractions' intensity builds, and this position also assists in widening the pelvic outlet. A woman's instinct is to find a position that assists her in dealing with the contraction, and often this action also enables the baby to rotate into a more favourable position (Jowitt, 2020; Lawrence et al., 2013; Leap & Hunter, 2016; Simkin et al., 2017).

Much has been written about the 'labour dance' (Akin et al., 2020; Toberna et al., 2020). As a midwife it is a privilege to watch a woman unrestricted by technology, rules and expectations of others, listening and responding as her body tells her. The dance may be evident by rhythmic rocking, hip circling and adjustments of position as the contractions exert their energy and power. As the labour moves forward, each woman's dance will adapt to the physiological changes that are occurring in her body. For example, a woman who has previously been pacing and swaying with contractions may suddenly need to be rocking backwards and forwards on her hands and knees. For others who have found the birthing pool or bath soothing, it may now be more comfortable to be leaning against a wall with pressure applied to the sacrum. The use of moist heat can be particularly effective. This can be provided by soaking hand towels in very hot water, then wringing them out and applying them at the start of a contraction. Where they are placed depends on where the woman is feeling her contractions most. An attentive support team will soon recognise the signs that a contraction may be beginning, and have the heat available before the contraction has reached its full intensity. The use of heat provides comfort and a positive sensation, which may assist a woman as she works with her contractions (Tarrats et al., 2019; Türkmen et al., 2020; Yazdkhasti et al., 2018).

Much of the midwifery support needed in labour is about reading the cues and suggesting positions and actions that will assist the constant shifts in each woman's experience. This may require the active involvement of supporters and the midwife by the provision of touch, massage, acupressure and physical support. It is also about trusting that the woman will find her own way and supporting, with patience, the time that the woman needs to do this.

REFLECTIVE THINKING EXERCISE

Think about the literature that identifies the 'presence' of the midwife during labour and birth.

- How are you 'present' for women in labour?
- How do you work with being 'present' and available to the woman but avoid being the watcher?
- What can you do to enhance your presence but not increase your activities?

Sustaining the midwife when providing support in labour

Providing continuity of care to a woman in labour can be an intensely satisfying experience for both the woman and her midwife and, as mentioned previously, research indicates that women prefer it to other models of care (Bradfield et al., 2019; Hildingsson et al., 2021; Olza et al., 2018; Perriman et al., 2018). For midwives, being with women in labour can be exhilarating and truly joyous but it is also challenging at times. Labour is a time when the midwife's energy and attention are focused and heightened for significant periods of time and, it cannot be emphasised enough, it is important to recognise one's own limitations when it comes to providing quality care for these extended periods of time. The issues around midwifery sustainability have been discussed at length in Chapter 16; however, some strategies that midwives use to ensure that they are able to effectively support women in labour include:

- involving the woman's support team in the physical as well as the emotional support
- taking the opportunity to rest too when there are lulls in the labour

- keeping hydrated and snacking regularly
- liaising with midwifery staff or practice colleagues for regular breaks—going to the toilet, going outside for some fresh air and a walk
- having a back-up midwife available to relieve for longer periods if required
- consulting regularly with midwifery colleagues for advice and debriefing
- being aware of reaching one's own limits and enabling a practice colleague with fresh energy to continue to provide care.

Physical assessment in active phase of labour

Throughout labour, midwifery assessment relies on integration of the following aspects:

- *observing the woman*—her demeanour, length and frequency of contractions, how she responds to them and the positions she adopts, interactions with support people
- *listening to the woman*—how she relates her labour story so far, fears or concerns, vocal / breathing responses during contractions
- *assessing the environment*—the effect of those present, lighting, temperature, general atmosphere
- *physical assessment*—baseline parameters of uterine activity (length, strength and frequency of contractions, abdominal palpation, cervical dilation and descent of the baby), the baby's reaction to labour (heart rate, reactivity, variability), vaginal loss, maternal responses to labour (pulse, temperature, blood pressure, level of hydration, level of pain, urinalysis).

In all labours, a midwife carries out continuous assessment of each woman with whom she works. Assessment and familiarity with the physiological signs that labour is progressing enable a midwife to determine that labour is progressing normally or to identify signs that complications may be developing and that other interventions are needed. There are several specific physical assessments that will be made by midwives with varying regularity throughout labour. These are measurement of contractions, assessment of vaginal loss, abdominal palpations, vaginal examinations, auscultation of baby's heart rate, and assessment of maternal urine, temperature, pulse, blood pressure and fluid balance. There is no evidence identifying how regularly many of these assessments should be carried out. Decisions regarding ongoing assessments should be made in response to the woman's own unique labour. From time to time midwives may use interventions such as artificial rupture of membranes but these should be considered with caution (Ndayisenga et al., 2021; Smyth et al., 2013; Watkins, 2021).

Contractions

Each woman will exhibit her individual pattern of contractions through her labour. However, in active labour which is progressing, contractions will increase in strength and intensity and in length and frequency. A midwife can assess tone, length and frequency of contractions by placing her hand on the woman's fundus and holding it there through several cycles of contraction and relaxation. The contraction can be timed from its beginning to end, and the length and frequency in each 10-minute period determined. It is useful for a student midwife to place her hand on a woman's fundus for 10-minute periods in order to become familiar with assessing contractions. The student will be able to feel the contraction beginning, often before the woman feels it as pain. In this way, student midwives will become familiar with the range of contractions felt and observed for different women.

If the pattern of contractions becomes irregular, this may be a sign that labour is slowing because of issues such as maternal exhaustion or poor positioning of the baby, or more commonly it may be that the woman has reached a plateau in labour that is normal for her and her labour will recommence in time (Davis, 2019). Where there is a change from an expected pattern, a midwife needs to make further assessments to determine the cause and possible midwifery actions. Usually such a diagnosis can be made only through the integration of several assessments of the wellbeing of mother and baby and the progress of labour. This may include assessing the birthing environment for disruptive influences, talking with the woman about any fears that she may have, as well as offering an abdominal palpation, a vaginal examination and auscultating the fetal heart rate. If the woman and her baby are well then often reassurance, offering a chance to change the environment (e.g. running a bath), encouraging food and / or fluids, offering the opportunity for rest and not focusing on time constraints will support the woman through this plateau until her contractions increase again.

Vaginal discharge

The development of or an increase in vaginal discharge can be a potential sign of labour progressing, although the amount and type of discharge will vary between women. A small amount of blood-stained mucus can indicate detachment of the membranes as the cervix dilates. Midwives will record when membranes rupture and assess the liquor for colour, amount and odour. Clear liquor is normal, whereas a green, brown or black discharge usually indicates meconium staining and may be associated with fetal distress. Often the membranes will rupture as the cervix nears full dilation, but this can occur earlier. A heavy, blood-stained mucus discharge may also indicate full dilation of the cervix. However, frank bleeding is always abnormal and needs to be further assessed and responded to appropriately.

Abdominal palpation

Alongside the assessment of uterine activity, an abdominal palpation can provide valuable information to assist the midwife to develop an understanding of how the labour is progressing. Palpation of the baby's position, presentation and descent into the pelvis early in the labour provides a baseline for ongoing assessment of the progress of the labour and auscultation of the baby's heart rate. Asking a woman about her impressions of her baby's position and movements during labour will assist the midwife in gaining valuable information prior to abdominal palpation. When undertaking an abdominal palpation, the midwife needs to consider and assess a number of factors (see following Clinical point). Abdominal palpation is a useful tool for assessing the progress of labour by defining descent and flexion of the presenting part and thereby avoiding unnecessary vaginal examinations.

CLINICAL POINT

Revision of palpation

Review Chapter 23, 'Working with women in pregnancy'.

- Consider:
  - consent from woman
  - maintaining privacy and dignity for the woman
  - religious and cultural considerations
  - hand washing
  - comfort measures:
    - encourage her to empty her bladder prior to examination
    - assist her to get into a comfortable position
    - wait for time between contractions to palpate
    - gentle touch.
- Abdominal palpation involves:
  - visual assessment
  - fundal assessment
  - lateral assessment
  - pelvic palpation
  - auscultation.
- Identify:
  - lie
  - presentation
  - position
  - engagement
  - descent
  - optimal position to hear and count baby's heart rate.
- Does the baby feel to be appropriate size for its gestation? Is the baby presenting head first? Is the head flexed? What position is the baby? Is descent appropriate for stage of labour and position of baby? Is the fetal heart rate within normal range?
- Compare descent of presenting part on abdominal palpation with descent of presenting part as assessed by vaginal examination.
- Assess tone, length and frequency of contractions.
- Share findings with the woman and document fully in notes.

CLINICAL POINT

Definitions

- *Effacement:* shortening and thinning of the cervical canal as the internal os dilates and forms part of the lower uterine segment (Fig. 25.1).
- *Dilation:* the external os (os uteri) increasingly dilates as a result of the contraction and retraction of the uterine muscles. In primigravidae, effacement of the cervix usually precedes dilation; in multigravidae, effacement and dilation normally occur simultaneously. Full dilation has been achieved when the os uteri has dilated sufficiently to allow the baby's head to pass through.
- *Position:* comparison of the position of the fontanelles and sutures of the baby's head in relation to the woman's pelvis. In occipitoanterior positions, the posterior fontanelle is felt towards the anterior part of the pelvis. In occipitoposterior positions, the anterior fontanelle will be felt anteriorly. The position of the sagittal suture in relation to the oblique diameters of the woman's pelvis further clarifies the position. For example, when the sagittal suture lies in the left oblique diameter of the pelvis (from the left posterior quadrant to the right anterior quadrant) and the posterior fontanelle lies anteriorly to the right, the position is the right occipitoanterior (Fig. 25.2).
- *Station:* relationship of the presenting part to the ischial spines of the maternal pelvis (Fig. 25.3).

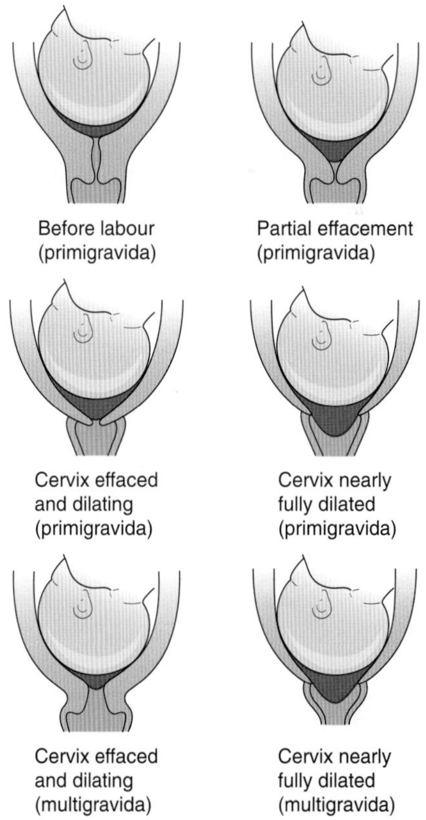

FIGURE 25.1 Effacement
(Based on Henderson & Macdonald, 2004)

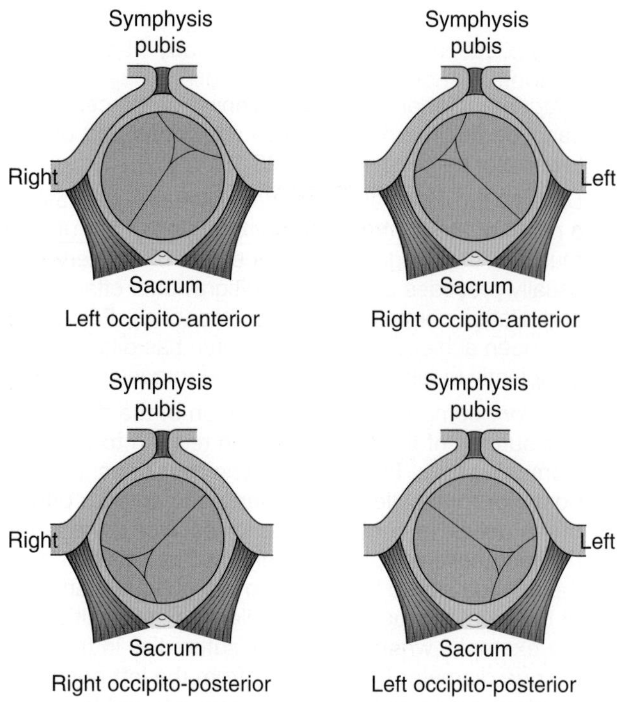

FIGURE 25.2 Position of the fontanelles and sutures of the baby's head in relation to the woman's pelvis
(Based on Henderson & Macdonald, 1988)

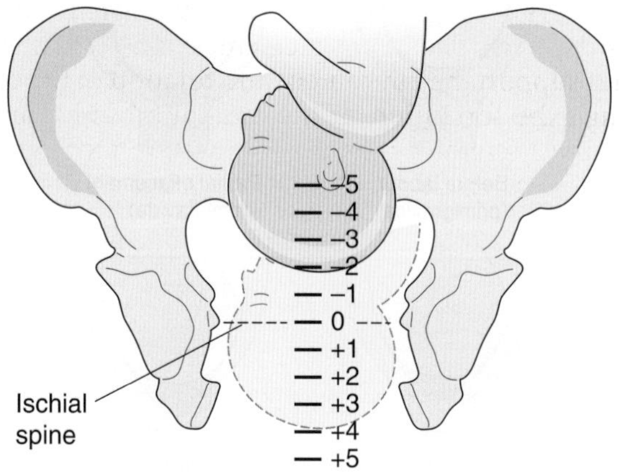

FIGURE 25.3 Relationship of the presenting part to the ischial spine of the maternal pelvis
(Based on Henderson & Macdonald, 2004)

Vaginal examinations

Routine vaginal examinations (VEs) are a common intervention in labour. They have become accepted as the definitive gauge of progress in labour, but the literature indicates that they are subjective and may be invasive, and that their benefit in normal labour is unproven and may cause harm. Recent studies have found a strong association between the number of vaginal examinations and neonatal sepsis (Christopher et al., 2019; Gluck et al., 2020; Nash, 2020). Even so, they are an important skill that midwives need to use judiciously. As part of a woman's individualised care, a VE may be appropriate. It is important for a midwife to have a sound rationale for why she would perform a VE and what information she hopes to obtain (Downe et al., 2013). When identifying the rationale for performing a VE during normal labour, it is helpful to consider whether there is any other way to identify the information. Will the information gained change the plan of care and do you need to know what is happening at this point? While some women find VEs unnecessarily intrusive, others may find the information gained valuable and be happy to have a VE performed if it is carried out sensitively (de Klerk et al., 2017). Developing the skills required for VE is an important part of being able to provide appropriate and effective midwifery care. The decision to perform a VE must be made in discussion with the woman and her consent documented along with the rationale for the examination.

CLINICAL POINT

Reasons to consider performing a vaginal examination in normal labour

- Woman's request
- Assessment of cervical effacement and dilation
- Confirmation of presentation, position and descent of the baby through the pelvis

Reasons to consider not doing a vaginal examination in normal labour

- Woman's consent declined
- History of sexual abuse
- Potential for introduction of infection for mother and baby
- Disruption to woman's focus and confidence
- Presence of other signs that labour is progressing

(Sources: Christopher et al., 2019; Downe et al., 2013; Gluck et al., 2020)

RESEARCH ACTIVITY

After familiarising yourself with the research relating to women's experiences of VEs identified earlier in this chapter, use the following questions to reflect on your own practice.

1. What do you take into consideration when offering VEs to a woman in labour?
2. What issues does this research raise for you in regard to your practice around VEs?

CLINICAL POINT

Performing a vaginal examination

- Preparation:
  - Explain to the woman the rationale for VE, what is involved, what she can expect to feel and how long it may take; gain consent.
  - Reassure the woman that the midwife will immediately discontinue the examination at the woman's request.
  - Maintain privacy and dignity for the woman.
  - Recognise and discuss religious and cultural considerations with the woman.
- Comfort measures:
  - encourage her to empty her bladder prior to examination
  - help her find a comfortable position
  - wait for time between contractions to examine
  - sensitive touch.
- Perform an abdominal palpation first to obtain comparative information, particularly in relation to descent and position of the baby.
- Position woman in semi-reclining position with knees raised and abducted (can also perform with woman lying on her side or on hands and knees, but students should gain experience with semi-recumbent position first).
- Explain all actions throughout the procedure.
- Wash hands and wear gloves; maintain sterile field and aseptic technique if the woman's membranes have ruptured.
- Observe vulva for any unusual features or any discharge, e.g. vulval varicosities, previous scarring, lesions (e.g. warts, herpes vesicles).
- Apply lubricant to forefinger and middle finger and gently insert into vagina.
- Note tone of vaginal muscles and pelvic floor, moisture (dryness may indicate pyrexia).
- Identify cervix and note consistency, effacement, position and dilation.
- Identify presenting part, feel for sutures and fontanelles to determine position of head in relation to pelvis, feel for moulding or caput succedaneum.
- Feel for spine and assess station of presenting part in relation to spine; feel for membranes—intact? Bulging forewaters or smooth? Note application of cervix to presenting part; note any unusual or abnormal features such as umbilical cord pulsation or vessels in the membranes.

After VE listen to the baby's heart and count the rate. Information gained:

- Assessment of vulva and vagina, identifying any abnormalities of tissues or discharge.
- Cervix—position (anterior, central, posterior, lateral):
  - consistency (soft, thick, firm, thin, stretchy)
  - effacement (non-effaced, partially or fully effaced)
  - dilation (os closed, 1–9 cm dilated, or fully dilated)
  - application of the cervix to the baby's head (loosely, moderately or well applied).
- Presenting part—cephalic:
  - position (anterior, lateral, posterior)
  - station in relation to ischial spine
  - presence/degree of caput/moulding.
- Membranes—intact or ruptured, bulging presence of liquor, colour, amount.

Findings from VE that, in conjunction with other midwifery assessments, indicate that labour is progressing normally:

- increasing descent, flexion and rotation anteriorly of baby's head in relation to the pelvis
- continued softening, effacement and dilation of the cervix
- increasing application of the cervix to the presenting part.

Following the examination, the findings should be discussed with the woman and the fetal heart rate assessed. Documentation would include all information gained from the procedure.

Artificial rupture of the membranes (amniotomy)

Intact membranes have an important physiological role during labour and birth. They protect the baby during labour from the potential for some infections and they play a role in relieving pressure on the baby during labour as well as during pregnancy. The intact membranes support the effacement and dilation of the cervix through the formation of the amniotic fluid filled sac sometimes referred to as the fore waters preceding the presenting part of the baby. The intact membranes have also been identified as having a role in the production and release of certain prostaglandins involved in the onset of labour (Smyth et al., 2013). Despite these benefits, artificial rupture of the membranes (ARM) is common and often performed without a clear clinical reason. Sometimes ARM is recommended in an attempt to accelerate labour. The supposition is that, with the membranes ruptured, the baby's head descends onto the cervix, causing more frequent and stronger contractions. ARM is also thought to release chemicals and hormones that stimulate contractions just as, conversely, the same is believed about intact membranes (Smyth et al., 2013). ARM also enables visualisation of the colour of the liquor. However, what commonly occurs following ARM is that the baby's head moves down and loses the manoeuvrability it once had with the support of the liquor-filled membranes. If the baby isn't in an optimal position, amniotomy may exacerbate this. It may also cause an increase in the intensity of the contractions, making them more difficult to cope with (Smyth et al., 2013). ARM is not a benign intervention and research shows that it can be harmful in a normal labour. Studies have identified that there is an increase in fetal distress and caesarean section following amniotomy in early labours, and these systematic reviews conclude that amniotomy should be reserved for labours that are not progressing normally (Ndayisenga et al., 2021; Watkins, 2020). These reviews demonstrate no evidence of shortening of the length of first stage of labour and a possible increase in caesarean section rates. Routine amniotomy is not recommended as part of standard labour management and care. A study by two midwife researchers in 2018 explored what shapes midwives' decision making around artificial rupture of membranes in low-risk labour (Mellor & Farry, 2018). From the results of this study the researchers created the HALO tool to encourage evidence-based practice around ARM. HALO provides midwives and allied professionals with evidence around the various forms of minimally invasive support measures that can help to avoid ARM in low risk labour. The authors of the tool have kindly agreed to some parts of the tool being reproduced here.

CLINICAL POINT

The HALO tool (Mellor & Farry, 2018)

Membranes matter—avoid ARM: This part of the tool provides midwives and others with the evidence to support avoidance of ARM in normal labours.

Before ARM think HALO: This part of the tool provides ideas for using minimally invasive measures to support normal labour and reduce the potential for unnecessary ARM.

H Hold off unless indicated
Hand over to a colleague and take a break

A Adjust maternal position regularly
Advocate for optimal environment

L Look after latent phase—warmth/TENS
Liquids—ensure good hydration

O Observe discretely—low lights, calm, quiet voice
Optimise oxytocin opportunities

(Source: Mellor & Farry, 2018. Text reproduced by kind permission of the authors.)

CRITICAL THINKING EXERCISE

Martha is in active labour with her fourth baby. She has been at the primary birthing unit for two hours and her contractions are slowly building in intensity. With her last three babies Martha has had her membranes artificially broken. She has a different midwife, Sue, this time and is asking that her membranes be broken because 'they don't break on their own' says Martha.

Read the Cochrane review by Smyth et al. (2013) with regard to amniotomy for shortening spontaneous labour.

- How would the findings of the review influence the decisions Sue will make with Martha?
- What information would Sue share with Martha with regard to her request to have her waters broken?

Listening to the baby's heart rate

The baby's heart rate is listened to during labour to confirm its presence, rate and how it responds to the labour process. It is important to identify any indicators of hypoxia in the baby. In normal labour, the appropriate method for listening to the baby's heart rate is intermittent auscultation (Alfirevic et al., 2017; NZCOM, 2020; RANZCOG, 2019). Intermittent auscultation is achieved by listening at intervals using a monaural stethoscope (Pinard) or a hand-held Doppler device (Sonicaid). This is most effective with the constant presence of an attentive midwife who is able to assimilate information regarding the woman and her baby's wellbeing through a combination of assessments (Martis et al., 2017; Maude et al., 2016). Using a Pinard stethoscope, the midwife can hear the heart rate as a contraction is finishing. This will confirm the rate and detect any slow recovery back to the baseline. For some women, using a Pinard to listen throughout a contraction may be uncomfortable, and the heart sounds may not be audible. A Doppler device can be used during a contraction and the heart rate can be heard without the woman needing to adjust her position. A Doppler device can also be used for women labouring in water (if the transducer is water resistant).

Intermittent auscultation enables regular, direct contact between the midwife and the woman. It provides an opportunity for the midwife to reassure the woman and her supporters, and provides encouragement (Maude et al., 2016).

The heart rate is determined by listening to and counting the beats for 60 seconds immediately after the end of a contraction. The rate is documented as a single number of beats per minute, not a range. The baseline heart rate refers to the heart rate present between periods of acceleration or deceleration, and is considered normal between 110 and 160 b.p.m. (NZCOM, 2020). The heart rate will usually remain steady or accelerate during contractions. Decelerations of the heart rate during contractions may be associated with umbilical cord compression or compression of the baby's head as it descends through the pelvis; this may be more likely when the membranes are not intact. Decelerations where the heart rate returns to the baseline immediately the contraction ceases are not generally associated with hypoxia (Alfirevic et al., 2017). Counting the heart rate during and immediately following a contraction provides the midwife with a clear indication of the baby's response to the labour (Martis et al., 2017; Maude et al., 2016).

CLINICAL POINT

Recommended monitoring in an uncomplicated pregnancy

For a woman who is healthy and has had an otherwise uncomplicated pregnancy, intermittent auscultation should be offered and recommended in labour to monitor fetal wellbeing (Alfirevic et al., 2017; Martis et al., 2017).

There are no studies that confirm the frequency of auscultation necessary to maintain safety. The New Zealand College of Midwives practice guide recommends 15–30 minute intervals during active labour (NZCOM, 2020). It also suggests listening after every contraction and pushing effort once the cervix is fully dilated. Increased monitoring is recognised as being appropriate from the transition phase until the birth of the baby. The midwife will document her assessment of the baby's wellbeing, including the heart rate, each time she listens. The frequency of monitoring the baby's heart rate throughout the labour in relation to outcome is not widely researched and there is a need for further studies in this area.

In the absence of clear evidence the NZCOM guidelines (2020) suggest the following for practitioners to consider but they also stress that consideration should be given to maternal preference and priorities.

In the active stages of labour, intermittent auscultation is undertaken (with the woman's permission) after a contraction, for a minimum of 60 seconds, and at least:

- every 15–30 minutes in the first stage
- every 5 minutes in the second stage or after every contraction.

Continuous electronic fetal monitoring (EFM) should be offered and recommended in pregnancies previously monitored with intermittent auscultation:

- if there is evidence on auscultation of a baseline less than 110 b.p.m. or greater than 160 b.p.m.
- if there is evidence on auscultation of abrupt or gradual decelerations
- if any intrapartum risk factors develop.

Current evidence does not support the use of admission cardiotocography (CTG) in low-risk pregnancy and it is therefore not recommended.

There are often variations in a **baby's heart rate** during the different phases of labour. These may be due to, for example, maternal position, dehydration, overheating and baby's head compression during transition and the pushing stage. The midwife needs to take these into consideration and, if possible, institute changes and recheck the heart rate response (Maude et al., 2016). Any persistent abnormal recordings are an indication for more-frequent observations, which may include continuous EFM and consultation with another midwife or an obstetric specialist. (For more detail about EFM see Ch. 39)

RESEARCH ACTIVITY

Read the NZCOM (2020) practice guidelines on Intermittent Auscultation for the Assessment of Intrapartum Fetal Wellbeing and consider the following questions.

1. What does the current research relating to intermittent fetal heart auscultation identify, and is this reflected in the NZCOM guidance for practice?
2. How do you currently monitor the fetal heart rate during a normal labour and birth?
3. Does the NZCOM practice guidance reflect your current practice or the protocol at the facility in which you work?

Maternal responses to physiological changes of labour

Assessment in active labour includes baseline urinalysis, blood pressure, temperature, pulse recordings and fluid balance. While there is little evidence available to indicate the value in routinely monitoring these recordings in a normal labour, having baseline information is useful for ongoing comparison, particularly if the labour develops complications. For example, ketones in urine and increasing pulse and temperature may indicate that the woman is becoming dehydrated; if not addressed, dehydration can lead to alterations in contractions and a slowing of labour. Fluid balance does not need to be formally recorded, but the midwife needs to be alert to keeping the woman hydrated through labour and preventing dehydration (Ciardulli et al., 2017). Where a woman is not passing urine frequently, the midwife needs to consider whether the woman has been drinking sufficiently.

Despite the lack of evidence about frequency of these assessments, most midwifery texts recommend regular observations at a variety of intervals and more frequently if problems present. This may be due to the fact that, in most countries, midwifery care is fragmented and the midwife and woman are unlikely to have already established a relationship in pregnancy. **Continuity of carer** allows a more individualised approach to physical assessment and recordings.

Nevertheless, there are some situations in normal labour that may warrant more frequent monitoring. These include:

- prelabour rupture of membranes
- recent history of vaginal infections
- invasive procedures, including VEs, bladder catheterisations
- irregularity of fetal heart rate (NZCOM, 2020).

REFLECTIVE THINKING EXERCISE

When thinking about your own practice and the interventions you might use:

- What do you know about what the evidence identifies about each intervention's effect on physiological birth?

- What information do you share with the woman before you proceed? Use your documentation at this time to inform your reflection.

ONGOING ASSESSMENT OF PROGRESS IN LABOUR

Having facilitated a supportive environment, taking into account the wishes of the labouring woman and the physical context of where she will birth, assessment of her progress in labour will require the midwife to be present and 'with' the woman. We have already discussed the importance of viewing each woman's labour as particular to her, rather than trying to 'fit' her labour into a standardised format. The holistic nature of midwifery care means being aware that 'the woman's emotional and physical reactions to labour may be the drivers and signs of progress and that interruption to or intervention of women's instinctual behaviours may delay or slow labour' (Dixon et al., 2013, p. 16).

As labour advances, her contractions will change. From being able to talk through some contractions and having a connection with what is going on around her, a woman in a progressing labour will begin to concentrate with each deeper sensation and may require support to work through each contraction. If her movements are unrestricted she can be encouraged to adopt positions in which she feels most comfortable. Encouraging her to empty her bladder regularly will aid her comfort, as well as providing an opportunity for finding alternative positions. Women who have the choice to be upright will have greater contraction intensity and efficiency and are less likely to require pharmacological pain relief (Gupta et al., 2017; Ibrahim et al., 2020). However, it is important to keep a balance between rest and activity. Some women will need periods of inactivity during the not-uncommon plateaus of labour to recharge and refocus their energy levels (Davis et al., 2019; Gaskin, 2003).

CLINICAL POINT

Facilitating a woman's ongoing labour

- Check how the woman is feeling about the labour and what form of support she wants from you.
- Avoid arbitrary time limits.
- Follow the birth plan in consultation with the woman as appropriate.
- Assess her wellbeing, including her emotional and behavioural responses.
- Consider assessing blood pressure, temperature, pulse and urinalysis—look for signs of dehydration and take appropriate action.
- Assess contractions, lie, presentation and descent of the baby—look for signs of continual progress and follow up any indication of delay such as lack of descent of the baby, and slowing of contractions.
- Discuss the need, or not, for a VE. If a VE is done, look for increasing dilation, anterior position of baby, continual descent and rotation through pelvis.
- Assess the baby's wellbeing, including heart rate—look for continual reassuring signs and follow up any non-reassuring patterns such as decelerations, tachycardia or bradycardia.
- If membranes have ruptured, check the colour of liquor—follow up any non-reassuring signs such as meconium.
- Facilitate the partner/supporter's involvement as per care plan.
- Encourage the woman to move into whatever positions she feels comfortable in.
- Encourage the woman to drink regularly and to eat if she wishes.

Documentation

It is important that the midwife collates and documents comprehensive assessments of the woman's and baby's health and wellbeing (NZCOM, 2021). This serves three main purposes:

- to be able to review and assess the progress of labour
- to provide an accurate diary of events for the woman to read, refer to and keep
- to provide a legal document that illustrates the information and rationale for the care given, and the subsequent events and outcomes.

For the midwifery notes to assist in assessment of progress, they should be a time-based diary of events permitting a detailed documentation of all assessments of the woman and her baby. Documentation provides evidence of midwifery decision making and, as such, the notes should contain as much information as possible. In contexts where partograms are used routinely, additional information must be recorded as the partogram does not provide enough on its own.

Partograms

Partograms have been shown to be an efficient means of exchanging information about labour progress between teams of caregivers. However, in a continuity-of-carer setting and where there is a spontaneous normal labour, the efficacy of the partogram has not been proven (Lavender et al., 2018). Partograms provide a visual display of only part of the woman's progress in labour and they assume that there will be VEs and charting of cervical dilation. They are a structured graphical representation (with alert and action lines) and may rely too much on a strict protocol of action. Partograms can be an agent for regimenting labour rather than supporting the woman's individual process. Observational studies have shown improved outcomes with the use of partograms when the labour is not progressing normally (Lavender et al., 2018). However, there is no evidence to suggest that there are any benefits to using partograms in physiologically normal labours. Research identifies that the parameters of normal labour need to be redefined to more accurately reflect women's actual experiences (Oladapo et al., 2018). Oladapo et al. concluded in their study that labour duration and cervical dilation rates were slower than the parameters traditionally used to define normal labour progress. The researchers challenge the overly stringent assessment of labour using the partogram based on Friedman's work. They recommend revision of existing active labour time frames to reflect more accurately the wide variety of women's labour experiences.

Woman-centred midwifery notes

The comprehensive nature of the labour notes means that they need to clearly document and describe midwifery care, advice and consultations. They should be written in a narrative style that is woman centred and provides the story of events as they unfold. The notes will outline information discussed with the woman and the rationale for the decisions made. The story of the labour and birth is an invaluable aid for later reflection on the birth with the woman. Professional midwifery care requires reflection on practice, and comprehensive notes support this process. Although some may view constant and concurrent documentation as time consuming and tedious, it need not be (NZCOM, 2021).

CLINICAL POINT

- Involve the supporters in the woman's care to free you for short periods to document events.
- Write something every 15–30 minutes—e.g. how the woman is feeling, the positions she is using, frequency/strength/length of contractions, vaginal discharge, input from supporters, baby's heart rate.
- If you use abbreviations, explain their meaning when first used and keep the notes in a form that can be understood by the woman and her family.
- If at times you are unable to write full notes, jot down brief reminders and times of significant events—e.g. rupture of membranes, vaginal examinations, fetal heart rate recordings—and update more comprehensively as soon as possible.
- Clearly note references to the woman's care plan and whether there are any changes to this plan. Document details of the discussion with the woman, and the rationale and consent for any decisions or birth plan changes.

LABOUR: TRANSITION PHASE TO BIRTH

Most labouring women and midwives are aware of a transitional period between the first stage of labour and the time when active maternal pushing efforts begin (Bjelke et al., 2019). Changes in the woman's behaviour, body language and vocal responses towards the end of the active phase of labour may indicate this transition stage. This often tumultuous period can challenge the woman and her supporters, and the midwife needs to guide and support them through the intensity of this time (Box 25.3).

Box 25.3 Supporting a woman through the challenges of transition

- Having confidence and belief in the woman's ability helps to strengthen the woman and her supporters.
- Recognise that this process is taking the woman to the edge of her ability to cope and she will need continuous, focused support.
- The constant presence and reassurance of the midwife will reduce the chance of resorting to the use of pharmacological interventions at a time when the woman is at her most vulnerable.

A woman's responses to this change in her labour may include increasing restlessness, breathing rhythm changes, shaking, vomiting, and a feeling of panic and of being engulfed by the process. The contractions relentlessly roll from one into the next, giving the woman no time to focus as she had earlier. Often at this time, women will vocalise that they 'can't do this anymore' and plead to the midwife and supporters to 'help me'.

CLINICAL POINT

Characteristics of transition to full dilation of the cervix

- The woman may feel she has lost control and have feelings of panic.
- She may say she cannot carry on, and ask for help.
- She may ask for pain relief.
- She may vomit or feel nauseous and be shaking.
- There may be a heavy 'show' of blood-stained mucus.
- She may have beginning sensations of pressure in her bowel or the urge to push—can be variable.
- For some women, labour slows down and she can rest or may even sleep.

There is no clear time frame for the transition period. For some women it can be a few hours and for others a matter of just a few contractions. Occasionally, women find that the contractions begin to ease off, and will benefit from this sudden calm in their labour and may even sleep. It is once again important to reassure the woman that this lull in her labour is very normal and that it is her mind and body preparing her for the next stage and the birth of her baby. If this happens, it is often a good time for the supporters to get a break, get some fresh air, go to the toilet, eat and drink before they are needed again. Midwives may often feel a need to 'do something' when the labour slows after a torrent of strong contractions and, as is also the case in misunderstood latent phase, it can be a time when unwarranted interventions are introduced, such as ARM and VE. Patience and trust are the hallmarks of an effective midwife and as long as mother and baby are both well they should not be interfered with. As the woman's cervix becomes fully dilated and the baby descends further, the woman's contractions and her responses give cues to the midwife that the woman is moving closer to the birth of her baby (Bjelke et al., 2019).

FOURTH DECISION POINT IN LABOUR

Second stage or birth to skin-to-skin

At this stage there will be a number of signs that the woman is ready to birth her baby. These cues may include the following:

- a pushing urge at the peak of a contraction
- the urge to push accompanied by deep, throaty sounds
- the woman tells you that she is feeling pressure or wants 'to push'
- blood-stained vaginal mucous discharge
- anal dilation
- possible spontaneous rupture of membranes
- perineal distension caused by pressure from the presenting part and/or intact membranes.

If a woman is experiencing urges to push but the other cues do not become apparent, it would be appropriate to consider a VE to confirm descent and position of the presenting part and dilation of the cervix.

These sensations are often very intense and can be challenging for the woman. This is a time for the midwife to reassure the woman and explain what is happening for her and her baby. It is important for the midwife to communicate calmly and clearly with the woman. Helping the woman to focus on and trust what her body is telling her enables her to work with these powerful sensations and find the positions that help her most effectively.

As the contractions become increasingly expulsive, most women will experience stronger urges to push. Urges to push may vary in frequency and intensity. Supporting spontaneous, involuntary pushing means that the woman pushes only when the contraction has built up and she is unable to resist the pushing urge. Spontaneous pushing is characterised by short periods of breath holding followed by expiratory grunts. This is often referred to as **non-directed pushing**, and has been found to result in shorter second stages, a reduction in maternal fatigue and fetal distress, and less intervention (Bjelke et al., 2019; Lemos, 2017).

Upright positions for pushing are most effective in assisting women to birth their babies. Using upright positions enables women to remain mobile, and they often prefer them (Gupta et al., 2017). There are a number of physiological advantages in being upright (Gupta et al., 2017; Healey et al., 2020; Zang et al., 2021) (see following Clinical point). Upright birth positioning appears to occur more often within certain models of care, and certain birth settings, compared with others. The preferences for positions, and the philosophies of health professionals, are also reported to impact upon the position that women adopt during birth. The facilitators and inhibitors of physiological birth position, impact of birth settings, how midwives and women perceive physiological birth positions, and how beliefs are translated into practice all need to be researched (Badi, 2019; Healy et al., 2020).

CLINICAL POINT

Advantages of being upright for birth

- Reduces risk of aortocaval compression, which means maximising oxygen availability for the woman and baby
- Gravity assists the baby into the optimal position and aids descent through the pelvis
- Stimulates stronger and more efficient uterine contractions
- Increases the diameter of the pelvic outlet
- Shorter second stage
- Fewer episiotomies
- Woman able to tolerate pain more easily
- Supports women's sense of control

(Sources: Gupta et al., 2017; Healy et al., 2020; Lemos, 2017; Zang et al., 2021)

CLINICAL POINT

Effective positions/places for pushing

- Squatting—using support people and/or furniture
- Kneeling—using cushions, mats, beanbags
- Sitting—on the toilet or birthing stool
- Standing—leaning against furniture, wall, people, tree
- Use of pool or bath—buoyancy of water supports upright positions

CRITICAL THINKING EXERCISE

Consider the labour environments in which you are with women.

1. What can you do to facilitate upright positions for women in labour?
2. What equipment is available to you and how could you adapt it to support the woman to be upright?

The second stage of labour has traditionally been subjected to strict time frames in the mistaken belief that this will benefit the mother and baby. Focusing on the purely physical aspects of birthing denies recognition of the complexities involved. This has led to a variety of interventions in response to the urgency that has developed around the birthing process. These interventions include directed or coached pushing, VEs, ARM, episiotomy and assisted or operative delivery. Arbitrary time frames have not been found to improve outcomes, and have subjected women and their babies to procedures that may have been unnecessary and at times caused harm (Bjelke et al., 2019, Kopas, 2014).

Previous studies have investigated the outcomes for well women and their babies where the pushing stage has exceeded the traditional time frames. These traditional limits have restricted primiparous women to 2 hours and multiparous women to 1 hour to birth their babies. Research shows that women and babies come to no harm where pushing efforts have exceeded these time limits (Lemos et al., 2017).

A MIDWIFE'S STORY

Maia and Tom are having their first baby and at 40 weeks, Maia has gone into spontaneous labour. She has laboured well at home with the support of Tom and her midwife Ali. They are planning to birth at the primary unit so must drive there once labour is well established. After only 4 hours, Maia's labour has suddenly advanced and Maia has the urge to push and goes to the toilet and shuts the door. She is now actively pushing but won't get off the toilet.

- As her midwife what would be your first priority at this stage?
- Is transfer appropriate at this stage or will you plan for a home birth?
- What do you need to do to make preparations for the baby's birth?
- What support do you need and what will you be asking them to do?

Facilitating a supportive birthing environment

The midwife has an important role in facilitating the birth of the baby by ensuring that the environment is appropriate and supportive of this physiological, psychological, emotional and spiritual process. It is necessary to consider the following:

- the woman's plan, desires and dreams for the birth of her baby
- privacy—phone off the hook, doors closed, curtains pulled, note on the door saying 'not to be disturbed'
- warmth—room temperature, warm towels for the baby, pool temperature comfortable for the woman
- comfort—positional techniques, hot towels, warm compresses, encouraging words
- space in which to use a variety of positions and props (e.g. pool, bath, mats, pillows, beanbags, birth stools, mirror)
- involvement of partner and supporters—supplying drinks to the woman, cool cloth for her face, massage or acupressure, applying hot towels, physical support for the woman, encouraging words
- unobtrusive presence of a second midwife who is known to the woman, is supportive of her birth plan and familiar with the safety equipment
- preparation of birthing and safety equipment—oxygen, suction, infant Ambubag, uterotonics, cord ties/clamps, scissors, availability of intravenous cannulation equipment and fluids.

Facilitating effective pushing efforts means that the midwife recognises when it is appropriate to make suggestions for the woman to try a variety of positions. This may be in response to recognition that efforts so far have resulted in little change in the descent of the presenting part of the baby. Identifying a lack of progress usually results from a combination of assessments. These may include:

- the woman stating that 'nothing has changed'
- no obvious anal dilation or perineal distension, and no presenting part visible
- abdominal palpation to identify the degree of descent of the presenting part in relation to the pelvic brim
- VE to confirm presentation, assess cervical dilation, define position, and assess station and the development of caput and moulding.

If lack of progress has been identified, sometimes simple changes to the woman's position may be all that is required to enable the labour to advance. The midwife can then guide the woman into more upright, open positions to enhance rotation and descent of the baby. This can be achieved, for example, by the use of supported squatting, sitting on the toilet or birth stool, or standing. Enabling the woman to see the effect of her pushes using a mirror can be very encouraging and energising as the presenting part becomes visible.

As the presenting part descends with contractions, it advances with the assistance of expulsive pushing efforts. It will initially advance, then recede between contractions. This process is necessary to enable the woman's tissues to accommodate the presenting part and also support gentle moulding of the baby's head. The use of hot compresses on the perineum and vulva can provide some soothing comfort at this time and is associated with lower rates of perineal trauma (Aasheim et al., 2017; Magoga et al., 2019). As the presenting part distends the vulva and perineum and then doesn't recede, the woman may experience intense burning and stretching. Hot compresses or perineal massage may provide some relief, and the midwife's calm, clear reassurance will be helpful (Aquino et al., 2020; Magoga et al., 2019). At this time the woman and her supporters will benefit from a relaxed, calm and unhurried atmosphere as the birth becomes imminent.

The midwife can encourage the gradual birth of the baby's head by suggesting that the woman breathes gently, pants or gives gentle, small pushes. With the intention of reducing perineal trauma, the midwife may have her 'hands on' or 'hands poised' to prevent rapid extension of the baby's head (Begley et al., 2019a; Pierce-Williams et al., 2021). Traditionally, midwives have been taught to apply digital pressure to the occiput to maintain flexion and reduce tissue damage. There is no evidence to support this practice at every birth; however, a midwife needs to be poised to support the baby's head if it appears to be advancing rapidly or if there is an indication of possible perineal trauma. Evidence has shown that hands off or poised is associated with fewer episiotomies and third-degree tears but that there was no difference between either hands on or off with regard to first or second-degree perineal tears (Begley et al., 2019a; Pierce-Williams et al., 2021).

Once the baby's head is born there can be a resting period before the next contraction.

Ten to thirty percent of babies will have a nuchal cord and they are not associated with an increase in perinatal morbidity or mortality (Gupta et al., 2020; Peesay, 2017). Midwives have routinely used this time to check whether there is a nuchal cord. Women can find this procedure extremely painful. The potential for harm calls into question the usefulness of this action. If the cord is present it can be looped over the baby's head or rolled down over the baby's shoulders as the baby is born (Mercer et al., 2005). If the cord is wound tightly around the neck it has been common practice to clamp and cut the cord to release it. As this severs the baby's oxygen supply, this practice is being increasingly questioned and should be used with caution (Akkaya et al., 2017). In her seminal work midwife researcher Judith Mercer describes the somersault manoeuvre as a way to assist the birth of the baby while keeping the umbilical cord intact. Tight nuchal cords have been associated with shoulder dystocia, and depriving the baby of its vital oxygen supply will only aggravate an already serious situation (Mercer et al., 2005). Clamping and cutting the cord before the baby is born also alters the physiology of placental separation, commits the woman to active management procedures and denies the baby its full complement of blood volume.

With the next contraction, the baby's shoulders rotate into the anterior/posterior diameter of the outlet of the pelvis and the baby's head will turn to be in alignment with the body. As the woman pushes, the shoulders are birthed and the rest of the body follows. The degree of hands-on support and guidance the midwife needs to provide will depend on the woman's wishes, her birth plan and the position she is in. Upright positions reduce the need for the midwife to apply traction techniques for the birth of the shoulders. The woman may wish to reach for her baby and lift it to her or have the baby placed gently against her warm skin. It is not unusual for some women to need time before they touch and hold their baby. It is important that the baby is kept warm by skin-to-skin contact and gentle drying with warm towels, to maintain the baby's temperature and stimulate respirations. The towels should be replaced as soon as they are damp. These first few minutes of relief, exhilaration and delight are precious. This is a once in a lifetime experience and should not be interrupted but be honoured, cherished and protected whenever possible.

The physiological transition that occurs in the immediate post-birth period is an extension of the birth process. Midwives promote the newborn's transition to extrauterine life through skin-to-skin contact. The midwife needs to be alert to the wellbeing of the mother and baby during this time. An effective, skilful midwife is able to make careful assessments without interfering in these moments. Assessments should include:

- baby's colour, heart rate, initiation of respiration, muscle tone, reflex irritability (Apgar score at 1, 5 and 10 minutes) (Table 25.4)
- observing the woman's response to her baby
- observing the woman's general wellbeing and ensuring her comfort
- maintaining observations of blood loss and signs of separation of the placenta.

The Apgar score was devised by Virginia Apgar in 1953 and has since become the most commonly used quantitative measuring tool for assessing the wellbeing of the newborn baby (Levene et al., 1993).

Enabling the new family to savour the moments after the birth involves supporting the woman and her family to take the time they need as they greet their new baby. This time also allows the woman's physiological responses to continue unimpeded. The environment has an important role to play in supporting this process. A quiet room with only the parents' voices, low lighting and a warm atmosphere are all helpful at this time and support both the woman's and baby's hormonal responses promoting normal physiological processes. As the baby adjusts to the new environment, they may begin to look around,

Table 25.4 The Apgar score

	0	1	2
Heart rate	Absent	Slow (<100)	Fast (>100)
Respiratory effort	Absent	Slow and irregular	Good and crying
Muscle tone	Limp	Some flexion of extremities	Active
Reflex irritability	No response	Grimace	Cry/cough
Colour	Pale	Body pink, extremities blue	Pink

nuzzle the breast and display signs of being interested in suckling. It is important not to force this process, but to observe for these cues. The baby may bring their hands to their mouth and start mouthing or rooting for the breast. There is no specific time frame for this to occur, and research identifies that support during this 'biologically sensitive period immediately after the birth' has significant advantages for both the mother and the baby. An unhurried, non-interfering approach best achieves this (Moore et al., 2016).

FIFTH DECISION POINT IN LABOUR

The third stage

The woman holding her baby close or breastfeeding her baby encourages the release of oxytocin to facilitate the separation of the placenta and membranes. The birth of the placenta and membranes constitutes the third stage of labour. This process can be facilitated in one of two ways: either by supporting the physiological process or by using active management techniques (Table 25.5). While we have identified the basic components of each approach the research has identified that there are considerable differences in the application of these techniques (Begley et al., 2019b).

The premise of actively managing the third stage is that women have less blood loss and require fewer blood transfusions. Excessive blood loss is commonly defined as 500 mL or more and is referred to as a postpartum haemorrhage (PPH). There is, however, continued discussion suggesting that 1000 mL blood loss or symptoms of hypovolaemia may be of more significance when identifying a PPH (Begley et al., 2019b). In other areas of medicine, for example trauma units and operating theatres, the significance of blood loss relies on the individual's responses to the blood loss rather than on the actual amount. When women undergo a caesarean section it is common for there to be blood loss of more than 500 mL that is not referred to as a PPH. How much blood loss is normal for each particular woman following birth is not known. It would seem reasonable to be guided by the woman's physiological responses rather than be limited by arbitrary amounts that may have no bearing on the wellbeing of an individual woman.

The appropriate support for the third stage of labour where women have experienced a physiological labour and birth and have no risk factors for PPH is the subject of ongoing debate. Critics of earlier trials have identified a number of issues, including the inconsistency of the techniques used in the trials, the variety of uterotonic regimens, the trial setting, the confidence of the practitioners involved and the inclusion of women in the trials who could not be termed as 'low risk' (Begley et al., 2015). A 2019 systematic review (Begley et al., 2019b) investigating third-stage management has once again been unable to come to any definitive conclusions other than for woman at risk of blood loss of 1000 mL or more; the findings suggest active management techniques may be beneficial for these women. For all other women the researchers recommend they should be given information antenatally to enable informed decision making.

There is evidence supporting midwives' claims that a physiological third stage is a safe option for well women (Edwards & Wickham, 2018; Oishi et al., 2017; Reed et al., 2019).

Table 25.5 Facilitating the third stage

Physiological support	Active management
1. Do not disturb mother and baby's interaction—promote skin-to-skin contact. 2. Facilitate a calm quiet environment—no hurry. 3. Observe for signs of separation of the placenta. 4. Observe for blood loss. 5. Assist the woman into a comfortable and upright position for birthing the placenta. 6. Encourage the woman to push the placenta out. 7. Support the placenta and membranes as they are birthed. 8. Note the time. 9. Clamp and cut the cord after it has stopped pulsating or once the placenta is born. 10. Palpate the uterus to ensure it is contracted. 11. Estimate the blood loss. 12. Complete the documentation.	1. Minimise separation of mother and baby—promote skin-to-skin contact. 2. Administer uterotonic after birth of anterior shoulder or after birth of the baby. Syntocinon (synthetic oxytocin) 5–10 IU IM; Syntometrine 1 mL (0.5 mg ergometrine and 5 IU synthetic oxytocin) IM. 3. Clamp and cut the cord. 4. Feel for uterine contraction. 5. Apply controlled cord traction by winding fingers around cord (or using a clamp) and applying sustained downward traction; when the placenta is visible, apply upward traction to follow the curve of the birth canal. 6. While traction is applied, counterpressure is provided with the other hand placed above the symphysis pubis. 7. Note the time of delivery of the placenta. 8. Palpate the uterus to ensure it is contracted. 9. Estimate the blood loss. 10. Complete the documentation.

Note: Do not mix methods; do not stimulate the uterus by 'fundal fiddling' as this may lead to partial separation of the placenta and blood loss.

Supporting a physiological third stage of labour

A supportive, warm environment, low lighting, attention to the woman's comfort, a calm and quiet atmosphere and having the baby close to or feeding at the breast have all been found to encourage the spontaneous birth of the placenta (Beatson, 2020). The birth plan developed by the woman and her midwife will have identified preferences for the birth of the placenta and membranes. Where the labour and birth have proceeded normally with no intervention, it is reasonable to expect that the birth of the placenta and membranes will follow the physiological process uninterrupted (Beatson, 2020; Edwards & Wickham, 2018; Reed et al., 2019). This is referred to variously as expectant, physiological or natural care. It is important for the midwife to be alert to the amount of vaginal blood loss and its effects on the wellbeing of the woman. Usually there is very little blood loss until the placenta begins to separate from the wall of the uterus.

The midwife waits for the following signs of separation:

- uterine contractions
- slowing and cessation of umbilical cord pulsations
- lengthening of the umbilical cord
- gush of fresh blood or clots per vaginum
- placenta visible at the introitus of the vagina.

With the separation of the placenta, the woman will commonly experience low pelvic pain and heaviness as the placenta descends into the lower segment of the uterus. With contractions the woman may feel a pushing urge. She may find it helpful to be in an upright position to assist her to birth the placenta. The use of gravity and pelvic-opening positions can facilitate this. It may be helpful to reassure the woman that the sensations when birthing the placenta won't be as intense as when birthing the baby. Palpation of the uterus and / or application of traction to the umbilical cord are contraindicated during this process, as they are implicated in the potential for increased bleeding and retention of the placenta. As the placenta descends into the vagina, the midwife can assist the woman to birth her placenta gently so that trailing membranes can be eased out and not torn.

As part of the midwifery assessment of the woman's wellbeing, it is important to monitor vaginal bleeding and uterine contractility immediately after the placenta's birth. Women at this time will often experience a great sense of relief and comfort. With physiological support, the therapeutic use of uterotonic drugs, oxytocin and / or ergometrine are indicated only where there is increased or unexpected blood loss before or after the birth of the placenta or where the uterus is atonic.

The timing of cutting the umbilical cord after pulsation ceases (see following Clinical point) can be influenced by:

- the birth plan
- a short cord interfering with the woman's ability to hold the baby close to the breast
- waiting until the placenta is born
- plans for a lotus birth (Box 25.4)
- the woman's request to change position in order to birth the placenta.

Box 25.4 Lotus birth

Some families choose to leave the placenta attached to the baby until the cord separates. This is known as a **lotus birth**. The cord is not cut, and once the placenta is born it is dried, salted and wrapped in preprepared leakproof material. The wrapping is changed as needed and some also choose to place fresh rosemary or lavender next to the placenta. The cord dries within 24 hours and separates (with the placenta) from the baby within 2–5 days. Reasons for choosing a lotus birth include the following:

- The family must carry both the baby and the placenta, and so will tend to stay at home and rest.
- The cord falls off in a shorter time than when cut and requires no extra care.
- Some claim the baby is calmer and more in tune with her or his surroundings.
- It is thought to provide the baby with a natural, gentle transition to extrauterine life from being connected to the mother.

(Adapted from Rachana S. *Lotus Birth*. Victoria: Greenwood Press; 2000 Zinsser L, 2018)

REFLECTIVE THINKING EXERCISE

Consider your confidence with regard to supporting a physiological third stage.

Discuss with your practice colleagues how to develop your skills and confidence with regard to the physiological birth of the placenta and membranes.

CLINICAL POINT

Is clamping the cord necessary following a normal physiological labour and birth?

Delaying clamping, or not clamping until after the cord ceases pulsating or the placenta is born, facilitates transfusion of blood between the placenta and the baby. Studies have found that 'in term neonates, delayed cord clamping has been associated with decreased iron-deficient anaemia and increased iron stores with potential valuable effects that extend beyond the newborn period, including improvements in long-term neurodevelopment' (McAdams, 2014; see also Bruckner et al., 2021; Mercer et al., 2018).

Timing of cord clamping

The research would therefore indicate that it is better to mimic nature than to interfere with the intricate and complex design of the physiological neonatal transition (Bruckner et al., 2021; Mercer et al., 2018). There is a significant increase in the baby's circulation if the cord is not clamped immediately following birth (Davies & Richards, 2021). If the cord is clamped in the first few seconds of the birth, the distribution of blood between baby and the placenta is 67% and 33% respectively; if the cord is clamped 3 minutes after the birth, the baby receives 87% with 13% left with the placenta (Yao et al., 1969). This increased blood volume has positive consequences for the newborn owing to increased vasodilation and perfusion (Davies & Richards, 2021; Mercer et al., 2018).

Active management of third stage

Early cord clamping, the administration of uterotonic drugs and the application of controlled cord traction (CCT) are used to shorten the time between the birth of the baby and the birth of the placenta and membranes. This is referred to as **active management**, and the impetus for this is the prevention of PPH (Begley et al., 2019b) (see Table 25.5). Oxytocin is the first-choice uterotonic because of the low incidence of adverse side effects compared with uterotonics containing ergometrine. Studies have demonstrated that ergometrine is associated with nausea, vomiting and increase in blood pressure (Begley et al., 2019b).

If uterotonic drugs are used during labour, it is important to continue with the active management procedures of cord clamping and CCT, as the physiological process has been interfered with. Mixing active and physiological care has been associated with adverse effects for the woman and her baby.

Midwives should be aware that blood loss may initially appear to be minimal in active management. However, it is often the case that when the woman gets up for a shower after the birth, she passes a large clot, and may feel faint and exhibit signs of blood loss. Often this hidden blood loss is not recorded and is not recognised in the literature about active management.

A MIDWIFE'S STORY

Leilani is 15 years old and is one of eight children. She has just given birth to her first baby. As well as her midwife Sonya, she has her mother, her grandmother and five of her siblings in the birthing room. She has yet to birth her placenta and the cord is still attached. The baby is nuzzling at the breast, but Leilani's grandmother is insistent that the cord is cut so she can hold the baby and give Leilani a rest. There have been signs of separation as the cord has stopped pulsating and there has been a small amount of fresh bleeding. Leilani is embarrassed about showing her breasts in front of her family.

- What could midwife Sonya do to enable Leilani to birth her placenta?
- What physiological processes are required for the placenta to be born?
- How does the environment impact on the birth of the placenta?

Examination of the placenta and membranes

Careful and thorough inspection of the placenta and membranes will need to be undertaken soon after the birth. If there is evidence of retained products, it is important to be aware of this as it may predispose the woman to bleeding or infection. During the examination of the placenta it is ideal to include the woman and her family in this fascinating exploration and to explain your findings with them (Reed et al., 2019). The aim is to identify the following:

- condition of the placenta and membranes
- number of vessels in the cord, insertion site and presence of knots
- signs of absence of cotyledons, including vessels through the membranes
- completeness of the membranes.

Placenta traditions

For many families, from a variety of cultures, the way the placenta is cared for requires some form of ceremony. Before the birth it is a good idea to discuss with the family whether they have plans for the baby's placenta and membranes. For some they may prefer that the placenta is disposed of without any involvement from the family, but for others it may be seen as a symbol of life, spirit and individuality:

> *The Maori word for land, whenua, also means placenta. The whenua is placed in a specially prepared receptacle and buried in a particular location. This practice reinforces the relationship between the newborn baby and the land of their birth.*
> (Te Ahukaramū, 2012)

Some Aboriginal tribes also bury their placenta under a tree or an ant pit, and in Samoa when the placenta is buried close to home there is a belief that this will also keep the growing child close to home. For more placenta traditions, a useful website is: http://www.TeAra.govt.nz/en/papatuanuku-the-land/page4.

RESEARCH ACTIVITY

Two Masters of Midwifery theses investigate midwifery practices in relation to support for a physiological third stage and delayed cord clamping (Beatson, 2021; Hewitt, 2020).

Read these works and consider the following questions in relation to your own practice.

1. How may this research influence your understanding and practice concerning the role of the midwife in facilitating a physiological third stage of labour and delayed cord clamping?
2. In light of the evidence provided by this research, how will you share information with women in regard to their choices for the birth of their placenta and cutting of the cord.

Assessing injury to the woman's labial, vaginal and perineal area

Episiotomy should be avoided during a normal birth and every effort should be made to minimise perineal injury and discomfort (Jiang et al., 2017). Sometimes, however, a tear to the woman's perineum, vagina or labial area is unavoidable and it is the midwife's role to make a careful assessment of the degree of trauma to this area. The assessment does not need to be done immediately, as every effort should be made to establish bonding between the woman and her baby and to give them time to explore each other and initiate breastfeeding. (Ch. 28 provides information about assessment of perineal trauma and repair.)

RESEARCH ACTIVITY

A Cochrane Database of Systematic Review (Moore et al., 2016) identifies the importance of early skin-to-skin contact for mother and baby.

1. What are the benefits for mother and baby when enabled to have skin-to-skin contact during the first few hours after birth?
2. What actions do you or can you take to support undisturbed skin-to-skin contact for women and their babies?

Ongoing assessment

Following the birth of the placenta and the perineal assessment and repair, the midwife needs to estimate the blood loss sustained and its effect on the woman. This is calculated by measuring actual blood loss and making a visual assessment of blood-stained linen, combined with assessment of the woman's wellbeing, including measurements of pulse and blood pressure. The actual amount of blood loss estimated is subjective. Each woman's individual response will need to be carefully assessed by the midwife. Palpation of the uterus and assessment of the fundal height to confirm that it is contracted and central assures the midwife that the woman's body is responding appropriately. Encouraging the woman to palpate her own uterus and recognise when it is well contracted or otherwise enables her to take responsibility for her wellbeing and know when to ask for assistance.

EXAMINATION OF THE BABY

Assessment of the baby occurs from the moment she or he is born. Observing the baby in her or his mother's arms, the body movements, colour and alertness, allows the midwife to ensure that the baby has made an effective transition from unborn to newborn. The first hour or so of the baby's life will be spent in skin-to-skin contact with the mother and feeding at the breast (Buckley, 2014; Moore et al., 2016). At some stage following this, it is appropriate for the midwife to examine the baby and to discuss her findings with the parents. There is no reason why this examination would not occur in the parents' presence. It is important that the room is warm and that the baby does not become cold during this assessment. Wrapping the baby in soft warm towels and exposing only the part of the baby you are examining not only keeps the baby warm, but also helps to keep the baby calm. It is important to remember that the baby has just come from the warm, confined space of the mother's uterus. Babies will often cry if unwrapped and left naked, and this can be distressing for both the baby and the parents (Davies & Richards, 2018). (Information about full examination of the newborn baby can be found in Ch. 31.)

ONGOING CARE IN THE FIRST FEW HOURS

The woman has expended an enormous amount of energy and will need to eat and drink to help restore her energy. Some families may have a special meal ready to celebrate the birth; others may have cultural preferences about the type of food first consumed after the birth of a baby; yet others know they are hungry, but can't think what they would like to eat. Offering light food and fluids is helpful, and organising this can enable the midwife to give the new family some time to themselves.

When the woman is ready, she may like to have a shower or bath. It is important to assist the woman and ensure that she is feeling able to manage; she should not be left alone, but should be given the privacy that she requires. A wash in bed may be more helpful for a woman who is tired and lacking energy. A seat in the shower can provide support if the woman is feeling weak and tired. This is also a useful time for the woman to try to empty her bladder. Encouraging the woman to empty her bladder within an hour or two of the birth is important for a number of reasons:

- It confirms that the woman *can* empty her bladder and that there are no issues of retention of urine possibly caused by trauma and/or oedema.
- It reduces discomfort and may lessen the intensity of her afterpains.

- A full bladder can impede effective uterine contractions and therefore increase the potential for bleeding.
- Being upright can assist the expulsion of any clots that may have collected in the vagina / cervix.

As the birth process can sometimes result in a loss of bladder sensation initially, encouraging the woman to empty her bladder regularly (every 2–3 hours) in the first 12 hours or so after the birth assists the uterus to remain contracted. It also enables the woman to recognise that her bladder is filling. Emptying her bladder regularly, especially just prior to breastfeeding, can help reduce the severity of the 'afterpains' that many women experience in the early postpartum period.

Afterpains (postnatal uterine contractions) are more commonly associated with multiparous women and with breastfeeding, but women can experience afterpains whether or not they have had a baby before and regardless of how they are feeding their baby. There has been a tendency to dismiss these as a mild inconvenience. However, there is a wide variation in women's experiences of afterpains. Some women feel the afterpains to be mildly uncomfortable and others describe them as excruciating or not dissimilar to labour pains. As the uterus contracts there is also usually a concurrent increase in bleeding, and this may include some clots. The oxytocin release resulting from breastfeeding can strengthen afterpains and cause women to be fearful when latching their baby. It is helpful to explain to women what the afterpains are and what they achieve. For many women, afterpains settle after a few days, but they can last up to a week or so for others. In the initial period after the birth, applying heat to the lower abdomen can be comforting. Ensuring the bladder is empty and not creating pressure on the uterus will also help. Acknowledging that afterpains can be distressing is important for women who may be worried that something is wrong.

DOCUMENTATION

Documentation of the labour and birth process and the ongoing care provided is intended to give a comprehensive and accurate account of the woman and her baby's experience and wellbeing. The documentation provides a record of the care from a midwife's perspective but it also describes the process for the woman to reflect on and treasure as part of her birthing history. The documentation also supports the midwife and woman as they debrief such an incredible experience. Any plans, decision points and actions taken, as well as their outcome, should be recorded. The aim when documenting is to provide a written record of events *as they occur*. As mentioned previously, this may not be possible at all times, but relevant times and events can be noted and full records completed as soon as possible. All documentation written retrospectively should be acknowledged as such. In the first few hours after the birth, while the parents and baby enjoy their newfound relationship, there is often opportunity for the midwife to complete the appropriate documentation. This will include:

- a description of the labour and birth events with times included, plan of care, actions taken and outcome
- the woman's and baby's responses to the labour and birth and each other
- description of the birth of the placenta and membranes, the examination and any findings—whether normal or abnormal, blood samples taken and estimation of the woman's blood loss
- description of the assessment of perineal and vaginal trauma, and the process of any repair undertaken, including suture material and technique used—a diagram can be helpful
- assessment of the woman's and baby's wellbeing, including the results of any examinations undertaken, with attention drawn to any concerns and the midwife's actions in response to this
- timing of any drugs given, the reason for administration and response
- completion of any requirements for notification of birth, newborn records, maternity facility documentation
- the midwife's assessment of the woman's and baby's wellbeing prior to the midwife leaving the woman's home, or handing care over to postnatal ward staff, or the woman going home
- ensuring the woman and her family are aware of indicators regarding possible concerns that would warrant contacting the midwife
- any specific plans for the next 12 hours or so regarding rest, breastfeeding, self-care and contacting / accessing caregivers

For further support for your midwifery documentation, see the NZ College of Midwives Record Keeping Toolkit (NZCOM, 2021).

Conclusion

The essence of being able to provide appropriate midwifery support for women in physiological labour requires understanding of beliefs, values, attitudes and practices and how these may affect the woman. The importance of the midwife–woman relationship and its development over time cannot be overstated. This relationship enables the woman and the midwife to learn to understand one another, and the midwife to come to know what and who are important for this particular woman. This 'knowing' can enable the midwife to be 'with woman' in the full sense of the term.

Understanding the physiological process of labour and birth enables the midwife to recognise that each woman will respond in her own way. This encompasses the physical, psychological, emotional and spiritual dimensions. What is normal for one woman may be abnormal for another. Being present, and the quality of that presence, enables the midwife to support the woman in the way that is most appropriate for that situation. Not all women wish for a constant presence, but when they want the midwife they want her to be 'there'. Being in the room is not enough: it is important to listen and attend to the woman and her supporters. This is most easily achieved through continuity of care provided by a known caregiver. Words of praise, comfort, encouragement and reassurance are all valuable tools of the midwife who actually means them (Bradfield et al., 2019; Downe et al., 2018; Hildingsson et al., 2021; Olza et al., 2018).

Midwives can support women through labour and its ebbs and flows by being available to the woman, encouraging and comforting her and helping her support people to do the same. Labour and birth are challenging for most women and they require understanding and belief to work through the challenge. A compassionate midwife has much to offer labouring women. Labour can be affected by a multitude of issues, and the midwife who recognises the potential impact of these issues will be in a position to assist the woman.

There are a variety of assessment tools that midwives can use to identify that labour is progressing. The skilful midwife will use these tools in combination with her observations and knowing of the woman. Understanding the effect of mobility, positions, gravity and environment can enable the midwife to assist the woman through her labour, especially when it is hard work. Knowledge of what supports and what may adversely affect the physiological process are key skills for a midwife.

Review questions

1. What elements are important to include in a birth plan to enable you to provide effective support during labour?
2. When supporting a labouring woman in a hospital environment, what strategies, tools and techniques will you use to encourage her to be active and upright?
3. How would you support a woman who is in the latent phase of labour?
4. During a woman's labour and birth, what documentation are you required to maintain, what do you currently do, and how does this meet your professional and legal obligations?
5. What assessments will you make to identify that a woman is progressing normally in labour, other than vaginal examinations?
6. How will you assess fetal wellbeing in the first stage of labour, and what evidence supports your actions?
7. Read the *Cochrane Database of Systematic Reviews* (Lemos et al., 2017) regarding pushing in the second stage of labour; how would the findings influence how you would support women during the second stage of their labour?
8. How will you ensure that you have the skills and confidence to be able to appropriately support a woman to birth her placenta and membranes physiologically?
9. What are the advantages for mother and baby of delayed cord clamping?
10. What support does a midwife require to be able to provide a continuous, attentive presence during a woman's childbirth experience?

Online resources

All4Maternity: https://www.all4maternity.com.
Birth to Earth: http://www.birthtoearth.com.
Cochrane Library: https://www.cochranelibrary.com.
Homebirth Aotearoa: http://homebirth.org.nz.
Homebirth Australia: http://www.homebirthaustralia.org/.
Homebirth UK: http://www.homebirth.org.uk.
Joan Donley Research Database: https://portal.midwife.org.nz/research-search?mode=JDMRC.
Maternity Services Consumer Council: http://www.maternity.org.nz.
MIDIRS website: http://www.midirs.org/.
Midwife thinking: https://midwifethinking.com/.
Midwifery Today: http://www.midwiferytoday.com.
Ministry of Health (NZ): http://www.moh.govt.nz.
National Institute for Health and Care Excellence (UK): http://www.nice.org.uk.
New Zealand College of Midwives: http://www.midwife.org.nz.
Te Ara—the Encyclopedia of New Zealand: http://www.TeAra.govt.nz.

References

Aasheim V, Nilsen ABV, Reinar LM, et al. Perineal techniques during the second stage of labour for reducing perineal trauma. *Cochrane Database Syst Rev.* 2017;6(6):CD006672. doi:10.1002/14651858.CD006672.pub3. PMID: 28608597; PMCID: PMC6481402.

Abalos E, Chamillard M, Díaz V, et al. Progression of the first stage of spontaneous labour. *Best Pract Res Clin Obstet Gynaecol.* 2020;67:19–32. doi:10.1016/j.bpobgyn.2020.03.001.

Akin B, Saydam BK. The effect of labor dance on perceived labor pain, birth satisfaction, and neonatal outcomes. *Explore (NY).* 2020;16(5):310–317.

Akkaya H, Büke B, Pekcan MK, et al. Nuchal cord: is it really the silent risk of pregnancy? *J Matern Fetal Neonatal Med.* 2017; 30(14):1730–1733.

Alfirevic Z, Devane D, Gyte GML, et al. Continuous cardiotocography (CTG) as a form of electronic fetal monitoring (EFM) for fetal assessment during labour. *Cochrane Database Syst Rev.* 2017;(2):CD006066. doi:10.1002/14651858.

Aquino CI, Guida M, Saccone G, et al. Perineal massage during labor: a systematic review and meta-analysis of randomized controlled trials. *J Matern Fetal Neonatal Med.* 2020;33(6): 1051–1063.

Australian College of Midwives. *Midwifery Philosophy and Values.* Canberra: ACM; 2019. Online: https://www.midwives.org.au/midwifery-philosophy-values.

Ayerle GM, Schäfers R, Mattern E, et al. Effects of the birthing room environment on vaginal births and client-centred outcomes for women at term planning a vaginal birth: BE-UP, a multicentre randomised controlled trial. *Trials.* 2018;19(1): 641. doi:10.1186/s13063-018-2979-7. PMID: 30454075; PMCID: PMC6245933.

Beake S, Chang Y, Cheyne H, et al. Experiences of early labour management from perspectives of women, labour companions and health professionals: A systematic review of qualitative evidence. *Midwifery.* 2018;57:69–84.

Beatson D. Midwives' Facilitation of Physiological Placental Birth: A Delphi Study (Master's thesis). Dunedin: Otago Polytechnic; 2020. Online: https://online.op.ac.nz/assets/OPRES/MID-Beatson-2021-thesis.pdf.

Begley CM, Gyte GM, Devane D, et al. Active versus expectant management for women in the third stage of labour. *Cochrane Database Syst Rev.* 2015;(3):CD007412.

Begley C, Guilliland K, Dixon L, et al. A qualitative exploration of techniques used by expert midwives to preserve the perineum intact. *Women Birth.* 2019a;32(1):87–97. pmid:29730096

Begley CM, Gyte G, Devane D, et al. Active versus expectant management for women in the third stage of labour. *Cochrane Database Syst Rev.* 2019b;(2):CD007412. doi:10.1002/14651858.CD007412.pub5.

Bjelke M, Lendahls L, Oscarsson M. Management of the passive phase of the second stage of labour in nulliparous women-Focus group discussions with Swedish midwives. *Midwifery.* 2019;75:89–96. doi:10.1016/j.midw.2019.04.011.

Bradfield Z, Hauck Y, Duggan R. Midwives' perceptions of being 'with women': a phenomenological study. *BMC Pregnancy Childbirth.* 2019;19(363). doi:10.1186/s12884-019-2548-4.

Bruckner M, Katheria AC, Schmölzer GM. Delayed cord clamping in healthy term infants: More harm or good? *Semin Fetal Neonatal Med.* 2021;26(2):101221. doi:10.1016/j.siny.2021.101221.

Buckley S. *The Hormonal Physiology of Childbearing.* New York, NY: Childbirth Connection; 2014.

Carlsson IM. Being in a safe and thus secure place, the core of early labour: A secondary analysis in a Swedish context. *Int J Qual Stud Health Well-being.* 2016;11:30230. doi:10.3402/qhw.v11.30230.

Christopher U, Goldy SJ, Oral BJ, et al. Multiple vaginal examinations and early neonatal sepsis. *Int J Reprod Contracept Obstet Gynecol.* 2019;8:876–81.

Ciardulli A, Saccone G, Anastasio H, et al. Less restrictive food intake during labor in low-risk singleton pregnancies: a systematic review and meta-analysis. *Obstet Gynecol.* 2017;129(3): 473–480. doi:10.1097/AOG.0000000000001898.

Dahan O. The riddle of the extreme ends of the birth experience: Birthing consciousness and its fragility. *Curr Psychol.* 2021. doi:10.1007/s12144-021-01439-7.

Davies L, Richards J. Maternal and newborn transition: adjustment to extrauterine life. In: Davies L, McDonald S, eds. *Examination of the Newborn and Neonatal Health: A Multidimensional Approach.* 2nd ed. Edinburgh: Churchill Livingstone; 2021:100–122.

Davis DL, Creedy DK, Bradfield Z, et al. Development of the woman-centred care scale-midwife self report (WCCS-MSR). *BMC Pregnancy Childbirth.* 2021;21:523. doi:10.1186/s12884-021-03987-z.

Davis E, Harrison L, Arms S. *Heart and Hands: A Midwife's Guide to Pregnancy and Birth.* 5th ed. Berkeley, CA: Celestial Arts; 2019.

de Klerk HW, Boere E, van Lunsen R. Women's experiences with vaginal examinations during labor in the Netherlands. *J Psychosom Obstet Gynaecol.* 2017;1–6. doi:10.1080/0167482X.2017.1291623. [Epub ahead of print].

Devane D, Lalor G, Daly S, et al. Cardiotocography versus intermittent auscultation of fetal heart on admission to labour ward for assessment of fetal wellbeing. *Cochrane Database Syst Rev.* 2017;1:CD005122.

Dixon L, Skinner J, Foureur M. The emotional and hormonal pathways of labour and birth: integrating mind, body and behaviour. *J N Z Coll Midwives.* 2013;48:15–23. doi:10.12784/nzcomjnl48.2013.3.15-23.

Downe S. A proposal for a new research and practice agenda for birth. *Midwifery Digest.* 2000;10(3):337–341.

Downe S, Gyte GML, Dahlen HG, et al. Routine vaginal examinations for assessing progress of labour to improve outcomes for women and babies at term. *Cochrane Database Syst Rev.* 2013;(7):CD010088. doi:10.1002/14651858.CD010088.pub2.

Downe S, Finlayson K, Oladapo OT, et al. What matters to women during childbirth: A systematic qualitative review. *PLoS ONE.* 2018;13(4):e0194906.. doi:10.1371/journal.pone.0194906.

Fontein-Kuipers Y, de Groot R, van Staa A. Woman-centered care 2.0: Bringing the concept into focus. *Eur J Midwifery.* 2018;2. doi:10.18332/ejm/91492.

Friedman E. The graphic analysis of labour. *Am J Obstet Gynecol.* 1954;68(6):1568–1575.

Gaskin IM. *Ina May's Guide to Childbirth.* New York: Bantam; 2003.

Gluck O, Mizrachi Y, Ganer Herman H. et al. The correlation between the number of vaginal examinations during active labor and febrile morbidity, a retrospective cohort study. *BMC Pregnancy Childbirth.* 2020;246. doi: 10.1186/s12884-020-02925-9.

Guilliland K, Pairman S, Victoria University. *The Midwifery Partnership: A Model for Practice* (Monograph Series: 95/1). Wellington: Department of Nursing and Midwifery, Victoria University; 1995.

Guilliland K, Pairman S. *The Midwifery Partnership: A Model for Practice.* 2nd ed. Christchurch: New Zealand College of Midwives; 2010.

Guittier MJ, Othenin-Girard V, de Gasquet B, et al. Maternal positioning to correct occiput posterior fetal position during the first stage of labour: a randomised controlled trial. *BJOG.* 2016;123(13):2199–2207. doi:10.1111/1471-0528.13855.

Gupta JK, Sood A, Hofmeyr GJ, et al. Position in the second stage of labour for women without epidural anaesthesia. *Cochrane Database Syst Rev.* 2017;(5):CD002006. doi:10.1002/14651858.CD002006.pub4.

Gupta J, Sharma R, Gupta A. To study the effect of nuchal cord on perinatal outcome and mode of delivery in uncomplicated pregnancies. *Int J Clin Obstet Gynaecol.* 2020;4(5):137–143. doi:10.33545/gynae.2020.v4.i5c693.

Healy M, Nyman V, Spence D, et al. How do midwives facilitate women to give birth during physiological second stage of labour? A systematic review. *PLoS ONE.* 2020;15(7):e0226502.
Henderson C, Macdonald S, eds. *Mayes' Midwifery. A Textbook for Midwives.* 11th ed. Edinburgh: Baillière Tindall; 1988.

Henderson C, Macdonald S, eds. *Mayes' Midwifery. A Textbook for Midwives.* 13th ed. Edinburgh: Baillière Tindall; 2004.

Hewitt, T. Timing of Cord Clamping (TOCC): An Observational Study of Cord Clamping Practice in a New Zealand Maternity Hospital (Master's thesis). Dunedin: Otago Polytechnic; 2020. Online: https://researchbank.ac.nz/bitstream/handle/10652/5469/MID%20Hewitt%202019%20thesis%20%2B.pdf?sequence=4&isAllowed=y.

Hildingsson I, Karlström A, Larsson B. Childbirth experience in women participating in a continuity of midwifery care project. *Women Birth.* 2021;34(3):e255–e261. doi:10.1016/j.wombi.2020.04.010.

Hundley V, Way S, Cheyne H, et al. Defining the latent phase of labour: is it important? *Evidence Based Midwifery*. 2017;15(3): 89–94.

Ibrahim HA, Said HII, Elgzar WTI. Effect of upright and ambulant positions versus lying down during the active first stage of labor on birth outcomes among nulliparous women: randomized controlled clinical trial. *Front Nurs*. 2020;3:239–248.

Inde Y, Nakai A, Sekiguchi A, et al. Cervical dilatation curves of spontaneous deliveries in pregnant Japanese females. *Int J Med Sci*. 2018;15(6):549–556. doi:10.7150/ijms.23505.

Jiang H, Qian X, Carroli G, et al. Selective versus routine use of episiotomy for vaginal birth. *Cochrane Database Syst Rev*. 2017;(2):CD000081, doi:10.1002/14651858.CD000081.pub3.

Jowitt M. *Dynamic Positions in Birth: A Fresh Look at How Women's Bodies Work in Labour*. 2nd ed. London: Pinter and Marin; 2020.

Kobayashi S, Hanada N, Matsuzaki M, et al. Assessment and support during early labour for improving birth outcomes. *Cochrane Database Syst Rev*. 2017;(4):CD011516, doi:10.1002/14651858.CD011516.pub2.

Lavender T, Cuthbert A, Smyth RMD. Effect of partograph use on outcomes for women in spontaneous labour at term and their babies. *Cochrane Database Syst Rev*. 2018;(8): CD005461. doi:10.1002/14651858.CD005461.pub5.

Lawrence A, Lewis L, Hofmeyr GJ, et al. Maternal positions and mobility during first stage labour. *Cochrane Database Syst Rev*. 2013;(8):CD003934, doi:10.1002/14651858.CD003934.pub3.

Leap N, Hunter B. *Supporting Women for Labour and Birth: A Thoughtful Guide*. Abingdon, UK: Routledge; 2016.

Lemos A, Amorim MM, Dornelas de Andrade A, et al. Pushing/bearing down methods for the second stage of labour. *Cochrane Database Syst Rev*. 2017;(3):CD009124. doi:10.1002/14651858.CD009124.pub3.

Levene MI, Tudehope DI, Thearle MJ. *Essentials of Neonatal Medicine*. Oxford: Blackwell Scientific; 1993.

Lundborg L, Åberg K, Sandström A, et al. First stage progression in women with spontaneous onset of labor: A large population-based cohort study. *PLoS ONE*. 2020;15(9):e0239724. doi:10.1371/journal.pone.0239724.

McAdams RM. Time to implement delayed cord clamping. *Obstet Gynecol*. 2014;123(3):549–552.

McLachlan HL, Forster DA, Davey MA, et al. The effect of primary midwife-led care on women's experience of childbirth—the results of the COSMOS trial. *BJOG*. 2016;123(3):465–474. doi:10.1111/1471-0528.13713.

Magoga G, Saccone G, Al-Kouatly HB, et al. Warm perineal compresses during the second stage of labor for reducing perineal trauma: A meta-analysis. *Eur J Obstet Gynecol Reprod Biol*. 2019;240:93–98. doi:10.1016/j.ejogrb.2019.06.011. Epub 2019 Jun 15. PMID: 31238205.

Martis R, Emilia O, Nurdiati DS, et al. Intermittent auscultation (IA) of fetal heart rate in labour for fetal well-being. *Cochrane Database Syst Rev*. 2017;(2):CD008680. doi:10.1002/14651858.CD008680.pub2.

Maude RM, Skinner JP, Foureur MJ. Putting intelligent structured intermittent auscultation (ISIA) into practice. *Women Birth*. 2016;29(3):285–292

Mellor C, Farry A. HALO tool; artificial rupture of membranes. i3; Institute for innovation and improvement, Waitemata District Health Board, New Zealand; 2018. Online: https://i3.waitematadhb.govt.nz/assets/documents/our-work/fellows/HALO-Tool-References.pdf; https://i3.waitematadhb.govt.nz/assets/documents/our-work/fellows/HALO-Tool.pdf.

Mercer JS, Skovgaard RL, Peareara-Eaves J, et al. Nuchal cord management and nurse-midwifery practice. *J Midwifery Womens Health*. 2005;50:373–379.

Mercer JS, Erickson-Owens DA, Deoni SCL, et al. Effects of delayed cord clamping on 4-month ferritin levels, brain myelin content, and neurodevelopment: a randomized controlled trial. *J Pediatr*. 2018;203:266–272.e2. doi:10.1016/j.jpeds.2018.06.006

Miller YD, Armanasco AA, McCosker L. et al. Variations in outcomes for women admitted to hospital in early versus active labour: an observational study. *BMC Pregnancy Childbirth*. 2020;20:469. doi:10.1186/s12884-020-03149-7.

Moore ER, Bergman N, Anderson GC. Early skin-to-skin contact for mothers and their healthy newborn infants. *Cochrane Database of Syst Rev*. 2016;(11):CD003519. doi:10.1002/14651858.CD003519.pub4.

Mylod D. *Using a Birth Ball in the Latent Phase of Labour to Reduce Pain Perception; A Randomised Controlled Trial (Doctoral thesis)*. Bournemouth: Bournemouth University; 2020.

Nash K. Is it time for a more holistic assessment of labour progress? *BJM*. 2020;8(8). doi:10.12968/bjom.2020.28.8.457.

National Institute for Clinical Excellence (NICE). *Intrapartum Care: Care of Healthy Women and their Babies during Childbirth. NICE clinical guidelines*. London: NICE; 2014.

Ndayisenga JP, Mukamana D, Murekezi J, et al. Early routine amniotomy: an unnecessary procedure. *Res J Health Sci*. 2021;9: 77–81. doi:10.4314/rejhs.v9i1.9.

New Zealand College of Midwives (NZCOM). *A Keteparaha (Toolkit) Supporting and Enhancing Effective Midwifery Record Keeping in Aotearoa*. Christchurch: NZCOM; 2021.

New Zealand College of Midwives (NZCOM). *Handbook for Practice*. Christchurch: NZCOM; 2015.

New Zealand College of Midwives (NZCOM). *Philosophy and Code of Ethics*. Online: https://www.midwife.org.nz/midwives/professional-standards/philosophy-and-code-of-ethics/.

New Zealand College of Midwives (NZCOM). *Intermittent auscultation for the assessment of intrapartum fetal wellbeing practice guidance*. 2020. Online: https://www.midwife.org.nz.

Oishi T, Tamura T, Yamamoto U. Outcomes of blood loss post physiological birth with physiological management in the third stage of labour at a maternity home in Japan. *J N Z Coll Midwives*. 2017;53:23–29.

Oladapo OT, Diaz V, Bonet M, et al. Cervical dilatation patterns of 'low-risk' women with spontaneous labour and normal perinatal outcomes: a systematic review. *BJOG*. 2018;125(8):944–954. doi:10.1111/1471-0528.14930.

Olza I, Leahy-Warren P, Benyamini Y, et al. Women's psychological experiences of physiological childbirth: a meta-synthesis. *BMJ Open*. 2018;8:e020347. doi:10.1136/ bmjopen-2017-020347.

Olza I, Uvnas-Moberg K, Ekström-Bergström A, et al. Birth as a neuro-psycho-social event: An integrative model of maternal experiences and their relation to neurohormonal events during childbirth. *PLoS ONE*. 2020;15(7):e0230992.

Ozkan S, Kadoglu M, Rathfisch A. Restricting oral fluid and food intake during labour: a qualitative analysis of women's views. *Int J Caring Sci*. 2017;10(1):235.

Peesay M. Nuchal cord and its implications. *Matern Health Neonatol Perinatol*. 2017;3:28.

Perriman N, Davis DL, Ferguson S. What women value in the midwifery continuity of care model: A systematic review with meta-synthesis. *Midwifery*. 2018 Jul;62:220–229. doi:10.1016/j.midw.2018.04.011. Epub 2018 Apr 12. PMID: 29723790.

Philpott RH, Castle WM. Cervicographs in the management of labour on primigravidae 1. The alert line for detecting normal labour. *J Obstet Gynaecol Br Commonw*. 1972;79(7):592–598.

Pierce-Williams R, Saccone G, Berghella V. Hands-on versus hands-off techniques for the prevention of perineal trauma during vaginal delivery: a systematic review and meta-analysis of randomized controlled trials. *J Matern Fetal Neonatal Med*. 2021; 34:6:993–1001. doi:10.1080/14767058.2019.1619686.

Rachana S. *Lotus Birth*. Victoria: Greenwood Press; 2000.

Reed R, Gabriel L, Kearney L. Birthing the placenta: women's decisions and experiences. *BMC Pregnancy Childbirth.* 2019;19:140. doi:10.1186/s12884-019-2288-5.
Rota A, Antolini L, Colciago E, et al. Timing of hospital admission in labour: latent versus active phase, mode of birth and intrapartum interventions. A correlational study. *Women Birth.* 2018;31(4):313–318.
Royal Australian and New Zealand College of Obstetricians and Gynaecologists (RANZCOG). *Intrapartum fetal surveillance, Clinical guideline.* 4th ed. Melbourne, Australia: RANZCOG; 2019.
Sandall J, Soltani H, Gates S, et al. Midwife-led continuity models versus other models of care for childbearing women. *Cochrane Database Syst Rev.* 2016;(4):CD004667. doi:10.1002/14651858.CD004667.
Seitchik J. The management of functional dystocia in the first stage of labour. *Clin Obstet Gynaecol.* 1987;30(1):42–49.
Simkin P, Hanson L, Ancheta R. *The Labour Progress Handbook. Early Intervention to Prevent and Treat Dystocia.* New Jersey: Wiley Blackwell; 2017.
Singata M, Tranmer J, Gyte GML. Restricting oral fluid and food intake during labour. *Cochrane Database Syst Rev.* 2013;(8): CD003930. doi:10.1002/14651858.CD003930.pub3.
Smyth RMD, Alldred SK, Markham C. Amniotomy for shortening spontaneous labour. *Cochrane Database Syst Rev.* 2013;(1): CD006167. doi:10.1002/14651858.CD006167.pub3.
Studd J. Partograms and nomograms of cervical dilatation in management of primigravid labour. *BMJ.* 1973;4(5890):451.
Tarrats L, Paez I, Navarri I, et al. Heat application on lumbar and suprapubic pain during the onset of labour using a new abdominal two-pocket belt: a randomized and controlled trial. *Gynecol Obstet.* 2019;9:511.
Te Ahukaramū Charles Royal. 'Papatūānuku–the land-Whenua–the placenta'. *Te Ara—The Encyclopedia of New Zealand.* 2012. Online: http://www.TeAra.govt.nz/en/papatuanuku-the-land/page-4.
Toberna CP, Horter D, Heslin K, et al. Dancing during labor: social media trend or future practice?. *J Patient Cent Res Rev.* 2020;7(2):213–217.
Türkmen H, Oran NT. Massage and heat application on labor pain and comfort: A quasi-randomized controlled experimental study. *Explore (NY).* 2020;11:S1550-8307(20)30234-2. doi:10.1016/j.explore.2020.08.002.
Watkins A. *Artificial rupture of the membranes in labour.* Ausmed; 2020. https://www.ausmed.co.nz/cpd/articles/artificial-rupture-membranes-labour.
World Health Organization (WHO). *WHO recommendations: intrapartum care for a positive childbirth experience.* Geneva: World Health Organization; 2018. Licence: CC BY-NC-SA 3.0 IGO.
Wrønding T, Argyraki A, Petersen JF, et al. The aesthetic nature of the birthing room environment may alter the need for obstetrical interventions–an observational retrospective cohort study. *Sci Rep.* 2019;9:303. doi:10.1038/s41598-018-36416-x.
Yao AC, Moinan M, Lind J. Distribution of blood between infant and placenta after birth. *Lancet.* 1969;294(7626):871–873.
Yazdkhasti M, Moghimi Hanjani S, Mehdizadeh Tourzani Z. The effect of localized heat and cold therapy on pain intensity, duration of phases of labor, and birth outcomes among primiparous females: a randomized, controlled trial. *SEMJ.* 2018 ;19(8):e65501. doi:10.5812/semj.65501.
Zang Y, Lu H, Zhang H, et al. Benefits and risks of upright positions during the second stage of labour: An overview of systematic reviews. *Int J Nurs Stud.* 2021;114:103812.

Further reading

Chapman V, Charles C. *The Midwife's Labour and Birth Handbook.* Hoboken, USA: Wiley Blackwell; 2013.
Crowther S. *Joy at Birth: An interpretive, Hermeneutic, Phenomenological Inquiry.* Abingdon, UK: Routledge; 2021.
Davies L. *The Art and Soul of Midwifery: Creativity in Practice, Education and Research.* Edinburgh: Churchill Livingstone Elsevier; 2007.
Frye A. *Holistic Midwifery. A Comprehensive Textbook for Midwives in Homebirth Practice; Care of the Mother and Baby From the Onset of Labor Through the Hours After Birth.* Vol. II. 2nd ed. Oregon: Labrys Press; 2013.
Tikao K. *Iho—A Cord Between Two Worlds: Traditional Māori Birthing Practices (Master's thesis), Master of Science Communication).* Dunedin: University of Otago; 2013.
Walsh D, Byrom S. *Birth Stories for the Soul: Tales From Women, Families and Childbirth Professionals.* Cambridgeshire: Quay Books; 2009.

CHAPTER 26

Working with pain in labour

Nicky Leap

LEARNING OUTCOMES

Learning outcomes for this chapter are:

1. To describe some of the history and contested perspectives regarding pain in labour
2. To describe the evidence and benefits of 'working with pain' approaches to supporting women in labour
3. To engage in discussions with others about how to promote women's sense of confidence in their ability to cope with pain in labour.

CHAPTER OVERVIEW

This chapter explores the midwifery art of being with women in pain in labour. The advantages of promoting women's confidence in their ability to cope with pain are discussed in relation to evidence that supports this approach. Historical, psychosocial, cultural and feminist perspectives on pain in labour are presented in order to inform and highlight exemplary midwifery practice.

KEY TERMS

'being with' women
empowerment
'pain relief in labour'
promoting physiological birth
support in labour
working with pain
women's experiences of labour

INTRODUCTION

In discussing the midwifery art of **'being with' women** in pain in labour, this chapter explores the rationale for engaging with women and their families[a] around the role of pain in normal birth. While acknowledging that midwives must be prepared to support all women in labour, including those who choose to use pain medication, it is not the intention of this chapter to give midwives information about specific methods of 'pain relief' and their administration. Cochrane systematic reviews provide over 20 comprehensive analyses of relevant evidence, including overviews of 'pain management' in labour (Jones et al., 2012) and 'complementary and alternative therapies' (Smith et al., 2006), as well as 'labour hypnosis' (Madden et al., 2016), 'immersion in water' (Cluett & Burns, 2018), 'sterile water injections' (Derry et al., 2012), inhalation analgesia (Klomp et al., 2012), parenteral opioids (Smith et al., 2018) and 'epidural versus non-epidural or no analgesia' (Anim-Somuah et al., 2018). Midwives will also, no doubt, be mindful of guidelines that exist in their practice areas regarding 'pain relief' options and their administration.

For many there will be value in reading this chapter in conjunction with Chapter 25, in which Juliet Thorpe and Jacqui Anderson have provided a comprehensive guide to supporting women in labour. There are also handbooks that explore the practicalities of supporting labouring women using 'active birth' techniques (Chapman & Charles, 2017; Leap & Hunter, 2022; Simkin et al., 2017). An assumption has been made that midwives will be aware of the benefits of providing supportive strategies such as encouraging women to move around, find positions that feel right, use water and make noise if they wish. It is essential that midwives have these skills if they are to work with women in pain and encourage physiological birth.

In a culture where, increasingly, women are using epidural anaesthesia for pain management in labour,[b] it is also important that midwives are able to articulate why there is value in engaging with women around **'working with pain'** (Leap & Anderson, 2008; Sanders, 2015a, 2015b; Sanders & Lamb, 2014, 2017). Non-pharmacological methods of managing pain are associated with a reduction in obstetric interventions and with significant benefits for women and babies (Adams et al., 2015; Chaillet et al., 2014), and it is important to remember that pain-free labours are not associated with more positive experiences of labour for women (Anim-Somuah et al., 2018; Hodnett, 2002; Lindholm & Hildingsson, 2015). Furthermore, although many women expect their birth to be a significant and normal event, and one in which they can be proud of their abilities to embrace and manage pain (Downe et al., 2018; Rafalovich, 2016; Van der Gucht & Lewis, 2015; Whitburn et al., 2017, 2019), others are very frightened about the level of pain they might experience (Dencker et al., 2019; Fenwick et al., 2005; Haines et al., 2012; Wigert et al., 2020). In these circumstances, midwives can play a key role in understanding, recognising and addressing women's fears (Gutteridge, 2020; Otley, 2011; Whitburn et al., 2017, 2019).

Fear about pain and a loss of control in labour are related to an increase in the use of pharmacological pain relief, obstetric interventions and unhappy experiences of birth (Haines et al., 2012; Otley, 2011), with all the attending side effects and long-term increases in the risk of postnatal depression and post-traumatic stress disorder (Toohill et al., 2014). The potential for midwifery-led interventions and continuity-of-carer midwifery models to reduce the number of women experiencing birth trauma and post-traumatic stress disorder has been identified (Simpson & Catling, 2016). There is therefore an imperative to focus on strategies that can reduce women's fear and anxiety during pregnancy and labour and to explore ways of communicating that (en)courage women to believe in their abilities in the face of uncertainty—literally 'the promotion of courage' (Gutteridge, 2020; Leap & Hunter, 2022).

This chapter offers an overview of the evidence that midwives can draw on in order to engage with women around pain in labour, with a view to addressing anxieties and enabling situations in which women can feel more powerful and confident as a result of their experiences of pregnancy and birth. In order to promote situations in which this can happen, midwives can explore and appreciate the various meanings that may be associated with labour pain for individual women and their families (Mander, 2010; Thompson et al., 2019; Van der Gucht & Lewis, 2015; Whitburn et al., 2017, 2019). An understanding of how perspectives on the physiology of pain and the culture of **'pain relief in labour'** have evolved over the past century in high-income countries will provide a starting point.

HISTORICAL PERSPECTIVES ON PAIN IN LABOUR

A comprehensive history of the development of pain theories can be found in Melzack & Wall's groundbreaking work, *The Challenge of Pain* (Melzack & Wall, 1988). The traditional theory of pain is known as 'specificity theory'. Pain is seen as no more than a particularly complex signal, broadcast over nerves leading from the site of injury to the brain, as first suggested by Descartes in 1664 and modified by Muller in 1842 and then von Frey in 1894. Various theories on pain were developed in the first half of the 20th century, but a major breakthrough occurred in 1965 when Melzack & Wall proposed the 'gate control theory of pain'; this provided a conceptual framework for understanding how pain messages are filtered and facilitated or inhibited through a 'gate' in the spinal cord that modulates reception and responses (Melzack & Wall, 1965). In more recent years, Melzack (1999) proposed the 'neuromatrix' theory of pain, which retains key elements of the gate theory, but includes additional inputs from the brain. Memory, emotion, cultural factors, stress regulation, immune systems and past experiences all play a role in how the brain processes and synthesises genetic and sensory nerve impulses. The neuromatrix theory of pain can be used to enable understandings about the complexity of responses to pain; it can be a starting point for exploring the nature of labour pain and the beneficial effects of non-pharmacological methods of pain relief in labour (Lowe, 2002; Trout, 2004; Whitburn et al., 2017).

The notion of a systematic approach to 'pain control' in labour began in Edinburgh in the 1840s, with the experimental work of James Young Simpson (Caton, 1999). Simpson's introduction of inhalation anaesthesia in childbirth spawned a series of campaigns led by middle-class women demanding access to this resource. Such demands played a significant role in the move from home to hospital birth in the 20th century. Debates and concerns about the advisability of analgesia and anaesthesia, in terms of safety and possible physical and psychological consequences, have changed little since Simpson's day. The potential harmful side effects of drugs and the social value of pain versus the preservation of meaning in childbirth when pain is removed continue to be hotly debated issues (Caton, 1999) that affect how women approach labour pain.

In the early 1930s, Grantly Dick-Read published *Childbirth Without Fear: the Principles and Practice of Natural Childbirth* (Dick-Read, 1933). This book launched the concept of eliminating the cycle of 'fear, tension and pain' through counteractive education and training. Gentle, coached breathing and relaxation, with the emphasis on collaboration with a coach, were to play a vital role in keeping the woman on course in the teachings of the natural childbirth movement and later the 'psychoprophylaxis' movement in Europe and North America. In the latter decades of the 20th century, the mechanistic focus of psychoprophylaxis increasingly gave way to the psychosexual approach, a model that sees acceptance of labour as purposeful within the highly charged, significant act of giving birth, with its far-reaching sequelae for women's lives (Kitzinger, 2015). In the 1980s, this approach became incorporated into that of the Active Birth movement, which drew on activities and philosophies associated with the yoga tradition in teaching women to develop 'all of their bodily resources for giving birth, to follow their own instincts and to take full control of the childbirth experience' (Balaskas, 1992, back cover).

At the same time as the Active Birth movement was gaining momentum, a new dimension to understanding pain in labour—one incorporating neurohormonal physiology—was introduced by Michel Odent (1984), who proposed that intrinsic opiates, such as the endorphins released by marathon runners, enable labouring women to enter a state of consciousness that enhances the progress of labour as well as providing a way of coping with pain. Odent drew on the work of Newton and colleagues (Newton & Peeler, 1968; Newton et al., 1966) in suggesting that privacy, intimacy and non-disturbance are required to enable the delicate balance of hormonal cascades to interact and promote effective physiological processes. Odent (1984, p. 14) described the 'virtually ecstatic state' induced by endogenous opiates where women labour undisturbed as something that has always been sensed. This 'sense' of women having some 'inbuilt' coping mechanism has probably always been familiar to midwives in the absence of any physiological explanations, as described here by a retired midwife who practised in Britain in the 1930s:

> *I think myself that the system has a certain amount of sedative in itself that it releases at a time like that. I'm sure it has, because I've seen people that looked as if they were half sozzled—and they didn't have anything! Just looked like somebody 'gone'—and they hadn't had any dope.*
>
> (Leap & Hunter, 2013, p. 165)

The familiarity of women disappearing into their own world in strong labour meant that midwives and childbirth educators embraced the theory of the body's own pain-modifying substances as 'Nature's reward' (Ginesi, 1996, p. 9). A full scientific description of the role of endogenous opioids in spontaneous labour is needed if 'endorphin' theory is to be given widespread credence. However, it is thought that incoming impulses of pain stimulate the release of encephalins, dynorphins and endorphins in the dorsal horn of the spinal cord and that these opioid peptides have the ability to inhibit the sensations of pain carried by neurons to the brain. It is likely that oxytocin plays an equally important role in reducing pain as part of a complex interplay of neurohormonal cascades that promote the physiology of birth, breastfeeding and attachment. Australian GP and author Sarah Buckley (2015) has outlined evidence suggesting the profound importance of respecting and promoting this hormonal physiology in the ways in which we provide maternity care. This includes understanding the potential effect of the physical environment on neurohormonal physiology (Foureur, 2008; Foureur et al., 2010; Hammond et al., 2013, 2014a, 2014b).

Since the second half of the 20th century, challenges to the concept of managing labour pain with anaesthesia and analgesia have tended to concentrate on 'non-pharmacological methods of pain relief' (Simkin, 1989), with a nuanced shift in emphasis over the years to 'non-pharmacological pain management strategies' (Sanders & Lamb, 2017) and the use of 'comfort measures' in labour (Simkin, 2015). With the development of antenatal education came a belief that midwives should be preparing women for labour by giving them 'informed choice' about all the 'methods of pain relief'.

In recent decades, the offering of what Leap (2000) has referred to as the 'menu' of various methods of 'pain relief' has been associated with the notion of a woman's right to make 'informed choices' about all aspects of her care. This approach requires practitioners to adopt a systematic way of explaining the advantages and disadvantages of each method 'on the menu' so that the woman may make appropriate choices, usually in advance of labour. The potential problem with this approach is that the person providing the information influences the decisions that women make and women may receive a message that some form of pharmacological pain relief in labour is usually necessary (Leap & Edwards, 2006). This message might be subtle but it can underpin the use of decision-making aids for pain relief (Raynes-Greenow et al., 2007, 2010) and the ways in which maternity services provide information for pregnant women—for example, consider the messages that women might receive if accessing the NHS Choices website on 'pain relief in labour'.[c] It has been suggested that the current approach of asking pregnant women to make decisions about the sort of pain relief they might like ahead of labour needs reconsideration; it may be more useful to engage in discussions about women's values, expectations and preferences and how these might affect the ways they would respond to any given situation that might arise (Lally et al., 2014).

Drawing on research and experience regarding women's positive birthing experiences, midwives are increasingly articulating an approach that involves building women's confidence in their ability to find ways to deal with labour pain through drawing on their own resources with appropriate support (Karlsdottir et al., 2014; Leap & Anderson, 2008; Leap et al., 2010a; Sanders, 2015a, 2015b; Sanders & Lamb, 2014). The rationale for this 'working with pain' approach is supported by evidence (Leap et al., 2010b); it is based on the notion that pain is purposeful in promoting normal birth and that the 'triumph' women experience after a drug-free labour can have far-reaching consequences for how they feel about their capabilities as women and as mothers (Karlsdottir et al., 2014; Leap, 2010; Leap & Anderson, 2008; Leap et al., 2010a; Van der Gucht & Lewis, 2015). Experienced midwives have suggested that most women can manage the pain of uncomplicated labour but that women are more likely to need pharmacological help for the pain associated with malposition and dystocia (Leap, 2000).

WOMEN'S PERSPECTIVES ON PAIN IN LABOUR

As identified in two important overviews of literature related to women's experiences of labour pain (Thomson et al., 2019; Whitburn et al., 2019), these experiences vary widely; they are complex and influenced by factors beyond the physical functions of labour. The experience of pain itself may be mediated by physical, psychological, spiritual, social and cultural factors, including tradition, anxiety, emotional associations, the position of the baby in utero, and levels of preparation and support (Mander, 2010). A woman's state of mind during labour can also influence how she gives meaning to her experience of pain in labour—those who stay focused and accepting of pain tending to report more positive experiences than do those who become distracted and catastrophise about pain (Whitburn et al., 2014). Social interactions and support for women in labour can also affect the meaning that women ascribe to labour pain: where women are encouraged to see it as purposeful and productive (as opposed to threatening), they are more likely to draw on their inner resources for managing pain and to report positive experiences (Whitburn et al., 2017).

Women have identified how much they value support for coping with labour pain and access to different ways of reducing or managing pain (Downe et al., 2018; Karlsdottir et al., 2014; Lundgren & Dahlberg, 1998, 2002; Ross-Davie & Cheyne, 2014; Van der Gucht & Lewis, 2015). In a number of studies, women have expressed satisfaction with the midwifery care they received when the midwife was 'present' in the room, offering support and information (Ross-Davie & Cheyne, 2014; Ross-Davie et al., 2014). They also valued feeling respected and commented on the sense of trust that evolved, even when they had not met the midwives prior to labour (Berg et al., 1996, 2012).

Culturally diverse groups of women have described childbirth as a difficult but empowering experience leading to a sense of achievement and a feeling of pride in their ability to cope with intense pain (Callister et al., 2003; Dickenson et al., 2003; Halldorsdottir & Karlsdottir, 1996; Karlsdottir et al., 2014; Leap et al., 2010a; Lundgren & Dahlberg, 1998; Niven & Murphy-Black, 2000). In contrast, women who have had obstetric interventions, particularly those who had unknown attendants, have described increased anxiety and pain and less emphasis on their active participation in birth (Callister et al., 2003).

Effective forms of pain relief are not necessarily associated with greater satisfaction when women evaluate their experience of birth (Anim-Somuah, 2018; Heinz & Sleigh, 2003; Hodnett, 2002; Kannan et al., 2001; Waldenström et al., 2004). Studies have repeatedly shown that the quality of support and the caregiver relationship are so important to women that they override the influences of age, socioeconomic status, ethnicity, childbirth preparation and the physical birth environment; the influence of pain, pain relief and intrapartum medical interventions on subsequent satisfaction are not as obvious, direct or powerful as the influence of the attitudes of the caregivers who provide **support in labour** (Hodnett, 2002).

With this in mind, it has been proposed that increases in epidural use may be associated with fragmented and unsupportive maternity care as well as a culture imbued with the dominance of biomedical discourse over other knowledge disciplines (Newnham et al., 2016, 2018; Walsh, 2009). Practice regarding epidurals, narcotics and elective caesarean section varies greatly regionally, between different maternity units and according to practitioner employment status, with particularly high rates in the private obstetrics sector (Dahlen et al., 2012; Roberts et al., 2000). Variations appear often to be related to institutional or professional opinion factors rather than to population factors or individual women's choices (Hodnett, 2002).

Women who express a desire to have a normal birth often cite concerns about the side effects associated with the use of opioids and epidurals as a major source of motivation (Henry & Nand, 2004). Although epidural analgesia is very effective in reducing pain, it can be associated with a range of increased risks for women, including having difficulty passing urine, fever, and very low blood pressure, as well as prolonged labour, fetal malposition, augmentation and instrumental vaginal birth (Anim-Somuah et al., 2018; Newnham et al., 2016). The use of opioids is associated with harmful effects on the mother's birth experience, longer labours, compromise of the baby and difficulties in initiating and sustaining breastfeeding (Bai et al., 2013; Burchell et al., 2016). Furthermore, although such drugs induce sedation and may therefore give caregivers the impression of having relieved pain, women overwhelmingly report on how ineffective opioids are in providing pain relief (Bricker & Lavender, 2002; Olofsson et al., 1996; Smith et al., 2018). Such concerns sit within wider debates about the potential public and psychological health impact of rates of intervention that are above those indicated by current evidence (Dahlen et al., 2012; Davis et al., 2011; Tracy & Tracy, 2003).

The particular nature of labour pain

The Association of Radical Midwives (UK) has always paid tribute to the value of learning from women's accounts of their births and, since its inception in 1978, its newsletter has consistently published birth stories written by women. An example is the moving account by Agnes Kotreba (1994), who gave birth after a fast labour before her midwives arrived. Her account acknowledges aspects of loneliness, potential death, images of water, and the physical and mental challenges of pain that are common themes elsewhere:

> *Dear God, how many more hours? I especially don't let myself panic or drown in this tidal wave which breaks my entrails and comes from a distance like the sound of a plane, intensifying until it gets intolerable, and then nothing—nothing, no pain whatsoever. I'm like cleansed, surprised, pulverized—Will I have the strength to endure the next attack? ... I twist myself in pain ... I think I emit a sound ... so far I am unable to show my suffering, it's my business, my biggest intimacy, my most complete and total nudity.*
>
> (Kotreba, 1994, pp. 16–17)

When considering such accounts, Vangie Kelpin (1992) suggests that it is not useful to compare labour pain to any other pain. She also questions the validity of fragmenting our understanding by analysing the pain of labour within different theories such as physical, psychological, sociological and cultural perspectives. She suggests that such approaches militate against the understanding of the nature of 'painfulness' as lived by women and mothers and that the inwardness of the birth experience is an opportunity to be attentive to:

> *... the deep significance of the momentous quality of the pain ... As we are surrounded by the deep sense of inwardness, we are forced to recognize our independence, our loneliness, our selfhood. To be conscious of our own existence. This actual self-consciousness exposes to us our wholeness, our strengths and our endurance.*
>
> (Kelpin, 1992, p. 101)

The pain of labour is constructed by Kelpin as an expression of 'the narrow gateway leading to release in the expanse of life' (p. 101). The release she describes with the birth of the baby is given the significance of change from 'self-as-world' to 'baby-as-world' where a new pain comes with the awe of focusing on a new being. Kelpin quotes Phyllis Chesler (1979, p. 281): 'Being born with motherhood is the sharpest pain I've known' and uses words like 'relief', 'disbelief', 'joy' and 'exhilaration' to describe the excitement and poignancy of the new baby's presence (p. 102).

Many women say that labour pain is quite different from any pain that is associated with injury or trauma, but that this is hard to explain in concrete terms. In her important study of pain, Elaine Scarry (1985) states that the person in pain may experience pain as 'the most vibrant example of what it is to have certainty': pain is 'effortlessly grasped', while for the onlooker the other person's pain is so elusive that it could be seen as 'the primary model of what it is to have doubt'; here, 'what is effortless is not grasping it' (Scarry, 1985, p. 4):

> *Pain can be seen as capable of bringing about an absolute split between one's own sense of reality and that of another person, even when in close proximity [as during labour].*
>
> (Scarry, 1985, p. 4)

This concept is significant for midwives who sit alongside women in pain; they can respond to cues given by the woman in order to offer support and suggestions, but primarily the midwife's role is to help the woman identify her own spontaneous coping strategies (Escott et al., 2004, 2009) and to be alert to aspects of care and the environment that disrupt these (Spiby et al., 2004).

It has been suggested that midwives consistently underestimate the intensity of pain experienced by women in labour (Chamberlain et al., 1993). This may be a coping mechanism on the part of midwives as the onlookers of pain. Scarry (1985) suggests that doubting a person in pain as an 'unreliable narrator' amplifies their suffering (pp. 6–7). However, recognising the severity of pain that a woman is experiencing during labour does not necessarily equate to the need to offer pain relief. In fact, women identify that when they are in pain any offer of pain relief is irresistible and potentially undermines their confidence in their ability to cope without using pharmacological pain relief:

> *I didn't really want an epidural. That wasn't what I was saying. What I wanted was something magic that no one's ever thought of before, that you were going to quickly invent right then to make it all better. But I really didn't want an epidural. It was an expression of my pain.*
>
> (Leap, 1997, p. 49)

Midwives and women have talked about the significance of the particular nature of pain in labour: its rhythms, the fact that it has a positive, finite goal, and that it stops as soon as the baby is born and then cannot be recalled.

But who can remember the pain [of childbirth], once it's over? All that remains of it is a shadow, not in the mind even, in the flesh. Pain marks you but too deep to see. Out of sight, out of mind.
(Atwood, 1987, p. 135)

Keeping in mind the particular nature of labour pain helps midwives resist the temptation to offer what is often described in healthcare as 'adequate pain relief', as explained here by a midwife:

Afterwards, I'm still emotionally and physically wrecked and they've moved on completely. It's like, through a fog they can remember the time they were pleading for an epidural but they've moved on. So that's been significant for me just in terms of women's ability to recover or move on or have a different agenda in a very short space of time. And that's given me enormous confidence to … just be there … and not see pain as long-term damage.
(Leap, 1997, p. 48)

AVOIDING ASSUMPTIONS ABOUT WOMEN'S EXPERIENCES OF PAIN IN LABOUR

Pain is never the sole creation of our anatomy and physiology; it emerges only at the intersection of bodies, minds and cultures.
(Morris, 1991, p. 1)

As midwives we constantly need to think about how our own 'bodies, minds and cultures' might affect our attitudes and responses to pain in labour. Hannah Dahlen (2010) suggests that the starting point for dealing with women's fear of childbirth is to examine our own fear and how this might potentially contribute to **women's experiences of labour** and escalating interventions. This concept is intrinsically linked to our exploring how we feel when we are alongside women who are finding contractions really painful and the decisions we make about what is appropriate support. Similarly, our own attitudes, values and assumptions can influence how we predict the ways women will experience labour.

Whilst we all tend to use stereotypes in order to interact with labouring women in ways we hope are appropriate, a study by Green and colleagues (1990) highlighted the common labour ward stereotypes of the 'well-educated, middle class NCT type' and the 'uneducated, working class woman'. Contrary to the assumptions of the midwives, they found that women in these stereotyped groups were equally likely to want to avoid pharmacological pain relief in labour; women who were less educated had the highest expectations that birth would be a fulfilling experience and were more likely to resist handing over control to staff.

Experienced midwives are aware of the pitfalls in deciding who will or will not cope with the pain of normal labour:

Women constantly shock me and I think I've learnt from those women. You could sit there and think, 'She's a hopeless case, she said her pain threshold's really low'—and all you've got to do is tell her she's doing well, that it's normal and allow her to get on with it in her own way, and I think she will.
(Leap, 1997, p. 44)

Stereotyping can also occur when midwives attempt to apply an understanding of the psychological factors that might be influencing women's experiences of pain in labour. Joan Raphael-Leff (1986) has drawn on psychotherapeutic practice in suggesting that conscious and unconscious attitudes or 'orientations' to pregnancy, labour and motherhood will affect whether women see labour as a 'natural event' or a 'depleting, medical event', and that this in turn will affect their experience of labour pain. She encourages midwives to identify the psychological factors that may assist them in recognising and acknowledging individual women's needs in labour. Some midwives feel that they should work out the deep psychological processes affecting the women they care for and that they should identify and help women get rid of the 'baggage' that might impede the process of childbirth—a practice that has been questioned (Leap, 2010; Oakley, 1980). Concerns have been expressed about the disempowering effect that such approaches can have on women where there is a shift in the midwife's role from empathetic listener to a more interventionist psychological role (Gosden, 1996; Gosden & Saul, 1999).

It is also important never to assume that a woman will respond to labour pain in a culturally determined way. As explored in Chapter 10, midwives constantly have to challenge our instinctive tendencies to engage in ethnocentric assumptions, particularly when working with people from Indigenous communities.

Bowler (1993) showed how midwives are in danger of stereotyping women according to their cultural background. In her study, she demonstrated how midwives dismissed Asian women in pain as 'making a fuss about nothing' because they were perceived to have a low pain threshold. This assumption led to women receiving less support than that offered to other women and pain relief being withheld. The racist notion that all women who share a particular culture are the same can mask the needs of individual women and lead to poorer service provision.

A book describing Māori women's experiences of pregnancy and birth, *Ukaipo* (Rimene et al., 1998), highlighted communication as an area where possible misunderstandings could arise. One woman pointed to the fact that nodding the head after receiving information from a midwife does not necessarily indicate understanding. Sometimes it is merely an effort to try to please or just to acknowledge that the information has been heard.

It is through *listening to women* that professionals may develop an understanding of the complex meanings that women attribute to labour pain. This may be significant in how midwives engage with women, and in particular how we facilitate discussions about labour in pregnancy and reflections afterwards (Mander, 2010).

Ultimately, being with women in labour requires us to be aware of the highly individual conditioning and circumstances that will affect how women respond to contractions. Women who have been taught self-hypnosis or calm-birthing techniques may breathe their way through contractions; at the other end of the spectrum are women who find the best way to respond is to run around the room roaring. The skill of the midwife is to be 'clueful' and open to the myriad of ways that women manage labour:

> *Our expertise as midwives rests in our ability to watch, to listen and to respond to any given situation with all of our senses. This will include the conscious and subconscious 'knowing' that has been generated from our experience and learning. It also involves a 'cluefulness' as we respond to the overt and covert clues from women and their worlds. The skill lies in knowing when to inform, suggest, act, seek help and, most importantly, when to be still or when to withdraw and remove ourselves. Our belief in a woman's inherent ability to be her own and her baby's expert should underpin all of these responses.*
>
> (Leap, 2010, p. 22)

PAIN IN LABOUR AND THE NOTION OF EMPOWERMENT

> *To have experienced birthing pain offers the possibilities of self knowledge, knowledge of our limitations and capabilities, knowledge of new life, as mother and of our place in the mysterious cycle of human life: birth, death and rebirth. As we birth our children, we, in a sense, birth ourselves. We are mothers, like our mothers, and our daughters after us.*
>
> (Kelpin, 1992, p. 103)

The notion of women 'being born' with their babies is described by one respondent in a study of young, single women who developed strategies in order to have children. This young woman described how the birth led her to make significant changes in her life, in particular in relation to her own parents. In spite of an extremely traumatic labour and birth, she reported:

> *It was about the best thing I ever experienced. I was totally amazed. The labour was like I had died ... I had just died. The minute she came out, I was born again. It was like we'd just been born together.*
>
> (Lewin, 1985, p. 135)

In her 'germinal' (feminist alternative to seminal)[d] text Adrienne Rich (1976) advises caution when it comes to the metaphor of 'I am a woman giving birth to myself'. She suggests that, for most women, there has always been a distinct lack of choice and very little consciousness around childbirth, let alone personal growth. Historically, women have always been told how they should feel about labour pain, from the classic victimisation of 'Eve's curse' to the 'ecstatic fulfillment' of the natural birth movement (p. 156). Rich makes a plea for us to view childbirth as challenge rather than pain, 'as one way of knowing and coming to terms with our bodies, of discovering our physical and psychic resources' (p. 157), as 'one experience of liberating ourselves from fear, passivity and alienation from our bodies' (p. 184). She suggests that there are far-reaching implications in highlighting the need for women to be attended by midwives who respond to a woman's distress in labour as a cry for active care and support, rather than as a demand to have pain taken away or numbed.

Andrea Robertson (1996, p. 19) sees the universality of pain in labour as a bond between women, 'a fundamental truth that confirms our special biological role and affirms the importance of our contribution to society'. Feminists may find Robertson's biological reductionism difficult, especially when she refers to women's bodies as 'designed to be as efficient as possible' and describes 'the very few failures ... necessary to ensure reproductive success amongst strong breeding stock' (Robertson, 1996, p. 19). Nevertheless, she makes an impassioned plea for reclaiming pain in labour. She sees its role as vital in stimulating hormonal responses that allow a biological function to take place with optimum efficiency, while at the same time promoting the 'innate sexuality' of the experience of labour. The body's 'natural painkillers' can be released and a positive emotional climate is ensured for the meeting of mother and child (Robertson, 1996, p. 19). In a later study, Robertson (2004) describes 'transition' (the name given to the end of the first stage of labour, when women are generally expressing most difficulty with pain) as 'the moment of truth' and suggests that 'it may be very important to allow women to have the experience of conquering an overwhelming personal crisis, to promote confidence and self-esteem in the new mother' (Robertson, 2004, p. 92).

> *Submission to the all-consuming and overwhelming nature of birth and the weathering of the inherent pain of labour is an empowering process for a woman, and one that should not be denied unless critical for her own well-being or that of her baby.*
>
> (Robertson, 2004, p. 88)

Kathryn Allen Rabuzzi (1994) was originally inspired to write about the potential 'ecstasy' of birth after an unanticipated 'natural' birth in the late 1950s which left her with a quest to find out more about the extraordinary and unanticipated feelings of 'dying, being born, and giving birth' and the accompanying sensations of 'outward and inward expansion' (Rabuzzi, 1994, p. vii). She claims that, in order for women to reframe the deeply acculturated belief that childbirth is painful and dangerous, they need to see pain as something to conquer rather than something posing a threat to conquer us. This way, she suggests, its meaning though not its intensity may change, although she recognises that there is a potential problem with reconceptualising around 'control' when many midwives propose a 'letting go' approach to labour (Rabuzzi, 1994, pp. 98–105).

Whatever the circumstances in which women give birth, there is no doubt that 'strong, competent, capable mothers who trust themselves and know their inner strength' (Katz-Rothman, 1996, p. 254) are ideally placed to rise to the challenges of new motherhood. This can affect early attachment and ongoing parenting relationships, which are critical to the long-term health of individuals. Positive attachment can have far-reaching consequences: children who are securely attached as infants tend to develop stronger self-esteem and better self-reliance as they grow older, leading to independence and confidence. These children also tend to perform better in school, have successful social relationships and experience less depression and anxiety (Redshaw, 2006).

PAIN IN LABOUR AND THE MIDWIFE–WOMAN RELATIONSHIP

There is strong evidence that continuity of caregiver throughout pregnancy, labour and birth reduces the amount of pain relief that women have during labour and increases their satisfaction with their maternity care (Forster et al., 2016; McLachlan et al., 2012; Sandall et al., 2016). This may be due to the relationship of trust that develops and the ability of midwives to enable situations where both the woman and her midwife/midwives feel confident and positive when approaching birth (Leap et al., 2010a; Walsh & Newburn, 2002). In situations where there is not necessarily a midwifery relationship that has developed through pregnancy, women who have continuous support from a female caregiver who is not a professional during labour are less likely to use pharmacological pain relief and are more likely to have a spontaneous vaginal birth (Bohren et al., 2017). It may be that midwives who work in situations that do not enable continuity of care are more likely to have to deal with the demands of the institution; they are less likely to be able to concentrate on intensive support of the woman than is a lay person, such as a 'doula', who knows the woman and is focused on helping her to find her inner resources in coping with pain without resorting to pharmacological pain relief (Bohren et al., 2017).

Where midwives work with women throughout pregnancy, labour and the postnatal period they are able to engage in discussions with individual women around grappling with uncertainty and the potential challenges of labour. The midwife's interpretation of pain is a key factor in these discussions. She[e] may convey the message that the pain of labour is a safe and purposeful pain that many women find manageable. Women are more likely to feel they can cope with labour if they are able to conceptualise labour pain as productive and purposeful; conversely, where they interpret pain as threatening they are more likely to have negative feelings and turn to pharmacological pain relief (Whitburn et al., 2017). In an Australian study, women identified that, during labour, the words and actions of people around them had a profound positive influence on the way they handled pain in labour—where people around them were known, trusted and calm, women felt safe and emotionally supported (Whitburn et al., 2017).

The midwife can explain that the sensations of contractions are different from other types of pain, such as the pain of injury. For many women who have not experienced labour, it is reassuring when the midwife explains that a contraction is a strong muscular activity that 'builds to a peak, starts to fade, lasts about a minute and then fades into a rest'; this has been coined 'the midwifery wave' owing to the associated hand movements that midwives worldwide tend to use when explaining this to women (Leap & Hunter 2022 p. 74).

In high-income countries, pain generally has negative connotations—it represents trauma, disease or stress, and something fearful, to be avoided or alleviated—and it is therefore a challenge for midwives to help women (re) frame their understanding of pain. Given the high rates of epidural anaesthesia in Australia and Aotearoa New Zealand,[b] the task of enabling situations where women embrace the pain of labour as part of a normal, physiological event is particularly challenging (Fenwick et al., 2005).

Where a midwife is able to provide continuity of care through pregnancy, she has the opportunity to engage with the people the woman has chosen to support her during labour, and explain to them the rationale for not automatically trying to take away pain in labour. This is particularly effective where midwives are able to visit the woman's home towards the end of pregnancy and make plans for the labour and birth, possibly sharing photographs of women in labour (Kemp & Sandall, 2010). This visit to the woman's home provides an ideal opportunity to talk about how being alongside the woman in pain might affect her supporters. The concept of decision making about the place of birth during labour can be explored, with a clear message that it is safe to stay at home when labour is progressing well and where the midwife is well supported to provide this service in the woman's home by staff in a referral hospital.

The approaches to engaging with women and their birth supporters described here are often in conflict with institutionalised pressures to ensure that women are informed about the full range of 'pain relief' options in order to make an 'informed choice'. It has been suggested that women are not prepared adequately for the amount of pain they will experience, with many women ending up having an epidural who had not wanted one (Halls, 2008; Lally et al., 2008). When responding to recommendations that women should be better informed about labour pain and 'pain relief' (Lally et al., 2008; Raynes-Greenow et al., 2007, 2010), midwives are challenged to find ways to ensure that the underlying message they are giving still reinforces belief in the women's ability to cope with pain in normal labour without having an epidural (Leap & Anderson, 2008).

The sorts of phrases that midwives use to encourage women in labour are often incorporated into antenatal preparation classes for self-hypnosis in labour (Semple & Newburn, 2011)—such as 'hypnobirthing' and 'calm birth'—as the phrases are deliberately steeped in positive messages to the subconscious, for example:

- Your body will tell you what to do.
- Every contraction will bring you closer to meeting your baby.

- When the contraction fades away you can forget about it because it has done its job and brought you closer to your baby.
- Between contractions there's a nice long rest.
- You can allow your labour to progress at just the right rate for you.
- Contractions are a wonderful power working for you.
- You can give birth to your baby safely and comfortably, trusting your body.

It is likely that the success or failure of any plans for wanting to avoid pharmacological pain relief in labour that women might have are vulnerable to the actions and attitudes of the caregivers they have during labour. There is strong evidence that women are less likely to use epidurals when they have continuous support in labour (Bohren et al., 2017), in midwifery-led care (Sandall et al., 2016) and where they give birth at home or in 'alternative hospital settings' where epidurals are not immediately available (Bohren et al., 2017; Hodnett et al., 2012). Common elements of this care include emotional support, information about labour progress and advice regarding comfort measures (Simkin, 2015). In fact, continuous support has been viewed in itself as a form of pain relief, specifically as an alternative to epidural anaesthesia (Dickenson et al., 2003) because of concerns about the deleterious effects of epidural anaesthesia on labour progress.

Individual women's responses to contractions are likely to change as labour progresses. In Chapter 25, the authors have discussed how support can be adapted at each stage of this process. As a straightforward labour unfolds, the midwife can provide encouragement and reinforce the notion that what the woman is feeling is entirely normal and appropriate. Many women benefit from praise and the expression of quiet confidence that all is well. Phrases using the woman's name, such as, 'Well done, Sarah' and 'You're doing really well, Sarah' spoken quietly after each contraction characterises the 'midwifery muttering' (Leap, 2010) that can have a steadying effect on a woman. This is particularly important if the woman is doubting her ability to cope. It is not uncommon to hear women reflect on their labours and say, 'She believed in me when I didn't believe in myself' and 'I didn't think I was doing well, but my midwife said I was doing well so I thought, "Well I must be doing OK then!"' (Leap et al., 2010a). Similarly, women's partners value the reassurance of the midwife's steadying voice and demeanour. This is important given the potential distress of seeing a partner in pain and the suggestion that men's experiences of labour are significantly improved where their partner has an epidural (Capogna et al., 2007).

Women can be encouraged to 'tune out' and concentrate on meeting each contraction and then seeing it off with a steadying deep breath, rather than interacting with their surroundings. This approach is described here by an experienced midwife:

> *I think [the first part of the labour] is often the most difficult part because they're very intellectually 'there'. They are having to mastermind and intellectualise the process and cope with it on that level. Once they get further up the track in their labour, then they go into 'dozy land' when the endorphins are released and I think it's an easier phase. They capitulate to the process, whereas at the beginning they are often intellectually trying to mastermind it. Once they capitulate and allow the process to go, then I think they usually deal with it a lot better. I often say 'You are not alone. There will be hundreds of women out in the world doing exactly what you are doing right now. This is a really big journey in your life but it is a journey women have made since time began.'*
>
> (Vague, 2003, p. 74)

It is easier to encourage women in their abilities to cope with labour when there is a trusting relationship that has been established during pregnancy; however, many midwives who meet the woman for the first time in labour are skilled at developing trust and 'working with pain'. Students express their appreciation of working alongside and learning from midwives and doulas who support women in this way (Berg et al., 1996, 2012). The quality of this support extends to women who choose or need to have pharmacological pain relief in labour.

In New Zealand the majority of women have a midwife as their lead maternity care provider and have reported on the value of this continuity of care (Ministry of Health, 2014). In Australia, student midwives are often the only healthcare practitioners providing individual women with continuity of care (as part of their education in continuity-of-care/follow-through experiences); women have identified how important that was for them in terms of the support they received for managing pain in labour (Browne & Taylor, 2014; Rolls & McGuinness, 2007; Tickle et al., 2016). Ultimately, the experience of labour—particularly the kind and unkind things that people say when a woman is facing uncertainty and pain—is never forgotten (Leap & Hunter, 2013; Simkin, 1991, 1992). In the words of midwifery lecturer Rachel Smith in her message to students (Leap & Hunter, 2022, p. 266):

> *You have stepped into a woman's life at the most vulnerable time of her life . . . into a situation where 60 or 70 years later, she will remember everything you said to her, everything you did, how you made her feel . . . You can make a difference for every woman who crosses your path.*

CRITICAL THINKING EXERCISE

In pairs, discuss how you would respond to a pregnant woman who says, 'I'd like to manage labour without an epidural or any drugs but I probably won't succeed as I've got a low pain threshold'. Practise your responses with each other, taking it in turns to be the pregnant woman. Together, write a script of a conversation that might ensue when a woman says this, to include all the messages that you think might help her to build her confidence in her abilities to manage pain in labour with appropriate support.

REFLECTIVE THINKING EXERCISE

Consider the following questions in relation to your own practice.

1. How do I discuss labour pain with pregnant women and their families?
2. What messages might I be giving about 'working with pain' and/or 'pain relief'?
3. Am I clear about the evidence regarding the potential unwanted side effects of pharmacological pain relief?
4. How do I respond when women in uncomplicated labour plead for an epidural?
5. How do I explore women's experiences of pain in labour in order to inform my practice?

Conclusion

Midwives and students have an important role to play in fostering women's belief that they will be able to cope with the pain of normal labour, and this has potential consequences for women in terms of **empowerment** and avoiding the unwanted consequences of obstetric intervention. Where a woman chooses pharmacological pain relief, or if an epidural is necessary due to complications, the way in which the midwife engages with the woman around her experiences of labour is equally important. As studies repeatedly show that the relationships, interactions and support are what matter to women, rather than the degree of pain itself, there is an imperative to engage with women and their supporters about pain in labour, including during pregnancy and reflecting afterwards in a process of learning together.

Review questions

In pairs, small groups or on your own:

1. List positive words and phrases that women might use to describe 'labour pain'.
2. Describe 10 ways in which you would assist a woman to 'work with' labour pain.
3. How might you respond if a colleague says, 'In this day and age, no woman should have to have pain in labour'?
4. How might a woman's responses to pain in labour help you understand the progress she is making?
5. How might you explain to a pregnant woman the role of endorphins and oxytocin in normal labour?
6. How might the ideas expressed in research on the effect of the environment on the neurohormonal physiology of labour affect a woman's experience of pain in labour and the support you might provide for her?
7. Give five examples of the way in which pain in labour has been interpreted historically.
8. How do you think the pain of labour differs from postsurgical pain?
9. List phrases you might use when describing pharmacological and non-pharmacological methods of 'pain relief' to a pregnant woman—without adopting a 'menu approach'.

NOTES

a. The words 'woman' and 'women' are used in this chapter. This in no way means to undermine or exclude people who give birth who do not identify as women. 'Families' is used in a similar way to the New Zealand concept of 'whānau' to mean the network of significant people to whom the woman turns for support during her experience of pregnancy, birth and new motherhood.

b. In 2019, 32% of women in Australia (Australian Institute of Health and Welfare, 2021) and 27% of women in New Zealand (Ministry of Health, 2021) had an epidural for pain management during labour.

c. For critique: *NHS Choices: Pain Relief in Labour*: https://www.nhs.uk/conditions/pregnancy-and-baby/pages/pain-relief-labour.aspx.

d. Sheila Kitzinger (2015) encouraged the use of the word 'ovular', rather than 'seminal' in order to address the sexist roots of language, but Sara Wickham (2017) has suggested that 'germinal' may be a more appropriate alternative, since it encompasses both egg and sperm.

e. The female pronoun is used here as the majority of midwives are women. This is not intended to exclude or undermine men who are midwives.

Online resources

Buckley SJ. Hormonal Physiology of Childbearing: Evidence and Implications for Women, Babies, and Maternity Care. 2015. Online: https://www.nationalpartnership.org/our-work/resources/health-care/maternity/hormonal-physiology-of-childbearing.pdf

Leap N, Dodwell M, Newburn M. Working With Pain in Labour: An Overview of Evidence. Evidence Based Briefing Paper. 2010. Online: https://www.nct.org.uk/sites/default/files/related_documents/Research%20overview-%20Working%20with%20pain%20in%20labour_6.pdf

Simkin P. Comfort in Labour: How You Can Help Yourself to a Normal Satisfying Childbirth. 2015. Online: http://www.nationalpartnership.org/research-library/maternal-health/comfort-in-labor-simkin.pdf.

References

Adams J, Frawley J, Steel A, et al. Use of pharmacological and non-pharmacological labor pain management techniques and their relationship to maternal and infant birth outcomes: examination of a nationally representative sample of 1,835 pregnant women. *Midwifery*. 2015;31:458–463.

Anim-Somuah M, Smyth RMD, Cyna AM, et al. Epidural versus non-epidural or no analgesia for pain management in labour. *Cochrane Database Syst Rev*. 2018;(5):CD000331, doi:10.1002/14651858.CD000331.pub4.

Atwood M. *The Handmaid's Tale*. London: Virago; 1987.

Australian Institute of Health and Welfare (AIHW). *Australia's Mothers and Babies 2019*. 2021. Online: https://www.aihw.gov.au/getmedia/bba093ef-a623-4cfd-818b-1bb5af9f0d20/Australia-s-mothers-and-babies.pdf.aspx?inline=true.

Bai DL, Wu KM, Tarrant M. Association between intrapartum interventions and breastfeeding duration. *J Midwifery Womens Health*. 2013;58(1):25–32.

Balaskas J. *Active Birth: The New Approach to Giving Birth Naturally*. Harvard: Harvard Common Press; 1992.

Berg M, Lundgren I, Hermansson E, et al. Women's experience of the encounter with the midwife during childbirth. *Midwifery*. 1996;12:11–15.

Berg M, Olafsdóttir OA, Lundgren I. A midwifery model of woman-centred childbirth care—in Swedish and Icelandic settings. *Sex Reprod Healthc*. 2012;3:79–87.

Bohren MA, Hofmeyr GJ, Sakala C, et al. Continuous support for women during childbirth. *Cochrane Database Syst Rev*. 2017;(7):CD003766, doi:10.1002/14651858.CD003766.pub6.

Bowler I. Stereotypes of women of Asian descent in midwifery: some evidence. *Midwifery*. 1993;9:7–16.

Bricker L, Lavender T. Parenteral opioids for labour pain relief: a systematic review. *Am J Obstet Gynecol*. 2002;186(5):94–109.

Browne J, Taylor J. 'It's a good thing…': women's views on their continuity experiences with midwifery students from one Australian region. *Midwifery*. 2014;30(3):e108–e114.

Buckley SJ. *Hormonal Physiology of Childbearing: Evidence and Implications for Women, Babies, and Maternity Care*. 2015. Online: https://www.nationalpartnership.org/our-work/resources/health-care/maternity/hormonal-physiology-of-childbearing.pdf.

Burchell T, Coster S, Norman I. The effect of intrapartum pethidine on breastfeeding: a scoping review. *Evid Based Midwifery*. 2016;14(2):49–56.

Callister LC, Khalaf I, Semenic S, et al. The pain of childbirth: perceptions of culturally diverse women. *Pain Manag Nurs*. 2003;4(4):145–154.

Capogna G, Camorcia M, Stirparo S. Expectant fathers' experience during labor with or without epidural analgesia. *Int J Obstet Anesth*. 2007;16(2):110–115.

Caton D. *What a Blessing She Had Chloroform: The Medical and Social Response to the Pain of Childbirth From 1800 to the Present*. New Haven: Yale University Press; 1999.

Chaillet N, Belaid L, Crochetiere C, et al. Nonpharmacologic approaches for pain management during labor compared with usual care: a meta-analysis. *Birth*. 2014;41(2):122–137.

Chamberlain G, Wraight A, Steer P, eds. *Pain and its Relief in Childbirth: The Results of a National Survey Conducted by the National Birthday Trust*. Edinburgh: Churchill Livingstone; 1993.

Chapman V, Charles C. (eds). *The Midwife's Labour and Birth Handbook*. 4th Edition. Chichester: John Wiley & Sons; 2017.

Chesler P. *With Child: A Diary of Motherhood*. New York: Thomas Y Crowell; 1979.

Cluett ER, Burns E, Cuthbert A. Immersion in water during labour and birth. *Cochrane Database Syst Rev*. 2018;(5):CD000111, doi:10.1002/14651858.CD000111.pub4.

Dahlen H. Undone by fear? Deluded by trust? Commentary. *Midwifery*. 2010;26(2):156–162. doi:10.1016/j.midw.2009.11.008.

Dahlen HG, Tracy S, Tracy M, et al. Rates of obstetric intervention among low-risk women giving birth in private and public hospitals in NSW: a population-based descriptive study. *BMJ Open Access*. 2012;5:e001723.

Davis DL, Baddock S, Pairman S, et al. Planned place of birth in New Zealand: Does it affect mode of birth and intervention rates among low-risk women? *Birth*. 2011;38(2):111–119.

Dencker A, Nilsson C, Begley C., et al. Causes and outcomes in studies of fear of childbirth: a systematic review. *Women Birth*. 2019;32(2): 99–111.

Derry S, Straube S, Moore RA, et al. Intracutaneous or subcutaneous sterile water injection compared with blinded controls for pain management in labour (Review). *Cochrane Database Syst Rev*. 2012;(1):CD009107. doi:009110.001002/14651858.CD14009107.pub14651852.

Dickenson J, Paech M, McDonald S, et al. Maternal satisfaction with childbirth and intrapartum analgesia in nulliparous labour. *Aust N Z J Obstet Gynaecol*. 2003;43(6):463–469.

Dick-Read G. *Childbirth Without Fear: The Principles and Practice of Natural Childbirth*. London: Heinemann; 1933.

Downe S, Finlayson K, Oladapo OT, et al. (2018). What matters to women during childbirth: a systematic qualitative review. *PLoS ONE*. 2018;13(4):e0194906.

Escott D, Spiby H, Slade P, et al. The range of coping strategies women use to manage pain and anxiety prior to and during first experience of labour. *Midwifery*. 2004;20(2):144–156.

Escott D, Slade P, Spiby H. Preparation for pain management during childbirth: the psychological aspects of coping strategy development in antenatal education. *Clin Psychol Rev*. 2009;29: 617–622.

Fenwick J, Hauck Y, Downie J, et al. The childbirth expectations of a self-selected cohort of Western Australian women. *Midwifery*. 2005;21:23–35.

Forster DA, McLachlan HL, Davey M-A, et al. Continuity of care by a primary midwife (caseload midwifery) increases women's satisfaction with antenatal, intrapartum and postpartum care: results from the COSMOS randomised controlled trial. *BMC Pregnancy Childbirth*. 2016;16:28.

Foureur M. Creating birth space to enable undisturbed birth. In: Fahy K, Foureur M, Hastie C, eds. *Birth Territory and Midwifery Guardianship: Theory for Practice, Education and Research*. Edinburgh: Heinemann/Elsevier; 2008:57–77 (Ch. 5).

Foureur M, Davis DL, Fenwick J, et al. The relationship between birth unit design and safe, satisfying birth: developing a hypothetical model. *Midwifery*. 2010;26(5):520–525.

Ginesi L. Physiology and birth—a personal view. *Midwifery Matters*. 1996;68:8–11.

Gosden D. Dissenting Voices: Conflict and Complexity in the Home Birth Movement in Australia (MA thesis). Sydney: Anthropology Department, Macquarie University; 1996.

Gosden D, Saul A. Reflections on the use of psychotherapy in midwifery. *Br J Midwifery*. 1999;7(9):543–546.

Green JM, Kitzinger J, Coupland V. Stereotypes of childbearing women—a look at some of the evidence. *Midwifery*. 1990;6(3):125–132.

Gutteridge K. (ed). *Understanding Anxiety, Worry and Fear in Childbearing: A Resource for Midwives and Clinicians*. Switzerland: Springer; 2020.

Haines HM, Rubertsson C, Pallant JF, et al. The influence of women's fear, attitudes and beliefs of childbirth on mode and experience of birth. *BMC Pregnancy Childbirth*. 2012;12:55.

Halldorsdottir S, Karlsdottir SI. Journeying through labour and delivery: perceptions of women who have given birth. *Midwifery*. 1996;12(2):48–61.

Halls KL. Maternal satisfaction regarding anaesthetic services during childbirth. *Br J Midwifery*. 2008;16(5):296–301.

Hammond A, Foureur M, Homer CSE, et al. Space, place and the midwife: exploring the relationship between the birth environment, neurobiology and midwifery practice. *Women Birth*. 2013;26:277–281.

Hammond A, Foureur M, Homer CSE. The hardware and software implications of hospital birth room design: a midwifery perspective. *Midwifery*. 2014a;30:825–830.

Hammond A, Homer CSE, Foureur M. Messages from space: an exploration of the relationship between hospital birth environments and midwifery practice. *HERD*. 2014b;74(4):81–95.

Heinz SD, Sleigh MJ. Epidural or no epidural anaesthesia: relationships between beliefs about childbirth and pain control choices. *J Reprod Heal Infant Psychol*. 2003;21(4):323–333.

Henry A, Nand S. Women's antenatal knowledge and plans regarding intrapartum pain management at the Royal Hospital for Women. *Aust N Z J Obstet Gynaecol*. 2004;44(4):314–317.

Hodnett ED. Pain and women's satisfaction with the experience of childbirth: a systematic review. *Am J Obstet Gynaecol*. 2002;186(5):S160–S172.

Hodnett ED, Downe S, Walsh D. Alternative versus conventional institutional settings for birth. *Cochrane Database Syst Rev*. 2012;(8):CD000012. doi:10.1002/14651858.CD000012.pub4.

Jones L, Othman M, Dowswell T, et al. Pain management for women in labour: an overview of systematic reviews. *Cochrane Database Syst Rev*. 2012;(3):CD009234.pub2.

Karlsdottir SI, Halldorsdottir S, Lundgren I. The third paradigm in labour pain preparation and management: the childbearing woman's paradigm. *Scand J Caring Sci*. 2014;28(2):315–327.

Katz-Rothman B. Women, providers and control. *J Obstet Gynecol Neonatal Nurs*. 1996;25(3):253–256.

Kelpin V. Birthing pain. In: Morse J, ed. *Qualitative Health Research*. London: Sage; 1992:93–103.

Kemp J, Sandall J. Normal birth, magical birth: the role of the 36-week birth talk in caseload midwifery practice. *Midwifery*. 2010;26:211–221.

Kitzinger S. *A Passion for Birth: My Life: Anthropology, Family and Feminism*. London: Pinter and Martin; 2015.

Klomp T, van Poppel M, Jones L, et al. Inhaled analgesia for pain management in labour. *Cochrane Database Syst Rev*. 2012;(9):CD009351, doi:10.1002/14651858.CD009351.pub2.

Kotreba A. The birth of my child at home, Monday 9th November 1992. *Midwifery Matters*. 1994;60:16–17.

Lally JE, Murtagh MJ, Macphail S. More in hope than expectation: women's experience and expectations of pain relief in labour. A review. *BMC Med*. 2008;6:7. doi:10.1186/1741-7015-6-7.

Lally JE, Thomson RG, MacPhail S, et al. Pain relief in labour: a qualitative study to determine how to support women to make decisions about pain relief in labour. *BMC Pregnancy Childbirth*. 2014;14:6.

Leap N. *A Midwifery Perspective on Pain in Labour (MSc dissertation)*. London: South Bank University; 1997.

Leap N. Pain in labour: towards a midwifery perspective. *MIDIRS Midwifery Digest*. 2000;10(1):49–53.

Leap N. The less we do, the more we give. In: Kirkham M, ed. *The Midwife–Mother Relationship*. 2nd ed. Basingstoke: Palgrave Macmillan; 2010:17–36 (Ch. 2).

Leap N, Anderson T. The role of pain and the empowerment of women. In: Downe S, ed. *Normal Childbirth: Evidence and Debate*. 2nd ed. Edinburgh: Churchill Livingstone; 2008 (Ch. 2).

Leap N, Edwards N. The politics of involving women in decision making. In: Page LA, Campbell R, eds. The New Midwifery: Science and Sensitivity in Practice. 2nd ed. London: Churchill Livingstone Elsevier; 2006 (Ch. 5).

Leap N, Sandall J, Buckland S, et al. Journey to confidence: women's experiences of pain in labour and continuity of carer. *J Midwifery Womens Health*. 2010a;55(3):234–242.

Leap N, Dodwell M, Newburn M. Working with pain in labour: an overview of evidence. Evidence-based briefing paper. *New Digest*. 2010b;49:22–26. Online: https://www.nct.org.uk/sites/default/files/related_documents/Research%20overview-%20Working%20with%20pain%20in%20labour_6.pdf.

Leap N, Hunter B. *The Midwife's Tale: An Oral History from Handywoman to Professional Midwife*. 2nd ed. Barnsley, UK: Pen and Sword History; 2013.

Leap N, Hunter B. *Supporting Women for Labour and Birth: A Thoughtful Guide*. 2nd ed. London: Routledge; 2022:38–60.

Lewin E. By design: reproductive strategies and the meaning of motherhood. In: Homans H, ed. *The Sexual Politics of Reproduction*. London: Gower; 1985:123–138.

Lindholm A, Hildingsson I. Women's preferences and received pain relief in childbirth—a prospective longitudinal study in a northern region of Sweden. *Sex Reprod Healthc*. 2015;6(2):74–81. doi:10.1016/j.srhc.2014.10.001.

Lowe NK. The nature of labor pain. *Am J Obstet Gynecol*. 2002;186(5):S16–S24.

Lundgren I, Dahlberg K. Women's experience of pain during childbirth. *Midwifery*. 1998;14(2):105–110.

Lundgren I, Dahlberg K. Midwives' experience of the encounter with women and their pain during childbirth. *Midwifery*. 2002;18(2):155–164.

Madden K, Middleton P, Cyna AM, et al. Hypnosis for pain management during labour and childbirth. *Cochrane Database Syst Rev*. 2016;(5):CD009356. doi:10.1002/14651858.CD009356.pub3.

McLachlan HL, Forster DA, Davey MA, et al. Effects of continuity of care by a primary midwife (caseload midwifery) on caesarean section rates in women of low obstetric risk: the COSMOS randomised controlled trial. *BJOG*. 2012;119(12):1483–1492.

Mander R. *Pain in Childbearing and its Control. Key Issues for Midwives and Women*. 2nd ed. Chichester, UK: Wiley-Blackwell; 2010.

Melzack R. From the gate to the neuromatrix. *Pain*. 1999;82:S121–S126.

Melzack R, Wall P. Pain mechanisms: a new theory. *Science*. 1965;150:971–979.

Melzack R, Wall P. *The Challenge of Pain*. London: Penguin; 1988.

Ministry of Health (MOH). *Maternity Consumer Survey 2014*. Wellington, New Zealand: MOH; 2014. Online: https://www.health.govt.nz/publication/maternity-consumer-survey-2014.

Ministry of Health (MOH). *Report on Maternity web tool*. 2021. https://minhealthnz.shinyapps.io/report-on-maternity-web-tool/.

Morris D. *The Culture of Pain*. Berkeley: University of California Press; 1991.

Newnham E, McKellar L, Pincombe J. A critical literature review of epidural analgesia. *Evid Based Midwifery*. 2016;14(1):22–28.

Newnham E, McKellar L, Pincombe J. *Towards the Humanisation of Birth: A Study of Epidural Analgesia and Hospital Birth Culture*. London: Palgrave Macmillan; 2018.

Newton N, Peeler D. Effect of disturbance on labor. An experiment with 100 mice. *Am J Obstet Gynecol.* 1968;101(8):1096–1102.

Newton N, Foshee D, Newton M. Experimental inhibition of labor through environmental disturbance. *Obstet Gynecol.* 1966;27(3):371–377.

Niven C, Murphy-Black T. Memory for labor pain: a review of the literature. *Birth.* 2000;27(4):244–253.

Oakley A. *Women Confined: Towards a Sociology of Childbirth.* Oxford: Martin Robertson; 1980.

Odent M. *Birth Re-Born: What Birth Can and Should Be.* London: Souvenir Press; 1984.

Olofsson C, Ekblom A, Ekman-Ordeberg G. Lack of analgesic effect of systematically administered morphine or pethidine on labour pain. *BJOG.* 1996;103(10):968–972.

Otley H. Fear of childbirth: understanding the causes, impact and treatment. *Br J Midwifery.* 2011;19(4):215–220.

Rabuzzi KA. *Mother With Child: Transformations Through Childbirth.* Bloomington: Indiana University Press; 1994.

Rafalovich A. Pain is the club: identity and membership in the natural childbirth community. *Qual Sociol Rev.* 2016;12(3): 100–116.

Raphael-Leff J. Facilitators and regulators: conscious and unconscious processes in pregnancy and motherhood. *Br J Med Psychol.* 1986;59:43–55.

Raynes-Greenow CH, Roberts CL, McCaffery K, et al. Knowledge and decision-making for labour analgesia of Australian primiparous women. *Midwifery.* 2007;23(2):139–145.

Raynes-Greenow CH, Nassar N, Torvaldsen S, et al. Assisting informed decision making for labour analgesia: a randomized controlled trial of a decision aid for labour analgesia versus a pamphlet. *BMC Pregnancy Childbirth.* 2010;10:15. doi:10.1186/ 1471-2393-10-15.

Redshaw M. First relationships and the growth of love and commitment. In: Page LA, Campbell R, eds. *The New Midwifery: Science and Sensitivity in Practice.* 2nd ed. Edinburgh: Churchill Livingstone/Elsevier; 2006:21–47 (Ch. 2).

Rich A. *Of Woman Born: Motherhood as Experience and Institution.* London: Virago; 1976.

Rimene C, Hassan C, Broughton J. *Ukaipo: The Place of Nurturing Maori Women and Childbirth.* Dunedin: University of Otago; 1998.

Roberts C, Tracy S, Peat B. Rates for obstetric intervention among private and public patients in Australia: population based descriptive study. *BMJ.* 2000;321:137–141.

Robertson A. The pain of labour. *Midwifery Today.* 1996;37:19–42.

Robertson A. *The Midwife Companion: The Art of Support During Birth.* 2nd ed. Sydney: Birth International; 2004.

Rolls C, McGuinness B. Women's experiences of a follow through journey program with bachelor of midwifery students. *Women Birth.* 2007;20:149–152.

Ross-Davie MC, Cheyne H. Intrapartum support: what do women want? A literature review to identify how far the nature of labour support shapes women's assessment of their birth experiences. *Evid Based Midwifery.* 2014;12(2):52–58.

Ross-Davie MC, McElligott M, Little M, et al. Midwifery support in labour: how important is it to stay in the room? *Pract Midwife.* 2014;17(6):19–22.

Sandall J, Soltani H, Gates S, et al. Midwife-led continuity models versus other models of care for childbearing women. *Cochrane Database Syst Rev.* 2016;(4):CD004667, doi:10.1002/14651858. CD004667.pub5.

Sanders R. Midwifery facilitation: exploring the functionality of labor discomfort. Commentary. *Birth.* 2015a;42(3):202–205.

Sanders R. Functional discomfort and a shift in midwifery paradigm. *Women Birth.* 2015b;28:e87–e91.

Sanders R, Lamb K. An exploration of the benefits and drawbacks of intrapartum pain management strategies. *Br J Midwifery.* 2014;22(9):394–401.

Sanders R, Lamb K. Non-pharmacological pain management strategies for labour: maintaining a physiological outlook. *Br J Midwifery.* 2017;25(2):2–9.

Scarry E. *The Body in Pain: The Making and Unmaking of the World.* Oxford: Oxford University Press; 1985.

Semple A, Newburn M. *Research overview: self-hypnosis for labour and birth.* Perspective. 2011;Dec:16–20. Online: https://www.nct.org.uk/sites/default/files/related_documents/Research%20overview-%20Self%20hypnosis%20for%20labour%20and%20birth%20%282011%29_2.pdf.

Simkin P. Non-pharmacological methods of pain relief during labour. In: Chalmers I, Enkin M, Keirse M, eds. *Effective Care in Pregnancy and Childbirth.* Oxford: Oxford University Press; 1989:893–913.

Simkin P. Just another day in a woman's life? Women's long term perceptions of their first birth experience. Part 1. *Birth.* 1991; 18:203–210.

Simkin P. Just another day in a woman's life? Women's long term perceptions of their first birth experience. Part II: nature and consistency of women's long term memories of their first birth experience. *Birth.* 1992;19:64–68.

Simkin P. *Comfort in Labour: How you can Help Yourself to a Normal Satisfying Childbirth.* 2015. Online: http://www.nationalpartnership.org/research-library/maternal-health/comfort-in-labor-simkin.pdf.

Simkin P, Ancheta R, Hanson L. *The Labor Progress Handbook: Early Interventions to Prevent and Treat Dystocia.* 4th ed. Chichester, W Sussex: Wiley-Blackwell; 2017.

Simpson M, Catling C. Understanding psychological traumatic birth experiences: a literature review. *Women Birth.* 2016;29(3): 203–207.

Smith CA, Collins CT, Cyna AM, et al. Complementary and alternative therapies for pain management in labour. *Cochrane Database Syst Rev.* 2006;(4):CD003521, doi:10.1002/14651858. CD003521.pub2.

Smith LA, Burns E, Cuthbert A. Parenteral opioids for maternal pain management in labour. *Cochrane Database Syst Rev.* 2018; (6):CD007396. doi:10.1002/14651858.CD007396.pub3.

Spiby H, Slade P, Escott D, et al. Selected coping strategies in labor: an investigation of women's experiences. *Birth.* 2004;30(3): 189–194.

Thomson G, Feeley C, Moran VH, et al. Women's experiences of pharmacological and non-pharmacological pain relief methods for labour and childbirth: a qualitative systematic review. *Reproductive Health.* 2019;16:71.

Tickle N, Sidebotham M, Fenwick J, et al. Women's experiences of having a Bachelor of Midwifery student provide continuity of care. *Women Birth.* 2016;29(3):245–251.

Toohill J, Fenwick J, Gamble J, et al. Prevalence of childbirth fear in an Australian sample of pregnant women. *BMC Pregnancy Childbirth.* 2014;14:275.

Tracy S, Tracy M. Costing the cascade: estimating the costs of increased intervention in childbirth using population data. *BJOG.* 2003;110:717–724.

Trout KK. The neuromatrix theory of pain: implications for selected nonpharmacologic methods of pain relief for labor. *J Midwifery Womens Health.* 2004;49(6):482–488.

Vague S. Midwives' Experiences of Working With Women in Labour: Interpreting the Meaning of Pain (Master's thesis). Auckland: Auckland University of Technology; 2003.

Van der Gucht N, Lewis K. Women's experiences of coping with pain during childbirth: a critical review of qualitative research. *Midwifery.* 2015;31:349–358.

Waldenström U, Hildingsson I, Rubertsson C, et al. A negative birth experience: prevalence and risk factors in a national sample. *Birth.* 2004;31(1):17–27.

Walsh D. Pain and epidural use in normal childbirth. *Evid Based Midwifery.* 2009;7(3):89–93.

Walsh D, Newburn M. Towards a social model of childbirth. Parts 1 and 2. *Br J Midwifery*. 2002;10(8):476–481.
Whitburn LY, Jones LE, Davy MA, et al. Women's experiences of labour pain and the role of the mind: an exploratory study. *Midwifery*. 2014;30:1029–1035.
Whitburn LY, Jones LE, Davey MA, et al. The meaning of labour pain: how the social environment and other contextual factors shape women's experiences. *BMC Pregnancy Childbirth*. 2017;17:157.
Whitburn LY, Jones LE, Davey MA, et al. The nature of labour pain: an updated review of the literature. *Women Birth*. 2019; 32:28–38.
Wickham S. *The language of birth: crossing the Ts and promoting positivity*. The Practising Midwife, 20 January 2017 online supplement. 2017. Online: https://www.sarawickham.com/articles-2/the-language-of-birth-crossing-the-ts-and-promoting-positivity/.
Wigert H, Nilsson C, Dencker A, et al. Women's experiences of fear of childbirth: a metasynthesis of qualitative studies. *Int J Qual Stud Health Well-being*. 2020;15(1).

Further reading

Chapman V, Charles C. *The Midwife's Labour and Birth Handbook*. 3rd ed. Chichester, UK: Wiley-Blackwell; 2013.
Leap N, Hunter B. Approaches to pain in labour. In: *Supporting Women for Labour and Birth: A Thoughtful Guide*. 2nd ed. London: Routledge; 2022:38–60 (Ch. 2).
Simkin P, Ancheta R. Hanson, L. *The Labor Progress Handbook: Early Interventions to Prevent and Treat Dystocia*. 4th ed. Chichester, West Sussex, UK: Wiley-Blackwell; 2017.
Thomson G, Feeley C, Moran VH, Downe S and Oladapo OT. Women's experiences of pharmacological and non-pharmacological pain relief methods for labour and childbirth: a qualitative systematic review. *Reproductive Health*. 2019;16:71.
Whitburn LY, Jones LE, Davey MA, et al. The nature of labour pain: an updated review of the literature. *Women Birth*. 2019; 32:28–38.

CHAPTER 27

Using water for labour and birth

Megan Cooper and Shea Caplice

LEARNING OUTCOMES

Learning outcomes for this chapter are:

1. To describe some of the history of using water for labour and birth
2. To critique the literature and use this to inform and guide safe evidence-based midwifery care for women using water for labour and birth
3. To explore the holistic benefits of water for labour and birth from the perspectives of women and midwives
4. To demonstrate how water for labour and birth aligns with midwifery philosophy and practice
5. To address common fears and concerns surrounding the use of water for labour and birth
6. To outline the principles and considerations of safely supporting women to use water for labour and birth.

CHAPTER OVERVIEW

This chapter provides an overview of the use of water immersion for labour and birth. It tracks the history and development of the use of water immersion for labour and birth over the past three decades, reviews some of the most recent literature that informs practice, and explores the physiology, potential problems and issues related to practice. Women's perspectives on their experiences of using water for labour and birth and recommendations for the safe use of water immersion are included.

The key principles of a midwifery model of care that underpin this chapter are that:

- pregnancy and childbirth are normal life events for most women
- midwifery care is woman centred
- **continuity of care** should be provided throughout the entire childbearing experience
- the woman–midwife relationship is a **partnership** based on:
  - trust, reciprocity and respect for the expertise of both the woman and the midwife
  - the woman's personal knowledge of her health history being considered as important as that of the midwife's
  - both partners having equal status and shared meaning through mutual understanding
  - the sharing of knowledge and power between the partners.

KEY TERMS

anxiety
continuity of care
fear
pain perception
pain relief
partnership
physiological birth
relaxing effect
water birth
water immersion

INTRODUCTION

Since the early 1980s, water immersion for labour and birth has been recognised as an effective midwifery option to support women in seeking a physiological birth. In many hospitals across Australian and Aotearoa New Zealand it is now viewed as a standard option of mainstream maternity care. Not surprisingly, birth in water has been and continues to be a mainstay of midwives who support women to birth at home.

Despite greater acceptance for the practice, there remain many barriers to the use of water for labour and birth with this impacting on the informed decision-making process for women and midwives' ability to offer and support women who wish to use this effective option (Cooper, McCutcheon & Warland, 2017, 2019). Over many decades, questions have been asked about efficacy and safety of **water immersion** and, particularly, **water birth**. In response, women, midwives, doctors and researchers have attempted to answer these questions and advocate for greater access to water immersion in mainstream maternity care settings.

Controversy between professionals continues, with much debate over the perceived benefits and potential risks. However, both the Australian College of Midwives (ACM) and New Zealand College of Midwives (NZCOM) (2015) consider water immersion as a core midwifery skill that facilitates normality (ACM, 2013; Stephens, 2011). The Royal Australian and New Zealand College of Obstetricians and Gynaecologists (RANZCOG) takes a more cautious approach to both water immersion and water birth. Its current statement asserts there is much less support in the medical community for water birth in comparison to water immersion during labour (RANZCOG, 2021). RANZCOG calls for more research; however, it notes that research to date has shown there are some benefits for women and has not established any major problems with water immersion during labour. This guideline makes six consensus-based recommendations: the need for units offering water immersion and water birth to have protocols and guidelines for use; for staff to have appropriate training in water immersion for labour and birth, including management of emergencies; for women to have access to information antenatally to support informed decision making; that women who require continuous electronic fetal monitoring can still access water if telemetry is available; that staff must be trained in obstetric emergency management; and for audit of data relating to maternal and neonatal outcomes and demographics of users.

The use of water immersion in labour and birth is closely associated with the act of **physiological birth** and this is arguably important in light of the exponential rise in intervention over the last three decades. Many women wishing to avoid intervention and who are looking for a normal, natural option will seek out water immersion. They will often choose their place of birth (including home birth) or care provider in order to ensure that the option is available (Cooper & Warland, 2019). Demand for water immersion is increasing. This means there is a need for maternity care services to factor the availability of pools and hot water supply into the infrastructure of hospitals and for midwives to understand the principles that underpin safe water immersion practice.

Definitions of labour and birth in water

For the purposes of this chapter, the following definitions apply:

- *labour in water*—the submersion of a woman in a receptacle (bath, pool or tub) of warm water of sufficient depth (generally not higher than the woman's axilla) during the first stage of labour
- *water birth*—the submersion of a woman in a receptacle (bath, pool or tub) of warm water of sufficient depth (generally not higher than the woman's axilla) during the second stage of labour to ensure the baby is born entirely underwater before immediately being brought to the water surface.

While there is little difference in the two definitions and the option of water immersion is commonly discussed as the one practice, much of the research differentiates the use of water in first and second stages of labour. This has influenced research findings and perceived risks related to the practice.

For clarity, *water immersion* will be used when describing the use of water irrespective of the stage of labour, *labour in water* will be used when discussing water immersion in the first stage of labour and *water birth* will be used to describe water immersion during second stage.

THE HISTORY OF WATER IMMERSION

The first documented water birth was reported in a French medical journal in 1805. The woman, who was exhausted after 48 hours of labour, climbed into a warm bath to relax before birthing her child into the water shortly after (Church, 1989, cited in Richmond, 2003). While there is some evidence to suggest that water birth was a common luxury of Egyptian Pharaohs and the Minoans of Crete (Cooper, Warland & McCutcheon, 2013), it was rarely broached in the medical literature until Igor Tjarkovsky generated global interest in the 1960s. The Russian water-birth enthusiast claimed that birth in water improved the psychic abilities of the baby despite little evidence to prove his theory (Zimmerman, 1993, cited in Richmond, 2003).

In 1975, Leboyer's book *Birth Without Violence* described the use of water as a healing therapy for babies. Premised on the belief that birth is a profound event that influences the future development of the baby, he stressed the need for peace, quiet and gentleness at the time of birth. Leboyer (1975) proposed that birthing through water minimised exposure to harsh stimuli such as light and sound and facilitated a gentle transition earthside for the baby. Around the same time, French obstetrician Michel Odent observed that women were attracted to the use of the shower or bath when in labour. His first experience of water birth was with a woman who was so completely relaxed in the bath that the baby was born before she was able to get out (Lichy & Herzberg, 1993). Subsequently, Odent began to offer water birth to all women who experienced long labours. Unlike Tjarkovsky, Odent was interested in the benefits of water immersion for the woman.

The practice of labouring and birthing in water continued to gather momentum into the 1980s particularly within the home-birth community. Demand for 'water babies' increased in response to a spiritual movement that revealed the dolphin–human connection and the notion of rebirthing (Sidenbladh, 1983). Inspired by enthusiastic women and midwives, water immersion spread into birth centres and hospital maternity units in the 1990s. Women's experiences have continued to drive demand and popularity of water immersion to this day (Fig. 27.1).

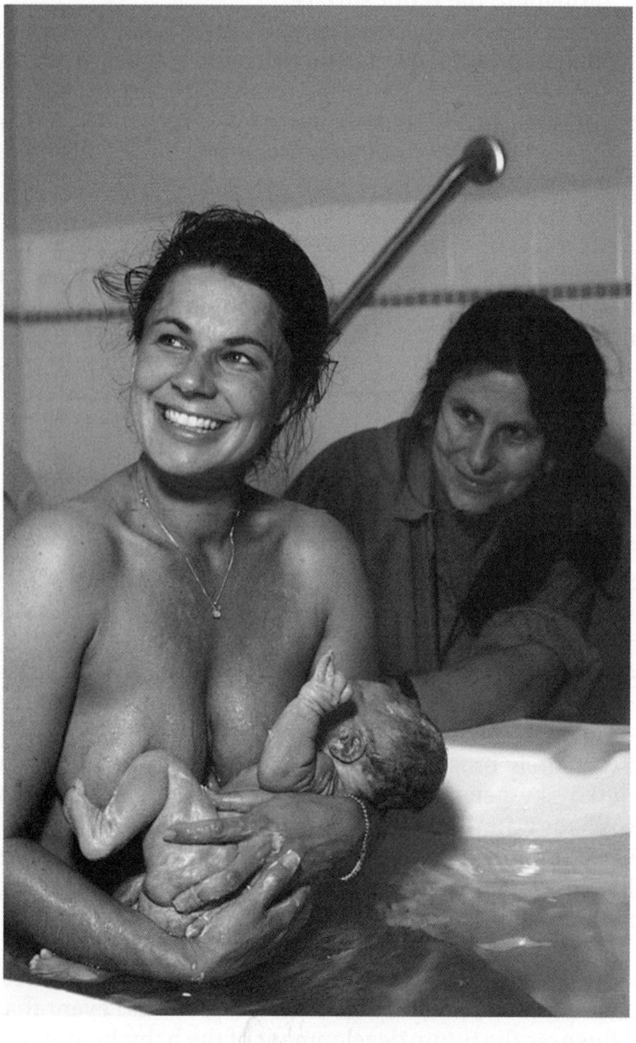

FIGURE 27.1 The growing popularity of water birth is largely due to the women who have experienced its benefits (Photograph copyright David Hancock.)

The first water births in New Zealand and Australia

The first of the modern water births in New Zealand occurred at Estelle Myer's Rainbow Dolphin Centre in Tutukaka on 17 March 1982. One woman is reported to have read an article on water birth and the experiments conducted by Igor Tjarkovsky motivating her to drive her house bus and three children to Tutukaka, intent on birthing in water. With the support of Estelle, friends, a midwife and a nurse, the woman birthed her baby, weighing 3.6 kg, into water, in a posterior position (her second persistently posterior baby), after 2.5 hours of labour. It is thought that this was the first water birth in the Southern Hemisphere, though Indigenous history may predate this if it existed in written form. Three years later, Estelle, in the company of six midwives, supported a Russian woman to birth her son into water in Sydney.

In Australia, water immersion has been occurring at planned home births attended by home-birth midwives since the early 1980s (Lecky-Thompson, 1989) and within hospital-based birth centres in Sydney and Melbourne since the early 1990s (Caplice, 2004a; Page, 1994). In New Zealand, Wanganui Hospital's maternity unit led the country by openly using water immersion for birth. The first documented water birth at Wanganui occurred in November 1989; between July 1991 and December 2000 there were a further 916 water births in the maternity unit (Young, 2001).

CLINICAL POINT

The first water births in Indigenous Australia and New Zealand

There is little early documented evidence of the practice of water birthing among the Indigenous women of Australia, although Odent (1990) says that some Aboriginal women on the Western coast of Australia first paddled in the sea, then gave birth on the beach. There are stories of traditional birthing practices among the Māori of New Zealand where water was used. It was common for babies to be born on beaches in the Te Kaha area (Binney & Chapman, 1986; Irwin & Ramsden, 1995), and Makereti records the use of water to facilitate birth of the whenua (placenta) when it was delayed (Makereti, 1986).

The incidence of water immersion

There remain no national data repositories that detail water immersion rates across Australia or New Zealand (Cooper, Warland & McCutcheon, 2018). For the most part, water immersion statistics are collected by individual institutions or jurisdictionally. However, much of these data are not publicly available and / or are inconsistent in measure and therefore the absolute incidence of water immersion is difficult to determine. This is further compounded by the fact that water immersion remains a mainstay of midwives who support women who are birthing at home. Unfortunately, these data are also not always collected or captured in population-wide statistics. During the 1990s and early 2000s, individual practice or facility audits reported a 65%–75% rate of pool use in labour (Banks, 1998; Cassie, 2002) and a 25%–38% water-birth rate throughout the 1990s and early 2000s (Banks, 1998; Fenton, 2004) while midwives in private practice in Australia report water-birth rates at home births of 60%–80% (Caplice, 2004b). These rates appear to have remained relatively consistent over time as reflected in Midwifery Practice Review statistics collected by the ACM (Personal communication, 2021).

In 2012, the New Zealand Midwifery and Maternity Providers Organisation (MMPO) reported pooled data from 532 midwives who provided care for 33,931 women (34,313 babies). This represented 55% of all births in New Zealand in 2012 (Dixon & Guilliland, 2014). The percentage of babies born into water was low at 7.2% (n = 2447) of all births (33,931), although 24% (7429) of women report using water immersion during labour. The incidence of water birth was not dissimilar from Maude and Kim's (2020) observational study which reported a 7.7% rate in one New Zealand District Health Board between February 2009 and March 2014.

The latest MMPO report published in 2016 suggests uptake had increased slightly with 26.8% (n = 7399) of the 30,165 women using water immersion for pain management during labour. Of those, 10.2% (n = 2806) gave birth in water (Daellenbach et al. 2016; http://www.mmpo.org.nz). Women who gave birth at home or at a primary facility had a higher proportion of water births (27.9% and 34.8% respectively) than those birthing at secondary or tertiary facilities. These numbers were up from the 2012 percentages at 23.9% and 24.9% respectively. This trend was also seen in secondary and tertiary facilities, which recorded an increase to 7.0% and 2.9% respectively, up from 4.8% and 2.6% in 2012 (Daellenbach et al. 2016). It is possible that the numbers of women using water immersion could be higher, owing to the fact that these reports do not reflect all births in New Zealand.

There is generally a lack of population data in Australia regarding the use of water for labour and birth. Data collected between 2000 and 2009 from Bankstown Hospital in Sydney revealed that 219 women birthed in water in this time frame, representing 1.2% of total births (approximately 18,000 births in 10 years) (Menakaya et al., 2013). The Sydney Royal Hospital for Women facility audits reported a water-birth rate of around 40% of the total births in the Birth Centre at the hospital, between 1992 when the practice first began and 2002. However, with the rise of intervention and the transition of the Birth Centre the water-birth rate for the last 5 years is around 9% (personal communication with RHW data manager). Following a survey of women in Queensland, Young and Kruske (2013) reported that 20% of women wished to use water immersion in 2009 but only 3% of those women actually gave birth in water. The latest policy directive from South Australia suggests that water births represented 1.7% of all births in 2015 and that this has been increasing since 2006 (SA Health, 2017). The most recent perinatal statistics from Queensland detail that 11.4% of the 34,308 women who gave birth in 2019 used water immersion (Queensland Health, 2020). Of the 13,767 who had a vaginal birth, 13.4% used water. However, these statistics do not differentiate between those who used water in labour versus those who had a water birth.

While some hospitals report a water-birth rate of 1%–2%, others report that the majority of women who access their service use water. Uptake appears to be higher in midwifery-led units and birth centres (Milosevic et al., 2019). A study published in 2013 found a 13% water-birth rate in an alongside Sydney birth centre between 1996 and 2008 (Dahlen et al., 2013). In a mixed methods study exploring practitioners' involvement in the development of Australian policies and guidelines related to water immersion (Cooper, 2017), one participant who worked in a midwifery-led birth centre stated:

> *We have a water immersion rate of 80% and a water birth rate of 60%. We have the highest intact perineum rate in the state according to the Mothers and Babies report 2010 (Response #42).*

There is a pressing need for population-level water immersion statistics to assist researchers, clinicians and women to make informed and evidence-based decisions surrounding its use. In the absence of these statistics, the current and growing evidence base reflects that water immersion offers equivalent, and in some cases better, outcomes when compared to land birth and other methods of pain relief. It is also associated with improvements in women's satisfaction and experiences of birth. All maternity facilities, birthing units and independent practitioners offering water immersion and birth should be collecting prospective outcome data.

USING WATER FOR LABOUR AND BIRTH: THE EVIDENCE

There is a paucity of high-level contemporaneous evidence for water immersion during labour and birth across the social sciences, midwifery, nursing and medical literature. Subsequently for this chapter many older references are still relied upon and remain pivotal to guiding practice.

In 1983, Odent published the outcomes of 100 water births at his alternative-birthing unit in Pithiviers, France. The article, which was published in *The Lancet*, was one of the first major medical publications to detail birth in water. While there was a consistent stream of research related to water immersion subsequent to this, there has been an expansion of research in the past five years, especially surrounding women's experiences.

Prior to more recent exploration of women's experiences, the majority of research related to water immersion has been empirical in nature and heavily focused on determining the safety of practice against land birth. Traditionally, research has been weighted according to the hierarchy of evidence with the randomised controlled trial (RCT) considered the 'gold standard' and the only true means of evaluating the effectiveness of an intervention. In times gone by, qualitative studies, that is, those that seek to explore experiences, perceptions and attitudes, have not placed high in the hierarchy of evidence but this is slowly changing. With the release of the COAG Health Council (2019) *Woman-centred care: Strategic directions for Australian maternity services*, there is now greater emphasis on the importance of informing practice and maternity services with woman-reported outcomes. In fact, a whole strategic direction is dedicated to 'respect[ing] women's choices, experiences and outcomes and us[ing] woman-reported data to inform quality improvement' in maternity care across Australia (p. 13). The literature base is now reflecting a more balanced examination of empirical and qualitative information that can assist policy makers, clinicians and women with respect to water immersion.

To date, there are still no large enough RCTs comparing birth in water with land birth, despite calls for such a study (Davies, 2010; Pinette et al., 2004). Some argue that this is due to the ethical issues of randomising women who hold strong views about their birth choices (Woodward & Kelly, 2004). While water immersion and, particularly, water birth continue to be challenged against the lack of sufficiently powered RCT, there have been 15 water immersion trials with a combined total of 3663 women to date; eight trials were specific to first stage, two have examined water birth, four have explored both first and second stage and one has compared immersion in early and late first-stage labour. Of the 15 trials, six were conducted between 1993 and 1998, six were undertaken in the first decade of the 21st century, and the last three were published between 2010 and 2015. The results of these trials have been examined in the latest Cochrane systematic review of water immersion with the intent of assessing the effects of water on women and their babies during each stage of labour (Cluett et al., 2018). Key findings from the review suggest that labouring in water probably results in less epidurals and has little to no effect on the rates of vaginal, instrumental or caesarean birth. Serious perineal tears were also not found to be different when comparing with women who did not use water immersion (Cluett et al., 2018). The difference in blood loss was not clear as evidence was of low quality but there was no apparent difference in neonatal infections or transfer to neonatal intensive care units (NICU). In second stage, Cluett et al. (2018) found little to no difference in rates of vaginal birth, however, determining whether water birth makes any difference to instrumental or caesarean births, transfer to NICU or infection rates was difficult given the quality of the evidence was low. The authors conclude by saying that there appears to be no difference in outcomes when comparing women who labour and give birth in water compared to those who do not.

While there has been a total of 15 trials over the last three decades, the numbers are small, and the trials vary in their design and methodology. As such, it is unlikely that a trial of the magnitude that Davies (2010) calls for will ever come to fruition.

Consequently, the safety of water immersion continues to be questioned in the absence of a large RCT, even though there remains little to no evidence that water immersion during labour and / or birth increases risk to healthy mothers and babies. Instead, research has highlighted that water immersion reduces the length of the first stage of labour and significantly reduces the need for pharmacological pain relief, and that women find it a positive experience and are highly satisfied (Feeley et al., 2021). Observational and cohort studies are also reassuring. The largest water-birth study, a retrospective population level examination of 6264 water births in the UK, found that birthing in water was not associated with lower Apgar scores or obstetric-anal sphincter injuries (Aughey et al., 2021). In fact, water birth was associated with a reduction in postpartum haemmorrhage and admission to the neonatal unit. This is the largest water-birth study to date.

PHYSIOLOGICAL EFFECTS

It is well established that water immersion has a calming and **relaxing effect** (Fig. 27.2). This is a consistent finding across multiple fields. Odent (1983) first described these

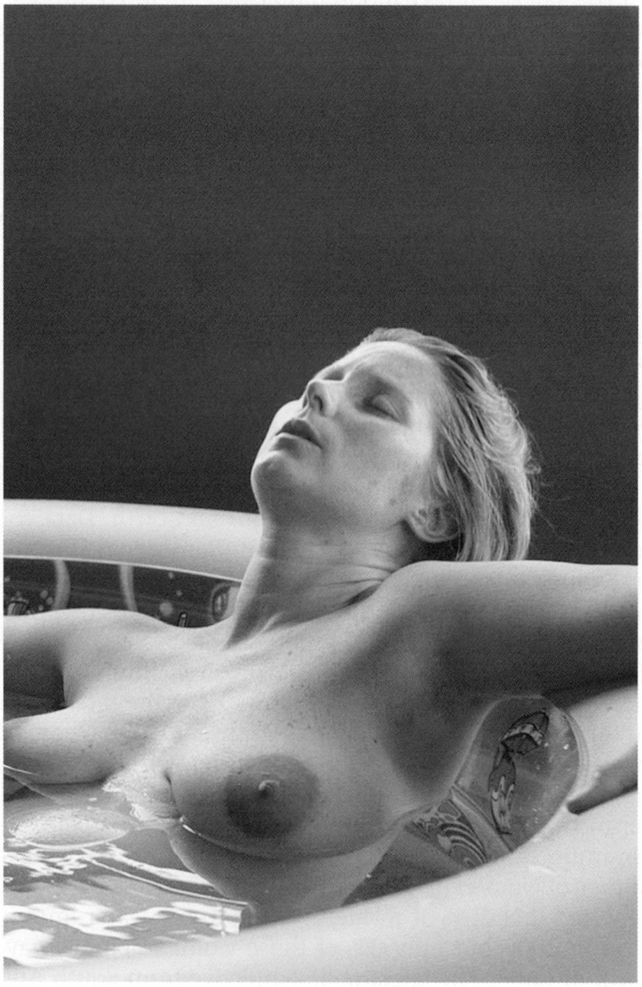

FIGURE 27.2 The relaxing effect of water immersion during labour (Photograph copyright David Hancock.)

benefits for women who were labouring after observing that they were not only less likely to require obstetric interventions but were also less likely to request exogenous pain relief. He noted that there was a tendency for women to 'fall asleep in a comfortable tub' (Odent, 1997, p. 415). The pain-relief effect of warm-water immersion is probably associated with an increased level of endorphins and catecholamines. Church (1989) also proposed that water immersion decreases **anxiety** owing to a reduction in adrenaline (epinephrine) levels and therefore uninhibited flow of natural oxytocins and endorphins. A natural balance of pain and relaxation is achieved, and labour progresses physiologically.

Much of the research to date has attempted to quantify the absolute effect of pain relief afforded to women who use water immersion during labour and birth. The prospective RCT by Cammu et al. (1994) found no statistical difference between the absolute values of labour pain between the two groups of women who ranked their pain on a Visual Analogue Scale (VAS). They reported that bathing provided no objective pain relief, but instead had a temporal pain-stabilising effect, possibly mediated through the improved relaxation experienced between contractions. This is thought to stimulate the closing of the gate for pain at the level of the dorsal horn (Cammu et al., 1994). This was further supported by the historical cohort study by Aird et al. (1997), who found that labouring in water offered women greater relaxation during the first stage of labour and better prepared them for second stage and birthing without assistance.

Water immersion is associated with both *hydrothermic* and *hydrokinetic* benefits. The *hydrothermic effect* relates to the conduction of heat from the warm water through the skin, leading to peripheral vasodilation. The resultant release of muscle spasm contributes to the reduction in pain (Brown, cited in Richmond, 2003). The *hydrokinetic effect* refers to the feeling of weightlessness often described by women (Deschênes, 1990). The combined effect of warmth and weightlessness contributes to women feeling more relaxed and less anxious (Ginesi & Niescierowicz, 1998).

The vasodilation of the peripheral blood vessels and the redistribution of blood flow when women are immersed in warm water during labour have been observed to contribute to a reduction in blood pressure (Benfield, 2002). A common concern has been that vasodilation and relaxation of uterine muscles might lead to an increased possibility of postpartum haemorrhage (PPH). However, numerous audits in maternity units that use immersion in water for labour and birth do not support this (Caplice, 2004b; Garland & Jones, 1997; Rosenthal, 1991). Similarly, it has been thought that the warm water may lead to an increase in maternal body temperature, which may negatively impact the neonate; however, Woodward & Kelly (2004) reported no difference in temperature in first or second stage between those who did and did not use water. It would seem that the natural processes already in place in the body are sufficient to counteract these theoretical problems (Richmond, 2003).

CLINICAL POINT

Relaxation and the effects of water immersion

Labouring in water promotes relaxation during the first stage of labour, enabling the woman to reach the second stage better prepared to give birth to her baby. Odent (1983) claims to have observed that water seems to help labouring women reach a certain state of consciousness where they become indifferent to what is going on around them. Odent continues to explore the biochemical and physiological effects of warm-water immersion and concludes that, 'when a parturient enters a bath at body temperature, there is immediate pain relief' (Odent, 1997, p. 415).

WATER IMMERSION AND MIDWIFERY PHILOSOPHY AND PRACTICE

At the core of their practice, midwives recognise and support labour and birth as normal, physiological processes and in this, they understand that women hold innate and intuitive knowledge about their body and their baby. As such, midwives equip themselves with a wide range of knowledge and skills in order to facilitate women to achieve a satisfying birth experience. Water immersion is just one of the options that midwives draw upon to support women towards attaining a normal, physiological labour and birth.

Overwhelmingly, midwives support the use of water immersion and this has been reflected in multiple studies. Cooper, Warland & McCutcheon (2018) surveyed 234 midwives and found that 94.4% and 84.3% strongly supported the options of water immersion and water birth, respectively. By clinical experience rated on a five-point Likert scale, midwives in this study highlighted that the greatest benefits of water immersion are that women are more relaxed, use less analgesia and have a more positive birth experience. Milosevic et al. (2020) highlighted that midwives working in midwifery-led units were highly supportive of water immersion and that the opportunity to facilitate the option had contributed to their want to work in a midwifery-led context:

> *I love pool births and that's half the reason I'm here. I think it just gives people immense pain relief, relaxation, and you just instantly see people relax as they get into it.*

THE ROLE OF WATER IMMERSION IN SUPPORTING PHYSIOLOGICAL BIRTH

There is growing evidence to suggest that water immersion increases the likelihood of normal, physiological birth (Burns et al., 2012). As such, women and midwives have come to see water immersion as a philosophy of non-intervention and a means of facilitating birth without pharmacological pain relief. Being with the woman, supporting and encouraging her through the transition phase and honouring her choices reduces maternal anxiety and the associated neurohormonal responses mean that women who are able to birth in a pool often do so without intervention. The benefits of labouring and birthing in water for women are reduced pain, increased functional diameter of the true pelvis, improved quality of contractions, increased release of endorphins, lessened need for analgesia and greater freedom of movement, as well as improved positioning through the different stages of labour (Chaichian et al., 2009; Mollamahmutoglu et al., 2012).

A secondary analysis of the Birthplace national prospective cohort study including 16,577 nulliparous women experiencing low-risk pregnancies (Lukasse et al. 2014), found that women who used water immersion in freestanding midwifery units were more likely to have a vaginal birth (RR 1.09; 95% CI 1.04–1.15) and as such, were less likely to experience an intrapartum caesarean section (RR 0.61; 95% CI 0.44–0.84). Another study by Liu et al. (2014) found similar results in that women in the conventional labour group were more likely to experience caesarean section (32.9% vs 13.2%, $p = 0.026$).

Midwives highlight the impact of water immersion on the rates of epidural and caesarean section. This was found by Cooper (2017) in phase two interviews of a larger study exploring Australian water immersion policies and guidelines and their impact on the practice:

> *It's quite empowering for the women when they get into the water, most often they relax and it's just enough to help them cope to get through to be able to achieve normal birth by themselves . . . so it's very empowering (Participant Eight).*

> *I really strongly believe that WI really does support normal labour. It does reduce your epidural rate . . . Certainly since we've used WI, our epidural rate has definitely dropped (Participant Eight).*

> *. . . our section rate is 10% and I would contribute part of that to the women having normal births and using water and non-pharmacological pain relief (Participant Nine).*

CLINICAL POINT

Reduction in the use of pharmacological pain relief

Increasingly, women want to find ways to manage the pain of labour naturally, thereby reducing the likelihood of requiring pharmacological pain relief. However, some women are unsure about their ability to go through a labour without some help, especially women having their first baby. 'I didn't want to use drugs if I could help it but then I'm such a "wuss" when it comes to pain' (Linda, in Maude, 2003, p. 93).

WOMEN'S EXPERIENCES OF WATER IMMERSION

In 2019, the COAG Health Council's *Woman-centred care: Strategic directions for Australian maternity services* detailed the strategies required to transform Australian maternity care provision. Cooper, Warland & McCutcheon (2013) acknowledge that in order to do so, women-reported outcomes must be acknowledged alongside empirical measures. While there has been a paucity of research examining women's experiences in the past, a recent expansion of literature reflects the significant benefits afforded to women by warm water immersion during labour and / or birth.

Of the quantitative studies conducted that have included an assessment of women's experiences, there is consistent finding that water immersion results in more positive childbirth experiences and greater satisfaction. In a prospective study, Lathrop et al. (2018) found that the water-birth group had a better experience when compared with those who had a conventional birth ($p < 0.001$) and a subgroup who had epidurals ($p = 0.002$). Lewis et al.'s (2018) exploratory study using critical incident techniques of 296 women found that 93 who had a water birth described birth as affirming, natural and empowering among other things. They also suggested that they had chosen water immersion for 'natural pain management', 'freedom to move' and to 'prevent pharmaceutical drug use' (p. 4). As part of a sequential exploratory mixed methods study, Cooper and Warland (2019) surveyed 740 women from Australia about their experiences of using water for labour and birth. Women rated water immersion benefits highly on 7-point Likert scales. The mostly highly rated benefits by option 'entirely agree' were 'sense of safety' (80.14%), 'an alert baby' (75.00%), 'a positive birth experience' (72.70%), 'water as soothing' (72.03%) and 'freedom of movement' (71.35%). When asked about their concerns, they most commonly selected extremely concerned against the options 'being told to get out of the bath when I did not want to' (n = 120/736, 16.30%), 'their contractions going away' (n = 76/736, 10.33%) and 'unsupportive staff' (n = 65/736, 8.83%).

Women's perspectives highlight that water immersion can lead to more choices, increased control, improved privacy, shelter and protection as well as a greater sense of relaxation. Their stories provide a rich source of knowledge about the use of water for labour and / or birth.

In 2020, Feeley et al. (2021) undertook a systematic meta-thematic synthesis to examine the views and experiences of women who had used water for labour and / or birth. Following analysis of seven qualitative studies, nine key findings were generated leading to the three main themes of *Liberation and self-emancipation*; *Synergy, transcendence and demarcation*; and *Thriving and transforming: birth and beyond*. Their findings echoed those of an earlier review by Clews et al. (2020). The following provides an overview of the findings from Feeley et al. (2021).

The pool is positively anticipated

Women positively anticipate entering the warm water during labour and birth (Maude & Foureur, 2007; Sprague, 2004; Ulfsdottir et al., 2018). They describe the need to be in water as reflected in the below quote:

There was a point where I had to get in there, and I guess it was a particular point in my labour where I went, I have got to be in that space NOW!!.

(Daisy, in Sprague, 2004)

This is true even where women did not give birth in water but were offered water immersion during labour (Ulfsdottir et al., 2018). They described water immersion as 'natural' and 'kind to the body'.

Water offers analgesic properties and the ability to cope with pain while enhancing control

A consistent finding across multiple studies is that women report warm water immersion as effective in 'cushioning' against the pain. They describe the experience as 'soothing' and 'relaxing' (Antonakou et al., 2018; Gonçalves et al., 2019; Hall & Holloway, 1997; Maude & Foureur, 2007; McKenna & Symon, 2014; Sprague, 2004; Ulfsdottir et al., 2018). However, rather than completely easing the pain, water immersion affords women the ability to manage the pain which in turn increases their sense of control over their birth experience. For many, this is the difference between coping or not coping:

I wouldn't have imagined myself in control but in labour it became important to me. I had to prove I could cope. The water somehow helped with this.

(Participant 5, in Hall & Holloway, 1997)

Women describe a synergy between mind and body (Ulfsdottir et al., 2018), and as such, are better able to cope with the pain (Antonakou et al., 2018; Gonçalves et al., 2019; Hall & Holloway, 1997; Maude & Foureur, 2007; McKenna & Symon, 2014; Sprague, 2004; Ulfsdottir et al., 2018). Water provides comfort and rest and, as described in the following quote, it 'softens' the impact of labour.

The contractions were stretched out and were less difficult to deal with in the water . . . It must have diffused the pain . . . I felt relaxed . . . I could actually stretch out and float. That was probably essential because I could relax very quickly . . . I could actually stretch out and rest . . . Water also decreased the intensity of the contractions . . . Water softened the whole thing and made it more bearable . . . it was much easier to cope with the pain.

(Claire, in Sprague, 2004)

Water increases buoyancy and freedom of movement

The physical benefits of water immersion are commonly described in terms of increased buoyancy and freedom of movement such that women are able to adopt positions of most comfort (McKenna & Symon, 2014; Ulfsdottir et al., 2018). This is particularly true for women who are of higher BMI (Sprague, 2004) or have a physical disability. The water alleviates feelings of 'heaviness' and 'clumsiness' as described in the following quote:

It's just being able to move and not be clumsy. Because in the end, I mean of the pregnancy, you are pretty heavy. So, I was really happy to be able to twist and turn and relax and the warmth. That is really nice and you can feel it in your whole body, so it was. . .and that is the greatest advantage. . .that you can move as you want to.

(Interview # 12, in Ulfsdottir et al., 2018)

Water immersion promotes safety, protection and privacy

The physical barrier of the pool is viewed positively by women in that it separates them from what is going on around them. The pool offers safety, separation and privacy from the clinical environment of the hospital that women can make their own (Gonçalves et al., 2019; Hall & Holloway, 1997; Maude & Foureur, 2007; McKenna & Symon, 2014; Sprague, 2004; Ulfsdottir et al., 2018). Despite being naked, they describe the pool as offering containment where they do not feel exposed or vulnerable (Sprague, 2004). This protection facilitates a positive mental state where women can focus on and listen to their bodies:

It was because the pool space was really safe . . . quite contained . . . it was dark, midnight dark . . . A place I could go to and feel safe, really safe . . . and thinking back, I am sure that made the difference.

(Rosa, in Sprague, 2004)

An altered state of consciousness

The protection, safety and comfort of warm water offers women the ability to go 'within' and as a result, they describe a distortion of time. They can focus on entering 'labour land' as a consequence of an altered state of consciousness (Maude & Foureur, 2007; Sprague, 2004; Ulfsdottir et al., 2018). Ulfsdottir et al. (2018) refers to this as a synergy between body and mind. Women often describe that the psychological benefits are as important, if not more important, than the physical.

Water shrunk everything down so that time stood still . . . there was this kind of bizarre gap in time when she was fully born, where I felt like I was looking into her soul or something, like this incredible, unexplainable sort of period of time that I have never felt before.

(Daisy, in Sprague, 2004)

The birthing pool mitigated against the clinical environment

The envelopment of the birthing pool not only provides comfort and privacy, but women also highlight that the pool itself shielded them from the harshness of the hospital environment (Gonçalves et al., 2019; McKenna & Symon, 2014; Sprague, 2004). They are able to enter a space that is less clinical. This not only affords psychological and physical benefits but also mitigates against intervention. As such, they can create their own territory which helps to promote a more home-like environment (Maude & Foureur, 2007).

Positive second stage

Women express joy and elation during the second stage in that they are able to receive their babies and lift them to their chests without any interruption (Gonçalves et al., 2019; Sprague, 2004; Ulfsdottir et al., 2018). Even if they do not receive their baby, they highly value the ability to watch the birth. In their mind, it is the ideal way to meet their baby. They also attribute an easier second stage to water due to the warmth and soothing sensation against their perineum making pushing easier (Gonçalves et al., 2019; Sprague, 2004; Ulfsdottir et al., 2018).

> *I was just making eye contact with her while she was in the water, just going, oh my god, this is like the thing of looking into me and looking into her . . . and oh, my god I am actually going to receive my own baby, and although my midwife was standing right beside me, I sort of felt like she knew that as well . . . and knowing that she would not lean over and grab her . . . and while I was waiting for the next contraction I was mildly freaking out about how excited I was that I was actually going to get her myself and how incredibly defining that was in our relationship, for me to just go, right now, you are my baby . . . to take her and bring her into the world . . . that is so major!!*
>
> (Daisy, in Sprague, 2004)

A positive and empowering birth experience

Women who use water during labour and / or birth describe their birth experience as 'wonderful', 'incredible', 'amazing' and 'extraordinary' among other words (Antonakou et al., 2018; Gonçalves et al., 2019; Maude & Foureur, 2007; McKenna & Symon, 2014; Sprague, 2004; Ulfsdottir et al., 2018). It often facilitates an experience that is beyond even their own expectations of a positive birth experience as reflected in the below quote:

> *My water birth was an absolutely wonderful thing, it was wonderful, it was extraordinary it was everything I wanted and a little more.*
>
> (M2, in Gonçalves et al., 2019)

Women commonly stated that they would opt for water immersion in their next birth after expressing feelings of 'victory' (Gonçalves et al., 2019; Sprague, 2004).

CLINICAL POINT

Women's perceptions of pain

Women's stories of their experiences of using water for labour and birth indicate that they do not necessarily use water to take the pain of labour away. Instead, they see water immersion as helping them to cope with pain, and to reduce their **fear** of pain and of childbirth itself (Maude, 2003). A woman in water may remain fearful and scared but is presented with the opportunity to relax in between contractions to the extent that her labour may progress more rapidly. Relaxation enables women who use water to focus internally on what is happening to them, their body and their baby.

Women's stories of using water for labour and birth have broadened our understanding of the meaning they make of the experience and have demonstrated that the efficacy of water immersion goes beyond measurable outcomes. It is also clear that women do not have to experience a water birth to experience the benefits water affords. Women experience mind–body connection owing to the liberation and emancipation of immersing in warm water, and are more attuned and aware of their physiological and psychological capabilities (Feeley et al., 2021; Ulfsdottir et al. 2018). Planning, preparation, education and anticipation of using water for labour and birth, supported by its safe and judicious use, creates an environment of relaxation, privacy and protection that enables and empowers women to maintain control (Feeley et al., 2021).

SAFETY AND EFFICACY OF USING WATER

Water immersion during labour and birth is practised globally by practitioners who employ a holistic approach to birth that supports women's choice. While most healthcare professionals agree that there is adequate evidence to support labouring in water there remain challenges to the option of water birth largely owing to questions of safety for the baby (Davies et al., 2015; Menakaya et al., 2013). This section examines the most commonly associated benefits and concerns related to water immersion.

Benefits

Immersion and duration of labour

A range of studies have documented a reduction in the duration of labour when water immersion is used. Garland & Jones (1997) analysed data from 209 primiparous women and 220 multiparous women and demonstrated a median and mean reduction in labour length for water birth. A retrospective case–control study by Otigbah et al. (2000) found that primigravidas having water births had shorter first and second stages of labour compared with controls ($p < 0.05$ and $p < 0.005$ respectively), reducing the total time spent in labour by 90 minutes (95% CI 31–148). A significantly shorter first stage of labour was also found following a review of 1600 water births (Thoeni et al. 2005). Similar results were found in a retrospective cohort study in Sweden when all water births ($n = 306$) at two maternity units were compared with conventional spontaneous vaginal births (n = 306) (Ulfsdottir et al., 2018). Labour duration in the water-birth group was shorter (6h 3min vs 7h 52min). These findings were echoed by Camargo et al.'s (2019) cross-sectional and quantitative study which found a statistically significant difference (p = 0.001) in length of labour when comparing water birth (n = 73) with birth outside of water (n = 31), while a statistically significant shorter second stage of labour (p = 0.03) was found in nulliparous women who gave birth in water compared to women who did not by Neiman et al.'s, (2020) US hospital-based retrospective cohort study.

Other studies showed no differences in length of labour. Burns et al. (2012) found that the mean length of labour for women using water immersion across three different birth settings was not statistically significantly different for either nulliparous (562–96 minutes) or multiparous (309–29 minutes) women. In their retrospective audit of water births compared with conventional vaginal births for low-risk women in a secondary-level hospital in Australia, Menakaya et al. (2013) found no statistically significant differences in the mean duration of first (350.65 minutes in primigravida and 222.67 minutes in multigravida) and second stages (51.3 minutes in primigravida and 20.28 minutes in multigravida) of labour. A similar result was found in a Turkish study of 102 participants (Uzunlar et al., 2021). There was no statistically significant difference found in labour duration between women who immersed in water during labour (n = 30) compared to those who had an epidural (n = 30) and those who had no pain relief (n = 42). Similarly, no definitive difference was found in labour duration when comparing water immersion with conventional birth in the latest Cochrane systematic review which included 15 studies and 3663 women (Cluett et al., 2018).

Of the RCTs conducted, Schorn et al., 1993 could not demonstrate a shorter labour in a prospective RCT of the use of warm water immersion by 93 women; however, the immersion was only for an average of 30–45 minutes while Cluett et al. (2004) found the mean duration of labour was similar in both groups in their RCT comparing water immersion with standard management for labour dystocia. However, there was no consistency in the measurement of labour commencement in any of these studies.

In a prospective clinical trial by Mollamahmutoglu et al. (2012), labour duration (first, second and third stage) was compared across three groups of primigravidas and multiparas—the water-birth group (n = 207), the conventional vaginal delivery group (n = 204) and the vaginal delivery with epidural anaesthesia group (n = 191). The water-birth group had a significantly reduced duration of second- and third-stage labour. However, the first stage of labour was shorter for the water-birth group when compared with the vaginal delivery with epidural analgesia but not the conventional vaginal delivery group (who had the shortest first-stage labour duration).

A more recent American descriptive correlational study by Snapp et al. (2020) found that the occurrence of prolonged first and second stages (p <0.001) was less in the water birth group (n = 10,252) contributing to a statistically significant difference for second stage compared to women who gave birth on land (n = 16,432).

Use of analgesia in labour

Water immersion is increasingly recognised as an effective pain relief option for women in labour and birth (Young & Kruske, 2012). In fact, the use of water immersion may offer women the opportunity to circumvent reliance on pharmacological pain relief. This is supported by Mallen-Perez et al. (2018) who found hydrotherapy during labour, when compared with traditional birth, was associated with statistically significantly lower pain at 30 and 90 minutes as well as during second stage.

Mollamahmutoglu et al. (2012) used the VAS scale to measure women's **pain perception** in their comparison of water birth, and conventional vaginal birth with and without epidural anaesthesia. They found that not only were VAS scores for the water birth group lower when compared with the conventional vaginal birth group, but they were also lower when compared with those who received epidural anaesthesia. As such, they assert that water immersion significantly reduces pain and the need for epidural / spinal anaesthesia in both primagravidas and multiparas. This in part could be due to the reduction in stress hormones and catecholamines, which inhibit oxytocin and labour progression in women (Cluett & Burns, 2009; Mollamahmutoglu et al., 2012).

Similarly, a retrospective case–control study by Otigbah et al. (2000) found there was a highly significant reduction in analgesia requirements in women having water births, with 38% of women in the water-birth group having no analgesia (95% CI 23.5–36.3, $p < 0.0001$) and 58% using only inhalation analgesia (nitrous oxide/ oxygen). Mallen-Perez et al. (2018) demonstrated that all women having their second baby who used hydrotherapy birthed without analgesia with this contributing to a statistically significant result (p = 0.007) when compared with the control group. Snapp et al. (2020), in their secondary analysis of the American Perinatal Data Registry between 2012 and 2017, also found that women who had a water birth were less likely to request pharmacological methods of pain relief.

Retrospective studies have also demonstrated that water immersion is associated with less analgesia use. Bailey et al. (2020) found that there was a statistically significantly lower uptake of narcotics in the water immersion group ($p < 0.001$) while Sidebottom et al. (2020) showed that epidural and intravenous pain medication was significantly lower in the water birth group ($p < 0.001$). A reduction in epidural use was also found in a prospective cohort study comparing 190 women who used water immersion with 190 women who did not in Ireland (15.9% vs 48.9%, OR 0.20, 95% CI 0.12 to 0.32) (Barry et al., 2020). The current Cochrane review of water immersion in labour and birth (15 trials involving 3663 women) reports a reduction in epidurals for women in water immersion compared with the control group (Cluett et al., 2018).

It could be argued that women choosing water immersion for labour and / or birth are often highly motivated towards achieving physiological birth and not using pharmacological pain relief; subsequently, the research needs to be viewed with this in mind.

Reduced intervention

At Southampton Hospital in England, Cluett et al. (2004) compared women who used water immersion during labour with those who had standard augmentation for dystocia and demonstrated that the women who used the birthing pool had significantly fewer epidurals, needed less assistance with giving birth and had fewer obstetric interventions.

Mollamahmutoglu et al. (2012) compared the incidence of interventions (induction and episiotomy requirements) across the three groups. Primigravida and multipara women in the water birth group had the lowest need for induction and episiotomy and, as such, the authors support the assertions of Ginesi & Niescierowicz (1998) that 'The positive physiological effects of hydrotherapy can facilitate the neurohormonal interactions of labour, reducing pain, and potentially facilitates the progress of labour' (Mollamahmutoglu et al., 2012, p. 47).

These findings are supported by more recent studies that have found that water immersion reduces the likelihood of intervention. For example, Ulfsdottir et al. (2017) found there were significantly fewer women in the water birth group who had an artificial rupture of membranes (13.7 vs 35.3%), an augmentation by oxytocin infusion (5.2 vs 31.3%) and internal cardiotocography (CTG) (11.1 vs 56.8%). Bailey et al. (2020) also showed that women who had a water birth were less likely to be augmented (7.5% vs 11.7%, $p = 0.03$) but were also less likely to be induced (11.4% vs 15.3%, $p = 0.04$) and have an actively managed third stage (44.9% vs 60.5%, $p < 0.001$).

Perineal trauma

Water birth is consistently associated with a lower incidence of episiotomy and a higher intact perineum rate when compared with land birth (Aird, 1997; Burke & Kilfoyle, 1995; Geissbuehler & Eberhard, 2000; Zanetti-Dallenbach et al., 2007b). Geissbuehler & Eberhard (2000) revealed an episiotomy rate of 12.8% in the water birth group compared with 35.4% in the land birth group. The episiotomy rate was five times higher in the control group in the study by Otigbah et al. (2000). This finding was more pronounced in a study by Lim et al. (2016) who found that 63.6% of women in the control group had an episiotomy compared to 0.85% in the water birth group ($p < 0.01$). A study by Snapp et al. (2020) also found a reduced incidence of episiotomy in the water birth group. One could argue, however, that there is no place for episiotomy in the practice of water birth, because if you are performing an episiotomy out of concern for the condition of the baby then you should not be continuing with a birth in water!

Many studies have shown that women experience equivalent, if not better, perineal outcomes when using water immersion. Otigbah et al. (2000) showed that primigravidae having water births had less perineal trauma ($p < 0.05$) while Menakaya et al. (2013) showed that more women in the water birth group had an intact perineum compared with women in the conventional vaginal birth group (40% vs 30%) but this was not statistically significant. Women in the standard birth group experienced higher-degree perineal trauma (third- and fourth-degree tears) more often and a statistically significant difference in episiotomy ($p = 0.001$). Another study that determined rates of perineal trauma, postpartum haemorrhage and 5-minute Apgar scores amongst low-risk women giving birth in a birth centre in water compared with six birth positions on land concluded that water birth did not demonstrate any disadvantage with regards to perineal trauma, Apgar scores and PPH (Dahlen et al., 2013).

Ulfsdottir et al. (2017) concluded there was a statistically significantly lower risk of second-degree tears in the water birth group. More recent research supports these findings in that women are more likely to experience an intact perineum and have similar rates of first- and second-degree perineal lacerations (Bailey et al. 2020). Second stage immersion was also found to reduce the risk of any type of perineal laceration (55.2%, 95% CI 50.1%–60.3% vs 70.1%, 95% CI 65.2%–74.6%, odds ratio 0.5, 95% CI 0.4–0.7) in Sidebottom et al.'s (2020) retrospective study.

Contrary to the above literature, a retrospective analysis by Cortes et al. (2011) examined the incidence of perineal trauma following a water birth versus a land birth and found that 2.5% of women who had a water birth experienced a third-degree tear versus 1.2% of the land birth group ($p > 0.05$, RR 1.9, 95% CI 0.58–6.23) despite a significantly shorter second stage of labour in the water birth group. The authors theorised that the higher incidence of third-degree tearing in the water birth group could be the shorter second stage of labour not allowing the muscular structures and connective tissue of the birth canal to prepare for the sudden transition of the baby through the perineum (Cortes et al., 2011). In a cohort study, Bovbjerg et al. (2016) reported that water birth is associated with an increase in genital tract trauma while a study by Aughey et al. (2021) found no difference in obstetric and sphincter injuries when comparing those who birthed in water and those who did not.

The higher rates of perineal trauma in some studies could be explained by the fact that women giving birth in water are enabled to have a more physiological or 'hands-off' second stage of labour such that access to and visibility of the perineum is limited. However, Mollamahmutoglu et al. (2012) contested the belief that conducting an episiotomy is preferable to third- and fourth-degree tears especially given that episiotomy rates were high in the non-water-birthing group and women who birthed in water had only minimal perineal tears. This was further supported by an Italian prospective observational study by Henderson et al. (2014) that found an increase in second-degree tears for nulliparas birthing in water, but this was offset by fewer episiotomies. Women who birthed in water did so in an 'upright position' (e.g., semi recumbent, squatting, kneeling or on all fours). They also experienced a hands-off birth whereby they received no assistance with the perineum or the baby's head. They also had a significantly higher rate of physiological third stage in comparison to the non-water birth group (all of whom had active management).

Concerns

Women contemplating birth in water need to know the possibility of adverse effects on the baby, in order to make an informed decision. The literature informs us that there are occasional poor outcomes that may be associated with birth in water, but it is important to note that it is not always clear whether these events can be definitely attributed to water immersion. This section discusses the most common concerns.

Water temperature

The temperature of water used in labour and for birth has caused concern in relation to fetal outcomes. In the late 1980s, temperatures of below 37°C were thought to stimulate the baby to breathe (Gradert et al., 1987; Lecky-Thompson, 1989; Lenstrup et al., 1987) and so pool temperatures were maintained at 37–8°C. However, in 1994, two cases of perinatal asphyxia were reported after the women were immersed in warm water during labour and it was thought that the temperature of the water had been a contributing factor even though this was never confirmed (Rosser, 1994).

Johnson (1996) explains that the fetus may be at increased risk when the mother experiences hyperthermia as physiologically the fetus has a baseline temperature 0.5–1°C higher than the maternal baseline. The fetal oxygen demands increase, making the baby susceptible to fetal distress. In response, guidelines often advise that the water is no warmer than 37.5°C due to the potential risk of birth asphyxia (Deans & Steer, 1995; Duley, 2001; Richmond, 2003). Contrary to this view, Charles (1998) postulated that a maternal temperature rise of up to 1°C may be beneficial to the baby due to increased oxygen transfer across the placenta; however, temperature thresholds were not defined to indicate what might be considered too hot.

Geissbuehler et al. (2002) measured maternal and neonatal temperatures following water birth and compared them with those of women and babies who birthed on land. The authors concluded that birth in water did not pose a thermal risk to either the woman or the baby. They concluded that women self-regulate their body temperature according to changes in the water temperature and argued that this was far superior to any water temperature guideline. In support of this, Tricia Anderson (2004) suggested that practitioners give up their obsession with the temperature of the water and instead focus on supporting the woman's physical comfort and ensuring that the woman has control over her environment. A joint Royal College of Obstetricians and Gynaecologists (RCOG) and Royal College of Midwives (RCM) statement on water immersion during labour and birth (2006) noted a wide variation in recommended water temperatures and supported the notion that there 'may be more benefit to allow women to regulate the pool temperature to their own comfort' (Alfirevic & Gould, 2006).

In practical terms, the midwife should assess the woman's temperature before she enters the pool and while she is immersed in addition to ensuring the water temperature is comfortable for the woman. It is useful to maintain an ambient room temperature that is comfortable for the woman and to have supplies of cool water or ice chips and access to a fan if the woman shows signs of dehydration or becomes too hot.

Maternal and neonatal infection

The theoretical risk of infection to either the woman or her baby remains a barrier to the widespread introduction of water immersion for labour and birth particularly for women with ruptured membranes. Waldenstrom & Nilsson (1992) conducted a non-randomised controlled study at the Stockholm Birth Centre comparing women who did and did not use the bath after ruptured membranes. They found no statistically significant difference between the groups with regard to infection, infant respiratory problems or symptoms of amnionitis in the woman. Robertson et al. (1998) conducted a medical review and found no association between the use of water immersion in labour and the development of chorioamnionitis and endometritis. Similarly, Geissbuehler & Eberhard (2000) analysed 7508 births and reported no statistically significant difference in infection rates between infants born in water and those born on land.

Michel Odent (2001) discussed bacteriological colonisation of babies at birth. He explained the concept of the 'race to the surface' used by bacteriologists, meaning that the first bacteria to reach a bacteria-free surface will be the likely rulers of the territory. Babies are born sharing the immunoglobulin G (IgG) antibodies of their mothers, and therefore it is beneficial for a baby to be colonised by the mother's bacteria. From a microbiological perspective, it would seem that birth in water is a positive action, in line with skin-to-skin contact. It is when babies come in contact with unfamiliar bacteria from caregivers and hospitals that the bacteria they are colonised by become potentially dangerous. This theory supports the idea that caregivers should stay out of the water unless absolutely necessary, but partners and siblings should not be discouraged, as they are likely to have similar bacterial colonisations to those of the mother (Fig. 27.3).

Five observational studies of 12,797 water births found either no maternal infection or no difference in maternal infection (Cammu et al., 1994; Eckert et al., 2001; Kausela et al., 1998; Rush et al., 1996; Schorn et al., 1993). In accordance with this, Geissbuehler et al. (2000) found higher rates of antibiotic use in land birth.

A study by Zanetti-Daellenbach et al., (2007a) comparing GBS-positive women who had a water birth with those who gave birth on land found that babies born in water were less colonised with GBS and, as such, they

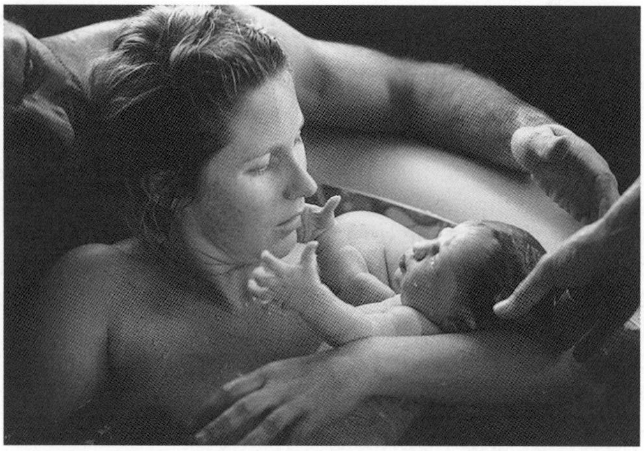

FIGURE 27.3 Partner support during a water birth
(Photograph copyright David Hancock.)

argued that GBS is not a contraindication for water birth. Burns et al. (2012) found no reported cases of maternal infection in their large prospective observational study (8924 women). Nor did Snapp et al. (2020) in the descriptional correlational study when examining maternal reproductive tract infections at six weeks postpartum.

Two epidemiological studies (Alderdice et al., 1995; Gilbert & Tookey, 1999) reported on neonatal morbidity including infection. Alderdice et al. (1995) surveyed Heads of Midwifery in England and Wales (4494 water births) and reported there were 51 incidences of neonatal morbidity including infection. In Gilbert & Tookey's 1999 study (4032 water births), two babies were reported to have evidence of infection. However, a review of the findings in Alderdice et al. (1995) and Gilbert & Tookey (1999) revealed that water birth could not be directly attributed as the cause of the infection symptoms (Young & Kruske, 2013).

Neonatal infection rates were rare and the rates of infection unchanged from earlier studies (Zanetti-Daellenbach et al., 2007b). Concerns proposed that neonatal infection could occur through contact with contaminated water (e.g., faecal matter, unclean pipes and hoses). One trial reported temperatures greater than 37.8°C as an indicator for infection and found no significant difference between those who had used water and those who had not (Eckert et al., 2001). Otigbah et al. (2000) compared water birth with land birth and reported no cases of neonatal infection and no differences in neonatal infection rates respectively. A prospective cohort study by Burns et al. (2012), which included 8924 low-risk women, reported that 35 babies in total (0.39%) had pyrexia or suspected infection; however, no babies had positive cultures. In Neiman et al.'s (2020) study, one neonate was septic following water immersion during labour while two required intravenous antibiotics. However, no neonates born via water birth required antibiotics nor were any diagnosed with sepsis.

At the First International Waterbirth Conference in London in 1995, it was concluded that the water diluted blood-borne viruses to the point where they became impotent and posed much less of a threat than the blood splashes that may occur in a land birth (Beech, 1996). Colombo et al. (2000) took pool-water samples from 14 different water births and measured the haemoglobin content to estimate the HIV viral load and concluded that the water had a diluting effect minimising the potential risk of HIV exposure to intact skin. However, in their opinion, the risk of nosocomial hepatitis B infection is significantly higher, and as such they recommend that all healthcare workers get vaccinated and that they wear gauntlet gloves while facilitating water birth. This was supported in the prospective observational study by Zanetti-Dallenbach et al. (2007b).

Vanderlaan & Hall (2020) undertook a systematic review of 47 cases from 35 articles of poor outcomes in neonates follow water immersion, 18 cases were related to infection. Non-waterborne pathogens including human herpesvirus, adenovirus, *Haemophilus parainfluenzae* and group B streptococcal meningitis were reported but the authors argued that there was no evidence to support that the water increased the transmission and, rather, there was evidence of vertical or other means of transmission in select cases. Waterborne infections including *Legionella pneumoniae* and *P. aeruginosa* were also reported and believed to be transmitted because of water aspiration. However, this was questionable in the *P. aeruginosa* cases given that the neonates were diagnosed with sepsis and meningitis rather than pneumonia. In the *Legionella pneumoniae* cases, the presentations were more consistent with transmission by aerolised droplets possibly due to water splashes as the babies were lifted from the water. In one case, the hospital was found to be infected with *Legionella*. A further nine cases were noted as suspected infections but were later believed to be a result of water aspiration. Seven resolved within 24 hours and besides elevated C-reactive protein values, all had normal laboratory results.

These findings support an earlier systematic review and meta-analysis undertaken by Vanderlaan and colleagues (2018) who determined that the odds of pneumonia and non-pneumonia infections were no different between babies born in water and those who are not.

The literature indicates that if pools/baths are adequately cleaned with soap and water and according to the infection control policies, then air dried, there is no increase in neonatal or maternal infection (Global Maternal/Child Health 2000, cited in Harper, 2000; Zanetti-Dallenbach et al., 2007b). Infection risks to babies appear to be caused primarily by Gram-negative organisms that colonise pump systems of spa baths and filling and draining hoses, and by inadequate bath-cleaning procedures (Vochem et al., 2001). Zanetti-Dallenbach et al. (2007b) stated that to reduce the risk of an infection with *Pseudomonas* the water tap should be fully opened for several minutes before filling the tub.

Third stage and blood loss

There have been no documented complications relating to the third stage being conducted in the bath, although Richmond (2003) hypothesised that there is an increased potential for postpartum haemorrhage associated with water birth owing to hyperaemia induced by warm water and the relaxing effect it has on uterine muscles. However, this has not been proven (Caplice, 2004b; Garland, 2002; Garland & Jones, 1997). In a study by Zanetti-Dallenbach et al. (2007b), women in all three study groups had a haemoglobin (Hb) assessment on admission and again at 2 days postpartum. The water birth group had higher Hb levels postpartum, which was not clinically significant and there were no statistical differences across the three groups. They concluded that the blood loss in water birth is comparable to that following a normal spontaneous birth.

Mollamahmutoglu et al. (2012) found that women having a water birth had a shorter third stage. They suggested that this could be explained by the hydrostatic pressure of the water, less perineal tears (or lesser severity) and a facilitated third stage.

A study of low-risk women in a secondary-level hospital in Australia reported that the average post-birth blood loss in the retrospective audit of water births compared to conventional vaginal births was 300 mL (Menakaya et al. 2013). There were no differences in the rates of postpartum blood loss between the two groups (Menakaya et al., 2013).

Nutter et al.'s (2014) analysis of 38 studies showed that the research generally confirms that water birth results in the same or decreased likelihood of PPH compared with land birth and, as such, presents no greater risk but may in fact decrease the risk of PPH. Research conducted after this review has supported Nutter et al.'s (2014) findings. Lim et al. (2016) reported no difference in estimated blood loss or postpartum haemorrhage when comparing women who had a water birth and those who had conventional vaginal births between 2010 and 2013. This was also found by Ulfsdottir et al. (2017) and Bailey et al. (2020). A recent study by Aughey et al. (2021) reported that women who birthed in water ($n = 6284$) had a statistically significantly reduced risk of experiencing a PPH of $\geq$ 1500 mL when compared with women who did not ($n = 39{,}824$) in their UK retrospective cohort study. However, they do note that they were not able to control for confounders such as slow labour progress and the bias of measuring blood loss in a birthing pool.

In comparison, Neiman et al. (2020) found that 3.4% of women who had a water birth experienced a PPH compared to only 0.9% of women who birthed on land, but this did not contribute to any difference in postpartum Hb or haematocrit levels between groups. Barry et al. (2020) also reported that the incidence of PPH (> 500 mL) was higher in the water birth group however, major PPHs (> 1000 mL) were not statistically significant. They also reported that a higher number of women in the water immersion group experienced a physiological third stage (28.9% vs 4.7%, OR 8.19; 95% CI 3.91 to 17.16). They also had two-fold increased incidence of babies over 4 kg (13.7% vs 5.3%, OR 2.85, 95% CI 1.34 to 6.10) and women who birthed in water were more likely to experience a third stage duration of more than 30 minutes compared to those who used water in labour (27.0% vs 3.3%, OR 10.73; 95% CI 3.13 to 36.80). These factors may have contributed to the higher PPH rate.

In recognising the difficulty of estimating blood loss following a water birth, Burns et al. (2019) implemented and evaluated an online learning tool to assist midwives in this skill. Their pre-test, post-test study revealed that the accuracy of blood loss estimations showed that midwives underestimated blood loss in the pre-test evaluations, but accuracy significantly improved at post-test 1 and this was largely sustained at post-test 2.

By majority policies and guidelines support women with low-risk pregnancies to use water, thereby reducing the likelihood of adverse events that may increase the risk of PPH. Midwives are also skilled in assessing women throughout labour and birth and recognising deviations from the woman's normal parameters and, as such, it would be expected that they would encourage the woman to leave the birthing pool where there is evidence of maternal and / or fetal compromise.

Maternal collapse

Maternal collapse is a common concern amongst midwives and those who oppose the introduction of using water immersion. This was found by Cooper, Warland & McCutcheon (2018) in a survey of 234 midwives about the most common concerns related to water immersion. It is, however, important to note that while maternal collapse was the most common concern, the most common response on the Likert scale was 'some concern'.

While women are buoyant in water, the need to evacuate them from the water presents challenges. Despite this, maternal collapse has rarely been recorded in the literature and this is likely due to the fact that women who use water are screened for their suitability and are encouraged to leave the pool or bath where there are signs of compromise (Young & Kruske, 2013). In any event, Young and Kruske (2013) suggest that all facilities have clear protocols in place for emergency management of maternal collapse, support staff in emergency drills and provide equipment to support the evacuation of women from the water.

Cord avulsion

Traction on the umbilical cord as the baby is lifted clear of the water may lead to cord avulsion or snapping, especially when the cord is short. Gilbert & Tookey's (1999) surveillance study and postal survey of perinatal mortality and morbidity among babies born in water identified snapped umbilical cords in five (out of 4032) which were probably the result of cord traction when bringing the babies to the surface rapidly. One of the five babies required a blood transfusion.

Cro & Preston (2002) reported on an audit following an instance of cord snapping at a water birth. They identified four cases of snapped umbilical cord out of 100 water births between September 1996 and March 2001. In three instances the cord was noted to have snapped while bringing the baby to the surface, and the ends were immediately clamped resulting in no adverse effects. In the fourth case, the snapped cord was discovered when it was noted that the baby was becoming paler and making reduced respiratory effort. A lot of blood was noted in the water. The baby required a blood transfusion and was discharged from hospital after 3 days. Follow-up at 8 weeks found the baby to be developing normally.

A large prospective observational study reported cord snap in 18/5192 water births compared with 2/3732 land births, with an overall rate of 0.22% (Burns et al., 2012). Three of the babies were admitted to a NICU and one baby had a transfusion. All were discharged home without problems. Ulfsdottir et al. (2017) also captured the incidence of cord avulsion in their retrospective cohort study and found no statistical difference between the water birth (n = 3/306) and non-water birth groups (n = 1/306) ($p = 0.8$). Similarly, no difference was found in the Neiman et al. (2020) retrospective cohort study. Barry et al. (2020) also reported cases of cord avulsion—one in the water birth group and one in the water immersion group. Neither baby suffered adversely nor were either transferred to the neonatal unit.

A review by Nutter et al. (2014) revealed that the rate of cord avulsion occurrences in water births is 2.4 per 1000 births. However, they found that a lack of data for comparison with land births makes it difficult to draw conclusions as to the relative frequency of cord avulsion.

Although it is a rare event, caregivers need to be aware of possible cord snap particularly when there is a short umbilical cord. The baby needs to be brought carefully and slowly to the surface to avoid undue traction on the cord. If the cord is short the woman is asked to stand. The midwife is advised to check the cord as soon as possible after birth.

Shoulder dystocia

Women who have experienced a shoulder dystocia in a prior birth and / or are at a perceived increased risk of shoulder dystocia in current birth are often precluded from accessing water immersion for labour and birth (SA Health, 2017). This is in spite of the fact that there is no effective or foolproof means via which to definitely predict shoulder dystocia. While there have been limited studies examining the incidence of shoulder dystocia and the associated outcomes with respect to water immersion, there is some argument that the benefits of buoyancy, ease of position changes, an upright position and women being more in control of their birth experience help as much as possible to mitigate any increased risk of shoulder dystocia. More recently, studies have reported the incidence of shoulder dystocia during water immersion as opposed to birth on land. Neiman et al. (2020) reported no statistical difference in the incidence of shoulder dystocia when comparing water birth, water immersion and land birth in their retrospective cohort study ($p = 0.441$). This supported Vanderlaan et al.'s (2018) findings in that they too found no difference in rates of shoulder dystocia between water and land births in their synthesis of four studies (OR 0.84 95% CI 0.43–1.63). In comparison, Snapp et al. (2020) found a statistically significant difference in rates of shoulder dystocia in their descriptional correlational study of 26,684 births in favour of birth in water (RR =0.41; 95% CI, 0.34-0.49). These studies suggest that the risk of shoulder dystocia is not increased by water immersion and instead, the benefits afforded by water may reduce the likelihood of this obstetric emergency.

Effects on the baby

Johnson (1996) describes in depth the physiology of fetal breathing in utero and the main factors that inhibit breathing in the newborn until she or he is lifted into air. Fetal breaths in utero are intermittent isometric movements with very little inspiration of amniotic fluid (Johnson, 1996). Approximately 24–48 hours prior to birth, in response to the increase in prostaglandin E_2 levels from the placenta, the fetal breathing movements slow down or cease. This decrease in fetal breathing movements allows more blood flow to the vital organs, including the brain. At birth, when the prostaglandin level is still high, the baby's breathing response is still slow—this is the first inhibitory response.

A second inhibitory response is related to acute hypoxia in the newborn. Babies are born experiencing a lack of oxygen in response to the birth process. This normal inhibition of breathing may be overridden if the baby becomes compromised in utero. Acute hypoxia causes apnoea and swallowing, and if severe and prolonged it will cause breathing and gasping (Fewell & Johnson, 1983).

Another important inhibitory component is the 'dive reflex'. Central to the physiology of the dive reflex is the larynx, which is covered with chemoreceptors (like taste buds). With application of foreign stimuli such as water to the larynx, these chemoreceptors initiate the closure of the glottis so that the water is swallowed and not inhaled (Harding et al., 1978). Johnson (1996) reports that, whereas substances such as water, non-species milks, isotonic alkalis and ammonia initiate the full diving response, physiological saline, amniotic fluid, lung and gastric fluids, urine, blood, meconium and milk from the same species at body temperature illicit little response when instilled to the larynx. Mollamahmutoglu et al. (2012) observed the diving reflex in all of the water birth newborns in their study. The authors state that aspiration due to failure of the diving reflex would occur only as a result of anaesthesia, severe asphyxia or poorly monitored pool temperature.

The last main factor thought to inhibit the newborn from initiating a breathing response while in water is environmental temperature. Johnson (1996) reported that maternal hyperthermia and resultant hyperthermia in the fetus may override the inhibition to breathe. Therefore, maternal hyperthermia or overheating should be avoided.

In light of births taking place in oceans, where the babies are reported to be born with no adverse effects, the suggestion that water should be kept close to maternal body temperature may not be necessary (Harper, 2002).

Birth under water is gentle and babies are not immediately subjected to the stimulants seen in standard births (i.e., light, noise, cold, gravity). Babies born in water are guided gently up to their mother's chest, often by the mother herself, and are held with their bodies still submerged in the warm water. They slowly start to adapt to extrauterine life whilst the cord continues pulsating and providing oxygen. They will start to breathe in their own time, and this can be after the 1-minute Apgar score is recorded, meaning the score is lowered. However, their heart rates and colour are usually scored as 2 during this time. This is reflected in a study by Menakaya et al. (2013). Babies in the water birth group had an Apgar score of 7 or less at 1 minute ($p = 0.05$), but there were no statistically significant differences in the 5-minute Apgar score between the two groups. There were eight admissions to the Neonatal Intensive Care Unit (NICU) from the water birth group compared with one from the standard group ($p = 0.023$). The reasons for these admissions were: observation (two after active resuscitation, one for apnoea and low birth weight, and one for shoulder dystocia), meconium aspiration (one baby), and three babies with feeding difficulties. One baby in the standard birth group was admitted to NICU with respiratory distress and required care for nine days (Menakaya et al., 2013). Mollamahmutoglu et al. (2012) found that Apgar scores were slightly lower in the water birth group but there was no difference in rate of admissions to the NICU between all groups. There were also no cases of neonatal infections or death.

Nutter et al. (2014) do not support the finding that babies born in water have lower 1- or 10-minute Apgar scores than non-water-birth babies; nor do they believe that are they at greater risk of infection or NICU admission. This was supported by a large cohort study comparing outcomes of 6534 babies born underwater, 10,290 babies not born underwater and 1573 planned water births that did not proceed (Bovbjerg et al., 2016). The authors concluded that the babies born under water experienced fewer negative effects than those born out of the water.

These findings have been echoed in more recent studies which have found no difference in mean Apgar scores and equivalent or reduced NICU admissions when water immersion is compared with conventional birth (Aughey et al. 2021; Bailey et al. 2020; Barry et al. 2020; Lim et al., 2016; Sidebottom et al. 2020, Vanderlaan et al. 2018). Sidebottom et al. (2020) found that NICU and special care nursery admission was significantly lower in the second stage immersion and suggested that this could be explained by the fact that the water immersion in labour group reflected a higher number of women who had left the pool due to medical indications. This was echoed in Aughey et al.'s (2021) retrospective cohort study which reflected an adjusted odds ratio of 0.65 (0.53,0.78) for NICU admission following water birth.

Potential near drowning

Nguyen et al. (2002) reported four cases of babies admitted to the neonatal unit following water births at hospital and home. These babies presented to hospital with moderate to severe respiratory distress and were reported to have water aspiration and subsequent pulmonary oedema, however, all babies improved over a 24-hour period. Similarly, Bowden et al. (2002) reported four admissions to a NICU after birth in water. The first case was suspected to have water inhalation; however, the discharge diagnosis was respiratory distress syndrome. The second baby developed seizures at eight hours of age and his discharge diagnosis was probable water intoxication after water birth. The third baby had a congenital abnormality diagnosed on day two. The fourth baby was admitted at four days of age with group B streptococcal meningitis not directly attributable to birth in water.

In response to these concerns, Pinette et al. (2004) conducted a retrospective review of the possible complications associated with water birth. They identified 16 citations that reported on neonatal complications that could be attributed to birth in water. The possible complications included freshwater drowning, neonatal hyponatraemia, hypoxic ischaemic encephalopathy and death, and, in response, the authors concluded that a large RCT is needed to measure adverse effects of water birth on the baby. However, Pinette et al. (2004) failed to mention that some of the complications had occurred after women had left the water prior to giving birth.

Concerns around water aspiration in babies born under water are not supported by the available evidence. A literature review seeking evidence for concerns expressed around water aspiration during water birth (Young & Kruske, 2013) failed to find a causal relationship between water birth and water aspiration symptoms. The number and type of studies where water aspiration was reported are small. There have been no RCTs using an association between water births and water aspiration as an outcome measure, but there have been four large prospective studies comparing water birth with land birth, accounting for 19,139 births of which 6457 were water births (Zanetti-Dallenbach et al., 2006).

Perinatal mortality and morbidity/adverse outcomes

The potential for increased perinatal morbidity and mortality associated with water immersion and water birth is low. The outcomes for women and babies using water immersion during labour and birth are comparable to those expected in any healthy childbearing population (Nutter et al., 2014).

A survey in England and Wales assessed the problems reported following births in water from 1992 to 1993. Of the 4834 births in water, it was reported that there were six stillbirths/neonatal deaths, none of which could be attributed to the use of water. The estimated mortality rate was 1.24 per 1000 live births (Alderdice et al., 1995). In 1999, Gilbert & Tookey compared the perinatal morbidity and mortality rates for babies born in water with those for babies born on land in the British Isles (surveillance study) and England and Wales (postal surveys). They found that perinatal mortality and risk of admission to special-care baby units did not differ across groups (Gilbert & Tookey, 1999).

More recent studies have concluded that there is no difference in neonatal death following water birth when compared with conventional births. This was the case in Vanderlaan et al.'s (2018) study. They suggested that the there has never been sufficient evidence to prove that water birth increases the risk of death based on their meta-analysis but acknowledge and highlight that this may be too few studies for a rare outcome. Similarly, Sidebottom et al. (2020) reported no statistical difference in the composite measure of adverse outcomes (e.g., sepsis, asphyxia, hypoxic ischemic encephalopathy or death) in the water immersion groups.

COVID-19 and other infectious diseases

In 2020, the first cases of COVID-19 were found in Australia and over the next few months, restrictions were implemented by authorities to reduce transmission amongst the community. The restrictions of social distancing and improved hygiene were effective but had marked implications for women during pregnancy and particularly during labour and birth. Social distancing measures resulted in limitations around support people and access to pain relief options including nitrous oxide and water immersion due to concerns around aerolisation of virus particles. In response, many maternity care services ceased the use of water immersion. In a survey undertaken by Cooper and King (2020) from the Australian College of Midwives, it was clear women were unhappy about this directive and many shared that they were seeking care by a privately practising midwife in order to have the birth that they wanted and to access water immersion. These findings reflected an earlier study by Dahlen et al. (2013).

Despite concerns surrounding the generation of aerolisation and potential increased spread of COVID-19, very few cases had been reported in women who were pregnant or birthing and women challenged the 'blanket' cessation of water immersion. A 'cautious' approach to nitrous oxide use was advised despite a higher risk of aerolisation, and yet a complete cessation of water immersion was imposed even though women who use water are generally calm and peaceful, and there is limited splashing of water.

In response, the ACM (2020) released an updated position statement with regards to water immersion and argued:

- COVID-19 is not a waterborne virus; it is transmitted through air via droplets (due to coughing, sneezing, breathing) or from surfaces that may be contaminated by said droplets; as such, the act of immersing in warm water during labour and / or birth is not likely to increase the risk of transmission, instead it may actually reduce it.
- A watery environment dilutes any potential risk of respiratory droplet and / or faecal contamination (Note: testing of faecal samples has been conducted in water due to the reduced risk of droplet and aerosol contamination). In fact, this is likely to reduce the risk compared with land birth.
- While COVID-19 may be found in faeces, there is currently no evidence of faecal–oral transmission.
- The physical barrier offered by the bath / pool assists with social distancing between the woman and those who are present for labour and / or birth including midwives and support people.
- Women who give birth in water commonly receive their baby and gently guide their baby to the surface, thereby reducing contact between the woman (and baby) and midwives (unless, of course, there is a need to intervene).
- Adherence to birth-pool cleaning protocols further reduces if not eliminates the risk of transmission to subsequent users.
- Midwives have ready access to personal protective equipment (PPE).

In the absence of research specifically addressing the use of water with regards to COVID-19 transmission, an individualised approach to water immersion with attentiveness to infection control, cleaning procedures and social distancing is unlikely to increase the risk of transmission.

In light of the above review of the evidence, preventing women from accessing water immersion during birth because of concerns about water aspiration, infection or other adverse events is generally not justified (Young & Kruske, 2013).

CLINICAL POINT

Key messages from research

- Women are highly satisfied with using water immersion for labour and birth.
- Women feel more in control during labour and birth, which ultimately leads to a more positive experience and reduced reliance on pharmacological pain relief.
- Outcomes and risks are similar for low-risk women who labour and birth in water and those who labour and birth in air.
- Witnessing and engaging with women who use water during labour and birth can often allay practitioner fears and anxieties. Midwives and other health care providers should have opportunities to experience water immersion.
- Midwives should actively seek and interpret research to inform their practice.
- Policies and guidelines do not often reflect the contemporary evidence base; midwives should actively engage in the development of policies and guidelines to ensure they reflect the evidence base and women's informed decision making.

CRITICAL THINKING EXERCISE

Alice is a healthy nulliparous woman who is thinking about a water birth. She seeks an answer to a question often put to her when she tells friends and family about her choice—could the baby drown? Formulate a response to this question in language that is easily understood.

USING WATER FOR LABOUR AND BIRTH: THE PRACTICE

Globally, there has been an increase in the number of women seeking to use water for labour and birth. In response to the increasing demand from women and midwives it has become more common to find water immersion facilities in maternity units at all levels. This is an attempt to provide a home-like environment that supports a more holistic approach to birth. Hodnett (2000) found that women who gave birth in home-like settings were less likely to use pharmacological pain relief, be augmented with oxytocin and experience fetal heart abnormalities. They were more likely to be mobile during labour and they were also happier with their care when compared with women who received standard care.

Women who make an informed decision to use water immersion for labour and birth are generally strongly motivated to labour without pain relief and medical intervention. When supported by a midwife throughout labour and birth, studies have demonstrated that women are less likely to need pain relief and they experience a decrease in the length of labour (Hodnett, 2000). Other research has concluded that the presence of a known midwife facilitates improved labour and birth outcomes and there is also good evidence to suggest that the combination of midwifery support and water immersion facilitates a positive, safe and satisfying birth experience (Feeley et al., 2021; Maude & Foureur, 2007; Otigbah et al. 2000).

There is emerging evidence to suggest that the practitioner's experience and support for water immersion directly influences their willingness to support and prompt the implementation of this option (Cooper, McCutcheon & Warland, 2019). In addition to this, it is now well established that midwives who hold any level of fear or anxiety with respect to water immersion and, especially, water birth are less likely to promote, offer or facilitate the option (Cooper, 2017). Midwives who are unfamiliar or opposed to water immersion for labour and birth appear to be more concerned about potential problems. Kitzinger (2009) talked about some hospital-based midwives being highly anxious about using birth pools and employing a 'protective gate-keeping' role to steer women away from making informed decisions. As such, they are less likely to undertake necessary training and professional development and avoid offering the option to women.

This is further complicated by the well-documented lack of support of water immersion from medical professionals. Many studies have highlighted that when compared with their midwifery counterparts, medical practitioners including obstetricians, paediatricians and anaesthetists are particularly concerned with the potential risks associated with water immersion, especially those related to the baby being birthed into water. As such, they argue that water immersion and, particularly, water birth are unnecessary (Cooper, McCutcheon & Warland, 2019)

In a critical analysis of Australian water immersion policies and guidelines, Cooper, McCutcheon & Warland (2017) highlighted that the landscape of maternity care in Australia remains heavily influenced by the biomedical paradigm. They stated:

> *the obstetric and biomedical view was that WI added additional risks to an already risk-laden process and therefore posed potential, possible and even theoretical threats to safety. Therefore, rather than the practice being offered / promoted, the practice of WI was instead restricted by compliance and obscure definitions of risk.* (p. 439)

Policies and guidelines were often not reflective of the contemporary evidence base and were written from a risk-averse approach such that they were viewed as reflecting authoritative opinions rather than the literature. Chapman (2004) who reviewed water birth protocols in New Zealand also found that there were inconsistencies in exclusion criteria across the documents and / or omissions of the contemporary evidence base, with this prompting the questions 'Who is formulating the protocols?' and 'What evidence supports the protocols?'. They argue this is likely to be detrimental to both women and care providers.

This was not dissimilar from studies by Newnham et al. (2015, 2017) who reflect the differences between the use of water as opposed to epidural anaesthesia and the culture of risk that means women often find it easier to access an epidural than water immersion. They discuss the pressure that women often feel to succumb to societal norms to avoid being labelled as irresponsible with this speaking to the stigmatisation of women who seek alternative to mainstream maternity care provision (Newnham et al., 2015). They argue that this has led to increasing rates and greater acceptance of medical intervention. Ultimately, midwives have to balance their role as advocates of women against their role as employees who are bound by hospital policies and guidelines. To describe this, they quote Bryers & van Teijlingen (2010, p. 493).

> *when a woman who has had a previous caesarean section chooses to have a waterbirth, the midwife is put in a difficult position: she may wish to support the woman, but to do so will mean that she . . . is practising outside the agreed clinical guidelines. Both the midwife and the woman will face considerable pressure from the dominant obstetric ideology; that this is not safe. However, the medical approach to this case is likely to see an epidural in labour as an acceptable*

risk because this is perceived as a technology which can be controlled by continuous monitoring; it is arguable whether this is 'an optimum level of care' but this is how it will be perceived as it is supported by the authoritative knowledge.

Infrastructural issues are likely a consequence of the lack of broader support for the option. Midwives have highlighted that often baths / pools are not available or are, in their minds, deliberately rendered unusable due to plugs going missing, a shortage of available hot water or women who do not wish to use water immersion being allocated to the only available rooms with pools / baths (Newnham et al., 2015; Russell, 2011; Seibold et al. 2010; Woodward, 2012). They also speak of the impact on them personally in terms of occupational health and safety when they are trying to access women while in the bath particularly in the event that they are required to evacuate women from the bath following a maternal collapse. Consideration to these factors and others such as appropriate personal protective equipment and cleaning protocols should be considered when implementing and offering water immersion. They should not be the factors that preclude women from accessing the option.

The challenges appear to be somewhat entrenched in the perception that water immersion is closely aligned to midwifery practice and, in the minds of medical practitioners, is still not supported by the level of evidence that would be expected of the biomedical and largely empirical evidence base. Even in light of this, midwives continue to advocate for water immersion and have taken it upon themselves to undertake research that directly addresses the challenges and concerns raised. They are largely the reason why there is an increasing evidence base to highlight the physical and psychological benefits of water immersion and greater high-quality data to mitigate against the safety concerns that are commonly raised. This reiterates the importance of midwives knowing how to both access and interpret research to support women in their choices and to actively play their role in improving labour and birth outcomes.

It is also important that midwives are aware of the key practices and principles that underpin the use of water immersion during labour and birth, and that they have the opportunity to witness women using water immersion (Young & Kruske, 2013). Both experience and ongoing professional development are recognised as important factors in increasing midwives' confidence and competence with respect to water immersion.

Skills and education of workforce

Young & Kruske (2012) highlight 'skill and education of the workforce as a key concern against the use of water birth' (p. 107). This is supported by Nicholls et al. (2016). The development of guidelines for practice needs to be supported by practice development for staff prior to implementation. A key component of informed choice regarding birth in water is that midwives are confident and competent in the practice so that they can provide advice and information to a woman that is unbiased and not contradicted.

One of the barriers to making water immersion more readily available is the inconsistencies in the education and training requirements of midwives when they are seeking to support women using water immersion. In Australia, midwives are generally required to undertake additional training in order to gain accreditation to facilitate water immersion and this is seen by many as another barrier to more widespread uptake (Cooper, Warland & McCutcheon, 2018, 2019). Many midwives have argued that water immersion is no different to the facilitation of another physiological birth and have questioned the necessity of accreditation requirements and that this is often why women are denied access. Some midwives have described long-term facilitation of water immersion in one venue only to be told that they must achieve accreditation in another facility before offering the option (Cooper, Warland & McCutcheon, 2019). In response, there have been calls for consistency in accreditation requirements on a national basis in Australia and for this to be offered as part of pre-registration midwifery courses, to ensure that midwives can offer water immersion regardless of their place of practice.

CLINICAL POINT

Continuous support in labour

Research supports the need for a continuous supportive presence with women during labour; this by itself has been shown to reduce the likelihood of medication for pain relief, a caesarean section or a forceps delivery (Maude, 2003; Maude & Foureur, 2007). For the women in these studies, to be able to labour and birth in water meant that they were required to form a relationship with a midwife who was philosophically in tune with them and would support their choices. There is a need for partnership and teamwork between women and midwives.

Water immersion policies and guidelines

Midwives are increasingly searching for the best available evidence to challenge and change many of the practices that have led to increasing rates of intervention and higher rates of surgical birth. They recognise that practice wisdom comes from many sources and, as such, use evidence generated from scientific inquiry, knowledge gained from clinical practice and the sharing of stories to inform their practice. This combination of evidence assists midwives to support women, through partnership, to receive thorough, unbiased information about choices for care, place of birth and caregiver, so that they can make truly informed decisions.

Most women know that they should avoid drugs and harmful substances during their pregnancies, yet the protocols for active management of labour often subject them to a range of medications and practices that precipitate into a cascade of intervention and ultimately lead to an operative birth. Indeed, women are reported to be confused by the ease of access to opiates for **pain relief** in labour rather than options to use non-pharmacological pain relief such as water immersion (Hirst, 2005, cited in Young & Kruske, 2012).

There is an evident inconsistency across policies and guidelines pertaining to the use of water immersion during labour and birth (Cooper, Warland & McCutcheon, 2018). The Northern Territory (NT), Australian Capital Territory (ACT), Queensland and Tasmania have no accessible current statewide policies that can support clinical guidelines. New South Wales (NSW) put out a policy directive entitled *Towards Normal Birth* in 2012, which included a recommendation that all maternity services offer access to water immersion in labour and that a state-wide policy should be published (NSW Health, 2010). To date, the NSW policy for the use of water for labour and birth remains unpublished. Western Australia (WA) and South Australia (SA) are the only states with statewide policies regarding water immersion for labour and birth (SA Health, 2017; WA Department of Health, 2009).

A review of policies and guidelines in Australia demonstrated that they were generally not reflective of the most up-to-date evidence and appear to be opinion-based. They neither promote nor facilitate women's informed decision making given they are largely written from a risk-minimisation stance. It has been suggested that a national approach to the development of maternity policies and guidelines may go a long way to overcoming some of these issues (Cameron & Ellwood, 2006). National review of the evidence base and widespread consultation will ultimately lead to high-quality guidance and water immersion becoming a more readily available and acceptable option.

Although guidelines will vary in each location, there are general principles that can be drawn from the literature regarding the considerations and benefits of using water for labour and birth. Two important considerations are:

- *The birthing family's attitude and expectations*—Education regarding the use of water for labour and birth is important antenatally to prepare women and their families. A woman's fear/anxiety about birthing in water may be a contraindication. However, with adequate education and preparation antenatally for the woman and her support team, fears can be allayed (Young & Kruske, 2013).
- *The midwife's attitude, experience and confidence in supporting women to use water for labour and birth*—Women who labour and birth in water should expect to be cared for by practitioners who have appropriate skills and education in the use of water immersion for labour and birth.

The benefits of using water for labour and birth are summarised in Box 27.1.

Box 27.1 Benefits of labour and birth in water

For the woman

- Warm water cradles, supports, relaxes, comforts and soothes, thereby reducing anxiety.
- It enables instinctive behaviour and increases the feeling of being in control, which in turn leads to a high degree of postnatal wellbeing.
- There is less operative delivery and perineal trauma.
- It provides buoyancy and increased mobility.
- It reduces pressure on muscles and vena cava (reduces blood pressure).
- It reduces the need for pharmacological pain relief.
- It provides a protected, secure birthing space.

For the baby

- The reduced maternal need for pharmacological pain relief reduces the side effects on the baby.
- Theoretically, the baby's first breath is gentle, as the air above the water is warm and humidified.
- Theoretically, it provides a smooth, trauma-free transitory passage for the baby.

For the midwife

- It provides the increasingly rare opportunity to witness and facilitate physiological birth.
- It develops and enhances the fundamental skill of working in partnership with women.
- It enables her to extend her knowledge base and participate in research into the use of water for labour and birth.

Who can use water for labour and birth?

Because each woman is an individual and her pregnancy is unique, her care should be individually negotiated through the partnership that forms between her and a known midwife. The midwife can assess the evidence base that informs the maternity unit policy for the use of water immersion for labour and birth, understand the women's needs, expectations and preferences, and then exercise clinical judgment in determining the woman's suitability for using water immersion.

Unfortunately, many maternity facilities have developed water-immersion and water-birth criteria that are too prescriptive and that inhibit autonomous midwifery practice. This appears to be more to do with risk minimisation rather than with what women want and this inhibits the woman's choice and autonomy (Cooper, McCutcheon & Warland, 2017). Some of these criteria are outlined in Box 27.2.

In some situations, the restrictions surrounding water immersion are so prescriptive that women will seek other options for their maternity care, with this including home birth supported by privately practising midwives. This

Box 27.2 Suggested criteria for water immersion and water birth

Criteria include:

- low-risk pregnancy >37 weeks (no adverse factors noted in maternal or fetal wellbeing during pregnancy or labour)
- the woman's choice to use water for labour and birth
- established labour
- no specific requirement for continuous fetal heart rate monitoring.

Some reasons why it may not be advisable for a woman to use the birth pool include the following:

- maternal temperature >37.5°C
- thick meconium staining of liquor
- recent use of a systemic opioid for analgesia
- most practitioners consider breech presentations and multiple pregnancies unsuitable for underwater birth; however, there is anecdotal evidence that these do occasionally occur both in hospitals and at home.

speaks to the importance of maternity care services consulting with consumers, engaging with the contemporary evidence base and incorporating infrastructure that supports women's preferences.

Midwives are well placed to negotiate and facilitate opportunities for the provision of water immersion. As reflected in studies by Cooper, McCutcheon & Warland (2021) and Woodward (2012) the implementation of water immersion in many venues has come to fruition because of the persistence and hard work of midwife champions who have listened to women and their preferences. While hard-fixed baths may be costly to implement, there are many portable pool options available which can present cost-effective options for implementing water immersion in maternity care venues.

Practicalities of facilitating water immersion

Facilitating water immersion in practice requires access to appropriate equipment, consideration of health and safety principles for women and practitioners, and understanding of the care that should be provided to women who are using water during labour and / or birth. A summary of equipment needed, health and safety considerations, recommendations for care and possible complications are given below.

Equipment

- Purpose-built birthing pool, portable birth pool, spa bath or inflatable paddling pool with firm sides
- A continuous supply of hot and cold water (temperature can be maintained by immersion heater or continuous supply of temperature-regulated water)
- Adequate supply of dry linen, especially towels
- Sieve—for keeping water as free of faecal contamination as possible
- Light source (e.g., waterproof torch or headlamp)
- Mirror
- Protective clothing (personal choice or according to hospital guidelines)
- Plastic waterproof support pillow or a rolled-up towel for head or arm support
- Portable delivery pack, oxygen and suction, oxytocics
- Waterproof Doppler unit and a Pinard stethoscope
- Portable nitrous oxide/Entonox as appropriate, though generally not at a home birth
- Foot stool
- Fan
- Bed or mattress nearby
- Easy access to emergency equipment for neonatal resuscitation and maternal collapse
- A water pump to drain water from the pool / bath (generally only needed in the case of a portable bath)
- Disposable liners (needed only in the case of a portable bath)

Work health and safety considerations

- Back care—midwife awareness required. A guideline for the removal of a collapsed woman from the water if required using a sling hammock. Although this is a rare occurrence, not having a plan for this is often a barrier to the introduction of birth in water in many units.
- Protective clothing:
  - long latex gauntlet gloves
  - knee pads or low stool
  - plastic aprons.
- Infection control:
  - cleaning of fixed bath / pool should follow strict protocols as developed by the hospital and disposable liners should be used in the case of portable pools
  - hoses and jets in the pool are not recommended. However, when hoses are required for filling pools, especially at home births, two different-coloured hoses, one for filling and one for emptying pools, must be used
  - an agreed policy for cleaning the birth pool (and hoses)
  - a system to alert caregivers to whether the pool has been cleaned such as a 'to be cleaned' sign
  - taps should be run on full for a few minutes before filling the pool/bath.
- Non-slip flooring/mats in pool/bath
- Electrical equipment kept away from 'wet' areas
- Adequate room ventilation
- Promotion of the safety and wellbeing of all, particularly children
- Attending staff should check skin integrity as per local guidelines regarding same

Care of woman and baby

During labour

- Advise and assist the woman to wait until she is in active labour before entering the pool.
- The water in the pool should be filled to the level of the woman's chest while she is sitting in the pool.
- Maintain the water temperature according to the woman's comfort.
- Do routine labour observations and fetal heart rate (FHR) recording according to local guidelines.
- Encourage the woman to drink as desired while in the water.
- As much as possible, keep faecal contamination of the water to a minimum.
- Encourage the woman to explore different positions in the pool.

During a birth in water

- The woman should not be left alone when in the water, and during the second stage the midwife should remain in the room.
- Attend to routine second-stage observations.
- Encourage physiological pushing. Physiological or non-directed pushing is less likely to tire the woman and her baby.
- A 'hands-off' technique by the midwife is advised when appropriate, supported by verbal guidance.
- A hands-off technique keeps tactile stimulation to a minimum (Johnson, 1996).
- The practice of checking for a nuchal cord is to be avoided. In most cases the nuchal cord can be loosened and disentangled under water as the baby is born (Burns & Kitzinger, 2000).
- The baby should be born completely under the water and brought gently to the surface, being careful to minimise unnecessary cord traction. The reported incidents of cord avulsion highlight the importance of minimising traction on the cord during birth. If the cord is short, then the woman is instructed and assisted to stand out of or above the water to receive her baby.
- Following the birth, do not allow the baby's head to resubmerge. It is important to communicate to the woman the need for the baby's head to remain above the water once born. This speaks to the importance of not filling the bath too much to ensure women can comfortably cuddle and hold their baby following birth without fear of them slipping back into the water.
- Routine observations and Apgar scores should be carried out on the baby. Experienced water-birth practitioners observe that babies born in water often appear more relaxed and quieter at birth.
- Maintain the baby's temperature by using a woollen bonnet (if available) and keeping the baby's body under the warm water. There is a need to maintain a neutral thermal zone for the baby and minimise oxygen consumption by reducing heat loss. Babies lose a lot of heat from their heads. Replace wet blankets with warm, dry ones as needed.
- Facilitate a physiological third stage, where the cord is left unclamped until the placenta and membranes are born. This is encouraged wherever possible. Active management may be used if indicated. There is no evidence to suggest that the third stage must be conducted out of the water (Burns & Kitzinger, 2000; Hastie & Fahy, 2009; Levy, 1990).
- The woman is assisted from the pool to a nearby couch or bed, as required, when she is ready. Ensure that she is kept warm following exit from the bath.
- Ensure the baby's warmth by drying thoroughly and maintaining skin-to-skin contact with the woman, as appropriate.
- Breastfeeding can occur in the bath if the mother is comfortable and the level of the water permits, otherwise it can be facilitated as soon as possible when the woman exits the water.

Complications

The midwife's clinical judgment is paramount. A woman who is fully informed and has a good relationship with her midwife will trust the midwife's judgment and immediately heed her advice to leave the water if there are any concerns for her safety or that of the baby. It is important for midwives to acknowledge that intuitive 'uneasy' feeling they may have even though there may not be any clinically evident signs of compromise. Midwives should be honest and open with the woman regarding their concerns and provide clear rationale for their decisions.

Possible complications include the following:

- *Fetal distress—FHR irregularity/abnormality*—In the case of a non-reassuring FHR and / or cardiotocographic (CTG) trace, the midwife should advise the woman to exit the bath (Johnson, 1996).
- *Meconium-stained liquor*—The woman is requested to leave the water if time permits and when she is able. If she is unable to exit the water in time, continue with the birth and follow protocols for management of meconium-stained liquor. The woman should leave the water immediately if thick meconium is observed (Enkin et al., 2000).
- *Slow progress in labour (any stage)*—Sometimes water immersion may slow labour. Assisting the woman from the water may remedy this situation (Eriksson et al., 1997). Encourage the woman to empty her bladder and remain upright and mobilising thereby allowing gravity to help contractions to re-establish. Returning to the water is still an option.
- *Use of narcotic analgesia*—Women who have been administered a systemic opioid for pain relief in labour need to be carefully assessed given the sedating effect of the medication on her and her baby.
- *Tight nuchal cord*—In the rare event that the cord needs to be cut, the woman is asked to stand out of the water. The cord must not be cut and clamped under water (Burns & Kitzinger, 2000).

- *Maternal hyperthermia*—This is to be avoided as it may lead to the overriding of the baby's normal inhibition of breathing (Johnson, 1996).
- *Episiotomy*—The most common indication for episiotomy is fetal distress. One could argue that there is no place for it in the practice of water birth as any concern for the baby's wellbeing should be an indication to request the woman leave the pool / bath to birth on land (Cluett & Burns, 2012).
- *Shoulder dystocia*—This is considered an emergency. When shoulder dystocia is diagnosed, the woman is assisted to stand up and place her leg on the side of the pool (this encourages hyperflexion of the leg, as in the McRoberts manoeuvre and may be all that is required to aid birth). Manipulation of the baby may initiate respirations or fetal distress and result in the baby gasping under water, therefore any manoeuvres should be performed out of the water.
- *Postpartum haemorrhage*—Owing to the difficulty of accurate estimates in water, blood loss is assessed simply as either >500 mL or <500 mL. A useful guide is how dark the water is getting and whether you can still assess the skin colour of the woman's thighs. Evidence of maternal compromise should prompt the midwife to advise and then assist the woman from the bath / pool (Harper, 2000).
- *Maternal collapse*—While maternal collapse in the bath is quite rare, particularly if the midwife is assessing the woman and advising the woman to leave the bath where there are signs of compromise, maternal collapse may still occur. Emergency evacuation drills and appropriate equipment to assist women from the bath in this event are essential.

CRITICAL THINKING EXERCISE

Sally has just given birth to the head of her baby under water in the bath when you notice signs of a shoulder dystocia. Describe some of the signs of shoulder dystocia and your management of the situation when a woman is in the bath/pool.

REFLECTIVE THINKING EXERCISE

Kiri is expecting her first baby. She is very healthy and carefully monitors her nutrition, exercise and rest. She is very keen to avoid any interventions in the normal process of labour and birth, and especially wants to avoid pharmacological pain relief. Reflect on the various alternative interventions available.

What information would you give her about the use of water for labour and birth to help her to make an informed decision?

Conclusion

History and several decades of research and literature have informed midwives' practice around the use of water for labour and birth. The aggregate results suggest that water birth is associated with high levels of maternal satisfaction, a reduction in the use of pharmacological pain relief, and an improved and more satisfying experience of childbirth. Water birth is also associated with decreased incidence of episiotomy and severe perineal lacerations and may contribute to reduced postpartum haemorrhage. There appears to be no increase in maternal or neonatal infection rates or nursery admissions after water birth.

Generally, there is a lack of published data in Australia and New Zealand on the use of water for labour and birth, but this is not indicative of its widespread usage. However, in spite of the paucity of RCTs on birth in water, water immersion for labour and birth does not appear to be associated with an increase in maternal or neonatal morbidity (Cluett et al., 2018). Outcomes compare favourably with those for any healthy childbearing population, and in some circumstances appear to be better. However, it is still argued that firm conclusions cannot be drawn about the safety and effectiveness of giving birth in water due to a lack of high-quality research, namely through RCTs and, as such, researchers and practitioners have called for further research and prospective auditing. However, Otigbah et al. (2000) asserted that 'until and unless formal and scientific evidence is available, water births should not be dismissed as being unacceptable' (p. 19). This view has been echoed by many researchers and professionals since these findings.

In response to the increasing demand from women and midwives, water-immersion facilities in maternity units have become more common. Women report that the use of warm water changes the dynamics of labouring and birthing, and gives them control over their experience. While being immersed in water does not necessarily take the pain away, it provides a release from the pain in the form of a warming, soothing, comforting and relaxing environment that helps facilitate the labour and birth process. As such, judicious use of water immersion may offer women the opportunity to experience a normal, physiological birth that is free from intervention.

As guardians of normal physiological birth, midwives need to seek opportunities to witness and practise water immersion and water birth. And in turn they must offer learning opportunities for midwifery students to experience and support women using water immersion. Midwives must also continue to access the emerging evidence base and use the information gained to inform their practice and challenge barriers that may prevent access to and uptake of water immersion in their context.

The use of water for labour and birth is a philosophy of non-intervention rather than a birth method. As the caesarean section rates increase, the option to use water is an opportunity for midwives to support women to birth physiologically and to experience the art of being 'with woman'.

Review questions

1. What are the key principles of a midwifery model of care that supports women in using water for labour and birth?
2. What do women like about using water for labour and birth?
3. The Cochrane Database of Systematic Reviews, updated in 2018, reported on 15 trials (3663 women) examining the effects of water immersion during labour. What conclusions did the reviewers reach?
4. What are the main mechanisms that inhibit breathing in utero to prevent the inhalation of water during a water birth?
5. What is the current thinking on the recommended temperature of the water during labour and birth?
6. Who can use water for labour and birth? When is it not advisable?
7. Discuss the research evidence associated with perineal trauma and the use of water immersion for labour and birth.
8. Describe the work health and safety considerations for the woman and the baby during a water birth.
9. Discuss a midwife's care of a woman and a baby during a water birth.
10. Describe how a midwife would assess a woman's blood loss during a water birth.

Online resources

Gentlebirth: http://www.gentlebirth.org/archives/watrbrth.html.
Sheila Kitzinger website: http://www.sheilakitzinger.com/WaterBirth.htm.
Waterbirth International: http://www.waterbirth.org.

Online learning

NSW Health Education and Training, Water Immersion for Labour and Birth:
https://www.heti.nsw.gov.au/education-and-training/courses-and-programs/water-immersion-for-labour-and-birth
Birth Spirit 'Waterbirth Workshop: An Open Access Resource':
http://www.birthspirit.co.nz/waterbirth-workshop-an-open-access-resource/.

References

Aird IA, Luckas MJM, Buckett WM, et al. Effects of intrapartum hydrotherapy on labour related parameters. *Aust N Z J Obstet Gynaecol.* 1997;37(2):137–142.

Alderdice F, Renfrew M, Marchant S, et al. Labour and birth in water in England and Wales: a survey report. *Br J Midwifery.* 1995;3(7):375–382.

Alfirevic Z, Gould D. Immersion in water during labour and birth. In: *Royal College of Obstetricians and Gynaecologists (RCOG)/ Royal College of Midwives Joint Statement No. 1*. Oxford: RCOG; 2006: 1–5.

Anderson T. Time to throw the water birth thermometer away? *MIDIRS Midwifery Dig.* 2004;14:3.

Antonakou A, Kostoglou E, Papoutsis D. Experiences of Greek women of water immersion during normal labour and birth. A qualitative study. *Eur J Midwifery.* 2018;2(7):1–8. doi:10.18332/ejm/92917.

Aughey H, Jardine J, Moitt N, et al. Waterbirth: a national retrospective cohort study of factors associated with its use among women in England. *BMC pregnancy and childbirth.* 2021;21(1):1–9, doi:10.1186/s12884-021-03724-6.

Australian College of Midwives. *Position Statement on the Use of Water During Labour and Birth.* Canberra: ACM; 2013. Online: https://18-midwives.cdn.aspedia.net/sites/default/files/uploaded-content/field_f_content_file/acm_position_statement_on_the_use_of_water_immersion_for_labour_and_birth_may_2013.pdf.

Australian College of Midwives. *ACM's updated position on use of water in labour.* Canberra: ACM; 2020. Online: https://www.midwives.org.au/news/acm-s-updated-position-use-water-labour.

Bailey JM, Zielinski RE, Emeis CL, et al. A retrospective comparison of waterbirth outcomes in two United States hospital settings. *Birth.* 2020;47(1):98–104. doi: 10.1111/birt.12473.

Banks M. Water birth pools—the essential labour aid! In: *Water Birth: Debunking the Myths.* Hamilton, NZ: Seminar Booklet; 1998.

Barry PL, McMahon LE, Banks RA,et al. Prospective cohort study of water immersion for labour and birth compared with standard care in an Irish maternity setting. *BMJ open.* 2020;10(12): e038080, doi:10.1136/bmjopen-2020-038080.

Beech BL. Water birth unplugged. In: *Proceedings of the First International Waterbirth Conference.* Cheshire: Books for Midwives; 1996:42–46.

Benfield RD. Hydrotherapy in labor. *J Nurs Scholarsh.* 2002;34(4): 347–52. doi:10.1111/j.1547-5069.2002.00347.x.

Binney J, Chapman G. *Nga Morehu—The Survivors.* Auckland: Oxford University Press; 1986.

Bovbjerg ML, Cheyney M, Everson C. Maternal and newborn outcomes following waterbirth: the midwives alliance of North America statistics project, 2004 to 2009 cohort. *J Midwifery Women Health.* 2016;61:11–20. doi:10.1111/jmwh.12394.

Bowden K, Kessler D, Pinette M, et al. Underwater birth: missing the evidence or missing the point? *Pediatrics.* 2002;112(4): 472–473.

Bryers HM, Van Teijlingen E. Risk, theory, social and medical models: a critical analysis of the concept of risk in maternity care. *Midwifery*. 2010;26(5):488–96. doi:10.1016/j.midw.2010.07.003.
Burke E, Kilfoyle A. A comparative study: water birth and bed-birth. *Midwives*. 1995;108:327.
Burns E, Kitzinger S. *Midwifery Guidelines for Use of Water in Labour*. Oxford: Oxford Brookes University, OCHRAD; 2000.
Burns EE, Boulton MG, Cluett E, et al. Characteristics, interventions, and outcomes of women who used a birthing pool: a prospective observational study. *Birth*. 2012;39(3):192–202. doi:10.1111/j.1523-536X.2012.00548.x.
Burns E, Hunter L, Rodd Z, et al. Developing and evaluating an online learning tool to improve midwives' accuracy of visual estimation of blood loss during waterbirth: An experimental study. *Midwifery*. 2019;68:65–73, doi:10.1007/s00192-019-04167-6.
Camargo JD, Varela V, Ferreira FM, et al. Perineal outcomes and its associated variables of water births versus non-water births: a cross-sectional study. *Revista Brasileira de Saúde Materno Infantil*. 2019;19:777–86. doi:10.1590/1806-93042019000400003.
Cameron J, Ellwood D. Choices, collaboration and outcomes in Australia. In: Symon A, editor. *Risk and choice in maternity care: an international perspective*. London: Elsevier Health Sciences; 2006.
Cammu H, Clasen K, van Wettere L, et al. 'To bathe or not to bathe' during the first stage of labor. *Acta Obstet Gynecol Scand*. 1994; 73:468–472.
Caplice S. *Waterbirth: Evidence for Practice (unpublished Master's thesis)*. Ultimo, NSW: University of Technology Sydney; 2004a.
Caplice S. Birth and water. *Presented at Birthing Normally Conference*. Sydney: Royal Hospital for Women; 2004b.
Cassie F. Water birth—a midwife's viewpoint. *N Z Midwifery News*. 2002;25:4–6.
Chaichian S, Akhlaghi A, Rousta F, et al. Experience of water birth delivery in Iran. *Arch Iran Med*. 2009;12(5):468–471.
Chapman, B. Waterbirth protocols: Five North Island hospitals in New Zealand. *J N Z Coll Midwives Journal*, 30, 20–24.
Charles C. Fetal hyperthermia risk from warm water immersion. *Br J Midwifery*. 1998;6(3):152–156.
Church L. Water birth: one birthing centre's observations. *J Nurse Midwifery*. 1989;34(4):165–170.
Clews C, Church S, Ekberg M. Women and waterbirth: A systematic meta-synthesis of qualitative studies. *Women Birth*. 2020;33(6):566–73. doi:10.1016/j.wombi.2019.11.007.
Cluett E, Burns E. Immersion in water in labour and birth. *Cochrane Database Syst Rev*. 2009;(2):CD000111, doi:10.1002/14651858.CD000111.pub3.
Cluett ER, Burns E. Immersion in water in labour and birth. *Cochrane Database Syst Rev*. 2012;(14):CD000111, doi:10.1002/14651858.CD000111.pub3.
Cluett ER, Burns E, Cuthbert A. Immersion in water during labour and birth. *Cochrane Database Syst Rev*. 2018;(5):CD000111, doi:10.1002/14651858.CD000111.pub4.
Cluett ER, Pickering RM, Getliffe K, et al. Randomised controlled trial of labouring in water compared with standard augmentation for management of dystocia in first stage labour. *Br Med J*. 2004;328(7435):314–317.
COAG Health Council. *Woman-centred care: Strategic directions for Australian maternity services*. Canberra: Department of Health; 2019. Online: https://www.health.gov.au/sites/default/files/documents/2019/11/woman-centred-care-strategic-directions-for-australian-maternity-services.pdf.
Colombo C, Pei P, Jost J. Water births and the exposure to HIV. *Pflege*. 2000;13(3):152–159.
Cooper M. *The exploration of water immersion policies/guidelines and the impact upon practice of labour and birth: a mixed methods study*. Adelaide, Australia: University of South Australia; 2017 (PhD thesis). doi:10.13140/RG.2.2.12503.80809.
Cooper M, King R. *Women's Experiences of Maternity Care at the Height of COVID-19*. Canberra: Australian College of Midwives; 2020. doi:10.13140/RG.2.2.25423.20648.
Cooper M, McCutcheon H, Warland J. A critical analysis of Australian policies and guidelines for water immersion during labour and birth. *Women Birth*. 2017;30(5):431–41. doi:10.1016/j.wombi.2017.04.001.
Cooper M, McCutcheon H, Warland J. Water immersion policies and guidelines: How are they informed? *Women Birth*. 2019;32(3):246–54. doi:10.1016/j.wombi.2018.08.169.
Cooper M, McCutcheon H, Warland J. 'They follow the wants and needs of an institution': Midwives' views of water immersion. *Women Birth*. 2021;34(2):e178–e187. doi:10.1016/j.wombi.2020.02.019.
Cooper M, Warland J. What are the benefits? Are they concerned? Women's experiences of water immersion for labor and birth. *Midwifery*. 2019;79:102541. doi:10.1016/j.midw.2019.102541.
Cooper M, Warland J, McCutcheon H. Diving in: a dip in the water of the labour and birth policy debate. *Essentially MIDIRS*. 2013;4(9):32–7.
Cooper M, Warland J, McCutcheon H. Water for labour and birth: getting back to the art of doing nothing. *MIDIRS Midwifery Digest*. 2017;21(1):53–8.
Cooper M, Warland J, McCutcheon H. Australian midwives views and experiences of practice and politics related to water immersion for labour and birth: A web based survey. *Women & Birth*. 2018;31(3):184–9. doi:10.1016/j.wombi.2017.09.001.
Cooper M, Warland J, McCutcheon H. Practitioner accreditation for the practice of water immersion during labour and birth: Results from a mixed methods study. *Women Birth*. 2019;32(3):255–62. doi:10.1016/j.wombi.2018.08.165
Cortes E, Basra R, Kelleher CJ. Waterbirth and pelvic floor injury: a retrospective study and postal survey using ICIQ modular long form questionnaires. *Eur J Obstet Gynecol Reprod Biol*. 2011;155:27–30. doi:10.1016/j.ejogrb.2010.11.012.
Cro S, Preston J. Cord snapping at waterbirth delivery. *Br J Midwifery*. 2002;10(8):494–497.
Daellenbach s, Gardner B, Dixon L, et al. *Report on New Zealand's MMPO Midwives Care Activities and Outcomes 2016*. Christchurch: New Zealand College of Midwives; 2016.
Dahlen H, Dowling H, Tracy M, et al. Maternal and perinatal outcomes among low risk women giving birth in water compared to six birth positions on land. A descriptive cross sectional study in a birth centre over 12 years. *Midwifery*. 2013;29:759–764.
Davies M. Waterbirths and the research required to assess the benefits versus the harms. *J Paediatr Child Health*. 2010;48(9):726–729. doi:10.1111/j.1440-1754.2010.01781.x.
Davies R, Davis D, Pearce M, et al. The effect of waterbirth on neonatal mortality and morbidity: a systematic review and meta-analysis. *JBI Database System Rev Implement Rep*. 2015;13(10):180–231. doi:10.11124/jbisrir-2015-2105. Online: https://journals.lww.com/jbisrir/toc/2015/13100.
Deans AC, Steer PS. Temperature of pool is important. *BMJ*. 1995; 311:390–391.
Deschênes L. L'hydrothérapie en obstétrique [Hydro-therapy in midwifery]. *Nurs Qué*. 1990;10(3):49–53.
Dixon L, Guilliland K. *Report on New Zealand MMPO Midwives Care Activities and Outcomes 2012*. Christchurch: New Zealand College of Midwives; 2014.
Duley LMM. Birth in water. In: *Royal College of Obstetricians and Gynaecologists (RCOG) Statement on Behalf of the Guidelines and Audit Committee of the RCOG*. Oxford: RCOG; 2001.
Eckert K, Turnbull D, MacLennan A. Immersion in water in the first stage of labor: a randomised controlled trial. *Birth*. 2001;28(2):84–93. doi: 10.1046/j.1523-536x.2001.00084.x.

Enkin M, Keirse M, Neilson J, et al. *A Guide to Effective Care in Pregnancy and Childbirth*. Oxford: Oxford University Press; 2000.
Eriksson M, Mattsson LA, Ladfors L. Early or late bath during the first stage of labour. Randomised study of 20 women. *Midwifery*. 1997;13:146–148.
Feeley C, Cooper M, Burns E. A systematic meta-thematic synthesis to examine the views and experiences of women following water immersion during labour and waterbirth. *J Adv Nurs*. 2021;77(7):2942–56. doi:10.1111/jan.14720.
Fenton D. Pukekohe Maternity Unit waterbirth audit 2002. *Midwifery News*. 2004;32:24–25.
Fewell JE, Johnson P. Upper airway dynamics during breathing and during apnoea in fetal lambs. *J Physiol*. 1983;339: 495–504.
Garland D. Collaborative waterbirth audit: supporting practice with audit. *MIDIRS Midwifery Dig*. 2002;12(4):508–511.
Garland D, Jones K. Waterbirth: updating the evidence. *Br J Midwifery*. 1997;5(6):368–372.
Geissbuehler V, Eberhard J. Water birth: a comparative study. A prospective study on more than 2000 water births. *Fetal Diagn Ther*. 2000;15:291–300.
Geissbuehler V, Eberhard J, Lebrecht A. Water birth: water temperature and bathing time—mother knows best! *J Perinat Med*. 2002;30:371–378.
Gilbert R, Tookey P. Perinatal mortality and morbidity among babies delivered in water: surveillance study and postal survey. *Br Med J*. 1999;319:483–487.
Ginesi L, Niescierowicz R. Neuroendocrinology and birth 1: stress. *Br J Midwifery*. 1998;6(10):659–663.
Gonçalves M, Coutinho E, Pareira V, et al. Woman's satisfaction with her water birth experience. In: Costa A, Reis L, Moreira A, eds. *Computer supported qualitative research new trends on qualitative research*. Springer Ltd; 2019:255–265.
Gradert Y, Hertel J, Lenstrup C, et al. Warm tub bath during labour. *Acta Obstet Gynecol Scand*. 1987;66:681–683.
Hall SM, Holloway IM. Staying in control: women's experiences of labour in water. *Midwifery*. 1997;14(1):30–6. doi:10.1016/S0266-6138(98)90112-7.
Harding R, Johnson P, McClelland M. Liquid sensitive laryngeal receptors in the developing sheep, cat and monkey. *J Physiol*. 1978;277:409–422.
Harper B. Water birth basics: from newborn breathing to hospital protocols. *Midwifery Today*. 2000;54:20–28.
Harper B. Taking the plunge: re-evaluating water birth temperature guidelines. *MIDIRS Midwifery Dig*. 2002;12(4):506–507.
Hastie C, Fahy K. Optimising psychophysiology in third stage of labour: theory applied to practice. *Women Birth*. 2009;22: 89–96.
Henderson J, Burns EE, Regalia AL, et al. Labouring women who used a birthing pool in obstetric units in Italy: prospective observational study. *BMC Pregnancy Childbirth*. 2014;14:17.
Hodnett E. Caregiver support for women during childbirth. *Cochrane Database Syst Rev*. 2000;(2):CD000199.
Irwin K, Ramsden I. Toi wāhine. In: *The Worlds of Maori Women*. Auckland: Penguin; 1995:1–143.
Johnson P. Birth under water—to breathe or not to breathe. *BJOG*. 1996;103(3):202–208. doi:10.1111/j.1471-0528.1996.tb09706.x.
Kausela P, Koivisto A-M, Heinonen PK. Warm tub bath during opening phase of labour. *Suom Laakaril*. 1998;11:1217–1221.
Kitzinger S. Letter from Europe: water birth: just a fad? *Birth*. 2009;36(3):258–260.
Lathrop A, Bonsack CF, Haas DM. Women's experiences with water birth: a matched groups prospective study. *Birth*. 2018;45(4): 416–23. doi:10.1111/birt.12362.
Leboyer F. *Birth Without Violence*. London: Mandarin; 1975.
Lecky-Thompson M. Water birthing. Celebrating a revolution in birth. In: *Proceedings of the Tenth National Homebirth Conference*. Sydney: Homebirth Access; 1989:115–122.
Lenstrup C, Schantz A, Berget A, et al. Warm tub during delivery. *Acta Obstet Gynecol Scand*. 1987;66:709–712.
Levy V. The midwife's management of the third stage of labour. In: Alexander J, Levy V, Roch S, eds. *Midwifery Practice: Intrapartum Care. A Research-Based Approach*. Basingstoke: Macmillan; 1990.
Lewis L, Hauck YL, Crichton C, Barnes C, Poletti C, Overing H, Keyes L, Thomson B. The perceptions and experiences of women who achieved and did not achieve a waterbirth. *BMC pregnancy and childbirth*. 2018;18(23):1–10. doi:10.1186/s12884-017-1637-5.
Lichy R, Herzberg E. *The Water Birth Handbook*. Bath: Gateway Books; 1993.
Lim KM, Tong PS, Chong YS. A comparative study between the pioneer cohort of waterbirths and conventional vaginal deliveries in an obstetrician-led unit in Singapore. *Taiwanese J Obstet Gynecol*. 2016;55(3):363–7. doi: 10.1016/j.tjog.2016.04.012.
Liu Y, Liu Y, Huang X, Du C, Peng J, Huang P, Zhang J. A comparison of maternal and neonatal outcomes between water immersion during labor and conventional labor and delivery. *BMC pregnancy and childbirth*. 2014;14(160):1–7. doi:10.1186/1471-2393-14-160.
Lukasse M, Rowe R, Townend J, Knight M, Hollowell J. Immersion in water for pain relief and the risk of intrapartum transfer among low risk nulliparous women: secondary analysis of the Birthplace national prospective cohort study. *BMC Pregnancy Childbirth*. 2014;14(60):1–11. doi:10.1186/1471-2393-14-60.
McKenna JA, Symon AG. Water VBAC: exploring a new frontier for women's autonomy. *Midwifery*. 2014;30(1):e20–5. doi:10.1016/j.midw.2013.10.004.
Makereti P. *The Old-Time Maori*. Auckland: New Women's Press; 1986.
Mallen-Perez L, Roé-Justiniano MT, Ochoa NC, et al. Use of hydrotherapy during labour: Assessment of pain, use of analgesia and neonatal safety. *Enfermería Clínica, English ed*. 2018;28(5):309–15. doi:10.1016/j.enfcle.2017.10.006.
Maude R. *It's beyond water: stories of women's experience of using water for labour and birth*. Wellington, NZ: Victoria University; 2003 (Master's thesis).
Maude R, Foureur M. It's beyond water: stories of women's experience of using water for labour and birth. *Women Birth*. 2007;20:17–24.
Maude RM, Kim M. Getting into the water: a prospective observational study of water immersion for labour and birth at a New Zealand District Health Board. *BMC pregnancy and childbirth*. 2020;20:312;1–12. doi:10.1186/s12884-020-03007-6.
Menakaya U, Albayati S, Vella E, et al. A retrospective comparison of water birth and conventional vaginal birth among women deemed to be low risk in a secondary level hospital in Australia. *Women Birth*. 2013;26:114–118. doi:10.1016/j.wombi.2012.10.002.
Milosevic S, Channon S, Hughes J, et al. Factors influencing water immersion during labour: qualitative case studies of six maternity units in the United Kingdom. *BMC Pregnancy Childbirth*. 2020;20(719):1–14. doi:10.1186/s12884-020-03416-7.
Milosevic S, Channon S, Hunter B, et al. Factors influencing the use of birth pools in the United Kingdom: perspectives of women, midwives and medical staff. *Midwifery*. 2019;79:102554. doi:10.1016/j.midw.2019.102554.
Mollamahmutoglu L, Moraloglu O, Ozyer S, et al. The effects of immersion in water on labour, birth and newborn and comparison with epidural analgesia and conventional vaginal delivery. *J Turk Ger Gynecol Assoc*. 2012;13(1):45–49. doi:10.5152/jtgga.2012.03.

Neiman E, Austin E, Tan A, et al. Outcomes of waterbirth in a US hospital‚Äêbased midwifery practice: a retrospective cohort study of water immersion during labor and birth. *J Midwifery Women's Health.* 2020;65(2):216–23. doi:10.1111/jmwh.13033.

Newnham EC, McKellar LV, Pincombe JI. Documenting risk: A comparison of policy and information pamphlets for using epidural or water in labour. *Women Birth.* 2015;28(3):221–7, doi:10.1016/j.wombi.2015.01.012.

Newnham E, McKellar L, Pincombe J. 'It's your body, but...'Mixed messages in childbirth education: findings from a hospital ethnography. *Midwifery.* 2017;55:53–9. doi:10.1016/j.midw.2017.09.003.

New South Wales Health. *Maternity—Towards Normal Birth in NSW.* 2010. Online: http://www1.health.nsw.gov.au/pds/ActivePDSDocuments/PD2010_045.pdf.

New Zealand College of Midwives (NZCOM). *The Use of Water in Labour and Birth.* Christchurch, NZ: NCOM; 2015.

Nguyen S, Kuschel C, Teele R, et al. Water birth—a near drowning experience. *Pediatrics.* 2002;110(2):411–413.

Nicholls S, Hauck Y, Bayes S, et al. Exploring midwives' perception of confidence around facilitating water birth in Western Australia: a qualitative descriptive study. *Midwifery.* 2016;33: 73–81.

Nutter E, Meyer S, Shaw-Battista J, et al. Waterbirth: an integrative analysis of peer-reviewed literature. *J Midwifery Womens Health.* 2014;59(3):286–319. doi:10.1111/jmwh.12194.

Odent M. Birth under water. *Lancet.* 1983;24(31):1476–1477.

Odent M. *Water and Sexuality.* London: Penguin; 1990.

Odent M. Can water immersion stop labour? *J Nurse Midwifery.* 1997;42(5):414–416.

Odent M. *The Scientification of Love.* London: Free Association Books; 2001.

Otigbah C, Dhanjal M, Harmsworth G, et al. A retrospective comparison of water births and conventional vaginal deliveries. *Eur J Obstet Gynecol Reprod Biol.* 2000;91:15–20.

Page A. *A midwives' perspective of water birth.* Melbourne: 1994 (unpublished study).

Pinette M, Wax J, Wilson E. The risks of underwater birth. *Am J Obstet Gynecol.* 2004;190:1211–1215.

Queensland Health. *Perinatal Statistics 2019 Annual Report Tables.* Brisbane: Queensland Health; 2020. Online: https://www.health.qld.gov.au/__data/assets/pdf_file/0024/1004964/tables2019.pdf.

Richmond H. Theories surrounding water birth. *Pract Midwife.* 2003;6(2):10–13.

Robertson PA, Huang LJ, Croughan-Minihane MS, et al. Is there an association between water baths during labor and the development of chorioamnionitis or endometritis? *Am J Obstet Gynecol.* 1998;178(6):1215–1221.

Rosenthal MJ. Warm water immersions in labour and birth. *Female Patient.* 1991;16:35–44.

Rosser J. Is water birth safe? The facts behind the controversy. *MIDIRS Midwifery Dig.* 1994;4(1):4–6.

Royal Australian and New Zealand College of Obstetricians and Gynaecologists (RANZCOG). *Warm Water Immersion During Labour and Birth. College Statement, C-Obs 24. 2021.* Online: https://ranzcog.edu.au/RANZCOG_SITE/media/RANZCOG-MEDIA/Women%27s%20Health/Statement%20and%20guidelines/Clinical-Obstetrics/Water-immersion-during-labour-and-birth-(C-Obs-24)_March-2021.pdf?ext=.pdf.

Royal College of Obstetricians and Gynaecologists (RCOG) and Royal College of Midwives (RCM). *Joint Statement No. 1.* London: RCOG/RCM; 2006.

Rush J, Burlock S, Lambert K, et al. The effects of whirlpool baths in labor: a randomized controlled trial. *Birth.* 1996;23:136–143.

Russell K. Struggling to get into the pool room? A critical discourse analysis of labor ward midwives' experiences of water birth. *Int J Childbirth.* 2011;1(1):52–60, doi:10.1891/2156-5287.1.1.52.

Schorn M, McAllister JL, Blanco JD. Water immersion and the effect on labor. *J Nurse Midwifery.* 1993;38(6):336–342. doi: 10.1016/0091-2182(93)90014-8.

Seibold C, Licqurish S, Rolls C, et al. 'Lending the space': Midwives perceptions of birth space and clinical risk management. *Midwifery.* 2010;26(5):526–31, doi:10.1016/j.midw.2010.06.011.

Sidebottom AC, Vacquier M, Simon K, et al. Maternal and Neonatal Outcomes in Hospital-Based Deliveries With Water Immersion. *Obstet Gynecol.* 2020;136(4):707. doi: 10.1097/AOG.0000000000003956.

Sidenbladh E. Waterbabies. London: Adam and Charles Black; 1983.

Snapp C, Stapleton SR, Wright J, et al. The experience of land and water birth within the American Association of Birth Centers Perinatal Data Registry, 2012–2017. *J Perinat Neonatal Nurs.* 2020;34(1):16–26. doi:10.1097/JPN.0000000000000450.

SA Health. *First Stage Labour and Birth in Water Clinical Directive.* 2017. Online: https://www.sahealth.sa.gov.au/wps/wcm/connect/ae527200465ec14d8572ff2e504170d4/First+Stage+Labour+and+Birth+in+Water_CD_v4_0.pdf?MOD=AJPERES&CACHEID=ROOTWORKSPACE-ae527200465ec14d8572ff2e504170d4-nDVkhnl.

Sprague AG. *An investigation into the use of water immersion upon the outcomes and experience of giving birth (Doctoral dissertation).* ACU Research Bank; 2004.

Stephens L. The need to support normality over non-evidence-based interventions. *Br J Midwifery.* 2011;19(11):686.

Thoeni A, Zech N, Moroder F. Review of 1600 water births. Does water birth increase the risk of neonatal infection? *J Matern Fetal Neonatal Med.* 2005;17(5):357.

Ulfsdottir H, Saltvedt S, Georgsson S. Waterbirth in Sweden—a comparative study. *Acta Obstetricia et Gynecologica Scandinavica.* 2017; 97. 10.1111/aogs.13286.

Ulfsdottir H, Saltvedt S, Ekborn M, et al. Like an empowering micro-home: a qualitative study of women's experience of giving birth in water. *Midwifery.* 2018;67:26–31. doi:10.1016/j.midw.2018.09.004.

Uzunlar Ö, Sert ÜY, Kadioğlu N, et al. The effects of water immersion and epidural analgesia on cellular immune response, neuroendocrine, and oxidative markers. *Turkish J Med Sci.* 2021; 51(3):1420–1427. doi:10.3906/sag-2009-181.

Vanderlaan J, Hall P. Systematic Review of Case Reports of Poor Neonatal Outcomes With Water Immersion During Labor and Birth. *J Perinat Neonatal Nurs.* 2020;34(4):311–23. doi:10.1097/JPN.0000000000000515.

Vanderlaan J, Hall PJ, Lewitt M. Neonatal outcomes with water birth: a systematic review and meta-analysis. *Midwifery.* 2018;59:27–38. doi:10.1016/j.midw.2017.12.023.

Vochem M, Vogt M, Doring G. Sepsis in a newborn due to *Pseudomonas aeruginosa* from a contaminated tub bath. *N Engl J Med.* 2001;345:378–379.

Waldenstrom U, Nilsson CA. Warm tub bath after spontaneous rupture of the membranes. *Birth.* 1992;19(2):57–63.

Western Australia Department of Health. *Operational State-Wide Policy for the Use of Water During Labour and/or Birth in WA Health Hospitals and Health Services.* Perth: Government of Western Australia, Department of Health; 2009.

Woodward JL. *The challenge of conducting a waterbirth randomised controlled trial (Doctoral dissertation).* University of Birmingham; 2012.

Woodward J, Kelly SM. A pilot study for a randomised controlled trial of waterbirth versus land birth. *BJOG.* 2004;111:537–545.

Young K, Kruske S. *Water Immersion in Queensland: Evidence, Access and Uptake.* Brisbane: Queensland Centre for Mothers and Babies, University of Queensland; 2012.

Young K, Kruske S. How valid are the common concerns raised against water birth? A focused review of the literature. *Women Birth*. 2013;2013(26):105–109.
Young L. *The Wanganui experience of waterbirth from July 1991 to December 2000 (unpublished clinical audit, Masters assignment)*. Palmerston North: Massey University; 2001.
Zanetti-Dallenbach R, Lapaire O, Maertens A, et al. Water birth, more than a trendy alternative: a prospective, observational study. *Arch Gynecol Obstet*. 2006;274(6):355–365.
Zanetti-Dallenbach RA, Holzgreve W, Hosli I. Neonatal group B *Streptococcus* colonisation in waterbirths. *Int J Gynaecol Obstet*. 2007a;98(1):54–55.
Zanetti-Dallenbach RA, Tschudin S, Zhong XY, et al. Maternal and neonatal infections and obstetrical outcome in water birth. *Eur J Obstet Gynecol Reprod Biol*. 2007b;134:37–43.

Further reading

Balaskas J. *The Water Birth Book*. London: Unwin Hyman; 2004.
Garland D. Waterbirth. *An Attitude to Care*. London: Books for Midwives; 2000.
Harper B. *Gentle Birth Choices*. Rochester, VT: Healing Arts Press; 1995.
Lichy R, Herzberg E. The waterbirth handbook. In: *A Guide to the Gentle Art of Water Birthing*. Bath: Gateway Books; 1997:1–120.
Napierala S. *Water Birth—A Midwives' Perspective*. Westport, CT: Bergin and Garvey; 1994.

Video

The art of birth. The story of four gentle births in water. Producers: Caplice S, Dusseldorp T. Australia: 2002.

CHAPTER 28

Perineal care and repair

Hannah G Dahlen and Holly Priddis

LEARNING OUTCOMES

Learning outcomes for this chapter are:

1. To understand the historical background to the midwife's role in perineal care and repair
2. To understand evidence-based methods for the prevention of perineal and pelvic floor damage and, in particular, midwifery strategies for minimising perineal trauma and improving second-stage comfort
3. To be able to identify the structures of the pelvic floor and its importance in midwifery practice
4. To identify degrees and types of perineal trauma and to understand what is in the scope of practice of a midwife, when to consult a more experienced practitioner and when to refer
5. To understand the principles of safe, effective perineal repair and when and how to perform an episiotomy
6. To be able to give women appropriate, compassionate, evidence-based advice regarding care of perineal trauma and pelvic floor in the immediate postpartum period.

CHAPTER OVERVIEW

Perineal trauma can have lifelong effects on the quality of women's lives. Midwives should try to minimise this trauma, and after correctly identifying it should be able to undertake perineal repair competently, using the best suturing techniques and materials, to minimise any associated short- and long-term morbidity. Prevention of perineal trauma, especially the most severe form of trauma (third- and fourth-degree tears), and improvement of second-stage comfort are important components of perineal care. The 'pelvic floor' is the term given to the structures that fill the outlet of the bony pelvis. These muscles have important functions, and disruption to their integrity can have serious consequences for a woman's health. It is important for a midwife to have an understanding of the structure and function of the pelvic floor muscles and perineal body in order to minimise damage and prevent long-term morbidity.

Care and advice given to the woman, following the birth, regarding her perineum and pelvic floor is often not evidence based and in some cases remains virtually absent. It is important for a woman to have the best possible support and advice in the postnatal period in order to be able to care for herself and ensure optimal perineal and pelvic floor muscle health. The midwife's role in giving support and evidence-based advice in the antenatal and postnatal periods can ensure that women minimise long-term morbidity, such as incontinence and sexual dysfunction.

KEY TERMS

episiotomy
faecal incontinence
labial lacerations
pelvic floor muscle exercises
pelvic organ prolapse
perineal pain
perineal trauma
suturing
urinary incontinence
vaginal and cervical lacerations
severe perineal trauma (third- and fourth-degree tears)

INTRODUCTION

These pages have not been written for those who lay them aside saying or thinking, 'much ado about a perineal tear!' They will have to come to terms with their own consciences.
(Ritgen, 1885, p. 321)

Both childbearing women and healthcare professionals place a high value on minimising **perineal trauma** and reducing potential associated morbidity (Australian Commission on Safety and Quality in Health Care, 2021). However, countries report wide variations in trauma rates and the rates also vary within individual countries; further variations exist among institutions and healthcare professionals (Australian Commission on Safety and Quality in Health Care, 2021; Australian Commission on Safety and Quality in Health Care and Australian Institute of Health and Welfare, 2017; Dahlen et al., 2015; Ministry of Health New Zealand Government, 2020b).

In Australia, 23% of women have an intact perineum, around 22% have a first-degree tear or vaginal graze and 30% have a second-degree tear, with 3% having a third- or fourth-degree tear (higher than average OECD countries rate) (5% of primiparous women) and 9% of women have some other form of laceration. Almost 1 in 4 mothers (24%) have an **episiotomy**, which is a substantial rise in the past decade, up from 14% in 2008 (AIHW, 2020).

In Aotearoa New Zealand the data on perineal outcomes is mostly given for primiparous women. The latest data indicates 26.5% of primiparous women have an intact perineum, 4.5% have a third- or fourth-degree tear without an episiotomy and 2.1% have a severe perineal trauma with an episiotomy (Ministry of Health New Zealand Government, 2020a). The proportion of women giving birth in New Zealand overall (both primips and multips) who had an episiotomy increased from 12.3% in 2009 to 16% in 2018; the reason for this increase is unknown. Like in Australia, it does not appear to be related to assisted birth, the rate of which has not increased over this time. Women who had an episiotomy were more likely to be primiparous (31.6%), of Indian (38.1%) or Asian (29.0%) ethnicity. There were large regional variations in episiotomy rates per District Health Board (2.7% Tairawhiti to 29.2% Auckland) (Ministry of Health New Zealand Government, 2020b).

Numerous factors have been suggested as potential contributors to perineal trauma, as have numerous solutions for minimisation of that trauma (Aasheim et al., 2017; Dahlen et al., 2015; Thornton & Dahlen, 2020). Some of these contributors and solutions are based on sound evidence, but many others are not. There is also evidence that incidence of perineal trauma was not always as high as it appears to be today, leading one to question contemporary second-stage management—both the complex package of care and the individual elements of that care (Dahlen et al., 2011; De Wees, 1889; Ritgen, 1885; Thacker & Banta, 1983).

Perineal preservation and perineal comfort during the second stage of labour are important goals in the practice of most midwives. Furthermore, both midwives and obstetricians are aware that perineal trauma is associated with significant short- and long-term morbidity for women following childbirth (Chang et al., 2018; Darmody et al., 2020). Women who have an intact perineum after the birth of their first baby have stronger pelvic floor muscles (as measured by electromyogram) and make a quicker muscle recovery than do women experiencing tears or episiotomies. Although perineal trauma has not been clearly associated with urinary incontinence, **severe perineal trauma (third- and fourth-degree tears)** has been shown to be associated with faecal incontinence (Linneberg et al., 2016; Luciano et al., 2020). Acute postpartum perineal pain is common among women who give birth vaginally and its severity is linked to that of the perineal injury (Dahlen & Homer, 2008a; East et al., 2012; Kenyon & Ford, 2004). **Perineal pain** can have both long- and short-term negative consequences for women's health and wellbeing (Fodstad et al., 2016; Jango et al., 2016). It can make everyday activities such as sitting, walking, voiding, defecating, providing self-care and caring for the baby, including breastfeeding, extremely difficult. It can also lead to relationship disharmony and sexual disorders that can lead to irritability, resentment, depression and maternal exhaustion (Priddis, Schmied, & Dahlen, 2014; Signorello et al., 2001; Steen & Marchant, 2001; Way, 2011).

Perineal pain experienced during the second stage of labour can also have an impact on how a woman views her birth experience. Women report that the advancement of the baby's head and stretching of the perineum in the minutes before giving birth are accompanied by pain that can be severe (Goutaudier et al., 2012), and this can lead to women remembering the second stage in a particularly negative light. In the developed world there has been a dramatic increase in caesarean section rates in the last decade even amongst low-risk women (Coates et al., 2021). Fear of the pain associated with labour as well as perineal injury are reported as reasons why women may request a caesarean section (Kolas et al., 2003; Tschudin et al., 2009). Methods of reducing pain and trauma during the second stage without having to resort to potentially harmful pharmacological pain relief or major abdominal surgery would be beneficial to women and indeed to society as a whole. It is curious to observe that much of the research on pain in labour has focused on the first stage, thus largely overlooking the pain associated with the actual birth (Sanders et al., 2005). This is why perineal care packages should always consider second-stage comfort as a key component.

Practitioners who are able to identify perineal trauma accurately and to repair the trauma in a timely and optimal manner can provide an overall enhanced experience of the birth for women as well as contributing to the reduction in long-term morbidity. Lastly, having an understanding of the evidence to support optimal postnatal care and advice for women regarding pelvic floor care can help enhance the wellbeing of women and reduce common morbidities in women's health, such as urinary and faecal incontinence.

HISTORICAL PERSPECTIVES

It is evident that in the distant past the perineum received great care and attention from midwives, with a strong focus on protection and preservation. With the advent of the man-midwife, the perineum became increasingly pathologised and a site for surgical interventions, such as episiotomy. In the last 30 years, however, there has been a re-emergence of care aimed at preserving and protecting the perineum (Dahlen et al., 2011).

The physician Soranus of Ephesus (98–138 AD) produced one of the most important treatises on obstetrics (Carter & Duriez, 1986). It was called *Gynaecology* and was written specifically for midwives (Temkin, 1956). One of the earliest writers to describe the care of the perineum, Soranus gave instructions that the midwife should support the perineum with a linen pad while the head is advancing and advised an attendant to stand behind the midwife's stool and place a 'pledget' underneath in order to restrain the anus and avoid the prolapse and rupture that can accompany straining (Temkin, 1956). Attempts to reduce perineal trauma, carry out repairs on it and improve comfort in the second stage appear to predate known written texts. For example, sutures may have been used for thousands of years, the eyed needle being invented somewhere between 50,000 and 30,000 BC (Mackenzie, 1973).

During the 11th century AD, Trota (or Trocta) became one of the first women to write a text on the subject of obstetrics (*Trotula*), although some historians propose that a man in fact wrote *Trotula*, or several men assuming a woman's name (Green, 2002; O'Dowd & Philipp, 2000). Trota's works draw heavily on the works of Soranus and again instruct the midwife to support the perineum with a linen pad. They also describe how to repair the trauma with silk sutures (Green, 2002; King & Rabil, 2005; Trotula, 1940). Graham (1950) writes that this is the first time in history that a complete perineal repair is recommended.

We are also provided with glimpses into the management of childbirth by well-known midwives, such as German midwife Justine Siegemund (1636–1706 AD), French midwife Louise Bourgeois (1563–1636 AD), Frisian midwife Catharina Schrader (1693–1740 AD) and English midwives Sarah Stone (1600s) and Elizabeth Nihell (1700s) (Dahlen, 2007a). Most of these midwives advocate protection of the perineum.

> *You certainly should not stretch or dilate anything with your fingers. This is a common mistake. This sharp stretching injures the woman's belly and causes swelling before the child gets that far and comes forth.*
>
> Siegemund (2005, p.74)

French midwife Madame du Coudray, known as the 'King's midwife', was famous for developing the first obstetric mannequin and for her tours around the French countryside educating midwives, with the King's blessing, between 1760 and 1783 (Gelbart, 1998). Like Siegemund, she warns against 'too much vaginal meddling . . . the best thing is to wait patiently, alert to all cues' (Gelbart, 1998, p. 33). Madame du Coudray, using her mannequin, spent many days teaching her students about 'natural delivery' and providing the students with techniques for facilitating the baby's 'slippery exit':

> *Although great science is not necessary in natural delivery there are still plenty of precautions to take during labor to ensure that favorable beginnings do not end badly.*
>
> (Gelbart, 1998, pp. 68–9)

Sir Fielding Ould altered care of the perineum dramatically in 1742 when he gave the first description of episiotomy. Although, no doubt, this practice was used only occasionally at first, eventually it became the most common form of obstetric surgery. At times, perineal care moved clearly away from prevention of perineal trauma into deliberate surgical intervention. This was accompanied by increased use of a supine birth position, forceps, obstetric anaesthesia and episiotomy, all of which led to poorer outcomes for women and their perineum.

There is evidence that perineal trauma was not always as common as it appears today, leading to questions around contemporary second-stage management. In the 1880s, De Wees, for example, reported only 51 lacerations in 1000 consecutive births (5.1%) (De Wees, 1889), and Ritgen described the exact length of 190 tears occurring during the births of 4875 women (3.9%) (Ritgen, 1885).

It has been observed that the rise in episiotomy rates in the United States was directly proportional to the move from birth at home to birth in hospital (Thacker & Banta, 1983). In the US in 1930, approximately 25% of women gave birth in hospital compared with 70% in 1945. The rate of episiotomy is thought to reflect this shift in the environment of birth and the resulting dominant surgical model of care (Thacker & Banta, 1983).

MIDWIVES AND PERINEAL REPAIR

In recent years, the role of the midwife has been extended to incorporate a broader range of clinical skills into practice. Perineal repair is one of these skills. Midwives are increasingly expected to undertake perineal repair on their own responsibility and to provide women with advice regarding perineal care. This falls within the scope of practice for a midwife (ICM, 2017).

The way that perineal repair is taught to midwives and the supervision, accreditation and frequency of updates for these healthcare professionals is managed differently in different organisations and under different models of care. For example, in midwifery-led units and birth centres, the proportion of midwives performing perineal repairs appears to be higher than in traditional labour ward settings (Dahlen, 2004).

Although the type of **suturing** material and technique of the repair is important, the skill of the operator has also been recognised as one of three main factors that influence the outcome of perineal repair (Royal College of Obstetricians and Gynaecologists (RCOG), 2015). The RCOG guideline states that practitioners who are appropriately trained are more likely to provide a consistent and high standard of perineal repair (RCOG, 2015). It also recommends 24-hour cover by an experienced practitioner to facilitate training and provide support and supervision (RCOG, 2015). Research has highlighted the deficiency and dissatisfaction among trainee doctors and midwives with their training in perineal anatomy and repair (East et al., 2014). Despite this, much perineal repair research is focused on suture material and technique rather than on skill or training.

In a study undertaken to explore Australian midwives' attitudes relating to perineal repair, respondents strongly supported the incorporation of perineal repair into midwifery practice (Dahlen & Homer, 2008b). The most important reason given for midwives undertaking perineal repair was that it provides continuity of care; the second most important reason was because it is part of their professional role. Three-quarters of respondents in the study felt that student midwives should have practical experience with perineal repair during their training. The study found that there was strong support for midwives and doctors to undertake perineal repair training together. In addition, there was support to move back to a collaborative and multidisciplinary approach where doctors and midwives teach and learn together. This would provide an opportunity for both professions to share skills and learn together, potentially enhancing collaboration and possibly leading to a greater consistency in practice.

The study also found that confidence in carrying out perineal repairs was associated with experience (Dahlen & Homer, 2008b). More-experienced midwives were more confident and enjoyed undertaking the procedure. This is reassuring for midwives who are beginners in perineal repair. It is important for midwives to know that the more skilled they become the more confident they will be and they will experience more satisfaction as a result. Experience also lessens worry about the quality of the procedure and the impact it has on women. All these factors can influence midwives' enthusiasm in learning this important skill. Reassurance is needed that practice not only makes perfect but also makes the skill more enjoyable and rewarding.

In New Zealand a survey aimed at identifying how midwives assess and manage second-degree perineal tears found that confidence to repair was directly related to years since midwifery qualification and self-employment (Cronin, 2014).

Whether working in Australia or New Zealand, most midwives will need to undertake additional skill acquisition and practice in order to gain confidence to perform perineal repair. When employed and prior to carrying out the procedure, the midwife should check with her / his employer regarding the prerequisites that may be required.

Risk factors for perineal trauma

Perineal trauma commonly accompanies vaginal birth, and can result from intentional trauma (episiotomy), non-intentional trauma (tears and grazes), or both. Trauma to the genital tract is more common in primiparous women and with operative vaginal births (Dahlen, Priddis, et al., 2013; Macarthur & Macarthur, 2004).

Numerous factors have been suggested as potential contributors to perineal trauma. These include maternal and fetal factors such as maternal nutritional status, body mass, parity, history of prior trauma, ethnicity, older age, abnormal collagen synthesis, baby's birth weight, fetal sex (male), fetal malposition and malpresentation. Second-stage management can also have an influence on perineal trauma and maternal comfort during the actual birth. These include continuous support, maternal position, style of pushing, techniques to relax the perineum, episiotomy, hand manoeuvres, perineal massage, vacuum versus forceps delivery, immersion in water and epidurals (due to the associated risk of instrumental birth) (Aasheim et al., 2017; Wright et al., 2021). Perineal trauma including severe perineal trauma is reported to be lower for women who give birth at home and in birth centres (Reitsma et al., 2020; Scarf et al., 2018) and higher for women who are attended by obstetricians (Dahlen, Dowling, et al., 2013 Dahlen, Priddis, et al., 2013;), with rates varying within professional groups and between individual clinicians.

There are also specific risk factors for severe perineal trauma that midwives need to be aware of (Box 28.1).

Box 28.1 Risk factors for severe perineal trauma

- Episiotomy (midline more likely than mediolateral)
- Birth in lithotomy position
- Epidural anaesthesia (due to increased operative delivery)
- Operative birth, particularly forceps delivery
- Accoucheur
- Prolonged second stage and use of oxytocin
- Primiparous women
- Malposition (e.g. occipito transverse or posterior position)
- Fetal birth weight
- Male sex
- Ethnicity (some ethnic groups, e.g. Asian women)

(Source: Dahlen, Priddis, et al., 2013)

Preventing perineal trauma and improving second-stage comfort

The evidence supports the application of perineal warm packs in the second stage of labour to reduce perineal trauma and increase comfort (Aasheim et al., 2017; Magoga et al., 2019). In addition, research suggests that the use of digital antenatal perineal massage, giving birth in an

Box 28.2 Summary of practices thought to influence perineal trauma and/or maternal comfort during the second stage of labour

Care that reduces perineal trauma and/or improves maternal second-stage comfort

Recommendations:

- Teach digital antenatal perineal massage in the last 6 weeks of pregnancy.
- Warm packs reduce severe perineal trauma and improve maternal comfort during the second stage.
- Giving birth in an upright (especially kneeling/all fours) or lateral position leads to increased maternal comfort during the second stage and to lower rates of episiotomy.
- Women should be advised to follow their own urges to push during the second stage.
- Slow down the birth of the baby using voice and hands if needed.
- Vacuum extractors should be used in preference to forceps, as they lead to less maternal trauma.
- Women should have support (constant caring companion) throughout labour and birth.
- Giving birth in a home-like environment, such as a birth centre, is protective against perineal damage.
- Giving birth at home leads to the lowest rates of perineal damage.
- Giving birth with midwives compared with obstetricians is associated with a reduced use of episiotomy.

Care that appears promising but needs further research in order to determine effect on perineal trauma and/or maternal second-stage comfort

Recommendations:

- Pelvic floor muscle training appears to be beneficial in reducing prolonged second stage and severe perineal trauma.
- Immersion in water during labour reduces the need for epidurals and maternal pain and therefore is potentially beneficial for perineal trauma and comfort.

Care with unknown effects on perineal trauma and/or maternal second-stage comfort

Recommendations:

- No conclusion can be drawn about the effectiveness of antenatal perineal stretching using a massaging device (Epi-No).
- No conclusion can be drawn about benefits or harms of perineal ice packs in the second stage.

Care that should be abandoned in light of the evidence that it does not reduce perineal trauma and/or improve maternal second-stage comfort

Recommendations:

- There is no evidence that lignocaine (lidocaine) spray reduces perineal pain during the second stage of labour.
- Episiotomy should be avoided unless there are compelling reasons, such as severe fetal distress.
- Women should be informed of the greater risk of instrumental birth associated with epidural usage and the associated perineal trauma risk.

(Source: Dahlen, 2007c)

upright or lateral position, advising women to follow their own urges to push during the second stage, facilitating a slow and gentle birth of the baby's head using hands poised/hands on as required, using a vacuum extractor in preference to forceps, restricting the use of episiotomy, avoiding an epidural where possible, supporting women throughout labour and birth, giving birth in a home-like environment or at home, and giving birth with midwives compared with obstetricians will all decrease the incidence of perineal trauma and/or increase second-stage comfort (Aasheim et al., 2017; Australian Commission on Safety and Quality in Health Care, 2021; Dahlen, Dowling, et al., 2013; Reitsma et al., 2020; Scarf et al., 2018). Pelvic floor muscle training undertaken antenatally can reduce the incidence of severe perineal trauma (Sobhgol et al., 2020). Several other clinical factors warrant further investigation, such as immersion in water (the evidence is mixed), and the use of perineal ice packs in the second stage, particularly where oedema is present. Research does not support the use of antenatal perineal stretching using a massaging device (Epi-No) (Brito et al., 2015) (Boxes 28.2–28.4).

ANATOMY AND PHYSIOLOGY OF THE PELVIC FLOOR

The anatomy of the female pelvic floor is complex and some find it daunting to learn; however, it is extremely

Box 28.3 Antenatal perineal massage instructions

- Perineal massage can commence at 34 weeks pregnancy if there are no contraindications (history of herpes, ruptured membranes, bleeding, etc.).
- You can use a water-based lubricant or non-scented oil like sweet almond oil to lubricate fingers.
- Introduce one to two fingers 3–4 cm into the vagina and apply and maintain pressure first downwards for 2 minutes and then for 2 minutes on each side of the vaginal entrance.
- Standing upright with one leg on a chair or toilet and using thumb/s is often easiest if arms are not long enough. Partners can also assist with the massage if the woman is comfortable with this.
- Even undertaking this once or twice a week seems to be effective.

(Source: Labrecque et al., 1999)

Box 28.4 Perineal warm compresses

- A clean jug or bowl is filled with 300 mL boiling water and 300 mL cool tap water. This gives a water temperature range over 15 minutes of between 45 and 59°C.
- A pad or cloth is soaked in the warm water and wrung out before being placed gently over the perineum during contractions. DO NOT PLACE OVER THE BABY'S HEAD.
- Wait until the baby's head is distending the perineum and the mother feels the stinging sensation to apply the warm compress. The temperature range of the perineal pad over 15 minutes is 38–44°C.
- The pad is resoaked to maintain warmth between contractions.
- The water in the jug needs to be replaced every 15 minutes until delivery to ensure significant warmth. NEVER ADD HOT WATER TO THE BOWL AS IT IS HARD TO DETERMINE TEMPERATURE WHEN GLOVES ARE ON AND THE PAD/CLOTH MAY ABSORB THE HOT WATER DIRECTLY AND CAUSE SCALDING.

(Based on the Warm Pack Trial Protocol, Dahlen, 2007c)

important that midwives have a sound understanding of the structures involved. This becomes critical when advising women about optimal pelvic floor health, identifying and repairing perineal trauma, and advising women about care following the birth. It is also important to refresh knowledge of the bony pelvis when learning about the pelvic floor, as ligaments and muscles (white line of fascia) supporting the pelvic organs originate from it.

The pelvic floor is made up of soft tissue that fills the bony outlet of the bony pelvis. It essentially forms a sling and extends from the skin of the vulva, perineum and buttocks below to the pelvic peritoneum above. The layers from the inside out include (Fig. 28.1):

- pelvic peritoneum
- pelvic fascia (parametrium), which thickens to form the supporting ligaments of the pelvic organs
- deep perineal muscles (levator ani)
- superficial perineal muscles
- subcutaneous fat
- skin.

The main functions of the pelvic floor are to:

- support the pelvic organs (vagina, uterus, ovaries, bladder and rectum)
- maintain intra-abdominal pressure during coughing, sneezing, vomiting and laughing
- aid defecation and micturition and maintain continence
- facilitate childbirth.

Pelvic peritoneum

The pelvic peritoneum lies over the uterus and ovaries. The front aspect forms the uterovesical pouch and this covers the upper surface of the bladder. Posteriorly it dips behind the vaginal fornix and forms the pouch of Douglas prior to passing over the rectum.

Pelvic fascia

The pelvic fascia consists of connective tissue that lines the pelvic walls and fills the spaces between the pelvic organs, and forms strong ligaments to support the uterus. It extends from the pelvic peritoneum and abdominal muscles above to the levator ani below. The main supporting ligaments are:

- *broad ligaments,* formed from the peritoneal covering of the uterine tubes; unlike the other ligaments, they do not have a supportive function
- *transverse cervical ligaments* (also known as the Cardinal or Mackenrodt's ligaments), which arise from the vaginal vault and the sides of the cervix and extend laterally in a fan-like structure to be inserted into the white line of fascia on the lateral pelvic walls; these form the main support for the uterus
- *uterosacral ligaments,* which are attached to the upper portion of the posterior wall of the cervix and extend upwards and backwards, encircling the rectum before attaching to the front of the second sacral vertebrae (sacrum); their main role is to support the uterus but also to keep it in its normal anteverted (forward-tilted) position
- *pubocervical ligaments,* fairly weak ligaments which originate in the cervix, pass under the bladder and attach to the pubic bone; they mainly provide support and stability for the bladder
- *round ligaments,* two bands of fibrous tissue enclosed in the peritoneum that originate near the fundus of the uterus; they pass between the folds of the broad

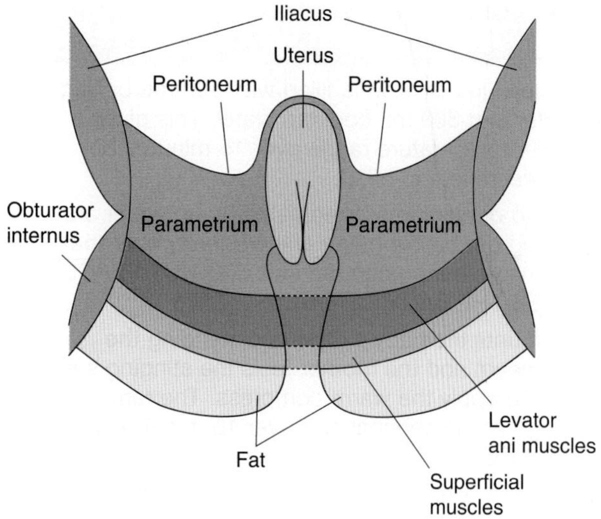

FIGURE 28.1 Tissue layers of the pelvic floor

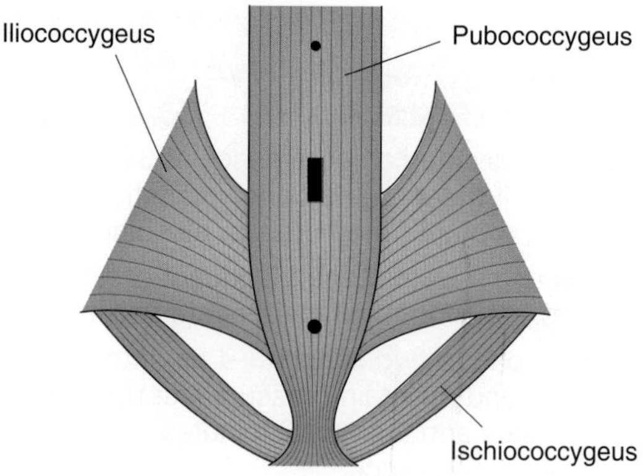

FIGURE 28.2 Deep muscles of the pelvic floor (levator ani muscles)
(Based on Nisbet & Rouse, 1992)

ligaments to the sides of the pelvis, through the inguinal canal and fuse with the labia majora. Their function is to maintain the uterus in the anteflexed (bent-on-itself) and anteverted (forward-tilted) positions (Kettle, 2005a).

Deep muscle layer

The deep muscle layer is around 3–5 cm in depth and is formed from a group of muscles known collectively as the levator ani. Each of these levator ani muscles arises from the internal lateral pelvic wall, the posterior aspect of the pubic bone, the white line of fascia and the ischial spine to converge midline. They pass backwards and downwards to meet in the upper vagina, perineal body, anal canal and the lateral border of the coccyx and lower part of the sacrum (Kettle, 2005a). This anatomical structure provides the hammock of strong muscle that supports the vaginal walls and uterus. The levator ani muscles also provide some support to the bladder and anal canal and counteract any increase in abdominal pressure. They are critical to the maintenance of the integrity and strength of the pelvic floor. They are divided into three main muscle groups (Fig. 28.2): the pubococcygeus and puborectalis muscles in the levator ani, the iliococcygeus muscles and the ischiococcygeus muscles.

- The *pubococcygeus muscles* are the most important part of the levator ani, in both size and function (Kettle, 2005a). Their main function is to provide support to the urethra, vagina and rectum as well as aiding micturition, defecation and constriction of the vagina during sexual intercourse. The pubococcygeus muscles form the anterior section of the levator ani. They originate from the anterior part of the obturator fascia and sweep backwards to form U-shaped structures around the urethra, vagina and anorectal junction. The muscle fibres pass downwards and backwards below the bladder on either side of the urethra, upper vagina and anal canal posteriorly, and then are inserted into the anococcygeal body coccyx (Kettle, 2005a).
- The *puborectalis muscles* form the most medial portion of the levator ani muscle and mark the transition from rectum to anus. They arise from the lower part of the symphysis pubis and converge with muscle fibres of the opposite side around the lower portion of the rectum. The strong sling that is so formed helps to maintain the forward angulation of the anorectal junction and plays a part in maintaining continence of faeces (Kettle, 2005a).
- The *iliococcygeus muscles* arise from the white line of pelvic fascia, and pass downwards and inwards to the anococcygeal body and coccyx. These muscles help to elevate the pelvic floor and are capable of rapid contraction.
- The *ischiococcygeus muscles* originate at the ischial spine and pass downwards and inwards to be inserted into the coccyx and lower sacrum. These muscles help to stabilise the sacroiliac and sacrococcygeal joints of the pelvis.

Superficial muscle layer

Although these muscles are small and contained in the superficial layer of the pelvic floor, they are critical to the overall function and strength of the pelvic floor. These muscles extend from the perineal body around the vagina to the clitoris (Fig. 28.3). They strengthen the sphincter action of the vagina and urethra, and play a part in sexual function (Kettle, 2005a). They are also the main muscles involved in perineal trauma.

- The *bulbocavernosus muscles* (also known as the bulbospongiosus) arise in the centre of the perineum, encircling the urethra and vagina, before inserting into the corpora cavernosa of the clitoris. Their main purpose is to constrict the vaginal orifice and to contribute anteriorly to the erection of the clitoris in sexual activity.

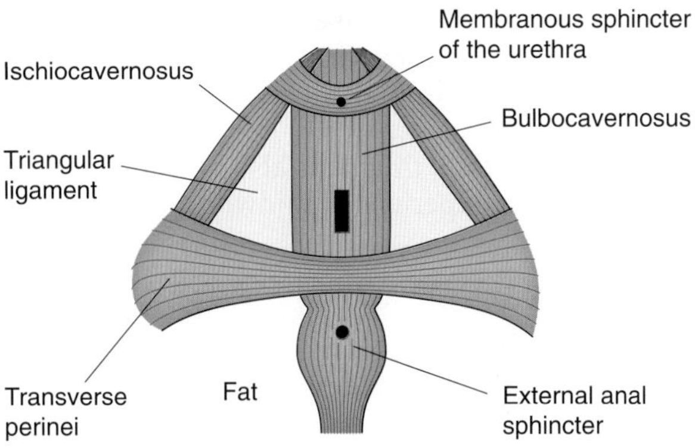

FIGURE 28.3 Superficial muscles of the pelvic floor
(Based on Nisbet & Rouse, 1992)

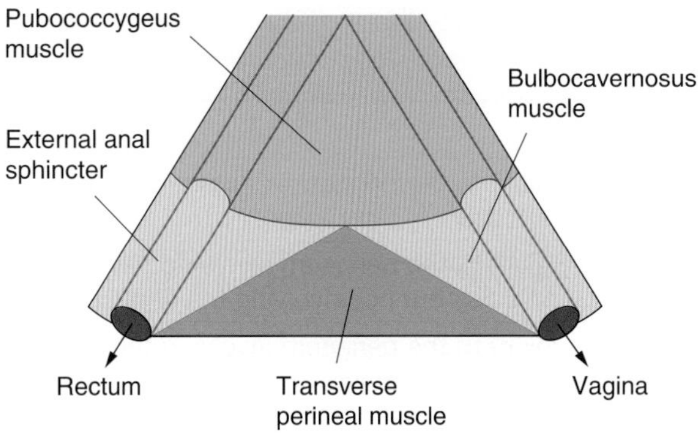

FIGURE 28.4 The perineal body
(Based on Nisbet & Rouse, 1992)

- The *ischiocavernosus muscles* are situated in the lateral boundary of the perineum; they originate in the ischial tuberosities and terminate in the clitoris. Some of the fibres interweave with the membranous sphincter of the urethra. Their main function is to maintain the engorgement of the clitoris.
- The *superficial transverse perinei* are muscles that pass from the ischial tuberosities to the perineal body and join with the bulbocavernosus in front. Their main function is to support the lower part of the vagina and to fix the central tendinous point of the perineal body.
- The *deep transverse perinei* are thin muscles that pass from each ischiopubic ramus to converge midline in the perineal body. Some of the fibres are inserted into the vagina and they contribute to stabilising the perineal body.
- The *external anal sphincter muscle* encompasses the anal opening and passes in front of the perineal body before attaching posteriorly to the coccyx. It controls the passage of faeces and flatus.
- The *membranous sphincter of the urethra* comprises two bands of muscle that originate at one of the pubic bones, passing above and below the urethra before inserting into the other pubic bone. It is capable of contracting to occlude the urethra (Kettle, 2005a).

The perineal body

The perineal body is a fibromuscular structure situated between the lowest third of the vagina in front, the anal canal behind and the ischial tuberosities laterally (Kettle, 2005a) (Fig. 28.4). It is a pyramid-like structure (approximately 3.5 cm in length), with the base of the pyramid being the skin. It is interlaced with the pubococcygeus, bulbocavernosus, superficial transverse perinei and external anal sphincter muscles. The lower part of the perineal body, where most of the superficial perineal muscles converge, is known as the *central point* of the perineum. This is the main area involved in perineal trauma. Some women have smaller perineal bodies, leading to what some midwives describe as a 'short perineum'. This has been implicated in increased severe perineal trauma (Dahlen, 2007a). The chief function of the perineal body is to control defecation and to stretch and flatten during childbirth.

Nerve, lymph and blood supply

The perineal branch of the third and fourth sacral nerves and the inferior rectal and pudendal nerve supply the pelvic floor. Lymph drainage is via the internal iliac glands, the blood supply is from the internal iliac and pudendal arteries, and venous drainage is into the corresponding veins.

Other

The final layer of the pelvic floor is composed of superficial fascia, fat and skin.

It is important for midwives to understand the underlying anatomy and physiology of the pelvic floor so that they can assist in maintaining its integrity during childbirth. A clear anatomical understanding is vital for repair of the pelvic floor, to achieve optimal outcomes for women.

The following sections outline the types of perineal trauma, and management during and after birth.

PERINEAL TRAUMA AND REPAIR

Degrees of perineal trauma

Perineal trauma can be caused by spontaneous perineal laceration, or intentionally by an episiotomy. Perineal trauma is generally divided into anterior and posterior trauma, of which there are four degrees (Table 28.1).

- Anterior trauma involves injury to anterior parts of the labia, vagina, urethra or clitoris.
- Posterior trauma is divided into:
  - first-degree trauma, which involves skin only
  - second-degree trauma, which involves the perineal muscles

Table 28.1 Degrees of spontaneous perineal trauma

Degree	Trauma
First	Injury to the perineal skin and/or vaginal mucosa
Second	Injury to the perineum involving perineal muscles but not involving the anal sphincter
Third	Injury to the perineum involving the anal sphincter complex • 3a—less than 50% of external anal sphincter (EAS) thickness torn • 3b—more than 50% of EAS thickness torn • 3c—both EAS and internal anal sphincter (IAS) torn
Fourth	Injury to perineum involving the anal sphincter complex (EAS and IAS) and anorectal mucosa

(Source: Royal College of Obstetricians and Gynaecologists. (2015). *The Management of Third- and Fourth-Degree Perineal Tears*. Green-top Guideline, 29, 11. ©Royal College of Obstetricians and Gynaecologists; reproduced with permission)

- third-degree trauma, which involves partial or complete disruption of the anal sphincter, now further divided into 3a, 3b and 3c
- fourth-degree trauma, which involves complete disruption of the external and internal anal sphincter, including the rectal mucosa.

Other types of trauma

Labial lacerations are often classified separately as labial grazes or tears. They tend to be fairly superficial tears that generally do not require sutures unless bleeding cannot be stopped, or they are deep or do not oppose well. Bilateral labial tears can be a concern for some midwives owing to the fact that the two sides may adhere to each other during healing. Suturing one side can help avoid this; alternatively, midwives can instruct women to make sure that the labia remain separated when bathing daily. If there are any doubts, then it is recommended to suture the lacerations.

Vaginal and cervical lacerations can cause serious postpartum haemorrhage if not identified and repaired in a timely manner. Both structures are very vascular, and careful inspection should be carried out after the birth to exclude this kind of trauma, which can be hard to see and can precipitate heavy blood loss. When examining the vagina following the birth, it is important not just to look but also to examine digitally, as vaginal tears can be hard to see when the rugae folds onto itself. Vaginal tears can also be high in the vaginal vault (high vaginal tear), and these can be easily missed but can lead to serious postpartum haemorrhage. Once detected, suturing should occur immediately. Cervical trauma tends to cause quite a bright blood loss and should be suspected if trickling continues (cervical tears tend to pump blood out). Cervical lacerations are more common with instrumental birth or births involving manipulations. An experienced obstetrician should carry out cervical suturing immediately to avoid excessive bleeding and cervical complications in subsequent pregnancies.

Clitoral and urethral trauma is also best repaired by an obstetrician or an experienced midwife.

Episiotomy

An episiotomy is a surgical incision made into the perineum, which if required should be performed only immediately prior to birth to enlarge the vaginal outlet and to assist the birth of the baby. The presenting part should be distending the perineum prior to performing the episiotomy and local anaesthetic should be given. It is in the scope of practice of a midwife to infiltrate the perineum and perform an episiotomy. The use of episiotomy should, however, be restricted to expediting the birth only when the presenting part is fully distending the perineum and when there is evidence of a non-reassuring fetal heart rate pattern. Other indications for an episiotomy include a rigid perineum which is preventing the birth occurring over an extended period of time or where there are indications that perineal trauma may be severe, such as 'button-holing'. There is no evidence to support the use of routine episiotomy in *any* circumstance, not even when there has been a previous third-degree tear. The practitioner *must* get verbal consent from the woman prior to performing an episiotomy.

There are three types of episiotomy:

- *Mediolateral episiotomy*—the incision starts in the midline of the fourchette and runs backwards to a point between the ischial tuberosity and the anus (Fig. 28.5). This type of incision appears to be less likely to extend to a third- or fourth-degree tear but is more painful during healing and tends to bleed more.
- *Midline episiotomy*—the incision is from the fourchette directly down towards the anus. It has been associated with less pain and bleeding, although there is an increased risk that it will extend to a third- or fourth-degree tear.

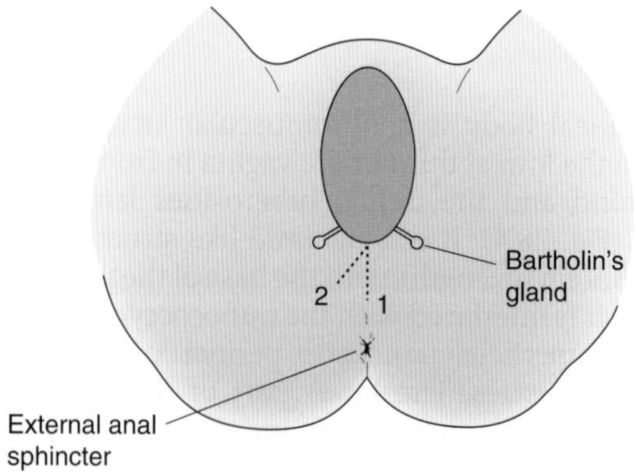

FIGURE 28.5 Types of episiotomy: 1 midline, 2 mediolateral (Based on Nisbet & Rouse, 1992)

- *Anterior episiotomy*—women with female genital mutilation (FGM) type 3 infibulations may require an anterior episiotomy and will often require a posterior episiotomy as well. You need to have training in anterior episiotomy in order to perform and repair it.

The structures involved when performing an episiotomy are similar to those involved in a second-degree tear, but there is a fundamental difference. When the perineum spontaneously tears it does so between muscle fibres, nerves and other structures, whereas when an episiotomy is performed it cuts *across* muscle fibres, nerves and other structures and follows an unnatural pathway. This is possibly why it is so much more painful and is associated with greater morbidity than a second-degree tear.

Infiltration of the perineum

Prior to performing an episiotomy, local anaesthetic should be administered. There are very few cases when there is not enough time to administer a local anaesthetic, and not doing so can lead to psychological trauma. Local anaesthetic such as lignocaine (lidocaine) 0.5% or 1% (10 mL) is most commonly used. Prior to infiltrating the perineum, the baby's head should be distending the perineum so that the muscles are as thin as possible. The area should be cleaned with an antiseptic solution. The midwife then inserts two fingers (gloved) into the vagina to protect the baby's head. The needle is inserted into the muscle layer in the area of the incision. The plunger of the syringe is withdrawn to ensure that the needle is not in a blood vessel. If blood is observed in the barrel of the syringe, the needle should be withdrawn slightly and re-inserted into another area of tissue, as local anaesthetic should never be injected into a blood vessel. The anaesthetic is then infiltrated into the muscle as the needle is withdrawn from the tissue (approximately 3–4 mL) in a 'fan- or feather-like' way. Just prior to the needle being completely withdrawn, the needle is re-inserted to the side of the incision site, where 2–3 mL of local anaesthetic are injected; this is repeated on the other side. Depending on how quickly the episiotomy needs to be performed, only one line of infiltration may be undertaken. Each time the midwife infiltrates, she must check to avoid blood vessels.

The infiltration should be performed a couple of minutes prior to the incision. Women with epidurals need to be assessed carefully, as the anaesthetic may have worn off and they may require local anaesthetic infiltration as well. Obstetricians sometimes perform a pudendal block prior to an instrumental birth.

Once the anaesthesia is effective, the midwife inserts the same two fingers into the vagina to protect the baby's head. An episiotomy is performed using blunt-ended Mayo scissors. These are opened: one blade is placed between the fingers and the other blade along the middle of the area where the lignocaine was introduced. A single confident cut, approximately 4 cm long (depending on the length of the perineum), is made, preferably during a contraction to minimise pain. A thin, well-stretched perineum is less likely to bleed. The midwife then removes the scissors quickly and prepares for the imminent birth of the baby's head. It is important to control the birth of the head, as rapid expulsion could extend the episiotomy. The woman should be encouraged to breathe the baby's head out at this point. If the baby is not born immediately, the midwife will need to apply pressure to any bleeding points in the incision to minimise blood loss.

Midwives and students can practise cutting an episiotomy using a tennis ball pushed to the opening of an old sock. Suturing an episiotomy is within the scope of practice of a midwife (see below).

Pelvic organ prolapse

When the pelvic floor muscles are overdistended, the musculature is sometimes unable to provide appropriate support for the organs. This can result in a prolapse of the pelvic organs. Those most at risk are grand multiparous women or women who have had a long, difficult labour and give birth to a large baby. Some women, however, seem to have no particular predisposing factors and may be genetically more prone to developing a prolapse than others. Women who have elective caesareans can still have **pelvic organ prolapse**.

Types of prolapse include:

- *uterovaginal prolapse*—the vaginal wall is weak and the uterus protrudes down into the vagina
- *cystocele*—the bladder bulges into the vagina owing to a weakened upper anterior vaginal wall
- *rectocele*—the rectum bulges into the vagina owing to a weakened posterior vaginal wall
- *cervical prolapse*—the cervix protrudes into the lower half of the vagina.

Depending on the severity, prolapses may require surgical intervention. The mode of birth for subsequent pregnancies would need to be carefully considered, to prevent further damage. Often the decision is made to repair the prolapse once the woman has completed her family.

To suture or not to suture?

In recent years, changes in perineal repair practice have been observed, particularly with midwives choosing not to suture certain degrees of perineal trauma. Unfortunately, there is no good evidence to date to help midwives make this decision, so caution must be taken and research needs to be undertaken urgently into this question.

A good rule of thumb is to suture when:

- there is bleeding that does not stop after a reasonable period of time with pressure
- the tear is ragged and may not approximate by itself
- the tear is greater than 1–2 cm in depth
- there are pockets or bulges in the tissue
- (most important of all) this is what the woman wants.

The small sample sizes in the trials to date on this issue (Fleming et al., 2003; Lundquist et al., 2000) are a limitation, and evidence from larger trials is needed.

Until this evidence is available, caution is needed as the evidence so far is not conclusive with regards to non-suturing of perineal trauma.

Midwifery responsibilities when repairing perineal trauma

Inspecting the perineum following the birth

After the placenta has been delivered, the midwife should make a thorough inspection of the vagina and perineum to determine the extent of any trauma. It is important that good lighting is used. The woman may need nitrous oxide for pain relief during the examination, as she may not yet have been given local anaesthetic. If the decision is made not to suture because there is only a first-degree tear or a small labial graze, the midwife should make sure that bleeding has ceased. It is recommended to recheck the trauma again in half an hour to make sure good haemostasis is achieved.

Once a perineal wound has been thoroughly inspected and the midwife is satisfied that the suturing is within her capabilities, the repair should be carried out as soon as possible under aseptic conditions. A lithotomy position is not generally required for suturing as long as there is good visibility, the woman is comfortable and the midwife is also comfortable.

The area is swabbed with an antiseptic solution. Sterile drapes are generally used, as it is a surgical procedure—unlike the birth where this is not required (Dahlen & Ryan, 2001). Sometimes a taped tampon is inserted into the vagina to prevent vaginal loss obscuring the wound in the vaginal vault and to help make it easier to see when suturing. If this is done, it is essential to count the tampon with the other swabs and to document that it has been inserted and when it has been removed. It is also a good idea to clip the end of the tape to the sterile drapes as a reminder that the tampon needs removing at the end.

Protection for the midwife

It is essential to ensure a good risk management approach when undertaking perineal repair. It is ideal to learn to suture wearing double gloves so that this becomes easy. If you normally wear size 6 gloves, then put a size 7 pair on first and a size 6 over the top. The larger gloves underneath fold over to give your fingertips some extra protection. If one layer of the gloves is damaged, the second layer may remain intact. It is also recommended that protective eyewear is worn, as it is not uncommon when injecting anaesthetic into the wound that it spurts back into the eyes. Lastly, don't forget your back. Make sure the bed is at the right height, you don't have to bend and twist too much, and the lighting is good.

Infiltration of the perineum with local anaesthetic

The quote 'being stitched up is worse than having the baby' (Willmott, 1980) is one that I use frequently when teaching this section of perineal repair. We well remember the days before midwives undertook perineal repair when some women would spend the whole time with their legs restrained in stirrups while they jumped and squealed through the repair. We hope those days are over.

A woman who is pain free will be able to relax, which makes suturing much easier. The most common anaesthetic used for infiltration of the perineum prior to suturing is lignocaine (0.5%–1%, 10–20 mL). A longer-lasting anaesthetic like bupivacaine (0.25%, 5–10 mL) can be used. Some local anaesthetics have adrenaline (epinephrine) added to them to prolong the duration of activity. Adrenaline can also serve a purpose in constricting blood vessels and making the wound easier to visualise during repair. It is very important to wait for this to work, which normally takes 4–5 minutes.

Women should be advised that inserting the local anaesthetic can sometimes be uncomfortable. Placing a lignocaine-soaked swab on the labia for a few minutes prior to infiltration of this sensitive part can reduce the discomfort a little. The addition of sodium bicarbonate to the anaesthetic will reduce pain on infiltration (1: 20 solution, e.g. 1 mL sodium bicarbonate to 20 mL lignocaine). If the woman has had an epidural it can be topped up prior to suturing, but she needs to be aware that it will then have to wear off before she is able to mobilise.

Prior to commencing suturing, test with a non-tooth forceps to ensure the local anaesthetic is effective. Check in regularly with the woman. Where trust is present and the woman knows the midwife will respond promptly to any discomfort, I find that women relax and focus on their baby quite easily during the repair.

Suture material

The ideal suture material should cause minimal reaction and be absorbed once it has served its purpose, which is to hold the tissue in apposition during the healing process (Kettle, 2005b). This enables the wound to heal by primary intention, controls the bleeding and minimises the risk of infection. When wound edges are brought together without too much tension then the healing process is optimally facilitated and the perineal trauma should heal within a couple of weeks.

Rapidly absorbed polyglactin 910 (Vicryl Rapide) is seen by many midwives to be the ideal suture material. It has the same properties as standard polyglactin 910 but the tensile strength is reduced owing to the sterilisation process, which is by gamma irradiation. The tensile strength (point when it breaks) of rapidly absorbed polyglactin 910 is reduced to between 10 and 14 days and it is fully absorbed by between 35 and 42 days. A prospective cohort study and three RCTs evaluated rapidly absorbed polyglactin 910 suture material. Vicryl Rapide led to a significant reduction in pain when walking at 10–14 days postpartum (Kettle, 2002). A systematic review on perineal care conducted by (Frolich & Kettle, 2015) described outcomes when comparing rapidly absorbed polyglactin 910 and standard polyglactin 910. The authors reported that rapidly absorbed polyglactin 910 may be more effective than standard polyglactin 910 at reducing analgesic use at 10 days postpartum; however, it appears to be no more effective than standard polyglactin 910 at reducing the number of women who report perineal pain at up to 3 months, or dyspareunia at up to 12 months. The largest trial also showed a reduction in pain in walking and reduction in suture removal in the Vicryl Rapide group (Kettle, 2002). However, although rapidly absorbed polyglactin 910 has some clear advantages over other polyglactin suture materials, in very large tears where tensile strength for a longer period would be optimal it might be wise to use the longer-lasting suture materials.

Suturing techniques

Perineal trauma is generally repaired in three stages. First the vagina is repaired, then the muscle layer, and finally the skin is closed.

The recommended technique now is a continuous non-locking suture used for all layers. A large RCT published in 2002 showed a significant reduction in perineal pain at 10 days when the loose non-locking stitch was used for all layers. For every six women sutured with this method, one less complained of pain at 10 days compared with those sutured with the interrupted method (Kettle, 2002). Suture removal was also significantly less frequent with the continuous non-locking suturing. The women in the continuous non-locking group often reported not knowing that they were sutured. A Cochrane systematic review showed that continuous suturing techniques for perineal closure, compared with interrupted methods, are associated with less short-term pain, need for analgesia and suture removal as well as using less suture material (Kettle et al., 2012). The Ipswich childbirth study (Gordon et al., 1998; Mackrodt et al., 1998) compared two-stage suturing (suturing only the vagina and muscle and leaving the skin) with a traditional three-stage approach (suturing vagina, muscle and skin). It found that the two-stage approach was associated with a small reduction in dyspareunia at 3 months postpartum; however, it has been suggested that further research is required to evaluate whether there is an increased risk of wound gaping, which may be unacceptable to women (Frolich & Kettle, 2015).

Undertaking the repair

A full description of how to undertake perineal repair can be found in the accompanying Skills Book (De-Vitry Smith & Bayes, 2022). However, regardless of the suturing method used, there are some basic principles that need to be applied (Kettle, 2005b):

- Carry out the perineal repair as soon as possible after the birth to minimise infection and blood loss.
- Prior to commencing the repair, check all the equipment and count and document the number of swabs. This needs to be repeated at the end of the repair as well.
- Undertake the repair under aseptic conditions.
- Make sure there is a good source of light so that the extent of the injury and structures involved can be clearly visualised.
- Make sure that good support and supervision are available before undertaking the repair. If in doubt ask for assistance.
- Handle perineal tissue gently with non-toothed forceps.
- Bleeding points need to be identified and sutured to prevent haematoma formation.
- It is important to repair the muscle layer competently, to prevent dead spaces that can lead to haematomas forming and infection developing.
- A minimal amount of suture material should be used.
- Don't overtighten sutures as this can cause the tissues to become hypoxic and delay healing.
- The suture at the apex of the wound is very important, as it provides the anchor for the procedure. It is important to know that the apex has been reached, to prevent ongoing bleeding. Sometimes there are several apexes and each needs suturing.
- The vaginal epithelium is closed with a continuous running suture, which starts at the apex of the wound and finishes at the hymenal remnants; this is then taken through into the deeper muscle layer (Fig. 28.6).
- The deep and superficial muscle layers are closed with continuous running sutures (Fig. 28.7).
- Finally, the skin is closed with continuous subcuticular sutures. The sutures are placed in the subcutaneous tissue instead of in the nerve-rich superficial skin, pulling the edges together. At the top of the wound the suture material is taken through into the vagina and tied off to the last vaginal suture (Fig. 28.8).
- Sutures at the beginning and end of the repair need to be tied securely but not too bulkily, using a square surgeon's knot at the beginning and a loop or Aberdeen knot at the end.
- It is important to make sure that good anatomical restoration of the perineal tissues is achieved.
- On completion of the suturing, if a vaginal tampon has been inserted this needs to be removed and the vaginal vault needs to be inspected.
- A finger is then inserted into the rectum to ensure that no sutures have been placed in this area and the

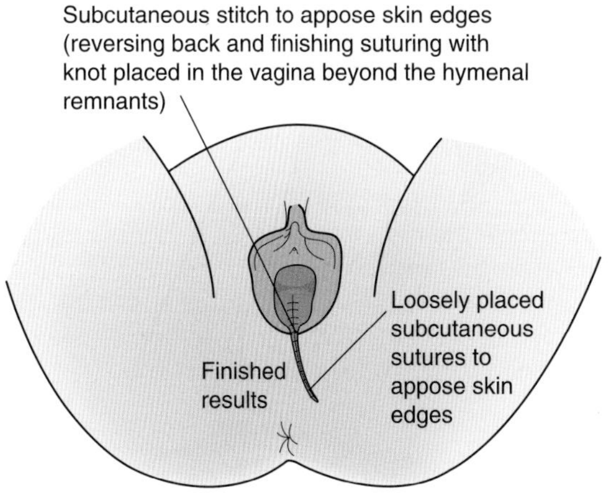

FIGURE 28.6 Continuous non-locking repair of vagina

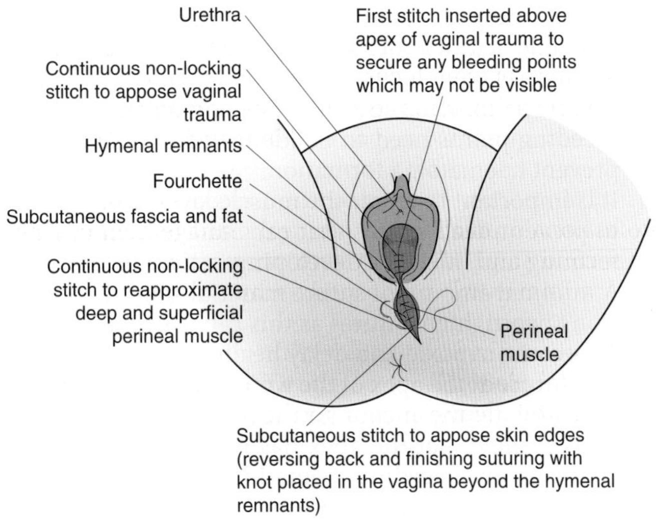

FIGURE 28.7 Continuous non-locking repair of perineal muscles

sphincter feels intact. This can be uncomfortable, so an explanation should be given.

- Accurate documentation is vital and should involve:
  - a description, and if possible a diagram, of the tear
  - the type and amount of anaesthetic infiltrate used
  - the type and size of suture material used
  - the technique used for the repair
  - the count of all sponges and sharps before and after the repair
  - the findings of the vaginal and rectal examination
  - advice given to the woman regarding postnatal care.
- Offer women a chance to view their perineum in a mirror. Many women do want to look, and a woman who feels involved and in touch with her body at this point may well remain feeling involved and in touch with her body. Using the continuous subcuticular method of repair also gives an aesthetically pleasing result.
- Inform the woman of the extent of the trauma, pain relief she can use, dietary considerations, importance of rest, personal hygiene, pelvic floor exercises and avoidance of constipation.

CRITICAL THINKING EXERCISE

If a woman asks not to be sutured what information would you give her and what are your professional responsibilities?

Severe perineal trauma

Only an experienced obstetrician or senior registrar supervised by a senior obstetrician should suture third- and fourth-degree tears, ideally in an operating theatre under spinal / epidural or general anaesthetic. Some indications that the woman may have sustained an anal injury are an absence of anal puckering around the anterior aspect of the anus (between 9 and 3 o'clock), and a tear that extends to the anal margin. If concerned then insert the

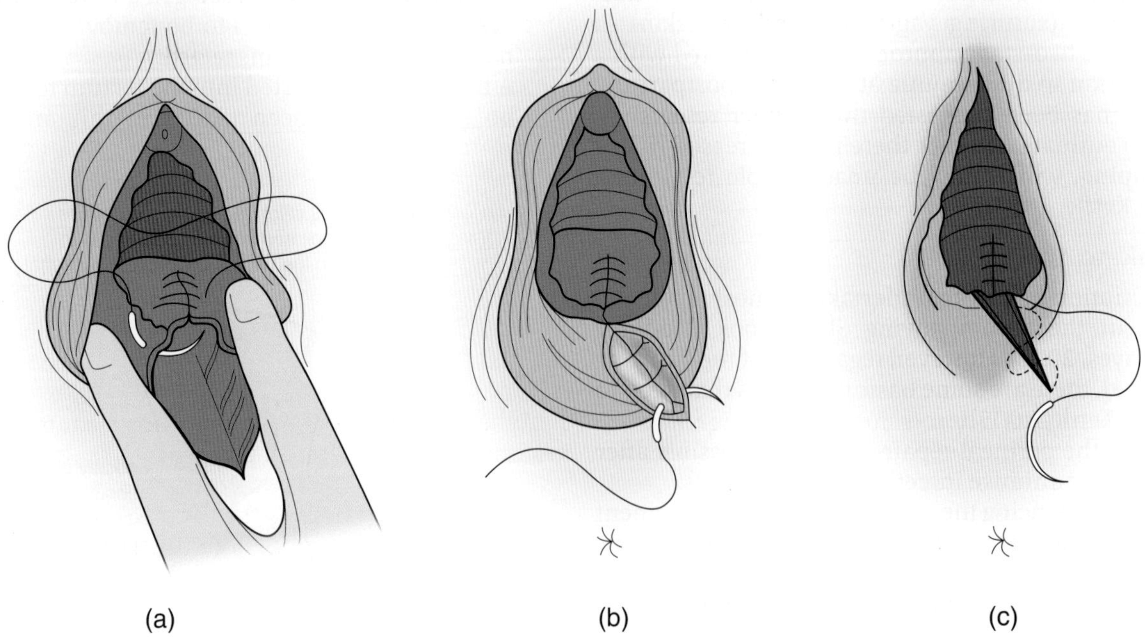

FIGURE 28.8 The three stages of perineal repair: (a) repair of the vagina; (b) repair of the perineal muscle; (c) repair of the skin

index finger into the woman's anus (obviously after explaining the procedure and gaining consent) and ask her to squeeze. If the external anal sphincter is torn, the separated ends can be observed to retract backwards towards the ischiorectal fossa. Damage to the internal anal sphincter is harder to detect but may be observed during a rectal examination (Kettle, 2005b).

Faecal incontinence and vesicovaginal fistula formation (where a hole is present between the bladder or urethra and vagina) are serious complications of severe perineal trauma and can have long-term physical and psychological effects. Postnatal follow-up with a medical practitioner is important to detect and prevent long-term sequelae. Best practice suggests that women with persistent anal problems should be referred for anal manometry, ultrasound scan and consultation with a colorectal surgeon (Kettle, 2005b). Counselling should be provided prior to another pregnancy.

Routine caesarean section is no longer recommended for all women who have experienced severe perineal trauma during a previous birth. Neither is routine episiotomy.

Compassionate care

The concept of compassionate care can be described as the ability of the health professional to commit fully to the experience of the person they are caring for, establishing and developing a connection that assists the health professional to feel empathy towards the experiences of the other (Burnell, 2009; Ménage et al., 2017; Priddis, Schmied, Kettle, et al., 2014; Roach, 2007). Tavernier (2006) explores the concept of compassionate care, relating empathy to 'presence' stating that when health practitioners are completely present they can facilitate increased feelings of trust and safety that result in positive physical and psychological outcomes for the person within their care as they feel understood, safe and in control owing to the 'presence' of the practitioner. In maternity care, Wagner (2000) describes the importance of compassionate care as 'humanizing birth', stating that:

> *... respecting the woman as an important and valuable human being and making certain that the woman's experience while giving birth is fulfilling and empowering is not just a nice extra, it is absolutely essential as it makes the woman strong and therefore makes society strong.*
>
> (Wagner, 2000, p. S25).

The principles of compassionate care are a requisite of midwives in New Zealand and threaded throughout the midwifery partnership relationship, the competencies of practice and standards of midwifery care (New Zealand College of Midwives, 2015).

The way women are cared for during the perinatal period has a direct impact on their capacity to understand and process their experience of perineal trauma, both positive and negative; it can also impact on their ability to manage any ongoing symptoms and related morbidities (Priddis, Schmied, & Dahlen, 2014; Priddis, Schmied, Kettle, et al., 2014). Research from Australia and the UK suggests that health professional education and training is often focused more on technical skill and less on providing compassionate care to women, particularly when undertaking perineal assessment and repair. This approach is demonstrated in a study conducted by East et al. (2014) examining the perceptions of health professionals' practices for perineal management during the second stage of labour, with one participant stating: 'One can never tell how a perineum will behave, therefore be poised, prepared and patient' (East et al., 2014, p.12). This statement describes the perineum as separate to the total physical and emotional form of the birthing woman, and demonstrates the medical separation of mind and body.

Women who experience severe perineal trauma have described feeling 'abandoned' by health providers and the healthcare system, and 'feeling like a piece of meat'—suggesting a lack of compassionate care (Priddis, Schmied, Kettle, et al., 2014). Many women describe the experience of suturing as traumatic; feeling like they were being 'patched up' and being 'tortured' (Briscoe et al., 2015; Salmon, 1999). Further, studies have found that, whereas health professionals were more focused on technical skill rather than on providing compassionate care, women in contrast were more concerned with how they were cared for during suturing, and the way they were spoken to and followed up afterwards (Priddis, Schmied, & Dahlen, 2014; Priddis, Schmied, Kettle, et al., 2014). Women have described this as a time of feeling vulnerable and exposed; those who experienced severe perineal trauma stated that their birth was traumatic, with their trauma exacerbated by how they were treated. Lack of compassionate care contributes to a sense of disembodiment, social isolation and mental health issues (Priddis, Schmied, Kettle, et al., 2014). Good communication and coordinated systems are also necessary to ensure that women who have experienced severe perineal trauma feel supported. Compassionate and supportive care is a fundamental human right for all childbearing women but can be absent, deficient or undervalued in many hospitals (Dahlen et al., 2015). Although it is important to continue to find ways to reduce the incidence of perineal trauma including severe perineal trauma during birth, there is also a need for more focus on consistent guidelines to ensure ongoing supportive care is consistently available to women who experience severe perineal trauma. In addition there is a need to ensure that women receive compassionate, supportive and evidence-informed care (Priddis, Schmied, Kettle, et al., 2014) (Box 28.5).

When caring for women who sustain perineal trauma, health professionals need to be respectful of the woman and her needs, to ensure that she has privacy and dignity during the labour and birth, whilst being sutured and through into the immediate postpartum period. As required, interpreters should be used to ensure the appropriate and culturally sensitive transfer of information. Communication with the woman should be supported by evidence-based written information, which should include: risk factors for severe

Box 28.5 Principles of ensuring compassionate care

1. Be respectful
2. Ask the woman about her needs
3. Encourage questions and respond appropriately
4. Ensure privacy and dignity
5. Ensure a culturally appropriate interpreter (if necessary)
6. Clear communication
7. Evidence-informed care
8. Provide culturally sensitive information
9. Ensure consistent advice and information during follow-up

(Source: Priddis, Schmied, Kettle, et al., 2014)

perineal trauma, strategies to reduce the risk, management of severe perineal trauma, postnatal care and follow-up and prognosis. Women should be encouraged to ask questions, to ensure they understand what has happened, and follow up on any concerns they have about their health and wellbeing during the postnatal period. Women value the supportive presence of their care providers, who can facilitate feelings of safety, control and trust (Beck, 2006; Gibbins & Thomson, 2001; Halldorsdottir & Karlsdottir, 1996).

REFLECTIVE THINKING EXERCISE

- Take some time to reflect on the importance of compassionate care when providing care for a woman who has experienced perineal trauma. How might this look?
- A woman declines being transferred to theatre to repair a third-degree perineal tear as she does not want to be separated from her new baby. Considering the principles of compassionate care, how would you support the woman to achieve the best outcomes?

Summary

A skilful technique and a sensitive, evidence-based approach to perineal care and repair can dramatically improve women's experiences. Unfortunately there is very little research on the effects of skills on women's perineal outcomes and experiences. We all know that it is not just the junior doctor or midwife who should receive adequate training and supervision. Indeed, there are some very experienced obstetricians and midwives who refuse to change their habits or keep up with new evidence, or continue to follow the old adage that an episiotomy is much easier to suture and so continue to have high episiotomy rates.

Postpartum care of the woman with perineal trauma

All midwives know that postnatal care is considered the 'poor cousin' in the maternity service, and unfortunately this is once again true when it comes to the paucity of research on best practice in perineal care. It could be argued this is 'the poor cousin's poor cousin'! Myths still abound about ineffective practices like salt or Savlon baths and the use of hair dryers to aid with perineal healing.

The National Institute for Health and Care Excellence (NICE) in the United Kingdom have identified recommendations regarding routine postnatal care for women and perineal healing (NICE, 2021). See Box 28.6.

Midwives need to be aware of the following principles of evidence-based postnatal perineal care:

- Ice in the first 2–3 days can reduce oedema and improve comfort. Femé Pad gel pads are particularly good, reducing pain and oedema significantly at 5 and 10 days compared with no treatment or an ice pack (East et al., 2012; Steen & Marchant, 2007).
- There is no evidence of benefit from adding either salt or Savlon, or anything else, to the bathwater.
- Applications of witch hazel to the perineum to promote healing, and the use of homeopathic drugs such as arnica to reduce bruising, have not been fully evaluated.
- There is not enough evidence to evaluate the use of ultrasound in treating perineal pain or dyspareunia, or both, following childbirth (Hay-Smith, 2000).
- Application of lignocaine gel or aqueous 5% lignocaine spray is recommended in the literature, as long as they do not contain steroids, which can cause wound breakdown.
- Significant pain and swelling of the perineal area or in the labia may be a haematoma and immediate consultation and referral to an obstetrician are required.
- Women who do pelvic floor exercises are less likely to report perineal pain and feelings of depression at 3 months following birth.
- Paracetamol is the oral analgesic drug of choice for mild perineal pain.
- Oral ibuprofen for relief of perineal pain in women after an episiotomy or severe perineal trauma is effective.
- A stat dose rectally of 100 mg diclofenac provides effective analgesia that appears to be maintained into the second and third postpartum days, with women requiring less supplementary analgesia.
- Women need advice about a healthy balanced diet to maximise tissue healing and minimise constipation.

(National Institute for Health and Care Excellence (NICE), 2021)

Other useful tips

Labial lacerations or grazes can also be very painful in the first few days after birth, particularly when voiding. Women should be advised to keep the area clean and dry, and to part the labia to prevent adhesions/fusion. Pouring a jug of warm water over the genitals when urinating

Box 28.6 NICE Postnatal Care Guidance 2021

- At each postnatal contact, as part of assessing perineal wound healing, ask the woman if she has any concerns and ask about:
  - pain not resolving or worsening
  - increasing need for pain relief
  - discharge that has a strong or unpleasant smell
  - swelling
  - wound breakdown.
- Advise the woman about the importance of good perineal hygiene, including daily showering of the perineum, frequent changing of sanitary pads, and hand washing before and after doing this.
- Consider using a validated pain scale to monitor perineal pain.
- If the woman or the healthcare professional has concerns about perineal healing or if the woman asks for reassurance, offer or arrange an examination of the perineum by a midwife or a doctor.
- If needed, discuss available pain relief options, taking into account if the woman is breastfeeding.
- If the perineal wound breaks down or there are ongoing healing concerns, refer the woman urgently to specialist maternity services (to be seen the same day in the case of a perineal wound breakdown).
- Be aware that perineal pain that persists or gets worse within the first few weeks after the birth may be associated with symptoms of depression, long-term perineal pain, problems with daily functioning and psychosexual difficulties.
- Be aware of the following risk factors for persistent postnatal perineal pain:
  - episiotomy, or labial or perineal tear
  - assisted vaginal birth
  - wound infection or breakdown
  - birth experienced as traumatic.

(Source: NICE, 2021)

can also help to reduce the stinging. The use of an alkaliniser (e.g. Ural) for the first couple of days can reduce the acidity of the urine and lead to reduced stinging when urinating. This needs to be commenced immediately after the birth for maximum effect.

HIPPS

Extrapolation of the musculoskeletal injury management protocol RICE (*rest, ice, compression, elevation*) to perineal care is problematic for obvious reasons. Hence a different mnemonic has been developed for perineal care, called HIPPS—*hygiene, ice, pelvic floor exercises, pain relief* and *support* (Box 28.7) (Dahlen, 2004). Evidence identifies that perineal hygiene, ice and regular pelvic floor exercises are helpful. Women should have pain relief if they need it (NICE, 2015) and all new mothers need reassurance and support.

Box 28.7 HIPPS

H Hygiene—keep clean and dry
I Ice—first 48–72 hours
P Pelvic floor exercises—after first 48 hours
P Pain relief
S Support—all the time

(Source: Dahlen, 2004, based on evidence from Chiarelli & Cockburn, 1999)

CRITICAL THINKING EXERCISE

What is the advice you would give a woman who has had perineal trauma when it comes to her postnatal care?

Urinary and faecal incontinence

Urinary incontinence

Although many clinical studies have attempted to discover a particular obstetric event that causes **urinary incontinence**, no single event has been found responsible, suggesting that urinary incontinence arises from multifactorial physiological causes. Common reasons for urinary incontinence in women are stress incontinence and detrusor instability (AIHW, 2013). Urinary incontinence (or leaking urine) is a common and distressing disorder in women, with an estimated prevalence of 16%–58% of women between the ages of 10 and 80 years (AIHW, 2013; Avery et al., 2015).

There is evidence that many women have urinary incontinence prior to childbirth, and that this is a significant contributing factor to postpartum urinary incontinence (Frawley et al., 2017). In Australian research conducted by Stainton et al. (2005), 124 women were followed prospectively and the only variable to emerge as a statistically significant indicator for predicting those most at risk for developing postpartum urine leakage was a history of urine leakage prior to the first pregnancy. Women with an antenatal history of leakage were four times more at risk of leaking urine 1 year after giving birth than women without previous urine leakage (Stainton et al., 2005). More recent studies have reported the onset of urinary incontinence occurring during pregnancy for primiparous women, with statistics ranging between 18.6–75% (McKinnie et al., 2005; Sangsawang, 2014; Sangsawang & Sangsawang, 2013). Postpartum incontinence would appear to be more prevalent in those predisposed to it.

Incontinence rates of 20%–30% have been reported for women at 3 and 12 months postpartum (Thom & Rortveit, 2010), with reports that for those women who experience urinary incontinence at 3 months postpartum, 76.4% of women continued to experience urinary incontinence up to 12 years following the birth (MacArthur et al., 2016).

A Cochrane systematic review found that pregnant women without prior urinary incontinence who were randomised to intensive antenatal **pelvic floor muscle exercises** (PFME) were less likely to report urinary incontinence in late pregnancy and up to 6 months postpartum than women randomised to no PFME or usual antenatal care (Woodley et al., 2020). Postnatal women with persistent urinary incontinence 3 months after birth who received PFME were less likely to report urinary incontinence 12 months after birth than women who did not receive treatment or received usual postnatal care. The treatment effect seems greater with a more intensive program. Faecal incontinence was also reduced at 12 months after birth, with women receiving PFME being about half as likely to report faecal incontinence as those who did not (Woodley et al., 2020).

Faecal incontinence

Although **faecal incontinence** is less common than urinary incontinence, it is particularly distressing. Women may experience involuntary loss of solid stool, liquid stool or flatus. Prevalence is difficult to estimate, both because there is no standard definition and because sufferers are reluctant to admit to faecal incontinence. Estimates of the prevalence of incontinence of stool (faecal incontinence) in primiparous women range from 2% to 6% (Baydock et al., 2009; Woodley et al., 2020). When involuntary loss of flatus in addition to stool (anal incontinence) is taken into account, this rate can be from 13% to 27% (Johannessen et al., 2015; MacArthur et al., 2013). Estimates of faecal urgency (inability to hold on to stool for 15 minutes) are higher still. An Australian study of women at high risk of faecal incontinence and its precursors (instrumental birth, large baby >4000 g) showed that by 12 months 2.6% had solid stool incontinence, 4.9% had liquid stool incontinence, 24.4% had flatal incontinence, 10.9% had soiling and 14.8% had faecal urgency. Overall, 32.4% had at least one of these precursor symptoms (Chiarelli et al., 2003).

Pelvic floor muscle exercises

An ode to the perineum
The bigger the tear the more it hurts.
The bigger the baby the more she works.
But if she exercises a bit before,
And after the birth a whole lot more,
Then strong will be her pelvic floor.

(Dahlen, 2007b)

Box 28.8 PFME routine: 'the knack'

- Aim for 6–10 pelvic floor muscle exercises with a 6–10-second hold twice a day (each woman will be able to hold and repeat exercises at different rates—these need to be individually tailored):
  - Squeeze your back passage (anus) together as if you are stopping yourself from passing wind.
  - Squeeze your front passage (urethra) together as if you need to stop the flow of urine.
  - Lift both together and hold for a count of 6–10.
  - Repeat 6–10 times.
- Use reminder triggers (red stick-on dots): shower, teeth, meals, queues, etc.
- Develop 'The knack' functional bracing—grip up before coughing, sneezing, lifting or bending.
- Practise good bladder habits.

(Source: Miller et al., 1998)

Pelvic floor muscle exercises should commence during pregnancy and continue for the rest of a woman's life. As stated earlier in the chapter, when done antenatally they can also reduce the incidence of severe perineal trauma (Sobhgol et al., 2020). Some women are at particular risk, such as those with a previous history of incontinence, giving birth to a large baby, or having had an operative delivery. Research has shown that women who undertake regular pelvic floor exercises following a ventouse or a baby >4000 g have a reduced incidence of incontinence at 3 months postpartum (Chiarelli & Cockburn, 2002).

'The knack' is one of the most effective ways to encourage good pelvic floor health (Box 28.8).

It is important that women do not see incontinence as a normal event during and after pregnancy, regardless of their cultural or social background. The midwife should educate women about pelvic floor health and ask open questions about incontinence. It is important for the midwife to explain to women the anatomy and physiology of the pelvic floor, as many women do not understand the location and structures of this important area of their body. The use of diagrams or a model is advisable. The use of pelvic floor muscles during childbirth should be outlined, as well as their long-term function. Lack of discussion about this important issue has led to many women living with unnecessary discomfort and morbidity. Increasingly, midwives are being taught to undertake pelvic floor assessments (with vaginal examination) to make sure that women are performing the PFME correctly. All midwives should see this as a core responsibility.

Conclusion

As midwives providing woman-centred care, we must see perineal care and repair as one of the core components of our role and a serious professional responsibility. In doing this, we can help turn things around 'one birth at a time'. Childbirth and perineal trauma are linked, and the midwife plays an important role in providing advice and support that could help prevent perineal trauma, properly identify and repair the trauma in a timely and sensitive manner if it occurs, and provide women with the correct advice and support in the postnatal period.

In order to do this, the midwife needs an understanding of the best evidence available, a comprehensive understanding of the anatomy and physiology involved, and the development of clinical skills that make her competent at perineal repair. The prevention of long-term morbidity for women is possible only if this knowledge is gained and updated on a regular basis. Midwives who are skilled in perineal repair can provide full continuity of care to women and make sure the repair is done in a timely, sensitive manner.

Finally, practice does 'make perfect'. If you wait until you're an expert, you will never master this skill. Make sure that you have good support and believe you can do it; and remember, the more you practise the easier it gets and the more you begin to enjoy your new-found skills. Most importantly, you will experience the satisfaction of being able to provide woman-centred continuity of care for the women you care for.

Review questions

1. Explain why it is important for a midwife to have the skills to undertake perineal repair.
2. List evidence-based strategies for the prevention of perineal trauma and improvement of second-stage comfort.
3. List some of the risk factors for severe perineal trauma.
4. List the structures and explain the function of the pelvic floor.
5. Explain the importance of the perineal body and its relationship to the pelvic floor.
6. Provide a definition for each of the following: first-, second-, third- and fourth-degree perineal trauma.
7. What perineal traumas are outside the scope of practice of a midwife to repair?
8. List the main types of prolapse of pelvic organs.
9. Describe the elements of postnatal perineal care that make up HIPPS.
10. Describe how you would teach women pelvic floor exercises using 'the knack'.
11. Describe how midwives can demonstrate compassionate care when providing care for women who have experienced perineal trauma.

Online resources

Royal College of Obstetricians and Gynaecologists research services guidelines: https://www.rcog.org.uk/en/guidelines-research-services/guidelines/gtg29/.

References

Aasheim V, Nilsen ABV, Lukasse M, et al. Perineal techniques during the second stage of labour for reducing perineal trauma. *Cochrane Syst Rev*. 2017. doi:10.1002/14651858.CD006672.pub3.

AIHW. *Australian Mothers and Babies 2018*. Perinatal statistics series no. 35. Cat. no. PER 100. Canberra: AIHW; 2018.

Australian Commission on Safety and Quality in Health Care (ACSQHC) and Australian Institute of Health and Welfare (AIHW). *The Second Australian Atlas of Healthcare Variation*. Sydney: ACSQHC; 2017.

Australian Commission on Safety and Quality in Health Care (ACSQHC). *Third and Fourth Degree Perineal Tears Clinical Care Standard*. Sydney: ACSQHC; 2021. Online: https://www.safetyandquality.gov.au/sites/default/files/2021-04/perineal_tears_ccs_v3.pdf.

Australian Institute of Health and Welfare (AIHW). *Incontinence in Australia*. Canberra: AIHW; 2017.

Avery JC, Mayer AJB, Duggan PM, et al. 'It's our lot': how resilience influences the experience of depression in women with urinary incontinence. *Health Sociol Rev*. 2015;24(1):94–108. doi:10.1080/14461242.2015.1007512.

Baydock SA, Flood C, Schulz JA, et al. Prevalence and risk factors for urinary and fecal incontinence four months after vaginal delivery. *J Obstet Gynaecol Canada*. 2009;31(1):36–41. doi:10.1016/S1701-2163(16)34051-8.

Beck C. Pentadic cartography: mapping birth trauma narratives. *Qual Health Res*. 2006;16(4):453–466. doi:10.1177/1049732305285968.

Briscoe L, Lavender T, O'Brien, et al. A mixed methods study to explore women and clinician's response to pain associated with suturing second degree perineal tears and episiotomies [PRAISE]. *Midwifery*. 2015;31(4):464–472. doi:10.1016/j.midw.2014.12.010.

Brito LGO, Ferreira CHJ, Duarte G, et al. Antepartum use of Epi-No birth trainer for preventing perineal trauma: systematic review. *Int Urogynaecol J*. 2015;26(10):1429–1436.

Burnell L. Compassionate care: a concept analysis. *Home Health Care Manage Pract*. 2009;21(5):319–324.

Carter E, Duriez T. *With Child: Birth Through the Ages*. Mainstream Publishing Company; 1986.

Chang SR, Lin WA, Lin HH, et al. Sexual dysfunction predicts depressive symptoms during the first 2 years postpartum. *Women Birth*. 2018;31(6):e403–e411. doi:10.1016/j.wombi.2018.01.003.
Chiarelli P, Cockburn J. The development of a physiotherapy continence promotion program using a customer focus. *Aust J Physiother*. 1999;45(2):111–119.
Chiarelli P, Cockburn J. Promoting urinary continence in women after delivery: randomised controlled trial. *Br Med J*. 2002;324:1241–1247.
Chiarelli P, Murphy B, Cockburn J. Fecal incontinence after high risk delivery. *Am Coll Obstet Gynecol*. 2003;102(6):1299–1305.
Coates D, Donnolley N, Henry A. The attitudes and beliefs of australian midwives and obstetricians about birth options and labor interventions. *J Midwifery Womens Health*. 2021; 66(2):161–173. doi:10.1111/jmwh.13168.
Cronin R. *New Zealand Midwives' Management of Perineal Trauma during Childbirth: A Survey of Practice (Unpublished Master's thesis)*. University of Wellington; 2014.
Dahlen H. Perineal Repairs by Midwives in the Delivery Ward and Birth Centre of Royal Prince Alfred and Canterbury Hospital: An audit. *Unpublished*.
Dahlen H. *Literature Review of Factors that Influence Perineal Trauma and Maternal Comfort During the Second Stage of Labour. Reduction of Perineal Trauma and Improved Perineal Comfort during and After Childbirth: The Perineal Warm Pack Trial (Unpublished PhD thesis)*. Sydney: University of Technology: 2007a.
Dahlen H. Postnatal Perineal Care: The Poor Cousin's Poor Cousin. Presentation at a perineal seminar, Sydney.
Dahlen H. *Reduction of Perineal Trauma and Improved Perineal Comfort During and After Childbirth: The Perineal Warm Pack Trial (Unpublished PhD Thesis)*. Sydney: University of Technology; 2007c.
Dahlen H, Homer C. Perineal trauma and postpartum perineal morbidity in Asian and non-Asian primiparous women. *J Obstet Gynecol Neonatal Nurs*. 2008a;37:455–463.
Dahlen H, Priddis H, Schmied V, et al. Trends and risk factors for severe perineal trauma during childbirth in New South Wales between 2000 and 2008: a population-based data study. *BMJ Open*. 2013;3(5):e002824. doi:10.1136/bmjopen-2013-002824.
Dahlen H, Ryan M. Challenging birth rituals: To swab and drape or not? *Birth Issues*. 2001;10(2):50–52.
Dahlen HG, Dowling H, Tracy M, et al. Maternal and perinatal outcomes amongst low risk women giving birth in water compared to six birth positions on land. A descriptive cross sectional study in a birth centre over 12 years. *Midwifery*. 2013;29(7):759–764. doi:10.1016/j.midw.2012.07.002.
Dahlen HG, Homer C. What are the views of Australian midwives in relation to perineal repair? *Women and Birth*. 2008b;21(1): 27–35.
Dahlen HG, Homer CSE, Leap N, et al. From social to surgical: historical perspectives on perineal care during labour and birth. *Women Birth*. 2011;24(3):105–111. doi:10.1016/j.wombi.2010.09.002.
Dahlen HG, Priddis H, Thornton C. Severe perineal trauma is rising, but let us not overreact. *Midwifery*. 2015;31:1–8.
Darmody E, Bradshaw C, Atkinson S. Women's experience of obstetric anal sphincter injury following childbirth: an integrated review. *Midwifery*. 2020;91:1–9. doi:10.1016/j.midw.2020.102820.
De Wees WB. Relaxation and management of the perineum during parturition. *JAMA*. 1889;13:804–808.
East C, Lau R, Biro MA. Midwives' and doctors' perceptions of their preparation for and practice in managing the perineum in the second stage of labour: a cross-sectional survey. *Midwifery* (in press). Online: http://www.sciencedirect.com.ezproxy.uws.edu.au/science/article/pii/S026661381400179X.
East CE, Sherburn M, Nagle C, et al. Perineal pain following childbirth: prevalence, effects on postnatal recovery and analgesia usage. *Midwifery*. 2021;28(1):93–97. doi:10.1016/j.midw.2010.11.009.
Fleming VEM, Hagen S, Niven C. Does perineal suturing make a difference? The SUNS trial. *BJOG*. 2003;110(7):684–689. Online: http://www.blackwell-synergy.com/doi/abs/10.1046/j.1471-0528.2003.02353.x.
Fodstad K, Staff AC, Laine K. Sexual activity and dyspareunia the first year postpartum in relation to degree of perineal trauma. *Int Urogynecol J*. 2016;27(10):1513–1523.
Frawley J, Sibbritt D, Steel A, et al. Complementary and conventional health-care utilization among young Australian women with urinary incontinence. *Urology*. 2017;99:92–99. doi:10.1016/j.urology.2016.07.060.
Frolich J, Kettle C. Perineal Care. *BMJ Clinical Evidence*. 2015;10.
Gelbart NR. *The King's Midwife: A history and mystery of Madame du Coudray*. London: University of California Press; 1998.
Gibbins J, Thomson AM. Women's expectations and experiences of childbirth. *Midwifery*. 2001;17:302–313.
Gordon B, Mackrodt C, Fern E, et al. The Ipswich Childbirth Study: 1. A randomised evaluation of two stage postpartum perineal repair leaving the skin unsutured. *BJOG*. 1998;105(4):435–440. doi:10.1111/j.1471-0528.1998.tb10130.x.
Goutaudier N, Séjourné N, Rousset C, et al. Negative emotions, childbirth pain, perinatal dissociation and self-efficacy as predictors of postpartum posttraumatic stress symptoms. *J Reprod Infant Psychol*. 2012;30(4):352–362. doi:10.1080/02646838.2012.738415.
Graham H. *Eternal Eve*. London: William Heinemann Medical; 1950.
Green MH, ed. *The Trotula*. Philadelphia: University of Pennsylvania Press; 2002.
Halldorsdottir S, Karlsdottir SI. Journeying through labour and delivery: perceptions of women who have given birth. *Midwifery*. 1996;12: 48–61.
Hay-Smith EJ. Therapeutic ultrasound for postpartum perineal pain and dyspareunia. *Cochrane Database Syst Rev*. 2000;(2): CD000495.
International Confederation of Midwives (ICM). *International Definition of a Midwife: Revised and adopted at Toronto Council Meeting*. International Confederation of Midwives. Online: http://www.internationalmidwives.org/index.php?module5ContentExpress&func5display&ceid59&bid522&btitle5ICM%20Documents&meid511.
Jango H, Langhoff-Roos J, Rosthoj S, et al. Mode of delivery after obstetric anal sphincter injury and the risk of long-term anal incontinence. *Am J Obstet Gynaecol*. 2016;214(6):733.e1–e13.
Johannessen HH, Wibe A, Stordahl A, Sandvik L, Mørkved S. Anal incontinence among first time mothers – What happens in pregnancy and the first year after delivery? *Acta Obstet Gynecol Scand*. 2015;94(9):1005–1013. doi:10.1111/aogs.12689.
Kenyon S, Ford F. How can we improve women's postbirth perineal health? *MIDIRS Midwifery Dig*. 2004;14(1):7–12.
Kettle C. Continuous versus interrupted perineal repair with standard or rapidly absorbed sutures after spontaneous vaginal birth: a randomised controlled trial. *Lancet*. 2002;359: 2217–2223.
Kettle C. Anatomy of the pelvic floor. In C. Henderson & D. Bick (Eds.), *Perineal Care: An international issue*. Quay Books.
Kettle, C. (2005b). The management of perineal trauma. In Henderson C, Bick D, eds. *Perineal Care: An International Issue*. Quay Books MA Healthcare; 32–57.
Kettle C, Dowswell T, Ismail KMK. Continuous and interrupted suturing techniques for repair of episiotomy or second-degree tears. *Cochrane Database Syst Rev*. 2012;(11):CD000947. doi:10.1002/14651858.
King ML, Rabil A. The other voice in early modern Europe: introduction to the series. In: Tatlock L, eds. *The Court Midwife*. Chicago: University of Chicago Press; 2005:xi–xxxi.

Kolas T, Hofoss D, Daltveit AK. Indications for caesarean deliveries in Norway. *Am J Obstet Gynecol.* 2003;188:864–870.
Labrecque M, Eason E, Marcoux S, et al. Randomized controlled trial of prevention of perineal trauma by perineal massage during pregnancy. *Am J Obstet Gynecol.* 1999;180(3 Pt 1):593–600.
Linneberg S, Leenskjold S, Glavind K. A five year follow-up of women with obstetric anal sphincter rupture at their first delivery. *Eur J Obstet Gynecol Reprod Biol.* 2016;205:315–319. doi:10.1016/j.ejogrb.2016.06.018.
Luciano L, Bouvier M, Baumstarck K, Vitton V. Is the extent of obstetric anal sphincter injury correlated with the severity of fecal incontinence in the long term? *Tech Coloproctol.* 2020;24(1):49–55. doi:10.1007/s10151-019-02128-1.
Lundquist M, Olsson A, Nissen E, Norman M. Is it necessary to suture all lacerations after a vaginal delivery? *Birth.* 2000;*27*(2):79–85. doi:10.1046/j.1523-536x.2000.00079.x.
Macarthur AJ, Macarthur C. Incidence, severity, and determinants of perineal pain after vaginal delivery: a prospective cohort study. *Am J Obstet Gynecol.* 2004;*191*:119–204.
MacArthur C, Wilson D, Herbison P, et al. Faecal incontinence persisting after childbirth: a 12 year longitudinal study. *BJOG.* 2013;*120*(2):169–179. doi:10.1111/1471-0528.12039.
MacArthur C, Wilson D, Herbison P, et al. Urinary incontinence persisting after childbirth: extent, delivery history, and effects in a 12-year longitudinal cohort study. *BJOG.* 2016;123(6): 1022–1029. doi:10.1111/1471-0528.13395.
Mackenzie D. The history of sutures. *Med Hist.* 1973;17:158–168.
Mackrodt C, Gordon B, Fern E, et al. The Ipswich Childbirth Study: 2. A randomised comparison of polyglactin 910 with chromic catgut for postpartum perineal repair. *BJOG.* 1998;105(4): 441–445. doi:10.1111/j.1471-0528.1998.tb10131.x.
Magoga G, Saccone G, Al-Kouatly HB, et al. Warm perineal compresses during the second stage of labor for reducing perineal trauma: a meta-analysis. *Eur J Obstet Gynecol Reprod Biol.* 2019;93–98. doi:10.1016/j.ejogrb.2019.06.011.
McKinnie V, Swift SE, Wang W, et al. The effect of pregnancy and mode of delivery on the prevalence of urinary and fecal incontinence. *Am J Obstet Gynecol.* 2005;193(2):512–517. doi:10.1016/j.ajog.2005.03.056.
Menage D, Bailey E, Lees S, et al. A concept analysis of compassionate midwifery. *J Adv Nurs.* 2016;73(3):558–573. doi:10.1111/jan.13214.
Miller JMA, Miller JA, DeLancey JO. A pelvic muscle precontraction can reduce cough related urine loss in selected women with mild SUI. *J Am Geriatrics Soc.* 1998;46(7):870–874.
Ministry of Health New Zealand Government. *New Zealand Maternity Clinical Indicators 2018.* New Zealand: Ministry of Health New Zealand Government; 2018.
Ministry of Health New Zealand Government. *Report on Maternity Web Tool.* New Zealand Ministry of Health New Zealand Government; 2020b.
National Institute for Health and Care Excellence (NICE). *Postnatal Care up to 8 Weeks After Birth.* 2015. Online: https://www.nice.org.uk/guidance/cg37.
National Institute for Health and Care Excellence (NICE). *Postnatal Care.* Online: www.nice.org.uk/guidance/ng194.
New Zealand College of Midwives. *Midwives' Handbook for Practice* (5th ed.). New Zealand College of Midwives; 2015.
Nisbet M, Rouse B. *Perineal Repair.* Melbourne: Davis and Geck. Cynamid Australia Pty; 1992.
O'Dowd MJ, Philipp E. *The History of Obstetrics and Gynecology.* The Parthenon Publishing Group Inc; 2000.
Priddis H, Schmied V, Dahlen H. Women's experiences following severe perineal trauma: a qualitative study. *BMC Women's Health.* 2014;14(32):1–11.
Priddis H, Schmied V, Kettle C, et al. "A patchwork of services" – caring for women who sustain severe perineal trauma in New South Wales – from the perspective of women and midwives. *BMC Pregnancy Childbirth.* 2014;14(236):1–14. doi:10.1186/1471-2393-14-236.
Reitsma A, Simioni J, Brunton G, et al. Maternal outcomes and birth interventions among women who begin labour intending to give birth at home compared to women of low obstetrical risk who intend to give birth in hospital: a systematic review and meta-analyses. *EClinicalMedicine.* 2020;21:100319. doi:10.1016/j.eclinm.2020.100319.
Ritgen G. Ueber sein Dammschutzverfahren. Monatschrift fur Geburtskunde u. *Frauenkrankh.* 1885;6:321–347.
Roach MS. *Caring: The human mode of being.* CHA Presses de l'ACS; 2007.
Royal College of Obstetricians and Gynaecologists (RCOG). *The Management of Third- and Fourth-degree Perineal Tears.* Green-Top Guideline no. 29. London: RCOG; 2015:11.
Salmon D. A feminist analysis of women's experiences of perineal trauma in the immediate post-delivery period. *Midwifery.* 1999;15(4):247–256.
Sanders J, Peters T, Campbell R. Techniques to reduce perineal pain during spontaneous vaginal delivery and perineal suturing: a UK survey of midwifery practice. *Midwifery.* 2005;21(2):154–160.
Sangsawang B. Risk factors for the development of stress urinary incontinence during pregnancy in primigravidae: a review of the literature. *Eur J Obstet Gynecol Reprod Biol.* 2014;178:27–34. doi:10.1016/j.ejogrb.2014.04.010.
Sangsawang B, Sangsawang N. Stress urinary incontinence in pregnant women: a review of prevalence, pathophysiology, and treatment. *Int Urogynecol J.* 2013;24(6):901–912. doi:10.1007/s00192-013-2061-7.
Scarf VL, Rossiter C, Vedam S, et al. Maternal and perinatal outcomes by planned place of birth among women with low-risk pregnancies in high-income countries: a systematic review and meta-analysis. *Midwifery.* 2018;62:240–255.
Siegemund, J. *The Court Midwife.* The University of Chicago Press; 2005.
Signorello L, Harlow B, Chekos A, et al. Postpartum sexual functioning and its relationship to perineal trauma: a retrospective cohort study of primiparous women. *Am J Obstet Gynecol.* 2001;184(5):881–890.
Sobhgol SS, Smith CA, Dahlen HG. The effect of antenatal pelvic floor muscle exercises on labour and birth outcomes: a systematic review and meta-analysis (Review). *Int Urogynecol J.* 2020;31(11):2189–2203. doi:10.1007/s00192-020-04298-1.
Stainton MC, Strahle A, Fethney J. Leaking urine prior to pregnancy: a risk factor for postnatal incontinence. *Aust N Z J Obstet Gynaecol.* 2005;45(4):295–299.
Steen M, Marchant P. Aleviating perineal trauma: the APT Study. *RCM Midwives Journal.* 2001;4(8):256–259.
Steen M, Marchant P. Ice packs and cooling gel pads versus no localised treatment for relief of perineal pain: a randomised controlled trial. *Evidence Based Midwifery.* 2007;5(1):16–22.
Tavernier SS. An evidence-based conceptual analysis of presence. *Holist Nurs Pract.* 2006;20(3):152–156.
Temkin OT. *Soranus, Gynaecology.* The Johns Hopkins University Press; 1956.
Thacker SB, Banta HD. Benefits and risks of episiotomy: an interpretative review of the English language literature, 1860–1980. *J Obstet Gynecol Br Commonw.* 1983;64(6):322–338.
Thom DH, Rortveit G. Prevalence of postpartum urinary incontinence: a systematic review. *Acta Obstet Gynecol Scand.* 2010;89(12):1511–1522. doi:10.3109/00016349.2010.526188.
Thornton JG, Dahlen HG. The UK Obstetric Anal Sphincter Injury (OASI) care bundle: a critical review (Review). *Midwifery.* 2020;90:102801. doi:10.1016/j.midw.2020.102801.
Trotula. *Diseases of Women.* London: Ward-Ritchie Press; 1940.

Tschudin S, Alder J, Hendriksen S, et al. Previous birth experience and birth anxiety: predictors of caesarean section on demand? *J Psychosom Obstet Gynaecol.* 2009;30(3):175–180. doi:10.1080/01674820902789233.

Wagner M. Fish can't see water: the need to humanise birth in Australia. 2000. Online: https://birthinternational.com/article/birth/fish-cant-see-water/.

Way S. A qualitative study exploring women's personal experiences of their perineum after childbirth: expectations, reality and returning to normality. *Midwifery* (in press). 2011. doi:10.1016/j.midw.2011.08.011.

Willmott J. Too many episiotomies. *Midwives Chron.* 1980;93: 46–48.

Woodley SJ, Lawrenson P, Boyle R, et al. Pelvic floor muscle training for preventing and treating urinary and faecal incontinence in antenatal and postnatal women. *Cochrane Database Syst Rev.* 2020;(5). doi:10.1002/14651858.CD007471.pub4.

Wright A, Nassar AH, Visser G, et al. FIGO good clinical practice paper: management of the second stage of labor. *Int J Gynecol Obstet.* 2021;152(2):172–181. doi:10.1002/ijgo.13552.

Further reading

Henderson C, Bick D, eds. Perineal Care: An International Issue. Wiltshire, UK: Quay Books; 2005.

De-Vitry Smith S-A & Bayes S. *Skills for Midwifery Practice ANZ Edition*, 2nd ed. Sydney, Australia: Elsevier; 2022.

CHAPTER 29

Overview of physiological changes during the postnatal period

Sally Baddock

LEARNING OUTCOMES

Learning outcomes for this chapter are:

1. To describe the change in maternal hormone levels following the birth of the baby
2. To describe the processes of involution and of healing at the placental site
3. To provide a physiological rationale for blood and fluid loss during the puerperium
4. To describe the changes which occur in the cervix, vagina and vulva in the puerperium
5. To compare physiological changes in the maternal body systems during pregnancy and during the postnatal period, particularly the renal, haematological and cardiovascular changes
6. To outline the hormonal control of lactation during pregnancy and the puerperium.

CHAPTER OVERVIEW

This chapter focuses on the physiological processes associated with the postnatal period or puerperium. The puerperium refers to the 6–8 weeks following birth when the reproductive organs return towards a non-pregnant state, and lactation begins. Many of the physiological, anatomical and endocrine changes in this period occur in the first 10–14 days as hormone levels adjust following birth of the placenta. While the reproductive organs heal and regain a shape and structure similar to before pregnancy, other systems of the body that had changed to support pregnancy now also return to their former function. These processes are the focus of this chapter. An understanding of the physiology underpinning these changes should help a midwife assess the wellbeing of the woman and baby. Further readings are provided at the end of the chapter for a more in-depth exploration of specific topics.

KEY TERMS

cellular barrier
decidua
endometrium
exfoliation
haemostasis
hypercoagulability
involution
lactogenesis
myometrium
regeneration

INTRODUCTION

The postnatal period is also known as the *puerperium*. This is the time following the birth, when the woman's body adapts to a non-pregnant state. This involves recovery from the physical effects of pregnancy, labour and birth, and a longer-term physiological adjustment as the changes that maintained and supported pregnancy and labour are no longer required. It is also the phase when infant-feeding practices and mother–child relationships are established. The physiology underpinning these changes is presented in this section. Body systems are described separately, but it should be remembered that systems do not work in isolation but rather are integrated in a complex manner.

HORMONAL CHANGES

The placental hormones human placental lactogen (hPL), human chorionic gonadotrophin (hCG), the oestrogens (estrogens) and progesterone control maternal physiology in pregnancy to provide an optimal environment for fetal development. The return of the body systems to a non-pregnant state is largely governed by the removal of the placental hormones. Following birth of the placenta, metabolism of circulating hormones and hormone stores results in a rapid drop in placental hormone levels. These changes are illustrated in Fig. 29.1. Human placental lactogen is absent from the plasma within 1–2 days and human chorionic gonadotrophin by 3–4 weeks. Oestrogens and progesterone levels drop quickly with the removal of the placenta and reach basal levels by 7 days (Blackburn, 2017). Ovarian production rises slowly over the first 2 weeks. During pregnancy, progesterone inhibits the direct effect of prolactin on the breast and inhibits lactogenesis. However, after birth with the decrease in progesterone and increase in prolactin, lactogenesis II can occur (Blackburn, 2017). Nipple stimulation maintains prolactin levels but, even in breastfeeding women, prolactin surges are reduced after 6 weeks (Blackburn, 2017). In non-breastfeeding women, prolactin levels drop significantly after birth, but are maintained above normal for 3–4 weeks even in the absence of suckling (Johnson, 2013).

INVOLUTION OF THE UTERUS

The uterus is well contracted at the end of the third stage and rises over the following hours to the level of the umbilicus. The uterus reduces in size over the next few days and weeks through a process termed ***involution*** (Fig. 29.2). This is facilitated by the release of oxytocin from the posterior pituitary, which continues after the birth of the placenta and membranes. It stimulates strong intermittent contractions of the uterus, leading to collapse of the uterine cavity, which no longer contains the fetus, and thus to realignment of the uterine walls in apposition to each

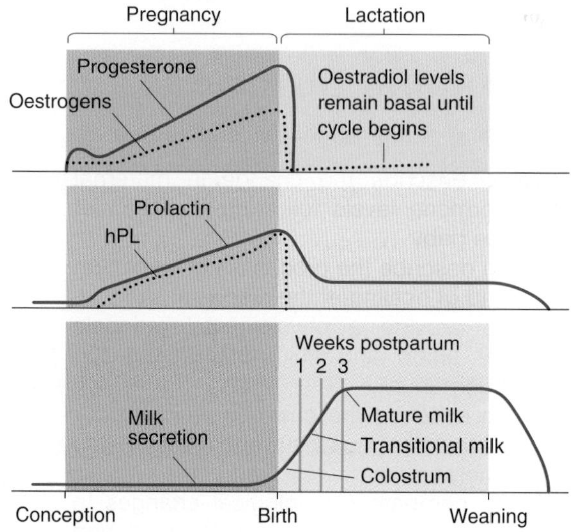

FIGURE 29.1 Sequence of hormone changes in the maternal circulation that underlie the onset of lactation in women
(Adapted from Johnson & Everitt, 2000)

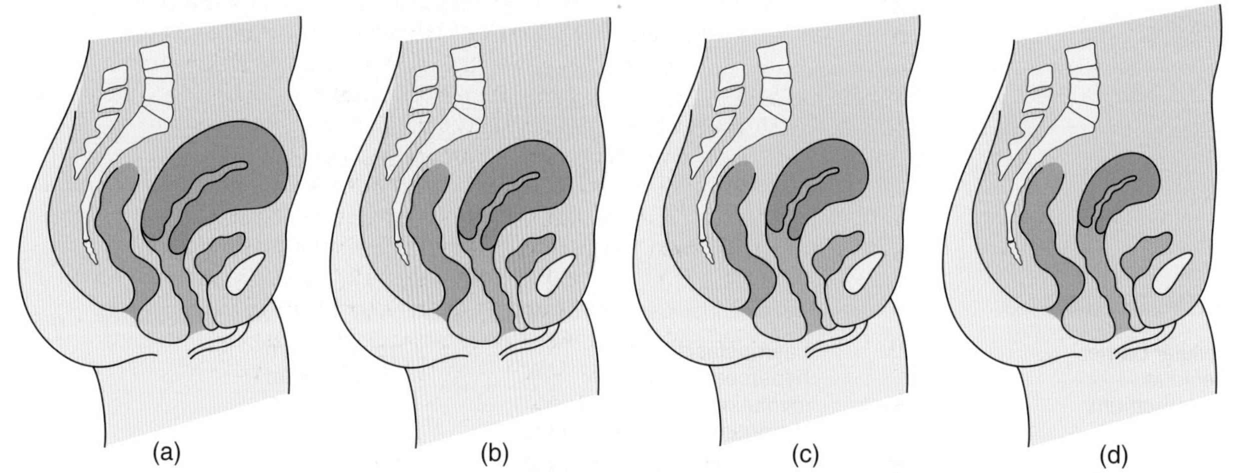

FIGURE 29.2 Involution of the uterus
(From Stables & Rankin, 2005)

other (Blackburn, 2017). This aids the process of **haemostasis** (stoppage of bleeding) and also reduces the size of the uterus immediately following birth.

The uterus is reported to be retroverted and empty in the early puerperium, to contain fluid and debris in the cavity in the middle part of the puerperium, and to be empty and anteverted in the late puerperium (Belachew et al., 2012). After birth the length of the uterus is 20 cm and felt at the level of umbilicus. Involution, as shown by 3D ultrasound study, is rapid in the first 2 weeks (Wataganara et al., 2015). After 1 week it is midway between the umbilicus and symphysis pubis. After 2 weeks it is at the level of the symphysis. By the end of the 6th week it is 7.5 cm long, with no significant difference to the prepregnant length, regardless of gestational number (Hawkins et al., 2014). The height of the fundus usually decreases by about 1 cm/day, and by 10 days the fundus cannot be palpated abdominally as the uterus has descended into the pelvis (Blackburn, 2017). The uterus decreases from 1 kg to about 350 g in the first 2 weeks following birth and then decreases more slowly over the next 6 weeks to approximately 60–80 g (Belachew et al., 2012; Blackburn, 2017). This process involves a reduction in the thickness of the **myometrium**, a shedding of the **decidua** and regeneration of the **endometrium**. Although the exact mechanisms involved are unclear, the rapid withdrawal of the placental hormones appears to facilitate the changes. Retained placental fragments or pelvic infection can slow involution (Blackburn, 2017).

Breastfeeding and parity have been demonstrated not to affect involution and this process occurs independently of thinning of the endometrium (Wataganara et al., 2015).

Changes to the myometrium

Withdrawal of oestrogen reduces protein synthesis in the muscle fibres. Blood flow is reduced to the myometrium as the uterus contracts and compresses the uterine blood vessels. The resulting ischaemia aids in destruction of myometrial cells. Proteolytic enzymes digest superfluous actin and myosin protein in the muscle cells by a process termed autolysis. The *size* of the muscle cells is reduced, without a significant decrease in the *number* of cells (Blackburn, 2017). The products of autolysis, as well as excess fibrous and elastic tissue, are engulfed by macrophages—a process called phagocytosis. A proportion of fibrous and elastic tissue remains within the uterus and increasing amounts may remain following further pregnancies; thus the uterus never returns fully to the prepregnant state (Rankin, 2017).

Shedding of the decidua

The upper portion of the spongy endometrium is sloughed off with the birth of the placenta and is shed as part of the postpartum vaginal blood loss (see later section) in the first few days of the puerperium. This assists the uterus to reduce in size and undergo involution. The placental site is left as a large wound.

Regeneration of the endometrium

In the first 2–3 days following the birth, the epithelial lining differentiates into two layers: a superficial layer and a basal layer. A **cellular barrier** to infection is formed by the superficial layer of granulation tissue and by the invasion of leucocytes (macrophages and lymphocytes) that enter the area to clean up the debris and microbes. This layer breaks down through necrosis, and is shed as postpartum vaginal blood loss over the next 4–6 weeks. **Regeneration** of the decidual layer surrounding the placental site takes 2–3 weeks, and by 16 days this layer is similar to the non-pregnant endometrium in the proliferative phase of the menstrual cycle (Blackburn, 2017). The placental site heals gradually over 6–7 weeks (Blackburn, 2017). Large blood vessels that supplied the intervillous spaces are blocked by invading fibroblasts. Healing occurs by **exfoliation** without the formation of scar tissue. Endometrial tissue heals inwards from the edges of the placental site and upwards from the endometrial glands.

Afterpains

Contraction of the uterine muscles is felt as 'afterpains' for 4–7 days and is strongest 12–24 hours postpartum, especially in multiparous women. These contractions facilitate the process of involution. Afterpains may occur in association with breastfeeding, owing to the release of oxytocin and uterine contractions, or they may occur independently of breastfeeding. For some women these contractions are very intense and may be similar to the severity of labour pains (Marchant et al., 2000). These women may require analgesics. There is little research on the subject, but one study showed that high-frequency transcutaneous electric nerve stimulation (TENS) was successful in reducing pain and discomfort of postpartum uterine contractions (Olsen et al., 2007). A Cochrane review of 28 studies from middle- and high-income countries, with a primary outcome of *adequate pain relief due to uterine cramping after birth as reported by women*, found moderate to low certainty of evidence that NSAIDs, paracetamol and opioids were likely better than placebo at reducing pain. Almost half the studies excluded breastfeeding women, and thus results are not generalisable to breastfeeding women. Due to the very low certainty of evidence (based on one small study), it was not possible to conclude if TENS was better than no TENS at providing pain relief or whether other forms of pain relief provided benefit (Deussen et al., 2020).

POSTPARTUM VAGINAL BLOOD LOSS (LOCHIA)

Postpartum vaginal blood loss (formerly referred to as lochia) (Marchant et al., 1999) refers to the discharge from the vagina in the weeks following birth. A prospective survey of 524 women in the United Kingdom who self-reported blood discharge identified considerable variation (Marchant et al., 1999). In this study, the median loss was 21 days while a quarter of the women reported vaginal loss after 28 days and up to 6 weeks after the birth, and 6% of women reported vaginal loss from 6 weeks and up to 12 weeks postpartum. A systematic review of 18 studies reported average blood loss as lasting from 24 to 36 days, although blood loss beyond 6 weeks was not unusual. The review highlighted the variability in how blood loss was measured and thus the difficulty in defining usual blood loss volume (Fletcher et al., 2012).

Fluid loss changes in appearance over time. Whereas Marchant et al. (1999) reported that women most consistently identified the fluid loss as red/brown in colour, three phases of fluid loss have been described by others (Fletcher et al., 2012). Postpartum vaginal fluid loss is described as initially red or dark brown with a fleshy smell and is discharged for the first few days, up to a week. This fluid contains mainly blood and pieces of chorionic villi from the placental site, shreds of amnion and chorion, leucocytes, epithelial cells, vernix, lanugo and meconium. During the second and third weeks the discharge tends to change to a pinkish-brown colour, and contains blood, mucus, erythrocytes, leucocytes, microorganisms and superficial decidual cells. Following this, a whitish-yellow discharge continues until 3–6 weeks postpartum. It is similar in composition to the pinkish fluid loss but does not contain erythrocytes (Blackburn, 2017). Self-reporting by women suggests that the differentiation into these phases may not be this clear (Marchant et al., 1999). Findings by Sherman et al. (1999) also supported greater variation in patterns of postnatal blood loss and longer duration than classically reported (median 36 days +/− 7.5 days). Data from the diaries of 39 women who matched the colour of their lochia to colour-graded slides supported the sequence of rubra to serosa to alba with a longer rubra phase associated with higher parity and not breastfeeding but no association with gestational age at birth or baby weight at birth. Further discussion of postnatal vaginal blood loss can be found in Chapter 31.

This fluid, which is lost postpartum, is sterile until it reaches the vagina. However, it is an excellent medium for the growth of bacteria. Puerperal infection may result from the invasion of endogenous organisms (those that are normally present in the woman's body), or from exogenous organisms introduced to the woman's body from elsewhere (e.g. from another person). The woman is particularly vulnerable to infections during the puerperium owing to the open wound at the placental site, the tissue trauma associated with labour and the excellent culture medium provided by the decidua and blood lost postpartum via the vagina (Rankin, 2017).

CRITICAL THINKING EXERCISE

In a UK study, Marchant et al. (1999) collected data from 524 women, using structured diaries, concerning postnatal vaginal loss on days 2–10, 14, 21 and 28 and again at 3 months. Forty-nine of the 161 primiparous women reported being either surprised or shocked at the amount of blood loss they experienced. Twenty-two per cent of the women reported that they had been worried about their vaginal blood loss during the period 28 days to 3 months (Marchant et al., 2000).

1. What are the underlying reasons for the blood loss?
2. What information could you share with women to give them realistic expectations?
3. What is normal blood loss during the puerperium?

CRITICAL THINKING EXERCISE

Cochrane reviews report evidence quality as part of their findings; for example, there is low to moderate quality of evidence for NSAIDs, paracetamol and / or opioids being more effective than placebo for providing pain relief due to postpartum uterine contractions (Deussen et al., 2020).

1. Identify factors that might contribute to the label of low quality of evidence.
2. Consider whether these factors could be improved in the studies previously cited to provide higher quality evidence. What ethical or practical considerations might provide challenges?

REFLECTIVE THINKING EXERCISE

Think about how you would explain to a woman why blood and fluid loss often occurs for up to 6 weeks after birth, and sometimes longer. How could she differentiate between normal and abnormal loss?

SOFT TISSUE HEALING

The soft tissues of the cervix and vagina undergo healing during the puerperium.

Cervix

Immediately after vaginal birth, the cervix appears stretched, swollen and bruised, and may have lacerations. The cervix loses its bruised, swollen appearance within 48 hours and becomes shorter and firmer as collagen and proteoglycans form (Blackburn, 2017). Magnetic resonance imaging (MRI) of eight women after uncomplicated vaginal births indicated the mean length of the cervix was 5.6 cm within 30 hours of birth and 2.9 cm at 6 months (Willms et al., 1995). A further study, using optical evaluation of the cervix obtained from digital photos taken with an endoscopic camera of 275 women, showed that the surface area of the ectocervix increased during pregnancy to 75% more than prepregnancy size and then returned to the prepregnant ectocervix area during the postpartum period (40–60 days after birth) (Qian et al.,

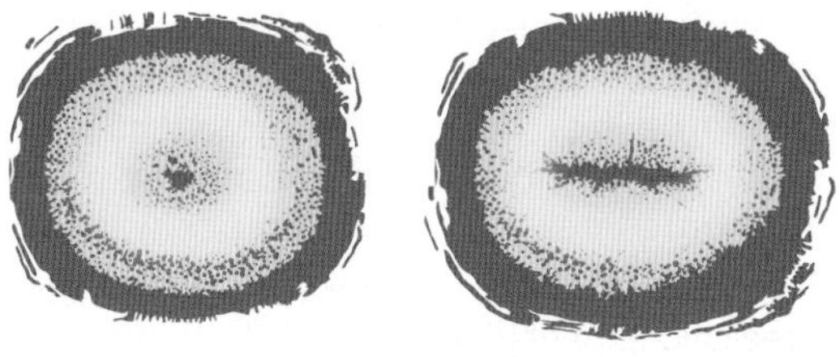

FIGURE 29.3 Re-formation of the external os: (a) nulliparous cervix; (b) parous cervix
(From Coad & Dunstall, 2005)

2016). The cervix also returns to a more rigid state. By day 2 or 3 the cervical os, while constricted, is still partially dilated by 3–4 cm and this reduces to approximately 1 cm dilation by 1 week, then becoming a small slit by 4 weeks (Blackburn, 2017). However, the cervix never returns fully to its prepregnant state, as illustrated in Fig. 29.3.

Vagina and vulva

The elevated progesterone levels during pregnancy cause increased vascularity of the vagina and vulva. These structures and the perineum are susceptible to bruising and oedema during labour. Immediately postpartum, the vaginal wall is stretched, bluish and swollen but regains its tonicity rapidly. Rugae reappear by 3–4 weeks. The vaginal mucosa is fragile for the first few weeks, but generally heals by 6–10 weeks (Blackburn, 2017). Submucosal venous congestion can take the entire puerperium to clear up. Small lacerations heal quickly but larger ones may need sutures to prevent haemorrhage and to aid healing.

Following birth the perineal tissues are stretched and may have lacerations. If the perineum is torn or cut (episiotomy), sutures may be inserted (see Ch. 28). Lacerations can make micturition extremely uncomfortable for 24–48 hours. During the first week, marked healing usually occurs in the perineal area (Rankin, 2017). Sexual intercourse can be painful or challenging for some time after birth because of healing from trauma. A questionnaire delivered to 2490 women in a population-based cohort in Sweden reported women who had tears in the vagina or in the perineum were approximately 1.5 times more likely not to have sexual intercourse by 6 months postpartum compared with women without such trauma. Women with tears in the external anal sphincter and rectum were over twice as likely not to have sexual intercourse by 6 months postpartum but by 1-year follow-up there was no statistically significant difference between groups (Radestad et al., 2008).

Although considerable healing of the perineum occurs during the puerperium, this may present a simplified picture. Findings from a prospective cohort of 229 Australian women having a vaginal birth identified that 74% experienced perineal pain at week 1. Subsequently, the pain resolved for many women, but 16% reported pain that was intermittent up to 8 weeks and 5% reported persistent perineal pain during weeks 1–8 (Cooklin et al., 2015). For many women this process can extend over a far greater time span—as reported in a study in the United Kingdom of 482 women where 87% at 12 months postpartum identified at least one index of perineal morbidity, such as stress and urge incontinence, flatus incontinence, sexual morbidity and dyspareunia (Williams et al., 2007). This topic is explored in more detail in Chapter 28.

Changes in the puerperium are not limited to the reproductive structures. During this time major changes also occur to other body systems. Key changes to the renal, cardiovascular, respiratory and gastrointestinal systems are described in the next section. (Readers are referred to the Further reading list at the end of the chapter for more in-depth explanations.)

CRITICAL THINKING EXERCISE

Considerable healing needs to take place following birth, for example around the placental site and any damage to the perineum and external genitalia. Identify some lifestyle choices that a midwife could discuss with a woman following birth that might facilitate this healing.

CRITICAL THINKING EXERCISE

A survey of 1800 pregnant women in Australia suggested 50% consulted a complementary and alternative medicine (CAM) practitioner during their pregnancy (Steel et al., 2012); this is supported by other studies suggesting 20%–60% engagement by women in CAM during pregnancy or childbirth (Holden et al., 2015; Johnson et al., 2016). Only 50% of these women disclose their use to conventional providers despite limited evidence on safety and effectiveness (Holden et al., 2015). An example is placentophagy or placentophagia—the postpartum ingestion of the placenta, which is supported by anecdotal reports; however, Farr et al. (2018) report no clinical benefits but do identify potential risk of infection from poorly prepared encapsulated supplements. There is also considerable anecdotal evidence as to the efficacy of CAM—for example, anecdotal and survey reports suggest the use of seaweed, arnica, St John's wort and herbal therapies to promote healing of the perineum (Bayles, 2007; Gilpin-Blake & Elliot, 2001; Holst et al., 2011).

What questions would you consider when trying to identify if these therapies were suitable to use in your practice? How would you find the answers?

RENAL SYSTEM

Following the birth and with the loss of progesterone, the renal system is able to revert to non-pregnant anatomy and physiology. The dilation of the renal tract is resolved and peristaltic action returns to normal. The bladder returns to its non-pregnant position—although there can be a loss of tone owing to the displacement and stretching during pregnancy and labour (Rankin, 2017).

With the removal of oestrogen from the system there is an increase in diuresis, which reduces body fluid volume. The decrease in oxytocin also facilitates this fluid loss, as oxytocin has an antidiuretic effect. The diuresis is greatest between 2 and 5 days after birth; however, trauma associated with birth may conversely lead to urine retention during this time (Blackburn, 2017). Fluid and electrolyte balance is usually returned to non-pregnant levels by 21 days. Removal of the accumulated fluid by diuresis returns plasma osmolality to non-pregnant levels.

The other parameters of the renal system, such as the renal plasma flow, glomerular filtration rate and plasma creatinine, return to non-pregnant levels by approximately 6 weeks postpartum (Blackburn, 2017). Glycosuria and proteinuria associated with pregnancy also resolve during this time.

REFLECTIVE THINKING EXERCISE

During the first 2–5 days following birth it is normal for a marked diuresis to occur. However, this time can also be associated with urinary retention.

What factors could account for urinary retention, and what strategies could you as a midwife discuss with the woman to decrease the impact of these factors?

Urinary tract

In the first few hours after birth, micturition may be difficult owing to several factors. Reflex suppression of detrusor muscle activity—that is, loss of muscle tone in the bladder—can reduce bladder emptying. Urethral sphincter spasm due to traumatised levator ani muscles and oedema caused by bruising of the bladder base and urethra during labour can interfere with normal micturition.

Dilation of the urinary tract clears within 6 weeks in most women, though in some this may take up to 12 weeks. Urinary tract infection is more likely in the latter group (Blackburn, 2017). Overstretching of the pelvic floor muscles during birth can lead to damage to nerves and ligaments, which can lead to prolapse or urinary or faecal incontinence. Pelvic floor exercises postpartum assist in retoning muscles and may reduce incontinence problems (Dumoulin & Hay-Smith, 2008; Radzimińska et al., 2018). In a randomised controlled trial, improvement in the level of postpartum urinary incontinence was as effective in women provided with only written instructions as in women who were provided with supervised prenatal pelvic floor muscle training (Fritel et al., 2015). Biofeedback pelvic floor muscle training has been investigated as a strategy to intensify pelvic floor muscle training to improve continence outcomes, but no difference was identified between this and basic pelvic floor muscle training (Hagen et al., 2020). This is an area of ongoing research to optimise outcomes for women.

CARDIOVASCULAR SYSTEM

Cardiac output increases significantly immediately after birth, as blood is returned to the systemic circulation from the uterus as it contracts, and the placenta as it buckles. Venous return to the maternal heart also improves after birth with the relief of inferior vena cava compression. This results in autoinfusion into the systemic circulation. Immediately after birth there is an increase in cardiac output to approximately 60%–80% of prelabour levels, but then a sharp decline within 10 minutes to levels that are maintained over the next days and weeks. The cardiac output returns to non-pregnant levels between 2 and 4 weeks postpartum (Blackburn, 2017); it remains elevated for longer if the woman is breastfeeding. However, if there is a greater blood loss than normal (e.g. postpartum haemorrhage or because of caesarean section), or if dehydration is present, then the cardiac output may not increase.

The extra blood volume acquired during pregnancy compensates for blood loss at the birth. Blood loss and diuresis in the first few days result in a decreased plasma volume. After 3 days, mobilisation of interstitial fluid can then lead to a transient increase in plasma volume and resultant haemodilution. Haemoglobin levels return to non-pregnant levels at about 4–6 weeks following the birth (Blackburn, 2017). The number of platelets increases in the first few days, then gradually falls to non-pregnant levels.

In the last 4 weeks of pregnancy, the levels of fibrinogen, plasminogen and coagulation factors II, VII, VIII and X rise significantly, resulting in a state of **hypercoagulability**. This facilitates rapid blood clotting at birth and reduces the risk of haemorrhage. With the birth of the placenta, fibrinolytic inhibitors are removed, and after 1–3 hours fibrinolytic activity (breakdown of blood clots) increases to normal (Blackburn, 2017). Lysis of fibrin deposited in the placental bed leads to a rise in fibrin degradation products (FDPs). As FDPs interfere with the formation of stable blood clots, there is an increased risk of coagulation disorders immediately after birth. There is also a secondary increase in various clotting factors (fibrinogen, factor V and factor VIII) during the first week, which enhances coagulability. All clotting factors gradually return to non-pregnant levels over the first 2 weeks, but changes to flow velocity and diameter of the deep veins may take up to 6 weeks to return to non-pregnant levels. Overall there continues to be an increased risk of thromboembolism through the puerperium.

CRITICAL THINKING EXERCISE

Compare the physiology of a non-pregnant woman with that of a woman who has just given birth. What physiological changes during pregnancy assist the pregnant woman to withstand bleeding from the placental site? Identify clinical signs that would suggest the woman is not compensating adequately.

CRITICAL THINKING EXERCISE

With the birth of the placenta there is a rapid decrease in placental hormones. This initiates many changes in the body, for example to the gastrointestinal system, the kidneys and the cardiovascular system. What are some of the key implications these changes have for the woman in the immediate postpartum period?

CLINICAL POINT

Deep vein thrombosis (DVT)

The risk of DVT is increased when any two of the following occur: stasis of blood flow, state of hypercoagulation and immobility. All three of these factors are likely to occur during pregnancy and the early puerperium, increasing the risk of DVT.

RESPIRATORY SYSTEM

Oxygen consumption increases 15%–25% during pregnancy (Lotgering et al., 1991) to meet fetal and placental needs and the demand from increased maternal tissues, and then increases 40%–60% during labour and increases by 200% during each contraction in labour (Blackburn, 2017). Oxygen consumption drops back to normal levels once birth of the baby and placenta occurs, and more gradually as maternal tissues return to normal (Blackburn, 2017). During pregnancy, progesterone increases the sensitivity of chemoreceptors to carbon dioxide and thus stimulates some degree of hyperventilation. Hyperventilation can lead to a decrease in the partial pressure of arterial carbon dioxide (P_aCO_2) and thus to respiratory alkalosis (Blackburn, 2017; Lotgering et al., 1991). As progesterone levels drop in the puerperium, dyspnoea and hyperventilation disappear and P_aCO_2 increases to normal. Following birth of the baby, full inflation of the lungs is again possible with removal of compression by the uterus (Rankin, 2017).

GASTROINTESTINAL SYSTEM

Following the birth and with the drop in circulating progesterone levels, the smooth muscle tone throughout the body returns, the woman's appetite increases, and gastric tone and motility return (Rankin, 2017). Heartburn and constipation resolve, although in the first few days there can be an increase in gas distension due to the reduced gastrointestinal muscle tone and motility (Blackburn, 2017). Often prior to labour or during the birth, the rectum has been evacuated and the first bowel movement can take 2–3 days to occur following the birth, as the effects of the progesterone diminish (Blackburn, 2017). Haemorrhoids will take some time to disperse and can become more oedematous immediately in the first few days, owing to pressure on the rectum and anus during the birth (Blackburn, 2017). Liver enzymes return to non-pregnant levels within 2–3 weeks (Blackburn, 2017).

LACTOGENESIS

The puerperium also sees the initiation of lactation. A brief account of the underlying hormonal changes is presented here.

In breastfeeding women, nipple stimulation during suckling initiates the *neuroendocrine reflex,* which stimulates the secretion and release of prolactin from the anterior pituitary gland and oxytocin release from the posterior pituitary gland (Figs. 29.4, 29.5). Although prolactin levels increase throughout pregnancy, **lactogenesis** is prevented by the presence of oestrogen and progesterone. With the drop in levels of progesterone following birth of the placenta, prolactin is effective at stimulating milk synthesis. Suckling stimulates the release of prolactin to maintain milk production, although in the absence of suckling the prolactin levels remain above prepregnant levels and limited milk production may continue for up to 4 weeks after birth (Johnson, 2013).

Oxytocin stimulates myometrial contraction and ejection of milk during lactation. Within 1 minute of nipple stimulation there is a rise in the blood levels of oxytocin, which remain elevated throughout the stimulation and then fall to normal levels about 6 minutes after stimulation ceases. The milk let-down reflex can occur in response to other stimuli, such as the sound of a baby crying. This reflex is also susceptible to inhibition by various types of psychological and physical stress, for example worry and uncertainty about breastfeeding. The mechanism is unclear, but may involve inhibition of oxytocin release or reduced delivery of oxytocin to myoepithelial cells. This latter mechanism could be a result of mammary vasoconstriction due to sympathetic nervous system involvement (Johnson, 2013).

Although lactogenesis is usually inhibited by elevated levels of progesterone during pregnancy, there are many examples of breastfeeding an infant during pregnancy, but little objective research reported (Madarshahian & Hassanabadi, 2012;). One small study of 68 women breastfeeding in the third trimester provided evidence that lactation-pregnancy overlap could have a negative effect on early infant weight gain (Marquis et al., 2002) but more research is needed. Lactogenesis can also be induced in women who have not been pregnant. Lactogenesis is explored in more detail in Chapter 32.

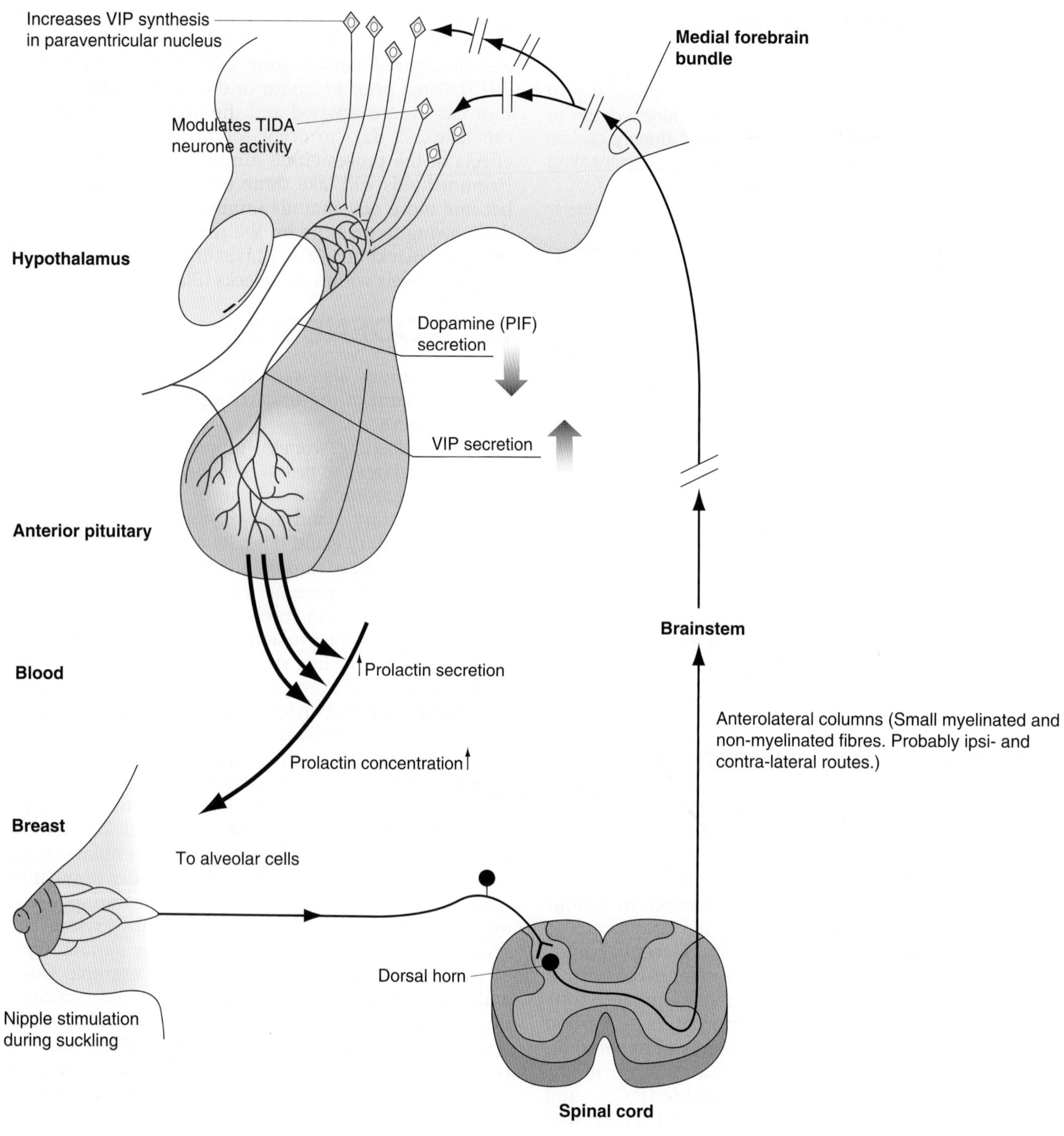

FIGURE 29.4 Somatosensory pathways in the suckling-induced reflex release of prolactin. PIF = prolactin-inhibiting factor; TIDA = tuberoinfundibular dopaminergic; VIP = vasoactive intestinal peptide

(Republished with permission from Johnson MH, Everitt BJ. *Essential Reproduction* (3rd ed). Oxford: Blackwell Scientific; 1988; permission conveyed through Copyright Clearance Center, Inc.)

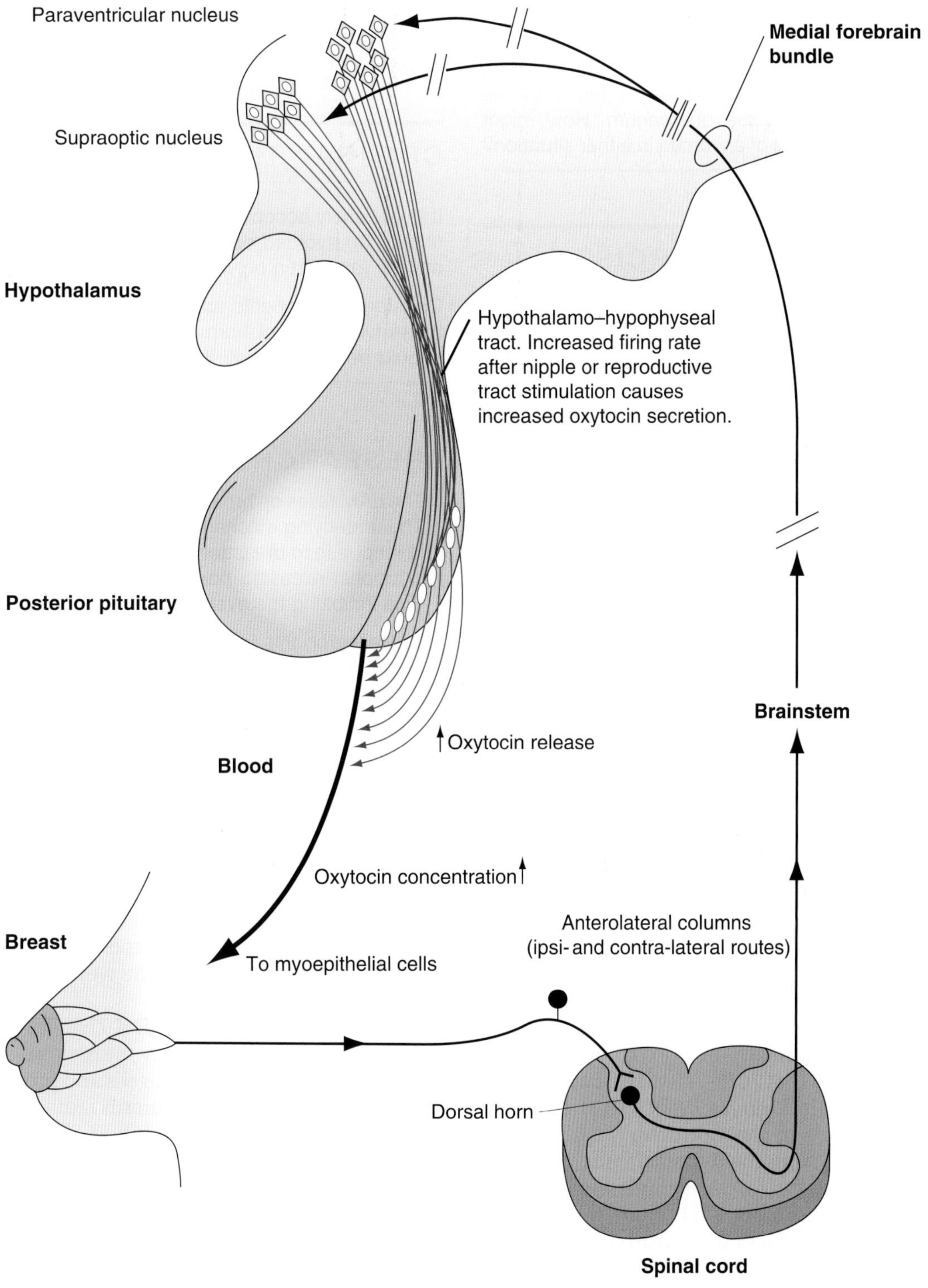

FIGURE 29.5 Somatosensory pathways in the suckling-induced reflex release of oxytocin
(Republished with permission from Johnson MH, Everitt BJ. *Essential Reproduction* (3rd ed). Oxford: Blackwell Scientific; 1988; permission conveyed through Copyright Clearance Center, Inc.)

CRITICAL THINKING EXERCISE

Consider physiological differences between a breastfeeding woman and a non-breastfeeding woman in terms of the physiological changes during the puerperium. How might these factors affect the needs of a woman in either situation?

CRITICAL THINKING EXERCISE

There is evidence from randomised control trials to suggest that skin-to-skin contact with healthy term infants in the early postpartum period improves breastfeeding initiation, breastfeeding duration and maternal–infant interactions, and reduces infant crying. In late pre-term infants it has also been shown to improve cardiorespiratory stability, temperature control and blood glucose levels (Moore et al., 2007). However, the skin-to-skin and control environments in studies are often very different, producing very diverse outcome measures that are difficult to combine in analysis.

1. Identify factors that you feel could confound results when trying to measure outcomes as identified above—i.e. what factors other than skin-to-skin contact might account for the differences?
2. Suggest a biologically plausible mechanism to explain increased breastfeeding initiation and duration following skin-to-skin contact.

RETURN OF MENSTRUATION AND OVULATION

There is considerable variation among women as to when menstruation and ovulation return, but it is generally found that breastfeeding delays the resumption of the reproductive cycle. A systematic review of the literature identified that most non-lactating women do not ovulate until 6 weeks postpartum and that 20%–70% of first menses are preceded by ovulation (Jackson & Glasier, 2011). Prolactin reduces the effectiveness of gonadotrophin-releasing hormone (GnRH) released from the hypothalamus, which in turn decreases the release of follicle-stimulating hormone (FSH) and luteinising hormone (LH) from the anterior pituitary. Prolactin also reduces the sensitivity of ovarian follicles to FSH and LH. Although lactation is associated with decreased fertility, menses is not a reliable indicator of ovulation. Some women ovulate prior to the resumption of menses, whereas others experience anovulatory menstrual cycles (Blackburn, 2017). However, an Australian study of 624 fully breastfeeding women identified a median duration of amenorrhoea of over 8.5 months. No amenorrhoeic, breastfeeding woman became pregnant in the first 6 months leading the authors to conclude that the lactational amenorrhoea method (LAM) was effective (Gross et al., 2002). However, studies have illustrated that for LAM to be effective, a woman must be exclusively or nearly exclusively breastfeeding and a Cochrane review published in 2015 estimated the typical use failure rate of LAM to be 0.45– 7.5% (Van der Wijden & Manion, 2015).

CRITICAL THINKING EXERCISE

It is generally accepted that the combined contraceptive pill should be avoided during lactation, whereas the use of the minipill (progestin only) is widely accepted.

Consider the benefits and risks to the mother and baby of these two types of hormonal contraceptives. What factors should be considered? What is the underlying physiology?

RESEARCH ACTIVITY

The LAM relies on breastfeeding as a contraceptive method. The underlying mechanism is a result of prolactin, released in response to breastfeeding, inhibiting the release of gonadotrophin-releasing hormone from the hypothalamus and thus inhibiting the ovarian cycle.

1. Research this topic and identify the breastfeeding guidelines around maintaining effective inhibition of the ovarian cycle.
2. Identify potential barriers to the success of this method in New Zealand and Australia.

SUMMARY OF KEY LEARNING POINTS

- The postnatal period (puerperium) is the 6–8 weeks following the birth when the woman's body adapts to a non-pregnant state.
- Anatomical and physiological changes of the puerperium are largely governed by the removal of the placental hormones hCG, hPL, oestrogens and progesterone.
- The process by which the uterus reduces in size to being a pelvic organ is called involution. This involves a reduction in protein synthesis resulting from the removal of oestrogen, destruction of actin and myosin fibres by autolysis, and removal of the products of autolysis by phagocytosis.
- A cellular barrier to infection is formed at the placental site by a superficial layer of granulation tissue. Regeneration of the decidual layer surrounding the placental site takes 2–3 weeks and at the placental site takes 6–7 weeks.
- 150–400 mL of fluid / blood are generally lost through the vagina over the 3–6 weeks following birth. Over time it changes in composition and appearance.
- Healing of soft tissue damage to the cervix, vulva and vagina also occurs during this time.
- Body systems other than the reproductive system also undergo changes during the puerperium.

- Dilation of the renal tract and peristaltic action return towards normal as progesterone levels decrease, but micturition may continue to be difficult in the hours following the birth. Removal of oestrogen leads to diuresis.
- Blood loss of 500–1000 mL may occur at birth. Autoinfusion into the systemic circulation occurs with contraction of the uterus and relief of vena cava compression. A state of hypercoagulability continues during the first 2 weeks as the levels of coagulation factors remain high. High levels of FDPs increase the risk of coagulation disorders.
- Oxygen consumption returns to normal as demands reduce and as progesterone levels decrease.
- Functioning of the gastrointestinal system returns to a non-pregnant state as progesterone levels drop.
- Prolactin levels increase throughout pregnancy; however, lactogenesis is prevented by oestrogens and progesterone. With the drop in level of these hormones following birth of the placenta, prolactin is effective at stimulating milk synthesis. Nipple stimulation results in release of prolactin and oxytocin. Oxytocin stimulates the milk let-down reflex.
- Breastfeeding is associated with decreased fertility via its inhibition of the ovarian cycle. Prolactin reduces the effectiveness of GnRH released from the hypothalamus, which in turn decreases the release of FSH and LH from the anterior pituitary.

Conclusion

In conclusion, the puerperium is a time of major physiological change, largely as a result of the birth of the baby and placenta. Hormones drive the changes over these 6–8 weeks. Involution of the uterus and associated structures of the reproductive system occurs, and maternal physiology largely returns to a non-pregnant state. Further to this, physiological and anatomical adjustments continue to support lactation.

Review questions

1. Describe the changes in the level of the pregnancy hormones following birth and explain why these changes occur.
2. With regard to healing at the site of placental separation, explain what is meant by the term ‘cellular barrier’.
3. Outline the process of healing at the placental site.
4. Describe how you would explain to a woman why micturition may be difficult following birth.
5. Provide a physiological explanation for the increased risk of thrombosis during the first 2 weeks of the puerperium.
6. Following birth of the baby, the oxygen needs of the woman decrease, yet cardiac output increases. Account for the increase in cardiac output and outline the mechanism that returns cardiac output to non-pregnant levels.
7. Explain why heartburn and constipation usually resolve in the puerperium.
8. Compare one physiological change to the cardiovascular system in pregnancy with that during the puerperium.
9. Name the hormone that is responsible for milk production. Explain why milk production does not occur during pregnancy.
10. Describe the normal physiological mechanisms that protect a woman from postpartum haemorrhage following the separation of the placenta from the uterine lining.

Acknowledgement

The work of Lesley Dixon, who contributed to the writing of this chapter in the first edition, is acknowledged with thanks.

Online resources

Kahn Academy: the Kahn Academy has YouTube videos on the basic physiology of the puerperium: https://www.khanacademy.org.

National Institute for Health and Care Excellence (NICE) guidelines: Postnatal Care. 2021: https://www.nice.org.uk/guidance/ng194.

NZCOM Cochrane summaries for midwives: https://www.midwife.org.nz/research/cochrane-summaries-for-midwifery.

NZCOM consensus statement: *Breastfeeding.* 2002, updated 2009, 2016: https://www.midwife.org.nz/midwives/professional-practice/consensus-statements/.

NZCOM consensus statement: *Complementary Therapies.* 2000, updated 2009, 2018 Online: https://www.midwife.org.nz/midwives/professional-practice/consensus-statements/.

World Health Organization (WHO) 2015 Integrated management of pregnancy and childbirth (IMPAC): http://www.who.int/maternal_child_adolescent/documents/impac/en/.

References

Bayles B. Herbal and other complementary medicine use by Texan midwives. *J Midwifery Womens Health.* 2007;52(5):473–478.

Belachew J, Axelsson O, Mulic-Lutvica A, et al. Longitudinal study of the uterine body and cavity with three-dimensional

ultrasonography in the puerperium. *Acta Obstet Gynecol Scand.* 2012;91(10):1184–1190.
Blackburn S. *Maternal, Fetal and Neonatal Physiology: A Clinical Perspective.* 5th ed. Saunders?Elsevier; 2017.
Coad J, Dunstall M. *Anatomy and Physiology for Midwives.* Edinburgh: Elsevier Churchill Livingstone; 2005.
Cooklin AR, Amir LH, Jarman J, et al. Maternal physical health symptoms in the first 8 weeks postpartum among primiparous Australian women. *Birth.* 2015;42(3):254–260.
Deussen AR, Ashwood P, Martis R, et al. Relief of pain due to uterine cramping/involution after birth. *Cochrane Database Syst Rev.* 2020;10, CD004908, doi:10.1002/14651858.CD004908.pub3.
Dumoulin C, Hay-Smith J. Pelvic floor muscle training versus no treatment for urinary incontinence in women. A Cochrane systematic review. *Eur J Phys Rehabil Med.* 2008;44(1):47–63.
Farr A, Chervenak FA, McCullough LB, et al. Human placentophagy: a review. *Am J Obstet Gynecol.* 2018;218(4), 401.e401–401.e411. doi:10.1016/j.ajog.2017.08.016.
Fletcher S, Grotegut CA, James AH. Lochia patterns among normal women: a systematic review. *J Womens Health (Larchmt).* 2012;21(12):1290–1294. doi:10.1089/jwh.2012.3668.
Fritel X, de Tayrac R, Bader G, et al. Preventing urinary incontinence with supervised prenatal pelvic floor exercises: a randomized controlled trial. *Obstet Gynecol.* 2015;126(2):370–377.
Gilpin-Blake D, Elliot S. A natural alternative to suturing. *Midwifery Today Int Midwife.* 2001;60:32.
Gross BA, Burger H; WHO Task Force on methods for the natural regulation of fertility. Breastfeeding patterns and return to fertility in Australian women. *Aust N Z J Obstet Gynaecol.* 2002;42(2): 148–154.
Hagen S, Bugge C, Dean SG, et el. Basic versus biofeedback-mediated intensive pelvic floor muscle training for women with urinary incontinence: the OPAL RCT. *Health Technol Assess.* 2020;24(70):1–144. doi:10.3310/hta24700.
Hawkins LK, Missmer SA, Correia KF, et al. Assessment of pregnancy-associated, within-woman change in uterine length. *J Matern Fetal Neonatal Med.* 2014;27(10):989–993.
Holden SC, Gardiner P, Birdee G, et al. Complementary and alternative medicine use among women during pregnancy and childbearing years. *Birth.* 2015;42(3):261–269.
Holst L, Wright D, Haavik S, et al. Safety and efficacy of herbal remedies in obstetrics—review and clinical implications. *Midwifery.* 2011;27(1):80–86.
Jackson E, Glasier A. Return of ovulation and menses in postpartum nonlactating women: a systematic review. *Obstet Gynecol.* 2011;117(3):657–662.
Johnson MH. *Essential Reproduction.* 7th ed. Chichester, UK: John Wiley; 2013.
Johnson MH, Everitt BJ. *Essential Reproduction.* 3rd ed. Oxford: Blackwell Scientific; 1988.
Johnson MH, Everitt BJ. *Essential Reproduction.* 4th ed. Oxford: Blackwell Scientific; 2000.
Johnson PJ, Kozhimannil KB, Jou J, et al. Complementary and alternative medicine use among women of reproductive age in the United States. *Womens Health Issues.* 2016;26(1):40–47.
Lotgering FK, van Doorn MB, Struijk PC, et al. Maximal aerobic exercise in pregnant women: heart rate, O_2 consumption, CO_2 production, and ventilation. *J Appl Physiol.* 1991;70(3):1016–1023.
Madarshahian F, Hassanabadi M. A comparative study of breastfeeding during pregnancy: impact on maternal and newborn outcomes. *J Nurs Res.* 2012;20(1):74–80.
Marchant S, Alexander J, Garcia J. A survey of women's experiences of vaginal loss from 24 hours to three months after childbirth (the BLiPP study). *Midwifery.* 1999;18:21–24.
Marchant S, Alexander J, Garcia J, et al. How does it feel to you? Uterine palpation and lochial loss as guides to postnatal 'recovery'. 2—The BLiPP study (blood loss in the postnatal period). *Pract Midwife.* 2000;3(7):31–33.
Marquis GS, Penny ME, Diaz JM. Postpartum consequences of an overlap of breastfeeding and pregnancy: reduced breast milk intake and growth during early infancy. *Pediatrics.* 2002; 109(4):e56.
Moore E, Anderson G, Bergman N. Early skin-to-skin contact for mothers and their healthy newborn infants. *Cochrane Database Syst Rev.* 2007;(3):CD003519, doi:10.1002/14651858. CD003519.pub2. Online. http://www.thecochranelibrary.com.
Olsen MF, Elden H, Janson ED, et al. A comparison of high- versus low-intensity, high-frequency transcutaneous electric nerve stimulation for painful postpartum uterine contractions. *Acta Obstet Gynecol Scand.* 2007;86(3):310–314.
Qian X, Jiang Y, Liu L, et al. Changes in ectocervical surface area in women throughout pregnancy compared to non-pregnant and postpartum states. *J Matern Fetal Neonatal Med.* 2016;29(22): 3677–3681.
Radestad I, Olsson A, Nissen E, et al. Tears in the vagina, perineum, sphincter ani, and rectum and first sexual intercourse after childbirth: a nationwide follow-up. *Birth.* 2008;35(2):98–106.
Radzimińska A, Strączyńska A, Weber-Rajek M, et al. The impact of pelvic floor muscle training on the quality of life of women with urinary incontinence: a systematic literature review. *Clin Interv Aging.* 2018;13:957–965. doi:10.2147/cia.s160057.
Rankin J. *Physiology in Childbearing With Anatomy and Related Biosciences.* 4th ed. Edinburgh: Elsevier; 2017.
Sherman D, Lurie S, Frenkel E, Kurzweil Y, Bukovsky I, Arieli S. Characteristics of normal lochia. *Am J Perinatol,* 16(8), 399–402. doi:10.1055/s-1999-6818.
Stables D, Rankin J. *Physiology in Childbearing With Anatomy and Related Biosciences.* 2nd ed. London: Elsevier; 2005.
Steel A, Adams J, Sibbritt D, et al. Utilisation of complementary and alternative medicine (CAM) practitioners within maternity care provision: results from a nationally representative cohort study of 1,835 pregnant women. *BMC Pregnancy Childbirth.* 2012;12:146.
Van der Wijden C, Manion C. Lactational amenorrhoea method for family planning. *Cochrane Database Syst Rev.* 2015(10): CD001329, doi:10.1002/14651858.CD001329.pub2.
Wataganara T, Phithakwatchara N, Komoltri C, et al. Functional three-dimensional sonographic study of the postpartum uterus. *J Matern Fetal Neonatal Med.* 2015;28(18):2221–2227.
Williams A, Herron-Max S, Knibb R. The prevalence of enduring postnatal perineal morbidity and its relationship to type of birth and birth risk factors. *J Clin Nurs.* 2007; 16(3):549–561.
Willms AB, Brown ED, Kettritz UI, et al. Anatomic changes in the pelvis after uncomplicated vaginal delivery: evaluation with serial MR imaging. *Radiology.* 1995;195(1):91–94.

Further reading

Blackburn S. Adaptations in major body systems in the pregnant woman, fetus, and neonate. In: Blackburn S, eds. Maternal, *Fetal and Neonatal Physiology: A Clinical Perspective.* 5th ed. Saunders/Elsevier; 2017:215–537 (Unit II).
Blackburn S. Postpartum period and lactation physiology. In: Blackburn S, eds. *Maternal, Fetal and Neonatal Physiology: A Clinical Perspective.* 5th ed. Saunders/Elsevier; 2017:142–159 (Ch. 5).
Carfoot S, Williamson P, Dickson R. A systematic review of randomized controlled trials evaluating the effect of mother / baby skin-to-skin care on successful breast feeding. *Midwifery.* 2005; 21(1):71–79.
Cooklin AR, Amir LH, Jarman J, et al. Maternal physical health symptoms in the first 8 weeks postpartum among primiparous Australian women. *Birth.* 2015;42(3):254–260.

Duarte-Guterman P, Leuner B, Galea LAM. The long and short term effects of motherhood on the brain. *Front Neuroendocrinol.* 2019;53:100740. doi:10.1016/j.yfrne.2019.02.004.
Holst L, Wright D, Haavik S, et al. Safety and efficacy of herbal remedies in obstetrics—review and clinical implications. *Midwifery*. 2011;27(1):80–86.
Howie L, Rankin J. The puerperium. In: Rankin J, eds. *Physiology in Childbearing With Anatomy and Related Biosciences.* 4th ed. Edinburgh: Elsevier; 2017:587–596 (Ch. 56).
Johnson MH. Lactation. In: Johnson MH, eds. *Essential Reproduction.* 7th ed. Chichester, UK: John Wiley; 2013:297–308 (Ch. 18).
Johnson MH. Postnatal care. In: Johnson MH, eds. *Essential Reproduction.* 7th ed. Chichester, UK: John Wiley; 2013:309–322 (Ch. 19).
Qian X, Jiang Y, Liu L, et al. Changes in ectocervical surface area in women throughout pregnancy compared to non-pregnant and postpartum states. *J Matern Fetal Neonatal Med.* 2016;29(22): 3677–3681.

CHAPTER 30

Supporting women becoming mothers

Lesley Dixon and Virginia Schmied

LEARNING OUTCOMES

Learning outcomes for this chapter are:

1. To identify the physical, emotional and social responses and the changes in roles that occur within relationships during the parenting transition
2. To identify the frameworks which guide midwifery practice when undertaking postnatal care
3. To describe the role of the midwife in assessing maternal health and wellbeing during the postpartum period
4. To outline the individual, holistic assessment of the physical, emotional and psychological health required for each woman to support parental adaptation during the postnatal period
5. To identify normal physical postpartum health and common discomforts that may affect the woman's health postnatally
6. To identify the importance of appropriately concluding the midwife–woman partnership, ensure ongoing healthcare provision and the legal and professional requirements for documentation and storage of the woman's health record.

CHAPTER OVERVIEW

The birth of a baby is usually accompanied by a range of experiences and emotions associated with the transition to parenthood. The arrival of a baby is usually a joyous occasion. Even so, there are many adjustments and adaptations required to accommodate the needs of a highly dependent infant. This chapter considers some of the theories that underpin our understanding of parental transition and adjustment for both parents and families. By understanding the complex interrelationships that strengthen optimal transition, midwives are better able to support parents to meet the challenges that parenting brings.

Postnatal care and the midwife's role in assessing maternal health and wellbeing in the postnatal period are discussed. In a partnership model of midwifery care, there will be continuity of care and a holistic approach to assessing a woman's health, with equal emphasis on the physical, emotional, spiritual and social aspects of a woman's wellbeing. Midwifery support and care that recognises a woman's cultural heritage, existing knowledge, practices and values will support the woman to have a positive experience in becoming a mother.

The postnatal period is also the time to conclude the midwife–woman partnership with referral to other health providers for ongoing healthcare.

KEY TERMS

afterpains
involution
lochial
micturition
Midwifery Standards Review
parental transition
perineum
postnatal period
social and emotional support
women's experiences

INTRODUCTION

This chapter focuses on supporting women during the **postnatal period**, with breastfeeding and newborn health discussed in Chapters 31 and 32. It commences with an overview of various theories relating to **parental transition** and identifies the complexity of this transitional process for the woman and her partner, her baby and other members of her family. The aims and principles of postnatal care and women's needs during this time are discussed along with the woman's response to the physiological, emotional and psychosocial changes of the postnatal period, and practical aspects of assessment and support. Chapter 41 focuses on complications in the postnatal period that can result from pathophysiology and Chapter 35 identifies the importance of the woman's psychosocial health and wellbeing. Caring for women during the postnatal period involves being aware of the physical, emotional and social adaptations that women make, how these are interrelated and the factors or conditions that influence adaptation. The postnatal period is a time of maximum change and growth for women and families as they complete the transition to parenthood.

PARENTAL TRANSITION

What is transition?

Transition is generally understood to be the process of change from one state or condition to another (https://en.oxforddictionaries.com/definition/transition). For women, becoming a mother is a time of major change and adaptation not just for her but also her partner/family/whānau. Whether it is a first baby or an addition to the current family, once a baby is born there is a change in roles for all members of a family. Each person needs to adapt and change to accommodate the needs of the baby. For the mother, this changing role can affect her own personal identity and understanding of herself, as well as her status and social role, whilst for couples and larger families there are changes within existing relationships. This process of transition is often considered to be a time of increased vulnerability and stress for the family as each member adapts to their new role (Mazzeschi et al., 2015, p. 17). Transition and adaptation can be improved when there is preparation and positive emotional, physical and social support during this time.

Theories of parental transition

Attachment theory was first conceptualised during the 1960s by John Bowlby, who argued that babies are born with innate biological programming to form attachments as a means of supporting their survival (Bowlby, 1969). Attachment was described as an emotional bond that connected the baby with the mother or a maternal figure and acted as a secure base ensuring that the baby was protected and nurtured and had its social and emotional needs met. Bowlby (1969) believed that disruption of this maternal/baby attachment led to emotional difficulties for the baby and antisocial behaviour during child development; this is discussed more fully in Chapter 35. Building on this work, Rubin, an American nurse academic, conceptualised a series of tasks that could be identified in both pregnancy and the postnatal period and that once achieved would support women to attain the mothering role (Rubin, 1984). These tasks were focused on ensuring attachment and keeping the baby safe alongside the formation of the maternal identity.

The concept of a maternal role was further developed by Mercer, who identified the transition to motherhood theory as the move to a personal state where the mother experiences confidence, competence and a sense of harmony in how she performs her role (Mercer, 1986). The primary components of this theory are the developmental and interactional steps which occur over a period of time, during which the mother bonds with the infant, acquires competence in general caretaking tasks, and then comes to express joy and pleasure in her role as a mother.

Mercer (2006) identified four stages of transition to motherhood; these were:

- commitment, attachment and preparation
- acquaintance, learning and physical restoration
- moving towards a new normal
- achievement of maternal identity.

Parratt & Fahy (2011) argue that this transition to motherhood theory is linear, unidirectional and uses humanistic and paternalistic concepts of the mothering role, which does not reflect a woman's lived experiences. They continue that the experience of childbirth and becoming a mother is complex and influenced by the woman's culture and context; it can be contradictory, sometimes distressing and often a powerful experience.

Schmied & Lupton (2001) similarly challenged accounts of pregnancy as a series of 'stages' of separation or 'polarisation' between mother and fetus during pregnancy, finding in an Australian study that many women describe the relationship with their unborn baby as ambiguous and uncertain, fluctuating rather than linear.

Bowlby's attachment theory has defined a parent–child bond as emotional and based on survival behaviours but is limited by its focus on the behaviour of the individual mother. More recently other family theories have superseded this one-dimensional view with an understanding that the family is a dynamic system in which each member has an impact on child rearing.

Becoming a mother

Over the past two decades, researchers have continued to examine women's accounts of the transition to motherhood. Nelson (2003) synthesised a number of these studies, describing the mothering processes of 'engagement' and 'growth and transformation'. The synthesis indicated that women were overwhelmed and largely unprepared for the transition to motherhood (Nelson, 2003) and that remains the case for many today (Andersson & Hildingsson, 2016;

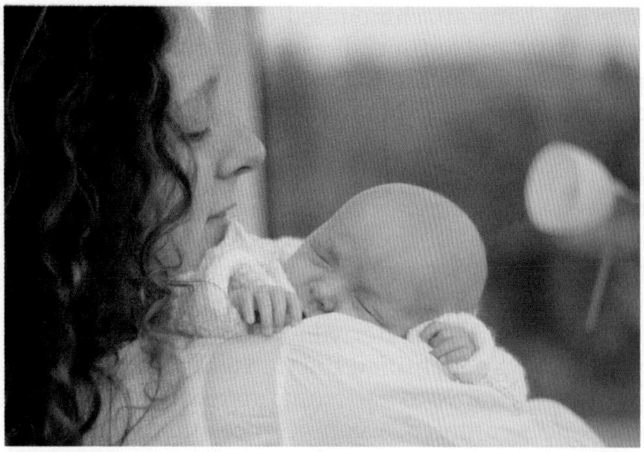

FIGURE 30.1 Maternal transitions

Henderson et al., 2016). To feel like mothers, women had to be involved or 'engaged' in mothering on a daily basis for some time (Fig. 30.1). Many conflicting emotions were characteristic of early motherhood, including intense love, joy, excitement, pride, fear, frustration, shock, tension, uncertainty, insecurity, helplessness, confusion and guilt (Nelson, 2003). One Australian study included in this synthesis articulated the journey of becoming a mother as dynamic and moving from 'realising'—a stage where women recognised the enormity of caring for their infant, felt 'unready' for the change in themselves and their lives, and 'drained', 'alone' with a sense of 'loss' in the early months of motherhood—to a stage of 'working it out' where they described themselves as a mother and the one who knows best what their baby needs. However, the majority of studies in high-income countries like Australia and Aotearoa New Zealand are conducted with white, middle-class women. The experiences of women from different cultural and linguistic backgrounds and for Aboriginal and Māori and Pacific Islander women may well be very different.

Marginalised women such as migrants and refugees may experience the contradictions and pressures of motherhood in different ways. Studies of motherhood amongst non-Western cultures emphasise the high regard within which mothers are held—they are popularly referred to, for example, as 'the light of the home' (Benza & Liamputtong, 2017). In many cultures motherhood is understood to come naturally, provide fulfilment and be empowering when it offers status within the family and social context. Liamputtong (2006) described the 'transformation of self' experienced by South-East Asian women living in Australia. Several discourses of the 'good mother' were evident in her research, particularly mothers' role as the 'keepers of morality' holding an ethic of care and responsibility for others, especially their children. Motherhood was not easy for these women and, combined with difficulties resulting from migration, motherhood became a double burden. Migrant mothers also valued their cultural heritage and often felt responsible for carrying on the beliefs of their homeland, as illustrated in this quote: 'There is a lot of pressure on women that come here. You are carrying so much. You are carrying the culture of Sudan' (Baird, 2012, p. 17).

CRITICAL THINKING EXERCISE

Understandings of motherhood are diverse and mothering practices are embedded in different cultural contexts. Consider the different cultures/ethnic groups within your own region and reflect on the expectations of women as they become mothers. How do these differ depending on culture/ethnicity?

Becoming a father

In contemporary Western societies, becoming a father is viewed as life enhancing, an opportunity for personal transformation as a man constructs his role as a good father (Ives, 2014). In line with this powerful Western discourse, men hold a strong desire to be 'authentically engaged' in the pregnancy (Chin et al., 2011; Fenwick et al., 2012; Goodman, 2005), birth (Johansson et al., 2015), and as a new father (Chin et al., 2011; Goodman, 2005). However, as for women, the transition to fatherhood can be very stressful (Chin et al., 2011; Premberg et al., 2008).

Men prepare for 'active' involvement in labour and birth and parenting, typically by attending antenatal appointments and classes (May & Fletcher, 2013; Steen et al., 2012). Yet studies (Elmir & Schmied, 2016; Ives, 2014; Johansson et al., 2015; Steen et al., 2012) confirm that men are more often than not on the periphery during labour and birth. Steen et al. (2012, p. 430) stated that 'men are genuinely struggling with the need to balance their own unknown and uncertain journey to fatherhood with the desire to provide some certainty and support for the journeying mother'.

Men report a lack of support for them in their new role and that they need more information on parenting, baby care and relationships in the antenatal period (Lewington et al., 2021).

Neural–biological processes and parenting

Beckes et al. (2015) suggest that there is a neurobiological basis for social attachment and relationships and attempt to define how these overlap with physiological systems. Their theory postulates that the neural systems are strongly involved in relationships, attachment and pair-bond behaviour. The theory is based on Bowlby's (1969) theory of attachment and argues that humans are innately social beings, which has an impact on psychological and physical wellbeing. They continue that attachment behaviour has a neurobiological driver, with physical contact between two bodies creating bidirectional sensory stimulation, designed to support homeostasis (equilibrium).

Following birth, women undergo major hormonal shifts with an increase in the neurohormones oxytocin and prolactin, both of which are linked to the development of maternal behaviour (Gordon et al., 2010). Oxytocin has been implicated in a number of social, affiliative and pair-bonding as well as parenting behaviours (Abraham et al., 2014; Bell et al., 2014; Gordon et al., 2010). It seems that it is not just women who have an increase in oxytocin during parental transition. Gordon et al. (2010) explored oxytocin levels of 160 co-habiting couples in the first postpartum weeks and at 6 months. The plasma oxytocin levels of both parents were measured and interactions between each parent and their infant were observed and coded for parenting behaviour. They found that parental oxytocin levels increased for both parents across the time span of the study with no difference between maternal and paternal plasma oxytocin levels. The oxytocin levels of the husband and wife were interrelated. For women, maternal oxytocin was related to affectionate parenting behaviour (affectionate touch, singing and talking to the baby), whereas for the father the oxytocin levels corresponded to stimulatory parenting behaviours (object presentation and stimulatory touch). Both styles of interaction increased oxytocin levels for the parents.

Abraham et al. (2014) also explored the interaction between oxytocin and parenting behaviour with a group of 89 couples using magnetic resonance imaging (MRI) to measure the parental brain response. This study involved heterosexual couples where the mother was the primary caregiver and homosexual fathers where the father was a primary caregiver. They found a parental caregiving neural network which was mainly consistent across parents and which integrated the functioning of two systems. These were the emotional-processing network and the sociocognitive network. Mothers showed greater activation in the emotional-processing network whereas fathers had greater processing in the sociocognitive network, which were both linked through oxytocin and behaviour. Those fathers who were primary caregivers exhibited higher emotional processing similar to the mothers. For all fathers, time spent providing childcare correlated with brain changes.

These studies demonstrate that there are physical and neurobiological changes that occur for both parents following the birth of a baby. These adaptations occur in response to neurohormones and result in changes within the brain's neural pathways for both the primary caregiver and their partner. It is theorised that these adaptations are necessary to support parental adaptation.

Determinants of parenting theory

Belsky (2014) has identified a theory which he argues can provide an understanding of how parental wellbeing, infant behaviour and parental stress and support can influence parenting behaviours. He identified three domains of parenting as: (a) the psychological resources of the parents, (b) the characteristics of the child and (c) the contextual sources of stress and support (Fig. 30.2). Each of these domains has an influence on determining parenting behaviour.

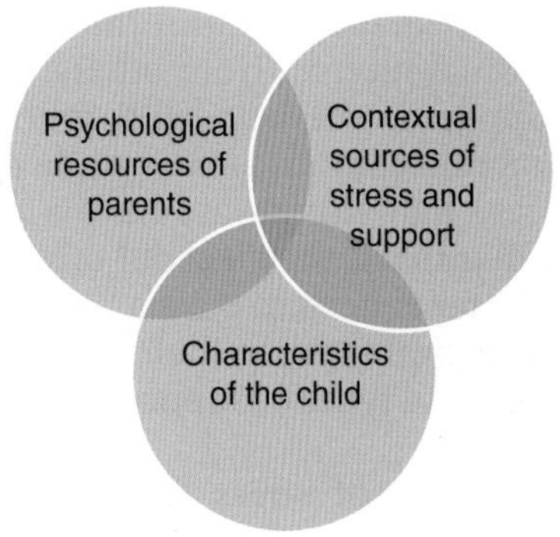

FIGURE 30.2 Belskys' determinants of parenting theory domains (Adapted from Belsky, 2014)

This model argues that parental functioning is influenced and determined by each of these concepts, which are cumulative and interact with each other—in that it is not just one but each of them that can have an influence either positively or negatively on the other domains and together they influence how parents transition and behave as parents.

The psychological resources of the parents

This concept assumes that there are linkages between the parent's psychological wellbeing and their ability to parent, with the parent's own experiences as a child having some impact on their parenting. Belsky (2014) argues that a mature healthy personality is able to provide sensitive parental care which is optimal for child development.

The characteristics of the infant

It is clear that some infants can have more challenging behaviours than others and that this may influence the parenting relationship. There is often difficulty in separating whether the temperament of the child can negatively affect parenting or whether it is the negative parenting that causes negative characteristics in the child. However, Belsky argues that it is the 'goodness of fit' that is most important in determining the parental relationship—in that characteristics that one individual may find difficult to cope with (e.g. frequent crying) another may not and this is dependent on the parent's own expectations and experiences.

Contextual sources of stress and support

Social support is an important element and influence on the psychological and physical health of an individual. Belsky (2014) contends that support is positively related to parental functioning. He categorises support as emotional support, physical support and social expectations.

Emotional support is the love and interpersonal acceptance an individual receives from others; physical or instrumental support is the help with routine tasks and childcare; social expectations are the guide to appropriate behaviour. These may not always have a positive influence on the individual if they feel out of step with others around them. Parents need to have a social network that has similar ideological views to their own for it to be supportive. Each of these types of support can influence how parents behave.

The main sources of stress which can undermine parental confidence and competence are those related to the marital relationship, social networks and employment/work. Having a child has been found to be a major stress for parents (Vismara et al., 2016). Parents' relationships are one of the key factors that influence parenting because they also have an impact on the general psychological wellbeing of the individuals.

Social isolation has been identified as a potential risk for poor parenting; however, as previously discussed, social support needs to be congruent with the individual's ideological views, otherwise it can have a negative impact and cause increased stress. Work is another potential source of stress for both parents and is dependent on work status and economic drivers. Maternal employment may increase or reduce stress depending on the individual.

Belsky (2014) argues that these determinants of parenting are integrated, so that it is not just one individual factor that has a negative impact on parenting but rather that each of these determinants can be mediated by the others. Optimal child development involves parenting that treats the child as an individual, and supports developmentally appropriate autonomy (Belsky, 2014). It is important to note that this will vary across cultures with different expectations in collectivist societies such as in New Zealand Māori and Australian Aboriginal communities compared with many Western societies (Lohoar et al., 2014). However, Belsky (2014) stresses that psychologically intrusive, manipulative or coercive parenting can result in suboptimal psychological infant development and behaviours.

Family structures

Belsky's work has identified the changing context of family structures and need for a better understanding of the fluid, complex and dynamic relationship between couples and within the family and how they influence parenting behaviour. In modern Western societies, family arrangements are becoming more complex with high rates of divorce, co-habitation, single parents, same-sex parents and blended families. It is becoming more common for men as fathers to be increasingly involved in home and family life. 'Co-parenting' is a term that refers to ways in which parents (whether married, living together or living apart) work together in their parental roles (Feinberg, 2002). Feinberg (2002) suggests that there are four basic components of co-parenting that often need to be considered by parents in their parenting role: (a) support versus undermining, (b) differences in childrearing issues and values, (c) division of parental work and (d) management of family interactions.

Supportive co-parenting involves parents supporting, acknowledging and respecting each other's contributions, decisions and authority. Parents also need to consider how they manage their potential differences in childrearing philosophy, values and expectations, with major disagreements linked to increased child behavioural problems. Division of parental work involves couples working together in an equal partnership to identify a fair and acceptable division of parenting work that works for them. Management of family interactions involves the balance of conflict and coalitions as the parents work together in their parental role.

The co-parenting relationship can be generalised to any relationship between two parental figures—so this could be couples, 'blended' families, a mother–grandmother relationship or gay/lesbian couples.

Co-parenting and involved fatherhood, however, may not be expected in other cultures where women and men continue to have more traditional parenting roles. Without traditional forms of family support in a new country, migrant women and men may have to take on new roles when they become parents and this can be stressful (Williams et al., 2012). In some studies, fathers talk about sharing parenting decisions with their partner (Lewington et al., 2021). Others, however, emphasised their traditional role as the decision maker, and yet another group felt the women made the decisions (Shorey et al., 2017). This change in roles may impact negatively on the couple's relationship contributing to poor mental health in this vulnerable time for women.

REFLECTIVE THINKING EXERCISE

Thinking about the families you have been involved with, consider the different family arrangements you have seen.

- Who provides the mother with emotional and practical support?
- How do the partners work together in their parenting role?
- How is the role of the father influenced by sociocultural context?

Emotional availability theory

Emotional availability theory is described as a way of understanding relationship dynamics with an explanation of relationships as having a bidirectional influence for the participants (Saunders et al., 2015). Emotional availability for adults refers to 'the ability of two people to share a healthy emotional connection' (p. 2). When considering the parent–child relationship, Saunders et al. (2015) identified four dimensions they considered important: sensitivity, structuring, non-intrusiveness and non-hostility (*sic*). Sensitivity involves behaviour that creates and maintains a healthy emotional connection to the infant. Structuring refers to the capacity of the parent to teach and guide. Non-intrusiveness refers to enabling the child to take the lead in play and avoiding interfering. Non-hostility refers to the adult being able to regulate his/her own negative emotions and not express these to the child. For the infant-to-adult connection there is a need for infant responsiveness to the adult and involvement, in that the child will respond to the adult cues and involve the adult in their play. Emotional attachment theory suggests that these dimensions can serve as an indicator in the quality of parent–child relationships.

The differing theories of parental transition provide different perceptions on how parents change and adapt to their new role. A summary of the key points of these theories is provided in Table 30.1.

Parental role changes

The introduction of a new baby into a couple's life increases stress within their relationship owing to the major and sustained life-role changes, unfamiliar childcare tasks, fatigue due to interrupted sleep, financial implications and greater potential for work–family conflict (Fillo et al., 2015). Many couples will be unfamiliar with childcare before becoming parents and are likely to be uncomfortable and lacking in confidence in their abilities to care for a child. Whilst couples may have experienced stress within their relationships in the past, childcare-related stress is a new challenge that needs to be navigated together. A baby requires immediate attention and is mostly unpredictable in when they will eat, settle or sleep. This unpredictability can often lead to the parents feeling a loss of control as they can no longer plan their daily activities and the baby's needs replace their own desires and needs. This lack of control is ongoing and continually changing.

The division of parental work has been explored by several authors. Fillo et al. (2015) explored the contribution to childcare over the first two years of parenthood for 137 American couples. They found that, despite these couples identifying a fair division of household labour (close to 50:50 in their study), women were more likely to do most of the childcare tasks (70:30). Kotila et al. (2013) used time diaries over a 24-hour workday and non-workday when babies were 3 and 9 months old to explore how parental work was divided between 182 dual-earner families. This American study found that these parents were highly involved with their babies but that mothers provided more positive engagement and routine childcare than the fathers. The fathers were available and accessible but spent more time in a 'helper' role. These discrepancies in time spent with the child begin early and demonstrate that gender divisions in parenting work continue despite an expectation of equality and shared parenting.

Table 30.1 Summary of transition theories

Theory	Key points
Transition to motherhood	Four stages: 1. Commitment, attachment preparation 2. Acquaintance, learning and physical restoration 3. Moving towards a new normal 4. Achievement of maternal identify
Neural–biological processes and parenting	Neural systems and neurohormones strongly involved in the development of relationships, attachment and bonding
Determinants of parenting	Three domains each of which has an influence on how parents behave: 1. Psychological resources of the parents 2. Characteristics of the child 3. Contextual sources of stress and support
Family structures	Co-parenting—involves parents working in an equal partnership to: 1. Support each other and not undermine 2. Discuss their differences in parenting issues and values 3. Agree on the division of parental work 4. Manage family interactions
Emotional availability theory	A way of understanding relationship dynamics with the ability of two people to share a healthy emotional connection. Has four dimensions: 1. Sensitivity—creating and maintaining emotional connection with infant 2. Structuring—teaching and guiding the infant 3. Non-intrusiveness—enabling the child to lead interactions 4. Non-hostility—parents manage and regulate their own emotions so negative emotions not expressed

A similar pattern emerged in the analysis of the Longitudinal Study of Australian Children (LSAC). For couple parents with children aged under 5 years, it is estimated that, per day:

- mothers spent 5.1 hours on childcare and 3.8 hours on household work
- fathers spent 2.2 hours on childcare and 1.3 hours on household work.

Although fathers contribute slightly more when the mother is in part-time or full-time employment, mothers continue to contribute almost double the amount of time in childcare and household work (Baxter, 2012).

Why is optimal parental transition important?

Babies need frequent engagement in developmentally appropriate parenting activities to facilitate their early socioemotional development (Kotila et al., 2014). A fuller discussion on the importance of early infant socioemotional development is provided in Chapter 35.

Not all families manage parental transitions well, with an increase in family stress resulting in an increased risk of divorce or an exit from a cohabiting relationship (Osborne et al., 2012). Family instability can have an impact on both the mother's and the child's physical and psychological health. In their study using data from the American Fragile Families and Child Wellbeing study, Osborne et al. (2012) not surprisingly found that women who transitioned to marriage or co-habitation with their child's father experienced a decline in material hardship, whereas those that exited in a co-habiting or marital relationship experienced decreased social support, increased material hardship, depression and parenting stress.

Preparation for parental transition

Supporting parents in their transition to parenting is important to the emotional, physical and psychological health of the parents, the baby, siblings and the extended family. Many couples experience a decline in their relationship as the family undergoes a cycle of disorganisation and re-organisation to reach a level of equilibrium (Entsieh & Hallstrom, 2016). Relationships during this time can be fragile with deterioration in relationship confidence, dedication, conflict management and problem intensity (Doss et al., 2014). Interventions have been designed to help support and buffer new parents by increasing knowledge of birth and baby care so as to provide a sense of competence and control. Antenatal education is frequently criticised as focusing too much on the labour and birth and not enough on the preparation for early parenting and childcare. In their synthesis of the needs of parents for early parenthood preparation, Entsieh & Hallstrom (2016) found that parents wanted antenatal education to involve the partners and to provide early and realistic information about parenting skills. In addition, the ability to learn from peers and other new parents (as guest speakers) was important, as was the ability to discuss the potential changing dynamics of their couple relationship prior to the birth of the baby.

Eira Nunes et al. (2020) conducted a systematic review and metanalysis of studies to examine the efficacy of co-parenting programs on outcomes related to children's adjustment, parents' wellbeing, and quality of the co-parenting, romantic, and parent–child relationships.

They found modest support for the efficacy of co-parenting programs impacting co-parenting, parent–child relationship, couple relationship, and parents' wellbeing. Programs offered a range of interventions including psychoeducational, skills training in communication, and co-parenting support. Parents in these studies found value in development of co-parenting and sharing their own experiences with each other and with peers.

Transition for other family members—especially siblings

When a baby is born and welcomed into the family there is an impact on other family members and specifically siblings. This transition can be disruptive and stressful with some children experiencing strong negative reactions to the new baby. Young children experience the transition to siblinghood in a variety of ways; they are often interested in the newborn and will assist with care but they may also show signs of distress. Parents are frequently concerned about sibling rivalry and want to ensure the firstborn's acceptance of a new sibling by supporting cooperation and sharing.

Kolak & Volling (2013) explored the contribution of the existing sibling's characteristics and co-parenting as a means of determining the child's adjustment after a sibling birth. They found that, for most children, there was an increase in externalising behaviour such as acting out, aggression, non-compliance and defiance following the birth of a sibling. For a small subset of children there was an increase in internalising behaviour—in that they became more withdrawn and anxious in the month following the birth of the sibling. Importantly, they found that co-parenting behaviour was able to mediate these transitions when there was cooperative co-parenting. Parental conflict and undermining behaviour may undermine children's emotional security, their feelings of safety and their social interactions. Undermining co-parenting behaviour was identified as higher levels of competition, displeasure and coldness between parents. High levels of supportive co-parenting were protective and appeared to buffer the child's reaction regardless of the child's temperament. They argue that differences in child temperament will require different strategies to meet the individual child's needs.

Song & Volling (2015) explored how the first-born child's temperament predicted their cooperative behaviour in response to their mother's request for help during a nappy change when the new sibling was 1 month in age. They found that supportive co-parenting moderated the association between the child's temperament and their cooperative behaviour. Children who were identified as having low soothability levels exhibited low levels of cooperation but this was moderated when both parents were supportive and the father was involved. Father's involvement may protect the sibling after the birth by compensating for the declining maternal attention and caregiving due to the needs of the newborn sibling. Hence it appears that it is not just the child's temperament but also the parents' relationship that can have an impact on how a sibling responds to a new baby.

REFLECTIVE THINKING EXERCISE

Consider the parenting education provided in your region and identify whether the education does any of the following:

1. Actively engages partners.
2. Provides realistic information (particularly related to breastfeeding).
3. Teaches specific parenting skills—changing nappies, settling babies, etc.
4. Supports parents to learn from peers and other new parents.
5. Provides an ability to discuss couple relationships and changes.

Summary

This section has presented an overview of transition to parenting concepts—to motherhood, to co-parenting and to a secure and attached family. A secure and caring environment is known to provide the best circumstances for brain, cognitive, social and emotional development for the baby. The early years set the foundations of lifelong health and wellbeing outcomes. It is critical, therefore, that all families are provided with opportunities to nurture and care for their infant with appropriate support and assistance available, particularly in the days and weeks following birth. The evidence clearly demonstrates that this is a time of great change—for women, their partners, babies and families. By understanding how the couple's relationship, their own upbringing and expectations and the characteristics of the baby influence and impact on transition, midwives are better able to provide support to parents during this time.

WOMEN'S NEEDS FOLLOWING THE BIRTH

It is clear that the first few days and weeks following birth is a period of major adjustment for the woman and her family, with many first-time mothers identifying difficulty or distress as they create their new identity as a mother (Emmanuel et al., 2011; Henderson et al., 2016). Parents report feeling insecure and unprepared for the sudden change that having a baby has on their daily routines. In modern society there are many families with little social support, and increasingly isolated nuclear families living away from the help, assistance and reassurance of their own families. Feeding newborns and identifying their needs can be difficult especially if there has been little contact with babies previously.

Women have also articulated what they want and need from postnatal care. Overwhelmingly, women report that they value individualised attention and care from midwives and other staff who are compassionate, positive and friendly (Burns & Schmied, 2017; Fenwick et al., 2010; Ménage et al., 2017; Seefat-van Teeffelen et al., 2011). Women have also identified the need for reassurance, assessment of physical and emotional health, information, advice and support on self-care and baby care following the birth (Alderdice et al., 2020). The most important aspect of postnatal care is having a midwife sit and listen to a woman's needs and concerns, ensuring that she is at the centre of making decisions about her care and that of her baby (Burns & Schmied, 2017; Fenwick et al., 2010). In an Australian longitudinal survey, researchers found that women need appropriate acknowledgement and support with an emphasis on maternal role development to facilitate their transition into motherhood (Emmanuel et al., 2011). Other researchers particularly emphasise the **social and emotional support** women require following the birth of their babies, most particularly if they have had a complicated or traumatic birth (Fenwick et al., 2013; Thomson & Downe, 2016). Postnatal care can meet this gap by supporting the woman and her baby's health and wellbeing in the days and weeks following birth and ensuring a smooth transition to parenting for the woman and her family, with as much emphasis placed on the psychological and emotional processes as on the physiological processes.

CRITICAL THINKING EXERCISE

Consider the following questions:

1. Where is the best place for a woman to recover following the birth? Give your reasons.
2. Is there an optimal length of stay on a postnatal ward? What do you think it should be? Give your reasons.
3. How long do women stay in your local maternity facility? What is the average hospital stay? Is there an ability to stay longer or shorter, depending on the woman's needs?

Phases of the postnatal period

Lambermon et al. (2020) in their integrative review of maternal self-care needs, identified a conceptual framework to demonstrate the women's numerous and diverse activities and needs in the early postpartum period. The authors used Orem's (1985) self-care theory (a state in which a person can maintain life, health and wellbeing) and reviewed nine studies about **women's experiences** of postnatal care. They identified three themes described as universal (basic activities of daily living such as having sufficient sleep and regular meals), developmental (adapting to the role of parent and the needs of the baby) and healthcare needs (dealing with physical pain and discomfort). They found that women need individualised care that supports the woman's physical health and emotional health as they recover from the birth and adapt to their new maternal role.

Regional workshops held in New Zealand in 1993 involving lay experts and health professionals identified that women's needs change during the postnatal period (NACCHDSS, 1993). Four phases were identified: (1) the first few hours, (2) the early days, (3) the early weeks and (4) completing the transition to parenthood. Each phase has different characteristics and each woman will go through these phases at her own pace (NACCHDSS, 1993). These two concepts have been blended in Fig. 30.3 to identify and demonstrate the needs of women as they recover from the birth and adapt to their new role during the postnatal period.

In phases 1 and 2, physical recovery is a main focus and priority for most women, along with childcare tasks (nappy changing, bathing, dressing) and being able to breastfeed the baby. Women will often ignore their own needs in order to respond to their baby's needs and will often miss sleep and meals even though sleep deprivation and unhealthy eating behaviour are known to have an effect on health and wellbeing (Lambermon et al., 2020). Ensuring that women are able to get sufficient

Women's needs during the post-partum period

Universal self-care needs Phases 1–2 First few hours and days	Healthcare needs Phases 1–2 First few hours and days	Development self-care needs Phase 3–4 Early weeks to completion of transition
• Sleeping • Eating • Personal hygiene • Resuming normal activities	Dealing with: • Pain and discomfort following the birth • Tiredness and lack of sleep • Physical changes • Learning to breastfeed • Judging illness of self or baby	• Finding a new routine • Taking care of the baby • Taking care of other children • Taking up the role of mother • Re-establishing role as partner • Resuming usual household activities (shopping, cooking etc.)

Self-care agency influencers
• Personal characteristics—culture, number of children • Physical and emotional wellbeing • Support from health professionals • Support from partner • Support from family and friends • Preparation prior to postpartum period • Expectations of postpartum period

(Adapted from Lambermon et al., 2020)

FIGURE 30.3 Women's needs during the postpartum period
(Adapted from Lambermon et al., 2020)

rest, regular meals and attend to their own hygiene needs is an important component of early postpartum midwifery care. Women also need reassurance about their physiological wellbeing, supported in a comfortable environment, and should be pain free. High levels of physical discomfort can cause emotional distress and lessen the ability to cope with the physical and emotional changes. At this time the midwife needs to be aware of normal physiology and should be able to give practical help and advice.

During phase 3, as a woman's physical recovery and parenting role progresses, she will gain confidence in her ability to care for herself and her baby. At some point the emotional aspects of the changes to her social world will start to have an impact. Changes to family dynamics and her personal role will become more apparent. Being able to talk about how she feels is an important part of the coping process; listening, understanding and reassuring may be of more value to the woman than physical assessment at this time (Kurth et al., 2016). A midwife will need to discuss support and, if necessary, help the woman to identify where support can be obtained, from groups that are culturally appropriate for her. Each interaction that a midwife has with a woman and her family should be seen as an opportunity to enhance the woman's self-knowledge and learning, as well as promoting health, confidence and independence.

Phase 4, the completion of the transition to parenthood, involves a woman and her family accepting the change in family dynamics and shared responsibility for the baby with increasing confidence. The timing of this may be variable and dependent on the woman, her family and the social support around her.

The aims of postnatal care

Postnatal care has been described as 'the individualised care provided to meet the needs of a mother and her baby following childbirth' (National Institute for Health and Care Excellence (NICE), 2013, Introduction), with relational continuity from a supportive midwife able to make a significant contribution and influence a woman's coping process (Boyle et al., 2016; Danbjørg et al., 2015). A number of guidelines and studies have described the principles and aims of postnatal care provision and are summarised in Box 30.1 (National Advisory Committee on Core Health and Disability Support Services (NACCHDSS), 1993; NICE, 2015; State of Victoria, 2012; WHO, 2013).

The provision of postnatal care varies internationally and is frequently undervalued, with many countries focusing their resources on care provision during the pregnancy and labour and birth and limiting postnatal care provision to hospital postnatal care only. The World Health Organization (WHO) identify the postnatal period as the 'most neglected' and argue that it is a critical phase in the lives of mothers and their newborn babies (WHO, 2013). They have set out a series of recommendations designed to improve the quality of postnatal care and reduce maternal and neonatal morbidity and mortality for low- and middle-income countries (see Box 30.2).

Box 30.1 Aims of postnatal care summarised

- To promote the physical and psychological health and wellbeing of the woman and her baby including recovery from the pregnancy, labour and birth
- To establish good infant-feeding practices including support and education for breastfeeding
- To foster positive maternal–child relationships
- To strengthen the mother's confidence in herself and her ability to care for her baby in her own social, cultural and family situation

Care should be provided in a way that:

- ensures all women and their families are treated with compassion, respect and dignity at all times with privacy needs considered
- seeks and respects the views, beliefs and values of the woman, her partner and her family in relation to her care and that of her baby at all times
- ensures the woman is in control of the pace and framework of events, including planning the timing and content of each postnatal care contact so that care is flexible and tailored to meet her social, clinical and emotional needs and those of her baby and family.

(Sources: Ball, 1994; NACCHDSS, 1993)

Box 30.2 WHO recommendations for postnatal care (2022)

- Women and their baby receive postnatal care in a healthcare facility for at least 24 hours following birth.
- There should be a minimum of three home postnatal contacts after the birth.
- If the birth is at home, then there should be a home visit following the birth within 24 hours along with a further three home visits.

(Source: WHO, 2022)

FRAMEWORKS FOR MIDWIFERY CARE

In New Zealand, postnatal care continues until 6 weeks with ongoing support after this provided by Well Child services. In the majority of Australian states and territories, women and their families are offered a home or clinic visit by the child and family health nursing service between 2 and 4 weeks following the birth. The minimum specifications for postnatal care in New Zealand have been defined (Box 30.3) with each woman entitled to at least this level of care (MOH, 2007).

The New Zealand College of Midwives (NZCOM), in its *Handbook for Practice* (NZCOM, 2015), outlines decision points that can be used to help identify times when there should be full midwifery assessments during the postnatal period. Each decision point summarises the assessments that should be made, investigations that should be performed, possible treatments, legal requirements, and health information and education that should be shared. The timing of decision points should be based on individual need, but the first decision point should occur within the first 24 hours of the birth (NZCOM, 2015). Subsequent decision points should be every 24–48 hours until the woman is confident in her home environment (NZCOM, 2015) (Box 30.4).

Ideally, the midwife would decide, on an individual basis with each woman, the frequency and length of visits that are required and when these visits should cease (MOH, 2007). There are many aspects of a mother's or baby's health that may indicate the need for more-frequent visits.

There are no similar specifications for minimum levels of care in Australia and care varies across states and territories depending on the models of maternity and midwifery care available to women. The NICE (2006, 2015) guidelines for postnatal care are often used to inform improvements in the provision of postnatal care in many states/territories; a summary is provided in Box 30.5. These guidelines outline the care that should be provided at every contact and then specific care within the first 24 hours, first week and weeks 2–8 following birth and these are used by some maternity services to inform care in Australia.

In Australia, opportunities for postnatal visiting in the woman's home after discharge from hospital are limited according to models of care and funding. Midwives who have gained accreditation as an 'eligible midwife' and have a Medicare provider number are able to offer women a Medicare rebate for short and long postnatal visits for

Box 30.3 Postnatal care in New Zealand

As described in Chapter 2, all pregnant women within New Zealand are expected to choose a practitioner as their lead maternity carer (LMC) as per Section 88 (MOH, 2021). The LMC is responsible for ensuring that all the following services are provided and that the provision of services is documented for both the mother and baby:

(a) postnatal consultations at mutually agreed times of the day to assess and care for the woman and baby in a maternity facility and at home until six weeks after birth, including:
  - (i) liaison and consultation with the woman and the maternity facility services regarding the timing of discharge of both mother and baby; and
  - (ii) one consultation at the woman's home before the end of the day after discharge from the maternity facility; and
  - (iii) at least seven postnatal consultations in total, including a minimum of five consultations conducted in the woman's home; and
  - (iv) if there is an exceptional circumstance that results in a postnatal consultation not being conducted in the woman's home, this reason must be clearly documented by the LMC; and

(b) as part of the consultations in clause (a):
  - (v) examinations of the baby consistent with the requirements of the Well Child Tamariki Ora Schedule, and
  - (vi) examinations of the woman at clinically appropriate times and before referral to the woman's primary care provider; and

(c) as a part of the consultations in clause (a), the provision of care and advice to the woman, including:
  - (vii) assistance with and advice about breastfeeding and the nutritional needs of the woman and baby; and
  - (viii) assessing for risk of postnatal distress, depression and family violence, with appropriate advice and referral (where services are available); and
  - (ix) providing appropriate information and education about screening; and (iv) offering to provide or refer the baby for the appropriate screening tests specified by the Ministry of Health and receive and follow up the results of these tests as necessary; and
  - (x) providing Ministry of Health information on immunisation and the National Immunisation Register and provision of any appropriate or scheduled immunisations consented to; and
  - (xi) providing access to services as outlined in the Well Child Tamariki Ora Schedule; and
  - (xii) providing advice regarding contraception; and
  - (xiii) providing parenting advice and education; and

(d) review and update the care plan and document progress, care given and outcomes, and ensuring that the maternity facility has a copy of the care plan if the woman is receiving in-patient postnatal care.

up to 6 weeks after birth, but at this point there is no set minimum or maximum number of visits.

Different countries have individual legislation and expectations regarding the time frame for formal postnatal care, as well as differences in frequency of home visits, so it is difficult to make comparisons about what constitutes the optimal amount of postnatal care.

Postnatal care in hospital

The majority of women in both Australia and New Zealand give birth in a hospital facility; therefore postnatal care commences for most women in hospital.

In many high-income, resource-rich countries, postnatal hospital stays have become shorter resulting in

Box 30.4 Decision points in postnatal care

First decision point in postnatal period—up to and including the first 24 hours postpartum

This timing provides an opportunity for the midwife to reflect on the birth experience with the woman and assess the health and wellbeing of the woman and her newborn baby. Facilitate and assist her transition to parenthood.

Information shared

- Facilitate mother–baby relationship whilst also continuing observation of the woman and her baby immediately postpartum.
- Provide an opportunity to discuss general wellbeing and need for rest.
- Guide and assist with breastfeeding/infant support, support parents getting to know their baby and provide parenting information.
- Provide education for the woman about self-care related to recovery from birth—changes to breasts whether breastfeeding or not, uterus involution, blood loss, bladder, perineum.
- Give information to support baby's care related to overall wellbeing of baby including safe sleeping.
- Reinforce information already provided if there are concerns about the woman or her baby and how to call for assistance.

Assessment and observation of the woman and her baby

- Physical assessment and observations of the woman, history to date and postnatal plan in discussion with the woman in relation to her ongoing plan of care.
- Physical assessment and observations of the baby occurs following skin to skin and first feed when the baby appears well at birth.
- Discuss outcome of assessments with the woman and her partner/support persons and discuss her ongoing care requirements.
- Following assessment and review, facilitate access to investigations and treatment for the woman or her baby as discussed and agreed in her care plan.

Subsequent decision points in postnatal period every 24–48 hours until woman feels confident in her home environment

This timing provides the opportunity to support and encourage the woman's independence while also ensuring the wellbeing of the woman and her baby.

Health information, education and referrals discussed with the woman

- Need for rest and for ongoing support.
- Discussion about the birth and an opportunity to reflect on outcome.
- Assess breastfeeding/infant feeding, getting to know the baby and parenting information.
- Education for the woman about self-care related to recovery from birth.
- Identify with the woman when, how and who to call for assistance.
- Information given for baby's care related to overall wellbeing of baby.
- Self-care for the woman, for example contraception, immunisation, nutrition and exercise, and mental health.
- Referral to GP, Well Child/Tamariki Ora, other health professionals, other community agencies as appropriate/necessary.

Assessment and observation of the woman

- Assess and review the woman's health status.
- Discuss with the woman outcomes of the assessment and any plans that eventuate from it.

Assessment and observation of the baby

- As per the Well Child/Tamariki Ora Schedule and as required, assess and review the baby's health status and discuss with the mother outcomes of this and plans that may eventuate.
- Observe the baby during an entire feed—breast or bottle.
- Following each assessment and review, facilitate access to investigations and treatment for the woman or her baby as discussed and agreed in the care plan with her.

(Source: NZCOM, 2015)

Box 30.5 The NICE guidelines for routine postnatal care

- A documented, individualised postnatal care plan should be developed with the woman ideally in the antenatal period or as soon as possible after birth. This should include:
  - relevant factors from the antenatal, intrapartum and immediate postnatal period
  - details of the healthcare professionals involved in her care and that of her baby, including roles and contact details
  - plans for the postnatal period
  - review at each postnatal contact.
- There should be local protocols about written communication, in particular about the transfer of care between clinical sectors and healthcare professionals. These protocols should be audited.
- Women should be offered relevant and timely information to enable them to promote their own and their baby's health and wellbeing and to recognise and respond to problems.
- At the first postnatal contact, women should be advised of the signs and symptoms of potentially life-threatening conditions and to contact their healthcare professional immediately or call for emergency help if any signs and symptoms occur.
- All maternity care providers (whether working in hospital or in primary care) should implement an externally evaluated, structured program that encourages breastfeeding, using the Baby Friendly Initiative as a minimum standard.
- At each postnatal contact, women should be asked about their emotional wellbeing, what family and social support they have and their usual coping strategies for dealing with day-to-day matters. Women and their families / partners should be encouraged to tell their healthcare professional about any changes in mood, emotional state and behaviour that are outside of the woman's normal pattern.
- At each postnatal contact, parents should be offered information and advice to enable them to assess their baby's general condition, identify signs and symptoms of common health problems seen in babies and contact a healthcare professional or emergency service if required.

(Source: NICE, 2006, 2015)

women going home within 24–48 hours of the birth (Henderson et al., 2016; Kurth et al., 2016; Ministry of Health (MOH), 2013).

A meta-analysis of 15 studies exploring the effects of early postnatal discharge on infant outcomes found that if women and their babies are discharged less than 48 hours after a vaginal birth and less than 96 hours after a caesarean birth the baby was more likely to be readmitted to hospital within 28 days when compared to standard discharge (Jones et al., 2020).

In Australia, data from the AIHW (2016) demonstrates a trend to earlier postnatal discharge with more women being discharged earlier (less than 5 days post birth), and in 2018 the median postnatal hospital stay for mothers was 2 to 3 days.

REFLECTIVE THINKING EXERCISE

Thinking about the strategies for supporting postnatal women in a hospital, consider what could be done in your local maternity hospital to facilitate and increase opportunities for midwives to spend time with women.

Postnatal care at home

In New Zealand it is usual for women to receive home visits from the midwife lead maternity carer (LMC) following hospital discharge until 6 weeks following the birth. The Section 88 contract specifies that each woman should receive a minimum of 5 home visits following the birth (MOH, 2021).

In 2016, 71.5% of women received between 6 and 9 home postnatal visits from midwives, with 14.1% receiving between 10 and 14 visits (NZCOM & Midwifery and Maternity Providers Organisation (MMPO), 2018). The 2014 *Maternity Consumer Survey* (MOH, 2015) found that most women felt that they had received the right number of visits but this did vary depending on the number of visits they had received (83% positive response with up to 6 visits, 96% positive response with 7–12 visits and 95% positive with 13 or more visits). It appears that between 7 and 12 visits over the 6-week postnatal period provided the most positive response from women.

In Australia, most women who birth in public hospitals in urban and regional Australia will be offered one or more home visits by a midwife depending on her needs and when she was discharged. In many instances these visits cease by 5 days at which point the family's care is transitioned to the maternal child and family health nursing service (Brodribb & Miller, 2015). Women experiencing midwifery care in the home are often more satisfied with their postnatal care in comparison with those cared for in the hospital (McLeish et al., 2020), particularly if that care is provided by a known midwife (Danbjørg et al., 2015). Practical advice and tips for supporting women postnatally at home are provided in Box 30.6.

Box 30.6 Helping women at home

Practical ways of helping women at home include:

- Ask friends, partners and family to help with household tasks; foster the idea that this should be normal within our society (Bick et al., 2009; McQueen & Mander, 2003).
- Be flexible about visits but ensure they are regular, giving a date and time for next visit.
- Have sufficient time set aside to listen, understand, reassure and give positive feedback.
- Discuss types of social support—how much does she have, is it enough and, if not, how can she recruit more?
- Encourage the woman to accept a lower standard of tidiness and cleanliness within the house.
- Discuss the benefits of exercise, which can improve mood level and reduce tension and anxiety. A short walk every day or several times a week can be helpful (Bick et al., 2009).
- Encourage women to have frequent short rests during the day (Bick et al., 2009).
- Encourage healthy eating and ensure that dietary needs are being met (Bick et al., 2009).
- Encourage discussion of problems or other concerns, such as finances, family relationships, or lack of personal time. These may affect how a woman feels and copes (Symon et al., 2003).
- Explain that 'perfect mothers' are a myth and that she only needs to be 'good enough'.

CRITICAL THINKING EXERCISE

You arrive to visit Cindy who is now 2 weeks postnatal with her third baby. All has been going well and Cindy has been well supported by her family and friends following the birth. When you arrive at the house, there is no one home. It looks like she has forgotten your appointment. What do you do next? When will you visit Cindy again?

CRITICAL THINKING EXERCISE

1. When you are in clinical practice observing postnatal care, how many home visits are women receiving?
2. Are there differences between women depending on their adaptation?
3. What is the key focus of each visit?
4. Are the visits individualised to the needs of each woman?
5. Are women happy with the amount of postnatal care they have received?
6. What do you think is the optimal number of postnatal visits following hospital discharge for best outcomes?

Box 30.7 The New Zealand Maternity Consumer Survey (2015)—summary of postnatal care responses

Individual aspects of the postnatal care received at home were also positively rated:

- the physical checks carried out on their baby (76% were very satisfied)
- the way in which their background, culture, beliefs and values were respected (75%)
- the way in which their decisions, views and choices were respected (72%)
- the advice they received from their midwife about caring for their baby (72%)
- their midwife listening to them (72%)
- the advice from their midwife about caring for themselves (71%)
- the way their midwife responded to their needs (71%).

Women were least likely to be very satisfied with the physical checks completed on themselves (67% were satisfied or very satisfied).

(Source: Research New Zealand, 2014. Maternity Consumer Survey, Wellington, Ministry of Health New Zealand)

Women's experiences of postnatal care

The 2014 New Zealand *Maternity Consumer Survey* surveyed the experiences of 4000 women who gave birth in New Zealand between December 2013 and February 2014 (MOH, 2015). In this report, 70% of women reported that they remained in hospital for at least 24 hours after the birth of their baby, with 45% staying longer than 48 hours (see Box 30.7). First-time mothers were more likely to stay longer. The majority of women (80%) reported that they were satisfied/very satisfied with the postnatal care they received during their hospital stay. A further 89% reported feeling satisfied/very satisfied with the care they received from their midwife during the first weeks after the baby's birth. There were no statistical differences between women who responded based on their ethnicity but women with disabilities reported lower levels of satisfaction with hospital postnatal care.

In Australia, women are less satisfied with postnatal care than with other aspects of maternity care (Brown et al., 2005; Todd et al., 2017). A recent survey of 886 Australian women indicated that 65% rated antenatal care as 'very good', 74% rated birth care as 'very good' and 58% rated postnatal care as 'very good'. The survey findings indicated that being 'always or almost always' treated with kindness and understanding was the factor most strongly associated with a 'very good' care rating. The survey also found that the highest satisfaction was amongst women who received care in one of two standalone midwifery-led units (Todd et al., 2017).

Australian and international research indicates that midwives have limited opportunity to provide adequate emotional support following the birth (Fenwick et al., 2010; Schmied & Bick, 2014) and women have also described the in-hospital environment as noisy, with concerns voiced about lack of privacy and constant interruptions, making the hospital not conducive to rest and recovery (Morrow et al., 2013; Schmied & Bick, 2014). Given these reports about in-hospital postnatal care, it is interesting that the prime reason women in Australia (McLachlan et al., 2009) and elsewhere give for staying in hospital is the 24-hour support. When presented with a number of options for home-based care, many women still indicate their preference for a longer hospital stay (Danbjørg et al., 2015; Kurth et al., 2016; McLachlan et al., 2009; Zadoroznyj et al., 2015). This reflects the perceived need by women, particularly first-time mothers, for 24-hour professional support. Indeed, women report feeling pressured to leave hospital before they felt ready, and not having enough time to rest and recover (Zadoroznyj et al., 2015). Researchers report that the information provided to women is rarely individualised to women's specific concerns.

Based on these negative reports, particularly of in-hospital care, many midwives and services have developed and trialled strategies to improve hospital-based postnatal care in Australia and the UK. These strategies have included:

- providing opportunities for women to plan for the postnatal period through discussion visits with midwives in the third trimester (Bick et al., 2012; Yelland et al., 2009)
- the development of consumer-written information focusing on the postnatal period (McKellar et al., 2006; Yelland et al., 2009), including maternal health, baby care and sources of support and advice after discharge
- introduction of new hand-held records to prompt evidence-based individualised care, with emphasis on undertaking routine physical observations and examinations only after the first postnatal contact based on the women's individual needs (Bick et al., 2012)
- midwifery mentoring and professional development opportunities—skill enhancement programs including communication skills training were considered an important component of most studies (Bick et al., 2012; Schmied et al., 2008; Yelland et al., 2009)
- re-organisation of staff rotation and administrative support has also been trialled.

For example, Schmied et al. (2008) and Morrow et al. (2013) implemented organisational and environmental changes intended to allow midwives to spend more time with women and to facilitate increased rest for women. Strategies included structuring care and administrative tasks so that midwives were able to provide each woman they cared for with an uninterrupted time (20–30 minutes) of individualised care, support and education. The allocation of this time was supported by the establishment of a breakfast and parenting room with an allocated midwife available to facilitate parent-led discussions, particularly in relation to infant feeding and parenting support/advice. Overall, however, these models do little to address the fragmentation of care across antenatal, birth and postnatal periods. Box 30.8 identifies other strategies which may support women during their hospital stay.

Increasingly, maternity services in Australia are introducing an antenatal and postnatal continuity-of-care model without intrapartum care. This ensures that the woman receives care from a known midwife in the postnatal period, however there are few evaluations to date of this model of care and midwives report not having sufficient time in the postnatal period to address breastfeeding concerns (Cummins et al., 2021).

Box 30.8 Helping women in a maternity facility

Practical ways of helping women within a maternity facility environment include:

- Promote a restful and caring atmosphere from all staff.
- Ensure regular meals and drinks are provided; have snacks readily available.
- Promote maternal and family contact with the baby.
- Control noise so that women can sleep/rest at appropriate times (Ockenden, 2000).
- Provide consistent help and advice regarding baby care; use positive feedback.
- Provide consistent help and advice regarding breastfeeding (Ockenden, 2000).
- Discuss pain and provide appropriate help with pain be it pharmacological or non-pharmacological management (Ockenden, 2000).
- Give frequent praise and reassurance.
- Promote a family-friendly facility, and encourage family and friends to visit and provide extra support.
- Many women when stressed, tired or in pain find a warm bath relaxing and refreshing. Lavender oil in the bathwater appears to aid this relaxation and may be helpful as a way of reducing stress, helping to alleviate muscle fatigue and promoting the feeling of being cared for. Research suggests that having a bath can relieve perineal discomfort and other aches and pains, but that it does not reduce high levels of pain or improve healing of the perineum; adding salt or a disinfectant to the bath has not been proven to have any more benefits than bathing in water alone (Bick et al., 2009).

ASSESSMENT OF WOMEN'S HEALTH

The midwifery partnership model, which encompasses continuity of care, enables the building of a supportive relationship between a midwife and a woman and her family throughout pregnancy and childbirth (Guilliland & Pairman, 2010). This relationship continues to be important during the postnatal period, when there is a time of physical recovery and emotional adaptation to parenthood. Even when continuity of care is not feasible or possible, the midwife still has an important role in supporting the woman and her baby during the postnatal period. Assessment of a woman's health includes assessment not only of her physical recovery, but also of her emotional responses to the demands of parenthood and of the social supports that she has to help with these changes, as identified in Box 30.9 (NICE, 2015). Henderson et al. (2016) argue that emotional distress and / or depression following childbirth is an understandable response to the difficulties of motherhood. Having good social support, realistic expectations of the difficulties of the mothering role and practical help with childcare can reduce the likelihood of becoming depressed following birth (Fahey & Shenassa, 2013; Leahy-Warren & McCarthy, 2011).

Box 30.9 Assessing parental and emotional attachment

- Home visits should be used as an opportunity to promote parent- or mother-to-baby emotional attachment
- Assessment for emotional attachment should be carried out at each postnatal contact
- Women should be encouraged to develop social networks as this promotes positive mother–baby interaction
- Group-based parent-training programs designed to promote emotional attachment and improve parenting skills should be available to parents who wish to access them
- Healthcare providers should offer fathers information and support in adjusting to their new role and responsibilities within the family unit

(Adapted from National Institute for Health and Care Excellence (NICE, 2015). *Postnatal Care up to 8 Weeks After Birth.* Clinical Guideline. Retrieved from http://nice.org.uk/guidance/qs37)

PHYSICAL ASSESSMENT OF MATERNAL HEALTH

It is important to remember that following birth the woman and her baby form a dyad, and what influences one will influence the other. Therefore, if the woman is unwell, uncomfortable or unhappy this will have an effect on the baby and vice versa. When providing postnatal care it is necessary to take this into account with most women needing help, support and reassurance with their parenting skills and to understand the needs of their baby. Hence postnatal care involves assessment of both the mother's and the newborn's health and wellbeing and the midwife's discussion will cover both during her postnatal visits—whether in the hospital or at home. For the purposes of this textbook, postnatal care has been separated into supporting women becoming mothers and newborn health to ensure a comprehensive examination of the issues.

In the first few hours and days following birth (phases one and two), a midwife needs to ask specific questions related to the woman's physical recovery, in order to establish whether there are any problems or concerns that might otherwise not be voiced. In New Zealand there is a guideline which identifies the specific observation and assessment required in the first hour following birth (Table 30.2; MOH, 2012).

Table 30.2 Maternal assessment in the hour following birth
Mother's overall sense of wellbeing and mobility
Facilitate skin-to-skin support and assess bonding of mother, partner family / whanau and baby
Palpate uterine height, position and tone
Observe blood loss
Monitor temperature, pulse, respirations, blood pressure and level of consciousness (frequency will depend on the woman's health)
Urine output
Assess bleeding from lacerations, episiotomy or caesarean section wound
Assess pain relief requirements
Provide IV fluids and medications if prescribed
Assess block levels if epidural / spinal was used during birth
(Source: MOH, 2012)

Following the birth, the baby is often the focus of attention and a woman's health can become secondary. Childbirth is a time when intimate areas of a woman's body become a focus of attention, and some women may feel uncomfortable with this and reluctant to volunteer information about their private body functions. Taking time to talk about a woman's health and feelings is an important way of reinforcing the need for the woman to look after herself and of the normality of the physiological changes she is experiencing. The physical postnatal assessment has been a routine part of postnatal care and this has historically been done as a top-to-toe check—ideally starting with the woman's emotional and psychological health and moving through each system of the body to assess each individual woman's physical recovery and identify any ill-health. This section focuses on the physical health assessment.

Breasts and feeding

The mother and baby have a symbiotic relationship with each other. An important aspect of the postnatal assessment is a discussion about the breasts, breastfeeding and any breast discomfort. This is discussed more fully in Chapter 32. Issues with breastfeeding or newborn behaviour can have an effect on the mother's psychosocial health and do need to be discussed fully.

The uterus, blood loss and afterpains

Involution of the uterus

A midwife will normally palpate the uterus shortly after the expulsion of the placenta, to ensure that there is a reduction in size of the uterus and an overall contraction of the uterus. The uterus can be felt as a hard round or ovoid structure at about the level of the woman's umbilicus, or sometimes just below. The fundus of the uterus should be central and feel firm to the touch. During the postnatal period the uterus reduces in size and it has been a common practice for the midwife to palpate a woman's uterus to check for **involution** on a regular basis during the postnatal period until the fundus is no longer palpable outside the pelvis. A tender or painful uterus can be a sign of infection or retained products of conception, as can slow involution, which is known as sub-involution (Blackburn, 2013). The uterus can also be tender to the touch and slower to involute following a caesarean section (Blackburn, 2013).

The NICE (2006, 2015) guidelines on postnatal care in the United Kingdom advise that routine palpation is unnecessary unless the vaginal loss becomes excessive (which may indicate postpartum haemorrhage), has an offensive odour, or the woman is feeling unwell and has a pyrexia, which may indicate uterine infection.

Marchant and colleagues (2003) argued that women can self-assess the condition and involution of their uterus in the postpartum period. As part of the larger Blood Loss in the Post Partum (BLiPP) study (Marchant et al., 1999), they asked women whether they had felt for their own uterus since the birth of the baby. The majority of women had not done so (67%) but 31% had tried to feel their own uterus; some had been unable to find it (15%). Others had tried but were unsure what they were feeling (49%), and 36% were able to describe the position, size and texture.

Palpation of a woman's uterus provides an opportunity to discuss the signs of normal involution and demonstrate how to do this herself. Advising women on how to palpate their own uterus early in the postpartum period promotes an understanding by women of their own body and returns the ability to monitor their own health to each woman. It can also provide an opportunity to discuss the signs and symptoms of postpartum haemorrhage and the midwife can provide an explanation of how to palpate the uterus (rub up a contraction), should this occur, along with stressing the importance of accessing professional help. It also provides an opportunity to discuss signs and symptoms of uterine infection, and the need to contact the midwife for a fuller assessment. Both are important when women are at home or going home in the early postpartum period.

Descriptions or measurements, when done, need to be consistently and accurately recorded, whether recorded by the midwife or by the woman during the postpartum period.

Vaginal blood loss

In the first hour following birth the midwife should observe and assess the woman's blood loss and physical condition in order to exclude primary postpartum haemorrhage (MOH, 2012). It is important for a midwife to discuss with the woman the blood loss following birth and what would constitute normal or excessive bleeding.

If there are concerns regarding excessive blood loss at any time, the midwife should check the blood pressure and pulse; a rapid pulse and low blood pressure would confirm that the blood loss is affecting the maternal physiology.

Assessing normal vaginal blood loss is subjective, and the volume of blood loss is difficult to measure when it occurs over several days and weeks. Immediately after the birth, women should expect the vaginal blood loss to be heavy and this may continue for the first few days (Bick et al., 2009). It is also normal for blood loss to be heavier following breastfeeding. The amount of blood loss should start to diminish over the first few days, but the duration of blood loss is variable (Bick et al., 2009). It is not unusual for women to pass blood clots as part of vaginal fluid loss; the size and frequency of these clots need to be described as these may indicate excessive or prolonged bleeding. Marchant (2003) suggests that using familiar items to identify and record the size of clots can be a useful guide in assessing the extent and size of blood clots and the extent of postpartum bleeding. Another method of determining the extent of postpartum blood loss is by how frequently a woman changes her sanitary pad, although this has to be interpreted with some caution, as some pads are more absorbent than others and some women will change pads more frequently depending on their hygiene requirements. Changing sanitary pads frequently because of full pads (several times in an hour) would be an indication of heavy, possibly excessive, vaginal bleeding.

Each woman is an individual and will have different expectations of vaginal blood loss following the birth; the midwife needs to use and integrate all these methods to obtain an overall picture of the woman's blood loss and to assess whether it is a problem for that woman.

Women may be reluctant to discuss vaginal loss, so it is important for midwives to discuss the subject during postnatal visits and to reassure women if they are concerned about the amount or continuation of blood loss. Asking women to describe their vaginal loss and listening to concerns related to the amount of blood loss is useful in determining whether the amount of vaginal blood loss is extensive and life threatening or within normal expectations. Documentation of the nature of the blood loss needs to be reflective of the woman's words and experiences. Recording the blood loss in the woman's words will also increase the participation of the woman in monitoring her health, as well as aiding in the detection of ill-health (Marchant et al., 2003).

CLINICAL POINT

Secondary postpartum haemorrhage

Secondary postpartum haemorrhage is defined as any abnormal or excessive bleeding from the uterus between 24 hours and 12 weeks after giving birth (Alexander et al., 2002). The cause is thought to be the retention of fragments of the placenta or membranes, or both, in the uterus potentially causing infection or preventing the uterus from contracting. Incidence is considered to be approximately 0.5%–2% of births in developed countries. For further information see Chapter 41.

Signs and symptoms

- Sudden and profuse blood loss or persistent increased blood loss
- Faintness or dizziness
- Low blood pressure and tachycardia

An increase in blood loss along with uterine tenderness and/or raised temperature could indicate endometritis or retained products of conception, and would require referral to a medical practitioner. If a woman is feeling unwell and an infection is suspected, the midwife should always take the temperature and pulse as part of her assessment to check for pyrexia and tachycardia.

CRITICAL THINKING EXERCISE

When considering blood loss following birth, how do you think it should be recorded? How do women describe their blood loss to you? Do women discuss blood loss spontaneously or does the midwife always ask?

Afterpains

Many women experience cramping and uterine pains following the birth which are generally called '**afterpains**'; they are more common in multiparous women, with frequency increasing with parity, but can also be experienced by primiparous women (Deussen et al., 2020). Afterpains are uterine contractions that can last for 4–7 days following the birth but are strongest in the first hours / days following birth. They are experienced as abdominal cramping and are frequently described as painful although the intensity of the pain varies for each woman. The pain is related to contraction and retraction of the uterine myometrium, which is caused by the release of oxytocin following birth and during breastfeeding. Afterpains can cause a significant level of pain that can be debilitating and distressing with the pain described as 'aching' and 'grinding' and, for some women, 'excruciating' (Jangsten et al., 2011). The afterpains can start within 2 hours of the birth and are often most intense in the first 12–24 hours and during breastfeeding. Acknowledging this pain and discussing ways of alleviating the pain is an important aspect of providing care.

CLINICAL POINT

Afterpains

The following practical support for women with afterpains was identified through audit and a review of the literature by midwives working at Rangiora Hospital (New Zealand) (Waite, 2002). Practical advice includes:

- frequent emptying of the bladder
- regular oral analgesia
- gentle massage of the fundus by the mother
- a heat pack applied to the abdomen
- applying pressure to the abdomen by the mother lying on her stomach with a pillow against the lower abdomen

However, none of the above has strong evidence to support its use because there is a lack of high-quality research evidence.

RESEARCH ACTIVITY

The information provided in the list above has been accumulated through practice experience and has not been evaluated. Midwives and women have found these measures helpful as a means of alleviating afterpains non-medically. Further research is required to ascertain the most effective methods of alleviating afterpains.

How would you undertake research to investigate this area further? What research designs could be used?

A Cochrane systematic review of the relief of afterpains compared different types of analgesia to determine what works best for afterpains (Deussen et al., 2020). The review included 28 randomised controlled trials involving 2749 women, although 11 of the 28 studies excluded breastfeeding women. The results indicate that non-steroidal anti-inflammatory drugs (NSAIDs) such as aspirin and naproxen were better than a placebo or opioids at relieving the pain. Paracetamol may be as effective as NSAIDs, with aspirin and naproxen not recommended when breastfeeding. Alternative therapies such as herbal analgesia and transcutaneous electrical nerve stimulation (TENS) did not have sufficient evidence to provide certainty of benefit. There are more studies being undertaken which may help to increase the certainty of evidence going forward.

Bladder, bowel and perineal health

Bladder function

Immediately following the birth, a full bladder will prevent the uterus from fully contracting and can cause heavier vaginal blood loss and increase severity of afterpains. Women should be encouraged to pass urine as soon as possible after the birth and to micturate every 2–3 hours in the first day. Over-distension of the bladder can lead to permanent injury. The timing of when women pass urine following the birth should be recorded, with an expectation that the woman should void within 6 hours of the birth (Bick et al., 2009; NICE, 2006, 2015). A study reviewing the effects of regional anaesthesia on the urinary bladder following birth in 120 women found that, for the women who had a normal birth without regional anaesthesia (epidural), the urge to void returned within a median of 2 hours (range 46–397 min) (Foon et al., 2010). For the women who had a normal birth with regional anaesthesia, sensation returned at a median of nearly 4 hours (234 min, range 95–382 min); however, for women who had an elective caesarean section under spinal anaesthesia, the median time to return of sensation was more than 6 hours (374 min, range 172–692 min). It is clearly important that women who have had regional anaesthesia have careful follow-up by the midwife to ensure that the bladder does not become distended and normal **micturition** has resumed.

Most women experience increased diuresis following the birth and for up to 2–5 days. There may be stinging during micturition owing to grazes around the vulval area or perineal damage. There may also be some oedema around the urethra, giving the woman less control when passing urine or making it difficult to pass urine. For those women who have had a urinary catheter inserted during labour and birth, once the catheter has been removed the midwife should document the time and volume of first micturition to ensure full bladder function has returned. Asking women about frequency and control of bladder function will identify urinary problems and will often lead to discussion of pelvic floor muscle exercises, perineal healing and adequate fluid intake.

Following the birth, women should be encouraged to do pelvic floor muscle exercises regularly. A Cochrane review found that nearly a third of women leaked urine following the birth and nearly 10% had some form of faecal incontinence (Woodley et al., 2020). Pelvic floor muscle training was found to be beneficial for women—whether done during the antenatal period or postnatally. The purpose of pelvic floor muscle exercises is to strengthen the peri-vaginal and perianal musculature which increases the woman's control. Doing pelvic floor exercises can prevent urinary incontinence at 6 months (Woodley et al., 2020). Early structured pelvic floor exercises can prevent the onset of urinary incontinence in late pregnancy and reduces the risk following the birth. If urinary incontinence persists, women should be advised to seek specialist help (see Ch. 28).

Bowel function

Bowel movement can occur within 24 hours of the birth but can also be delayed for up to 3 days following the birth. This is due to the pregnancy hormones aiding bowel evacuation prior to labour and/or during birth. Constipation can be a problem for some women following the birth with symptoms including pain, discomfort, straining and a hard stool (Turawa et al., 2020). A Cochrane review evaluated the effectiveness and safety of interventions for preventing constipation during the postnatal period (Turawa et al., 2020). The review included five randomised controlled trials involving 1208 women. Four trials compared the giving of a laxative versus a placebo, whilst one trial compared a laxative with a stool-bulking agent and laxative for women who had surgery for a third-degree tear. The authors report insufficient evidence on the effectiveness and safety of using laxatives to be able to draw conclusions on their ability to prevent constipation. In addition there was no evidence of difference in constipation when laxative and a stool-bulking agent were used following third-degree tear surgery compared to a laxative only. There have been no trials looking at the provision of advice on diet and physical activity to prevent constipation.

Perianal pain and haemorrhoids are common during late pregnancy and following birth due to hormonal changes during this time (Lamb & Sanders, 2015). Haemorrhoids are the result of swollen veins around the anus becoming prolapsed and causing pain. Women may describe perianal discomfort, itching, burning, mucous discharge, sharp or dull pain which increases with defecation, painful protrusion at the anus and bleeding (Poskus et al., 2014). For further information see Chapter 41 on complications after birth.

Following birth, haemorrhoids can become worse owing to the pressure on the tissue during birth; they can take some time to resolve. There is an increased incidence of haemorrhoids following a forceps birth, a longer second stage and vaginal births of heavier babies (Bick et al., 2009; Poskus et al., 2014). Constipation and haemorrhoids are emotive issues and require sensitive discussion during pregnancy and in the days following the birth (Lamb &

Sanders, 2015). Avoidance of constipation is important as it can make haemorrhoids more extensive and painful. As the effects of progesterone decrease, haemorrhoids should improve, but for a small number of women haemorrhoids can continue for up to a year after the birth and will often recur and be worse with subsequent pregnancies (Williams et al., 2007). If the haemorrhoids are severe, swollen, extensively prolapsed or there is rectal bleeding there should be a referral to a health specialist for a full assessment (NICE, 2006, 2015).

Perineal care

Following birth, many women will experience some pain, swelling or tenderness in the **perineum**. A systematic review (Manresa et al., 2019) identified that:

- 42% of women with an intact perineum experienced perineal pain at 2 days following a vaginal birth; this reduced to 11% at 4–10 days following the birth
- 64.3% of women with first-degree perineal trauma experience pain at 2 days following birth decreasing to 25.5% on day 10
- 50–69% of women with second-degree trauma or episiotomy experienced perineal pain at 2 days, which reduced to 27% between 4–10 days.

Levels of pain are subjective, but women who have had some degree of perineal trauma (such as a tear or episiotomy) are more likely to have higher levels of perineal pain, which can last up to 3 months following birth (Manresa et al., 2019). A painful perineum can have a negative impact on a woman, because she may be unable to move freely, sitting can be uncomfortable and caring for her baby becomes more difficult, marring her enjoyment of the early motherhood experience. Recognition and acknowledgement that perineal pain is distressing is important, along with discussion about different methods of alleviating the pain and support of the choice that is culturally valid for the woman. (For a fuller discussion of perineal pain and healing, see Ch. 28.)

Where trauma has occurred, midwives should always check the perineum and assess the healing regularly until they are sure that full healing has occurred. Marchant et al. (2003) suggest that the level of perineal discomfort experienced or the degree of anxiety exhibited by women may mirror the progress of healing. A physical assessment of healing and exclusion of haematoma should always be considered, if perineal pain is increasing or the woman is concerned (Bick et al., 2009).

CRITICAL THINKING EXERCISE

Linda is a 34-year-old woman who has just had her second baby. It was a spontaneous birth and she had a second-degree tear. You visit her at home on her second day following the birth and she is complaining that her 'bum' is sore. What would you do next? What are the possible causes of the pain? What advice would you give her?

Sexual health and contraception

Sexual health, sexual desire and the resumption of sex following the birth is influenced by a range of factors and are often topics that can be difficult for some women and midwives to discuss. Transition to parenthood involves changes and adjustments to the couple's relationship and includes the resumption of their physical sexual relationship. Women have identified several factors that affect their sexuality and sexual patterns following birth. These include changes to body image, sleep deprivation and changing lifestyles. Woolhouse et al. (2012) found that the changes to lifestyle following birth affected sexual intimacy and sexual relationships. In their Australian study they interviewed 18 women between 2.5 and 3.5 years following a first birth. They found that extreme tiredness, changing lifestyles and body image affected the women's sexual desire and libido. Women felt guilt and feelings of failure as a result of these changes. They concluded that it is important for couples to stay connected and find ways to have quality time together and work as a team in the transition to parenthood.

Each woman and her partner will have an individual response to the changes that occur following childbirth. These changes can lead to a deepening of intimacy and a stronger relationship, or alternatively may lead to sexual problems and difficulties which over time can have an impact on the couple's relationship. It is important that midwives discuss sex and sexuality during the postnatal period.

Women experiencing pain during sexual intercourse (dyspareunia) should be referred to their general practitioner for ongoing support and treatment. For further discussion on dyspareunia see Chapter 41.

Discussing sex and sexuality will naturally lead to a discussion about contraception.

When should contraception begin again?

Contraception counselling should be a routine part of antenatal care so that women have a contraception plan identified prior to the birth (Ministry of Health, 2020a). If the woman is not, or is partially, breastfeeding then contraception needs to begin prior to the first ovulation following birth. Menses can begin as early as day 35 to day 40 postpartum. Ovulation would have happened 12–16 days prior to this. Therefore, the contraceptive method for women who have resumed intercourse should begin before day 21. Women should be advised to aim for an interval of 12 months or more between pregnancies so as to reduce the risk of preterm birth, low birthweight and small for gestational age babies (Ministry of Health, 2020a). This is especially important for women who have had a caesarean section. Most methods of contraception can be started immediately following the birth apart from the combined oral contraceptive pill. A fuller discussion of contraception is provided in Chapter 34.

Nutrition and weight loss following birth

Food is often associated with caring and nurturing, as well as social occasions. Women need to be well nourished following the birth, so regular meals and fluids will help to promote health and wellbeing. Most women will resume eating their normal diet and should eat when hungry. Breastfeeding requires an increase in calories, so women will often have an increased appetite during lactation.

The return to pre-pregnant weight is gradual and for most women can take up to 6–12 months, although for between 14% and 20% of women there may be an increase in weight after the birth (Lovelady, 2011). For most women, breastfeeding helps with weight loss following the birth, but this appears to be less effective in women who are obese (BMI >35 kg/m^2) (Lovelady, 2011). New Zealand and Australia have high rates of obesity (Australian Government, 2020; Ministry of Health, 2020b). Excessive weight gain during pregnancy and/or postpartum weight retention are risk factors that can lead to obesity in women (Ministry of Health, 2014). Midwives should advise women of the benefits of weight loss and discuss healthy eating, activity and breastfeeding as strategies for encouraging a return to pre-pregnancy weight following the birth (Ministry of Health, 2014). The UK NICE (2010) guidelines provide information on weight management before, during and after the birth; Box 30.10 identifies the information provided for the postpartum period.

Box 30.10 A summary of the NICE guidelines on weight management for before, during and after birth advise the following

- Midwives should encourage women to breastfeed and reassure that eating a healthy diet along with regular moderate-intensity physical activity will support a gradual weight loss and not adversely affect the quality of breast milk.
- During the postpartum period midwives should provide advice on healthy eating and physical exercise that is individualised to each woman and her family. This advice will need to take into account the woman's role within the family and how she can be supported by her partner and wider family.
- Women who are overweight or obese should be asked if they have concerns about their weight and would like further support and refer them to appropriate community-based services.

For more information about healthy eating and exercise postpartum see Chapter 21.

(Source: NICE, 2010)

Cardiovascular health

All women should receive active and ongoing assessment of their physiological health in the immediate postnatal period (1 hour) (Ministry of Health, 2012). Immediately following the birth, it is usual to take a baseline temperature, pulse and blood pressure. It is now advised that blood pressure is measured again within 6 hours of the birth to exclude preeclampsia (NICE, 2006, 2015). While there is little evidence to support the routine taking of temperature, pulse and blood pressure on a daily basis, there should always be individual decision making regarding the necessity of these physical observations. For women who are admitted to a hospital (postnatal ward) following birth some regions of Australia and New Zealand have introduced a maternity early warning system (MEWS). This involves the use of an adult vital signs chart which uses eight vital sign parameters specific to maternity to calculate an early warning score. This then triggers a response based on the local hospital escalation pathways so that the woman's condition is managed appropriately. The frequency of observations depends on the woman's health assessment. Women who have had hypertension and/or preeclampsia during their pregnancy should have their blood pressure monitored for four days, followed by weekly blood pressure measurements (MOH, 2022). In many Australian maternity services, women who have had hypertension in pregnancy will be required to have a 4-day stay in hospital for monitoring of blood pressure. A recent UK study demonstrates that guidelines for postnatal management of hypertension in pregnancy are not routinely implemented, particularly the postnatal follow-up after discharge (Bick et al., 2020). Women need to be encouraged to attend for follow-up appointments with GPs and cardiovascular specialists. Temperature and pulse should be taken if there are concerns regarding postpartum infection at any time during the postpartum. Pyrexia, a respiratory rate of more than 25 breaths per min and tachycardia are indicative of postpartum sepsis (Health Quality & Safety Commission NZ, 2018) (see Ch. 41 for more detail).

CLINICAL POINT

Signs and symptoms of uterine infection

- Pyrexia—temperature above 37.5°C
- Rigors
- Abdominal pain
- Offensive vaginal loss
- Excessive blood loss

This is discussed further in Chapter 41.

The cardiovascular system returns to a near pre-pregnant state rapidly following the birth. If there has been excessive bleeding at any time, an assessment of haemoglobin level is important and necessary to determine

Box 30.11 Research summary—diagnosing anaemia

A New Zealand study explored the diagnosis and treatment of anaemia amongst 21 midwives and 189 women who met the criteria for anaemia at registration (Calje & Skinner, 2017). The study found that 22.8% (n = 43) of the women had haemoglobin tested following the birth, 38 women had a blood loss of more than 500 mL and, of these, 28 (73%) had their haemoglobin tested. All five women with a blood loss of more than 1500 mL had a haemoglobin test. Overall 21 out of the 43 tested had a haemoglobin level of less than 100 g/L, with seven (33.3%) prescribed iron.

whether iron therapy is required. Additionally, if a woman has had low iron levels prior to the birth, postpartum assessment of haemoglobin should be undertaken. Signs of postpartum anaemia include pallor, tiredness, dizziness, loss of appetite and oedema (East, 2012). Low iron levels can have a long-term effect on the woman's health postpartum and may lead to increased incidence of postpartum depression. If the woman is diagnosed as being iron deficient then treatment will be necessary; the type of treatment is dependent on the haemoglobin level and may vary from oral iron to intravenous iron therapy or blood transfusion (Breyman et al., 2011) (Box 30.11).

Provision of anti-D immunoglobulin for Rhesus-negative women

To prevent isoimmunisation for the mother and Rhesus haemolytic disease of the newborn (as discussed in Ch. 22), women who are Rhesus negative, and their babies, should be assessed to see whether there is a need for anti-D immunoglobulin administration. This is done by taking blood from the placenta immediately following the birth for the direct Coombs test (level of maternal antibodies in cord blood) and taking blood from the mother for the Kleihauer test (number of fetal cells in maternal blood). If indicated, anti-D should be administered to the mother *within 72 hours* of the birth to reduce the risk of RhD alloimmunisation. A dose of 625 IU is recommended with additional doses indicated dependent on the volume of fetomaternal haemorrhage although consultation with a transfusion medicine specialist is recommended if a dose of more than 1250 IU is indicated (https://www.nzblood.co.nz/assets/Transfusion-Medicine/PDFs/111G130.pdf). If anti-D immunoglobulin has not been provided within this time span a dose given within 10 days may provide some protection (NZ Blood, 2013). Midwives need to be alert and ensure that all Rhesus-negative women receive these tests and treatment if required.

Administration of rubella

Women who are not immune to rubella can be immunised following the birth and prior to discharge from hospital with the measles–mumps–rubella (MMR) vaccine provided. This can be given alongside the anti-D as long as separate syringes and sites are used. If not given simultaneously, the MMR should be given 3 months after the anti-D has been given (NICE, 2006, 2015). Women should be advised that pregnancy should be avoided within 1 month of having the MMR.

Assessment for deep vein thrombosis

In the first few days following birth, many women may get swollen ankles even when they may not have had ankle oedema in pregnancy; this is due to physiological changes in the renal system (discussed in Ch. 29). Elevation and reassurance that oedema is transitory is generally all that is required. Deep vein thrombosis (DVT) is a blood clot that occurs in the veins of the leg. Pregnancy and birth can predispose to venous thromboembolism because of the increased coagulability of the platelets. Early ambulation helps to reduce the risk of deep vein thrombosis or pulmonary embolism. The midwife needs to be aware of the signs and symptoms of both these complications and refer to a medical practitioner if she has any concerns (see Ch. 41).

It is usual to check for pain, redness or swelling in the legs on a regular basis to rule out deep vein thrombosis and thrombophlebitis. This assessment will often lead to discussions regarding ankle oedema and promotion of health through exercise. This is also an opportune time to identify whether the woman has returned to smoking and to discuss the increased risk of thromboembolism when smoking. It is also important to discuss the need to provide a smoke-free environment for the baby, along with strategies for smoking cessation or reduction for those women/families who smoke.

CLINICAL POINT

Thromboembolism

- Encourage mobilisation as early as possible—as appropriate to the birth.
- If a woman has calf pain, redness or swelling she should be immediately referred for assessment for deep vein thrombosis.
- If a woman has shortness of breath or chest pain she should be immediately referred for assessment for pulmonary thromboembolism.

For more information see Chapter 41.

Regular exercise following birth

Women should be supported to consider incorporating regular exercise into their daytime routines both before and after the birth. Exercise is increasingly being recognised as important—not just for weight control, but also for its effects on mood. Increased levels of postpartum depression were found in women who did not engage in antenatal exercise (Guida et al., 2012). A small randomised controlled trial undertaken in Australia found that women who received an 8-week mother and baby program which included specialised exercise had significant improvements in wellbeing scores and less depressive symptoms following the birth compared with women who were not randomised to this intervention (Norman et al., 2010). The NICE guidelines for weight management (2010) advise that, for women who have had a normal pregnancy and birth, a mild exercise program of walking, pelvic floor muscle exercises and stretching can begin immediately following the birth, but high-impact activity should not be resumed too soon after the birth. For women who have had complex pregnancies and caesarean births, physical activity should not be resumed until after the 6–8-week check. Midwives need to emphasise the importance for women to undertake pelvic floor exercises, regardless of type of birth, during the postpartum period. For more information on how to do pelvic floor exercises see Chapter 21.

Summary

The midwife needs to discuss and assess the physical recovery of each woman during the postnatal period and ensure that any follow-up appointments and referrals are attended to. Discussion can lead to identification of support and treatment for particular problems, as well as reassuring each woman of the normality of her experience.

EMOTIONAL AND PSYCHOSOCIAL RESPONSES TO CHANGE

Maternal mood and emotions

As discussed at the start of this chapter, the transition from pregnancy through the birth to becoming parents is a challenging time for a mother, her partner and the wider family. A range of emotions is felt in the postpartum period, and many women describe relief, euphoria, joy, pleasure, and also vulnerability, despair, fear and concern. These emotions will vary depending on the woman, the birth, her own life experiences, family roles and history, all of which will influence her adjustment to the new or expanded responsibilities of becoming a mother.

Hormonal influences or 'baby blues' (phases 1 and 2)

Following the birth, many women feel high or elated and are very happy to socialise with their visitors, friends and relatives. This high mood often turns to a low mood at some point in the first few days following birth, and the characteristic tearfulness, anxiety and irritability are often called the 'baby blues' or the 'postnatal blues' (NICE, 2018). Despite a great deal of research, the cause is still unknown, although one theory is that it occurs because of the decrease in oestrogen and progesterone levels along with changes in the blood electrolyte balance and in the balance of serotonin and dopamine (neurotransmitters) (Rankin, 2017). It is estimated that 50%–80% of women experience this mood swing, which is generally transient and lasts only a few days (Dennis & Hodnett, 2007).

For women who experience the blues, there is a tendency for mood swings, tearfulness, and exhaustion or to feel overwhelmed, along with increased discomfort and pain levels. It often coincides with the onset of full lactation and unsettled behaviour in the baby. Midwives need to make women aware of the signs and symptoms of the 'baby blues', and help the women to rest and have family support and ensure physical comfort (such as food, fluids, and being pain free and able to get some sleep) at this time to promote wellbeing (NICE, 2006).

Some women may exhibit a continued period of low mood following the birth; this may be tied to increased levels of anxiety and/or antenatal anxiety/depression. It is important that the midwife is able to discuss this with the woman and screen for postpartum depression. The Edinburgh Postnatal Depression Scale (EPDS) and the Postpartum Depression Screening Scale (PDSS) are two tools that midwives can use to assess for possible pathological postnatal distress/depression before making appropriate referral for specialist care (for more in-depth discussion see Ch. 35).

CRITICAL THINKING EXERCISE

You are visiting Kelly, who is 3 days postpartum following a normal birth at the local birthing unit. She was discharged home this morning and appeared to be recovering well until today. During your visit she is tearful and upset. She says she feels tired and aches 'everywhere'. The baby is feeding frequently and isn't settling between feeds. Kelly's partner has gone out to get some food and do some other errands.

1. What are the issues causing Kelly to be upset?
2. What is the midwife's role in this situation?
3. When will you plan to visit again?

Emotional support, physical support and social expectations (phase 3)

As discussed at the start of this chapter, the transition to motherhood is challenging for many women. Some describe being in an 'in between' space as they develop a new self-identity as a mother / parent and redefine relationships within their own cultural context (Finlayson et al., 2020). The first few months can be blurred by tiredness, an overwhelming feeling of responsibility and constantly being available for their baby. In their recent synthesis of literature Finlayson et al. describe that woman want to feel 'cared for', to be seen as individuals and for their needs as well as their baby's needs to be recognised and met by health professionals and others close to them (Finlayson et al., 2020).

Social support is imperative for postnatal health and wellbeing. Studies that follow women over time consistently demonstrate that those who have social support, including positive partner relationship, family support and a peer network, have better mental health in the first year after birth (Giallo et al., 2017; Ginja et al., 2018; Herbell & Zauszniewski, 2019; Vaezi et al., 2019). Leahy-Warren et al. (2012) suggest four components of support, *emotional, informational, appraisal* and *instrumental*. The effectiveness of social support depends on the perceived need and effectiveness and on the relationship between the giver and receiver of the support. Not all have easy access to support; for example, migrant women and others in marginalised groups describe being alone, isolated and often fearful (Leahy-Warren et al., 2018; Prevatt & Desmarais, 2018; Schmied et al., 2017). Social relationships can provide women with a supportive resource during transition periods as well as promoting a sense of self-worth and psychological wellbeing (Tani & Castagna, 2017). One well-tried community strategy is new parents' groups and these peer-support initiatives have been evaluated positively by parents for the social support they offer (McLean et al., 2020). Over the past decade or so, women are increasingly turning to technology to access social support, many joining online communities. However, a recent systematic review of the literature did not find that pregnancy-specific platforms enhanced the perceived social support, wellbeing and self-efficacy of pregnant women (Ginja et al., 2018).

REFLECTIVE THINKING EXERCISE

Tanya is a single teenage mother living with her family. She has been well supported by her own mother during the first few weeks postnatally, but now she says she is feeling lonely, all her friends are at school and she has no one to talk to. Her mother is increasingly providing care for the baby.

How would you support Tanya in her mothering role? What groups are there in your area that could help support Tanya?

A study from the United Kingdom exploring loneliness found that any life transition can be a key trigger for loneliness (British Red Cross & Co-Op, 2016). This study found that young new mothers (18–25 years) had an increased risk of loneliness. These young mothers may have had good social connections prior to the birth but they experienced diminishing support from family and friends over the months following the birth. They perceived negative 'judgments' from older mothers and others in the community about their choice to have a child at a young age. This lack of understanding undermined the woman's confidence, raised their anxiety levels and stopped them from engaging with others.

Partners have also identified changes in emotional health with men describing stress, exhaustion, poor concentration and irritability in the first year following the birth of the baby (Darwin et al., 2017). Darwin et al. (2017) interviewed 42 first-time fathers in the UK, finding that they felt the need to support their partner and protect their partnership as an important part of navigating fatherhood.

Midwives have an important role to play in offering formal social support to women. Schmied et al. (2011) conceptualised this as occurring along a continuum from authentic presence at one end, perceived as effective support, to disconnected encounters at the other, perceived as ineffective or even discouraging and counterproductive. A trusting relationship, organisational systems and services that offer models of continuity of midwifery care or peer support models are more likely to facilitate authentic presence, because these models foster relationship building. Added to the challenge for health professionals of fragmented services, however, are staff shortage and duplication or multiplication of tasks, which mitigate against giving time and being with women, and professionals may learn to cope by conveying temporal pressure to women (Schmied et al., 2011).

It is important that midwives ask women about their support network and discuss strategies to ensure that the support provided by family and friends is what women need. Midwives can support women by trying to make motherhood a special time in which a new mother feels valued and cared for; by providing care based on individual need with a balance between reassurance, support and physical monitoring, they can also help women to establish their own support networks (Ockenden, 2000; Podkolinski, 1998).

Birth stories and debriefing

In the first few days following birth, most women will tell their family and visitors about their labour and birth. Often the story is told repetitively and with incredible detail, as the woman sorts out what happened and when. There may be differences between the woman's perceptions of the labour and birth and the perceptions of the caregivers, which can be explored through discussions. Women prefer to discuss their birth experience with the midwife who was present during the birth where possible, regardless of how normal or complex the birth was (Dahlberg et al., 2016). These birth stories are retained for many years and will be told at different times around pregnancy and births of friends and relatives. It is important that a midwife is aware of women's need to assimilate the events of the births and takes time to discuss with each woman her perceptions of the birth, what was said and done, who was present, and the order of events.

This helps the woman to build a picture of her labour and birth. Ideally, the midwife who attended the birth will talk through the birth with the woman; but if this is not possible another midwife can assist a woman with this by reference to notes and by giving the woman time to talk.

In building her picture of the birth, a woman draws on her own experiences, comments and discussions with the people who were present during her labour and birth, and the documentation and timelines provided for her by her midwife through the midwifery notes. Lyons (1998) suggests that, in writing notes and in talking through birth stories, a midwife should focus on the positive qualities shown by the mother, especially in situations where the mother may have a sense of failure or disappointment. A Cochrane review explored the effects of debriefing interventions compared with standard postnatal care as a way of preventing psychological trauma following birth (Bastos et al., 2015). This review found little high-quality evidence of benefit or harm from debriefing as a preventative for psychological trauma. More research is needed into the importance of debriefing—not just as a way to prevent psychological harm but also as a way of supporting an improved understanding for the woman and her family about her labour and birth.

Spiritual and cultural health

Supporting the woman's spiritual needs requires a full understanding of the woman's spiritual health. This is enhanced through continuity of care from the midwife along with active listening. Some women can articulate these clearly; others require gentle, persistent delving if the midwife detects spiritual pain. The midwife might not feel qualified to support the woman in spiritual difficulty but through the woman's family she can involve the woman's own spiritual guides.

Like spiritual health, cultural health also requires care and sensitivity. In New Zealand, healthcare professionals are expected to develop and meet standards of cultural competence (*Health Practitioners Competence Assurance Act 2003, 2003*) and the midwifery profession has embraced the frameworks of cultural safety, midwifery partnership and Tūranga Kaupapa as outlined in Chapter 11. Midwives must acknowledge and respect cultures that may be different from the dominant culture or from their own in order to provide individualised and woman-centred care.

The Australian *National Competency Standards for the Midwife* (Nursing and Midwifery Board of Australia (NMBA), 2018a) state that a midwife ensures practice is culturally safe by planning, implementing and evaluating strategies for providing culturally safe practice for women, their families and colleagues. In practice this is demonstrated by the midwife incorporating knowledge of cross-cultural and historical factors into practice, demonstrating respect for differences in cultural meanings and responses to health and maternity care, recognising the specific needs of Aboriginal and Torres Strait Islander women and their communities, and recognising and respecting customary law.

Ending the midwife–woman partnership (phase 4)

Although the length of time that midwives care for women in the postnatal period may vary between New Zealand and Australia, the principles of bringing the midwife–woman relationship to a close are the same. The focus is on holistic completion of the midwife–woman partnership through thorough assessments of mother and baby, clear communication and debriefing on care and smooth transfer of care to Well Woman and Well Child providers as appropriate. The midwife signals the closure of the relationship in advance and negotiates with 'the completion of the midwifery partnership with the woman' (Standard Nine of the NZCOM Standards for Practice (NZCOM, 2015, p. 26). Standard 2 of the Nursing and Midwifery Board of Australia *National Competency Standards for the Midwife* (NMBA, 2018a) identifies that the midwife 'concludes professional relationships in a way that differentiates the boundaries between professional and personal relationships' (p. 4). The parting between midwife and woman / whānau should be signalled at the first introductory visit with an explanation on how the partnership begins, and when it conventionally ends. The professional boundaries of the midwife–woman relationship are well defined in the ICM *International Code of Ethics for Midwives* (2008). Women should be reminded of the approaching conclusion of the relationship at the beginning of the postpartum period and again when setting the final discharge visit. The timing of this should be about the woman's readiness (or not) for discharge.

At the final discharge visit the midwife is required to fully assess both maternal and newborn health (Box 30.12). The midwife's approach to the final assessment should be a holistic one, seeking information on the woman's current health status and following up on issues that have arisen in the weeks since the birth (e.g. with regard to the woman's physical, emotional and psychosocial health). It is important to attend to any outstanding social health (e.g. legal or support) issues. These may include transport needs, budget services, legal services (e.g. around immigration status), interpreter services, low-cost counselling options and new mothers' groups. Also consider issues such as whether the woman plans to return to work and, if so, how she will continue breastfeeding and manage care of her family. Those mothers who plan to return to work or study prior to their baby reaching 6 months may need advice and support to continue breastfeeding exclusively or fully.

The midwife contributes to the woman's emotional health when she concludes the partnership in a timely, respectful and mutually satisfying way that meets the woman's expectations. A formal conclusion to the midwife–woman relationship allows the midwife to 'write the ending of the story with each woman'.

REVIEWING AND ASSESSING THE WOMAN'S HEALTH PRIOR TO DISCHARGE FROM CARE

In New Zealand, under Section 88 of the New Zealand Public Health and Disability Act 2000, the LMC is responsible for conducting comprehensive examinations of both mother and baby prior to discharge and transfer of the baby to a Well Child provider (MOH, 2007). Box 30.13 provides a set of questions which help to identify the

Box 30.12 Final postnatal visit, NZCOM decision point

This timing provides for the completion of the midwifery relationship and feedback about the care given.

Women's information shared from assessment and examination

- Review history to date with the woman including pregnancy, labour and birth and postnatal recovery.
- Assess and review the woman's physical health status and discuss with her outcomes of this assessment and any health issues that are ongoing, ensuring the woman has follow-up if needed.
- Assess the woman's emotional wellbeing and family/whānau support.

Full physical and developmental assessment of baby

- Assess and review baby's health status and discuss with the mother the outcomes of this including those of any screening investigations that have been conducted to date. Include partner/whānau as woman wishes.
- Ensure the baby has follow-up if needed in relation to this assessment and review if there are any concerns.
- Also consider:
  - whether the baby has been seen by Well Child/Tamariki Ora service
  - observing the baby during an entire feed—breast or bottle
  - weighing the baby prior to discharge depending on previous timing of weight and measurements
  - parenting discussion
  - reinforcing public health messages, e.g. immunisation, safe sleeping, family violence, smoke-free environments.

Health information shared

- Cervical screening.
- Contraception.
- Appointment with general practice/Well Child/Tamariki Ora by 6 weeks for the baby for examination/immunisation.
- Self-care, including nutrition and exercise, rest and support, signs of postnatal depression
- Discuss local support groups that may be of interest to the woman.
- Discuss Midwifery Standards Review and consumer feedback.
- Confirm this is the end of midwifery care but ensure the woman knows when and how to seek assistance now the midwifery relationship is completed.

Box 30.13 Final physical assessment questions to identify a full return to health and to support ongoing referral to other healthcare providers

- Are there any concerns related to breastfeeding?
- Has the uterus involuted completely or is it still palpable abdominally? Is there any pain or tenderness?
- If there is a caesarean scar, has it fully healed?
- Has the vaginal bleeding stopped? If there is bleeding, is it **lochial** or menstrual?
- If there has been any perineal, vaginal wall or labial damage (sutured or not), how well healed is this area? Use a good light and gloved hands to inspect the area.
- Does the woman have any concerns regarding bowel and/or urinary function or incontinence?
- Was the woman diagnosed with gestational diabetes? If so ensure that the primary healthcare provider (GP) is informed so that they can offer screening for type 2 diabetes at 3 months postpartum using HbA_{1c} (MOH, 2014). Make sure the woman also has this information.
- Was there a hypertensive disorder of pregnancy? Has it now resolved? If not, ensure ongoing care and communication with the woman's general practitioner (MOH, 2018).
- What is her activity level? Does she feel unusually fatigued? Have you assessed for anaemia?
- Was she a smoker before pregnancy? What is her smoking status at discharge?
- Are there concerns related to family violence—has she been screened again postnatally?
- Psychosocial health—are there concerns related to anxiety or depression?
- Is she adapting to her parenting role well?
- Does she have support? Does she feel supported?
- Does she need immunisation for rubella for herself?
- Is she on the cervical screening register; does she need cervical screening?
- Have you discussed sexual health and contraception?

health and ongoing support needs of the woman to help the midwife in her referral to other healthcare providers. The expectation is that the midwife will continue her responsibility to provide care until 6 weeks postpartum. Many women will meet with the Well Child provider at some time between 4 and 6 weeks so the timing of the discharge visit may vary.

In Australia at this time there is no similar mandatory requirement for midwives in Australia. Nevertheless, Australian midwives do conduct assessments of women and babies prior to discharge from maternity services.

Family violence screening

Domestic and family violence is a complex issue that spans all socioeconomic strata. Women should be screened for family violence during pregnancy (see Ch. 23) and again during the postnatal period at a suitable time prior to discharge. In New Zealand this is between 1 and 6 weeks postpartum, in Australia this is often undertaken by the maternal child and family health nurse between 1 and 4 weeks postpartum. It is important to ensure screening occurs in a safe environment for the woman (without the partner). If family violence is disclosed at any time, the midwife needs to consider the safety of the woman and her family. In addition, if there are concerns about undisclosed family violence, the midwife should consider sharing her concerns with other agencies / health professionals (GP, Well Child provider). For more information on family violence see Chapter 35.

Cervical screening

Cervical screening is a program of regular diagnostic investigation of cervical cytology among a population of women. Some midwives use the final discharge visit to offer the woman a cervical smear if it is due. In Australia, only midwives who have been credentialled in performing smears are able to undertake these. Regardless of whether a smear is taken, the discharge visit is an appropriate time to provide information about the importance of ongoing cervical screening and address any questions the woman may have. It is important that midwives are familiar with their college's consensus guidelines and updates.

Well Woman referral

Although New Zealand women can choose midwife-only care during pregnancy and childbirth, they will need to determine whether they want to be referred to a GP following the completion of their maternity care. Midwives should ensure that both the woman and her GP have summary documentation of the woman's maternity care. The College of Midwives and Royal New Zealand College of General Practitioners have produced a standardised form for referral (Fig. 30.4). Some women may choose not to be referred to a Well Woman care provider or may choose an organisation such as the family planning clinic for their ongoing sexual healthcare.

In Australia, at discharge from maternity services, a summary of the woman's maternity care and health of her baby (discharge summary) is sent to the woman's GP and to the maternal, child and family health nursing services. Practices vary across states and territories and between public and private hospitals. For example, in a national survey of midwives, 77.4% indicated that their maternity service referred women to maternal child and family health nursing services and around 50% referred them to general practice (Psaila et al., 2014). In Queensland, discharge summaries were most commonly sent to GPs (83%), and less commonly to child and family health nurses (52%). Discharge summaries were usually disseminated within 1 week of discharge (87%), but did not capture any information about care provided by domiciliary services (Jenkinson et al., 2014). Both these studies indicated significant gaps in the information provided in discharge summaries, particularly in psychosocial and cultural information, and post-discharge advice (Jenkinson et al., 2014; Psaila et al., 2014).

Documentation: health record

Maintaining an accurate record of clinical health is a fundamental part of midwifery practice and enhances the provision of care (NZCOM, 2021). The New Zealand College of Midwives has developed a toolkit (keteparaha) designed to support and enhance midwifery record keeping in Aotearoa. This describes a healthcare record as 'an identified individual's health and the health care they received (NZCOM, 2021, p. 6). Health records may be on paper or online and held by an organisation, service provider or the consumer themselves. In Australia, similar health records are maintained and increasingly there is a move towards electronic record keeping—for example, e-maternity in New South Wales—but this varies across states and territories.

When providing maternity care, midwives are required to: 'maintain purposeful, ongoing, updated records and make them available to the woman and other relevant persons' (NZCOM Standard four, 2015, p. 21). Similarly in Australia, the *National Competency Standards for the Midwife* (standard 3) require the midwife to 'engage in timely consultation, referral and documentation' and 'uses relevant processes to identify, document and manage complexity and risk' (Nursing and Midwifery Board of Australia, *National Competency Standards for the Midwife*, 2018b, p. 4).

In New Zealand, midwives are encouraged to provide women with a copy of her maternity notes during care and at discharge from care. Principles are that the woman will have a complete record of the maternity care, with relevant information shared securely with other providers.

It is important that documentation of care is clear and comprehensible to women, with abbreviations and medical jargon avoided or explained. Language used should be professional non-judgmental and positively phrased. All clinical information and midwifery assessments,

POSTNATAL

Please ensure that the completed form is sent to the GP (below) and the Well Child provider by four weeks postpartum, and that a copy is given to the woman.

Date ____________________ Planned date of discharge from LMC ____________________

Dear Dr ____________________

I am writing to update you on my client and her baby who have been in my care.

Name ____________________ DOB __________ NHI __________

Address ____________________ Home telephone __________

____________________ Mobile number __________

____________________ Alternative contact number __________

Partner/family/social support ____________________

Pregnancy summary ____________________

Birth summary (including mode of birth) and postnatal period ____________________

Parity __________ Contraception ____________________

Baby's name ____________________ DOB __________ NHI __________

Sex __________ Gestation __________ Apgar score __________

Birth weight __________ Last recorded weight __________ Date __________

Newborn baby summary ____________________

Newborn metabolic screening ❑ Yes ❑ No

Newborn hearing screening ❑ Yes ❑ No

Red eye reflex done ❑ Yes ❑ No

Vitamin K ❑ IM Oral ❑ 1st ❑ 2nd ❑ 3rd ❑ Declined

Baby's feeding ❑ Exclusive breastfeeding ❑ Fully breastfeeding ❑ Partially breastfeeding ❑ Artificial feeding

Well Child provider notified ❑ Yes ❑ No

Summary of ongoing maternal and baby needs and referrals made ____________________

❑ I will follow up this summary with a phone call.

If you have any further questions please feel free to contact me.

Lead maternity carer ____________________

Contact details ____________________

FIGURE 30.4 Referral to GP/Well Child provider form (© New Zealand College of Midwives, https://www.midwife.org.nz/forms)

decisions and interventions should be recorded with enough detail to inform colleagues who may be sharing care and provide proper evidence of the care, including informed decision-making processes. Women should be provided with a copy of their notes, results of tests and any referral letters written to their general practitioner, Well Child provider or other specialist.

Retention of documentation

In New Zealand records must be kept safe for a period of 10 years (New Zealand Legislation, 1996). In Australia this period is usually 21 years, although there are differences across states and territories depending on local legislation. 'Safe' includes protecting the records from unauthorised access and locking them securely within fireproof and waterproof containers. If the woman wasn't provided with a copy of her maternity records, then she must always know where to find her records during the midwife's guardianship of them. When midwives cease to practise, those records in their care must be transferred to a nominated organisation or service provider. It is also required that midwives nominate in their wills the appropriate transfer or disposal of these documents in the event of their death.

Midwifery standards review

In New Zealand at the final discharge visit the midwife should offer the woman the opportunity to provide feedback through a consumer feedback questionnaire. This will involve explanation of the **Midwifery Standards Review** (MSR) and the role of the consumer feedback. Feedback can be provided either online (from the College of Midwives website, https://portal.midwife.org.nz/consumer-feedback) or on paper and the woman can remain anonymous if she chooses. This feedback enables a woman to provide her perspective on the midwifery care she has received and what this experience has meant for her. The feedback contributes to the midwife's MSR process and enables the women's views to be taken into consideration when the midwife reflects on her practice.

In New Zealand, MSR has been developed to provide a systematic process that enables the midwife, whatever her practice setting, to reflect on her midwifery practice with two reviewers—one midwife colleague and one consumer of midwifery services, each of whom has been specifically educated to do this work for the New Zealand College of Midwives. The design of the process reflects the midwifery profession's partnership with women, as well as the requirement for the midwife to be professionally accountable to herself, the women for whom she cares, and the profession (NZCOM, 2012). Undertaking MSR at least every 3 years is a Midwifery Council recertification requirement.

In Australia, the Midwifery Practice Review process is part of the continuing professional development program, MidPLUS, developed by the Australian College of Midwives, and launched in September 2007 (Griffiths & Homer, 2008). Once a woman is discharged from care, the midwife's obligation is governed by the Nursing and Midwifery Board of Australia *Midwife Standards for Practice* (NMBA, 2018b).

Conclusion

The postnatal period is the final transition, a time of major life change and one of potential stress as a woman becomes a mother and a couple becomes a family. Support from family, friends and healthcare professionals is important and can affect the emotional wellbeing and coping ability of each individual. How a woman adjusts to her new role will depend on her previous experiences, her family and her social roles, as well as the birth itself. Postnatal care should help women achieve a smooth transition into motherhood with as much attention given to women's psychological and emotional adaptations as to their physical recovery.

Assessment of maternal wellbeing is based on knowledge of the physiological, psychological and social changes in the postnatal period and how these may affect the woman's recovery. Sharing knowledge and experience with women enables and supports them to monitor their own health. There is need for flexibility, sensitivity and understanding from midwives when providing postnatal care.

Women have traditionally helped each other following childbirth by helping with domestic chores or caring for other children. There should be a focus on encouraging women to seek practical help and support at home from family, friends and community support groups, so that women are not expected to manage alone. As women go through each phase of the postnatal period in their own time, the focus of the midwives' visits will change. Providing support to women is about giving practical help, advice, positive feedback and praise. It needs to be done in a sensitive and caring way, which is individual to each woman and her family. Women value the support of a midwife whom they know and who has established their confidence and trust.

The final discharge visit in New Zealand is made by the midwife on conclusion of midwifery care at an appropriate time between 4 and 6 weeks. Both the woman and the baby must be thoroughly assessed and appropriate referrals should be made to Well Child and Well Woman services for ongoing healthcare. Documentation should be completed and health records appropriately stored. This visit concludes the midwife–woman partnership and it is an important opportunity to ensure that any physical, social or emotional health concerns are addressed.

Becoming a mother is challenging, exciting, and difficult; it involves physical, social, and emotional changes that women can manage successfully when provided with good care and support.

Review questions

1. Why is it necessary for a midwife to understand parental transition?
2. Identify and describe the aim of postnatal care.
3. How can a midwife promote promote optimal postnatal care in a hospital facility or at home?
4. Identify and describe the four phases of the postpartum period.
5. Discuss the physical assessment that a midwife should undertake during a postnatal visit.
6. Identify the emotional and social adaptations that a woman and her partner make in the first few weeks after the birth of a baby.
7. How can midwives support women during the postnatal period?
8. Outline a holistic health assessment of the woman at 6 weeks postpartum.
9. What professional obligations do midwives in your country have in relation to documentation and care of health records?
10. Explain the key aspects of how midwives complete the midwife–woman partnership relationship.

Online resources

National Institute for Health and Care Excellence (NICE), postnatal care: http://www.nice.org.uk/.

New Zealand support groups for fathers: http://fatherandchild.org.nz/.

Parents' Centres New Zealand Inc.: http://www.parentscentre.org.nz/parenting.

Plunket postnatal groups: http://www.plunket.org.nz/plunket-near-you.

Primary Clinical Care Manual. 8th ed.: https://www.health.qld.gov.au/rrcsu/.

Raising Children Network—The Australian parenting website: https://raisingchildren.net.au/.

Raising Children Supporting Parents—A New Zealand parenting website https://raisingchildren.org.nz/.

References

Abraham E, Hendler T, Shapira-Lichter I, et al. Father's brain is sensitive to childcare experiences. *Proc Natl Acad Sci USA*. 2014;111(27):9792–9797.

Alderdice F, McLeish J, Henderson J, et al. Women's ideal and real expectations of postnatal care during their first pregnancy: An online survey in England. *Midwifery*. 2020:89:102815. doi:10.1016/j.midw.2020.102815.

Alexander J, Thomas P, Sanhera J. Treatments for secondary postpartum haemorrhage. *Cochrane Database Syst Rev*. 2002;(1):CD002867.

Andersson E, Hildingsson I. Mother's postnatal stress: an investigation of links to various factors during pregnancy and postpartum. *Scand J Caring Sci*. 2016;30(4):782–789. doi:10.1111/scs.12305.

Austin M-P, Highet N, Expert Working Group. *Mental Health Care in the Perinatal Period: Australian Clinical Practice Guideline*. Melbourne: Centre of Perinatal Excellence; 2017.

Australian Government. *Overweight and Obesity: An Interactive Insight*. Australian Institute of Health and Welfare; 2020. Online: https://www.aihw.gov.au/reports/overweight-obesity/overweight-and-obesity-an-interactive-insight/contents/what-is-overweight-and-obesity.

Baird MB. Well-being in refugee women experiencing cultural transition. *ANS Adv Nurs Sci*. 2012;35(3):249–263.

Ball J. *Reactions to Motherhood: The Role of Postnatal Care*. 2nd ed. Hale: Books for Midwives; 1994.

Bastos M, Furuta M, Small R, et al. Debriefing interventions for the prevention of psychological trauma in women following childbirth. *Cochrane Database Syst Rev*. 2015;(4):CD007194, doi:10.1002/14651858.CD007194.pub2.

Baxter JA. Fathering across families: how father involvement varies for children when their father has children living elsewhere. *J Fam Stud*. 2012;18(2–3):187–201.

Beckes L, Ijzerman H, Tops M. Toward a radically embodied neuroscience of attachment and relationships. *Front Hum Neurosci*. 2015;9:266. doi:10.3389/fnhum.2015.00266.

Bell AF, Erickson EN, Carter CS. Beyond labor: the role of natural and synthetic oxytocin in the transition to motherhood. *J Midwifery Womens Health*. 2014;59(1):35–42, quiz 108. doi:10.1111/jmwh.12101.

Belsky J. *Social–contextual determinants of parenting*. Encyclopedia on Early Childhood Development; 2014. Online: http://www.child-encyclopedia.com/sites/default/files/textes-experts/en/654/social-contextual-determinants-of-parenting.pdf.

Benza S, Liamputtong P. Becoming an 'Amai': meanings and experiences of motherhood amongst Zimbabwean women living in Melbourne, Australia. *Midwifery*. 2017;45:72–78. doi:10.1016/j.midw.2016.12.011.

Bick D, MacArthur C, Winter H. *Postnatal Care: Evidence and Guidelines for Management*. 2nd ed. London: Elsevier; 2009.

Bick DE, Murrells T, Weavers A, et al. Revising acute care systems and processes to improve breastfeeding and maternal postnatal health: a pre and post intervention study in one English maternity unit. *BMC Pregnancy Childbirth*. 2012;12(1):41.

Bick D, Silverio SA, Bye A, et al. Postnatal care following hypertensive disorders of pregnancy: a qualitative study of views and experiences of primary and secondary care clinicians. *BMJ Open*. 2020;10:e034382. doi:10.1136/bmjopen-2019-034382.

Blackburn ST. *Maternal, Fetal, and Neonatal Physiology: A Clinical Perspective*. 3rd ed. St Louis, MO: Elsevier; 2013.

Bowlby J. *Attachment: Attachment and Loss*. Vol. 1. New York: Basic Books; 1969.

Boyle S, Thomas H, Brooks F. Women's views on partnership working with midwives during pregnancy and childbirth. *Midwifery*. 2016;32:21–29. doi:10.1016/j.midw.2015.09.001.

Breyman C, Bian X, Blanco-Capito L, et al. Expert recommendations for the diagnosis and treatment of iron-deficiency anemia during pregnancy and the postpartum period in the Asia-Pacific region. *J Perinat Med*. 2011;39(2):113–121.

British Red Cross, Co-Op. *Trapped in a Bubble: An Investigation into Triggers for Loneliness in the UK*; 2016. Online: http://www.redcross.org.uk/~/media/BritishRedCross/Documents/What%20we%20do/UK%20services/Co_Op_Trapped_in_a_bubble_report_AW.pdf.

Brown SJ, Davey M-A, Bruinsma FJ. Women's views and experiences of postnatal hospital care in the Victorian Survey of Recent Mothers 2000. *Midwifery*. 2005;21(2):109–126.

Brodribb W, Miller Y. Which mothers receive a post partum home visit in Queensland, Australia? A cross-sectional retrospective study. *Aust Health Rev*. 2015;39(3):337–343. doi:10.1071/AH14055.

Burns E, Schmied V. "The right help at the right time": positive constructions of peer and professional support for breastfeeding. *Women Birth*. 2017;30(5):389–397. doi:10.1016/j.wombi.2017.03.002.

Calje E, Skinner J. The challenge of defining and treating anemia and iron deficiency in pregnancy: a study of New Zealand midwives' management of iron status in pregnancy and the postpartum period. *Birth*. 2017;44(2):181–190.

Chin R, Hall P, Daiches A. Fathers' experiences of their transition to fatherhood: a metasynthesis. *J Reprod Infant Psychol*. 2011;29(1):4–18. doi:10.1080/02646838.2010.513044.

Cummins A, Griew K, Devonport C, et al. Exploring the value and acceptability of an antenatal and postnatal midwifery continuity of care model to women and midwives, using the Quality Maternal Newborn Care Framework. *Women Birth*. 2021;35(1):59–69. doi:10.1016/j.wombi.2021.03.006.

Dahlberg U, Haugan G, Aune I. Women's experiences of home visits by midwives in the early postnatal period. *Midwifery*. 2016;39:57–62. doi:10.1016/j.midw.2016.05.003.

Danbjørg DB, Wagner L, Kristensen BR, et al. Intervention among new parents followed up by an interview study exploring their experiences of telemedicine after early postnatal discharge. *Midwifery*. 2015;31(6):574–581. doi:10.1016/j.midw.2015.02.007.

Darwin Z, Galdas P, Hinchliff S, et al.; Born and Bred in Yorkshire (BaBY) team. Fathers' views and experiences of their own mental health during pregnancy and the first postnatal year: a qualitative interview study of men participating in the UK Born and Bred in Yorkshire (BaBY) cohort. *BMC Pregnancy Childbirth*. 2017;17(1):45. doi:10.1186/s12884-017-1229-4.

Dennis CL, Hodnett ED. Psychosocial and psychological interventions for treating postpartum depression. *Cochrane Database Syst Rev*. 2007;(4):CD006116, doi:10.1002/14651858.CD006116.pub2.

Deussen A, Ashwood P, Martis R, et al., Relief of pain due to uterine cramping / involution after birth (Review). *Cochrane Database Syst Rev*. 2020;(10):CD004908. doi:10.1002/14651858.CD004908.pub2.

Doss BD, Cicila LN, Hsueh AC, et al. A randomized controlled trial of brief coparenting and relationship interventions during the transition to parenthood. *J Fam Psychol*. 2014;28(4):483–494. doi:10.1037/a0037311.

East M. Post partum anaemia. Are we vigilant enough? *Pract Midwife*. 2012;15(6):37–39.

Eira Nunes C, de Roten Y, El Ghaziri N, et al. Co-parenting programs: A systematic review and meta-analysis. *Fam Relat*. 2020;70(3):759–776. doi:10.1111/fare.12438.

Elmir R, Schmied V. A meta-ethnographic synthesis of fathers' experiences of complicated births that are potentially traumatic. *Midwifery*. 2016;32:66–74. doi:10.1016/j.midw.2015.09.008.

Emmanuel EN, Creedy DK, St John W, et al. Maternal role development: the impact of maternal distress and social support following childbirth. *Midwifery*. 2011;27(2):265–272. doi:10.1016/j.midw.2009.07.003.

Entsieh AA, Hallstrom IK. First-time parents' prenatal needs for early parenthood preparation—a systematic review and meta-synthesis of qualitative literature. *Midwifery*. 2016;39:1–11. doi:10.1016/j.midw.2016.04.006.

Fahey JO, Shenassa E. Understanding and meeting the needs of women in the postpartum period: the perinatal maternal health promotion model. *J Midwifery Womens Health*. 2013;58(6):613–621. doi:10.1111/jmwh.12139.

Feinberg M. Coparenting and the transition to parenthood: a framework for prevention. *Clin Child Fam Psychol Rev*. 2002;5(3):173–195.

Fenwick J, Butt J, Dhaliwal S, et al. Western Australian women's perceptions of the style and quality of midwifery postnatal care in hospital and at home. *Women Birth*. 2010;23(1):10–21. doi:10.1016/j.wombi.2009.06.001.

Fenwick J, Bayes S, Johansson M. A qualitative investigation into the pregnancy experiences and childbirth expectations of Australian fathers-to-be. *Sex Reprod Healthc*. 2012;3(1):3–9. doi:10.1016/j.srhc.2011.11.001.

Fenwick J, Gamble J, Creedy D, et al. Women's perceptions of emotional support following childbirth: a qualitative investigation. *Midwifery*. 2013;29(3):217–224. doi:10.1016/j.midw.2011.12.008.

Fillo J, Simpson JA, Rholes WS, et al. Dads doing diapers: individual and relational outcomes associated with the division of childcare across the transition to parenthood. *J Pers Soc Psychol*. 2015;108(2):298–316. doi:10.1037/a0038572.

Finlayson K, Crossland N, Bonet M, et al. What matters to women in the postnatal period: A meta-synthesis of qualitative studies. *PLoS ONE*. 2020;15(4):e0231415.

Foon R, Toozs-Hobson P, Millns P, et al. The impact of anaesthesia and mode of delivery on the urinary bladder in the postdelivery period. *Int J Gynaecol Obstet*. 2010;110(2):114–117.

Giallo R, Pilkington P, McDonald E, et al. Physical, sexual and social health factors associated with the trajectories of maternal depressive symptoms from pregnancy to 4 years postpartum. *Soc Psychiatry Psychiatr Epidemiol*. 2017;52(7):815–828.

Ginja S, Coad J, Bailey E, et al. Associations between social support, mental wellbeing, self-efficacy and technology use in first-time antenatal women: data from the BaBBLeS cohort study. *BMC Pregnancy Childbirth*. 2018;18(1):441. doi:10.1186/s12884-018-2049-x.

Goodman JH. Becoming an involved father of an infant. *J Obstet Gynecol Neonatal Nurs*. 2005;34(2):190–200. doi:10.1177/0884217505274581.

Gordon I, Zagoory-Sharon O, Leckman JF, et al. Oxytocin and the development of parenting in humans. *Biol Psychiatry*. 2010;68(4):377–382. doi:10.1016/j.biopsych.2010.02.005.

Griffiths M, Home C. Developing a review process for Australian midwives: a report of the Midwifery Practice Review project process. *Women Birth*. 2008;21(3):119–125. doi:10.1016/j.wombi.2008.05.001.

Guida J, Sundaram S, Leiferman J. Antenatal physical activity: investigating the effects on postpartum depression. *Health*. 2012;4(12):1276–1286.

Guilliland K, Pairman S. *The Midwifery Partnership, A Model for Practice*. 2nd ed. Christchurch, NZ: New Zealand College of Midwives; 2010.

Health Practitioners Competence Assurance Act 2003; 2003 (reprinted 7 March 2017). Online: http://www.legislation.govt.nz/act/public/2003/0048/latest/DLM203312.html.

Health Quality & Safety Commission NZ. *Preventing Maternal Morbidity: Is it Sepsis? Know the Signs and What to Do*. Health Quality & Safety Commission; 2018.

Henderson A, Harmon S, Newman H. The price mothers pay, even when they are not buying it: mental health consequences of idealized motherhood. *Sex Roles*. 2016;74(11):512–526. doi:10.1007/s11199-015-0534-5.

Henderson J, Alderdice F, Redshaw M. Factors associated with maternal postpartum fatigue: An observational study. *BMJ Open*. 2019;9(7): e025927. doi: 10.1136/bmjopen-2018-025927.

Herbell K, Zauszniewski J. Stress experiences and mental health of pregnant women: the mediating role of social support. *Issues Ment. Health Nurs.* 2019;40(7):613–620.

International Confederation of Midwives (ICM). *International Code of Ethics for Midwives*. 2008, reviewed 2014. Online: https://internationalmidwives.org/assets/uploads/documents/CoreDocuments/CD2008_001%20V2014%20ENG%20International%20Code%20of%20Ethics%20for%20Midwives.pdf.

Ives J. Men, maternity and moral residue: negotiating the moral demands of the transition to first time fatherhood. *Sociol Health Illn*. 2014;36(7):1003–1019. doi:10.1111/1467-9566.12138.

Jangsten E, Bergh I, Mattsson L, et al. Afterpains: a comparison between active and expectant management of the third stage of labor. *Birth*. 2011;38(4):294–301.

Jenkinson B, Young K, Kruske S. Maternity services and the discharge process: a review of practice in Queensland. *Women Birth*. 2014;27(2):114–120. doi:10.1016/j.wombi.2013.12.001.

Johansson M, Fenwick J, Premberg Å. A meta-synthesis of fathers' experiences of their partner's labour and the birth of their baby. *Midwifery*. 2015;31(1):9–18. doi:10.1016/j.midw.2014.05.005.

Jones E, Taylor B, MacArthur C, et al. Early postnatal discharge for infants: A meta-analysis. *Pediatrics*. 2020;146(3):e20193365. doi:10.1542/peds.2019-3365.

Kolak AM, Volling BL. Coparenting moderates the association between firstborn children's temperament and problem behavior across the transition to siblinghood. *J Fam Psychol*. 2013;27(3): 355–364. doi:10.1037/a0032864.

Kotila LE, Schoppe-Sullivan SJ, Dush CM. Time in parenting activities in dual-earner families at the transition to parenthood. *Fam Relat*. 2013;62(5):795–807. doi:10.1111/fare.12037.

Kotila LE, Schoppe-Sullivan SJ, Kamp Dush CM. Infant characteristics and parental engagement at the transition to parenthood. *Infant Behav Dev*. 2014;37(4):787–799. doi:10.1016/j.infbeh.2014.09.002.

Kurth E, Krahenbuhl K, Eicher M, et al. Safe start at home: what parents of newborns need after early discharge from hospital—a focus group study. *BMC Health Serv Res*. 2016;16:82. doi:10.1186/s12913-016-1300-2.

Lamb K, Sanders R. Constipation and haemorrhoids: A midwifery perspective for the childbearing continuum. *Br J Midwifery*. 2015; 23(3):171–177.

Lambermon F, Vandenbussche F, Dedding C, et al. Maternal self-care in the early postpartum period: An integrative review. *Midwifery*. 2020;90:102799. doi: 10.1016/j.midw.2020.102799.

Leahy-Warren P, McCarthy G. Maternal parental self-efficacy in the postpartum period. *Midwifery*. 2011;27(6):802–810. doi:10.1016/j.midw.2010.07.008.

Lewington L, Lee J, Sebar B. "I'm not just a babysitter": Masculinity and men's experiences of first-time fatherhood. *Men Masc*. 2021;24(4):571–589. doi:10.1177/1097184X21993884.

Liamputtong P. Motherhood and "moral career": discourses of good motherhood among southeast Asian immigrant women in Australia. *Qual Sociol*. 2006;29(1):25–53.

Lohoar S, Butera N, Kennedy E. *Strengths of Australian Aboriginal Cultural Practices in Family Life and Child Rearing*. CFCA paper no. 25; 2014. Online: https://aifs.gov.au/cfca/sites/default/files/publication-documents/cfca25.pdf.

Loutzenhiser L, Mcauslan P, Sharpe DP. The trajectory of maternal and paternal fatigue and factors associated with fatigue across the transition to parenthood. *Clin Psychol*. 2015;19(1):15–27. doi:10.1111/cp.12048.

Lovelady C. Balancing exercise and food intake with lactation to promote post-partum weight loss. *Proc Nutr Soc*. 2011;70(2): 181–184.

Lyons S. Post-traumatic stress disorder following childbirth: causes prevention and treatment. In: Clement S, eds. *Psychological Perspective on Pregnancy and Childbirth*. Edinburgh: Elsevier; 1998 [Ch. 7].

Marchant S. Transition to motherhood: from the woman's perspective. In: Stewart M, ed. *Pregnancy, Birth and Maternity Care: Feminist Perspectives*. London: Books for Midwives; 2003:71–85.

Marchant S, Alexander J, Garcia J, et al. A survey of women's experiences of vaginal loss from 24 hours to three months after childbirth (the BLiPP study). *Midwifery*. 1999;15(2):72–81.

Marchant S, Alexander J, Garcia J. How does it feel to you? Uterine palpation and lochia loss as guides to post natal recovery. In: Wickham S, ed. *Midwifery: Best Practice*. Vol. 2. London: Elsevier; 2003:132–135.

May C, Fletcher R. Preparing fathers for the transition to parenthood: recommendations for the content of antenatal education. *Midwifery*. 2013;29(5):474–478. doi:10.1016/j.midw.2012.03.005.

Manresa M, Pereda A, Bataller E, et al. Incidence of perineal pain and dyspareunia following spontaneous vaginal birth: a systematic review and meta-analysis. *Int Urogynecol J*. 2019;30: 853–868.

Mazzeschi C, Pazzagli C, Radi G, et al. Antecedents of maternal parenting stress: the role of attachment style, prenatal attachment, and dyadic adjustment in first-time mothers. *Front Psychol*. 2015;6:1443. doi:10.3389/fpsyg.2015.01443.

McKellar LV, Pincombe JI, Henderson AM. Insights from Australian parents into educational experiences in the early postnatal period. *Midwifery*. 2006;22(4):356–364.

McLachlan HL, Gold L, Forster DA, et al. Women's views of postnatal care in the context of the increasing pressure on postnatal beds in Australia. *Women Birth*. 2009;22(4):128–133. doi:10.1016/j.wombi.2009.04.003.

McLean K, Edwards S, Mantilla A. A review of community playgroup participation. *Australas J Early Child*. 2020:45(2);155–169.

McLeish J, Harvey M, Redshaw M., et al. First-time mothers' expectations and experiences of postnatal care in England. *Qual Health Res*. 2020;30(12):1876–1887.

McQueen A, Mander R. Tiredness and fatigue in the postnatal period. *J Adv Nurs*. 2003;42(5):463–469.

Ménage D, Bailey E, Lees S, et al. A concept analysis of compassionate midwifery. *J Adv Nurs*. 2017;73(3):558–573. doi:10.1111/jan.13214.

Mercer R. *First-time Motherhood: Experiences From Teens to Forties*. New York: Springer; 1986.

Mercer RT. Nursing support of the process of becoming a mother. *J Obstet Gynecol Neonatal Nurs*. 2006;35(5):649–651.

Ministry of Health (MOH). *Primary Maternity Services Notice 2007*. Wellington: Ministry of Health; 2007.

Ministry of Health (MOH). *Primary Maternity Services Notice 2021*. Wellington: Ministry of Health; 2021.

Ministry of Health (MOH). *Observation of Mother and Baby in the Immediate Postnatal Period: Consensus Statements Guiding Practice*; 2012. Online: https://www.health.govt.nz/publication/observation-mother-and-baby-immediate-postnatal-period-consensus-statements-guiding-practice.

Ministry of Health (MOH). *Maternity Services—DHB-Funded Primary Maternity Facility Tier Level Two Service Specification*; 2013. Online: https://www.midwife.org.nz/pdf/resources/DHBFundedMaternityFacilityT2.pdf.

Ministry of Health (MOH). *Screening, Diagnosis and Management of Gestational Diabetes in New Zealand: A Clinical Practice Guideline*; 2014. Online: https://www.health.govt.nz/publication/screening-diagnosis-and-management-gestational-diabetes-new-zealand-clinical-practice-guideline.

Ministry of Health (MOH). *Maternity Consumer Survey 2014*. 2015. Online: https://www.health.govt.nz/publication/maternity-consumer-survey-2014.

Ministry of Health (MOH). *Diagnosis and Treatment of Hypertension and Pre-Eclampsia in Pregnancy in New Zealand: A Clinical Practice Guideline*; 2018. Online: http://www.health.govt.nz/publication/diagnosis-and-treatment-hypertension-and-pre-eclampsia-pregnancy-new-zealand-clinical-practice.

Ministry of Health (MOH). *Guidance for Healthy Weight Gain in Pregnancy*. Wellington: Ministry of Health; 2014.

Ministry of Health (MOH). *New Zealand Aotearoa's Guidance on Contraception*. Wellington: Ministry of Health; 2020a.

Ministry of Health (MOH). *New Zealand Health Survey*; 2020b. Online: https://minhealthnz.shinyapps.io/nz-health-survey-2019-20-annual-data-explorer/_w_29cafb30/#!/.

Ministry of Health (MOH). *Diagnosis and Treatment of Hypertension and Pre-Eclampsia in Pregnancy in New Zealand: A Clinical Practice Guideline*; 2022.

Morrow J, McLachlan H, Forster D, et al. Redesigning postnatal care: exploring the views and experiences of midwives. *Midwifery*. 2013;29(2):159–166. doi:10.1016/j.midw.2011.11.006.

National Advisory Committee on Core Health and Disability Support Services (NACCHDSS). *Care of Mother and Baby After Normal Delivery*. Wellington: NACCHDSS; 1993.

National Institute for Health and Care Excellence (NICE). *Postnatal Care: Routine Postnatal Care of Women and Their Babies*. NICE clinical guidance CG37. Leicester: NICE; 2006. Online: https://www.rcpch.ac.uk/sites/default/files/asset_library/Research/Clinical%20Effectiveness/Endorsed%20guidelines/Postnatal%20Care%20%28NICE%29/Postnatal%20guideline%20-%20NICE%20guideline.pdf.

National Institute for Health and Care Excellence (NICE). *Weight Management Before, During and After Pregnancy*. NICE public health guidance 27. Leicester: NICE; 2010. Online: https://www.nice.org.uk/Guidance/PH27.

National Institute for Health and Care Excellence (NICE). *Postnatal Care*. Quality standard [QS37]. 2013, updated 2015. Online: https://www.nice.org.uk/guidance/qs37/chapter/introduction.

National Institute for Health and Care Excellence (NICE). *Postnatal Care up to 8 Weeks After Birth*. NICE clinical guideline CG37 updated; 2015. Online: https://www.nice.org.uk/guidance/CG37.

National Institute for Health and Care Excellence (NICE). *Antenatal and postnatal mental health: The NICE guidelines on clinical management and service guidance, updated edition*; 2018. Online: https://www.nice.org.uk/guidance/cg192/evidence/full-guideline-pdf-4840896925.

Nelson AM. Transition to motherhood. *J Obstet Gynecol Neonatal Nurs*. 2003;32(4):465–477.

New Zealand Blood. *Use of Rh-D Immunoglobulin During Pregnancy and the Post Partum Period*; 2013. Online: https://www.nzblood.co.nz/assets/Transfusion-Medicine/PDFs/USE-OF-RH-D-IMMUNOGLOBULIN-DURING-PREGNANCY-AND-THE-POST-PARTUM-PERIOD-111G130.pdf.

New Zealand College of Midwives (NZCOM). *Midwifery Standards Review Handbook*. Christchurch, NZ: New Zealand College of Midwives; 2012.

New Zealand College of Midwives (NZCOM). *Midwives Handbook for Practice*. 5th ed. Christchurch: New Zealand College of Midwives; 2015.

New Zealand College of Midwives (NZCOM), Midwifery and Maternity Providers Organisation (MMPO). *Report on New Zealand's MMPO Midwives Care Activities and Outcomes 2016*; 2018. Online: https://www.midwife.org.nz/pdf/JDMRC/mmpo%202012%20for%20web.pdf.

New Zealand College of Midwives (NZCOM). *A Keteparaha/Toolkit: Supporting and Enhancing Effective Midwifery Record Keeping in Aotearoa*; 2021. Online: https://www.midwife.org.nz/wp-content/uploads/2021/06/Keteparaha-Toolkit-Record-keeping-June-2021.pdf.

New Zealand Legislation. *Health (Retention of Health Information) Regulations*; 1996. Online: https://legislation.govt.nz/regulation/public/1996/0343/latest/DLM225650.html.

Norman E, Sherburn M, Osborne R, et al. An exercise and education program improves well-being of new mothers: a randomised controlled trial. *Phys Ther*. 2010;90(3):348–355.

Nursing and Midwifery Board of Australia (NMBA). *National Competency Standards for the Midwife*; 2018a. Online: http://www.nursingmidwiferyboard.gov.au/Codes-Guidelines-Statements/Codes-Guidelines.aspx.

Nursing and Midwifery Board of Australia (NMBA). *Midwife Standards for Practice*. 2018b. Online: http://www.nursingmidwiferyboard.gov.au/Codes-Guidelines-Statements/Professional-standards/Midwife-standards-for-practice.aspx.

Ockenden J. After the birth is over ... rest and support for the new mothers. *Pract Midwife*. 2000;3(11):10–13.

Osborne C, Berger LM, Magnuson K. Family structure transitions and changes in maternal resources and well-being. *Demography*. 2012;49(1):23–47. doi:10.1007/s13524-011-0080-x. doi:10.1080/02646838.2014.956301.

Parera N, Liolitsa D, Lype S, et al. Phlebotonics for haemorrhoids (Review). *Cochrane Database Sys Rev*. 2012;8. doi:10.1002/14651858.CD004322.pub3.

Parratt JA, Fahy KM. A feminist critique of foundational nursing research and theory on transition to motherhood. *Midwifery*. 2011;27(4):445–451. doi:10.1016/j.midw.2010.02.012.

Podkolinski J. Women's experience of postnatal support. In: Clement S, eds. *Psychological Perspectives on Pregnancy and Childbirth*. Edinburgh: Elsevier; 1998 [Ch. 11].

Poskus T, Buzinskiene D, Drasutiene G, et al. Haemorrhoids and anal fissures during pregnancy and after childbirth: A prospective cohort study. *BJOG*. 2014;121:1666–1672.

Premberg A, Hellström AL, Berg M. Experiences of the first year as father. *Scand J Caring Sci*. 2008;22(1):56–63. doi:10.1111/j.1471–6712.2007.00584.x.

Prevatt BS, Desmarais S. Facilitators and barriers to disclosure of postpartum mood disorder symptoms to a healthcare provider. *Matern Child Health J*. 2018;22(1):120–129. doi:10.1007/s10995-017-2361-5.

Psaila K, Kruske S, Fowler C, et al. Smoothing out the transition of care between maternity and child and family health services: perspectives of child and family health nurses and midwives. *BMC Pregnancy Childbirth*. 2014;14:151. doi:10.1186/1471-2393-14-151.

Rankin J. *Physiology in Childbearing with Anatomy and Related Biosciences*. 4th ed. London: Elsevier; 2017.

Research New Zealand. *Maternity Consumer Survey*, Wellington, Ministry of Health New Zealand; 2014.

Rubin R. *Maternal Identity and the Maternal Experience*. New York: Springer; 1984.

Saunders H, Kraus A, Barone L, et al. Emotional availability: theory, research, and intervention. *Front Psychol*. 2015;6:1069. doi:10.3389/fpsyg.2015.01069.

Schmied V, Bick D. Postnatal care—current issues and future challenges. *Midwifery*. 2014;30(6):571–574.

Schmied V, Black E, Naidoo N, et al. Migrant women's experiences, meanings and ways of dealing with postnatal depression: A meta-ethnographic study. *PLoS ONE*. 2017;12(3): e0172385. doi: 10.1371/journal.pone.0172385.

Schmied V, Cooke M, Gutwein R, et al. An evaluation of strategies to improve the quality and content of hospital-based postnatal care in a metropolitan Australian hospital. *J Clin Nurs*. 2008;18(3):1850–1861.

Schmied V, Donovan J, Kruske S, et al. Commonalities and challenges: a review of Australian state and territory maternity and child health policies. *Contemp Nurse*. 2011;40(1):106–117.

Schmied V, Lupton D. The externality of the inside: body images of pregnancy. *Nurs Inq*. 2001;8(1):32–40. doi:10.1046/j.1440-1800.2001.00088.x.

Seefat-van Teeffelen A, Nieuwenhuijze M, Korstjen I. Women want proactive psychosocial support from midwives during transition to motherhood: a qualitative study. *Midwifery*. 2011;27(1):e122–e127. doi:10.1016/j.midw.2009.09.006.

Shorey S, Dennis C, Bridge S, et al. First-time fathers' postnatal experiences and support needs: A descriptive qualitative study. *J Adv Nurs*. 2017;73(12):2987–2996.

Song JH, Volling BL. Coparenting and children's temperament predict firstborns' cooperation in the care of an infant sibling. *J Fam Psychol*. 2015;29(1):130–135. doi:10.1037/fam0000052.

State of Victoria, Department of Health. *Postnatal Care Program Guidelines for Victorian Health Services*. Melbourne: Victorian Government, Department of Health; 2012. Online: http://docs2.health.vic.gov.au/docs/doc/715A53A28AA4E8CACA257ACC006D257E/$FILE/121022%20Postnatal%20care%20guidelines_web.pdf.

Steen M, Downe S, Bamford N, et al. Not-patient and not-visitor: a metasynthesis fathers' encounters with pregnancy, birth and maternity care. *Midwifery*. 2012;28(4):362–371. doi:10.1016/j.midw.2011.06.009.

Symon A, Glazener CM, MacDonald A, et al. Pilot study: quality of life assessment of postnatal fatigue and other physical morbidity. *J Psychosom Obstet Gynaecol*. 2003;24(4):215–219.

Tani F, Castagna V. Maternal social support, quality of birth experience, and post-partum depression in primiparous women. *J Matern Fetal Neonatal Med*. 2017;30(6):689–692. doi:10.1080/14767058.2016.1182980.

Thomson G, Downe S. Emotions and support needs following a distressing birth: scoping study with pregnant multigravida women in North-West England. *Midwifery*. 2016;40:32–39. doi:10.1016/j.midw.2016.06.010.

Todd AL, Ampt AJ, Roberts CL. "Very good" ratings in a survey of maternity care: kindness and understanding matter to Australian women. *Birth*. 2017;44(1):48–57. doi:10.1111/birt.12264.

Turawa EB, Musekiwa A, Rohwer AC. Interventions for preventing postpartum constipation. *Cochrane Database Syst Rev*. 2020;(8):CD011625, doi:10.1002/14651858.CD011625.pub3.

Vaezi A, Soojoodi F, Banihashemi A, et al. The association between social support and postpartum depression in women: A cross sectional study. *Women Birth*. 2019;32(2):e238–e242. doi:10.1016/j.wombi.2018.07.014.

Vismara L, Rolle L, Agostini F, et al. Perinatal parenting stress, anxiety, and depression outcomes in first-time mothers and fathers: a 3- to 6-months postpartum follow-up study. *Front Psychol*. 2016;7:938. doi:10.3389/fpsyg.2016.00938.

Waite J. Report on Rangiora Hospital afterpains audit: feedback on a midwifery led initiative. *Midwifery News*. 2002;24:28.

Williams A, Herron-Marx S, Hicks C. The prevalence of enduring postnatal perineal morbidity and its relationship to perineal trauma. *Midwifery*. 2007;23(4):392–403.

Williams R, Hewison A, Stewart M, et al. 'We are doing our best': African and African-Caribbean fatherhood, health and preventive primary care services, in England. *Health Soc Care Community*. 2012;20(2):216–223. doi:10.1111/j.1365-2524.2011.01037.x.

Woodley S, Lawrenson P, Boyle R, et al. Pelvic floor muscle training for preventing and treating urinary and faecal incontinence in antenatal and postnatal women. *Cochrane Database Sys Rev*. 2020;6(5):CD007471. doi:10.1002/14651858.CD007471.pub4.

Woolhouse H, McDonald E, Brown S. Women's experiences of sex and intimacy after childbirth: making the adjustment to motherhood. *J Psychosom Obstet Gynaecol*. 2012;33(4):185–190. doi:10.3109/0167482x.2012.720314.

World Health Organization (WHO). *WHO Recommendations on Postnatal Care of the Mother and Newborn*; 2013. Online: http://apps.who.int/iris/bitstream/10665/97603/1/9789241506649_eng.pdf?ua=1.

World Health Organization (WHO). *WHO Recommendations on Maternal and Newborn Care for a Positive Postnatal Experience*; 2022. Online: https://www.who.int/publications/i/item/9789240044074.

Yelland J, Krastev A, Brown S. Enhancing early postnatal care: findings from a major reform of maternity care in three Australian hospitals. *Midwifery*. 2009;25(4):392–402.

Zadoroznyj M, Brodribb WE, Young K, et al. 'I really needed help': what mothers say about their post-birth care in Queensland, Australia. *Women Birth*. 2015;28(3):246–251. doi:10.1016/j.wombi.2015.03.004.

Further reading

Allison J. *The Golden Month: Caring for the World's Mothers After Childbirth*. Auckland: Beatnik; 2015.

Blackburn ST. *Maternal, Fetal, and Neonatal Physiology: A Clinical Perspective*. 4th ed. St Louis, MO: Elsevier; 2013.

Fahy K. An Australian history of the subordination of midwifery. *Women Birth*. 2007;20(1):25–29.

Fauconnier A, Goltzene A, Issartel F, et al. Late post-partum dyspareunia: does delivery play a role? *Prog Urol*. 2012;22(4):225–232.

Forster DA, McLachlan HL, Rayner J, et al. The early postnatal period: exploring women's views, expectations and experiences of care using focus groups in Victoria, Australia. *BMC Pregnancy Childbirth*. 2008;8(1):27.

Forster DA, McLachlan HL, Yelland J, et al. Staffing in postnatal units: is it adequate for the provision of quality care? Staff perspectives from a state-wide review of postnatal care in Victoria, Australia. *BMC Health Serv Res*. 2006;6(1):83.

Gethin A, Macgregor B. *Helping Your Baby to Sleep: Why Gentle Techniques Work Best*. Sydney: Finch Publishing; 2007.

Stewart M, ed. *Pregnancy, Birth and Maternity Care: Feminist Perspectives*. London: Books for Midwives; 2004.

Wickham S, ed. *Midwifery: Best Practice*. Vols. 1–5. London: Elsevier; 2003–2009.

CHAPTER 31

Supporting the newborn

Lorna Davies and Sally Baddock

LEARNING OUTCOMES

Learning outcomes for this chapter are:

1. To optimise the physiological transition from intrauterine to extrauterine life in the early neonatal period
2. To carry out newborn assessments and identify the normal, variations and deviations of normal and plan appropriate action around these findings
3. To support the woman and her family to recognise normal behaviour and development in the baby
4. To practise midwifery within a woman-centred, partnership-based framework that incorporates decision points for newborns during the first 6 weeks of life
5. To reflect critically upon the legal, ethical and professional implications surrounding the health and wellbeing of the newborn.

CHAPTER OVERVIEW

This chapter introduces the newborn baby within the context of the mother–baby dyad. It explores the significant role that the midwife plays in facilitating and supporting a new mother in the care of her baby throughout this transitional period. Although the chapter will focus on the health and wellbeing of the baby, it will explore some of the factors that may affect this status and explain the knowledge and skills that midwives require in assessing the wellbeing of the baby, including the newborn physical assessment. In addition, the most common minor complications that may affect the health and wellbeing of the neonate will be addressed.

KEY TERMS

antenatal influences
care of the newborn
midwifery support
mother–baby dyad
newborn assessment
normal growth and development
physiological transition following birth
sleep
social interaction
transition to extrauterine life

INTRODUCTION

The title of this chapter, 'Supporting the newborn', may at first glance suggest that the support for the baby is provided by the midwife. However, the most important role of the midwife in relation to the baby is to provide support to equip the woman with the skills and knowledge that she needs in order to provide the specific care and support for her baby during the first few days and weeks of life. The transition from womb to world for the newborn involves complex interactions between biological, physiological, behavioural, social and environmental factors. The mother likewise undergoes a similar transitional experience. The **mother–baby dyad** is the optimal 'econiche' providing a mutually reciprocal environment that leads to improved health and wellbeing for both (Buckley, 2015). There are essential skills and knowledge that the midwife requires in relation to this area of practice; however, in a situation where both mother and baby are healthy and well, any actions or interventions on the part of the midwife should be carried out only with the fully informed consent of the parents following robust information sharing.

Antenatal influences

Monitoring the health and wellbeing of the newborn is not something that begins at birth, but rather is part of a continuum which it could be argued begins before the baby is even conceived.

During pregnancy the midwife has the opportunity to work with women to enhance the potential for the health and wellbeing of the baby long before the woman is ready to birth. In the past decade or so, there has been an increasing focus on the importance of the uterine environment in supporting optimal fetal development and future health outcomes (Fleming et al., 2018; Roura & Arulkumaran, 2015). Behaviours such as smoking, drinking alcohol and taking recreational drugs have been associated with less-than-optimal outcomes for some time. Other lifestyle factors such as obesity and exposure to environmental toxins in the workplace and the home are also targeted as causes of less-than-optimal health sequelae. Additionally, scientific evidence is increasingly demonstrating that the emotional wellbeing of a woman during pregnancy may have an impact on the health and wellbeing of her baby. Prolonged levels of stress in pregnancy resulting from any number of factors including, for example, poverty, depression or family violence can produce excessive cortisol production, which causes preterm birth and low birth weight (Hoffman et al., 2016; Latendresse, 2009). It may also impact on the mother's ability to form a meaningful attachment with her baby and this can equally have long-term effects on the health of the baby for life (Davies, 2017). It is important therefore that midwives do not isolate episodes of care, but remain aware that what happens during the period before birth may have a significant effect on the long-term health of the baby.

THE TRANSITION TO EXTRAUTERINE LIFE

Allowing labour to begin spontaneously is beneficial for numerous reasons. Labour onset is mediated by many factors including hormonal messages between the mother and baby that signal both physiological and psychological readiness for birth (Buckley, 2015). Importantly, for the baby this means its organs, specifically its lungs, brain and gastrointestinal system, are mature and ready to function (Hillman et al., 2012). Exposure to intrapartum maternal hormones and the process of labour itself further enhance a successful transition to newborn life. Sarah Buckley explains how babies born after a drug-free spontaneous labour differ from those exposed to medicalised births. She states that they are more alert at birth, demonstrate normal newborn behaviour, breastfeed more successfully, require less specialist care and have lower rates of food allergies. Others report similar findings, specifically fewer Apgar scores less than 7 and fewer admissions to neonatal intensive care units for assistance with breathing (Buckley, 2015).

The transition from intrauterine to extrauterine life is a remarkable physiological event. It involves a series of finely evolved modifications that will enable the newborn baby to take its first metaphorical steps towards independent life. This transition begins as the woman goes into labour and the neurohormonal cascade that follows prepares the baby for independent life. A midwife who has a strong knowledge and understanding of physiological processes will support the woman to labour and birth with minimal intervention, as discussed in Chapter 27. By encouraging non-pharmacological strategies for helping the woman to cope with her labour the midwife will benefit the baby, who is more likely to be alert and responsive in the important hours following birth. Ensuring the cord is not clamped and cut unnecessarily early and allowing the placental transfer to take place gently will ensure that the baby will benefit in terms of cardiorespiratory transition and receive its full quota of blood, which will possibly prevent anaemia developing as the baby moves into infanthood and childhood (Davies & Richards, 2020).

Babies are affected by active management because early clamping of their cord, which is part of the process of active management of the birth of the placenta, removes approximately 80 mL of their cord blood from their vascular system—resulting in lower birth weights, increased rates of anaemia in the first 6 months of life, bradycardia in the first 1–2 minutes of life and reduced hospital mortality (Davies & McDonald, 2020; Fogarty et al., 2017). It is now recommended that cord clamping is delayed for at least 1–3 minutes in all births (World Health Organization, 2019). Ideally the midwife will wait until the cord is white and flaccid to ensure that placental transfusion is complete; the optimal way of achieving this is to separate the cord from the placenta after the latter has been birthed.

CRITICAL THINKING EXERCISE

When it is not possible to achieve a normal physiological birth for whatever reason, the midwife should be considering strategies to bring the woman closer to this 'default' position. What measures might you take as a midwife to bring the woman as close to the default birth position of normal physiological birth as possible?

The idea that the baby is an 'independent being' once born is seriously misguided because the baby is still hugely reliant on its mother to meet its needs. Human babies are born in a very immature state in relation to other mammalian species, and some writers have suggested that the early days, weeks and months of life are actually an extension of intrauterine life (Verbiest et al., 2017). This would suggest that babies are designed to remain in close contact with their mother in an econiche where all of its needs can be met. It is the mother who primarily activates the physiological activity of her baby from thermoregulation to metabolic adaptation, and from appetite to level of activity (Davies & Richards, 2020). If this is not possible, then a 'mother figure' or figures are able to provide care for the baby, although it is believed that the plasticity of the structure of the brain of the baby does not occur in the same way as it does when the mother and baby are coupled. The neurological 'wiring and firing' that takes place in the early hours, days and weeks in the life of a newborn is most effective when the baby is provided with love and security by its own mother (Bergman, 2014). In his classic work, Shore (1997) argues that the baby is primed to receive sensory input in order to develop more advanced neural systems. At birth the baby has more synapses than at any other time during life and this 'window of opportunity' is crucial in terms of establishing neural pathways (Lagercrantz, 2015). The initial sensory needs of a baby are smell and touch, both of which are achieved by ensuring that skin-to-skin contact takes place for long periods in the early postbirth period (Buckley, 2015). Therefore it is imperative that midwives seek out ways of ensuring that mother and baby remain together wherever they can and remember that the physical needs of the baby are only part of a complex and dynamic biological process (Davies, 2017).

Close contact between mother and baby in the hours following birth not only lays down the blueprint for effective physiological responses in the baby, but also fosters attachment and promotes development that may have significance for lifelong health and wellbeing. When left undisturbed, human mothers demonstrate 'species-specific behaviour' (Bergman, 2014). The mother generally 'explores' her baby first using her fingertips to feel the baby's head, fingers and toes. She then strokes the baby's body with her hand before cuddling the baby into her arms with the baby facing her. She establishes eye contact and talks to her baby, looking for support from her partner and significant others, including the midwife. Unless otherwise indicated, the parents should be the people who confirm the sex of the baby as part of this 'unveiling' of their baby. Generally, from the moment of birth, infants are sentient beings, alert and aware of their surroundings, and able to respond to those present and to the environment. The baby is particularly familiar with the voice of its mother at birth and rapidly gains a recognition of her unique scent. Evidence suggests that the baby usually takes about 45–55 minutes to find the way to its mother's breast using the primal reflexes such as stepping, crawling, grasping and, of course, rooting for the first latch and feed (Mulupuru et al., 2019; see Ch. 32). After this feed they will generally sleep for anything up to 6 hours (Widström et al., 2011).

It is important to recognise that women's partners are also neurohormonally primed to safeguard the relationship of mother and baby. When fathers feel empowered to actively engage during pregnancy and birth, synergistic neurohormonal activity will result and they will respond to the behaviours of their partner and baby activating an appropriate protective paternal response (Feldman, 2012).

The baby's responsive behaviours therefore induce responses from both parents, which calls forth a response from the baby. A neurobehavioural feedback loop is therefore established and the resulting interactions develop the bond between parents and child that is essential for the ongoing development of the baby (Davies, 2017).

REFLECTIVE THINKING EXERCISE

In order to best prepare for this optimal start to life for the baby, the midwife needs to prepare and maintain a birthing environment that acknowledges the importance of the intrapartum experience whatever the setting.

Consider how you might prepare the birthing environment to optimise the physiological transition of the newborn baby in the following settings:

- the woman's home
- a midwifery-led birthing unit
- a tertiary hospital birthing room
- a caesarean section theatre.

PHYSIOLOGICAL TRANSITION FOLLOWING BIRTH

Within a birth environment that provides warmth, safety and privacy the baby is able to make essential physiological adaptations to ensure that respiratory and cardiovascular function is initiated and maintained. A warm habitat (preferably the mother) in conjunction with access to colostrum will allow the baby to thermoregulate, control metabolic processes, take in adequate nutrition, eliminate wastes and ward off infection (Davies & Richards, 2020). It is important that the midwife has a good knowledge of this transitional physiology in order to ensure that a safe transition is occurring. In this section these activities are explored and how best midwives may offer support, if necessary, is considered.

Respiratory function

The preparation for independent respiration commences in utero when surfactant is produced from around 32 weeks gestation. Surfactant comprises phospholipids and specialised protein molecules that reduce the surface tension of the alveolar fluid at the air–alveolar interface, and contribute to the elasticity of lung tissue (Lee & Slutsky, 2016). Fetal breathing movements increase with gestation and remain an intermittent process until extrauterine respirations are established. What remains unclear is the exact mechanisms responsible for this onset of respirations, although increase in oxygen tension and clamping the umbilical cord appear to facilitate the process. Synthesis of surfactant is thought to be affected by acidosis and/or hypothermia (Pramanik & Rosenkrantz, 2020).

First active breath

The respiratory and cardiovascular changes that occur immediately after birth happen simultaneously and are mutually dependent (Davies & Richards, 2008). The factors initiating the first breath and lung expansion are thought to be the result of a combination of some or all of the following factors: uterine contractions in the second stage of labour (Mercer & Skovgaard, 2002), compression of the chest wall during birth and the recoil of the chest wall immediately after birth and chemoreceptor stimulation by reduction in oxygen and increase in carbon dioxide in the blood (McEwan, 2017a); other external stimuli such as cold, light, noise and touch are secondary triggers for the baby to take the first breath.

At the first inspiration produced by the contraction of the diaphragm, the baby closes off its glottis in order to prevent gaseous loss and to sustain positive intrathoracic pressure (LoMauro & Aliverti, 2016).

Following birth the respiratory rate of the baby rises to around 60 breaths per minute. The peak respiratory rate occurs at 1 hour in most newborns and remains relatively constant over the following 6 hours. Pauses in breathing are common and irregular breathing patterns occur most frequently during active sleep (Barrett et al., 2012).

Lung fluid

Lung fluid is not surfactant. It is a clear fluid that facilitates cell proliferation and differentiation. Prior to labour, production of lung fluid is reduced. At birth the lungs' primary function changes from secretion of fluid to the absorption of gases. It is possible that the catecholamine surge at birth is the final trigger for this change (LoMauro & Alvietti, 2016). Lung perfusion, which commences in late labour and continues after birth, facilitates the absorption of lung fluid from the alveoli by osmosis (Mercer & Skovgaard, 2002). At birth, the remaining lung fluid (approximately 80–100 mL) is either expelled through the upper airways or absorbed through temporarily more permeable alveolar epithelium into the interstitial tissue (Michaelides, 2017a). Within 2 hours of the birth of a healthy term neonate about 80% of the fluid has been reabsorbed, and it is completely absorbed from the alveoli within 12–24 hours. The fluid is absorbed from the interstitial tissue into the pulmonary vasculature and lymphatic drainage over the next few days (McEwan, 2017a).

At birth the neonate demonstrates shallow, irregular breathing with irregular pauses between breaths usually lasting 5–15 seconds. Pauses of less than 20 seconds are not usually of clinical concern (McDonald, 2020). Babies normally have an average respiratory rate of 40 breaths/minute (the range is 30–60 breaths/minute), although the rate may be elevated in the first 2 hours after birth (Davies & Richards, 2020). Breathing is diaphragmatic—the chest and abdomen rise and fall together. Such symmetry confirms that the lungs and diaphragm are functioning correctly. While an elevated respiratory rate is a sign that the baby is unwell, tachypnoea cannot be assessed without taking the baby's other behaviours into account, such as recent crying, feeding or sleeping (Tappero & Honeyfield, 2018). As a result of the need to breathe and feed simultaneously, babies are generally obligate nose breathers and do not switch spontaneously to breathing through the mouth when nasal obstruction occurs (Alvo et al., 2021).

Cardiovascular transition

The cardiovascular adaptations that occur at birth are more fully discussed in a maternal/neonatal or neonatal physiology textbook such as Blackburn (2017). In brief, the temporary fetal structures that support the fetal circulation are reversed after birth. These structures are the foramen ovale, ductus arteriosus, ductus venosus and hypogastric arteries. The increase in catecholamine release encouraged by birth stimulates increased cardiac contractility and output (McEwan, 2017a).

Pulmonary oxygenation of blood

In uterine life, 5%–10% of cardiac output enters the pulmonary circulation in order to meet pulmonary cellular growth and nutrition needs. High pulmonary vascular resistance and the patent ductus arteriosus ensure that the remainder of the cardiac output enters the arterial system. Blood with high oxygen levels is blended and shunted to the organs of greatest need such as the coronary arteries and brain (Singh & Tissot, 2018).

At birth, adjustments must be made to the baby's circulation so that deoxygenated blood flows to the lungs for oxygenation. This involves several mechanisms. The expansion of the lungs and associated lowered pulmonary vascular resistance which occurs with the first breath enables virtually the entire heart's output to enter the pulmonary circulation. Oxygenated blood returning to the heart via the pulmonary veins increases the pressure within the left atrium (Singh & Tissot, 2018). This triggers the closure of the foramen ovale.

Closure of the foramen ovale and the ductus arteriosus

In the first 24–48 hours following birth, the detection of flow murmurs, which are innocent heart murmurs, may indicate incomplete closure of the foramen ovale. This may persist until the pressures stabilise enabling the foramen to remain closed. In the initial days after birth, the closure can benignly reverse. For example, if pulmonary vascular resistance is high because the baby is crying, the foramen may temporarily reopen as a result of the increased resistance and transient cyanotic episodes may occur (Hooper et al., 2015).

The ductus arteriosus is usually functionally closed by 8–10 hours after birth, but will not anatomically close for several more months. Indeed, before pressures stabilise, a temporary reverse shunt through the ductus arteriosus may persist for a few hours, which can be heard as a 'flow murmur'. In some babies the ductus has been shown to be only intermittently patent for up to 3 days after birth (Blackburn, 2017).

Thermoregulation

Before birth, the temperature of the infant closely follows the mother's temperature. After birth, thermal exchange with the environment and a gradient transfer from the internal organs to the body surface of the baby and the surrounding air lead to a rapid fall in its body temperature (Davies & Richards, 2020). Newborn babies are sustained within a narrow range of core (internal) body temperatures that are generally about 36.5–37.5°C (Blackburn, 2017). The baby uses a number of mechanisms to balance heat loss and heat production in order to maintain its core temperature within a wide range of environmental temperatures. Balancing heat loss and gain is known as *thermoregulation*. The range of ambient temperatures that maintains a baby's core body temperature using minimum oxygen consumption at a minimum metabolic rate is called the *thermoneutral range* (Blackburn, 2017).

At birth, thermoregulatory mechanisms are not fully developed, although they become progressively more efficient within a relatively short period. However, the initial limited response to temperature changes in the first 24 hours of life means that babies are particularly susceptible to losing heat during this time and are therefore more prone to hypothermia. By 24–48 hours of age, healthy term neonates are able to increase their heat production up to 2.5 times in response to cold; however, they still remain susceptible to environmental temperature changes (Box 31.1). Until the mechanisms controlling thermoregulation (and heat loss in particular) stabilise, the thermoneutral range of babies is at a higher environmental temperature than that of older children and adults. Therefore, during the first weeks of life, rooms need to be kept warm and/or extra clothing and blankets may be required (Blackburn, 2017).

Box 31.1 Neonatal features contributing to heat loss or conservation

Neonatal features contributing to heat loss

- Large surface area to mass ratio (approximately three times greater than in adults). In particular, a baby's head (the major heat loss area in a clothed baby) comprises a larger proportion of the body than that of an adult
- Less subcutaneous fat
- Thin epidermis
- Blood vessels closer to the skin, so changes in the ambient temperature more readily influence the circulating blood, thereby influencing the temperature-regulating centre in the hypothalamus
- Decreased ability to shiver

Neonatal features contributing to heat production

- Decreased ability to sweat
- Flexed posture, which conserves heat by reducing exposed surface area
- Non-shivering thermogenesis

(Sources: Blackburn, 2013; Michaelides, 2017b)

Midwifery action to support thermoregulation

As discussed earlier, following birth healthy term babies should be placed against their mother's body skin-to-skin as soon as possible and for as long as possible as the primary measure to reduce heat loss. The baby should be gently dried and covered with a warm blanket to maintain their temperature. A mother's body conducts direct warmth to the baby, and the blanket traps a layer of warm, insulating air around the baby (Blackburn, 2017). The warmth generated from the mother minimises the need for the baby to use energy needed for other transitional processes on maintaining body temperature (Davies & Richards, 2020). Evidence suggests that there may be 'thermal synchrony' between mother and baby when skin-to-skin is practised (Ludington-Hoe et al., 2006). This would further contribute to energy conservation, which may assist in stabilising the heart and respiratory rate of the baby (Ebisch et al., 2012).

Skin-to-skin is the practice of having undisturbed time between a mother and baby in the immediate period after birth, also referred to as the 'Golden Hour', and as often as desired in the immediate postnatal period regardless of whether a woman intends to breastfeed or not (Bigelow & Power, 2020). Skin-to-skin benefits both the mother and baby. For a mother, having her baby skin-to-skin elevates the release of hormones such as prolactin, beta-endorphin and oxytocin, which are respectively associated with breastfeeding, analgesia, and attachment and nurturing interactions (Kostandy & Luddington-Hoe, 2016; Liu et al., 2015; Moore et al., 2016). All of these hormones are released in higher amounts compared with mothers who experience a delay in skin-to-skin, such as in caesarean births or when routine neonatal procedures take precedence (Bigelow & Power, 2020).

Skin-to-skin supports the baby in its transition to newborn life. It provides a thermoneutral environment thereby facilitating regulation of glucose metabolism, respiration and stabilisation of the heart rate (Moore et al., 2016). These babies appear to cry less, have lower stress levels as measured by cortisol, establish a microbiota that reflects maternal rather than hospital flora, have enhanced breastfeeding initiation and are breastfed for longer in the first year of life (Davies & Richards, 2020).

CRITICAL THINKING EXERCISE

Heat conservation

There are four ways in which babies can lose heat from their body surface (Blackburn, 2017):

1. evaporation
2. convection
3. conduction
4. radiation.

Which method(s) of heat loss is/are prevented by each of the following heat conservation methods?

- Placing the baby in immediate skin-to-skin contact with the mother.
- Drying the baby thoroughly immediately after birth (this also encourages the onset of respiration).
- Encouraging the mother to initiate skin-to-skin contact on an ongoing basis.
- Prewarming any hats, blankets and clothing prior to the birth.
- Prewarming the resuscitation area.
- Maintaining the temperature in the birthing room at >25°C.
- Replacing wet blankets or towels after drying the baby.
- Not bathing the baby until temperature has been stable for at least 2 hours (usually after the first 24 hours).
- Not placing the bassinet against windows, outside walls or doorways.
- In cooler environments, keeping the baby's head covered and body well wrapped.

(Source: Davies & Richards, 2020)

CLINICAL POINT

Conserving heat and keeping babies warm

There are multiple studies that demonstrate that babies who experience skin-to-skin contact immediately after birth are more likely to thermoregulate effectively (Moore et al., 2016; Widström et al., 2019). This is the single most effective way of ensuring that babies are able to conserve heat.

Hats applied at birth for small and pre-term infants have proved effective in reducing heat loss from the head in cool environments or when heat loss is a concern (Davidson et al., 2012; Michaelides, 2017b). However, it has been suggested that the presence of a hat on a healthy term baby in a warm room when it is enjoying skin-to-skin with its mother may interfere with the olfactory signals embodied in maternal/newborn scents. These sensory cues act as primary mediators in the attachment process (Lundström et al., 2013). The key role of the midwife therefore should be to actively encourage skin-to-skin contact and to ensure that the thermal environment of the room in conjunction with the maternal thermal habitus is thermoregulatory sufficient by careful monitoring of the baby at this time.

While warm towels, blankets and clothing are needed, overly tight wrapping prevents the movement that generates heat. The baby's clothes should not be too tight. It is better to use several thin layers than one or two thick layers (natural fabrics 'breathe' better than synthetics).

Bathing and temperature maintenance

Babies do not need to be bathed immediately after birth unless there is a risk of vertical transmission of an infection from the mother, such as hepatitis B or HIV. Bathing soon after birth increases the risk of hypothermia, and therefore it would be prudent to wait until the temperature of the baby has stabilised, usually after the first 24 hours (Davies & Richards, 2020).

Midwifery actions regarding bathing the baby

- Antenatal discussion about baby's first bath.
- Bath the baby in a draught-free room.
- Ensure the ambient temperature is 25–28°C.
- The baby's temperature should be within the normal range.
- Water temperature should be 36.7°C (similar temperature to skin when tested with the inside surface of an adult's wrist).
- Warm the towels and clothing.
- Do not expose the baby unnecessarily (e.g. keep wrapped in a towel while bathing the head).
- Dry the baby promptly and thoroughly, especially the hair and in the folds of the skin.

(Trotter, 2020)

The other important factor in maintaining thermoregulation is breastfeeding, as breast milk provides fuel for the baby's metabolic processes. Skin-to-skin contact appears to influence neurobehavioural responses making rooting and latching easier to achieve (Widström et al., 2019).

Impaired thermoregulatory control

Neonatal hypothermia

Following birth, the immature thermoregulatory system of the baby leaves the infant vulnerable to changes in environmental temperature (Davies & Richards, 2020). If the temperature of the baby falls below 36.5°C, there is a risk of hypothermia. Prevention is the best treatment and this can be achieved by following the actions outlined above. A mildly hypothermic baby (36–36.5°C) can generally be warmed without difficulty by nestling the baby against the mother skin-to-skin (and covering with a blanket) in a warm (>25°C) room (Michaelides, 2017b). If this is not possible or the baby continues to lose heat then a paediatrician should be informed.

Untreated hypothermia can result in generalised vasoconstriction that includes the pulmonary vessels. Pulmonary vasoconstriction results in decreased pulmonary perfusion that affects pH, P_aO_2 and P_aCO_2 levels. Increased P_aCO_2 and decreased P_aO_2 and pH levels result in respiratory acidosis. Consequently the baby will exhibit signs of respiratory distress (McEwan, 2017b). Underscoring the need for active steps to prevent heat loss is the fact that in newborn babies there is an interrelationship between thermoregulation, oxygenation and normal glycaemia. Normal function/levels in each of these metabolic processes support normal function/levels in the others. Therefore, the development of hypothermia, hypoxia or hypoglycaemia puts the baby at risk for development of the other two conditions (Fig. 31.1, Boxes 31.2, 31.3).

Neonatal hyperthermia

Hyperthermia is a temperature above 37.5°C and although it is much less common than hypothermia in the newborn, it can be as harmful as hypothermia if ignored. The most common cause of neonatal hyperthermia is underestimation of the effect of the environmental temperature on the baby (e.g. putting the bassinet next to a heater). However, babies can develop hyperthermia in response to an infection or occasionally an underlying medical condition and so any indication of a raised temperature must be carefully monitored. Research has reported a possible association between sudden unexpected death in infancy (SUDI) and the presence of *Staphylococcus aureus* (Blackwell et al., 2015). Blackwell's study notes that hyperthermia is one of the symptoms associated with the presence of staphylococcal endotoxins.

In general, it is important to assess the situation systemically rather than relying solely on temperature as a guide. Medical consultation is warranted when the baby's temperature is above 37.5°C without an obvious environmental cause, such as direct sunlight in a well-heated room, or when the baby has a lower temperature but is exhibiting other signs of being unwell such as not feeding. Similarly, consultation would be made if the temperature has not returned to normal within an hour of correcting an environmental cause (Michaelides, 2017b).

If the baby has overheated as a result of environmental factors, the baby should be slowly cooled by removing excessive layers of clothing, exposing its hands to the air and using a single blanket or sheet for cover. Extremes

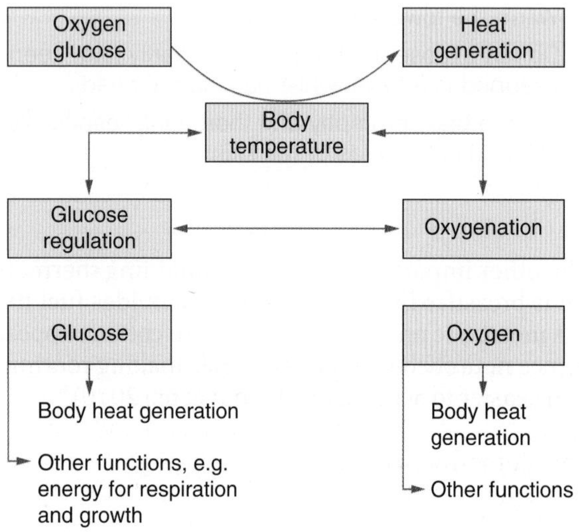

FIGURE 31.1 Interrelationship between temperature regulation, glucose concentration and respiration
(Source: based on Davies & MacDonald, 2020)

Box 31.2 Relationship between hypothermia, hypoxia and hypoglycaemia in neonates

- Healthy neonates have limited stores of glycogen and brown fat and are vulnerable to rapid heat loss.
- Pre-term infants have less glycogen stores and brown fat and greater vulnerability to heat loss than term babies.
- Hypothermia leads to brown fat lipolysis to restore the temperature. The process consumes oxygen and glycogen.
- Hypoglycaemia leads to mobilisation of glycogen stores to restore serum glucose levels. The process of converting glycogen to glucose requires oxygen and heat. Glycogen stores are depleted.
- Hypoxia leads to anaerobic methods of oxygen production. These inefficient processes require heat and glucose. Glycogen stores are depleted.

(Based on Davies & Richards, 2020)

Box 31.3 Clinical alert

Clothed babies who become hypothermic in an appropriately warm environment need *very prompt* medical assessment and investigation, especially for infection. In these circumstances the low temperature is likely to indicate a serious illness (usually an infection) rather than an environmental cause for the hypothermia.

Referral must not be delayed

A low (or raised) temperature may be the only sign of early onset group B streptococcal infection. Unexpected hypothermia in an otherwise well baby is always abnormal.

(Based on Davies & Richards, 2020)

such as removing all covers or cool bathing must be avoided, as rapid cooling can precipitate excessive heat loss and shock (Michaelides, 2017b).

Haemopoietic system

Haemoglobin concentration

The fetal circulation enables fetal blood to be oxygenated at the placental site and to be transported to the brain and other vital organs as efficiently as possible. This is assisted by high concentrations of fetal haemoglobin (HbF), a type of haemoglobin that has a higher affinity for oxygen than does adult haemoglobin. After birth the neonate is exposed to higher oxygen levels associated with breathing air. As the red cells with fetal haemoglobin are haemolysed, they are replaced by cells containing adult haemoglobin with a lower affinity for oxygen. Neonatal red blood cells have a shorter lifespan than adult cells, and as they are destroyed this produces elevated serum bilirubin levels and physiological jaundice in some babies (Deken & Meeks, 2020) (see below).

The haemoglobin level is initially high (180–200 g/L), and 50%–85% of this is fetal haemoglobin. The levels decrease gradually, with changes apparent in the first week after birth, and fall to approximately 120 g/L by 3 months of age. Conversion from fetal to adult haemoglobin, which is commenced in utero, is completed in the first 1–2 years of life (Davies & Richards, 2020).

Physiological jaundice

Physiological jaundice occurs as a result of the normal breakdown of red blood cells which contain HbF that is no longer required. In a healthy baby the liver is immature and thus unable to process circulating bilirubin until approximately 2 weeks following the birth (Deken & Meeks, 2020).

Physiological jaundice is a very common phenomenon in the newborn, occurring in more than 60% of term babies. It usually appears at about 72 hours of age, peaks at 4 days and declines over the next week (Deken & Meeks, 2020). As long as the baby is alert, has good muscle tone, is feeding well, passing urine normally and is content between feeds, no action is required other than to patiently wait for the jaundice to dissipate (Box 31.4). It is believed that this benign form of jaundice may bestow specific benefits that trigger protective mechanisms in the newborn including antioxidant and antibiotic properties (Gazzin, 2016).

Box 31.4 Clinical alert

Women are sometimes told to expose the baby to the sun to 'treat' physiological jaundice. However, in countries such as Australia and New Zealand that have high ultraviolet levels this is not recommended as the radiation can lead to melanoma development (Ghazi et al., 2012) as well as the risk of sunburn. Babies should therefore never be placed in direct sunlight.

Pathological jaundice

There are, however, occasions when hyperbilirubinaemia reaches elevated levels which can lead to acute bilirubin encephalopathy or bilirubin-induced brain injury. Careful assessment and monitoring of any signs of jaundice in the first weeks of life is therefore important to exclude any potential pathology. Jaundice may additionally be the only sign of bacterial infection (Deken & Meeks, 2020). See Chapter 42 for pathological causes of jaundice and for treatment methods.

CLINICAL POINT

Assessing jaundice

Jaundice progresses from the 'baby's head to the toes. As a rule of thumb, the further down the body the jaundice has progressed, the higher the serum bilirubin level. The Kramer rule is a visual assessment tool that has an accuracy value of 86.27% (Aprillia et al., 2017; see Kramer's rule, Fig. 31.2). Daily assessment and monitoring of the skin colour, muscle tone, alertness, feeding patterns, urinary output and sleeping behaviours of the baby will assist in determining whether an estimation of serum bilirubin is warranted. It is very important not to rely on skin colour alone. A dehydrated baby, for example, will exhibit the lethargy and poor urine output related to the lack of fluids while still only mildly yellow, whilst babies who are alert and feeding well with good muscle tone and urinary output may be quite yellow looking but be well.

- Serum bilirubin estimation in a term baby is warranted if:
  - the baby is less than 48 hours of age
  - the baby is jaundiced (any degree of yellowness) and sleepy and/or feeding poorly and/or has a reduced urinary output.
- If the jaundice persists for longer than 7–10 days, look at the condition of the baby overall and consider the possibility of breast milk jaundice (see Ch. 32).
- Remember that the level of jaundice in darker-skinned babies is more difficult to assess. Check the sclera of the eyes and/or blanch the baby's gums with a gloved finger. The depth of the yellow discoloration provides additional information.

Note: Assess the baby in natural light where possible.

Red blood cells, haematocrit and leucocytes

Neonatal red blood cells (RBCs) have a lifespan of 80–100 days, approximately two-thirds of the lifespan of adult RBCs. In the first few days of the baby's life, the haematocrit (packed-cell volume, PCV) may increase above fetal levels as a result of placental transfusion and diminished extracellular fluid volume. The RBC count ($5–7 \times 10^{12}$/L) and haematocrit levels (55%) decrease gradually during the first 2–3 months of life. The leucocyte or white blood cell (WBC) count is usually high by conventional standards ($1–25 \times 10^{9}$/L) but decreases rapidly. An elevated level of immature neutrophils is usually an indicator of infection.

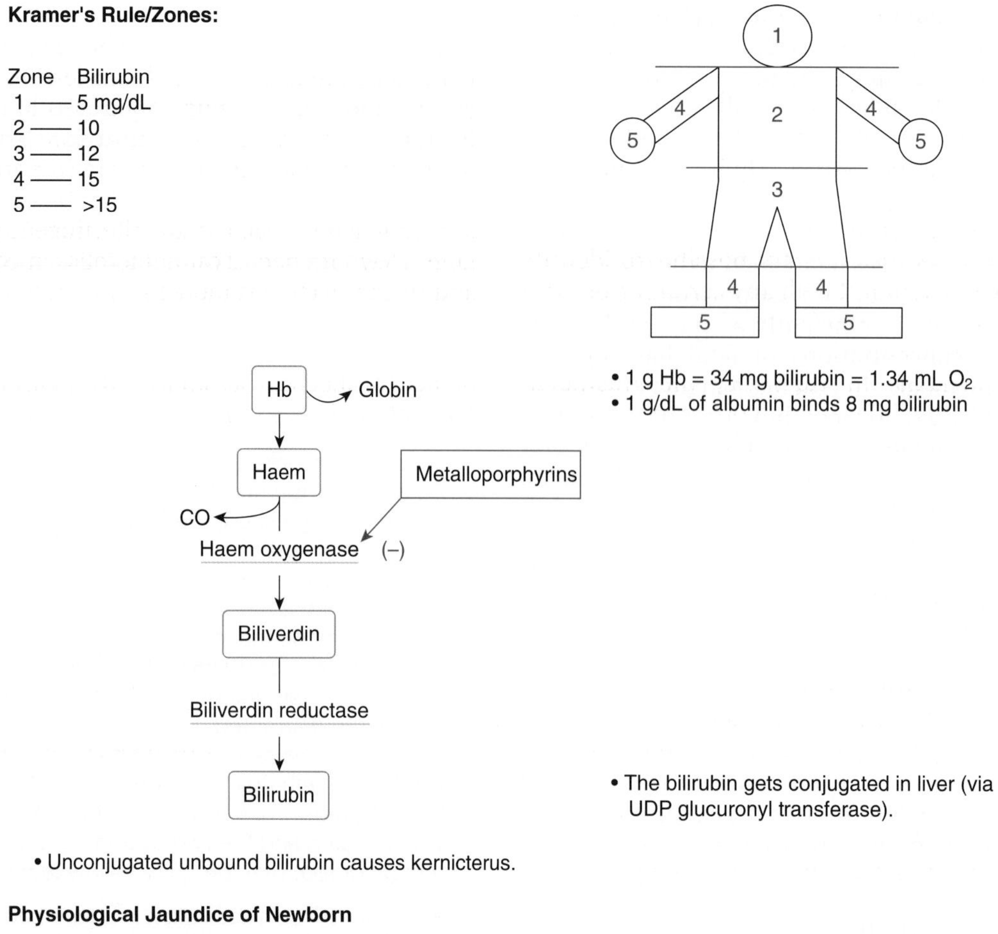

FIGURE 31.2 Kramer's rule.
(Source: Adapted from Neonatal Directorate Management Committee.)

Clotting factors and vitamin K synthesis

Vitamin K is essential in order to synthesise the functional forms of coagulation factors II, VII, IX, and X in the liver of the baby. It would seem that limited placental transfer of vitamin K leaves the baby depleted of some required components in the clotting mechanism (Lippi & Franchini, 2011). Colonisation of the intestine by the bacteria that synthesise vitamin K does not occur until feeding is established. Therefore, blood clotting is to all intents and purposes impaired in the first week postpartum while levels of vitamin K-dependent clotting factors are low (Blackburn, 2017; Michaelides, 2017a). It is unclear why newborn infants have reduced levels of vitamin K-dependent clotting factors; it has been postulated that this may be related to fetal growth regulation (Blackburn, 2017). If vitamin K is not administered parenterally, the natural course is for the vitamin K levels to decrease initially as maternally acquired vitamin K is used. Neonatal vitamin K stores then increase gradually over the first month (Blackburn, 2017).

Vitamin K deficiency bleeding

A rare but serious condition that occurs in some babies is vitamin K deficiency bleeding (VKDB). VKDB can occur as early onset (<48 hours), classic (2–7 days) or late onset (1 week to 6 months) (Blackburn, 2017). The natural prevalence of the classic form is 0.25% to 1.5% (250–1500 per 100,000) babies (Marchelli et al., 2018).

Breastfed babies are seen to be at more risk of haemorrhagic disease than formula-fed infants because formula contains vitamin K. However, it is difficult to predict which babies will develop VKDB, as babies without specific risk factors can develop classic VKDB (Zurynski et al., 2020). Because of these factors, prophylactic vitamin K at birth is recommended to prevent VKDB (Blackburn, 2017). It has been suggested that it is not likely to be an abnormally low milk concentration of vitamin K that creates the potential for the problem of VKDB, but rather a low cumulative intake of breast milk in the first week or so of life (Dekker & Bertone, 2019). This holds a pertinent message for midwives and others supporting women in their early endeavours to breastfeed.

Routine vitamin K prophylaxis

VKDB is a rare disease but it is becoming more prevalent, especially in countries such as the UK and Aotearoa New Zealand where parents may choose to decline the administration of Vitamin K for their babies (Zurynski et al., 2020). The World Health Organization strongly recommends routine prophylaxis of 1mg intramuscular (IM) vitamin K for all babies. Oral multi-dose vitamin K is an alternative but the efficacy and reliability of oral administration is inferior, particularly in relation to late onset VKDB (Visser et al., 2011). It is probable that vitamin K prophylaxis is not needed at birth by every baby; nevertheless, because it is not possible to identify those who do need vitamin K with any certainty, prophylaxis is policy in most maternity services. The NZCOM Consensus Statement (2001, updated 2016) supports vitamin K prophylaxis. In Australia, the Australian College of Midwives (ACM) were part of a joint statement recommending that all babies should be given vitamin K prophylactically (National Health and Medical Research Council (NHMRC), 2010).

Dosage

- A single dose (1 mg) of IM vitamin K at birth effectively prevents classic VKDB (Zurynski et al., 2020).
- The effectiveness of IM vitamin K in the prevention of late VKDB has been established (Sankar et al., 2016).
- An updated systematic review to identify studies exploring the value of oral administration vs IM is long overdue. The last Cochrane review on this in 2000 compared IM with oral routes of administration of vitamin K (Puckett & Offringa, 2000). Evaluation of 11 randomised controlled trials (RCTs) identified that if administered soon after birth a single dose of IM vitamin K, compared with a single oral dose, provided higher plasma levels of vitamin K in the first few weeks of life when the risk of VKDB is highest. However, multiple doses of oral vitamin K resulted in higher plasma levels at 2 weeks and 2 months than did a single IM dose.
- Local policies relating to the administration of oral vitamin K may differ. The three-dose regimen is common. The doses are usually spread across the first 6 weeks of life (e.g. at birth, 1 week and 6 weeks) (Dekkerand Bertone, 2019).

There is a need for further research on the administration of vitamin K for babies at birth not least because there is no universal dosage currently. The possible adaptive relationship between low levels of vitamin K and the infant's microbiome has been raised as possible reason for low levels in the newborn (Domingo-Bellez et al., 2019). Additionally there is an argument that premature cord clamping may have impacted on the coagulation levels in the baby, which may have increased the prevalence of VKDB. There is currently an interest in whether maternal supplementation could improve vitamin K in breastfed infants. However, there is currently insufficient evidence to recommend this as an alternative (Dekker & Bertone, 2019).

In the meantime, midwives are advised to focus on their local policies and to watch for any further developments.

Immunological adaptations

Functional immaturity of the immune system and lack of exposure to common microorganisms at birth mean that babies are very vulnerable to infections, particularly respiratory and gastrointestinal infections. Antibody-mediated and cell-mediated immunity, the inflammatory response and complement factors are all different in newborn infants. Newborn babies cannot localise infections very well, and so an infection is more likely to become systemic. The immaturity of the gut defence mechanism increases the likelihood of both gastrointestinal infection and later development of allergies (Blackburn, 2017; Weström et al., 2020). A key player in immunological defences is the microbiome.

Microbiome

The importance of the microbiome is now incontrovertible. Our microbiota is a unique ecosystem that is composed of bacteria, bacteriophage, fungi, protozoa and viruses (Pickard et al., 2017). It responds to and may alter as a result of a range of factors including genes, culture, nutrition, medication, age and BMI, among others. These alterations can effect changes within our bodies and thus alter our health status (Wen & Duffy, 2017).

Both commensal and pathogenic microorganisms colonise extensively in the baby during birth, although there is evidence that the microbiome of the fetus begins in utero (Collado et al., 2016). Colonisation ensues following exposure to maternal vaginal and faecal bacteria, the mother's skin, and eventually from other people and the general environment (McEwan, 2017b). When a baby is born vaginally, the bacteria most commonly resemble those present in the maternal vaginal microbiota and include *Lactobacillus, Prevotella* and *Sneathia* (Fettweis et al., 2019). Following caesarean section, the microbiota is very different with a lower bacterial diversity (Rutayisire et al., 2016). By understanding the development of the early life gut microbiota, we are able to access this short-lived window of opportunity to improve health outcomes for the baby regardless of modality of birth.

CLINICAL POINT

Prevention and assessment of neonatal infection

The newborn infant is particularly susceptible to infection because of its immature immune system. However, the risk of infection can be minimised if relatively simple measures are put in place. These include: ensuring that standard precautions are enforced by health professionals at all times, sharing information with parents about how to prevent infection through general hygiene measures such as hand cleansing and providing them with information about danger signals for infection (Box 31.5), keeping equipment used for the baby in closed containers and encouraging common-sense precautions such as keeping the baby away from people with colds, etc.

Midwives need to be able to recognise any risk factors for development of infection and monitor for signs of onset; have a good understanding of the subtle signs of infection in neonates, and particularly note that fever may not be present with an infection; and understand normal neonatal laboratory findings and recognise, and act on, changes that are associated with neonatal infection. In relation to the microbiome, there are specific actions that the midwife can encourage that may contribute to the gut integrity that will offer the newborn a whole host of benefits in terms of health and wellbeing (Dahlen et al., 2014; Kristensen & Henriksen, 2016; Matamoros et al., 2013). See Table 31.1.

Renal system

At birth the kidneys are structurally complete but functionally immature. There are limitations in the glomerular filtration rate capability and the ability to concentrate or dilute urine. Newborn babies have little renal reserve to cope with increased levels of solutes, which may occur in physiologically stressed or ill neonates (Michaelides, 2017a; Tappero & Honeyfield, 2018). The total body water

Box 31.5 Child sickness danger signals

Get help from a doctor *quickly* if your baby or young child shows any of these signs.

General:

- Cannot be woken or is responding less than usual to what is going on around them.
- Has glazed eyes and is not focusing on anything.
- Seems more floppy, drowsy or less alert than usual.
- Has a convulsion or fit.
- Has an unusual cry for 1 hour or more.
- Has been badly injured.
- There is a bulge in the groin which gets bigger with crying.

Temperature:

- Feels too cold or too hot (temperature 38.3°C or higher).
- Circulation and skin colour:
  - Body is much paler than usual or suddenly goes very white.
  - Nails are blue or big toe is completely white, or colour does not return to toe within three seconds of a squeeze.

Breathing:

- Goes blue or stops breathing.
- Breathes more quickly than normal or grunts.
- Is wheezing when breathing out.
- In-drawing of the chest is visible with each breath.

Vomiting and diarrhoea:

- Has vomited at least half the feed after each of the last three feeds.
- Has green vomit.
- Has taken less fluid than usual.
- Has passed less urine than usual.
- Has a large amount of blood in nappy.

(Source: Ministry of Health, 2016; http://www.health.govt.nz/your-health/pregnancy-and-kids/first-year/helpful-advice-during-first-year/baby-and-child-sickness-danger-signs https://creativecommons.org/licenses/by/4.0/)

Table 31.1 Supporting the microbiome

In pregnancy
Carry out a nutritional assessment and discuss gut health and its significance in pregnancy.
Consider colostrum harvesting prior to planned CS, if gestation diabetes is present or any other condition that may delay milk transfer for the baby.
Educate women and their partners about the benefits of breastfeeding in relation to the microbiome.
Discuss the importance of a physiological labour and birth as a means of optimising the physiological preparation of the gut environment for the baby.
During labour and birth
Encourage a 'default' approach where normal physiological birth is not possible, i.e. discussing with obstetric colleagues the possibility of labouring to some degree wherever possible in order to trigger the anti-inflammatory responses etc. of early labour.
During a CS request that antibiotics are not introduced until the baby has been born and the cord clamped.
In the early postnatal period
Practise skin-to-skin contact wherever birth has occurred as early as is practical.
Use harvested colostrum where necessary but continue to additionally put the baby to the breast.
Aim to assist the woman to establish breastfeeding as early as possible and ensure that as much support as the woman requires is available.
Support exclusive breastfeeding wherever possible.
Avoid bathing the baby for at least the first 24 hours and longer if possible.

content in newborn babies is a larger proportion of body fluid than in adults. The shift of intracellular fluid into the extracellular compartment after birth results in a diuresis that causes loss of 5%–10% of birth weight over the first week (National Guideline Alliance (UK), 2017). If the mother has received synthetic oxytocin to induce or augment labour, the baby is likely to experience a greater degree of diuresis owing to the antidiuretic effect of synthetic oxytocin.

Urine is normally passed within 24 hours of birth. Initially the newborn baby excretes as little as 30–60 mL in the first 48 hours of life. Volume and frequency increase with rising fluid intake. The urine has a low specific gravity, is straw coloured and is odourless. Until fluid intake increases, the urine may be cloudy from the presence of mucus or urates. Urates may cause pink or brick-red staining on the nappy. Whilst a common and normal finding in the first few days of life, the presence of urates in the urine of babies more than a few days old may indicate dehydration (Tappero & Honeyfield, 2018). When the bladder becomes full it is palpable abdominally. The kidneys may also be palpable. On micturition the direction and force of the stream of urine should be noted.

Gastrointestinal system

Stomach

At birth the cardiac sphincter and nervous control of the stomach are immature. The cardiac sphincter has transient episodes of relaxation that predispose to possetting (regurgitation). Sphincter muscle tone improves rapidly during the first week, while final maturity may take up to 12 months (Blackburn, 2017; Michaelides, 2017a). Projectile vomiting, especially appearing from approximately the end of the first week, may indicate congenital pyloric stenosis.

Liver

Physiological immaturity of the liver results in low production of hepatic glucuronyl transferase for the conjugation of bilirubin. This may result in transient physiological jaundice after 48 hours. Glycogen stores are rapidly depleted, and therefore early feeding is needed to maintain normal blood glucose levels and compensate for used glycogen. Liver function and colonisation of the intestine, both of which assist in the formation of vitamin K, are stimulated by feeding (Davies, 2020).

Glucose regulation

During pregnancy the fetus is in an environment in which glucose levels are consistently 60%–70% of maternal levels. During the third trimester, the fetus prepares for the transition primarily by storing glycogen, producing catecholamines and depositing brown fat (Cornblath & Ichord, 2000).

Following birth, as a result of intricate biochemical processes that facilitate metabolic transitional activity, a transient period of neonatal hypoglycaemia usually occurs. This is a physiologically self-limiting event in the case of healthy term neonates and is a normal part of the adaptation process once the maternal glucose supply has ceased (Hawdon, 2016). Midwives should be aware that early metabolic adaptation in the normal term baby is typified by active ketogenesis (the utilisation of ketone bodies for energy). This results in lower blood glucose levels than may previously have been considered 'normal' levels (Hewitt et al., 2005). There does not appear to be a definitive consensus concerning the normoglycaemic to hypoglycaemic cut-off point in the neonate. The key recognition is that there will be a preliminary fall in blood glucose in the 2–6 hours following birth and thereafter a slow but steady rise in the proceeding 24 hours (Hawdon, 2016).

Neonatologist Jane Hawdon (2013) recalls her experience of early research in this area and acknowledges that the fear of 'pathological' hypoglycaemia in the newborn was resulting in overdiagnosis of the condition and subsequent intervention. She concludes that this practice led to unnecessary and untimely intervention in the form of serial blood glucose measurements, affecting maternal confidence and resulting in supplementation of breastfeeding.

A more recent intervention is oral dextrose gel which has been hailed as a cost-effective and relatively low-level intervention with good outcomes. A recent evaluative randomised controlled trial revealed that the intervention did not reduce the number of NICU admissions for babies at risk but did reduce hypoglycaemia. It concluded that further long-term follow-up is needed to determine the clinical utility of the practice (Harding et al., 2021).

It should be noted however that, whilst healthy term babies are at low risk of developing hypoglycaemia, any situation before or after birth that has either prevented the accumulation of glycogen stores (e.g. pre-term birth or fetal growth restriction) or caused abnormal consumption of glycogen (e.g. fetal distress or hypothermia) increases the risk of hypoglycaemia. Satisfactory early feeding is particularly important for these babies and blood glucose levels may need to be monitored (Hawdon, 2016) (see Ch. 42).

CLINICAL POINT

Signs of neonatal hypoglycaemia

Signs are often vague and non-specific. They can include:

Hypothermia	Irritability	Tachypnoea / apnoea
Poor temperature control	Lethargy	Abnormal eye movements
Sweating	Hypotonia	Tachycardia
Poor suck or refusal to feed	Seizures	Congestive heart failure
Tremors	Cyanosis	Respiratory distress

(Adapted from British Association of Perinatal Medicine, 2017.)

Neurological system

Nervous system activity develops progressively in fetal life; however, although term babies are able to receive and process stimuli appropriate for neonatal development, the nervous system is still quite anatomically and physiologically immature. The brain is approximately a quarter of adult size and myelination of nerve fibres is incomplete. Such immaturity results in brainstem and spinal reflex activity predominating in the early months. Healthy term babies are capable of **social interaction**, which continues to develop as the brain continues to grow rapidly (Blackburn, 2017). The autonomic nervous system of the baby maintains homeostasis; however, instability of thermoregulatory processes in the early days and uncoordinated muscle movement reflect the incomplete state of neurological development. The presence of a wide range of reflex activities at varying ages is an indication of the normality and integrity of the neurological and muscular systems.

PHYSICAL ASSESSMENT OF THE NEWBORN

Although it is a physical assessment, the examination of the newborn should be completed using a holistic approach. In New Zealand the **newborn assessment** is a standard component of the Ministry of Health contract specifications for the provision of primary maternity care (MOH, 2007). This means that a midwife is expected to be able to carry out a full and comprehensive assessment of the essentially healthy baby including the assessments for hips, heart and eyes. If any problems are detected then the baby is referred to a paediatrician for further follow-up. In Australia the midwife's legal and professional responsibilities with regards to neonatal assessment vary according to state and local protocols. However, in many locations a medical practitioner is expected to perform a neonatal assessment within 24 hours of birth or before discharge from the maternity unit. Nevertheless, this does not preclude the midwife developing the skills of neonatal assessment. In the presence of continuity-of-care models the ability to take on this aspect of practice assumes greater significance and likewise rural practice has a greater need for such skills. In some countries, it feels as though the examination of the newborn has been accredited with some sort of expert status that requires a level of skill and responsibility over and above normal midwifery practice expectation. This is unfortunate because, far from being a mere physical assessment, the examination of the newborn is a wonderful opportunity to educate, inform and facilitate empowerment for women and their families.

The examination of the newborn should form part of an ongoing process of monitoring. An initial assessment should take place in the birthing room in the immediate postbirth period. This allows for observation of the baby as a whole, forms the baseline for future checks and provides an alert to areas of concern. This early assessment does not need to be carried out immediately after birth and can be left for an hour or so unless any problems are detected. It can be carried out at the bedside of the mother to avoid unnecessary separation, to facilitate information sharing regarding the health and wellbeing of the baby and to offer parents an opportunity to ask questions and to express any concerns.

The initial 'head-to-toe' assessment does not always include an examination of the hips. This may be completed when the baby is 24 hours old (Bahar et al., 2019). In addition, assessment of cardiovascular function and the red eye reflex is usually repeated 24 hours after the initial examination. These three areas are subject to significant change within the first few hours and a 24-hour lapse allows for the final adaptations in the cardiovascular system and for circulating maternal hormones to settle as this may have an effect, for example, on ligamentous laxity in the hips (Bahar et al., 2019). However, with the exception of these areas, the general principles that apply to the full neonatal examination also apply to ongoing assessments.

The examination of the baby, whether 24 hours or 6 weeks after birth, offers a good opportunity for the midwife to utilise health promotion and education skills. Women are usually receptive to any information that they are offered when it relates to their baby. A conversation during this important assessment could include the topics of skincare, choice of nappies, sleeping arrangements or bathing. It should, however, always be focused on getting the parents to consider their own solutions, rather than providing the answers.

History

It is always worth spending some time revisiting the family medical history prior to commencing the examination, even if the woman is well known to the midwife in a continuity-of-care model. It is not unusual for important information to surface once the baby has been born, even when the woman has been asked directly in the antenatal period.

Factors to take into account from the clinical record and the baby's parents include:

- the parents' appearance/stature—a small baby may merely reflect the size of the parents, for example
- genetic factors—any known family history
- environmental factors—known maternal exposure to teratogenic agents, smoking, recreational or prescription drugs, etc.
- social factors, maternal blood group, medical conditions
- pregnancy and intrapartum variations—such as intrauterine growth, liquor volume, fetal distress, maternal analgesia, intrapartum complications
- neonatal factors—Apgar score, birth weight (McDonald, 2020).

General rules for examining newborn babies (Box 31.6)

The assessment, like all assessments, should begin with observation. A great deal of information can be elicited by just looking before laying hands on the baby. Observe as much as possible before the baby is fully undressed.

Box 31.6 General rules for examining newborn babies

- The examination should always be undertaken with the consent of the baby's mother and in her presence.
- The assessment findings are communicated to the baby's mother or both parents at the time of the examination.
- Equipment should be checked before use and at hand. This should include:
  - light source (pen torch)
  - neonatal stethoscope
  - thermometer
  - ophthalmoscope
  - tape measure for head circumference
  - measuring mat for accurate length measurement.
- The environment where the examination is taking place should have adequate lighting (but not too bright) and be quiet and warm.
- The baby should be in a quiet, alert state.
- Endeavour to carry out the assessment as close to the mother as physically possible and involve her in the process.
- Be firm but gentle—babies feel insecure if not handled confidently. Smooth, gentle handling will give maximum information with minimum disturbance to the baby.
- Without compromising the thoroughness of the examination, minimise the time during which the baby is unclothed, to prevent chilling and disturbance.
- Use the same process every time so that nothing is missed.
- Examine the baby generally in a 'top-to-toe' direction.
- Pay particular attention to symmetry. Each side should be roughly the same—sounds, length, size, creases, muscle tone, flexion.

Exceptions to the 'top-to-toe' process are:

- It is usual to start with examination of the baby's heart and lungs while the baby is least disturbed and less likely to cry. Nearly all babies cry when naked for any length of time, so it would be advisable to listen to the heart and lungs before removing all of the baby's clothes.
- Examination of the hips for developmental dysplasia is uncomfortable for the baby and therefore best carried out at the end of the examination on a firm surface. Similarly, weighing the baby should be reserved until near the end of the examination (McDonald, 2020).

All of the head, the baby's general muscle tone and some of the reflexes can be observed while the baby is still clothed. The general appearance of the baby in relation to colour, position, posture, spontaneous activity, facial dysmorphia and length-to-leanness proportion can be taken into account. The behavioural state of the baby is also observable: is the baby irritable and crying, alert awake or sleeping peacefully?

The other important observation is how the mother is interacting with her baby. Is there evidence of attachment? Are they behaving in the way that you would expect of a mother/baby pairing? If things are not as they should be, it may be necessary to explore this further by engaging in conversation with the woman to establish how the relationship is developing.

General measurements (centile charts)

Every baby in all Australian states as well as New Zealand has an individual health record book that is maintained by all providers of healthcare during the first 2–5 years. These include centile charts to record the growth of the baby. In 2006, the World Health Organization published International Child Growth Standards. These growth charts are based on growth rates of babies who are exclusively breastfed for 6 months and continue to be breastfed after the introduction of solids. Consult the Well Child record book or the local area Department of Health website, as centile charts usually reflect the growth patterns of each country's population and therefore vary a little. Serial measurements of weight, length and head circumference are recorded in the clinical notes and/or on the centile charts in the baby's health record book. The centile charts provide a visual record that enables comparison of growth in the three measurement dimensions. Different centile charts are used for boys and girls. In healthy term babies, all three measurements parallel each other along the same centile curve (e.g. all following the 50th centile curve) (Fig. 31.3). Babies who have an initial measurement below the 3rd or above the 97th centile are carefully assessed to exclude underlying causes, as are babies with ongoing measurements that begin to fall below the initial centile curve. Referral to a medical practitioner for review is usually required in these circumstances.

Babies double their weight by 5–6 months and treble it by the end of the first year. After 6 months babies gain 100 g per week on average. The average length at birth is 48–52 cm. By 6 months, 8–10 cm is gained, and another 10 cm by the end of the first year. (See Ch. 32 for feeding and weight gain.)

In mid-2010, the Ministry of Health in New Zealand amended growth charts to include the following:

- new centiles—using nine centiles and extending from the 0.4th to the 99.6th centile
- no centile lines for 1–2 weeks of age—because most babies lose some weight and then regain it during the two weeks after birth
- a separate pre-term birth section
- an adult height prediction and BMI look up (MOH, 2015).

More recently Australia has made some changes such as excluding pre-term and small-for-gestational-age babies (Farmey et al., 2020).

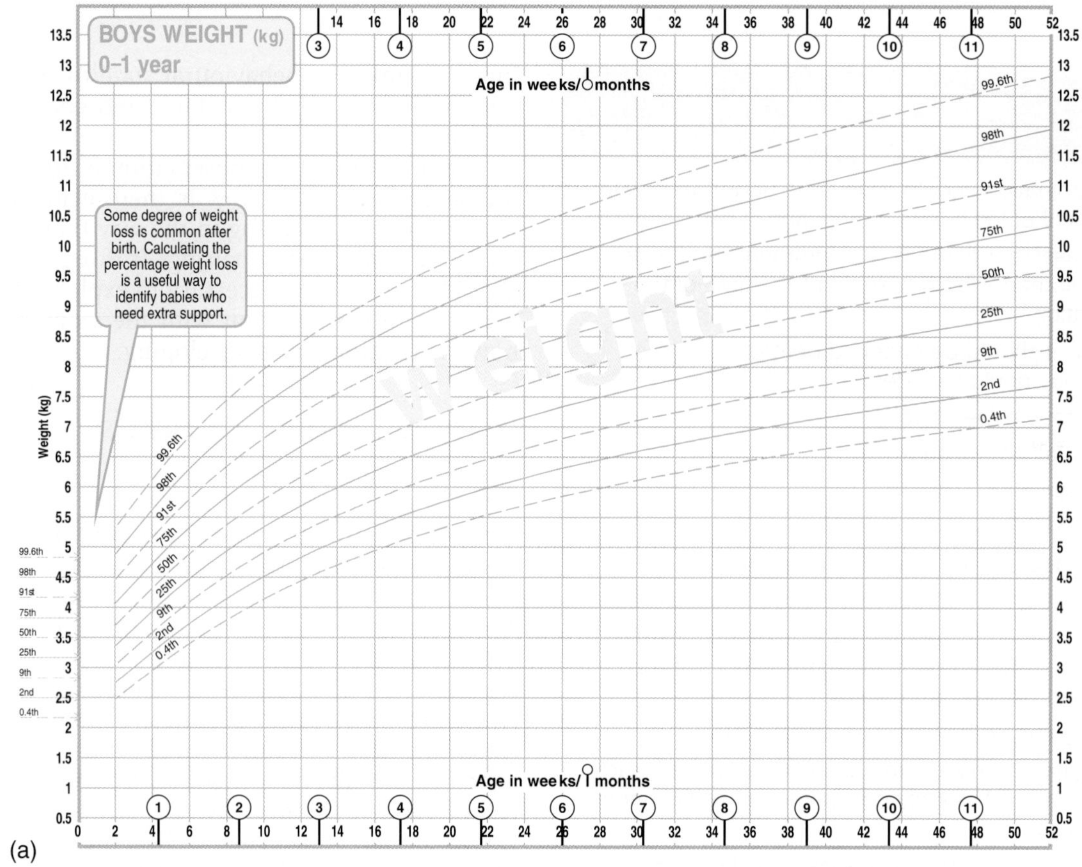

(a)

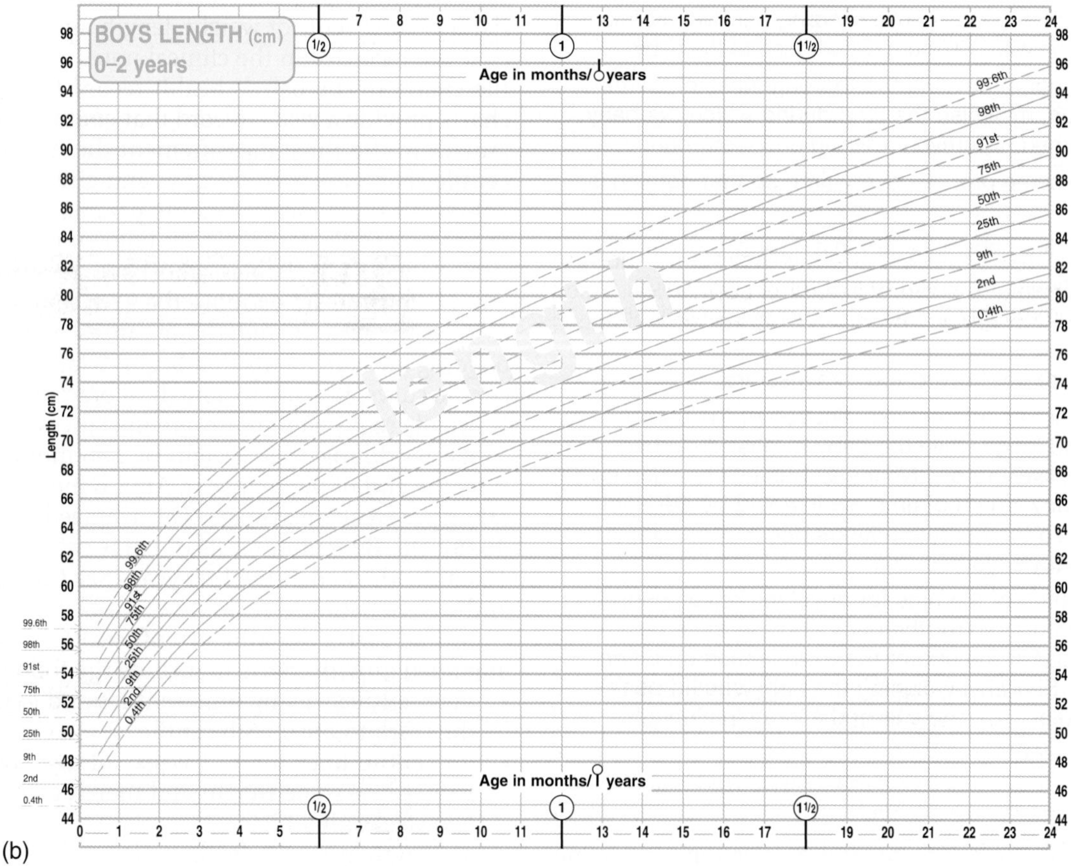

(b)

FIGURE 31.3 Growth charts: (a) head circumference from 24 weeks to 1 year (male); (b) length from 35 weeks to 1 year (male); (c) weight from 23 weeks to 1 year (male)
(Source: Adapted from Henderson & Macdonald, 2004)

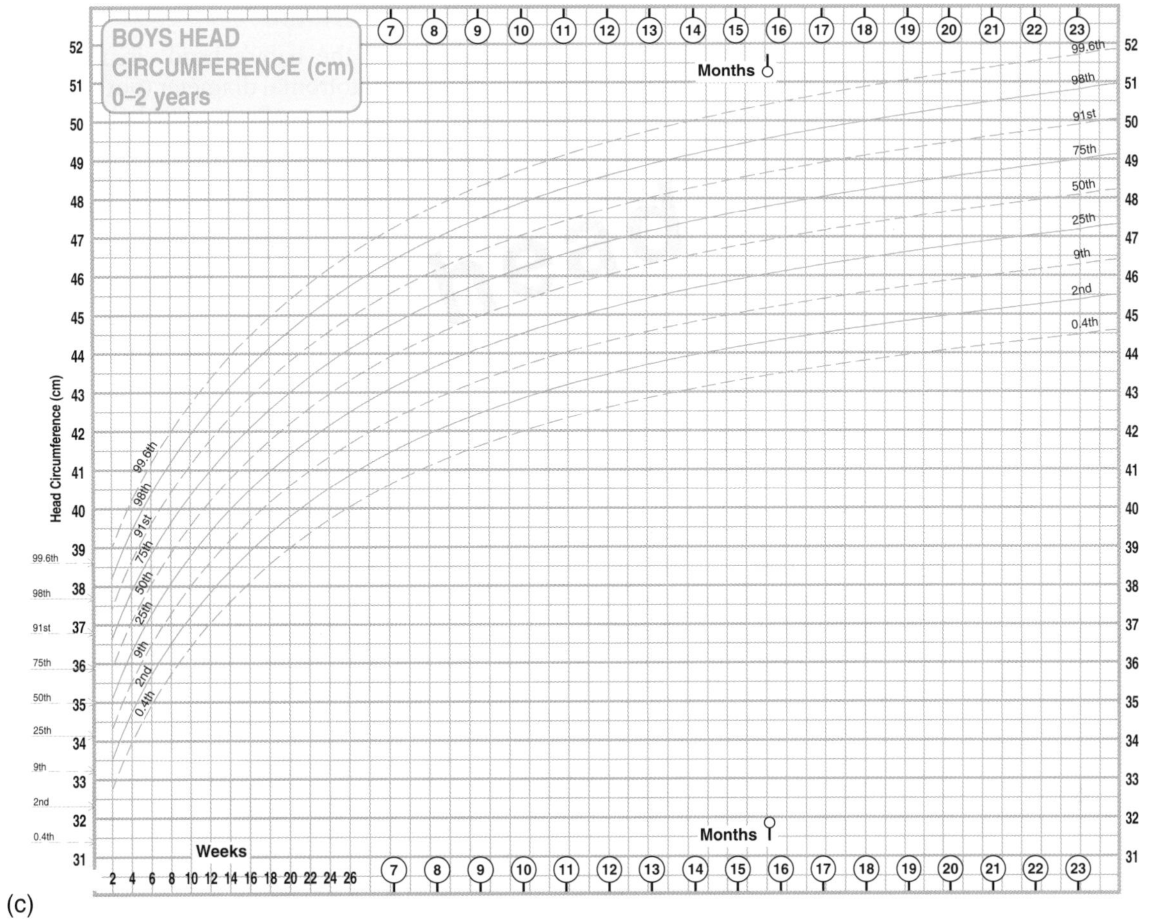

FIGURE 31.3 cont'd

In both countries the changes have been introduced in order to encourage a more accurate population-based centile chart that allows for some discrepancies such as initial weight loss as well as acknowledging the more specific needs of pre-term and SGA babies.

Crown-to-heel length

Local policy applies as to whether calibrated measuring equipment or a tape measure is used to assess length in the first few weeks of life. When a tape measure is used at the early examinations, this assessment is only an approximation. Calibrated equipment is required for accurate and reliable length measurement.

To use a calibrated box or mat (Fig. 31.4), the baby's head and feet must be flat against either end, which is quite difficult to achieve with newly born babies. Whichever method is used, the mother is usually asked to assist by holding the baby's leg(s) straight while the measurement is taken.

The average crown-to-heel length of a term baby at birth is 51 cm (MOH, 2015).

Weight

It may be prudent to weigh the baby towards the end of the assessment when clothes have been removed. To

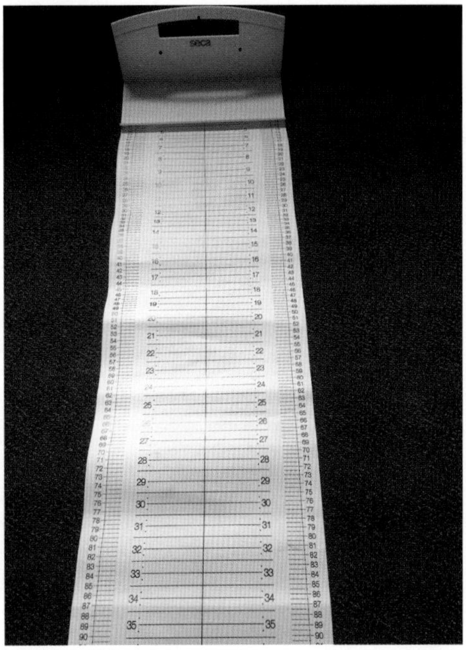

FIGURE 31.4 Calibrated mat for measuring crown–heel length

improve reliability it is preferable to use the same set of regularly maintained scales for serial weight measurements. Babies are generally weighed at birth, sometime towards the end of the first week, then weekly until 4–6 weeks old. The average birth weight of a term baby is 3500 g, although this may be higher or lower in some populations (MOH, 2015). Healthy term babies can lose 5%–10% of their birth weight due to physiological diuresis (Blackburn, 2017). In practice, a 7% loss is generally regarded as the alert point where a discussion with the mother about considering increasing feeding would be prudent. Because a midwifery assessment and feeding plan is made with the mother at 7% weight loss, referral to a medical practitioner is usually made at the point of 10% weight loss. The baby should have regained her or his birth weight by 10–14 days. Generally, term infants gain 30 g/day for the first 3 months (Blackburn, 2017). However, if a healthy term baby appears to be feeding well and is having six to eight wet nappies in 24 hours, this is a fairly good indication that the baby is feeding well. Babies who are not term, and/or not feeding well, and/or not exhibiting normal urinary output, need to have an appropriate plan of care in place (see Ch. 42).

Head circumference

Measurement of the baby's head circumference is taken around the occipitofrontal diameter (not the ears). The average head circumference for a term baby is 35 cm (MOH, 2015). There may be a discrepancy between the measurement at birth and that at the end-of-first-week assessment, as moulding can make an accurate initial assessment difficult.

Gestational age assessment

It is possible to make a general assessment of gestational age at birth as unexpectedly pre-term babies can make an appearance. The following signs would indicate that the baby is full term:

- Flexed limbs at rest (Fig. 31.5).
- The elbow does not reach the midline when the 'scarf sign' is assessed (Fig. 31.6).
- The ear promptly returns to the normal position when folded forwards and released.
- Cartilage and curves of the pinna are complete.
- Genitalia are well developed; in males, the scrotum is covered in rugae and testes are usually descended, and in females the labia majora completely cover the clitoris and labia minora.

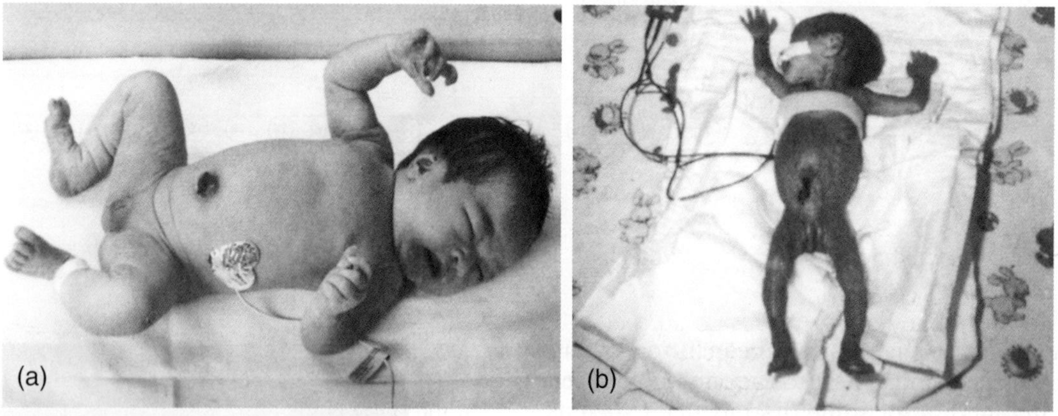

FIGURE 31.5 Posture: (a) term posture (flexed); (b) pre-term posture (extended)
(Source: Thureen et al., 2005)

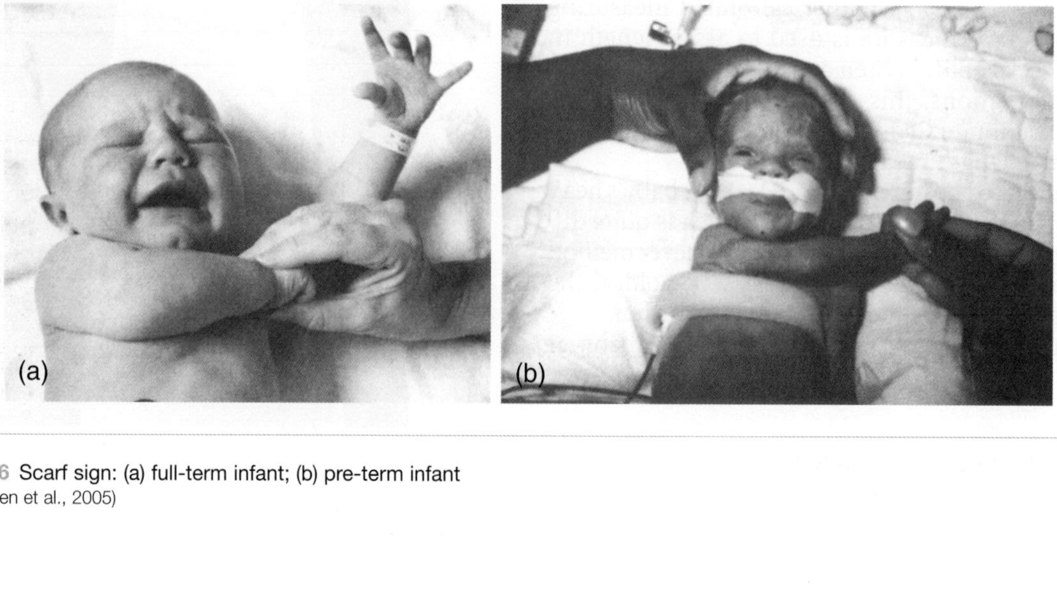

FIGURE 31.6 Scarf sign: (a) full-term infant; (b) pre-term infant
(Source: Thureen et al., 2005)

- In the first 12 hours there are creases over the whole of the sole of the foot.

Temperature

The temperature of the baby should be taken and recorded. As previously discussed, this is especially important at the initial examination when the baby is most vulnerable to hypothermia.

CLINICAL POINT

Sites for temperature assessment

- *Axillary temperature—this is the preferred site. Note:* In a hypothermic baby, the reading will be higher than the core as the area contains large areas of brown fat (Bliss-Holtz, 1991). As this may make recognition of hypothermia more difficult, behavioural and other physiological signs should also be assessed when the temperature is taken. The normal range for axillary temperature is 36.5–37.5°C.
- *Tympanic temperature*—This site has traditionally been considered less accurate for newborn babies. However, recent work in this area has suggested that the accuracy of non-contact infra-red tympanic thermometer measurement could make it worthy of consideration (Uslu et al., 2011).
- *Skin sites*—for a rapid general assessment of temperature, skin sites can be useful.
- Feeling the forehead or the back of the neck with the inside of the wrist can provide a quick check, to decide whether the baby needs extra clothing, for example.
- *Commercial 'spots' or 'tapes'*—used on the skin, these are a non-invasive method for taking the temperature that parents may find useful as the baby grows older.

Note: The newborn baby should never be subjected to rectal temperature readings. The introduction of a thermometer into the rectum can cause vagal stimulation and has been known to lead to collapse (Lunze & Hamer, 2012). It also carries the potential of perforation of the bowel wall (Lye & Densmore, 2018).

Examination of specific areas

Lungs

The respiratory rate (normal range: 30–60 breaths/min) should be counted when the baby is quiet or asleep and the rise and fall of the chest and abdomen should be observed (Table 31.2). They should rise and fall together. Counting respirations when the baby is clothed can be difficult. The following methods are practical ways to count the rate without disturbing the baby.

- Listen through the diaphragm of a stethoscope held a few centimetres from the baby's nose.
- Feel the rise and fall of the baby's abdomen through a hand placed on it.
- Always count for a full minute (initially, newborn respirations are frequently irregular).
- Assess the baby's colour.

Babies' heart sounds can be heard in many parts of the chest, so auscultate the lungs towards the lateral side of the chest to diminish the volume of the heart sounds. Focus on the breath sounds until the heart sounds are secondary to the breath. Then the breath sounds can be assessed.

Listen for air entry into both lungs. Note whether each side sounds similar.

CLINICAL POINT

Monitoring 'wet' lungs

Occasionally audible rales and/or rhonchi may be present at birth, which may be associated with lung fluid not yet reabsorbed. Rales are characterised by discontinuous clicking or rattling sounds whereas rhonchi are continuous low-pitched rattling lung sounds that sound like snoring.

If the baby is full term, healthy and alert, with normal respiratory and heart rates, good colour and muscle tone, recheck in 15 minutes. If the baby remains well and the

Table 31.2 Neonatal breathing patterns

	Normal variations	Outside normal variations (any or all of these)
Rate	40 breaths/min average; range 30–60 breaths/min (sleeping or quiet alert state)	More than 60 breaths/min (sleeping or in quiet alert state)
Rhythm	Regular and irregular periods Apnoea <20 seconds	Irregular breathing Apnoea >20 seconds
Chest/abdominal movement	Synchronised diaphragm and abdominal movement	Subcostal and/or intercostal in-drawing
Nose	Breathes through the nose, no nasal flaring	Flaring of nostrils
Sound	Silent	Expiratory 'grunt'
Colour	Pink	Pale/cyanosis

(See Ch. 42 for respiratory distress syndrome.)
(Source: Based on Davies & McDonald, 2020)

sounds continue to diminish, monitor every 15 minutes until they have gone. They should have largely cleared within an hour of birth. If there is persistent or fluctuating colour change (dusky, cyanosis) and tachycardia, tachypnoea, lethargy, reduced muscle tone and persistent or worsening lung sounds, refer to a medical practitioner.

Note: Transient tachypnoea of the newborn can occur in otherwise healthy babies (see Ch. 42).

Heart

The heart is examined for rate, regularity, heart sounds and the presence of murmurs. The baby is assessed for general signs that may indicate a cardiac anomaly—that is, variations in colour, raised respiratory rate, lethargy or poor feeding.

CLINICAL POINT

Auscultation of the lungs and heart

- Use a neonatal stethoscope wherever possible for optimal auscultation.
- Warm it in the hand before placing it on the baby's chest.
- Use smooth, gentle actions. If the baby is disturbed and cries, the sounds will not be audible.
- The part of the stethoscope used will vary, although the heart can be heard with both the bell and the diaphragm sides., However, the breath sounds are more clearly heard with the diaphragm. (McDonald, 2020)
- Focus on the heart sounds, which will minimise other sounds, but be aware of the breath sounds.
- When the heart sounds have your full attention the cardiac cycle can then be assessed.
- Count: rate and note regularity (110–150 beats minute).
- Listen to:
    - systolic (first) heart sound S_1 (lub)
    - diastolic (second) heart sound S_2 (dub)
    - the spaces in between the sounds.

Listening positions for cardiac assessment are shown in Fig. 31.7.

Heart murmurs

Heart murmurs are sounds that may be heard as: blood flow is disturbed as it crosses an abnormal valve; as it flows under pressure through a defect in either the atrial or ventricular septum; or sometimes when there is increased flow as it crosses a normal valve. The murmur reflects turbulent blood flow, typically from the pressure difference between adjacent cardiac structures. Cardiac murmurs in the neonate may be normal (physiological, benign, flow, transitional, etc.) or abnormal (pathological). Most newborns (90%) will have 'soft' murmurs which are transient and not associated with anomalies (Davidson et al., 2012). Murmurs can be classified according to their:

- location
- radiation
- timing (systolic, diastolic, continuous)

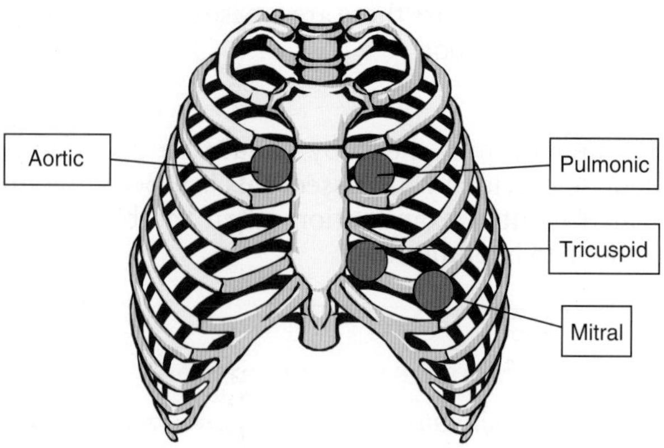

FIGURE 31.7 Listening positions for cardiac assessment

- intensity (1–6 systolic, 1–4 diastolic)
- pitch (high or low frequency)
- quality.

Murmurs are not heard if there is nothing to make the flow turbulent. Many serious cardiac malformations are silent, and therefore midwives need to always be observant for systemic signs of cardiac compromise—colour, respiratory rate, muscle tone, feeding problems, and so on (see Ch. 42). Flowing fluid does not make a noise if it is not under a lot of pressure. Think of the absence of noise when water flows through a wide-bore hose. When fluid is forced through a small opening, the pressure is raised and the resulting turbulence creates a noise. Think of the way water begins to hiss when pressure is increased by a thumb partially closing the opening of a wide-bore hose. Large defects in the atrial or ventricular septa allow the blood to flow through the defect with little or no change in pressure. Consequently there is no turbulence and no sound is made. Diagnosis of large cardiac anomalies is nearly always made through clinical observation of babies and their behaviour.

CLINICAL POINT

Important information for communicating in the event of consultation referral related to cardiac variations

The following information should be given and recorded in the documentation to enable a paediatrician to plan appropriate action:

- The general condition of the baby, especially colour, respiratory rate and feeding behaviour. (Major cardiac anomalies are either very soft or inaudible. These anomalies announce themselves as more general signs and symptoms.)
- The heart rate (normal 110–50 b.p.m.).
- Any additional sound(s):
    - nature—rumbling, breezy, whistling, creaking, rubbing
    - volume—soft, easily heard, loud
    - where the murmur is audible
    - in which part of the cardiac cycle the murmur is audible (e.g. with the systolic sound).

Midwives and women need to be aware that non-specific signs and symptoms such as pallor or failure to thrive may be the only indication of a silent cardiac defect that will become apparent at a later time.

Physiological flow murmurs are the most commonly heard murmurs at the initial examination. These should be reassessed in 24 hours. Most generally resolve by the examination at the end of the first week. However, until significant experience is gained, if any sound other than the normal systolic and diastolic sounds are heard, consultation with a medical practitioner is warranted.

Pulse oximetry

Many maternity units are now performing a SaO_2 on all babies prior to discharge—even if the baby is asymptomatic, as this is an effective way of identifying ductal-dependent lesions which may otherwise lie undetected but manifest in the presentation of a very unwell baby at 3–4 days postpartum.

There has been a strong drive in both Australia and New Zealand to introduce universal pulse oximetry screening. However, to date this has not been achieved in either country and adoption of such a strategy remains a state-by-state approach in Australia and a District Health Board decision in New Zealand. The economics of the implementation nationally and the fact that there is insufficient evidence to support a wholesale strategy through a sector-led quality improvement program have informed this outcome. Whether a scheme on the scale of that seen in the UK and US will eventually be introduced remains to be seen. In the meantime, it needs to be acknowledged that although pulse oximetry screening is a valuable and efficacious intervention, it does not replace the newborn clinical assessment for congenital heart disease. Auscultating for murmurs, detection of clinically visible cyanosis and palpation of pulses (femoral pulses in particular) remain an important part of the newborn and 6-week examination.

Head

After measuring the head circumference, the head is assessed for general shape, presence of moulding, microcephaly, macrocephaly, caput succedaneum, cephalhaematoma or a 'chignon' from vacuum delivery, cuts and abrasions, fetal scalp electrode or blood sample sites (Fig. 31.8). The sutures are palpated—they should be easily felt unless there is overriding of the bones associated with moulding. Note width, overriding or premature fusion of the sutures. The distribution and texture of hair is also noted—hair is usually silky and fine; coarse-textured hair is abnormal.

The anterior and posterior fontanelles are palpated—frequently the posterior fontanelle is often not palpable but does not anatomically close for 6–8 weeks. The anterior fontanelle often does not close until the child is 18 months of age. The anterior fontanelle should be flat; a sunken fontanelle is a late sign of dehydration, whereas a bulging fontanelle may indicate hydrocephalus or intracranial haemorrhage.

Positional plagiocephaly

Some babies always lie with their head in one position. This can lead to 'flattening' of the occiput that becomes more noticeable after 3–4 weeks. Positional plagiocephaly has become much more common since the introduction of back sleeping to prevent sudden infant death syndrome (SIDS). In the early stages, plagiocephaly is easily preventable, by varying the baby's head position. Mothers can be encouraged to turn their baby's head to one side during the day and to the other side at night, and discouraged from using car seats for seating outside of the car. Moulding helmet treatment may be necessary if the condition is undetected and untreated in the early stage. It is important to differentiate plagiocephaly from unilateral premature closure of the coronal suture (Michaelides, 2017a). (See section 'Care of the newborn' on 'tummy time'.)

Face

The face is examined for symmetry, placement of features, expression and shape.

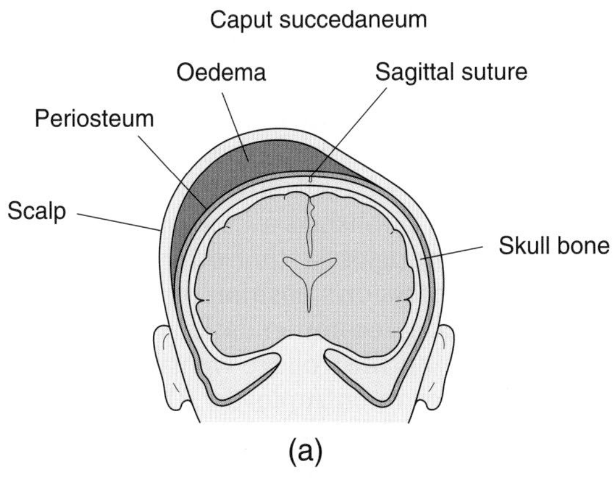

FIGURE 31.8 Characteristics of: (a) caput succedaneum; (b) cephalhaematoma
(Source: Based on Thureen et al., 2005)

Eyes

The eyes are examined to ensure the eyes are present; note symmetry, any discharge or swelling. The eyes should move; the baby will follow movement and gaze at the mother's face when held. The iris may be dark blue at birth but the colour may gradually change over the first 3–6 months. Tears are not usual for the first 2 months, although some babies have tears from birth.

The presence of subconjunctival haemorrhages (treatment not usually required) and the epicanthic fold (skinfold over the medial aspect of the eye) are recorded. This fold may be familial but is also seen in some congenital syndromes including Down syndrome.

Examination for the red reflex with an ophthalmoscope confirms the clarity of the lens and the presence of the retina. The red reflex may be seen on examination as the red pupils are seen in photographs taken without the 'red eye reduction' button on. Early and careful examination for the presence of red reflex is important because congenital cataract is sight threatening. The assessment must be undertaken soon after birth because it is recommended that babies with congenital cataract significant enough to affect sight have surgery before 6 weeks of age (Siderov, 2020). If the red reflex is not assessed by the examiner, it is important to record this in the health record so that the assessment can be undertaken at the next examination.

CLINICAL POINT

Assessing the red reflex

- Make sure that the baby is comfortable and awake either lying down or held by the parent.
- Darken the room if possible as it is easier to see the red eye reflex when the pupils are larger.
- Set the lens power to zero or about +1 to +2 (dioptres)
- Position yourself directly in front of the baby, approximately 45–50 cm away (or at arm's length).
- Hold the ophthalmoscope close to your own eye (keep glasses on if you need to although you can adjust the ophthalmoscope lens power).
- Vary the lens until a clear focus on the anterior eye is achieved.
- The red reflex should appear in the baby's pupil.
- The aperture can be adjusted so that it is large enough to enable you to view the red reflex in both eyes, which will give a stronger indication of symmetry in terms of intensity and colour.
- Note that the skin level of melanin in the baby will alter the degree of 'redness' viewed.

Note: Whichever method, individual or simultaneous elicits a red reflex should be recorded in the clinical notes.

(Source: Siderov, 2020)

Vision

Before the 6-week examination, parents should be asked whether they think their baby can see: 'Does their baby close his/her eyes against bright light, stare at people's faces when they are up close, turn towards light, smile at the parent without being touched or spoken to?' (Bowman, 2016).

Referral to an ophthalmologist or paediatrician is warranted for any of the following situations:

- *close relative with an eye tumour at birth or during infancy*
- *close relative with a congenital eye malformation*
- *rubella or contact with rubella or other congenital infection during pregnancy (e.g. toxoplasmosis)*
- *prematurity (<32 weeks gestation or <1250 g birth weight)*
- *eye malformations (absent red reflex, bulging eye, abnormal pupil); failure to fix or follow objects/movements; abnormal eye movements*
- *newborn seizures, encephalopathy, certain errors of metabolism*
- *trauma to the eye*
- *conjunctivitis that worsens or does not resolve.*

(Bowman, 2016)

Nose

The nostrils (nares) should be patent and the respiratory rate normal, and the baby should have no difficulty breathing (30–60 breaths per minute). Saline drops in small quantity can be used to clear the nares if the baby is 'snuffling'. Cotton buds may cause trauma if they are used to clear the nares.

Mouth

The baby's mouth should be pink and moist. The mouth opens symmetrically but is usually held closed at rest. The lips are complete and the philtrum present. A receding jaw is sometimes associated with feeding difficulties. The rooting reflex should be elicited by brushing the baby's cheek. The palate should be viewed with the use of a pen torch. The soft palate is carefully assessed, as small clefts can easily be missed. The gum lines are checked for completion and for premature dentition. The sucking reflex (preferably when feeding) is noted. At subsequent examinations, the mouth is examined for signs of *Candida* albicans infection (thrush). Oral thrush is seen as white plaques on the gums, inside of the cheeks or a white film over the tongue.

The presence of ankyloglossia or 'tongue tie' is documented. Treatment is not required unless the tongue cannot move upwards or cannot protrude over the bottom gum line and/or is significant enough to impede latching or sucking (see Chs 32 and 42). Thorough assessment should be made by a health professional specialised in such assessments to determine what, if any, treatment is required. NZCOM (2019) has published a Consensus Statement on 'Assessment of ankyloglossia' that outlines the New Zealand midwifery profession's position on assessment of ankyloglossia, including recommendations for scope of practice. It is available on the College website at: http://www.midwife.org.nz/wp-content/uploads/2019/05/Tongue-tie-Ankyloglossia.pdf. Each Australian State and Territory has slightly different guidelines. Useful information for both Australian and New Zealand readers can be found via the Australian Breastfeeding Association website 'Tongue tie': https://www.breastfeeding.asn.au/bf-info/tongue-tie.

Ears

The auditory canals should be checked for patency using a pen torch. The pinna should be flexible and cartilaginous. The upper edge of the pinna should be above or level with the outer corner of the eye. Low-set ears should act as an alert for other anomalies. It should be noted that moulding may affect these proportions at birth, which makes it important to recheck during the first-week examination.

Skin tags and spots occur most commonly in front of the ear lobe but can be found behind the ear. Skin tags are usually benign but may be associated with a bone deficit lying under the tag and may contain meningeal tissue. Skin tags may also be associated with renal and/or neurological anomalies. Medical consultation is warranted when skin tags are noted.

Hearing

In New Zealand, a universal newborn hearing screening and early intervention program is in place, details of which can be viewed at: https://www.nsu.govt.nz/health-professionals/universal-newborn-hearing-screening-programme. This is a national standardised program which is delivered across the country. It serves to develop policies and standards and provides monitoring and governance. Australia has a National Hearing Screening Committee with each state represented but each state has self-governance, which can lead to some variations in how the service is delivered. The Australian framework can be found at: http://www.health.gov.au/internet/main/publishing.nsf/Content/neonatal-hearing-screening.

Even if the baby has undergone screening and passed, hearing can change at any time and it is important for the parents to monitor hearing milestones along with other growth and development milestones. Therefore, parents should be asked whether they think their baby can hear before the 6-week examination. Questions such as: 'Does the baby startle to loud noise, and does she/he turn her/his head in the direction of localised noise, such as the mother's voice?'

> *Referral to a paediatrician, otolaryngeal specialist and/or audiologist is warranted for any of the following situations:*
> - *a close relative who has been deaf from early childhood*
> - *rubella or contact with rubella or other congenital infection during pregnancy (e.g. cytomegalovirus, CMV)*
> - *prematurity (<32 weeks gestation or <1500 g birth weight)*
> - *malformation of head or face, or other physical findings known to be associated with deafness*
> - *serum bilirubin levels that require exchange transfusion*
> - *Apgar score of 0–4 at 1 minute or 0–6 at 5 minutes or more than 5 days ventilation*
> - *bacterial meningitis*
> - *received ototoxic medications.*
>
> (MOH, 2012, p. 92)

Neck

The rooting reflex is elicited bilaterally to examine range and symmetry of movement. The head should move freely; creases should be symmetrical. Any webbing or cystic growths are noted; check creases for skin lesions.

Skin

The presence of jaundice, duskiness and pallor is noted. The amount of vernix caseosa (see Fig. 31.11a), lanugo and peeling (see below) is recorded. It is important to examine creases for heat rash and pustules, and the buttocks for nappy rash (bright red) or *Candida* rash, which may vary from pinky to bright red in colour and is often excoriated. This is associated with *Candida* lesions in the mouth and painful maternal nipples. Also examine for common variations and birthmarks.

The neonate's skin is thin and easily blistered or excoriated by friction, acid or alkaline substances and pressure. The epidermis is nonetheless an effective barrier in preventing infection, especially as the skin pH falls from an average of 6.4 at birth to a mean of 4.9 over the first few days (Trotter, 2020).

Lanugo, the fine soft downy hair that is more likely to be present if the baby is pre-term, and vernix caseosa, the waxy, cheese-like substance on the skin of the baby, should be noted and recorded. Vernix has antimicrobial properties and assists with thermoregulation in the early hours following birth. It should therefore be left in situ whenever possible and early bathing should be avoided. During the first week the skin on the hands and feet may peel, particularly if the baby is post-term. Peeling requires no treatment; application of oils or creams is not necessary (Blackburn, 2017; Michaelides, 2017a).

Common skin variations

Birthmarks need obstetric or paediatric assessment so that a treatment plan and ongoing parental support can be initiated (Figs 31.9 and 31.10).

The following skin variations are common and clear spontaneously without treatment (Fig. 31.11). Parents

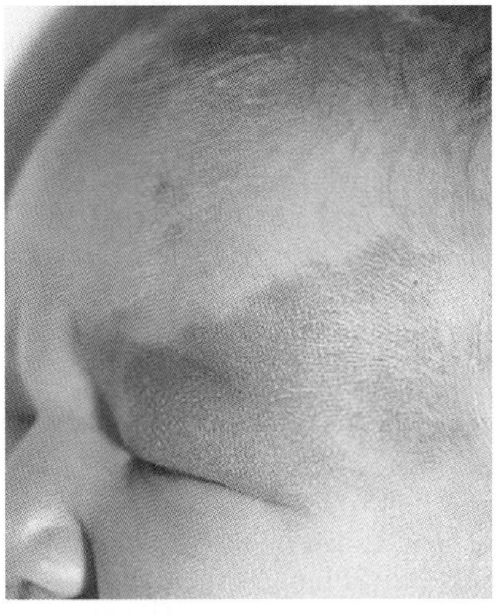

FIGURE 31.9 Port wine stain
(Source: Callen et al., 2000)

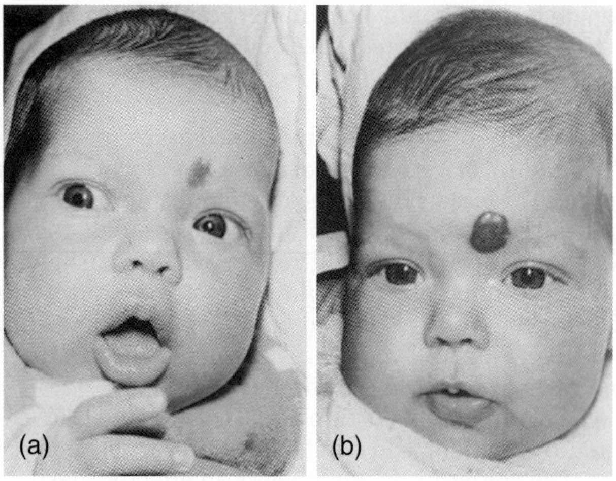

FIGURE 31.10 Strawberry naevus: (a) 4 days after birth; (b) 6 weeks after birth
(Source: Thureen et al., 2005)

may need reassurance that these are normal and do not need intervention:

- *Acrocyanosis* is the transitory bluish colour of the hands and feet seen in the first 2–6 hours after birth, before peripheral perfusion is fully established.
- *Superficial capillary naevi* (see Fig. 31.11) are pale reddish marks commonly called 'stork bites', seen on about a third of babies, on the eyelids, between the brows, on the nose and at the nape of the neck. They mostly disappear over the first year, although the marks at the nape of the neck sometimes persist.
- *Hyperpigmented macules (previously known as Mongolian blue spots)* (see Fig. 31.11) are bluish/black or bluish/grey areas primarily seen on the buttocks or lower back, although they can be found anywhere on the body. They are more readily visible in babies with darker skins, although they can be found within all ethnicities. They usually fade over the first year of life, although some persist to adulthood. They must be recorded to avoid any ambiguity about bruising of the area.
- *Milia* are exposed sebaceous glands on the face. They appear as raised white spots particularly on the nose. They disappear in the first 4–6 weeks after birth.
- *Erythema toxicum* (see Fig. 31.11) is a transient rash present in the first week of life. The spots are most commonly small, erythematous lesions with a white centre that look like pimples. They are not an infection; the fluid in the spots contains eosinophils, not pathogens. The rash can be quite extensive and the spots can run into each other, making large blotchy red patches on the baby's skin. The rash is usually aggravated by heat. It can be unsightly and cause anxiety for parents but as long as the baby is otherwise well there is no cause for concern. The rash usually clears in a few days.
- *Petechiae*, sometimes called traumatic cyanosis, are small, pinpoint haemorrhagic skin lesions, giving a dusky (bluish/grey) appearance to the face and head when there are multiple tiny petechiae in the skin. They usually disappear within 48–72 hours.
- *Subcutaneous fat necrosis* is a localised area of induration that is reddish and blotchy with a hardened area of fat underneath. Usually spontaneous, it can follow a forceps delivery when it is usually found over the zygomatic process on the baby's skull. It gradually disappears over several months (Rubin et al., 2015) (See also the Stanford University website: https://med.stanford.edu/newborns/professional-education/photo-gallery/skin.html.)

Chest

In a term infant the nipples should have approximately 6–7 mm of breast tissue. Engorgement of breast tissue as a result of circulating maternal hormones in both boys and girls may occur, and occasionally a milk-like substance may be seen. This is not an infection and will resolve naturally over 1–2 weeks as the level of maternal hormones decreases.

Umbilicus

The umbilical cord stump should be clean and dry and the clamp or other ligature should be checked to ensure it is secure. This can be removed after 48–72 hours. The cord should be examined for the presence of three vessels. A small number of babies with one umbilical artery have one or more associated congenital anomalies, usually cardiac, pulmonary or renal, especially renal agenesis (McDonald, 2020). At birth the cord is bluish-white and contains a variable amount of Wharton's jelly. As it dries out it shrinks and darkens to a yellow-brownish colour. The umbilical cord separates by a process of 'dry gangrene' that takes between 3 and 7 days.

Any sort of discharge including blood, serous or purulent drainage is abnormal and may indicate a problem (Tappero & Honeyfield, 2018). Redness at the base of the cord or umbilical 'flare' is usually associated with an infection, which requires urgent medical attention as the onset of neonatal septicaemia is a life-threatening complication. An umbilical hernia may be apparent if the abdominal muscles have not completely closed around the umbilicus. If this presents then a medical assessment is required to exclude exomphalos and patent urachus. Generally speaking, unless it is very large, an umbilical hernia does not usually require treatment and will close spontaneously by 2–3 years of age (Alexandre et al., 2021).

CLINICAL POINT

Umbilical cord care

The cord stump separates by saprophytic action; using antiseptics to clean the base of the cord interferes with this process so special cleaning or treatment is not required. Application of powders, antiseptic or alcohol wipes has been shown to delay cord separation (Trotter, 2020) and does *not* lead to a decrease in rates of infection.

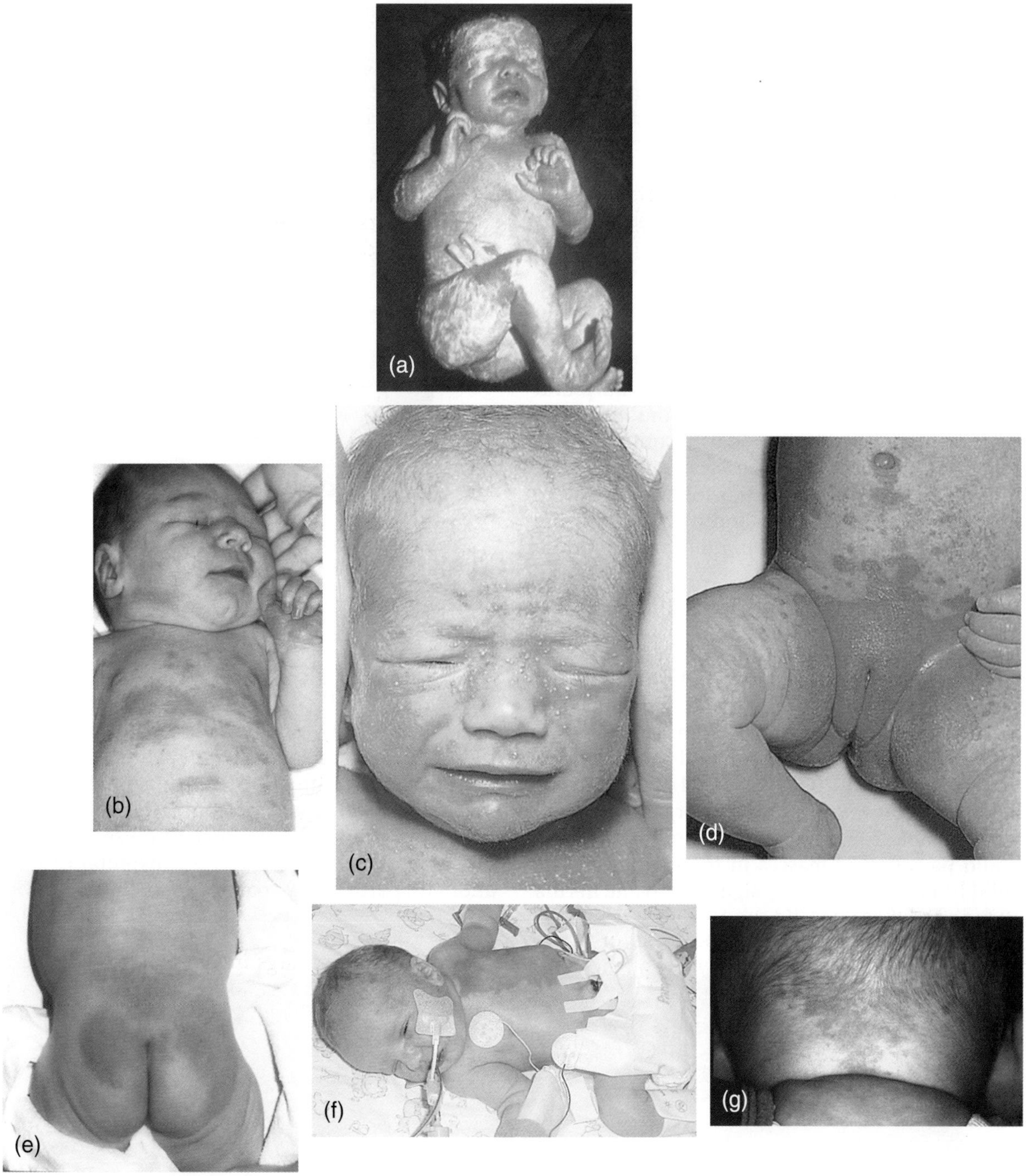

FIGURE 31.11 Skin variations: (a) vernix caseosa; (b) and (c) erythema toxicum; (d) *Candida* dermatitis; (e) hyperpigmented macules; (f) harlequin sign; (g) 'stork bites'
(Source: Thureen et al., 2005; photograph (g) Eichenfield LF 2015)

As the cord begins to separate it can become quite sticky around the base; the sticky material should be gently removed with a damp cotton bud and carefully dried. As the cord comes off there may be a *very small* amount of dark blood seen. This is normal but should present for only one or two nappy changes.

Occasionally the centre of the umbilicus has a small piece of raised, granulomatous flesh where the cord has separated which can rub on the baby's clothing and will not heal over. If this is the case, the stump can be referred for painless cauterisation.

Abdomen

Each quadrant of the abdomen should be auscultated for bowel sounds, which are present from approximately 1 hour after birth.

CLINICAL POINT

Palpating the abdominal organs

Palpation of the abdominal organs of the baby is an essential component of the assessment. The flat surface of the fingertips is used. The palpation moves from light to deep, watching the baby's face to detect discomfort. The examiner's other hand is placed on the back of the baby to provide a firm support. It may help to flex the baby's hip by raising the legs unilaterally to relax the abdominal muscles during palpation.

Liver

The inferior border of the liver should be palpable 1–2 cm below the costal margin in the midclavicular line and extends across the midline; the normal edge is 'sharp and soft' (McDonald, 2020). Start palpation at the iliac crest and work upwards towards the liver to come onto the liver border (Fig. 31.12). It is sometimes easier to use the edge of the thumb rather than the fingertips for this palpation. The spleen is not usually palpable and if it is felt on the left-hand side of the abdomen then a referral should be considered (Fig. 31.13).

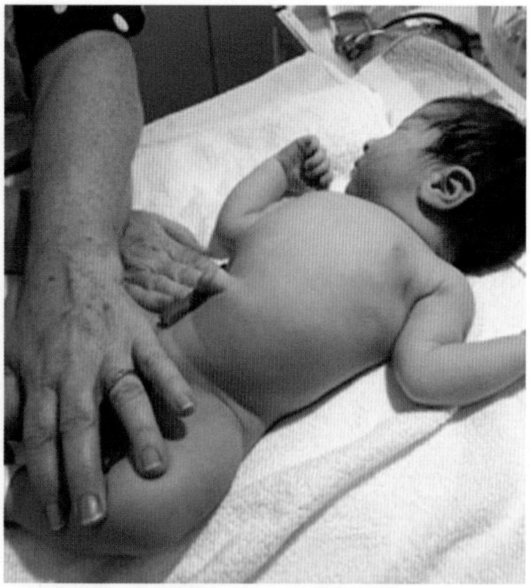

FIGURE 31.12 Abdominal palpation: liver
(Source: Davies L, McDonald S. *Examination of the Newborn and Neonatal Health.* 2nd ed. 2020. London: Elsevier; 2021: p. 26)

Kidneys and bladder

The kidneys are usually palpable in the first 24–48 hours. They are moderately firm and approximately 4.5–5.0 cm long. The right kidney may not be easily palpable. The kidney is palpated by placing the hand under the baby's flank and using deep, smooth abdominal pressure over the renal area (McDonald, 2020; Fig. 31.14).

The bladder becomes an abdominal organ when full and may be palpable 1–2 cm above the symphysis pubis. There should be no other masses in the abdomen. The groin should be examined for any sign of palpable hernia or undescended testicle.

Femoral pulses

Each pulse is individually assessed and then both left and right are assessed together to ensure that they are both present and that they beat in unison. The femoral and brachial pulses should be compared. Any difference between the two pulses, absence of pulse or asynchronous rate or pressure may indicate congenital cardiovascular anomaly, particularly coarctation of the aorta (McDonald, 2020).

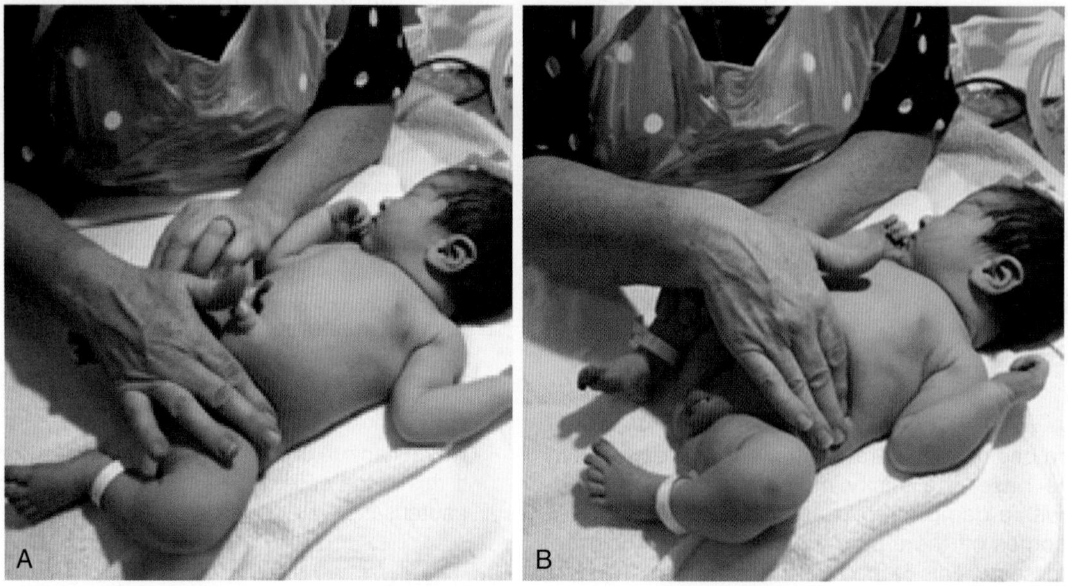

FIGURE 31.13 Abdominal palpation: spleen
(Source: Davies L, McDonald S. *Examination of the Newborn and Neonatal Health.* 2nd ed. 2020. London: Elsevier; 2021: p. 27)

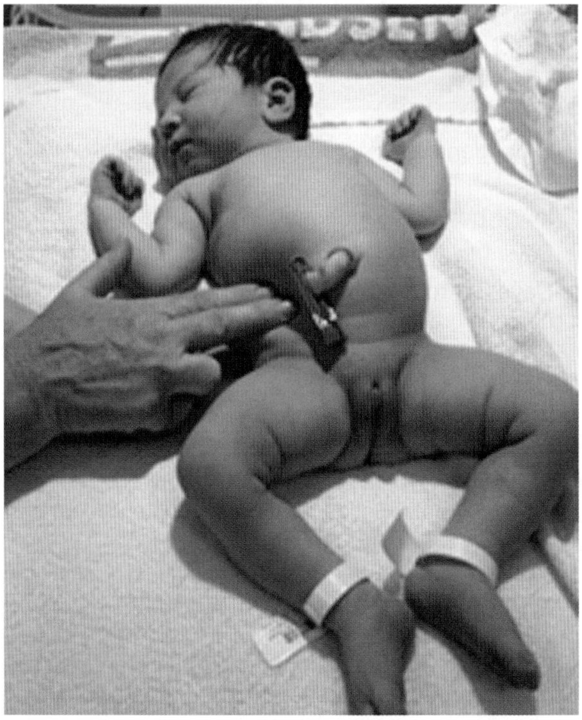

FIGURE 31.14 Abdominal palpation: kidneys
(Source: Davies L, McDonald S. *Examination of the Newborn and Neonatal Health.* 2nd ed. 2020. London: Elsevier; 2021: p. 27)

CLINICAL POINT
Palpating femoral pulses

With the baby lying flat, draw an imaginary line between the umbilicus and the normally flexed knees. The pulses are palpable where the line crosses the groin, in the groove between the leg muscle tendons (Fig. 31.15).

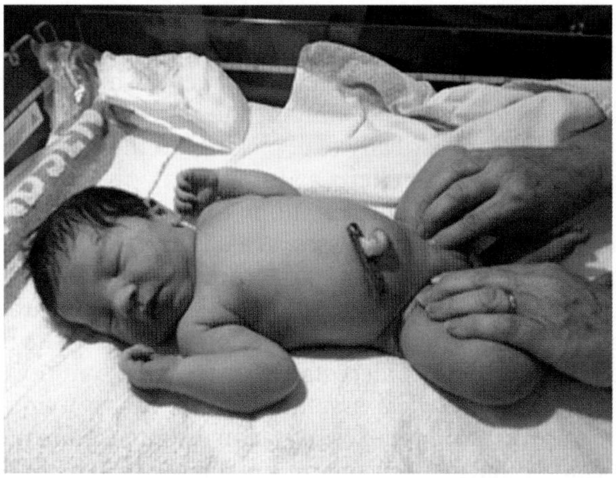

FIGURE 31.15 Femoral pulses
(Source: Davies L, McDonald S. *Examination of the Newborn and Neonatal Health.* 2nd ed. 2020. London: Elsevier; 2021: p. 27)

Limbs

Upper limbs

The symmetry of length, creases, flexion and muscle tone are assessed. The axillae and elbows are checked for abnormalities; the hands are opened to check for extra digits (polydactyly), skin tags or webbing between the fingers. The palms are examined to look for a single palmar crease that may be associated with Down syndrome (Davidson et al., 2012).

It is important to confirm symmetry and normal range of movement in the joints. *(Do not force the joints.)* The hands are normally held as loosely clenched fists.

Lower limbs

Again symmetry of length, creases, flexion and muscle tone is determined. The term baby has creases over more than two-thirds of the sole of the foot. Check for polydactyly, webbing and skin tags. The groin and popliteal spaces are examined for abnormalities. Symmetry and normal range of movement in the joints should be confirmed. Note that the knee joints often cannot be fully extended for the first few days (Johnston et al., 2003).

The term baby's feet should dorsiflex easily so that the upper surface of the foot almost touches or does touch the shin. Examine for signs of talipes equinovarus. *Do not force the foot.* If it will not naturally flex, refer the baby for paediatric or orthopaedic examination.

Spine and back

By turning the baby over the midwife can examine the spine by palpating the length of the spine and each of the vertebral spinous processes. If there appears to be a gap, a 'hairy' patch, or an area of thickened or differently textured skin over the spine, a referral is made to a paediatrician for exclusion of neural tube defect.

The cleft in the buttocks is examined; about 2–4% of babies have a dimple, usually at the top of the cleft (Starship Hospital, 2019). Ensure that the base of the dimple is sighted and that it is closed. The dimples are usually benign; however, very occasionally they are open to the meninges at the base, or it may be a congenital pilonidal sinus. If the base cannot be clearly seen or the dimple is deep, paediatric consultation is indicated. Dimples anywhere on the spine should always be medically assessed (see Ch. 42).

While examining the back, note the baby's posture when held in ventral suspension (see Neurological examination section and Fig. 31.16).

Visually check that the anus is patent and correctly positioned.

Genitalia

Female

The labia majora covers the clitoris and labia minora. The labia should be parted to examine the clitoris for appropriate size. The hymen will normally be perforated and this will be confirmed by the presence of a whitish

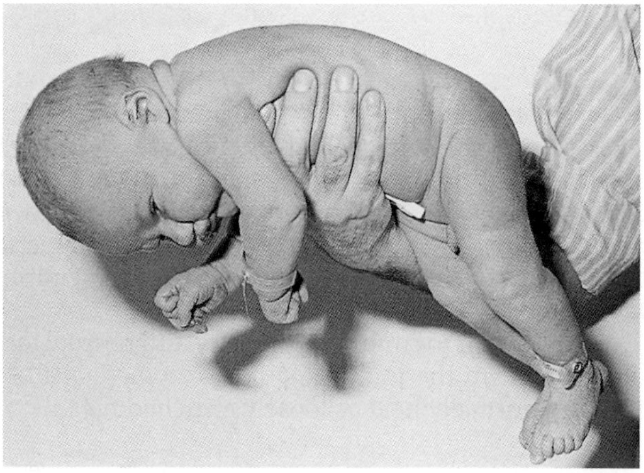

FIGURE 31.16 Ventral suspension
(Source: Fraser & Cooper, 2009)

discharge. A small quantity of blood-stained discharge in the first few days (pseudomenstruation), caused by the withdrawal of maternal hormones at birth, can sometimes occur (Baston & Durwood, 2017).

Male

The foreskin should cover the glans penis and should not be retracted. Hypospadias can be discounted by ensuring that the urethral opening is at the end of the penis and that the tissue is intact along the full length of the inferior surface.

The scrotum should be soft and rugaed. Hydrocoele (collection of fluid in the scrotum) is not uncommon but, whilst most resolve spontaneously, consultation is appropriate. Likewise, inguinal hernia should be excluded.

The scrotum should be gently palpated between the thumb and forefinger in order to locate the testes. They are firm, pea-like structures 1.5–2 cm long. The testes are sensitive to temperature and may retract to the inguinal canal when cold. It is not uncommon for one or both testes to have not descended. If they are not palpable in the scrotum, palpate the groin from the iliac crest to the external inguinal ring, where undescended testes are sometimes palpable. Babies with undescended testicle(s) need medical follow-up as it can take several years for the testes to descend. Testes that fail to descend are treated surgically in childhood.

Ambiguous genitalia

Gender should not be ascribed if there is any question of ambiguity and medical referral is required. Chromosomal analysis may be required as ambiguous genitalia are almost always associated with an underlying abnormality (Gordon, 2011).

Elimination

It is important to establish whether the baby has passed urine and meconium. The baby should have passed urine between two and five times in the first 24 hours, and meconium at least once.

CLINICAL POINT

Usual alterations to bowel motions

Breastfed babies

- Stool generally has little or no odour.
- Passing meconium is the main indicator that the lower bowel is functional.
- Days 1 to 2: meconium (dark green, sticky and unformed).
- Days 2/3 to 3/4: meconium → transitional stool (i.e. copious greenish-brown, loose stool). The baby's mother may need reassurance that this is not diarrhoea.
- Days 3/4 to approx. 10/12: mustard yellow, very loose, unformed stools, often only yellow fluid containing seed-like solid waste. Passed at almost every feed.
- Approx. day 10/12 onwards: mustard yellow, soft, loosely formed stools. Solids retain a seed-like appearance.
- After the first fortnight, breastfed babies generally pass a bowel motion two to three times a day. However, some exclusively breastfeeding babies may only pass a stool once every 3–5 days. As long as the baby is content, gaining weight, feeding well and passing normal amounts of urine, the baby is not constipated. These babies pass a large quantity of soft, non-constipated stool when they do have a bowel motion.

Formula-fed babies

- Stools have a sharp, distinctive odour.
- Meconium and transitional stool are passed as above.
- From 3–4 days onwards, stools are pale yellow, well formed and solids do not have a seed-like appearance.
- Formula-fed babies pass two to three stools a day.

Formula-fed babies do not exhibit the irregular pattern seen in some breastfed babies. If a formula-fed baby does not pass at least one bowel motion each day, the baby should be assessed for constipation.

Neurological examination

The neurological condition of the baby can be ascertained largely from astute observation and discussion with the mother about behaviour such as breastfeeding (Johnston et al., 2003). Many of the reflexes can also be viewed opportunistically (e.g. picking up the baby to undress him/her often elicits a Moro reflex).

The movements and reactions of the baby to stimuli change as gestation progresses. What is normal at 34 weeks is not normal at term. When interpreting the neurological examination, the baby's gestational age and state of arousal need to be taken into account (McDonald, 2020). The baby needs to be in a quiet alert state. The integrity and normality of the neurological system is tested by assessing the baby's posture and reflexes. Weak or absent responses may indicate immaturity or an abnormality.

Posture

- Supine—legs are semiflexed and the head turns to one side. The arms and legs recoil readily if extended and released. The elbow should not cross the midline when the arm is drawn across the chest and up to the neck (scarf sign, see Fig. 31.6).

- Prone—legs are more flexed and tucked up under the abdomen; the arms are held to the chest in a flexed position.
- Ventral suspension—when the baby is held up by the examiner's hand under the chest (Fig. 31.16), the body is semiflexed, the head is briefly extended in line with the spine, and the limbs are momentarily flexed.
- All limbs move spontaneously.

Rooting, sucking and swallowing

These are easily observed when the baby commences feeding. The rooting reflex is easily stimulated by brushing the baby's cheek or upper lip with a finger. The baby will turn towards the stimulus and open the mouth ready to suck. The suck–swallow–breathe pattern is coordinated and strong enough for adequate feeding from 36 weeks gestation.

Grasp reflexes

These can be elicited in both the hands and feet. They are strong enough in term neonates to briefly lift the baby away from the examination surface.

Traction response

When the baby is pulled forwards by the hands from supine to a sitting position, the elbows, knees and ankles flex (Fig. 31.17). The head lags behind the body. When the baby reaches the sitting position, the head falls onto the chest. The response reflects the development of flexor tone, which occurs at about 37 weeks gestation.

Asymmetric tonic neck reflex

The head is turned to one side while the baby is supine. The limbs on the side the baby is facing extend, while the limbs on the opposite side flex (Fig. 31.18). It is strong from 30 to 36 weeks, may not be seen in the early newborn period, and returns 4–6 weeks after birth. A very strong response at birth requires a medical consultation (Davidson et al., 2012).

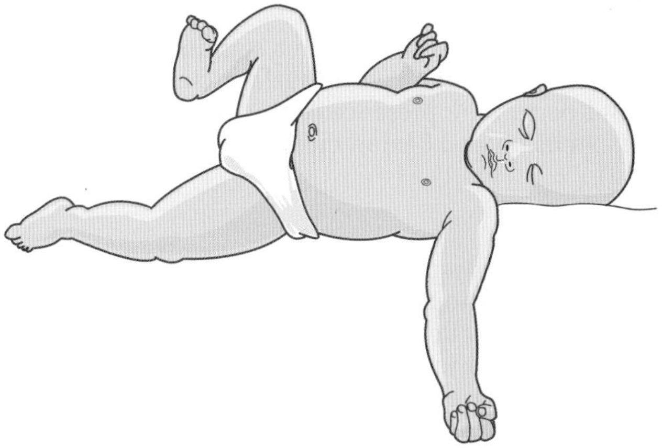

FIGURE 31.18 Tonic neck reflex
(Source: Thureen et al., 2005)

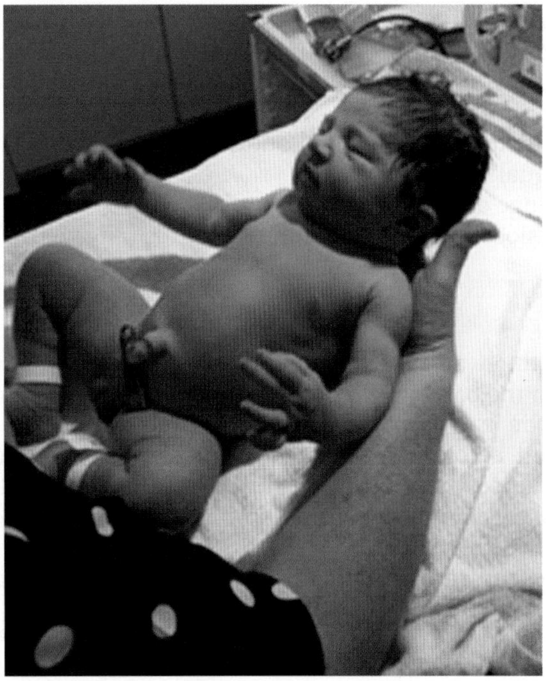

FIGURE 31.19 Moro reflex
(Source: Davies L, McDonald S. *Examination of the Newborn and Neonatal Health*. 2nd ed. 2020. London: Elsevier; 2021: p. 34)

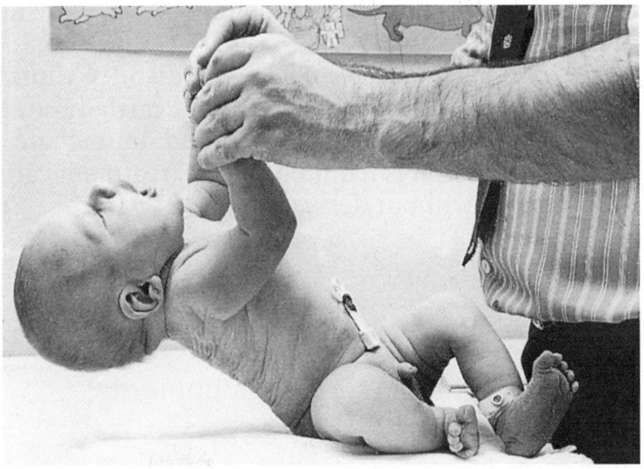

FIGURE 31.17 Traction response
(Source: Fraser & Cooper, 2009)

Moro reflex (startle reflex)

In response to a loud noise or sudden lowering of the head into the examiner's hand, the baby extends the arms, hands and fingers outwards and the knees flex (Fig. 31.19). The arms slowly return into the chest (like a hug).

Stepping response

When the baby is supported in a standing position with the soles of the feet on a firm surface, simulated walking should occur. The presence of this reflex indicates mature extension and flexion mechanisms (Davidson et al., 2012).

Hips

Developmental dysplasia of the hips (DDH) is a condition that can have serious consequences if not diagnosed and treated shortly after birth (see Ch. 42 for treatment). Clinical examination using Ortolani's and Barlow's tests are used extensively to screen the newborn and the procedure diagnoses most babies requiring orthopaedic assessment. When examiners are experienced, sensitivity is significantly improved. The tests have high specificity but a low sensitivity, resulting in false-positive results and subsequent overtreatment or false-negative results leading to late detection (Li et al., 2021). Ultrasound is used for screening in some centres. Two recent reviews of the research concluded that there is as yet insufficient clear evidence for or against general ultrasound screening of neonates for DDH (Shaw & Segal, 2016). Examine the hips for:

- symmetry of thigh and buttock creases
- equal leg length
- range of abduction
- dislocation or laxity of the hip joints ('clicky hips').

Symmetry of thigh and buttock creases, leg length

The thigh and buttock creases should be symmetrical when the baby is lying prone. (Note these when examining the baby's back, to minimise handling.) The legs should be of equal length. When the baby is lying flat with knees flexed, the height of both knees should be equal. Asymmetry and/or limited range of abduction may be signs of DDH. These assessments are unreliable alone and must be accompanied by the abduction/adduction tests (see below).

Abduction/adduction tests

Each joint should be physically assessed separately for dislocation or laxity. Two tests are normally used:

- *Ortolani's test* (Fig. 31.20) examines for the presence of a dislocated hip.
- *Barlow's test* (Fig. 31.21) examines the joints for laxity and the capability for the joint to dislocate with ease (see following Clinical point for procedures).

Findings:

- *Normal finding*—no movement is felt in the joint.
- *Joint laxity*—on examination the joint feels lax or unstable (i.e. 'gives' a little) but does not clunk. It may 'click' during the examination. Joint laxity at birth can be the result of the breech position in some babies, or may be related to a hormonal effect on the joint capsule, especially in baby girls. In most cases the joint capsule tightens over several days and the laxity disappears. Persistent joint laxity is abnormal. *All* babies with joint laxity are referred for medical assessment so that the state of the joint can be monitored and treatment commenced where necessary.
- *Dislocated or dislocatable hip(s)*—if a distinct 'clunk' is felt and/or heard when either test is carried out, the femoral head is dislocated or reduced. Immediate orthopaedic referral is required so that treatment can be commenced without delay (see Ch. 42).

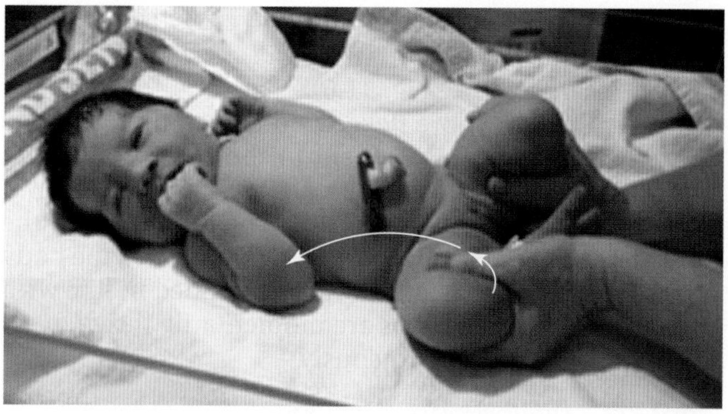

FIGURE 31.20 Ortolani's test
(Source: Davies L, McDonald S. *Examination of the Newborn and Neonatal Health*. 2nd ed. 2020. London: Elsevier; 2021: p. 33)

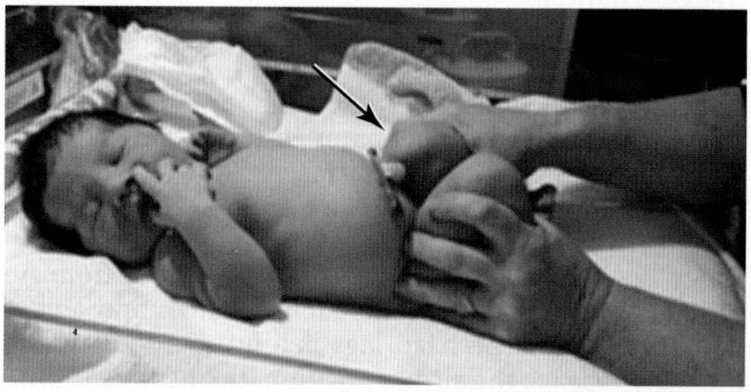

FIGURE 31.21 Barlow's test
(Source: Davies L, McDonald S. *Examination of the Newborn and Neonatal Health*. 2nd ed. 2020. London: Elsevier; 2021: p. 33)

CLINICAL POINT

Examining the hips for developmental dysplasia

In all cases *be gentle*. The pressure you apply to the baby's legs should be the same as you would apply in holding an egg. Excessive force is not needed. If the hip joint is unstable, it will move as the test is carried out. Repeated, vigorous manipulation of the neonatal hip is suspected to lead to subsequent instability so keep manipulation to the minimum needed for screening. Normal hip joints are stable.

Preparation

- Obtain consent from mother.
- Have the warm, relaxed baby lying flat on a warm, flat surface.
- Nappy should be off.

Do *not* attempt the examination if the baby is distressed as this will create resistance.

Barlow's test

Assess each hip separately.

1. Hold the knee and hip in a flexed position.
2. Place the thumb on inner surface of the thigh (inner trochanter), and the index and middle fingers over the greater trochanter of the femur.
3. Lifting the thigh, *adduct* the leg gently, and use the thumb to apply pressure laterally so that the femur is pushed downwards towards the bed. (The aim is to slide a dislocatable head of femur over the rim and *out of the acetabulum*.)
4. A positive result is a palpable clunk.
5. Record findings.

Ortolani's test

Each hip joint is assessed separately.

1. Stabilise the pelvis with the non-examining hand.
2. Hold each leg, place the thumb on the inner surface of the thigh, and the index and middle fingers over the greater trochanter of the femur.
3. Flex the knees and the hips 90°.
4. Lifting the thigh slightly, *abduct* the leg gently, applying pressure over the trochanter with the fingers. (The aim is to slide a dislocated head of femur over the rim and back *into the acetabulum*.)
5. A positive result is a palpable, often audible clunk.

(Sources: Michaelides, 2011; McDonald & Rose, 2020)

An excellent resource about DDH can be found at https://www.youtube.com/watch?v=AS-Z7_pbmjM.

Record of neonatal examination

The introduction of digital management systems for recording and reporting newborn assessment has changed practice in the past few years. However, paper-based materials for sharing information between health professionals and parents are still used for specific purposes, such as the New Zealand based 'Tamariki Ora/ Well Child Book'. Whatever system is utilised, it is important that the assessment is fully recorded. Table 31.3 shows some

Table 31.3 Recording results of neonatal examination

Clinical examination			Result*
Fontanelles	✓		
Eyes	✓	✓	Red reflex ✓✓
Nose/mouth	✓		Palate ✓
Ears	✓	✓	
Heart	✓		S_1✓ S_2✓ murmurs
Lungs	✓	✓	Air entry =
Abdomen	✓		Soft. Liver border 1 cm ↓ costal margin
Umbilicus	✓		3 vessels
Femoral pulses	✓	✓	Synchronous
Genitals	✓		♀
Hips	✓	✓	L & R stable
Back	✓		
Anus	✓		Patent
Legs/arms	✓	✓	Symmetrical
Reflexes, movements/tone	✓		Symmetrical
Skin	✓		Pink, peripheral acrocyanosis
Signature:	Date:		

*Record normal as ✓. Record abnormal as X. Not examined: leave blank.
(Source: Based on Davies & McDonald, 2008)

commonly used symbols for recording selected assessments. These records usually form part of a total record for the baby at birth and at subsequent assessment points.

CARE OF THE NEWBORN

Development: birth to 6 weeks

Initially babies have limited ways of communicating. Crying is the primary verbal means and non-verbal would include reflex responses such as sucking or rooting. They begin to smile between 4 and 6 weeks of age and begin to show signs of random 'cooing' when content. Random smiling may occur quite early, but smiling socially in response to an adult does not usually appear before 4 weeks, and often closer to 6 weeks. A baby will demonstrate restlessness if hot or uncomfortable.

Initially, babies move their arms and legs and can turn their head from side to side as they seek the breast. By 4–6 weeks, babies can generally turn their head from side to side and raise their head from the cot when in the prone position as they develop neck strength. The practice of 'tummy time' has become popular in recent years in the belief that it helps to develop neck, shoulder, back and arm strength and prevent plagiocephaly (flat-headedness). The practice involves placing the baby on their tummy for a few minutes leading up to 10–15 minutes at any one time. It has been suggested that babies are prevented from rounding out the back of their heads by being able to turn them from side to side because they spend too long in restrictive car seats, carriers and capsules which prevent them from head turning spontaneously. A study in 2013 concluded that babies do just as well when it comes to rolling over whether or not they spend time on their tummies (Darrah & Bartlett, 2013). This may be reassuring for the parents of babies who do not like tummy time and it may be worth suggesting that tummy time can also take place when the baby is enjoying skin-to-skin with its parents as well as lying alone on a mat on the floor. Babies should never be left alone on their tummies (SIDS and Kids, 2017).

Senses and perception

Habituation is the process whereby there is an initial response to a visual or auditory stimulus such as a loud noise, followed by diminishing response with repetition until the response disappears. Being able to ignore a noisy environment is a defence mechanism of the baby. Orientation is the neonate's ability to be alert to, follow and fixate on appealing, complex visual stimuli. Self-quieting ability refers to babies' capacity to quieten and comfort themselves (e.g. fist sucking) (Davidson et al., 2012).

Vision

Babies are sensitive to bright lights. They focus at a distance of 15–20 cm and show a preference for the shape of the human face and bold black-and-white patterns. They can briefly track a moving object by the end of the first week and can differentiate their mother's face from a stranger's by 2 weeks. Over the first 2 months, interest in colour and variety of patterns develops (Siderov, 2020). Interaction with the mother is developed through eye-to-eye contact.

Hearing

Newborn babies turn towards localised sound. High-pitched sound makes them blink or startle. They are comforted by low-pitched sounds such as the crooning noises mothers make to comfort a crying baby. They prefer the sound of their mother's voice to others' voices and prefer the human voice over other noise. After a few weeks, they mimic human speech patterns, moving in response (Blackburn, 2017).

Smell, taste and touch

Babies respond positively to the smell of human milk and can differentiate their mother's milk within a few days. They prefer a sweet taste and turn away from unpleasant smells.

They respond to being picked up, stroked and talked to. They can mimic facial expressions and hand movements made by adults by 12 days of age. Babies enjoy skin-to-skin contact, immersion in warm water, rocking, cuddling and stroking (Blackburn, 2017; Michaelides, 2017a). 'Pain in babies is expressed by brow bulging, eyelid squeezing, nasolabial furrowing and open lipped crying' (Gardner SL et al., 2020).

Sleep–wake states

Successive sleep–wake patterns vary considerably and the baby will take some time to demonstrate a consistent pattern. At first the baby wakes because of hunger; however, longer periods of wakefulness unrelated to hunger that meet the baby's social interaction needs begin to occur in the succeeding weeks.

In general, most newborns will **sleep** about 16–20 hours out of every 24 hours for the first few months. The depth and duration of sleep varies considerably from one baby to another (Leigh, 2016). At times during the day, the baby will be active and crying, or will lie quietly awake. A newborn usually sleeps 2–4 hours at a time and wakes up hungry. Understanding the baby's sleep–wake state can help mother and midwife identify cues so that they work with, rather than against, the baby's state of consciousness, so conserving energy (Box 31.7).

Crying

Term neonates usually cry without tears and generally for reasons of hunger, thirst or discomfort, although sometimes there is no obvious reason. Parents are able to differentiate the cry as they gain experience with their baby. Midwives have a role in supporting parents as they grow to understand the baby's individual pattern of communication and learn to comfort him or her.

Box 31.7 Behavioural observation of sleep–wake states in the newborn

Sleep states

- *Deep or quiet sleep*—eyes closed, no eye movements, respirations regular, hard to wake, occasional jerky movements
- *Active rapid eye movement* (REM)—eyes closed, rapid eye movements seen, respirations less regular, may be sucking movements, easier to wake, occasional random movements

Awake states

- *Drowsy—eyes* open or closed, eyelids may flutter, occasional smiling, smoother limb movements but may startle, minimal response to sensory stimulus and minimal motor activity
- *Quiet alert*—eyes open, alert and focused on source of stimulus, minimal motor activity, may or may not be fussing
- *Active alert*—eyes open, alert, generally active and reactive to a variety of stimuli and the surrounding environment, may or may not be fussing
- *Crying*—actively, may be hard to console, much muscular activity. It may be difficult to get a response, and the mother may need to 'bring baby down' to an active alert state for feeding

(Source: Davidson et al., 2012)

Ongoing midwifery care

Midwifery support and assessment until transfer of care to Well Child services

The main purposes of midwifery care are to support the mother to care confidently for her baby and to consider the baby's ongoing wellbeing and development. Every episode of care includes gathering information from the mother and any test results, examining the baby, sharing timely information and providing encouragement. Decision points subsequent to the initial assessment at birth are generally every 24–48 hours until the woman is confident in her own environment, and become weekly towards the end of the first 6 weeks. The final postnatal decision point, usually between 5 and 6 weeks, is more comprehensive and includes a full assessment and referral letters that mark the transfer of care from midwifery to Well Child care provider(s).

Information shared

Good history taking is the foundation of good midwifery practice. Information shared between the mother and the midwife about the baby's wellbeing and lactation and feeding patterns provides a mutual platform for planning future care. Just as information is highlighted in a timely fashion during pregnancy, discussing what the mother can expect to notice before the next visit and what to contact the midwife about forms part of each postnatal visit. In addition, this is the period that protection from infection and injury is discussed. Most of the local health department Well Child record books contain comprehensive information on an 'age and stage' basis. Midwives draw women's attention to pertinent sections in these books and provide any additional relevant sources such as websites/pamphlets at each visit. (See sections on Immunisation, Prevention of injury and Car safety in this chapter.)

Everyday assessment for mothers and midwives

The thriving baby

The baby should be content between feeds and have a wet nappy at every feed. After the first 24 hours, the baby should have six to eight wet nappies and regular bowel motions, usually two to three, every 24 hours. *Note:* Disposable nappies are designed to pull the moisture away from the baby's skin. It is sometimes quite difficult to tell whether the baby has passed urine just by looking at the nappy. Feeling the weight of a dry, unused nappy against the one removed from the baby helps to determine this. Disposable nappies full of urine feel heavy when 'weighed' in the hand.

The baby should appear well and feel warm to touch, including extremities. Breathing is not very noticeable (see normal variations in breathing, earlier in this chapter). Arms and legs are flexed and feel firm, with good muscle tone. The baby has a contented expression, not normally grimacing or frowning. There should be no signs of infectious skin lesions and the umbilical cord should be clean and dry (see Umbilical cord care, this chapter).

The midwife should ask the mother how the baby is, and *listen* to the answer. If the mother expresses concerns these should be taken seriously. Babies can become unwell very quickly and do not show signs of illness in the way that adults and older children do. Signs are often subtle, for example; a baby that has been feeding well then stops feeding or persistent low-grade jaundice (see Box 31.5 for warning signals).

Newborn metabolic screening programs

Both Australia and New Zealand undertake a population-based newborn metabolic screening program; all parents in both countries are offered screening for their baby and the vast majority of parents take up the offer. This involves the collection of blood from the baby for testing between 48 and 72 hours of age.

The blood sample taken from the heel of the baby is used to screen for a variety of congenital metabolic disorders and some endocrine disorders. These are all rare conditions, and early diagnosis and treatment can prevent serious complications including brain and organ damage.

In New Zealand, there are over 20 tests performed to detect metabolic disorders in the newborn. They fall into three groups:

- amino acid disorders (e.g. maple syrup urine disease and phenylketonuria)
- fatty acid disorders (e.g. medium-chain acyl-CoA dehydrogenase deficiency)
- other disorders (e.g. cystic fibrosis, hypothyroidism) (MOH National Screening Unit, 2010, updated 2017).

While most conditions tested for in Australia and New Zealand are the same, population differences mean that there are some variations between the countries. In Australia, the number of tests performed during the newborn metabolic screening test varies according to State and Territory government policy (it is possible to test for up to 30 diseases). However, the most common tests are the same as New Zealand. Please refer to the Ministry/Department of Health for the specific conditions that are screened for in local areas. The current websites are: Australia—https://www.health.gov.au/health-topics/pregnancy-birth-and-baby/newborn-bloodspot-screening; New Zealand—https://www.nsu.govt.nz/health-professionals/newborn-metabolic-screening-programme. Information for both health professionals and parents can be found there.

Newborn metabolic screening test blood spot collection

A capillary blood sample is collected from pricking the heel of the baby (please see following Clinical Point) and the blood is collected onto an absorbent card which is sent to a laboratory for analysis (MOH National Screening Unit, 2010). Advances in understanding of the development of indicator metabolites and the technology used for analysis means that we now recognise the importance of collecting the sample within the 48–72 hour period. Maple syrup urine disease and congenital adrenal hyperplasia, for example, can be fatal within 7–10 days of age. Therefore, timely collection and prompt dispatch of the filled collection cards is essential for timely analysis and availability of results. Forty-eight hours of protein feeding are no longer required prior to the blood being taken for testing in either country.

Both the specificity and sensitivity of the tests are good, but about 1 baby in every 100 will need a second blood test if the first test did not give a clear result and if so parents will be notified promptly. This is generally down to error in the collection process and a second test will almost always elicit a normal result.

The information leaflet provided to New Zealand mothers prior to obtaining consent makes the tests undertaken and the storage of information explicit. Australian consent forms contain similar information. Informed consent must be obtained for both sample collection and testing in both Australia and New Zealand.

CLINICAL POINT

Collecting a neonatal capillary blood sample

For estimation of blood glucose, serum bilirubin, full blood count and newborn metabolic screening blood test.

- The sample is collected from the heel.
- The foot must be lower than body.
- Recent international research has shown that circulation is not improved by heel warming (Box 31.8) and the practice has been discontinued. The Royal Australasian College of Physicians (Paediatrics and Child Health Division) guidelines recommend that parents put socks or bootees on the baby's feet and wrap the baby warmly before the blood sample is taken. It is also recommended that to relieve pain the mother holds and feeds the baby during the procedure, and that multisensory stimulation is employed.

Procedure

1. Alcohol-impregnated swabs should not be used prior to collecting a blood sample as the alcohol can affect the accuracy of the results (Johnson et al., 2019).
2. Avoid sensitive areas of the heel (see Fig. 31.22).
3. Puncture the outer aspect of the heel with a sterile disposable lancet (National Screening Unit, 2020). Automated lancets are preferable to manual ones and slicer lancets have been shown to be more effective than 'stabber' lancets.
4. Wipe away the first drop of blood with dry sterile gauze.
5. Depending on the test, either gently fill the microcapillary collection tube or allow blood to drop onto the

Box 31.8 Clinical alert

Never put the baby's foot in warm water or wrap in a warmed cloth. It is not necessary and it is *very* easy to seriously scald a neonate's sensitive skin.

(Source: NHS, 2016)

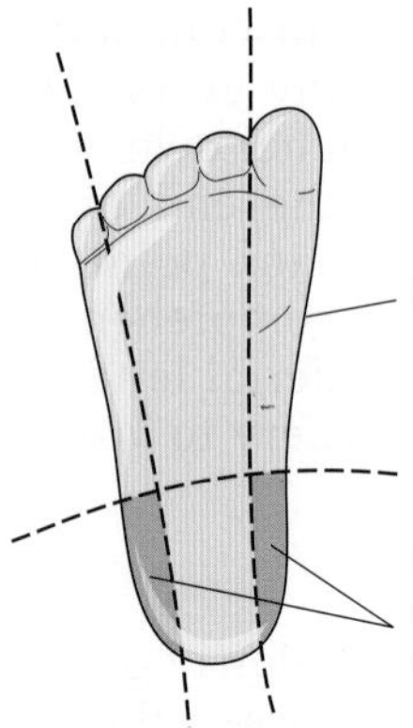

FIGURE 31.22 Heel puncture sites for neonatal blood sampling (Source: Fraser, 2009)

filter paper and ensure that the whole circle is filled with blood through the full thickness of the paper. Fill the collection paper from the reverse side.

6. Apply gentle pressure with gauze or a cotton wool ball until bleeding stops.
7. Label the specimen appropriately and send for analysis.

(For comprehensive information on collecting please refer to the National Screening Unit Guidelines (2010).)

Other information shared

Postnatal visits offer the opportunity for the midwife to share information using health education and health promotion strategies.

Warmth and hygiene

There is no 'right' way to bath a baby as long as the baby does not get cold in the process and does not suffer accidental immersion. Common-sense precautions such as a warm room, towels and clothes, getting all necessary equipment ready before starting and drying the baby thoroughly are simple ways to prevent chilling. Current evidence indicates that it is better not to use baby toiletry products such as shampoo or bubble bath for at least the first month of life, as there may be an association with the development of infant skin conditions (Trotter, 2020).

Parents are frequently encouraged to dress their baby in many layers of clothing. Generally, it is sufficient to use one layer more than the other people in the room are wearing. Babies do not sweat very effectively, and so can become overheated. Overheating while sleeping is also a risk factor for SUDI. The American Academy of Pediatrics (2016) states that the room temperature should be comfortable for a lightly clothed adult and the baby should be lightly clothed for sleep, with overbundling and covering of the face and head avoided, and should not feel hot to the touch. The nape of the neck is a good indicator of the overall temperature of the baby and it should feel warm rather than hot or cold when felt with the inside of the wrist.

CRITICAL THINKING EXERCISE

At an antenatal visit, a pregnant woman asks you what sort of clothes, what size and how many she needs for her baby. She also asks you whether she should use disposable or reusable nappies. Consider your reply. Where would you access the information the woman needs in your local community or maternity services?

Prevention of injury or accident and reducing the risk of SUDI

Common-sense precautions to prevent injury should be observed by midwives and parents. Babies should not be left unattended in cots with the sides down or on beds, chairs or tables. Parents and caregivers must be reminded never to leave the baby unattended in the bath even for a second (even if the parents are using bath aids). Bathwater should be tested to ensure it is not too hot before bathing the baby.

Reduce the risk of suffocation or SUDI by putting babies to bed on their backs. Keep the face clear. Make sure the mattress is firm and fits the cot snugly, with no gaps around the edges. Pillows are not required in bassinets and waterproof mattress covers need to be tightly fitting to avoid loose covers that may suffocate the baby. Babies should be put to bed in a cot or a bassinet. Waterbeds, car seats, sofas, chairs and bean bags are not suitable as beds for babies. Keep the bassinet or cot free of soft toys.

CLINICAL POINT

Bed sharing (by Sally Baddock)

Bed sharing or co-sleeping between babies and their mothers (and other family members) is a traditional practice in many cultures and is part of a chosen parenting style in others (Ball et al., 2016). Bed sharing is often seen as a way of facilitating breastfeeding and the majority of infants that bed share are breastfed (Ball et al., 2016; Blair et al., 2010). However, bed sharing is not a single coherent practice. Families follow varied practices and choose to bed share for different reasons and this may impact on the safety or otherwise of their sleeping arrangements (Baddock et al., 2000).

Parents who choose to bed share report ease of breastfeeding, reduced tiredness, emotional benefits and having a more settled baby (Ball et al., 1999; McKenna & Volpe, 2007) and observational studies report increased breastfeeding, increased maternal interactions and synchronisation of mother–baby sleep patterns during bed share sleep. Mothers and babies are also found to sleep facing each other, in close proximity and with the baby most often at the level of the mother's breast, facilitating breastfeeding (Baddock et al., 2006; McKenna et al., 1997). Fathers have not been shown to interact with the baby overnight in studies where the mother is also present (Baddock et al., 2007).

While bed share babies wake more often, total sleep time is similar to that of cot sleep babies, as cot sleepers tend to wake for longer at each waking (Baddock et al., 2004). Maternal checks are sometimes prompted by infant movements, but equally the mother self-initiates many checks through the night (Baddock et al., 2007; Ball, 2009). Further evidence suggests that child–parent proximity may have longer term influences on children's social, emotional and physical development (Mileva-Seitz et al., 2017).

The benefits of bed sharing seem to stem from the mother–baby partnership and the facilitation of breastfeeding. Non-breastfeeding mother–baby pairs may not derive the same benefits from bed sharing (Ball, 2006). This is supported by a study of low-income families in inner city Chicago at high risk of sudden unexpected death in infancy (SUDI) where bed sharing was common but breastfeeding was not (Hauck et al., 2003).

However, bed sharing is associated with an increased risk of SUDI in a number of circumstances and it is important that families are able to make informed decisions about infant place of sleep. Bed sharing with a mother who smoked during pregnancy has consistently been identified in international studies as increasing the risk of SUDI (Carpenter et al., 2004, 2013; Mitchell et al., 2017). The risk from maternal smoking is greater for bed share infants than for infants who sleep in a cot. It is possible that infants compromised by maternal smoking may not have adequate ventilatory (Campbell et al., 2001) or thermal (Tuffnell et al., 1995) responses to particular stresses arising in the bed-sharing environment. The increased risk may be from increased head covering that inadvertently occurs during bed sharing owing to the mobility of the bedding (Baddock et al., 2006; Ball, 2009), or it may be connected with the warmer environment associated with thicker adult bedding (Baddock et al., 2004). The close maternal contact in bed sharing may also expose infants to more effects from passive smoking—for example, nicotine has been shown to accumulate on furniture surfaces and bedding, even if the mother smokes only outside the house (Matt et al., 2004).

Other risk factors associated with bed sharing include recent maternal alcohol or drug consumption, maternal overtiredness, excessive bedding, household overcrowding and bed sharing with a premature infant or an infant age younger than 12 weeks (Blair et al., 1999, 2009; Carpenter et al., 2004, 2013). Sleeping on a couch, chair or waterbed with a baby increases the risk of SUDI, which is possibly due to the likelihood of the baby becoming trapped between the adult and furniture (Blair et al., 2009). Pillows or situations that might lead to wedging or trapping of the baby (e.g. between the bed and wall or between two mattresses) also pose a risk (Child and Youth Mortality Review Committee, 2013).

There continues to be debate about the risk of bed sharing when infants less than 3 months are breastfed and not exposed to risk factors such as maternal smoking. In a recent case–control study from New Zealand, the risk of SUDI when bed sharing in the absence of maternal smoking was 1.5 times that of not bed sharing but did not reach statistical significance, while that associated with the combination of bed sharing and maternal smoking was 38 times that of not bed sharing and not being exposed to smoking (Mitchell et al., 2017).

New Zealand Māori and Pacifika infants (Mitchell et al., 2017) and Australian Aboriginal and Torres Strait Islander infants (Panaretto et al., 2002; Young et al., 2017) are overrepresented in SUDI deaths. The combined risks of parental smoking and bed sharing are prevalent in these groups (MacFarlane et al., 2018; Tipene-Leach et al., 2010). In New Zealand, wahakura (woven flax baskets) and Pēpi-pods (plastic containers of similar size, fitted with mattresses and covers) have been developed to provide a safer bed-sharing option where maternal smoking and bed sharing are common and are now also distributed in Australia. Evidence suggests no significant differences in infant SUDI risk behaviours in wahakura or Pēpi-pods compared with bassinets and identifies an increase in sustained breastfeeding for those provided a wahakura (Baddock et al., 2017, 2018; Tipene-Leach et al., 2018). This suggests wahakura and Pēpi-pods are relatively safe and can be promoted as an alternative to infant–adult bed sharing. When the sleep device is handed over to the family the midwife has a targeted opportunity for sharing safe sleep messages and this has been identified as a key component of the intervention (McIntosh et al., 2018). This includes educating all people that care for baby, such as grandparents, other family members and childcare workers. Internationally a range of 'baby boxes' are available, based on the baby boxes first distributed in Finland (the Kela Maternity package) in the 1930s. They are often provided with free baby products and used to engage parents in safe sleep education but unlike the wahakura and Pēpi-pod are not necessarily designed for in-bed use, or supported by objective research (Bartick et al., 2018).

Maternal–infant bed sharing also commonly occurs in maternity units in hospitals but there are concerns about the safety of this practice in hospital beds. A study in the UK has provided evidence that clip-on-bassinets may provide a safer alternative to bed sharing, with similar benefits of maternal–infant proximity, increased breastfeeding and increased mothers' satisfaction with their postnatal experience in hospital (Ball et al., 2006). There is no research published to date investigating this type of sleeping arrangement in New Zealand or Australia.

The risks and benefits to the infant while bed sharing have been assimilated in a systematic review that included 59 publications with a focus on in-depth physiology and / or breastfeeding during bed sharing (Baddock et al., 2019). Most of the participants in this research were described as at low risk of SUDI and more research is needed to understand the responses of higher risk infants and of hazardous situations. However, such research poses many challenges.

In summary, factors that increase the risk of SUDI associated with bed sharing are grouped around a vulnerable baby (prematurity, young age, exposure to smoking), an impaired mother (alcohol, overtired) and the physical environment (overheating, hazardous bedding, sofa sleeping). Most authorities recommend that the safest place for babies to sleep is in a cot beside the parent's bed for the first 6 months (Mitchell, 2010). However, there are a variety of reasons that parents may choose to bed share and it is important that they are informed of the risks and benefits associated with this sleep arrangement. There is evidence to support that it is the circumstances of bed sharing that lead to the increased risk of SUDI, and not the bed sharing itself (Blair et al., 2009, 2013).

For current advice regarding safety measures to consider if families choose to bed share, check the following websites:

http://www.unicef.org.uk/Documents/Baby_Friendly/Leaflets/caringatnight_web.pdf

https://www.health.govt.nz/your-health/pregnancy-and-kids/first-year/first-6-weeks/keeping-baby-safe-bed-first-6-weeks

https://www.northlanddhb.org.nz/your-health/health-resources/sudden-unexpected-death-in-infancy-sudi/?url=/AboutUs/SUDIpreventionhealtheducation.aspx.

https://hapai.co.nz/content/national-sudi-prevention-coordination-service

Keep the baby's environment smoke free. Maternal smoking in pregnancy significantly increases the risk of SUDI. Ongoing smoke-free programs are in place in both New Zealand and Australia. The emphasis of these programs is to stop smoking in pregnancy and to keep the new baby's environment smoke free.

Breastfeed if at all possible. Protection from infection and risk reduction for SUDI are among the many benefits of breastfeeding.

Risk reduction campaigns, particularly those related to sleeping position, and quitting smoking have contributed to a significant decline in SUDI over the past 20 or so years in countries such as Australia and New Zealand. Nonetheless, women and families still need information and support to reduce the risk of SUDI, which midwives and other maternity care and Well Child care providers are well placed to provide. Resources for parents and midwives are accessible from Australian and New Zealand Ministries of Health, the Australian SIDS and Kids organisation and New Zealand's Change for our Children: http://www.changeforourchildren.nz/safe_start_programme/issues_forum. (See Ch. 42 for more extensive discussion of SUDI.)

Car safety

There is evidence that death or injury in a car accident can be prevented or minimised by appropriate restraint for age. In Australia and New Zealand it is illegal for any person to be unrestrained in a car. Newborns are restrained in car seats that are the correct size for newborns. In many areas, local health authorities or Well Child services provide an affordable hire service. Midwives should source local availability so that women can be given the required information.

Discharge from midwifery care and transfer to Well Child services

In New Zealand at the final postnatal visit, between 4 and 6 weeks, the midwife is expected to carry out the final comprehensive assessment for the baby, which includes a developmental assessment. The findings should be recorded in the clinical notes and the Well Child health record book. When the baby is transferred from midwifery care, there should be a seamless transfer of care to the agreed Well Child provider. It is the responsibility of the midwife to ensure that the health professionals providing ongoing care receive appropriate referral or transfer documents that should include the history of pregnancy, birth and the postnatal period. Information about feeding and behavioural patterns, as well as the baby's developmental and physical assessment, should be included. The Well Child health record book usually includes a written record as well as up-to-date measurements on the centile growth graphs and a record of assessments and any immunisations the baby may have received at birth. Most women will also hold a copy of their clinical notes. A referral letter should be written to the baby's general practitioner and a letter or referral form (depending on what is used locally) should also go to the Well Child provider service. Local practice may also include telephone notification that the baby has been discharged from midwifery care. Telephone referrals should be followed up with a full written referral.

Conclusion

Providing support for the newborn begins in the antenatal period when good midwifery care can help to ensure that the baby receives the best possible opportunity to grow, develop and prepare for its transfer to the external world.

The birth of the baby signals the transition from intrauterine to extrauterine life. This episode is characterised by a series of physiological adaptations which are usually orchestrated by behaviours initiated by both mother and baby. These adaptations should be supported by good midwifery care based around a sound knowledge of fetal and neonatal anatomy and physiology. The midwife needs to prepare a birthing environment where these physiological adaptations can occur in a safe, supported and undisturbed way, regardless of where the birth takes place, and this should be seen as a fundamental midwifery action.

Midwives need to develop and sustain knowledge and skills in order to undertake a comprehensive physical assessment of a newborn baby as this is within the scope of midwifery practice. This assessment will normally take place at several different points during the postnatal period, which means that a midwife needs also to develop skills around identifying the **normal growth and development** of the baby during this time. Recognition of normal features and/or behaviours in the baby will assist early identification of any deviations from normal that may require treatment and/or referral to a medical practitioner or other appropriate agency. The midwife needs therefore to be aware of appropriate modes of referral and of the availability of and access to a range of community groups and services relating to the newborn.

Indication that the baby is thriving needs to be shared with the parents and this conversation should be used to highlight areas for further discussion around issues relating to the health and wellbeing of the baby. For example, when examining the baby's umbilicus, the subject of cord care hygiene may be prompted, or if the temperature of the room is on the high side, a discussion around SUDI may ensue. Likewise a conversation about common variations in baby behaviours such as sleeping and crying is necessary as this may assist women in developing confidence as they learn to care for their newborn baby.

The ongoing monitoring of the health and wellbeing of the baby is the responsibility of the midwife for up to 6 weeks following birth. After the conclusion of the midwife/mother partnership, the transfer of care to Well Child services should provide a seamless transition ensuring a continuum of care for the baby. Good record keeping and interprofessional communication should ensure that healthcare providers can continue to provide individualised and contextualised care.

Supporting the newborn is a crucially important aspect in the role of the midwife. It does not start at a given point in the childbirth experience of a woman, but rather is embodied within the continuum of care throughout this time. The baby transits from intrauterine to extrauterine life as the woman moves into the role of new mother. Even if it is her second or subsequent baby, she is for this baby a new mother and the same principle of course applies equally to the partner as the father. Supporting the newborn requires specialised clinical skills and knowledge on the part of the midwife but equally relies on sound communication and interpersonal skills. Perhaps above all it requires a commitment to support the baby within the context of its family as a social entity. As a first-line support person during the introduction of a new family member, midwives are in a strong position to influence change which may lead to improvements in both short- and long-term health outcomes not just for the baby, but also for the mother, father and indeed the whole family.

Review questions

1. How does 'skin-to-skin' promote temperature stability?
2. How is privacy and quiet provided in the first hours after birth in maternity units?
3. What would be the result if one or more of the temporary structures in the fetal circulation failed to close after birth?
4. What is your local regimen for oral vitamin K prophylaxis?
5. How is the mother–baby relationship supported?
6. If you work in an area where the temperatures are extreme, what advice will you give to women about protecting their baby in very hot or very cold conditions?
7. What are the procedures in your local area if a lax hip joint is detected at birth? And at 1 week?
8. How will you differentiate a monilial rash from nappy rash on a baby's buttocks and groin? What advice will you give the mother? How are these rashes treated?
9. In your area, which conditions are tested for in the newborn metabolic screening? What is the incidence of these conditions? How are they treated?
10. What action will you take if one of the tests has a positive result?
11. In your area, what happens to the metabolic screening cards once the tests are completed?
12. What assessments will you make if a mother reports an unsettled and crying baby?

Online resources

Health ministries and departments

Australian Government, Department of Health and Ageing: http://www.health.gov.au/.

Department of Health, South Australia: http://www.sahealth.sa.gov.au/wps/wcm/connect/Public+Content/SA+Health+Internet/.

Department of Health, Western Australia: http://ww2.health.wa.gov.au.

Department of Health and Human Services, Tasmania: http://www.dhhs.tas.gov.au/.

New South Wales Health: http://www.health.nsw.gov.au/Pages/default.aspx.

New Zealand Ministry of Health: http://www.health.govt.nz/.

Queensland Health: http://www.health.qld.gov.au/

Immunisation sites

Immunisation Advisory Centre, New Zealand: http://www.immune.org.nz/.

National Immunisation Program Schedule (Australia): https://www.health.gov.au/health-topics/immunisation/when-to-get-vaccinated/national-immunisation-program-schedule.

NSW Multicultural Health Communication Service: http://www.mhcs.health.nsw.gov.au.

Other sites

Cochrane Collaboration, a major database of evaluations of the evidence for maternity care; accessible through libraries in education institutes and some hospitals: https://www.cochrane.org/.

New South Wales Government Centre for Genetics Education: http://www.genetics.edu.au/Publications-and-Resources/Genetics-Fact-Sheets/genetics-fact-sheet-users-guide.

New Zealand Ministry of Health National Screening Unit: http://www.nsu.govt.nz.

Stanford School of Medicine, Newborn nursery at LPH, Professional education, Photo Gallery: http://med.stanford.edu/newborns/professional-education/photo-gallery.html.

SUDI prevention information for parents and for health professionals: http://www.changeforourchildren.co.nz/; http://www.sidsandkids.org.nz/.

References

Alexandre G Troullioud LAG, Jaafar S, et al. Pediatric Umbilical Hernia. In: *StatPearls* [Treasure Island (FL): StatPearls Publishing; 2021. Online: https://www.ncbi.nlm.nih.gov/books/NBK459294/.

Alvo A, Villarroel G, Sedano C. Neonatal nasal obstruction. *Eur Arch Otorhinolaryngol.* 2021. Online: https://doi.org/10.1007/s00405-020-06546-y.

American Academy of Pediatrics Task Force on Sudden Infant Death Syndrome. Policy statement. The changing concept of sudden infant death syndrome: diagnostic coding shifts, controversies regarding the sleeping environment and new variables to consider in reducing risk. *Pediatrics.* 2016;138(5):e20162938.

Aprillia, Z., D. Gayatri, and F.T. Waluyanti, *Sensitivity, Specificity, and Accuracy of Kramer Examination of Neonatal Jaundice: Comparison with Total Bilirubin Serum. Compr Child Adolesc Nurs.* 2017;40(suppl 1):88–94.

Baddock SA, Day HF, Rimene CR. Bedsharing practices of different cultural groups. Paper presented at the SIDS 2000, 6th SIDS International Conference, Auckland, New Zealand: 2017.

Baddock SA, Galland BC, Beckers MGS, et al. Bed sharing and the infant's thermal environment in the home setting. *Arch Dis Child.* 2004;89:1111–1116.

Baddock SA, Galland BC, Bolton DPG, et al. Differences in infant and parent behaviors during routine bed sharing compared with cot sleeping in the home setting. *Pediatrics.* 2006;117: 1599–1607.

Baddock SA, Galland BC, Taylor BJ, et al. Sleep arrangements and behavior of bed-sharing families in the home setting. *Pediatrics.* 2007;119(1):200–207.

Baddock SA, Tipene-Leach D, Williams SM, et al. Wahakura versus bassinet for safe infant sleep: a randomized trial. *Pediatrics.* 2017;139(2.pii)e20160162. doi:10.1542/peds.2016–0162.

Baddock SA, Tipene-Leach D, Williams SM, et al. Physiological stability in an indigenous sleep device: a randomised controlled trial. *Arch Dis Child.* 2018;103(4):377–382.

Baddock SA, Purnell MT, Blair PS et al. The influence of bed-sharing on infant physiology, breastfeeding and behaviour: A systematic review. *Sleep Med Rev.* 2019;43:106–117.

Bahar K, Karapınar ED. Yılmazbaş P, et al. Risk factor assessment and a ten-year experience of DDH Screening in a Well-Child Population. *BioMed Res Int.* 2019: ID 7213681. doi:org/ 10.1155/2019/7213681.

Ball HL. Parent–infant bed-sharing behaviour. Effects of feeding type and presence of father. *Hum Nat.* 2006;17(3):301–318.

Ball H. Airway covering during bed-sharing. *Child Care Health Dev.* 2009;35(5):728–737.

Ball HL, Hooker E, Kelly PJ. Where will the baby sleep? Attitudes and practices of new and experienced parents regarding cosleeping with their newborn infants. *Am Anthropol.* 1999;101(1):143–151.

Ball HL, Ward-Platt MP, Heslop E, et al. Randomised trial of infant sleep location on the postnatal ward. *Arch Dis Child.* 2006;91(12): 1005–1010.

Ball HL, Howe D, Bryant IA, et al. Bed-sharing by breastfeeding mothers: who bed-shares and what is the relationship with breastfeeding duration? *Acta Paediatr.* 2016;105(6):628–634.

Barrett J, Wonch KE, Gonzalez A, et al. Maternal affect and quality of parenting experiences are related to amygdala response to infant faces. *Soc Neurosci.* 2012;7(3):252–268.

Bartick MC, Tomori C, Ball HL. Babies in boxes and the missing links on safe sleep: human evolution. *Matern Child Nutr.* 2018;14(2):e12544. doi:10.1111/mcn.12544.

Baston H, Durward H. *Examination of the Newborn.* 2nd ed. Abingdon, UK: Routledge; 2017.

Bergman NJ. The neuroscience of birth – and the case for zero separation. *Curationis.* 2014;37(2):1–4.

Bigelow AE. Power M. Mother–Infant Skin-to-Skin Contact: Short- and Long-Term Effects for Mothers and Their Children Born Full-Term. *Front Psychol.* 2020; 11:1921 https://www.frontiersin.org/article/10.3389/fpsyg.2020.01921

Blackburn ST. *Maternal, Fetal, Neonatal Physiology: A Clinical Perspective.* 5th ed. Maryland Heights, MO: Elsevier Saunders; 2017.

Blackwell C, Moscovis S, Hall S, et al. RJ Exploring the risk factors for sudden infant deths and their role in inflammatory responses to infection. *Front Immunol.* 2015 5 March. doi. org/10.3389/fimmu.2015.00044.

Blair P, Fleming P, Smith I, et al. Babies sleeping with parents: case-control study of factors influencing the risk of the sudden infant death syndrome. *BMJ.* 1999;319:1457–1462.

Blair PS, Sidebotham P, Evason-Coombe C, et al. Hazardous cosleeping environments and risk factors amenable to change: Case-control study of SIDS in south west England. *BMJ.* 2009; 339:b3666.

Blair PS, Heron J, Fleming PJ. Relationship between bed sharing and breastfeeding: longitudinal, population-based analysis. *Pediatrics.* 2010;126(5):e1119–e1126.

Blair PS, Fleming PJ, Ashmore S. A lack of data and questionable emphasis. *BMJ Open.* 2013;published online May 22.

Bliss-Holtz J. Determining cold stress in full term newborns through temperature site comparisons. *Sch Inq Nurs Pract.* 1991;5(2):113–123.

Bowman R. Assessing vision in a baby. *Community Eye Health.* 2016;29(93):16–17.

Buckley S. *Hormonal Physiology of Childbearing: Evidence and Implications for Women, Babies, and Maternity Care.* Washington DC: Childbirth Connection Programs: National Partnership for Women and Families; 2015. Online: http://www.nationalpartnership.org/research-library/maternal-health/hormonal-physiology-of-childbearing.pdf.

Callen JP, Greer KE, Paller AS, et al. *Color Atlas of Dermatology.* 2nd ed. Philadelphia: WB Saunders; 2000.

Campbell AJ, Galland BC, Bolton DPG, et al. Ventilatory responses to rebreathing in infants exposed to maternal smoking. *Acta Paediatr.* 2001;90(7):793–800.

Carpenter RG, Irgens LM, Blair PS, et al. Sudden unexplained infant death in 20 regions. *Lancet.* 2004;363:185–191.

Carpenter RG, McGarvey C, Mitchell EA, et al. Bed sharing when parents do not smoke: Is there a risk of sids? An individual level analysis of five major case–control studies. *BMJ Open.* 2013;3:5. pii:e002299. doi:10.1136/bmjopen-2012-002299.

Child and Youth Mortality Review Committee Te Ròpù Arotake Auau Mate o te Hunga Tamariki, Taiohi. *Special Report: Unintentional Suffocation, Foreign Body Inhalation and Strangulation.* Wellington: Child and Youth Mortality Review Committee; 2013.

Collado M, Autuva S, Aakko J et al. Human gut colonisation may be initiated *in utero* by distinct microbial communities in the placenta and amniotic fluid Nature. *Sci Rep.* 2016; 6:2312.

Cornblath M, Ichord R. Hypoglycemia in the neonate. *Semin Perinatol.* 2000;24(2):136–149.

Dahlen HG, Downe S, Kennedy HP, et al. Is society being reshaped on a microbiological and epigenetic level by the way women give birth? *Midwifery.* 2014;30(12):1149–1151.

Darrah J, Bartlett DJ. Infant rolling abilities—the same or different 20 years after the back to sleep campaign? *Early Hum Dev.* 2013;89(5):311–314.

Davidson MR, London ML, Ladewig PW. *Olds' Maternal–Newborn Nursing and Women's Health Across the Lifespan.* Boston: Pearson; 2012.

Davies L. Biobehavioural aspects of parenting. In: Rankin J, eds. *Physiology in Childbearing.* 4th ed. London: Elsevier; 2017:597–603.

Davies, L. Influences on the health of the newborn, before and during pregnancy. In Davies, L and McDonald S (eds) *Examination of the Newborn and neonatal health.* 2nd ed. 2020. London: Elsevier: 84–99 (Ch. 5).

Davies L, Richards J. Maternal and newborn transition: adjustment to extrauterine life. In: Davies L, MacDonald S, eds. *Examination of the Newborn and Neonatal Health.* Edinburgh: Churchill Livingstone; 2008:107–126 [Ch. 7].

Davies L, Richards J. Maternal and newborn transition: adjustment to extrauterine life. In: Davies L, MacDonald S, eds.

Examination of the Newborn and Neonatal Health. London: Elsevier; 2020:100–122 (Ch. 6).
Deken A,Meeks M. Neonatal jaundice: implications for newborn health. In: Davies L, McDonald S, eds. *Examination of the Newborn: A Multidimensional Approach.* London: Elsevier; 2020: 209–229 [Ch. 12].
Dekker R, *Bertone A Evidence on the Vitamin K Shot in Newborns.* Evidence Based Birth. Online: https://evidencebasedbirth.com/evidence-for-the-vitamin-k-shot-in-newborns/.
Dominguez-Bello MG, Godoy-Vitorino F, Knight R, et al. Role of the microbiome in human development *Gut.* 2019;68:1108–1114.
Ebisch SJ, Aureli T, Bafunno D, et al. Mother and child in synchrony: Thermal facial imprints of autonomic contagion. *Biol Psychol.* 2012;89(1):123–129.
Eichenfield LF, et al. *Neonatal and Infant Dermatology.* 3rd ed. Saunders; 2015.
Farmey AJ, Hyett JA, Schluter PJ, et al. New Australian birthweight centiles. *Med J Aust.* 2020; 213(2):79–85. doi:10.5694/mja2.50676.
Feldman R. Bio-behavioral synchrony: a model for integrating biological and microsocial behavioral processes in the study of parenting. *Parenting.* 2012;12(2–3):154–164. doi:10.1080/15295192.2012.683342.
Fettweis JM, Serrano MG, Brooks JP, et al. The vaginal microbiome and pretern birth. *Nat Med.* 2019;25:1012–1021. doi:10.1038/s41591-019-0450-2.
Fleming TP, Watkins AJ, Velazquez MA, et al. Origins of lifetime health around the time of conception: causes and consequences. *Lancet.* 2018;391(10132):1842–1852. doi:10.1016/S0140-6736(18)30312-X.
Fogarty M, Osborn DA, Askie L, et al. Delayed versus early umbilical cord clamping for preterm infants: a systematic review and meta-analysis. *Am J Obstet Gynecol.* 2017. doi:10.1016/j.ajog.2017.10.231.
Fraser DM, Cooper MA, eds. *Myles' Textbook for Midwives.* 15th ed. Edinburgh: Churchill Livingstone; 2009.
Gardner SL, Carter BS, Enzman-Hines MI, et al. *Merenstein and Gardner's Handbook of Neonatal Intensive Care.* 9th ed. St Louis: Elsevier; 2020.
Gazzin, S., et al., A Novel Perspective on the Biology of Bilirubin in Health and Disease. *Trends Mol Med.* 2016;22(9):758–768.
Ghazi S, Couteau C, Paparis E, et al. Interest of external photoprotection by means of clothing and sunscreen products in young children. *J Eür Acad Dermatol Venereol.* 2012;8(2): 1026–1030.
Gordon M. Examination of the newborn abdomen and genitalia. In: Lomax A, eds. *Examination of the Newborn: An Evidence Informed Guide.* Chichester, UK: Wiley Blackwell; 2011:134–151 [Ch. 7].
Harding J, Hegarty JE, Crowther CA, et al. Evaluation of oral dextrose gel for prevention of neonatal hypoglycemia (hPOD): a multicenter, double-blind randomized controlled trial. 2021. *PLoS ONE.* doi:10.1371/journal.pmed.1003411.
Hauck FR, Herman SM, Donovan M, et al. Sleep environment and the risk of sudden infant death syndrome in an urban population: the Chicago Infant Mortality Study. *Pediatrics.* 2003; 111(5/2):1207–1214.
Henderson C, MacDonald S. *Mayes' Midwifery.* 13th ed. London: Baillière Tindall; 2004.
Hawdon JM. Definition of neonatal hypoglycaemia: time for a rethink? *Arch Dis Child Fetal Neonatal Ed.* 2013 Sep;98(5):F382–3. doi:10.1136/archdischild-2012-303422. Epub 2013 May 3. PMID: 23645576.
Hawdon JM. Postnatal metabolic adaptation and neonatal hypoglycaemia. *Paediatr Child Health.* 2016;26(4):135–139.
Hewitt V, Watts R, Robertson J, et al. Systematic review: nursing and midwifery management of hypoglycaemia in healthy term neonates. *Int J Evid Based Healthc.* 2005;3(7):169–205.
Hillman NH, Suhas GK, Jobe AJ. Physiology of transition from intrauterine to extrauterine life. *Clin Perinatol.* 2012;39(4):769–783. doi:10.1016/j.clp.2012.09.009.
Hoffman MC, Mazzoni SE, Wagner BD, et al. Measures of maternal stress and mood in relation to preterm birth. *Obstet Gynecol.* 2016;127(3):545–552. doi:10.1097/AOG.0000000000001287.
Hooper S, te Pas A, Lang J, et al. Cardiovascular transition at birth: a physiological sequence. *Pediatr Res.* 2015;77:608–614. doi:10.1038/pr.2015.21.
Johnson R, Taylor W, de-Vitry Smith S et al. *Skills for Midwifery Practice.* Australia and New Zealand ed. Chatswood: Elsevier; 2019.
Johnston P, Flood K, Spinks K, eds. *The Newborn Child.* 9th ed. London: Churchill Livingstone; 2003.
Kostandy RR, Luddington-Hoe S. Kangarro care (skin-to-skin) for clustered pain procedures: case study. *World J Neurosci.* 2016;6(1):43–51.
Kristensen K, Henriksen L. Cesarean section and disease associated with immune function. *J Allergy Clin Immunol.* 2016;137(2):587–590.
Lagercrantz H. The conscious infant. In Lagercrantz H. *Infant brain development: Formation of the mind and consciousness.* Springer; 2015:86–98.
Latendresse G. The interaction between chronic stress and pregnancy: preterm birth from a biobehavioral perspective. *J Midwifery Womens Health.* 2009;54(1):8–17. doi:10.1016/j.jmwh.2008.08.001.
Lee, WL, Slutsky AS. Acute hypoxemic respiratory failure and ARDS. In Courtney Broaddus V, Mason RJ, Ernst JD, et al., eds. *Murray and Nadel's Textbook of Respiratory Medicine.* Philadelphia: Saunders; 2016.
Leigh B. *Six states of awareness for newborns.* 2016. Online: https://www.centreforperinatalpsychology.com.au/states-of-alertness/.
Lippi G, Franchini M. Vitamin K in neonates: facts and myths. *Blood Transfus.* 2011;9(1):4–9. doi:10.2450/2010.0034-10.
Li H, Shu L, Yu J, et al. Using Z-score to optimize population-specific DDH screening: a retrospective study in Hangzhou, China. *BMC Musculoskelet Disord.* 22;344 (2021). doi:10.1186/s12891-021-04216-6.
Liu M, Zhao L, Li XF. Effect of skin contact between mother and child in pain relief of full-term newborns during heel blood collection. *Clin Exp Obstet Gynecol.* 2015;42(3):304–308. doi:10.12891/ceog1831.
LoMauro A, Aliverti A. Physiology masterclass: Extremes of age: newborn and infancy. *Breathe (Sheff).* 2016;12(1):65–68. doi:10.1183/20734735.013315.
Ludington-Hoe SM, Lewis T, Morgan K, et al. Breast and infant temperatures with twins during shared kangaroo care. *J Obstet Gynecol Neonatal Nurs.* 2006;35:223–231. doi:10.1111/j.1552-6909.2006.00024.x.
Lundström JN, Mathe A, Schaal B, et al. Maternal status regulates cortical responses to the body odor of newborns. *Front Psychol.* 2013;4:597. doi:10.3389/fpsyg.2013.00597.
Lunze, K., Hamer, D. Thermal protection of the newborn in resource-limited environments. *J Perinatol.* 2021;32:317–324 (2012). doi:10.1038/jp.2012.11.
Lye PS, Densmore EM. Fever: Temperature Measurement. In: KleigmanR, Lye PS, Base D, eds. *Nelson Pediatric Symptom-Based Diagnosis.* 2018. Online: https://www.sciencedirect.com/topics/nursing-and-health-professions/rectal temperature.
MacFarlane M, Mitchell EA, Thompson JMD, et al. Smoking in pregnancy: a key factor for sudden infant death among Maori. *Acta Paediatr.* 2018. doi:10.1111/apa.14431.
McDonald S. The practical examination of the newborn. In: Davies, L McDonald S, eds. *Examination of the Newborn and Neonatal Health.* 2nd ed. London: Elsevier:6–38 [Ch. 2].
McDonald S Rose L. Newborn Screening and Immunization. In: Davies L, McDonald S, eds. *Examination of the Newborn and*

Neonatal Health. 2nd ed. London. Elsevier; 2020. 240–256 [Ch. 14].
McIntosh C, Trenholme A, Stewart J, et al. Evaluation of a sudden unexpected death in infancy intervention programme aimed at improving parental awareness of risk factors and protective infant care practices. *J Paediatr Child Health*. 2018;54(4):377–382. doi:10.1111/jpc.13772.
McKenna JJ, Mosko SS, Richard CA. Bedsharing promotes breast-feeding. *Pediatrics*. 1997;100(2/1):214–219.
McKenna JJ, Volpe LE. Sleeping with baby: an internet-based sampling of parental experiences, choices, perceptions, and interpretations in a western industrialized context. *Infant Child Dev*. 2007;16(4):359–385.
Marchelli MR, Santoro E, Marchesi A, et al. Vitamin K deficiency: a case report and review of current guidelines. *Ital J Pediatr*. 2018; 44(1):36.
Matamoros S, Gras-Leguen C, Le Vacon F, et al. Development of intestinal microbiota in infants and its impact on health. *Trends Microbiol*. 2013;21(4):167–173.
Matt GE, Quintana PJ, Hovell MF, et al. Households contaminated by environmental tobacco smoke: sources of infant exposures. *Tob Control*. 2004;13(1):29–37. doi:10.1136/tc.2003.003889.
Mercer JS, Skovgaard RL. Neonatal transitional physiology: a new paradigm. *J Perinat Neonatal Nurs*. 2002;15(4):56–75.
Michaelides S. The newborn baby: physiology, assessment and care. In: MacDonald S, Magill-Cuerden J, eds. *Mayes' Midwifery*. 14th ed. London: Baillière Tindall, Elsevier; 2011:567–600 [Ch. 41].
Michaelides S. Physiology, assessment and care of the newborn . In: MacDonald, Johnson G, eds. *Mayes' Midwifery*. 15th ed. London: Baillière Tindall, Elsevier; 2017a:705–740 [Ch. 42].
Michaelides S. Thermoregulation. In: MacDonald S, Johnson G, eds. *Mayes' Midwifery*. 17th ed. London: Baillière Tindall, Elsevier; 2017b:741–756 [Ch. 43].
Mileva-Seitz VR, Bakermans-Kranenburg MJ, Battaini C, Luijk MPCM. Parent-child bed-sharing: the good, the bad, and the burden of evidence. *Sleep Med Rev*. 2017;32:4e27.
Ministry of Health (MOH). *Section 88 Primary Maternity Services Notice 2007*. Wellington: Ministry of Health; 2007. Online: http://www.health.govt.nz/our-work/life-stages/maternity-services/primary-maternity-services-notice-section-88.
Ministry of Health (MOH). *Tamariki Ora, Well Child Health Book*. Wellington: Ministry of Health, Manatu Hauora; 2012.
Ministry of Health (MOH). Growth charts. In: Tamariki Ora, *Well Child Health Book*. Wellington: Ministry of Health; 2015. Online: https://www.health.govt.nz/our-work/life-stages/child-health/well-child-tamariki-ora-services/growth-charts.
Ministry of Health (MOH). *Baby and Child Sickness—Danger Signs*. 2016. Online: http://www.health.govt.nz/your-health/pregnancy-and-kids/first-year/helpful-advice-during-first-year/baby-and-child-sickness-danger-signs.
Ministry of Health National Screening Unit. *Guidelines for practitioners providing services within the Newborn Metabolic Screening Programme in New Zealand*. MOH: Wellington; 2010.
Mitchell EA. Bed sharing and the risk of sudden infant death: parents need clear information. *Curr Pediatr Rev*. 2010;6:63–66.
Mitchell EA, Thompson JM, Zuccollo J, et al. The combination of bed sharing and maternal smoking leads to a greatly increased risk of sudden unexpected death in infancy: the New Zealand SUDI Nationwide Case Control Study. *N Z Med J*. 2017; 130(1456):52–64.
Moore ER, Bergman N, Anderson GC, et al. Early skin-to-skin contact for mothers and their healthy newborn infants. *Cochrane Database Syst Rev*. 2016;(11):CD003519.
Mulupuru S, Siddu A, Murki, S et al. Breast crawl at birth, effect on breastfeeding rate and infant growth in infants delivered at an urban tertiary care public hospital: A randomized controlled trial. *J Neonatal Nurs*. 2019;25(5):236–239. doi:10.1016/j.jnn.2019.04.008.
National Health and Medical Research Council (NHMRC). *Joint Statement and Recommendations on Vitamin K Administration to Newborn Infants to Prevent Vitamin K Deficiencies in Infancy*. Canberra: Commonwealth of Australia; October 2010.
National Screening Unit. Newborn Metabolic Screening Programme (NMSP). *Guidelines for practitioners providing services within the Newborn Metabolic Screening Programme in New Zealand*. 2020. Online: https://www.nsu.govt.nz/pregnancy-newborn-screening/newborn-metabolic-screening-programme-heel-prick-test.
Neonatal Directorate Management Committee. *Jaundice. Clinical practice guideline*. 2011, updated 2017. Online: https://www.kemh.health.wa.au/services/nccu/npw/docs/3_hyperbilirrubinaemia_and_neonatal_jaundice.pdf.
New Zealand College of Midwives (NZCOM). A consensus statement: vitamin K prophylaxis in the newborn. *J N Z Coll Midwives*. 2001;23:33. Updated 2016. Online: https://www.midwife.org.nz/quality-practice/nzcom-consensus-statements.
New Zealand College of Midwives. *Assessment of Anklyglossia:* 2019. Online: http://www.midwife.org.nz/wp-content/uploads/2019/05/Tongue-tie-Ankyloglossia.pdf.
National Guideline Alliance (UK). *Faltering Growth – recognition and management*. London: National Institute for Health and Care Excellence (UK); 2017 September (NICE Guideline, No. 75.) Online: https://www.ncbi.nlm.nih.gov/books/NBK458459/.
NHS. *Guidelines for Newborn Blood Spot*. 2016. Online: https://www.scribd.com/document/327784256/2016-Guidelines-for-Newborn-Blood-Spot-NHS.
McEwan T. Adaptation to extrauterine life 1—respirations and cardiac functions. In: Rankin J, ed. *Physiology in Childbearing with Anatomy and Related Biosciences*. 4th ed. London: Elsevier; 2017a:501–512 [Ch. 48].
McEwan T. Adaptation to extrauterine life 2—gastrointestinal, metabolic, neural and immunological considerations. In: Rankin J, ed. *Physiology in Childbearing with Anatomy and Related Biociences*. 4th ed. London: Elsevier; 2017b:657513–520 [Ch. 49].
Panaretto K, Whitehall J, McBride G, et al. Sudden infant death syndrome in Indigenous and non-Indigenous infants in north Queensland, 1990–1998. *J Paediatr Child Health*. 2002;38(2): 135–139.
Pickard JM, Zeng MY, Caruso R, Núñez G. Gut microbiota: Role in pathogen colonization, immune responses, and inflammatory disease. *Immunol Rev*. 2017;279(1):70–89. doi:10.1111/imr.12567.
Pramanik AK, Rosenkrantz T. *Respiratory Distress Syndrome Medscape*. 2020. Online: https://emedicine.medscape.com/article/976034-overview.
Puckett RM, Offringa M. Prophylactic vitamin K for vitamin K deficiency bleeding in neonates. *Cochrane Database Syst Rev*. 2000;(4):CD002776, doi:10.1002/14651858.CD002776.
Roura LC, Arulkumaran S. Facing the noncommunicable disease (NCD) global epidemic—the battle of prevention starts in utero—the FIGO challenge. *Best Pract Res Clin Obstet Gynaecol*. 2015;29(1):5–14.
Rubin G, Spagnut G, Morandi F, et al. Subcutaneous fat necrosis of the newborn. *Clin Case Rep*. 2015;3(12):1017–1020. doi:10.1002/ccr3.4.
Rutayisire E, Huang K, Liu Y, et al. The mode of delivery affects the diversity and colonization pattern of the gut microbiota during the first year of infants' life: a systematic review. *BMC Gastroenterol*. 2016;16(1):86. doi:10.1186/s12876-016-0498-0. PMID: 27475754; PMCID: PMC4967522.

Sankar MJ, Chandrasekaran A, Kumar P, et al. Vitamin K prophylaxis for prevention of vitamin K deficiency bleeding: a systematic review. *J Perinatol.* 2016;36(suppl 1):S29–35. doi:10.1038/jp.2016.30. PMID: 27109090; PMCID: PMC4862383.

Shaw BA, Segal LS, Section on Orthopedics. Evaluation and referral for developmental dysplasia of the hip in infants. *Pediatrics.* 2016;138(6):e20163107. doi:10.1542/peds.2016-3107.

Shore R. *Rethinking the Brain: New Insights Into Early Development.* New York: Families and Work Institute; 1997.

Siderov J. The newborn eye: visual function and screening for ocular disorders. In: Davies L, MacDonald S, eds. *Examination of the Newborn and Neonatal Health.* London;Elsevier. 2020: 175–184 [Ch. 10].

SIDS and Kids. *Tummy time.* SIDS and Kids; 2017. Online: http://www.sidsandkids.org.nz.

Singh Y, Tissot C. Echocardiographic evaluation of the transitional circulation for the neonatologists. *Front Pediatr.* 2018;6(140).

Starship Hospital. *Back and scalp lesions in the newborn.* 2019. Online: https://www.starship.org.nz/health-professionals/back-and-scalp-lesions-in-the-newborn/.

Tappero EP Honeyfield ME. *Physical Assessment of the Newborn.* Springer; 2019.

Thureen PJ, Deacon J, Hernandez JA, et al, eds. *Assessment and Care of the Well Newborn.* 2nd ed. St Louis: Saunders; 2005.

Tipene-Leach D, Hutchison L, Tangiora A, et al. Sids-related knowledge and infant care practices among Māori mothers. *N Z Med J.* 2010;123(1326):88–96.

Tipene-Leach D, Baddock SA, Williams SM, et al. The Pepi-Pod study: Overnight video, oximetry and thermal environment while using an in-bed sleep device for sudden unexpected death in infancy prevention. *J Paediatr Child Health.* 2018;54(6):638–646.

Trotter D. Neonatal skincare and cord care implications for practice. In: Davies L, MacDonald S, eds. *Examination of the Newborn and Neonatal Health.* London Churchill Livingstone; 2020:230–29 [Ch. 13].

Tuffnell CS, Petersen SA, Wailoo MP. Factors affecting rectal temperature in infancy. *Arch Dis Child.* 1995;73(5):443–446.

Uslu S, Ozdemir H, Bulbul A, et al. A comparison of different methods of temperature measurements in sick newborns. *J Trop Pediatr.* 2011;57:418–23. doi:10.1093/tropej/fmq120.

Verbiest SB, Tully KP, Stuebe AM. *Promoting Maternal and Infant health in the 4th trimester: Zero to Three.* Online: https://beforeandbeyond.org/wp-content/uploads/2017/01/Zero-to-Three-Article-for-Dr.-Verbiest.pdf.

Visser DY, Jansen NJ, IJland MM, et al. Intracranial bleeding due to vitamin K deficiency: advantages of using a pediatric intensive care registry. Intensive Care Med. 2011. 37(6):1014–1020. doi:10.1007/s00134-011-2175-7.

Wen L, Duffy A. Factors influencing the gut microbiota, inflammation, and type 2 diabetes. *J Nutr.* 2017;14 7(7):1468S–1475S. doi:10.3945/jn.116.240754.

Weström B, Arévalo Sureda E, Pierzynowska K, et al. The immature gut barrier and its importance in establishing immunity in newborn mammals. *Front Immunol.* 2020;11:1153. doi:10.3389/fimmu.2020.01153.

Widström AM, Lilja G, Aaltomaa-Michalias P, et al. Newborn behaviour to locate the breast when skin-to-skin: a possible method for enabling early self-regulation. *Acta Paediatr.* 2011;100(1):79–85. doi:10.1111/j.1651-2227.2010.01983.x.

Widström AM, Brimdyr K, Svensson K, et al. Skin-to-skin contact the first hour after birth, underlying implications and clinical practice. *Acta Paediatr.* 2019;108:1192–1204.

World Health Organization. *Optimal Timing of Cord Clamping for the Prevention of Iron Deficiency Anaemia in Infants.* E-library of Evidence for Nutrition Actions (eLENA); 2019. Online: https://www.who.int/elena/titles/cord_clamping/en/.

Young J, Watson K, Craigie L, et al. Uniting cultural practices and safe sleep environments for vulnerable indigenous australian infants. *Aust Nurs Midwifery J.* 2017;24(9):37.

Zurynski Y, Grover CJ, Jalaludin B, et al. Vitamin K deficiency bleeding in Australian infants 1993–2017: an Australian Paediatric Surveillance Unit study. *Arch Dis Child.* 2020;105:433–438.

CHAPTER 32

Protecting, promoting and supporting breastfeeding

Carol Bartle and Elaine Burns

LEARNING OUTCOMES

1. Understand global, Australian and Aotearoa New Zealand initiatives to protect, promote and support breastfeeding
2. Recognise breastfeeding as a public health priority
3. Understand breast anatomy and physiology, mechanics of breastfeeding and infant suckling
4. Understand the composition of breast milk; recognise the nutritive, immunological, health and developmental advantages that breastfeeding and breast milk provide
5. Recognise the social, economic and environmental significance of breastfeeding and factors affecting women's decisions to breastfeed, including influence of families, culture, education/support, psychosocial health, inequity and economic pressures
6. Describe midwifery practices including communication skills, and women-centred respectful interactions, to support lactation and breastfeeding
7. Recognise breastfeeding challenges and describe evidence-based positive interventions to overcome complexity
8. Understand the implications of breastfeeding loss, why provision of information about all aspects of infant feeding is necessary, and implications of increasing use of infant formula (breast milk substitutes).

CHAPTER OVERVIEW

A position statement by the International Confederation of Midwives (ICM, 2005, 2017) highlights breastfeeding as an unequalled way of providing the ideal food for healthy infant growth and development, and an integral part of the reproductive process with important implications for maternal health. This chapter aims to describe breastfeeding from a midwifery standpoint, taking into consideration the social, political and global perspectives which underpin infant feeding. It establishes an evidence-based framework for supporting and assisting women who intend to breastfeed and for protecting and promoting breastfeeding.

KEY TERMS

barriers
breastfeeding self-efficacy
breastfeeding protection
breastfeeding support
breast milk substitutes
enablers
exclusive breastfeeding
lactogenesis
newborn behavioural sequences
oxytocin
prolactin
skin-to-skin
sustainability

INTRODUCTION

Breastfeeding is the optimal way to feed infants. It improves the short- and long-term survival, health and development of infants and children, as well as women's health. It is environmentally sustainable and contributes significantly to human capital development (Horta et al., 2007; Victora et al., 2016). The protection, promotion and support of breastfeeding is a global health priority and the World Health Organization recommend that infants be exclusively breastfed for the first 6 months after birth, with continuation of breastfeeding into the second year of life (and beyond) in combination with age-appropriate complementary foods (WHO, 2003). International, national and local programs and initiatives, such as the Baby-Friendly Hospital Initiative (BFHI), national breastfeeding strategies, breastfeeding support organisations and community peer support programs, alongside some legal or regulatory frameworks, support breastfeeding (McFadden et al., 2017; WHO, 2020a, 2017). Health economic analyses clearly demonstrate the value of supporting breastfeeding and the health and societal costs of not supporting breastfeeding (Pokhrel et al., 2014; Renfrew et al., 2012a; Smith, 2019a; Walters et al., 2019).

Global trends highlight an inverse relationship between increasing infant age and decreased rates of breastfeeding. In Australia and Aotearoa New Zealand, where the majority of women initiate breastfeeding, breastfeeding rates decline significantly by the age of 6 months (Australian Institute of Health and Welfare (AIHW), 2020; Castro et al., 2017; NZBA, 2020a; Public Health Association Australia, 2019). In Australia, the first National Infant Feeding Survey, conducted in 2010, revealed that more than 9 out of 10 women commenced breastfeeding, but by 5 months of age only 1–2 in 10 infants were exclusively breastfed (AIHW, 2011). Australian National Infant Feeding survey data has not been collected since 2010, however, a recent report from the Australian Feeding Infants and Toddler cross-sectional survey (OzFITS, 2021) has revealed a similar breastfeeding initiation rate of 93% and duration of exclusive breastfeeding to five months at 22% (Netting et al., 2022). The 2017–18 Australian Bureau of Statistics data revealed that more infants living in the highest socioeconomic areas were exclusively breastfed to 4 months compared to the lowest socioeconomic areas (AIHW, 2020). The median duration of exclusive breastfeeding in Aotearoa New Zealand was reported as being 4 months in a cohort of infants (n = 6685) enrolled in the Growing Up in New Zealand study (Castro et al., 2017). Exclusive breastfeeding rates for infants at discharge from maternity facilities in Aotearoa New Zealand have fallen since 2019 by 1.71% and in 2020 were reported as being 77.48%. (NZBA, 2020b).

Women's breastfeeding decisions are complex and influenced by self-confidence, self-efficacy, previous breastfeeding experiences, birth experiences, economics, family, culture, and social and professional support (Balogun et al., 2016; McFadden et al., 2017). Many barriers to breastfeeding exist at the societal rather than individual level, creating inequity in infant feeding choices. Because these influences are typically outside the control of many women (Brown, 2018b), women's 'choices' about their feeding methods have been described as an illusion of choice (Young, 2018). The Lancet Breastfeeding Series drew attention to the need for countries to scale up known interventions, policies, programs and supportive systems, from legal and policy directives to social attitudes and healthcare systems, to enable women to breastfeed (Rollins et al., 2016). Influences from a range of settings, including within families and healthcare systems, the availability of maternity leave, economics and workforce factors, supportive child care, community attitudes, and the breast milk substitute industry and marketing practices have been identified as **enablers** or **barriers** (Rollins et al., 2016).

Midwifery care is positively associated with breastfeeding initiation and duration (McFadden et al., 2017; Mortensen et al., 2019). The Global Strategy for Infant and Young Child Feeding (GSIYCF) highlights the evidence-based knowledge and clinical skills needed to support women to initiate and establish breastfeeding and to overcome challenges (WHO, 2003). Midwives can provide evidence-informed, sensitive and relational care, tailored to each breastfeeding journey, to support women to meet their goals for breastfeeding (Blix et al., 2019). From a midwifery perspective, recognising and understanding what influences decisions to initiate, continue or stop breastfeeding is essential (Brown, 2015; Groleau et al., 2013; McFadden et al., 2017). Findings from a cross-sectional survey showed that women want accessible, consistent, non-judgmental support and reassurance about infant feeding regardless of how they feed their babies (Cramer et al., 2021). There is a need to tailor services to support diverse communities to acknowledge traditional and familial practices to reduce breastfeeding inequalities (Cook et al., 2021). Cook et al. (2021) found that confidence and motivation were crucial facilitators of breastfeeding and mothers felt that interventions should seek to reassure and support throughout the whole breastfeeding journey

THE IMPORTANCE OF BREASTFEEDING

In terms of health and wellbeing, research has established the importance of breastfeeding and human milk for infants and mothers (Stuebe, 2009; Victora et al., 2016). The value of **exclusive breastfeeding** for 6 months and continued breastfeeding, in relation to improvements to infant and maternal health, nutritional, immunological, developmental, psychological, social, economic and environmental benefits, is significant (Bartick et al., 2017; American Academy of Pediatrics, 2012). Breastfeeding is also important to women who plan to breastfeed. Ayton et al. (2019) found that cessation of exclusive breastfeeding can be experienced as unexpected and devastating, leaving women with breastfeeding grief which was described as a prolonged sense of loss and failure. Women decide to breastfeed for a range of reasons. In a study by Brown (2016), women highlighted other factors, as well as health, that were important to them such as convenience, low cost, ease and emotional closeness.

Breastfeeding and infant and child health

During the first 6 months of life, the risk of morbidity and mortality due to infectious disease is lower among exclusively breastfed infants compared with partially breastfed infants (Bartick et al., 2017; Victora et al., 2016). Breastfeeding reduces the risk of gastrointestinal infections (Kramer & Kakuma, 2012), diarrhoea (Gribble, 2011) and rotavirus (Prameela & Vijaya, 2012), necrotising enterocolitis (Tudehope, 2013), otitis media (Sabirov et al., 2009), respiratory infections, asthma (Oddy, 2013) and malocclusion (Victora et al., 2016). Exclusive breastfeeding is associated with a reduced rate of childhood and adulthood obesity (Horta et al., 2015; Victora et al., 2016) and is a protective immunological mechanism against diabetes development in later life (Cardwell et al., 2012; Horta et al., 2015). Breastfeeding and breast milk intake are associated with a reduced risk of sudden unexpected death in infancy (SUDI) (Hauck et al., 2011; Taskforce on Sudden Infant Death Syndrome, 2016). Breastfed children show improvements in motor and social development (Michaelsen et al., 2009) as well as in cognitive performance (Victora et al., 2016), compared with non-breastfed children. Breast milk contains long-chain polyunsaturated fatty acids and studies have documented correlation of serum levels of these nutrients with brain growth and development (Huffman et al., 2011). Physical close contact between mother and infant during breastfeeding is considered to provide psychosocial stimulation associated with neurodevelopmental and neurobehavioural benefits (Belfort et al., 2016).

Breastfeeding and women's health

Initiation of breastfeeding after childbirth stimulates **oxytocin** release, which contracts the uterus, hastens involution and reduces the risk of postpartum haemorrhage (Riordan & Wambach, 2009). Breastfeeding prolongs lactational amenorrhoea, reducing fertility and increasing infant spacing, which reduces risks associated with short birth intervals (Kramer & Kakuma, 2012). Improvements to maternal health through breastfeeding are correlated to women's lifetime durations of breastfeeding (Bartick et al., 2017). A meta-analysis of 47 studies found that for each year a woman breastfeeds, the risk of invasive breast cancer is reduced by more than 4% (Collaborative Group on Hormonal Factors in Breast Cancer, 2002).

Longer term maternal health benefits include a risk reduction in development of premenopausal breast cancer (do Carmo et al., 2012), ovarian cancer (Feng et al., 2014; Su et al., 2013), type 2 diabetes (Gunderson et al., 2015; Stuebe, 2009) cardiovascular disease (Schwarz, 2013; Schwarz et al., 2009) and stroke (Jacobson et al., 2018). Lactation also plays a significant role in a woman's long-term metabolic health (Schwarz & Nothnagle, 2015). Postpartum depression risk increases if breastfeeding is not initiated, or if breastfeeding ceases prematurely (Bartick et al., 2017; Ip et al., 2009; Kendall-Tackett, 2007). Research suggests the importance of understanding women's breastfeeding intentions, as the highest risk of postpartum depression was found among women who had planned to breastfeed but found themselves unable to (Borra et al., 2015). This highlights the importance of providing **breastfeeding support** to women who plan to breastfeed and compassionate support for women who intended to breastfeed but did not actually breastfeed.

ANATOMY AND PHYSIOLOGY OF THE BREAST

It is important for midwives to understand the anatomy and physiology of lactation in women. The next section details breast development for breastfeeding and how breast milk is produced.

Breast development

Mammary gland development occurs over the woman's lifespan commencing during the embryonic period. Hormonal changes during puberty and pregnancy influence breast growth and tissue development, changing again with involution following breastfeeding cessation. **Lactogenesis** refers to the breast functioning as a secretory gland to synthesise and secrete breast milk. There are several phases in the development of the mammary gland. These include mammogenesis, lactogenesis stage I (secretory cell development), and lactogenesis stage II (secretory cell activation), lactogenesis III (or galactopoiesis) and involution (Wambach & Watson Genna, 2021).

Mammogenesis

Breast formation (mammogenesis) occurs during embryonic and fetal life commencing in the fourth or fifth week of gestation. After birth the female infant breast continues to develop a ductal structure but this discontinues around the second year. Breast growth and glandular tissue development are next accelerated during puberty under the influence of increased plasma levels of oestrogen, **prolactin** and luteinising, follicle-stimulating and growth hormones (Fig. 32.1). Pubertal growth of breast tissue includes the primary and secondary ducts and development of alveolar buds. The next stage of mammogenesis occurs during pregnancy where maturation of glandular tissue begins shortly after conception. There is steady breast growth during pregnancy due to the proliferation of the alveoli and ductule network. Breast blood supply increases, with blood vessels becoming more visible on the skin's surface (Wambach & Watson Genna, 2021). Early pregnancy breast changes occur under the

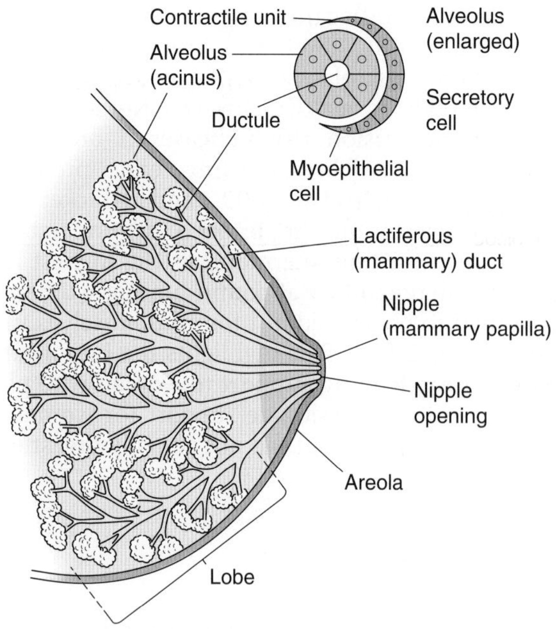

FIGURE 32.1 Structure of the female breast
(Reprinted from World Health Organization (2006), *Infant and Young Child Feeding Counselling: An Integrated Course*, p.19. © WHO)

influence of oestrogen, human placental lactogen (for areolar growth), glucocorticoids, human chorionic gonadotrophin (hCG), insulin, growth hormone, thyroid hormone, progesterone and prolactin (for nipple growth).

During pregnancy mature glandular tissue includes multiple interconnected alveoli each with a central duct surrounded by secretory cells and an external ring of contractile myoepithelial cells. Lobes of duct and multiple alveoli branches can be seen in a network similar to the roots of a tree (Wambach & Watson Genna, 2021). In each breast there are approximately 15–25 lobes containing 10–100 alveoli (Geddes, 2007). Each lobe has a central duct which opens to a nipple opening. The ducts become fuller and increase in diameter after the stimulation of milk ejection. The amount of adipose (or fat) tissue surrounding the lobes is variable between individuals and does not impact on either storage or production capacity of the woman's breast (Wambach & Watson Genna, 2021). The breast receives blood supply mostly from the internal mammary arteries and both the intercostal and thoracic arteries. The areola is the most sensitive part of the breast, followed by the skin and then the nipple. Hair follicles surround the areola. Montgomery tubercles or alveolar glands can be found on the areola and are thought to be 'scent organs' which help guide the infant to the areola (Doucet et al., 2012). During pregnancy the transition to milk production is called lactogenesis and this occurs in three stages.

Lactogenesis I

Lactogenesis represents the commencement of lactation and begins around 16 weeks of pregnancy. The development of the mammary gland accelerates from mid-pregnancy onwards, when circulating levels of progesterone, human placental lactogen and prolactin stimulate continued breast growth as myoepithelial cells of the alveoli mature and differentiate into secretory cells for milk production (secretory differentiation) (Hassiotou & Geddes, 2013) . At this time, colostrum droplets move through the cell membrane of the alveoli and collect within ductules. Pregnant women may notice small amounts of visible colostrum present in the latter stages of pregnancy. Circulating levels of progesterone released by the placenta, in addition to prolactin-inhibiting factor produced by the hypothalamus, prevent full milk secretion during pregnancy (Neville et al., 2001). Although a relatively rare occurrence, lack of breast growth during pregnancy may indicate reduced or impaired glandular tissue function, and this is a risk factor for lactation insufficiency (Arbour & Kessler, 2013).

Lactogenesis II

Lactogenesis II is characterised by increasing milk production and occurs at around days 2 or 3 until day 8 after birth (Wambach & Watson Genna, 2021). Lactogenesis II is stimulated by the rapid drop in progesterone following birth of the placenta, and the presence of prolactin.

Changes during lactogenesis II reflect secretory activation of the mammary gland (Pang & Hartmann, 2007). When progesterone levels drop, tight junctions within the mammary epithelium close which alters the composition of the breast milk from colostrum to transitional milk (Fig. 32.2). Following lactogenesis II, levels of sodium, chloride and protein in breast milk decrease and levels of lactose and milk lipids rise (Ballard & Morrow, 2013). Lactose functions as an osmolyte by drawing water into breast milk, and the rising lactose levels result in increased volume (Mirzaei-Aghsaghali & Fathi, 2012). Compositional changes of breast milk, maternal experience of breast fullness, and increased milk production are markers of successful lactogenesis II. Delayed lactogenesis II is associated with mother–infant separation and

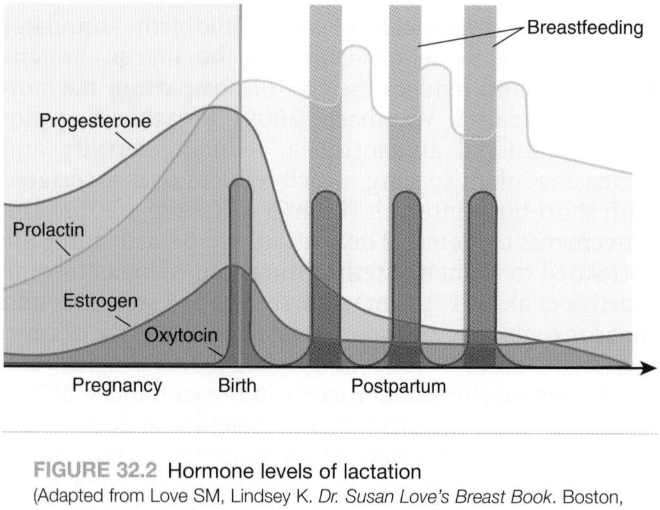

FIGURE 32.2 Hormone levels of lactation
(Adapted from Love SM, Lindsey K. *Dr. Susan Love's Breast Book*. Boston, Mass: Addison-Wesley; 1990.)

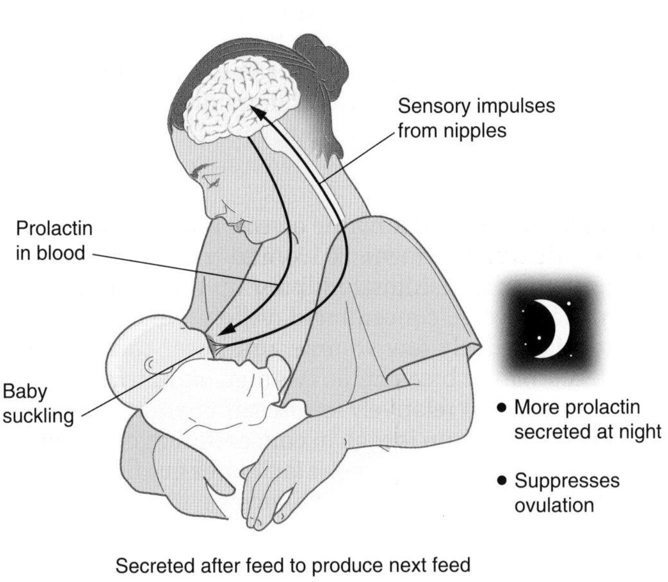

FIGURE 32.3 Prolactin reflex
(Adapted from World Health Organization (2009), *Infant and Young Child Feeding (IYCF): Model Chapter for Textbooks for Medical Students and Allied Health Professionals*, p. 11. Geneva: WHO.)

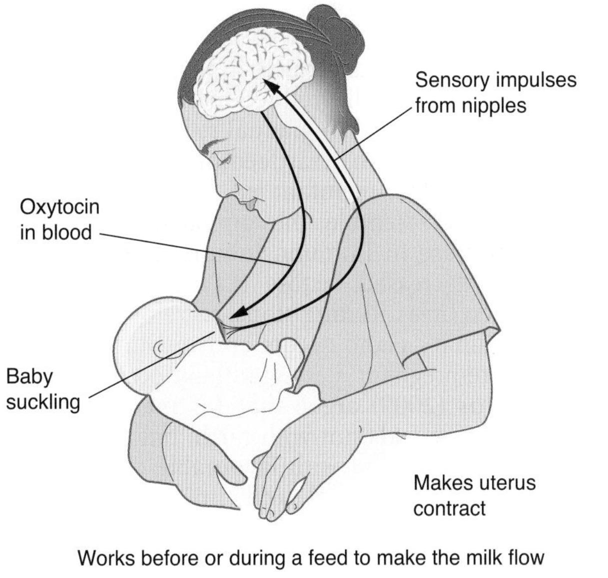

FIGURE 32.4 Oxytocin reflex
(Adapted from World Health Organization (2009), *Infant and Young Child Feeding (IYCF): Model Chapter for Textbooks for Medical Students and Allied Health Professionals*, p. 11. Geneva: WHO.)

maternal obesity. Other factors can include primiparity, prior breast surgery, age over 30, labour/birth factors, diabetes, postpartum haemorrhage, BMI and stress (Wambach & Watson Genna, 2021); Fig. 32.2).

The more often an infant suckles at the breast the more prolactin will be secreted by the anterior pituitary gland (Fig. 32.3). The concentrations in maternal blood stream double in response to infant sucking. Prolactin levels follow a circadian rhythm and are highest at night (Wambach & Watson Genna, 2021). The more often an infant feeds at the breast the higher the prolactin level in the blood stream (Cox et al., 1996). High levels of prolactin can delay ovulation, provided the woman is exclusively breastfeeding including night feeding during the first 5–6 months. Cigarette smoking can suppress prolactin levels as can anxiety and depression (Wambach & Watson Genna, 2021).

It is postulated that the more often the infant breastfeeds in the early days the more prolactin receptor sites develop within lactocyte cells in the alveoli. A higher amount of prolactin receptors is linked to higher breast milk volumes (Zuppa et al., 1988).

The hormone oxytocin is produced in the hypothalamus, stored in the posterior lobe of the pituitary gland, and its release stimulates myoepithelial cells in the alveoli to contract, which facilitates transport of breast milk towards the nipple (Fig. 32.4). Oxytocin is released in response to suckling and triggers the 'milk ejection reflex', also called the 'let-down reflex' (Wambach & Watson Genna, 2021).

Mothers may experience signs indicating an effective neurohormonal pathway during milk ejection reflexes. Although a breastfeeding mother may have numerous milk ejection reflexes during a feed, the initial reflex is the strongest, and newborns may obtain up to 50% of the entire feed volume during this reflex (Prime et al., 2011). Indicators include tingling sensations of the breast before or during suckling, spontaneous flow of milk when the newborn suckles or cries, changes in suckling patterns, and audible swallowing sounds during feeding. Oxytocin stimulates uterine contractions, so some women notice mild to moderate uterine afterpains, or increased lochia during breastfeeds. Oxytocin has important psychological effects associated with enhanced maternal feelings of infant affection. Britton et al. (2006) propose theoretical links between attachment security and breastfeeding, suggesting that women who breastfeed may display enhanced sensitivity and more secure infant attachments. Functional magnetic resonance imaging (fMRI) studies have mapped areas of the brain associated with maternal behaviour, and connections between breastfeeding and greater maternal–infant bonding and empathy have been found (Kim & Unger, 2010).

Lactogenesis III or galactopoiesis

Galactopoiesis marks a shift from endocrine (hormone based) control for breastfeeding to autocrine (at the breast) control. Lactogenesis III production and maintenance of mature breast milk occurs from approximately 2–6 weeks after birth. Although hormonal involvement continues to be influential, the synthesis of mature breast milk is primarily controlled at the breast by repeated milk removal (Wambach & Watson Genna, 2021). Over the first 6 months of lactation, basal prolactin levels decrease, despite daily breast milk production remaining relatively constant, which suggests the reducing control that prolactin has upon milk synthesis in established lactation (Cox et al., 1996).

Involution

If breastfeeding stops or reduces in frequency, peptides in breast milk inhibit cell production and milk-producing epithelial cells die, with a gradual reduction of milk volumes. The reduction in breastfeeding frequency, or weaning, may be mother or infant led. Breast milk produced during weaning resembles the composition of colostrum, with an increase in immunoglobulins, protein and sodium, and decreased lactose (Lawrence & Lawrence, 2011). When breastfeeding stops, secretory deactivation of the mammary gland occurs and involution of breast tissue to pre-pregnant state gradually occurs. Stuebe & Rich-Edwards (2009) argue that for maternal metabolism, pregnancy ends not with birth, but with weaning. Lactation is associated with favourable changes in adiposity, glycaemic control and lipid homeostasis in women, which continue after weaning (Gunderson et al., 2015; Much et al., 2016).

Breast storage capacity

Significant variations in storage capacity exist among women and also to some extent between the left and right breast of the same woman (Daly et al., 1993). Breast storage capacity determines how much milk can be stored in the breast before the shape of prolactin receptor sites is altered. Storage capacity influences the frequency of feedings required to satisfy infant requirements and maintain breast milk production. Women with smaller storage capacities store less milk before breast fullness and distension of prolactin receptor sites occur, and frequent breast drainage is necessary to prevent build-up of FIL and to maintain sufficient milk supplies. Women with larger storage capacities can store more milk before breast distension occurs and may feed less frequently before breast milk production is compromised (Kent et al., 2006). However, it is well established that breast size does not impact whether or not a woman can provide breast milk for her infant (Wambach & Spencer, 2021).

COMPOSITION OF BREAST MILK

Human milk is species-specific and uniquely suited to requirements of human infants. Breast milk is dynamic in nature, and slight compositional variations exist in response to frequency and length of an independent breastfeed, diurnal rhythms, stage of lactation, between mothers, and between populations of mothers (Ballard & Morrow, 2013). Human milk is integral in the developing infant immune system and contains live cells including T-cells, macrophages, lymphocytes, probiotics and immunoglobulins and stem cells and probiotic bacteria (Hassiotou & Geddes, 2013; Spencer & Francis, 2021). The macronutrient components of human milk are protein, lipids and lactose which are synthesised in the alveolar cells of the breasts. Approximately 12% of human milk contains solids (fats, carbohydrates, proteins, vitamins and minerals) and the other 88% is water (Spencer & Francis, 2021). Milk production begins with colostrum, followed by transitional milk and mature breast milk.

Colostrum

Colostrum is produced by the alveoli from 16 weeks gestation (Ballard & Morrow, 2013), and traces of colostrum are present in transitional milk for up to 14 days. Colostrum is a viscous, concentrated, yellow, white or orange liquid of relatively low volume and lower calorific content than mature breast milk. It is high in protein, sodium and minerals but relatively low in carbohydrates, fats and vitamins. Colostrum is high in concentration of immunoglobulin and growth factors, it facilitates gut flora growth and has laxative effects which aids in the excretion of meconium from the gut (Spencer & Francis, 2021). The macrophages, lymphocytes, neutrophils, antibodies and immune cells in colostrum assist in the protection of a newborn's fragile mucous membranes against microbes and viruses, by preventing entry, transport and proliferation (Ballard & Morrow, 2013). Towards the end of pregnancy women may be able to express small amounts of colostrum. During the first 24 hours after birth a full-term uncompromised infant will feed on average 4 or more times, which increases to 8 or more times in the next few days. Within the first 24 hours after birth the amount of colostrum available is approximately 37 mL (range 7–123 mL) (Hartmann, 1987). This increases over the first few days before lactogenesis II commences and the production of transitional milk.

When a mother births prematurely, the composition of her breast milk differs from that of milk for full-term infants. For the first 3 weeks following birth, premature milk reflects more of a colostrum composition and is generally higher in protein, minerals and immunoglobulins (Furber & Thompson, 2008). The specificity of premature breast milk increases immune protection, promotes gut maturation and improves neurodevelopmental outcome in the premature infant (Tudehope, 2013).

Transitional breast milk

Transitional breast milk is produced with the onset of lactogenesis II on day 3-4. Transitional milk shares the immunological characteristics of colostrum combined with the nutritive characteristics of mature milk (Ballard & Morrow, 2013). When compared with the composition of colostrum, transitional milk has higher levels of lactose, carbohydrate and fats. By 5 days after birth the amount of breast milk produced by the woman is approximately 500 mL/day (Cregan, et al., 2002). Women who have not had a baby before produce slightly less milk in the first week than multiparous women who produce approximately 140 mL/day more (Ingram et al., 2001). Factors that can improve the volume of milk produced include unrestricted feeding. Unrestricted breastfeeding in the first month after birth is a strong predictor of adequate milk output for the full duration of breastfeeding (Spencer & Francis, 2021).

Mature breast milk

The breast begins to synthesise mature breast milk from approximately 2 weeks after birth and milk is classified as being fully mature after 4–6 weeks. Mature milk is a rich, balanced fluid containing approximately 90% water and 10% proteins, carbohydrates, fats, vitamins and minerals. It is white/bluish in colour, has a slightly alkaline pH (7.0–7.45) and an average calorie count of between 65 and 70 kcal/100 mL (272 kJ/100 mL) (Spencer & Francis, 2021). The colour of mature breast milk can change depending on diet and consumption of brightly pigmented food. A one-month-old breastfed infant consumes approximately 750–800 mL of breast milk per day. Milk volume of mature milk is approximately 800 mL/day with a range of 550–1150 mL/day (Spencer & Francis, 2021). If milk volume falls below 300 mL/day, milk composition begins to reflect more of a colostrum profile, with increased amounts of protein and sodium and decreased amounts of lactose, calcium and zinc. Geographical location and dietary variations have been highlighted as influencers of compositional and immunological characteristics of mature milk. The caloric content of breast milk increases as the infant matures and can be higher in mothers of male infants than female (Galante et al., 2018). Birth weight does not reflect milk intake but infant weight at 1 month is a strong predictor of milk output (Neville & Oliva-Rasbach, 1987).

Foremilk and hindmilk

Frequency of breastfeeds and breast fullness appear to influence both the protein and the fat content, and these may vary within different ducts of the same breast, potentially reflecting within-breast variations in milk drainage (Murase et al., 2009). Foremilk is the milk ejected at the start of a feed and tends to be slightly lower in fat than the milk at the end of a feed however there is fat in all breast milk (Mizuno et al., 2009). As the infant breastfeeds, increase in fat content is gradual, increasing over time as the breast drains more fully. Despite maternal concerns about foremilk and hindmilk, it is the volume of milk consumed by the infant that determines weight gain. The amount of fat consumed daily by breastfed infants remains stable, independent of length of feed or feeding frequency. If infants are breastfeeding effectively, and feedings are not terminated too soon, they receive about the same amount of milk fat over the course of a day (Mizuno et al., 2009).

Nutritional properties of breast milk

Macronutrients are present in breast milk at a fairly stable level and the mother's dietary intake does not adversely impact this unless the mother is malnourished (Spencer & Francis, 2021). Maternal dietary intake can influence the amount of water-soluble vitamins such as B and C and calcium and copper (Allen & Hampel, 2019). Breast milk contains fats (lipids), carbohydrates (lactose), proteins, vitamins, minerals, immunoglobulins, amino acids and probiotics.

Fats (lipids)

The primary solid component of mature breast milk is the lipid (fat) component that provides 50% of the calorific requirements of infant energy needs. Approximately 98% of breast milk fats are triglycerides, which are broken down into fatty acids and glycerol (Blackburn, 2007). Long-chain polyunsaturated fatty acids, such as docosahexaenoic acid (DHA), are essential for the development of visual acuity and brain development, vitamin function and are essential in the formation of cell membranes and prostaglandins (Gibson & Makrides, 2001). Breast milk lipids help transport vitamins such as A, D, E and K.

Carbohydrates (lactose and oligosaccharides)

Carbohydrate in human milk is mostly lactose, which is a disaccharide made from two monosaccharides glucose and galactose and provides 40%–45% of infant energy requirements (Wambach & Spencer 2021). Carbohydrates enhance calcium absorption, promote growth of lactobacilli in the intestines, and reduce growth of gut pathogens (Spencer & Francis, 2021). Studies have identified unabsorbed lactose in the faeces of breastfed infants, which is thought to be associated with the softer stool consistency, as well as improved absorption of minerals throughout digestion (Han et al., 2011). Lactose will also readily metabolise to galactose and glucose. More than a hundred human milk oligosaccharides (HMOs) have been identified in breast milk and not every woman synthesises the same set of HMOs. HMOs are unconjugated glycans that are unique to human milk and significant to the infant microbiome. These anti-adhesive antimicrobials prevent pathogen attachment to infant mucosal surfaces and lower the risk of viral, bacterial and protozoan parasite infections (Bode, 2012).

Protein

Breast milk protein assists in providing optimal nutrition to breastfed infants, provides defence against infection and facilitates optimal development of important physiological functions. While breast milk proteins provide essential sources of amino acids to rapidly growing infants, they also support digestion and uptake of other essential breast milk nutrients. Approximately 0.8%–0.9% of breast milk is protein composed of whey and casein, which have variable ratios throughout lactation from 90:10 in early lactation, to 80:20 at about 6 weeks, to 50:50 in late lactation (Xiao-Ming, 2008). The breast milk whey:casein ratio is frequently cited within literature as being 60:40, which is an approximation over the entire duration of lactation. Whey is the more dominant constituent and relatively easy for the infant to digest. It contains albumins, enzymes, immunoglobulins and hormones. Whey enhances immune function, provides defence against bacteria, viruses and yeasts, and supports gut development and function (Lönnerdal, 2003). Casein, which is the smaller component, has a soft curd consistency and is less easily digestible. The whey:casein ratio in cow's milk is reversed, with approximately 80% casein and 20% whey (Lawrence & Lawrence, 2011).

Vitamins

Fat-soluble and water-soluble essential vitamins are available in breast milk to support cell growth and function, and are required for blood clotting, central nervous system development and skin integrity, to protect the retinas, and to mediate cell function. The amount of fat-soluble vitamins decreases and water-soluble vitamins increases in human milk as breastfeeding continues. Fat-soluble vitamin availability A, D, E, and K can be impacted by maternal diet (Wambach & Spencer, 2021). Vitamin K will start being made by the neonate after it has had a sufficient amount of breast milk. Supplementation is necessary to prevent haemorrhagic disease in the infant (Medves, 2002). There is a relationship between B group vitamins B_1, B_2, B_5, B_6, B_{12}, and the maternal diet (Kent, 2007) with vitamin B_{12} deficiencies found in breastfed infants if a mother is on a strict vegan diet (Wambach & Spencer, 2021). Vitamin D content of breast milk will depend on maternal vitamin D intake and stores. Vitamin D levels in breast milk are considered insufficient to meet the infant's requirements alone, although there is only limited evidence of significant vitamin D insufficiency in breastfed infants (UNICEF UK Baby Friendly Initiative, 2017). Bagnoli et al. (2013) suggest that supplementation of both mother and infant should be considered when exposure to sunlight is minimal.

Minerals

In the first 6 months of life, human milk contains the essential minerals required for electrolyte balance, and infant cell and organ function. Minerals in human milk are bound to digestible proteins and are also present in complex and ionised states making them readily bioavailable. Colostrum has eight times more zinc than mature milk. The levels of iron in breast milk are low and infants' main source of iron for the first 6 months comes from their own body stores (Greer, 2021). A study of iron deficiency in exclusively breastfed infants conducted by Raj et al. (2008) concluded that the small amounts of iron and lactoferrin in breast milk are readily absorbed. When combined with an infant's own iron stores, adequate levels of iron are maintained in the infant in the first 6 months. Concentrations of iron, zinc and copper decrease during lactation and from 6 months of age it is recommended that complementary foods be introduced to ensure sufficient micronutrient intake (Spencer & Francis, 2021).

Immunoglobulins

Immunoglobulins are proteins that boost immunologic response in the infant. Five immunoglobulins are present in breast milk: IgG, IgA, IgM, IgE and IgD. These antibodies offer protective responses to bacteria and viruses and support the infant's immune response. Secretory IgA in particular has significant immunologic importance for the infant (Spencer & Francis, 2021). Levels of secretory IgA are highest in colostrum (4 mg/mL) compared to mature milk (1 mg/mL) (Bernt & Walker, 2001). Mothers of infants who are unwell have been found to have higher IgA levels in breast milk (Feist et al., 2000).

Probiotics

Human milk contains bacteria including staphylococcus, streptococcus, lactobacillus, pseudomonas, and bifidobacterium in addition to macro and micronutrients (Spencer & Francis, 2021). These are live organisms that can colonise the infant gut and oral mucosa and offer substantial health benefits. Bacteria in breast milk creates a balanced microbiome with high amounts of gut bacteria but low diversity, when compared to infants who are formula fed who have lower amounts of gut bacteria but high diversity. A balanced microbiome leads to a stronger immune system (Gomez-Gallego et al., 2016).

An understanding of the anatomy and physiology of lactation, and the composition of breast milk, as discussed above is essential for midwives. With this knowledge midwives are well positioned to support breastfeeding women through education and supportive language and practices.

MIDWIFERY EDUCATION AND SUPPORT FOR BREASTFEEDING

Support and education during pregnancy

Women make infant feeding decisions before or during pregnancy. This is partially influenced by non-modifiable sociodemographic characteristics such as age, ethnicity, education and economics and by modifiable factors such as knowledge and access to support (Brodribb, 2019). Statistically, women who are older, have tertiary education and higher household incomes are more likely to breastfeed (AIHW, 2011). Factors impacting a woman's decision to breastfeed include whether they were breastfed themselves (Kornides et al., 2013), if their partner is supportive (Odom et al., 2014), if they have female role models who breastfed and if they are in a culture which promotes and supports breastfeeding (Girard et al., 2016; Roll & Cheater, 2016).

Support from healthcare professionals can impact on whether a woman initiates and continues to breastfeed (James et al., 2017). Cochrane review findings from more than 100 trials revealed that any extra support provided to breastfeeding women, by either health professionals or peers, increases the duration of breastfeeding to 6 months and beyond. This was especially effective if delivered in a face-to-face format and if there was a schedule of 4–8 visits (McFadden et al., 2017).

In the midwifery care context, breastfeeding education should occur throughout the continuum of women's childbearing experiences and be tailored to meet individual needs. Discussion should explore women's attitudes, expectations, knowledge and previous experiences of infant feeding during pregnancy, and provide opportunities for women to discuss their feelings in non-judgmental and safe environments. Education should be consistent and follow the updated BFHI Ten Steps to Successful Breastfeeding (UNICEF, 2018; Box 32.1). Recent research has revealed that women prefer to receive antenatal education by non-electronic means and women feel least prepared for breastfeeding and the post-birth period (Wright et al., 2020). Women want more information on what to expect with breastfeeding and strategies to recognise and overcome breastfeeding challenges (Buultjens et al., 2017).

Breastfeeding education during pregnancy should enable parental understanding of the importance of the mother–infant symbiotic relationship during breastfeeding as well as how to initiate breastfeeding, how to maintain milk supply, and how to recognise normal infant-feeding cues and behaviours. Reasons behind the recommendations for exclusive breastfeeding for the first 6 months of the infant's life should be explored during the antenatal period. Written resources and contact details for community breastfeeding support services are important components of formal or informal breastfeeding education activities (Renfrew et al., 2012b). Including partners and other family members in discussions is important, as well as wider familial and social support, because this is associated with increased breastfeeding duration (Brown & Davies, 2014; Mitchell-Box et al., 2013). Emotional support from fathers has been associated with greater breastfeeding initiation (Emmott & Mace, 2015).

Box 32.1 The Ten Steps to Successful Breastfeeding

The Ten Steps summarise a package of policies and procedures that maternity facilities providing maternity and newborn care should implement to support breastfeeding.

Critical management procedures

1.
   a. Comply fully with the International Code of Marketing Breast-milk Substitutes and relevant World Health Assembly resolutions.
   b. Have a written breastfeeding policy that is routinely communicated to all staff and parents.
   c. Establish ongoing monitoring and data-management systems.
2. Ensure that staff have sufficient knowledge, competence and skills to support breastfeeding.

Key clinical practices

3. Discuss the importance and management of breastfeeding with pregnant women and their families.
4. Facilitate immediate and uninterrupted skin-to-skin contact and support mothers to initiate breastfeeding as soon as possible after birth.*
5. Support mothers to initiate and maintain breastfeeding and manage common difficulties.
6. Do not provide breastfed newborns any food or fluids other than breastmilk, unless medically indicated.
7. Enable mothers and their infants to remain together and to practice rooming-in 24 hours a day.
8. Support mothers to recognise and respond to their infants' cues for feeding.
9. Counsel mothers on the use and risks of feeding bottles, teats and pacifiers.
10. Coordinate discharge so that parents and their infants have timely access to ongoing support and care.

* Step 4 has been expanded: 'Place babies in skin-to-skin contact with their mothers immediately following birth for at least an hour. Encourage mothers to recognise when their babies are ready to breastfeed, offering help if needed' (Source: WHO, 2018)

Midwifery support and education after birth

The first 2–6 weeks after birth represents a transitional period which requires additional support from midwives.

The skill of positioning the baby at the breast is not always instinctive to mothers. Breastfeeding is a learned skill developed through appropriate and timely education, observation of others, personal breastfeeding experience, practice and support (Brodribb, 2019). Midwifery support and communication during early breastfeeding establishment has the potential to enhance or hinder the establishment of breastfeeding and the mother–newborn connection.

Women have described breastfeeding support from health professionals along a continuum from disconnected encounters at one end through to authentic presence at the other (Schmied et al., 2011). Detrimental midwifery language and practices include a focus on breastfeeding as the mechanical transfer of nutrition rather than as a relationship between mother and infant (Burns et al., 2013). Negative language used to describe the breastfeeding infant can impact on the mother–infant relationship (Burns et al., 2016). The busy nature of the postnatal ward environment often demands efficiency-driven, task-orientated approaches to care (Hunter et al., 2015). However, this can lead to 'expert clinician', 'hands-on', 'breast-focused' communication (Swerts et al., 2016).

Evidence suggests the importance of self-efficacy to both breastfeeding initiation and duration. Self-efficacy is defined as confidence in the ability to breastfeed. A systematic review and meta-analysis examined the efficacy of an intervention, either educational or psychosocial, on **breastfeeding self-efficacy** and found that women with confidence in their breastfeeding capacity are more likely to breastfeed exclusively for a longer period and that breastfeeding self-efficacy decreases maternal perception of insufficient milk supply (Galipeau et al., 2018).

Relationship-based approaches to breastfeeding support reflect a style of communication that enhances mother–infant connection and supports ongoing breastfeeding. Confidence-enhancing midwifery practices begin with recognising the woman as the expert on her own body and her baby. Midwives who 'tune in' to the mother by getting to know her story, and support her to 'tune in' to her baby by recognising normal newborn signs of hunger or tiredness, effectively support women to be self-determining in decision making about infant feeding (Burns et al., 2013).

CRITICAL THINKING EXERCISE

- Reflect on what relational midwifery care means to you. What language and practices are used by midwives who develop rapport and connection with women in the postnatal period?
- Consider what steps you would take to ensure that the mother–infant relationship is prioritised in the postnatal period.
- Reflect on any negative language used to describe the infant in the postnatal period and consider how to reframe this into positive interpretations of newborn infant behaviour.

This next section highlights the areas of midwifery knowledge and practice that are important for breastfeeding support and the prioritisation of the mother–infant relationship.

Importance of the first 24–48 hours for breastfeeding

Infant-led latching

Education during pregnancy may give the impression that the infant is a passive participant within the breastfeeding relationship, and not take into account the role that neonatal feeding reflexes play in breastfeeding success (Colson et al., 2008). As described by Widström et al. (2011), breastfeeding reflexes are initially depressed following birth. When the infant is placed skin to skin in an upright position, between the mother's breasts, the infant is able to start the 'after-birth journey' towards the breast and transition through the nine distinct behavioural stages. If infants are supported to go through this process while in **skin-to-skin** contact with their mothers, this results in early and optimal self-regulation (Widström et al., 2011). Widström et al. (2011) describe the critical importance of not forcing infants to the breast, and of allowing infants to proceed through the nine steps at their own pace, with infant-led rest periods.

Klaus (1998) describes how newborns are independently able to crawl to their mothers' breasts within the first half to one hour after birth, if placed prone on their mothers' abdomens. This has now been termed the 'breast crawl' (UNICEF, 2007), and demonstrates the sensory, central, motor and neurobehavioural stages involved in baby-led attachment as described by Widström et al. (2011). Propelled by olfactory (smell of the mother), visual (darkness of the areola) and taste (amniotic fluid) signals, infant-led attachment promotes the central, motor and neuroendocrine components that are directly or indirectly involved with supporting effective breastfeeding establishment, and thus species continuation (Henderson, 2011; UNICEF, 2007).

Importance of skin-to-skin

Skin-to-skin contact is when the mother's naked chest and body is in contact with the infant's naked body. A blanket or dry towel is often placed on the baby's back. Ideally skin-to-skin contact begins at birth and should last continually until the end of the first breastfeed (Moore et al., 2012). Step 4 of the Ten Steps to Successful Breastfeeding includes skin-to-skin and it is promoted, encouraged and facilitated to support mother–infant physiology, attachment, bonding and the initiation of breastfeeding after the birth of an infant (Bystrova et al., 2003; Hunt, 2008; Ludington-Hoe et al., 2006). Oxytocin is released into the maternal circulation in response to skin-to-skin contact between mother and infant immediately after birth, and the pulses induced by this contact have been found to be longer lasting than those observed during labour and breastfeeding (Uvnäs-Moberg et al., 2014). Maternal release of oxytocin occurs when sensory nerves in the skin are activated by skin-to-skin contact, touch, warmth and stroking, and also by massage-like hand movements performed by the infant (Uvnäs-Moberg et al., 2014). Skin-to-skin contact with the mother may be particularly useful for infants who are disinterested in breastfeeding, as mother contact can rouse and stimulate sleepy infants to feed (Couread et al., 2006; Doucet et al., 2007) and skin-to-skin contact also has value for older infants with severe latching problems (Svensson et al., 2013). Skin-to-skin contact is initiated at birth, can be continued at any time in the post-birth period, and it may also be continued in the postnatal wards and the home environment. Mother–infant skin-to-skin care supports breastfeeding, with infants in skin-to-skin contact more likely to breastfeed successfully during their first feed (Aghdas et al., 2014; Moore et al., 2012). Skin-to-skin contact with the mother or father leads to a calmer infant who cries less (Brodribb, 2019).

Skin-to-skin contact is just as important for women after caesarean section as it is for women following normal birth. Women want their partner present at the caesarean section and to have their baby in skin-to-skin contact (Frederick et al., 2016). If separated after caesarean section women describe feeling disconnected from their baby and report multiple benefits when health professionals facilitate closeness and skin-to-skin contact with their baby in the operating theatre and recovery ward (Stevens et al., 2019). Some concerns have been expressed about skin-to-skin contact in the context of sudden unexpected postnatal collapse of the infant, although this is a rare occurrence. Safe positioning and observation of the infant during skin-to-skin, particularly when mothers are obese, very fatigued or have been sedated and/or if the infant has required resuscitation, is recommended, with a safe positioning check list suggested (Ludington-Hoe et al., 2014). Ludington-Hoe et al. (2014) also advise that information can be provided to parents and the family so they are aware of how to protect the infant airway during skin-to-skin contact.

The nine infant behavioural stages after birth

The mutual mother–infant early sensitive period includes pre-programmed behaviours for bonding and breastfeeding (Widström et al., 2019). Observational research on infants has established a detailed analysis of the **newborn behavioural sequences** that begin immediately after birth and end with the infant latching at the breast, suckling and then falling asleep (Widström et al., 2011). This work provides significant evidence of the importance of mother–infant skin-to-skin practices and how critical the period of time after birth is, and also demonstrates how easily the infant behavioural sequence can be derailed. Studies of data from four countries indicate that differences in newborn behaviours after birth are very small (Brimdyr et al., 2020). Uninterrupted skin-to-skin contact immediately after birth until after the first breastfeed has finished—at least an hour or more—supports the continuation of the physiological process of labour, birth and placental birth, and helps to restore and support physiological processes for mothers and babies who have had birth interventions. Uninterrupted does not mean unobserved, and midwives can quietly observe the process without interference, unless there is a clinical concern for the baby's wellbeing.

The nine newborn instinctual behavioural phases are: birth cry, relaxation, awakening, activity, resting,

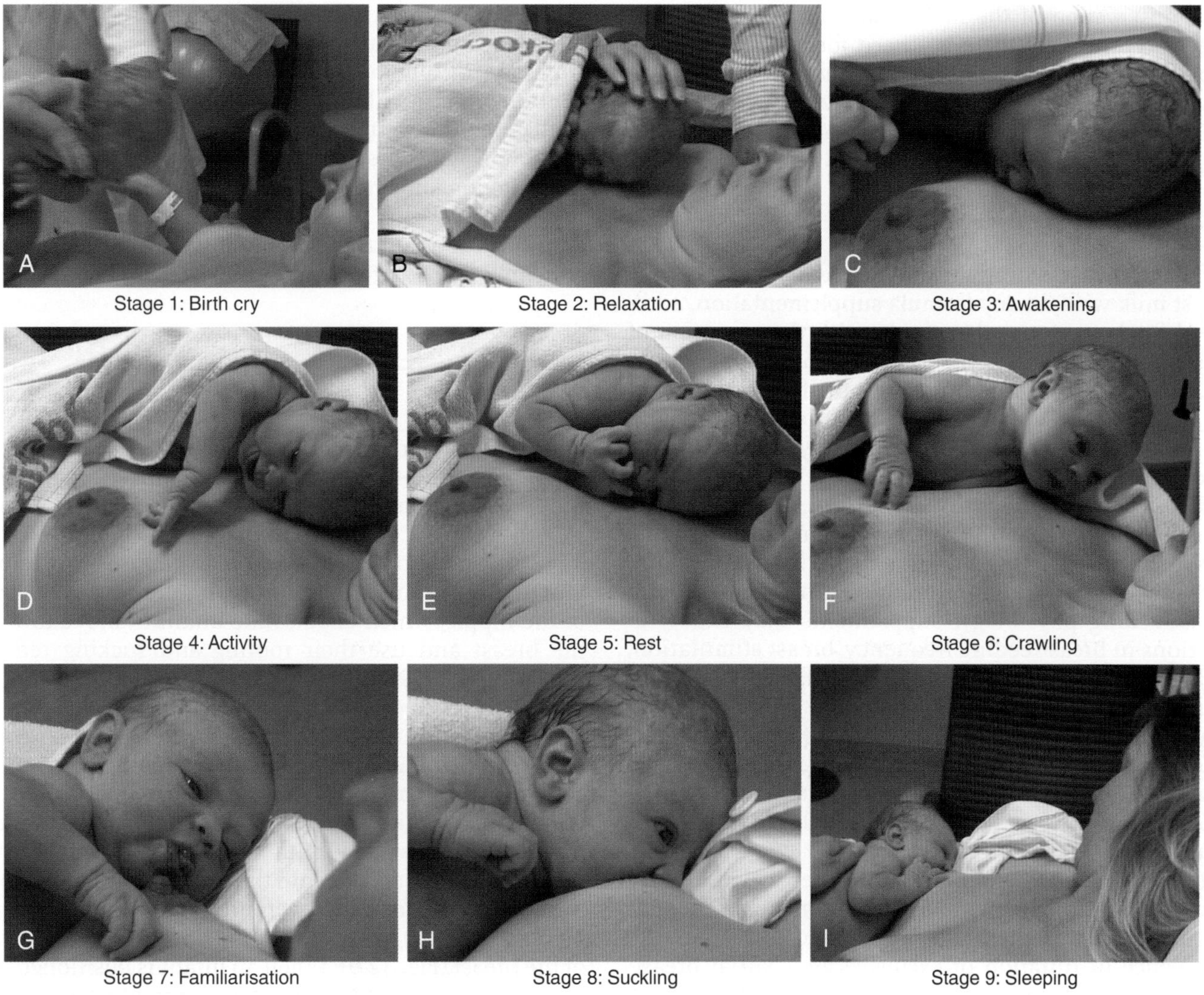

FIGURE 32.5 The nine newborn instinctual behavioural phases
(Dr Kajsa Brimdyr, Healthy Children Project)

crawling, familiarisation, suckling and sleeping (Fig. 32.5). Active stages are interspersed with rest periods, and during the rest/relaxation periods the infant does not demonstrate rooting reflexes. The quiet and inactive pauses are to be expected and need to be protected. If the newborn infant is disturbed during the relaxation periods, this can further delay progress through the nine stages and disrupt latch and suckling (Widström et al., 2019). A plausible hypothesis presented by Widström et al. (2020) proposes that the nine stages are developed and practised by the fetus in utero in the same specific order, indicating that the newborn has been learning this sequence in utero and is primed and prepared for this experience after birth.

Observation of all infants after birth will identify any infant, including those who appear to have had a relatively stress-free birth, who may be slower to coordinate and cue for a feed. Attention to time and space, observation and avoidance of interruption, such as weighing the infant, are recommended at this time (Widström et al., 2019). The priority for the first hour (or longer if necessary) is close observation of the mother and infant as the nine stages occur. Unless there is a need for intervention, the infant should not be removed from the mother's skin to be weighed until after the first breastfeed.

Importance of exclusive breastfeeding

Exclusive breastfeeding means the infant receives only breast milk without any formula supplementation, additional food, water or other fluids, with the exception of prescribed medications, including vitamin supplements. Exclusive breastfeeding throughout the first 6 months of life is associated with a decreased risk of morbidity and mortality compared with partial breastfeeding (Kramer & Kakuma, 2012).

The encouragement of 'infant-led' or 'responsive' breastfeeding enables the supply–demand requirements to synchronise. Giving additional fluids to the infant, such as water or infant formula, can interfere with breastfeeding physiology. Supplements may cause reductions in breastfeeding frequency, breast stimulation, breast milk production and breast milk removal. Supplementation with formula may reduce both the overall health effect of breast milk and breastfeeding (Meyers, 2009) and the overall duration of breastfeeding (Nevo et al., 2007). Supplementation is also associated with a reduction of maternal breastfeeding self-efficacy (Blyth et al., 2002).

Jaafar et al. (2016) found that pacifier use in healthy term breastfeeding infants started from birth, or after lactation is established, did not significantly affect the prevalence or duration of exclusive and partial breastfeeding up to 4 months of age. However, evidence to assess the short-term breastfeeding difficulties faced by mothers and long-term effect of pacifiers on infants' health is lacking. The revised and updated BFHI Ten Steps to Successful Breastfeeding (WHO/UNICEF, 2018) now supports the importance of counselling women on the use of pacifiers rather than completely restricting their use.

Importance of early initiation of breastfeeding

Early initiation and frequent breastfeeding opportunities are essential to support the physiology of lactation. The time after birth is described as a psychophysiological 'sensitive period' where future physiology and behaviour are programmed (Moore et al., 2012). Skin-to-skin contact, for at least an hour, increases breastfeeding and reduces the risk of hypoglycaemia and hypothermia (UNICEF, 2007).

Early initiation of breastfeeding reduces the risk of infection-related infant mortalities and increases the likelihood of exclusive and sustained breastfeeding (Edmond et al., 2007). Colostrum ingestion supports colonisation of the newborn gut, which reduces the infection risk. Unless medically indicated, any midwifery action, intervention or maternal–infant separation should be delayed until after the first breastfeed has occurred. Midwives should delay newborn care procedures such as weighing, examination and vitamin K administration until after the first hour (Sobel et al., 2011). Suckling in the first hour after birth is associated with an increase in bonding and attachment (Widström et al., 1990).

Positioning and latching at the breast

Positioning refers to the position of the infant relative to the position of the mother. It is the interface between the mother–infant body positions, and the infant's mouth-to-breast position, that supports effective latching. Whichever position the woman chooses it is important that the infant is held close, with the nose at the level of the nipple, which enables the infant to move towards the breast and use their rooting and sucking reflexes (Brodribb, 2019). Principles of correct positioning include: a relaxed and comfortable mother with breasts allowed to fall naturally forwards, the infant at the level of the breast (Fig. 32.6). Attachment or latching refers to the bringing of the infant to the breast. The infant's rooting reflex can be stimulated and this triggers the infant's mouth to open widely, with subsequent drawing of the nipple and breast tissue into the infant mouth (Fig. 32.7). The tongue is forward over the gums and under the areola (Fig. 32.8), with the chin placed on the underside of the breast (Fig. 32.9). When an infant is positioned and latched effectively at the breast, the nipple and surrounding breast tissue are drawn into an elongated shape that extends back to the junction of the hard and soft palate

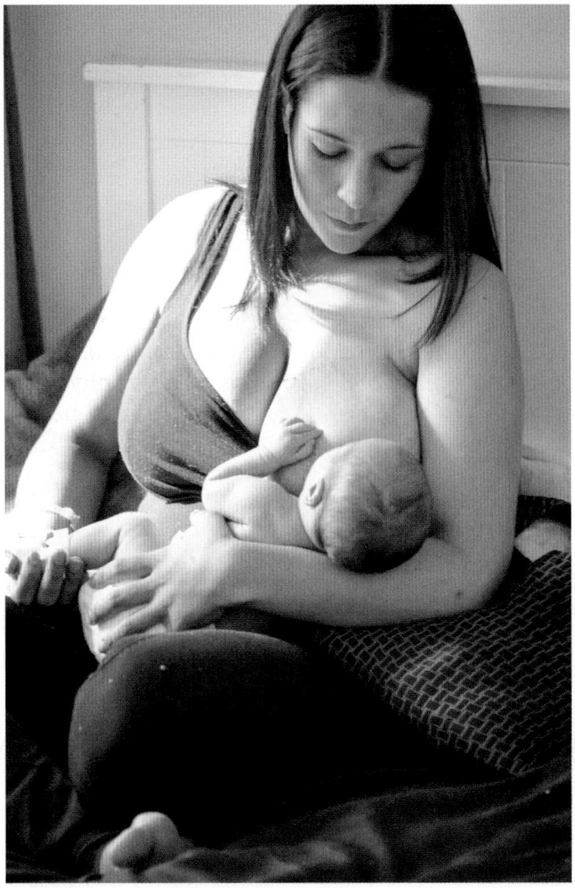

FIGURE 32.6 Mother–infant positioning
(Copyright: Charly Rose Photography)

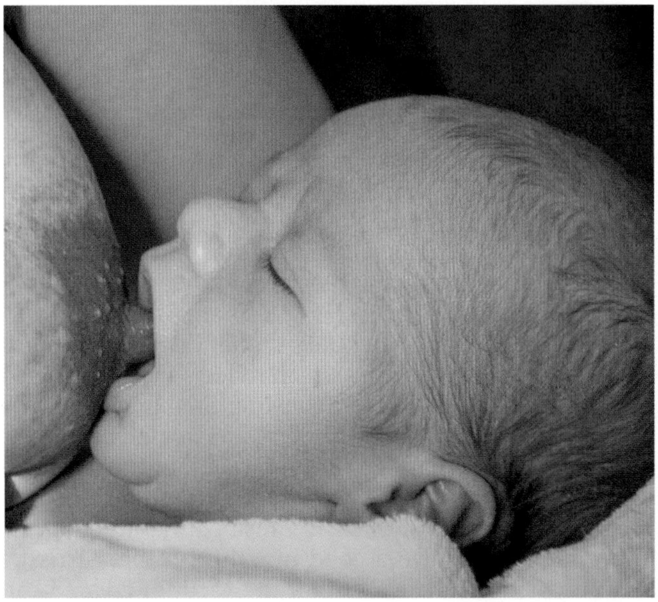

FIGURE 32.7 Wide-open mouth, head slightly extended, chin touching the breast
(Copyright: Charly Rose Photography)

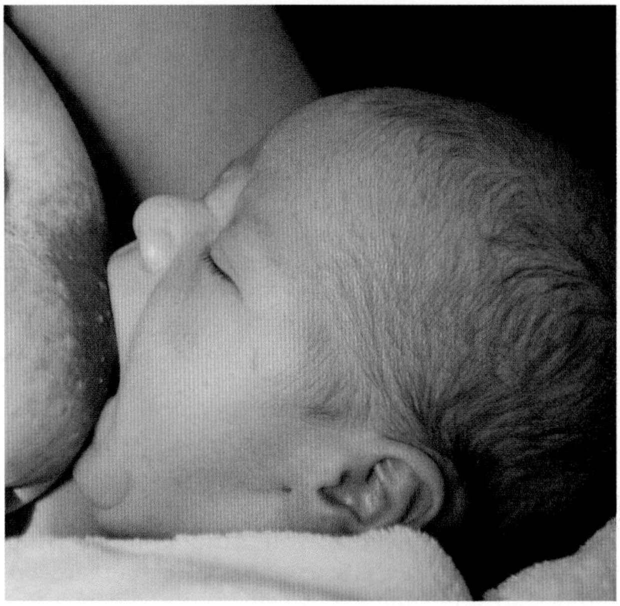

FIGURE 32.8 Anchoring bottom lip onto the areola
(Copyright: Charly Rose Photography)

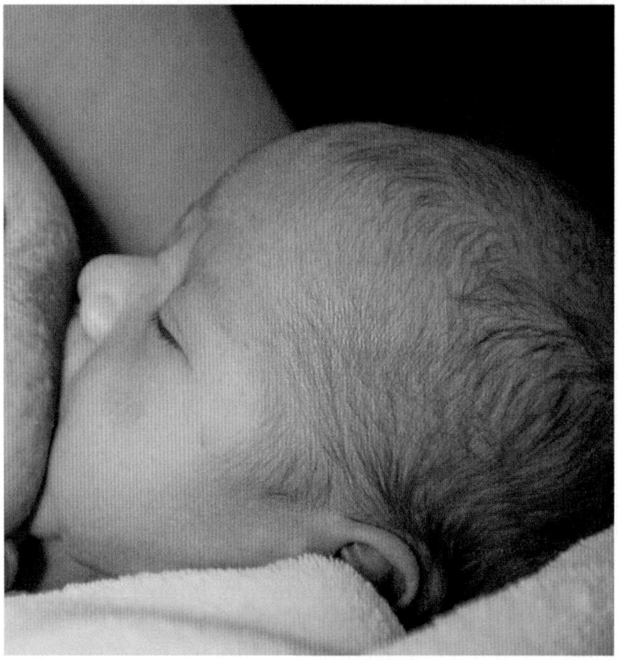

FIGURE 32.9 Infant–breast latching—nose free, chin touching breast
(Copyright: Charly Rose Photography)

(Brodribb, 2019) (Figs 32.10 and 32.11). Correct positioning is associated with breastfeeding success. A frequent reason cited by women for early breastfeeding cessation is nipple pain due to latching problems. The most common reasons for nipple pain include incorrect positioning and attachment, infection, tongue tie, oral anomaly,

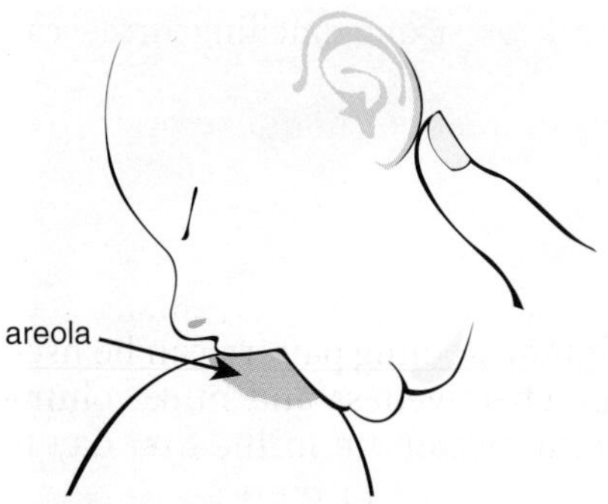

FIGURE 32.10 Correct attachment, external view
(Courtesy of Dr Jack Newman)

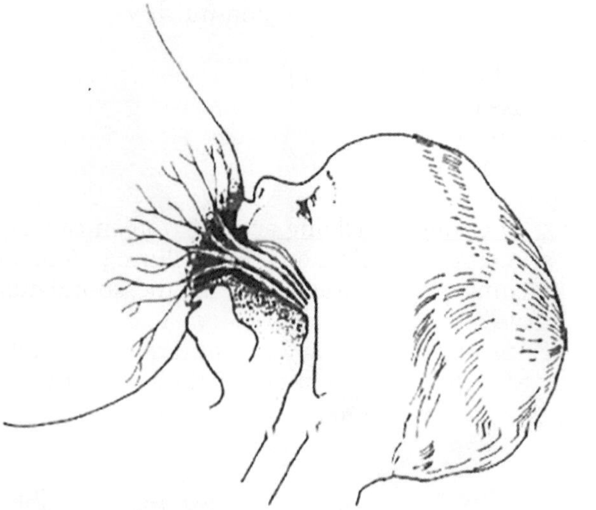

FIGURE 32.11 Correct attachment, internal view
(Source: Infant and Young Child Feeding Counselling: An Integrated Course. Session 3 How Breastfeeding Works. WHO, 2006, p. 19)

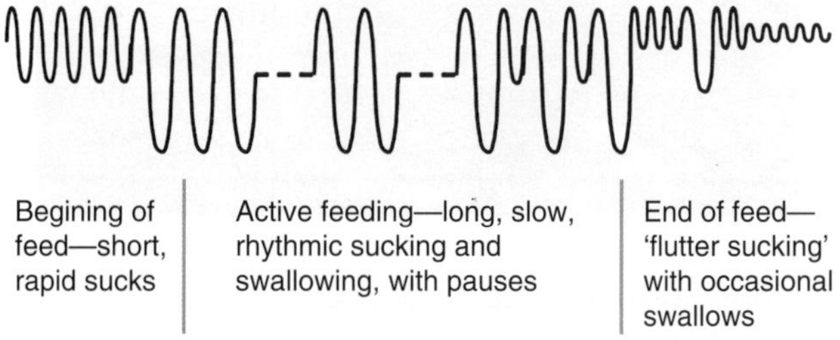

FIGURE 32.12 Suck–swallow pattern of a breastfeed
(Source: UNICEF UK Baby Friendly Initiative, 2011)

flat or inverted nipples, mastitis, and vasospasm (Kent et al., 2015). An alternative approach to standard positioning and attachment strategies promoted in breastfeeding education is biological nurturing (BN) (Colson et al., 2008). When BN is facilitated, the mother adopts a semi-reclined position with the infant placed prone on her chest, and the infant is supported to search for, locate and attach to the breast independently. Midwifery assessment of maternal–infant wellbeing and milk transfer during breastfeeds is an essential component of BN (Colson, 2005).

Responsive breastfeeding

Successful lactation requires a responsive infant-led approach and this is associated with increased breastfeeding duration (Brown & Arnott, 2014). 'Rooming-in' or continuous close maternal–infant contact, with minimal maternal–infant separation from birth, promotes a responsive breastfeeding style and has been associated with increased maternal–infant interactions and improved breastfeeding outcomes (Duma et al., 2013). Successful breastfeeding requires sensitive, reciprocal relationships between mothers and infants, and a responsive feeding approach supports this. Supporting mothers to provide environments sensitive to infants' cues where they can tune in with each other is important (UNICEF UK Baby Friendly Initiative, 2013). Infants who are ready to feed demonstrate feeding cues including visual attention to the mother with eye opening and eye contact, soft vocal sounds, rooting and sucking movements. An infant-led approach to breastfeeding may contradict pre-established parenting beliefs (Pak-Gorstein et al., 2009) and cultural ideology, such as prioritisation of early feeding and sleep routines (Brown & Arnott, 2014). A sensitive approach during discussion with parents supports the exploration and acknowledgment of personal and cultural beliefs regarding infant feeding and care.

Signs breastfeeding is progressing well

One of the most common questions asked of midwives in the early establishment phase of breastfeeding is: 'How can I tell if my baby is getting enough milk?' Supplementation with infant formula and/or breastfeeding cessation can be due to a perception of insufficient milk supply. Yet true insufficient milk supply is experienced by a very small minority of women (Noonan, 2011). Knowledge of the signs that an infant is getting sufficient milk intake can improve maternal confidence with breastfeeding (Kent et al., 2021) (Figs 32.11 and 32.12).

When latching at the breast is effective the infant applies a baseline vacuum, which reflects the seal formed by the mouth, prior to active suckling. Suckling should be free from friction as there is only a small extension of the nipple, once the infant applies the vacuum by the downward movement of the tongue. If the infant has only the nipple in their mouth this will cause pain to the mother. The infant must have a good mouthful of breast tissue and be positioned close so that the vacuum created can be maintained (Brodribb, 2019).

Suck–swallow pattern

When latching is effective a variation in suckling rate and pattern occurs in response to breast milk flow and volume. The first suckles are non-nutritive (stimulating) and are short, shallow, irregular and fast with short pauses, which stimulate a milk ejection reflex and trigger the release of breast milk from the alveoli into the ducts towards the nipple (Mizuno & Ueda, 2006). During a milk ejection reflex the infant's suckling pattern will change to nutritive (receiving milk) suckling, with slower, stronger, regular and longer suckling action. Women can experience numerous milk ejection reflexes during a feed. Effective latching plays a crucial role in the stimulation of breast milk synthesis and transfer of milk. Ineffective positioning and latching can initiate a cascade of negative events such as nipple pain and trauma with subsequent implications for breast milk supply (Graffy & Taylor, 2005). The suck–swallow pattern of a breastfed infant is illustrated in Fig. 32.12.

Unrestricted breastfeeding opportunities enable the infant to feed to individual need, which in turn balances breast milk supply throughout lactation. Every mother–infant breastfeeding dyad is unique, and wide variations in breastfeeding frequency and suckling duration have been identified both between different infants and in the same infant at different chronological stages. Variations in frequency and suckling duration illustrate the corresponding fit between a mother's unique breast anatomy and the similarly unique growth requirements of her infant (Wambach & Watson Genna, 2021). Feeding frequency alone is not a reliable enough indicator of infant milk intake, although mothers may erroneously associate increased feeding frequency as an indicator of low milk supply (Gatti, 2008). During the early months, many infants 'cluster feed', which means that feeding frequency increases over a period of time, typically in the evening (Nevo et al., 2007). Increased feeding clusters may be associated with times of rapid growth and development, which often occur around 2–3 weeks, 6 weeks and 3 months of age (Wilson-Clay & Hoover, 2008), and frequent feeding stimulates a temporary increase in milk production (West & Marasco, 2009).

Infant urine output

Urine output indicates normal renal function, and frequency of urination generally coincides with breast milk volumes at different lactation stages. Normal urine output should include at least one wet nappy in the first 24 hours and at least 2–3 between 24 and 72 hours (Watt & Mead, 2013). During this time, a 'rust-coloured stain' in the nappy may also be seen, which indicates uric acid crystals, or urates—generally considered a non-significant finding at this time (Lauwers & Swisher, 2011). Once lactogenesis II has occurred (around day 3), urination frequency and volume over a 24-hour cycle should increase daily, and by the fifth day a minimum of six to eight wet nappies with clear or pale urine over a 24-hour period is expected. After lactogenesis II, neonatal output is a strong indicator of weight alterations. For example, the newborn who displays an increased output will have increased weight gain, whereas the newborn with decreased urine output will display weight loss (Noel-Weiss et al., 2011). Scant, dark or strong-smelling urine can indicate poor fluid intake and subsequent infant assessment and breastfeeding evaluation should be prioritised (Laing & Wong, 2002).

Infant bowel habits

In the early weeks of breastfeeding, colour, consistency and frequency of the infant stooling pattern can be used to assess breastfeeding effectiveness and milk volume intake. A transition from meconium in the first day to green-brown, less-sticky motions in the second 24–48 hours will indicate the infant is digesting colostrum (den Hertog et al., 2012). Unformed bowel motions that are mustard yellow and may have the appearance of seeds or curds (the less-digestible curd in breast milk) are also a positive indicator of lactogenesis II (Noonan, 2011). Within the first 6 weeks of life, the median number of defecations per day is six (Tuc et al., 2008). Within the first month of life, the breastfeeding infant passes at least one substantial bowel movement every 24-hour period, with less-frequent bowel motions potentially indicating insufficient milk intake and warranting further evaluation (Noonan, 2011). Frequency of bowel motions decreases as the infant matures, which is associated in part with the change in milk composition as lactation is fully established. Wide variations in stool frequency beyond the sixth week of life are considered normal (Tuc et al., 2008).

Infant weight assessment

Weight assessment is often promoted as a reliable indicator of breastfeeding effectiveness, and weight loss patterns are often used as a foundation from which clinical decisions about infant-feeding care plans are made (Noel-Weiss et al., 2011). Noel-Weiss et al. (2011) highlight that some infant weight loss within the first 2 weeks of life is physiological and may not necessarily indicate ineffective breastfeeding. Physiological weight loss can be accounted for by the passage of meconium and loss of stored fluid through evaporation and excretion (Lauwers & Swisher, 2011). The provision of maternal intravenous fluids during labour also appears to influence neonatal output and infant weight loss within the first 24 hours after birth (Noel-Weiss et al., 2011).

Paul et al. (2016) suggest that the majority of newborns take more than a week to achieve birthweight and sometimes weeks longer. Infants who have had a caesarean birth on average take longer to regain their birth weight than those following normal birth. The National Institute for Health and Care Excellence (NICE UK) Faltering Growth Guideline (2017) advise that if infants have lost lose more than 10% of their birth weight in the early days of life, or they have not returned to their birth weight by 3 weeks of age, a referral to paediatric services is warranted, but only if there is evidence of illness, marked weight loss, or failure to respond to feeding support. Some infants, who have had a slow start to breastfeeding but are otherwise well, may take longer to return to birthweight than 14 days (Gonzalez-Viana et al., 2017).

Weight monitoring is only one indicator of the health and wellbeing of an infant (Brodribb, 2019). Noel-Weiss et al. (2011) and Noonan (2011) suggest that the reliance on weight assessments alone may result in midwives missing red flags, and inaccurately differentiating physiological from pathological weight loss. Weight assessment should be considered one assessment strategy incorporated within a holistic breastfeeding evaluation that includes the mother's experience of breast fullness, observing infant breastfeeding behaviour, observing milk transfer, and other indications of adequate infant hydration (Noonan, 2011). Kent et al. (2021) demonstrated that after support from health professionals women were able to identify the signs that their infant was receiving sufficient breast milk. This included waking for feeds, alertness when awake, number of wet nappies, attachment and sucking patterns, and recognising changes in firmness of the breast before and after feeding. Breastfeeding challenges such as delay in transitional milk production or nipple pain can impact on the positive signs that women are looking for. An understanding of breastfeeding challenges and how to overcome them is important for midwives.

Breastfeeding challenges

When the infant is able to effectively latch, suckle and obtain milk from the breast, and when breastfeeding opportunities are unrestricted, the majority of breastfeeding challenges can be prevented. Breastfeeding challenges experienced in the early postpartum period, such as nipple trauma or latching difficulties, are often cited by mothers as a primary reason for the early cessation of breastfeeding (Kent et al., 2015). Early support for challenges is essential to protect breastfeeding and support women to achieve their breastfeeding goals (Stuebe, 2014). Maternal, infant and breastfeeding assessments are essential for diagnosing breastfeeding challenges and identifying all confounding, contributing variables (Stuebe, 2014). When discussing breastfeeding challenges midwives must recognise the emotional impact of any alterations in bodily appearance of the woman's breasts, due to infection, engorgement or trauma, which will impact on her sense of self and her body image. Strategies to support the woman should be evidence based, negotiated with the woman, and documented within a clear plan of care, including follow-up arrangements (Wambach, 2021).

Birth and labour medications

Birth and early postnatal period environments have an impact on breastfeeding initiation and continuation (Brown, 2018a). If an infant has been exposed to labour medications, experienced an induction of labour, long labour, or has been born after an instrumental or caesarean birth, skin-to-skin care and facilitation of the instinctive behavioural sequences may support breastfeeding initiation. Medicated infants may demonstrate longer rest periods and take a longer time during the familiarisation stage. Evidence suggests that intrapartum exposure to the drugs fentanyl and synthetic oxytocin significantly decrease the likelihood of the infant suckling while skin-to-skin with the mother during the first hour after birth (Brimdyr et al., 2019).

Research findings about the effects of epidural anaesthesia and its effects on breastfeeding have been mixed despite evidence which suggests that exposure to fentanyl decreases the likelihood of the infant suckling while skin-to-skin during the first hour after birth (Brimdyr et al., 2015). Epidural medication readily crosses the placenta and fetal blood–brain barrier, and may depress neonatal feeding reflexes, and the half-life of epidural fentanyl in the maternal circulation is 2 to 2.5 hours (French et al., 2016). A systematic review (French et al., 2016) found conflicting research results. Assessing breastfeeding in the first few hours after birth and the use of an objective breastfeeding observation system were included in the recommendations. Epidurals may not have any long-term effects on breastfeeding if women are determined to breastfeed and have good support but may be challenging for women whose breastfeeding intentions are more vulnerable (Montgomery & Hale., 2012).

Research has indicated associations between caesarean births and early breastfeeding cessation (Hobbs et al., 2016). A literature review found that breastfeeding post-caesarean birth was negatively impacted by post-operative pain and a lack of support (Fielder, 2016). Delayed lactation is associated with caesarean birth and also linked to early cessation of breastfeeding (Kelly et al., 2020).

Nipple pain and trauma

Nipple pain, with or without evidence of trauma, is one of the most common breastfeeding challenges that women experience during early breastfeeding and is frequently cited as a reason for early breastfeeding cessation (Kent et al., 2015). Early nipple sensitivity is associated with infant suckling and stretching of nipple collagen fibres, with sensitivity generally lasting one minute and peaking between the third and sixth day postpartum (Morland-Schultz & Hill, 2008). Amir et al. (2015), in a study of 340 primiparous women, found that 79% of women experienced nipple pain and 58% experienced nipple damage. Effective early breastfeeding management is crucial to avoid early weaning (Kent et al., 2015). The most common factor related to nipple pain and/or damage is incorrect latching (Blair et al., 2003). Factors that may interfere with effective latching include ankyloglossia (tongue-tie), disorganised suckling (McClellan et al., 2012) and flat/inverted nipples. Nipple pain or trauma may occur as a consequence of breast engorgement, interstitial oedema, or nipple pathologies such as bacterial, fungal or herpes simplex infections, eczema or Raynaud's phenomenon (Amir et al., 2013). Persistent nipple pain is also described by women whose infants apply abnormally high intraoral pressure during suckling and milk transfer (McClellan et al., 2008). Thorough maternal, infant and breastfeeding assessments should be completed to identify predisposing or contributing factors; strategies should firstly manage nipple damage, but also focus on prevention of further complications (Strong, 2011). Independently achieving pain-free breastfeeding may be an essential strategy in protecting the breastfeeding relationship (Odom et al., 2013). Using an appropriate pain scale with descriptors of pain levels may be useful (Cadwell et al., 2004).

Applying expressed breast milk to the nipples may be equally or more beneficial than the application of ointments such as lanolin in the short-term experience of nipple pain (Dennis et al., 2014). If skin integrity is broken, moist wound-healing principles can be applied, although there is little evidence that nipple creams, ointments or moist dressings either heal damage or relieve pain (Morland-Schultz & Hill, 2008). Most topical nipple ointments do not appear to be associated with adverse effects, however, so the preferences of the individual woman can be supported (Morland-Schultz & Hill, 2008). If nipples appear infected or if healing is prolonged despite effective latching, bacterial or fungal infection should be considered (Amir et al., 2013). If nipple damage is persistent, or if exudate is present, a swab of the nipple wound may determine the causative organism and guide appropriate management strategies.

Breast engorgement

Some degree of breast fullness in the early postnatal period is considered normal and can be described as physiological. Around day 2 to 3 after birth an increased fullness in the breast is welcomed as it signals the commencement of lactogenesis II (Hoover et al., 2021). It can, however, be painful and lead to premature weaning, damaged nipples, mastitis and breast abscess (Mangesi et al., 2010). There is a difference between physiological and pathological engorgement. The former has been described as 'discrete' and as a positive sign of milk 'coming in', with no intervention being necessary apart from supporting effective latching and breastfeeding. Physiological engorgement results from interstitial oedema in the breast, and may be more significant if women have had intravenous fluids during labour (Hoover et al., 2021).

Secondary or pathological engorgement occurs once lactation has been established when the mother's milk synthesis exceeds milk removal. Secondary engorgement, which can occur throughout lactation, is usually due to sudden increase in milk synthesis, lymphatic and/or vascular congestion, or interstitial oedema, and can be triggered by ineffective or insufficient breast milk drainage, compression of breast tissue and/or obstruction of milk ducts (Smriti et al., 2008). Engorgement is often related to mother–infant separation, maternal or infant illness, supplementation or abrupt weaning.

Pathological or secondary engorgement is almost always preventable. With ineffective breast milk drainage and subsequent milk stasis, levels of FIL (feedback inhibitor of lactation) will collect within the milk, suppressing the release of prolactin and breast milk synthesis. Prolonged engorgement will also trigger apoptosis (cell death), which results in the involution of glandular breast tissue leading to milk reabsorption, collapse of alveolar structures, and cessation of milk production (Lawrence & Lawrence, 2011). Overdistension of the alveoli exerts pressure on surrounding breast tissue, exacerbating breast oedema by occluding vascular blood flow and increasing arterial pressure. When this occurs, connective tissue within the breast is compressed and lymphatic drainage is impeded, resulting in further breast oedema due to the build-up of interstitial fluid (Hoover et al., 2021).

Infant latching assessment and observation of a breastfeed should always be completed in situations where a breastfeeding complication occurs. Adequate and frequent milk removal will both prevent and manage engorgement (Berens & Brodribb, 2016). Thoroughly draining one breast as much as possible at each feed or alternating the first breast offered to the baby at the start of a feed may encourage better breast drainage (Smith, 2021).

Although difficulties with latching may not precede engorgement, oedema within the areola and breast may interfere with latching once breast engorgement occurs. If oedema extends into the areola, hand expression of small amounts of milk, or reverse pressure softening, may help. Reverse pressure softening temporarily moves interstitial fluid away from the areolar tissue by applying gentle positive pressure to soften a 2–5-cm area of the areola surrounding the base of the nipple, which temporarily moves some swelling slightly backwards and upwards into the breast (Berens & Brodribb, 2016; Cotterman, 2004). Efficacy of other treatments such as heat or cold therapy, cabbage leaves, ultrasound and analgesia has not been established but, as these interventions pose minimal risk, they can be used as pain relief measures if the mother desires (Mangesi & Dowswell, 2010). Although some interventions including hot/cold packs, acupuncture and cabbage leaves have been found useful, there is still insufficient evidence from trials (Mangesi & Zakarija-Grkovic, 2016).

Blocked milk ducts

A blocked milk duct is often characterised by a palpable, tender, pea-sized lump under the surface of the breast. It is usually composed of fatty plugs or small calcium stones collecting in localised areas of milk stasis owing to ineffective breast emptying (Lawrence & Lawrence, 2011). Blocked milk ducts usually occur without systemic symptoms such as localised redness, significant discomfort, pyrexia, malaise or other flu-like symptoms. Predisposing factors for blocked milk ducts include problems with latching, abrupt alterations to breastfeeding behaviours, copious oversupply of breast milk and engorgement (Campbell, 2006). Supplementation of feeds with bottles, use of pacifiers, inadequate emptying of the breast or skipping a feed can predispose women to a blocked milk duct (Wambach, 2021). Pressure on a part of the breast from clothing or carrying heavy bags that cross and compress the breast, has been implicated in the development of blocked milk ducts (Betzold, 2007).

Management of a blocked milk duct includes improving breastfeeding technique, encouraging unrestricted infant-led feeding, and identifying, eliminating and managing causative factors (Wambach, 2021). Assessment includes observation of a breastfeed and the tender area or lump. Recommendations include changing infant position, feeding from the affected breast first or applying a warm pack before the feed and a cold pack after the feed to reduce inflammation, and massaging the breast during the breastfeed (Brodribb, 2019). Use of hot or cold therapy and analgesics may alleviate maternal discomfort as may expressing under a warm shower. With effective treatment, the majority of blocked ducts resolve within 24–48 hours (Campbell, 2006). Dietary supplementation with the phospholipid emulsifier lecithin may emulsify the fatty blockage and augment breast drainage (Walker, 2009). Results of a retrospective case series suggest the potentially positive impact of the use of therapeutic ultrasound to help reduce blockage within a milk duct (Lavigne & Gleberzon, 2012). When resolution does not occur despite appropriate management strategies, diagnostic ultrasound investigation could be considered to exclude alternative breast pathology (Wambach, 2021).

Breast inflammation/mastitis

Inflammation of the breast, or mastitis, may occur with or without infection and has a variety of aetiologies, and possible presentations, ranging from the relatively benign blocked milk duct to the more invasive breast abscess (Betzold, 2007). Although mastitis can occur at any time during lactation, it is most common during the first 1–3 months postpartum (Amir, 2014; Brodribb, 2019). Women will typically describe a localised area of redness on one breast that is firm and tender. There may also be pyrexia (>38.5 °C), myalgia, malaise and flu-like symptoms if infective mastitis is present (Wambach, 2021). Infective mastitis occurs when bacterial colonisation occurs at the site of inflammation and *Staphylococcus aureus* is the most common organism which enters the breast through damaged nipples and colonises breast milk forced into interstitial tissue. Factors leading to ineffective milk removal, prolonged milk stasis, or supply–demand imbalances that occur in combination with nipple trauma, maternal stress, illness or malnutrition have all been implicated in the aetiology of mastitis (Betzold, 2007). Amir (2014) also adds illness in the mother or the infant, rapid weaning and blocked nipple pores to the list of predisposing factors.

First-line management strategies need to improve breast milk drainage from the affected breast. Frequent and regular breast drainage, by either breastfeeding or manual breast expression, in combination with strategies to improve latching should be encouraged. Management strategies also include reduction of maternal discomfort and breast inflammation with cold compresses, use of anti-inflammatory medication, and adequate rest, balanced nutrition and sufficient fluid intake (Betzold, 2007). Amir (2014) suggests starting breastfeeds on the affected breast, positioning the infant with the chin or nose pointing towards the blocked area to assist with drainage, massaging the breast during the feed with an edible oil or non-toxic lubricant, and expressing breast milk after a feed. Amir (2014) also points out there is no evidence of risk to the infant from continuation of breastfeeding.

Antibiotic therapy is often initiated when women have symptoms of systemic illness, or if symptoms do not improve within 12–24 hours. However, there is insufficient evidence for use of antibiotic therapy for mastitis, and also a need to conduct high-quality double-blinded RCTs to determine whether antibiotics should be used in this common postpartum condition (Jahanfar et al., 2013). The standard antibiotic used for mastitis is a penicillinase-resistant penicillin, or a cephalosporin, for a 6- to 14-day treatment (Jahanfar et al., 2013). Delayed or ineffective treatment of infective mastitis can result in the formation of a breast abscess. A breast abscess, which often presents with similar symptoms to mastitis, is a localised collection of pus within breast tissue (Dener & Inan, 2003), and diagnosis can be made by ultrasound. Treatment includes antibiotics, needle aspiration or surgical drainage of the abscess (Mass, 2004).

Flat or inverted nipples

Nipple inversion can present in two ways: retractile (or umbilicated) nipples, which may be everted by stimulation or manipulation, and invaginated nipples, where the nipple cannot evert. Nipple appearance alone cannot be considered an indicator of breastfeeding success (Wambach, 2021). The degree of inversion may not affect the ability of the infant to grasp the areola tissue and draw the nipple towards the back of the mouth. First-line management strategies could include recommendations to stimulate nipple erection with breast and nipple massage, application of a cold cloth, and brief episodes of hand or manual breast pump expression prior to attempting to breastfeed. If these strategies are successful and latching improves, the degree of inversion is likely to lessen with continued duration of breastfeeding. When first-line management strategies are exhausted, second-line strategies should be considered such as short-term use of silicone nipple shields, or finger, syringe or cup feeding (Wambach, 2021). Nipple shields have been associated with a decreased duration of breastfeeding (Pincombe et al., 2008), although the current body of evidence does not include mixed-method research designs to identify effects on breastfeeding duration (McKechnie & Eglash, 2010). Hanna et al. (2013) suggest that ultra-thin, silicone nipple shields may support mothers to continue breastfeeding who may have otherwise discontinued. Kreemer (2013) notes that compared with other second-line management strategies, nipple shields may facilitate direct breastfeeding and support women to retain a greater degree of control of their breastfeeding experiences. In a review of nipple shield use, Chow et al. (2015) found that the use of a nipple shield can maintain breastfeeding and provide a sense of accomplishment for the mother.

Lactation insufficiency

Lactation insufficiency occurs when the volume of breast milk does not provide sufficient nutrient and/or caloric requirements required for normal infant growth and development. There are two types of lactation insufficiency: primary and secondary. Primary insufficiency may occur when maternal pre-existing medical, anatomical or hormonal pathologies interfere with the normal process of breast development and lactogenesis (Arbour & Kessler, 2013; Hurst, 2007). Secondary insufficiency is more common and results from inappropriate breastfeeding management and/or infant-related problems (Hurst, 2007). A significant percentage of women report low milk supply and cite it as the primary reason for early cessation. Concern regarding milk supply was one of three central mediators of breastfeeding duration in a cohort of Queensland women (Newby & Davies, 2016). Li et al. (2008) found that perception of an unsatisfied infant was cited consistently as one of the top reasons in mothers' decisions to stop breastfeeding. Perception of low milk supply may be triggered by a lack of maternal confidence, misunderstanding of infant breastfeeding behaviours, prolonged periods of infant unsettledness, frequent night waking, or periods of increased feeding frequency (Huang et al., 2009; Otsuka et al., 2008). Galipeau et al. (2017) conducted a study with 123 breastfeeding mothers aimed at determining the relationship between perceived insufficient milk supply (PIMS) and actual insufficient milk supply (AIMS) and found no significant relationship between PIMS and AIMS. Maternal breastfeeding self-efficacy and number of feeds were related to PIMS at week 2, and skin-to-skin contact at birth and number of feeds were related to AIMS as measured by 24-hour milk production at week 2. Interventions aimed at increasing maternal confidence were recommended.

The inability of the breast to produce sufficient milk results from disruption to the glandular and ductal system within the breast and may be unilateral or bilateral depending on the underlying pathology. Maternal pre-existing medical conditions such as diabetes or polycystic ovarian syndrome may alter the hormonal balance required for the mammary tissue development, and may predispose towards mammary hypoplasia (Arbour & Kessler, 2013). If a woman does not experience breast growth and increased vascularisation during pregnancy, and if breasts are widely spaced, asymmetric or tubular in nature, mammary hypoplasia should be considered (Arbour & Kessler, 2013). Conditions such as pregnancy-induced hypertension or preeclampsia (Hurst, 2007), obesity, pre-pregnancy or gestational diabetes (Matias et al., 2014), significant anaemia, retained placental fragments, pituitary insufficiency disorders such as Sheehan's syndrome (Nommsen-Rivers et al., 2012), or gestational ovarian theca lutein cysts (Hoover et al., 2002) may result in delayed lactogenesis II and lactation insufficiency. Previous breast surgery, such as augmentation or reduction, mammoplasty or mastectomy, may compromise breast functionality if glandular tissue or ductal/nerve pathways are severed or disrupted, and are associated with higher incidences of lactation insufficiency (Cruz & Korchin, 2010; Michalopoulos, 2007). A detailed history should be taken when women report previous breast surgery.

Concerns about lactation insufficiency may reflect a social and cultural lack of trust and understanding of breastfeeding, and highlight the importance of tailored, contextual, woman-focused, evidence-based holistic breastfeeding education and support (Huang et al., 2009). A full evaluation of milk supply, breast fullness, infant latching, milk transfer, infant output and weight should be completed when there are concerns about lactation issues (Hurst, 2007).

Therapeutic management should involve improving position and latch, and increasing breast milk synthesis through unrestricted breastfeeding opportunities, mother–infant skin-to-skin contact, breast expression and possibly the use of galactagogues (Hurst, 2007). Morton (2009) and Morton et al. (2009) found that a three-pronged approach using hand expression, breast compression and a breast pump can maximise milk supply, particularly in cases of preterm birth. Infants may require supplementary feeds until the milk supply is providing sufficient nutritional and caloric requirements. The mother's own expressed breast milk (EBM) should be used as a first-line supplement when available, and donor breast milk or infant formula provided when EBM is not available. Depending on the cause of low supply, supplementation may be a temporary or a permanent solution. To support breast stimulation supplementary milk can be given via a supplementary nursing system if possible (Muresan, 2011). Additional breast stimulation with an effective electric breast pump can support the physiological release of prolactin and stimulate breast milk synthesis. As prolactin levels are highest 30 minutes following a breastfeed, expression at this time will stimulate further prolactin release and maximise milk synthesis potential (Hurst, 2007).

Galactagogues may support an increase in milk supply and are frequently recommended for therapeutic management of low milk supply when initial breastfeeding strategies have not been effective. Non-pharmaceutical galactagogues include herbs such as fenugreek, goat's rue, milk thistle, blessed thistle and homeopathic preparations (Academy of Breastfeeding Medicine Protocol Committee, 2011). Pharmaceutical galactagogues, typically domperidone and metoclopramide, are dopamine antagonists, which increase prolactin and stimulate milk synthesis (Lawrence & Lawrence, 2011). Prescribing pharmaceuticals for the purpose of increasing breast milk supply constitutes an 'off-label' use of the medication that raises ethical and professional questions for the individual midwife regarding the appropriateness of prescribing these medications. A cross-sectional study with 1876 respondents in Australia found that galactagogue use was common, with 60% of the breastfeeding women participants using lactation cookies (47%), brewer's yeast (32%) fenugreek (22%) and domperidone (19%). Perceived effectiveness was described as highest for Domperidone although over 23% of these users described experiencing multiple side effects compared to 3% for those taking the herbal remedies (McBride et al., 2021).

In another Australian study decisions to use galactagogues were made following concerns about milk supply and influenced by access to and quality of breastfeeding support, maternal agency and determination to provide breast milk (Zizzo et al., 2021). Individually tailored support is important to manage conflicting information. Evidence gaps about effectiveness and safety of galactagogues were also identified.

Ankyloglossia (tongue tie)

Ankyloglossia is a congenital condition in which the lingual frenulum (the tissue that attaches the tongue to the floor of the mouth) is thickened, tightened and/or shortened, which may restrict or impact on tongue mobility. If tongue mobility is restricted the infant latch is compromised (Hillan, 2008). Degrees of ankyloglossia vary and, while some infants breastfeed successfully, there may be challenges for a small percentage of infants. Poor latching at the breast may result in decreased breast stimulation and milk transfer, which will lead to decreased milk supply and potential infant slow weight gain. When infant tongue movement is compromised the mother may experience painful or damaged nipples, breast pain or mastitis (Edmunds et al., 2011). A careful functional assessment and visual inspection of the infant's oral cavity in addition to a breastfeeding assessment is an important midwifery competency. If clinically indicated a frenotomy, or the surgical release of the lingual frenulum, appears to be successful in decreasing some complications associated with tongue tie, and this may support continued breastfeeding (Edmunds et al., 2011).

The preterm infant: lactation and breastfeeding in neonatal intensive care

When birth occurs prematurely, there are difficulties with initiation, establishment and maintenance of lactation and breastfeeding, with mothers of preterm infants at higher risk of low milk supply and decreased rates of breastfeeding (Tudehope, 2013). The advantages of breast milk provision for the premature infant are compelling (Callen & Pinelli, 2005). Breast milk reduces the incidence of necrotising enterocolitis (NEC) (Herrmann & Carroll, 2014), and in a large prospective trial, breast milk-fed infants developed NEC 6 to 10 times less often than those fed formula exclusively, and 3 times less often if they were fed breast milk and formula (Lucas & Cole, 1990). Breast milk contributes positively to neurodevelopment in preterm infants (Padurara, 2018) and reduces the incidence of late-onset sepsis (Underwood, 2013). Neonatal diet is an important modifiable factor that can affect long-term cognitive outcome by prevention of neonatal infection/NEC. Human milk, mother's own and/or banked donor milk provides this important 'milk factor' protection (Lapidaire et al., 2021).

Palmquist et al. (2020) found that mothers of very-low-birth-weight infants in a NICU experienced physical and emotional trauma that impacted on their lactation experiences. Barriers to breastfeeding, such as infant–mother separation, stress and anxiety, and lack of accommodation close to the infant, are contributing factors to low milk supply and breastfeeding difficulties. Providing expressed breast milk has been described as a way for mothers to be connected to their NICU babies (Sweet, 2008) but Palmquist et al. (2020) found that mothers placed pressures on themselves to make milk so they could feel part of their infant's care. Midwives can provide information and support while recognising the need to acknowledge and mitigate structural barriers in the NICU.

Frequent removal of breast milk is essential to maximise milk synthesis. Women need support to initiate expressing as soon after birth as possible, and 8 to10 expressing episodes in 24 hours, including at least 1 during the night, are usually necessary (Brodribb, 2019). The aim is to establish a high milk yield (>750 mL/day) by the second postpartum week to reflect a normal pattern of lactation establishment (Meier, 2001). Mothers of preterm infants may increase their milk supplies by combining hand expression and breast compression techniques with pumping (Morton, 2009; Morton et al., 2009).

Non-nutritive sucking (NNS), using a pacifier or a parent's clean finger during tube-feeds, can be beneficial to infants in NICU who are partially or non-oral feeding, as it can build positive associations between sucking and sensations of a full stomach while potentially improving oral-motor skills and self-regulation (Nye, 2008; Pineda et al., 2019). Transition to oral feeding should be pleasurable for the infant and parents can learn to interpret their infant's signals for hunger, satiety or stress. Pauses during feeding episodes are necessary if infants are struggling with feeding and showing stress. Meier et al. (2007) found that immaturity, uncoordinated sucking and immature oral–motor tone impact on the ability of the infant to latch, sustain breastfeeds or facilitate milk transfer. Nyqvist (2008) challenged the narrative of immature sucking behaviour and demonstrated that very preterm infants have the capacity for early development of oral motor competence, sufficient for the establishment of full breastfeeding, if provided with early supported opportunities. It is important that immature suckling patterns (short sucking bursts with long pauses) are recognised as successful breastfeeding experiences no matter how short the duration, provided the infant is stable during the feed. Transition to mature sucking patterns occurs gradually at varying postmenstrual ages (Nyqvist, 2013).

Kangaroo-mother-care is critical to support positive long-term breastfeeding rates as well as infant growth and neurodevelopment (Mohammadi et al., 2021; Wang et al., 2021). Renfrew et al. (2010) identified effective interventions to support breastfeeding in NICUs such as kangaroo care skin-to-skin contact, double pumping, peer support for mothers in hospital and the community, multidisciplinary staff training and UNICEF Baby Friendly accreditation of the maternity facility. The Baby Friendly Hospital Initiative's Neo-BFHI has been developed to protect, promote and support breastfeeding in NICUs (Nyqvist et al., 2015; WHO/UNICEF, 2020).

CRITICAL THINKING EXERCISE

What strategies can midwives use to support women with the initiation, establishment and maintenance of lactation when mother–infant separation occurs? What recommendations could be suggested for the following?

- Expressing, safe storage and transport of breast milk
- Skin-to-skin contact/kangaroo mother-care
- Maximising milk production
- Maintaining lactation during maternal–infant separation and limited breastfeeding opportunities

Breastfeeding multiples

Advances in technology to support women experiencing infertility has led to an increase in multiple births (Smith, 2021). Breastfeeding two or more infants is possible and women can produce enough milk to sustain two to five infants (Szucs et al., 2010). The realities of breastfeeding twins or higher-order multiples can be challenging, and mothers of multiples require additional support (Smith, 2021). Midwives who demonstrate confidence in a woman's ability to breastfeed multiples can impact her capacity (Brodribb, 2019). There is a lack of good evidence about the best methods of supporting women who are breastfeeding twins or more (Whitford et al., 2017). The lived experience of women breastfeeding triplets was reported by Leonard (2000), who described the significant intensity that breastfeeding more than one infant creates. Mothers reported being continuously tired, stressed, thirsty, hungry and isolated from adult company (Leonard, 2000). Leonard (2002) recommended that mothers of multiples are provided with enhanced professional breastfeeding guidance. Strategies to promote breastfeeding amongst mothers of multiples should include breastfeeding peer and social support, and preparation discussions during pregnancy (Leonard, 2002).

Mothers of twins may produce twice the volume of milk of singletons, and mothers of triplets can produce more than 3 litres/day once lactation is well established (Brodribb, 2019). However, as twin and higher-order multiple births are often associated with prematurity, small for gestational age, and associated infant morbidities, breastfeeding initiation and establishment can present particular challenges (Smith, 2021). Breastfeeding each twin individually may be easier in the initial stage of breastfeeding when both the mother and infants are learning, or when infants have different sucking abilities, feeding patterns or equipment attached, such as continuous positive airway pressure (CPAP), monitors or intravenous (IV) lines. Breastfeeding both twins at the same time, when manageable, has the advantage of saving time and there is also a physiological advantage in that the more vigorous baby on one side may stimulate the let-down reflex for the other twin (Flidel-Rimon & Shinwell, 2006). Common positions for twin breastfeeding may include a 'double underarm hold' where one infant lies under each of the mother's arms, the 'double cradle hold' where each baby is held in a cradle position with their bodies crossing on the mother's abdomen, or a combination of the two where one baby is underarm and the other is in the cradle position. As long as the principles of correct positioning and attachment are followed, any position that works for the mother should be supported (Brodribb, 2019).

Breastfeeding aversion response (BAR)

The relationship between a breastfeeding mother and her newborn (or child) reflects a shared physically intimate connection that continues for as long as both desire. Challenges can arise which impact the mother–infant (or child) relationship during breastfeeding. One recently described phenomena is breastfeeding aversion response (BAR), which has been investigated by Melissa Morns and colleagues (2022). The phenomenon of BAR has been described by breastfeeding women as an 'involuntary', 'intense', 'overwhelming' and 'uncontrollable' urge to cease breastfeeding during a breastfeed. The triggers have been described as pregnant and/or tandem breastfeeding an older nursling, or feeding around the time of menstruation. Women described feeling conflicted when they wanted to continue breastfeeding for as long as the infant wanted but that the experience of BAR challenged their capacity. Commitment to achieving breastfeeding goals led women to prioritise their breastfeeding relationship over their own discomfort (Morns et al., 2022). More information and research is required to better understand the incidence and phenomenon of BAR and to inform health professional recommendations for women who experience this breastfeeding challenge.

Donor milk and human milk banking

The establishment of human milk banks is one of the most important primary healthcare activities for infants, especially preterm infants (Brodribb, 2019). Pasteurised human milk retains the nutritional and protective immune properties of breast milk and is protective against necrotising enterocolitis in preterm infants (Brodribb, 2019; Hartmann, 2017).

Outside of formal milk banking, women are sharing their milk on a more informal basis and since 2010, when the Canadian donor milk-sharing site 'Eats on Feets' launched, this largely private practice has become more mainstream and public. Walker & Armstrong (2012), the founders of 'Eats on Feets', also developed 'The four pillars of safe breast milk sharing', which is described as a resource for informed breast milk sharing. Gribble (2013), in her survey of peer-to-peer donors and recipients recruited via Facebook, found that one-half of the donors could not donate to milk banks because there were no local banks, or they did not qualify as donors. Other donors viewed the process of donating to milk banks as difficult, or they had philosophical objections to milk banking and an attraction to peer sharing. Critics of the outright condemnation of milk sharing by some health authorities suggest that information should be given to women to enable informed decisions, and to make milk sharing as safe as possible (Akre et al., 2011). The Australian College of Midwives (ACM) position statement on the use of donor milk supports the rights of babies to optimal nutrition, and the rights of women to make informed infant-feeding decisions, which includes using donor milk (ACM, 2014). The New Zealand College of Midwives developed a consensus statement supporting informed decision making regarding ethical and safe human milk sharing practices, and considers that the donation of human milk (as with donations of blood) is a gift rather than a commodity (NZCOM, 2019). The College does not support commercialisation of human milk, or exploitation of women donors for profit (NZCOM, 2019).

Wight et al. (2008) note that processed donor milk retains much of its nutritional and immunological value as opposed to preterm formula, which provides only basic nutrition. Although pasteurisation reduces some bioactivity, there are many significant components that remain extremely valuable for infants particularly within NICU settings (Ewaschuk et al., 2011; Hartmann, 2017; Peila et al., 2016). Pasteurisation of donated milk aims to ensure bacterial removal and virus inactivation while preserving as many bioactive proteins as possible (Hartmann et al., 2007). A study of microbiome analyses indicated that each mother has a unique microbiota (Cacho et al., 2017). This microbiota research indicated that live microbial reestablishment of pasteurised donor milk can be restored with the addition of small volumes of mother's own milk to donor milk samples (Cacho et al., 2017).

Human milk and donor human milk are positively associated with improved absorption and utilisation of nutrients owing to breast milk enzymes, faster gastric emptying, a faster reduction of gastric permeability, stimulation of gastrointestinal growth, motility and maturation, and faster attainment of enteral feeds (Assad et al., 2016; Wight et al., 2008). The protective effect of mothers' own milk, and donor milk, against necrotising enterocolitis and late-onset sepsis in NICU settings has been well documented (Boyd et al., 2007; Schanler, 2014; Wight et al., 2008).

Guidelines which cover recruitment of donors, collection, storage and handling of breast milk, administration and batch tracking, training and competencies of milk bank staff, information for donors, potential donors and parents, and clinical evidence for the use of donor milk and cost-effectiveness have been developed (NICE, 2010). Hartmann et al. (2007) developed best practice guidelines for donor milk banking in Australia. Donors to human milk banks are required to have medical and lifestyle screening, which may include questions about prescription medication, herbal medication, smoking and alcohol consumption, and a range of blood tests including HIV-1 and HIV-2 antibody (anti-HIV-1 and anti-HIV-2), human T-cell lymphotrophic virus 1 and 2 antibody (anti-HTLV-1 and anti-HTLV-2), hepatitis C virus antibody (anti-HCV), hepatitis B surface antigen (HBsAg), hepatitis B core antibody (anti-HBc) and syphilis antibody (Hartmann et al., 2007).

Because the recipients of donor human milk from milk banks are mainly extremely-low-birth-weight, very-low-birth-weight, low-birth-weight and growth-restricted infants (HMBANA, 2009), donors are also required to use strict hygiene methods during collection, storage and transport of their donated milk. Milk banks require a full informed consent process to be undertaken, both for the donor and also for the parents of the recipient infant.

Contraindications to breastfeeding

Medical contraindications—infant

There are a limited number of medical contraindications to breastfeeding. The lack of a particular enzyme in inherited metabolic disorders such as Phenylketonuria can impact exclusive breastfeeding (Brodribb, 2019). The metabolic disorder galactosaemia is a complete contraindication owing to a genetic inability of the body to process galactose. Exposure to galactose results in severe systemic toxicity, which may include multiorgan (liver, kidney, brain) impairment (Page-Goertz & Chevreux, 2021). Breastfeeding is contraindicated for infants with maple syrup urine disease and phenylketonuria, although some breastfeeding is possible under careful monitoring in cases of phenylketonuria (WHO/UNICEF, 2009).

Medical contraindications—maternal

There are very few medical conditions in the mother considered complete contraindications to breastfeeding (Lawrence, 2013). Permanent avoidance of breastfeeding is generally recommended for mothers with HIV infection in developed countries (MOH, 2016; DOH Australia, 2021). HIV infection is considered a contraindication in developing countries only if replacement feeding is acceptable, feasible, affordable, sustainable and safe (AFASS) (WHO/UNICEF, 2009). In some developing countries health authorities recommend breastfeeding for HIV infected mothers who are taking lifelong antiretroviral treatment. This is a weighing up of the lower risk of HIV transmission in mothers on antiretroviral treatment, compared with the increased risk of infant death from malnutrition, diarrhoea and pneumonia if not breastfeeding (World Health Organization, 2021).

The World Health Organization also recommends a temporary interruption of breastfeeding in situations where there is maternal active, untreated tuberculosis (TB), or active herpes simplex lesions on a breast or nipple. Guidelines from the New Zealand Ministry of Health recommend breastfeeding irrespective of a mother's TB status (MOH, 2010). The World Health Organization released guidelines about infant feeding in areas of Zika virus. There are no documented cases of Zika virus being transmitted to infants through breastfeeding and optimal breastfeeding practices are recommended (WHO, 2016a).

Medication

Only a small number of drugs are completely contraindicated when breastfeeding. These include lithium, oral retinoids, iodine, anticancer drugs amiodarone and gold salts (Hotham & Hotham, 2015). Although medications do transfer into human milk to some degree, the amount transferred is usually low and subclinical (Hale & Rowe, 2017). It is rarely necessary for the breastfeeding woman to discontinue breastfeeding (Burkey & Holmes, 2013; Jones, 2013). Hale & Rowe (2017) describe the mechanisms of drug entry into human milk. The amount of medication excreted into milk will depend on a number of kinetic factors; lipid solubility and molecular size of the drug; levels of the medication, and protein binding in the maternal circulation; the oral bioavailability in the infant and mother; and the half-life of the drug in the maternal and infant plasma compartments.

The risks of adverse effects on the infant can be mitigated by taking the medication immediately after breastfeeding. The level of medication in breast milk at the next feed will be very low if the drug is a short-acting medication (Hotham & Hotham, 2015). Drugs which translate to a relative infant dose of greater than 10%, (such as long-acting medications) are contraindicated in breastfeeding women; an example is lithium (Hotham & Hotham, 2015). It has also been reported that infants under 2 months of age are at a greater risk of adverse effects from small amounts of medication in breast milk when compared to infants over 6 months of age (Anderson et al., 2003).

Misuse of drugs should be avoided by breastfeeding women to avoid infant toxicity, and because the mother's ability to care safely for her infant will become compromised when intoxicated. However, maternal substance misuse is not a categorical contraindication to breastfeeding. Although breastfeeding women who smoke are advised to stop smoking, breastfeeding is recommended even if the mother does not stop smoking because breastfeeding offers immune protection for the infant, including a reduction in respiratory illness (Mennella et al., 2007). Alcohol passes freely into breast milk, and regular consumption or binge drinking is inadvisable. The Ministry of Health NZ and the National Health and Medical Research Council, Australia (NHMRC) advise the avoidance of alcohol when breastfeeding (MOH, 2018; NHMRC, 2020). Some breastfeeding women will choose to have an occasional glass of alcohol and it is important to provide information to minimise any potential risks to their breastfeeding infant/child from even small amounts of alcohol. If a woman chooses to drink a glass of alcohol it is important to breastfeed before consuming the alcohol and to wait for at least 2 hours after consuming alcohol before feeding again. It takes on average 2 hours to process one standard glass of alcohol (Hotham & Hotham, 2015).

Information on medication safety in pregnancy and lactation can be accessed from the Drugs and Lactation Database (LactMed), which is also available as a free app for mobile devices. The Australian Breastfeeding Association has a free 'Feed Safe' app available for download on smartphone devices (Australian Breastfeeding Association, 2021). Hale et al. (2007; 2021) have developed lactation risk categories, L1–L5, with L1 being compatible with breastfeeding and L5 hazardous.

CRITICAL THINKING EXERCISE

Consider common medications that may be prescribed or taken during breastfeeding. Identify medications from the following categories and consider what information you would give to a woman concerned about breastfeeding while on medication:

- cold or sinus medication
- antianxiety medications or antidepressants
- antibiotics
- herbal supplements (such as St John's wort, black cohosh or blessed thistle)
- pain medications.

What information could you provide to women about alcohol, nicotine and caffeine?

Considerations for infant feeding when supporting people who identify as (LGBTIQ+)

Midwives aim to be informed about the needs of all women in their care, and also need to be aware of clients who identify as lesbian, gay, bisexual, transgender, intersex and queer (LGBTIQ+), and how to support access to respectful maternity care free from discrimination and abuse. People who identify as LGBTIQ+ may need access to lactation support but can encounter barriers to information and assistance. Barriers to accessing healthcare have been found to include the fear of discrimination and stigma, difficulty disclosing sexual orientation and health professional lack of knowledge (Stewart & O'Reilly, 2017). Obedin-Maliver & Makadon (2016) point out that a positive psychological outcome will depend on the experience someone has from when they first present for care and this depends on the total experience being inclusive and affirming.

Midwifery care is relational, inclusive and respectful, and asking pregnant clients how they wish to be addressed, and how they wish to be referred to, is essential. Both gender-inclusive language and sexed language are important in maternity care. Gribble et al. (2022) discuss the importance of sexed language for effective communication in pregnancy, birth, lactation, breastfeeding, and newborn care, and the potential implications and risks of using desexed language. While it is important to be sensitive to individual needs when providing midwifery care, the avoidance of sexed terms in data collection, childbirth and pregnancy research, and government and organisational policies may be detrimental to the health and wellbeing of women and children.

The International Confederation of Midwives supports the right of all people to receive humanised and inclusive midwifery care regardless of their sexual orientation, gender identity or gender expression (ICM, 2017). A protocol for non-traditional lactation support has been developed by the Academy of Breastfeeding Medicine (ABM) (Ferri et al., 2020).

Breast milk substitutes (infant formula and baby milks)

Although some parents do make the decision to use formula milks, many mixed-feed (breastfeeding/formula) because of breastfeeding challenges and barriers which include lack of timely support and the influence of formula marketing. Formula marketing has a significant effect on breastfeeding decisions, rates and durations, and a direct effect on public and population health outcomes (Baker et al., 2016; Baker et al., 2021; Hastings et al., 2020).

There is no robust evidence to support the addition of novel ingredients in formula such as docosahexaenoic acid (DHA) and arachidonic acid (AA) (Jasani et al., 2017; Verfuerden et al., 2020), although misleading nutrition and health claims are made (Berry & Gribble, 2017; Kent, 2014). There is also little evidence that hydrolysed formula has any role in feeding healthy infants although it has been recommended for the prevention of allergy for about 30 years (Genuneit & Boyle, 2021).

Formula is recommended only until the infant is 1 year of age. Stage 1 products can be used up until 1 year, but follow-on formula marketing causes confusion for parents and has a negative impact on breastfeeding (WHO, 2013). Studies suggest a direct correlation between marketing strategies for follow-on formulae and other formula products, and the perception and subsequent use of these products as **breast milk substitutes** (Berry et al., 2010; WHO, 2013).

Powdered infant milks are not sterile, and best practice reconstitution and preparation instructions are essential. The main organisms of concern are *Salmonella* and *Cronobacter sakazakii* (European Food Safety Authority, 2004). Cronobacter species is linked to sepsis and meningitis in newborn and preterm infants (Silano et al., 2016). Optimal guidelines to reduce risk to infants from bacterial infection recommend the reconstitution of powdered infant formula with water at no less than 70°C, as this temperature effectively destroys these bacteria (Silano et al., 2016; WHO, 2007).

Parents who plan to use formula/bottle-feed need access to clear, up-to-date, non-commercial information about products and bottle-feeding from midwives and/or other health workers, which includes how to prepare feeds safely and the importance of a responsive feeding style which promotes closeness and cue-based feeding for all infants (UNICEF UK Baby Friendly Initiative, 2016). The Ten Steps to Successful Breastfeeding also apply to parents using formula products, and maternity facilities should provide appropriate policies for staff and parents. Skin-to-skin contact after birth, rooming in, staff support, responsive feeding, management of formula feeds and referral to community supports are relevant for parents using formula. Parents express the need for more information but report experiencing barriers to accessing professional support (Appleton et al., 2018). Additional non-judgmental support from health professionals for parents who use formula can be provided in a way that does not undermine breastfeeding.

REFLECTIVE THINKING EXERCISE

- The majority of women initiate breastfeeding following birth, but many discontinue exclusive breastfeeding relatively quickly. Breastfeeding support through peer and community services is associated with increasing breastfeeding duration.
- What resources and/or services are available for breastfeeding women in your community and how are women referred to them?

GLOBAL INITIATIVES TO PROTECT, PROMOTE AND SUPPORT BREASTFEEDING

International policies and initiatives have been established in an endeavour to support women, and to increase rates of breastfeeding initiation, exclusivity and duration globally (Gupta et al., 2019; Hocking et al., 2019; Lubold et al., 2019; Rollins et al., 2016; Walker, 2007; Zakarija-Grković et al., 2020). These include the beginning of the WHO/UNICEF partnership for protecting, promoting and supporting breastfeeding and development of the BFHI. (See Table 32.1 for a summary of global initiatives).

- *Innocenti Declaration (1990/2005)*—WHO/UNICEF and various key health and global policy makers meet in Innocenti, Italy to set targets for the promotion and support of breastfeeding.
- *The Global Strategy for Infant and Young Child Feeding (2003)*—the GSIYCF provides guidance on all aspects of infant and young child feeding and is intended to be a guide for action, identifying the responsibilities and accountability of organisations including governments, health services, health professional and voluntary organisations, employers, educational institutions, child care services and the media.
- *The World Breastfeeding Trends Initiative (WBTi)*—Australia established a WBTi group in 2017 and released the first report in 2018. The WBTi Australia report is the first to explicitly incorporate gender-responsive budgeting approaches and the principles of the WBCi (World Breastfeeding Costing Initiative) tool into the analysis and assessment (WBTi Australia, 2018).

Table 32.1 Global initiatives to protect, promote and support breastfeeding

Title	Organisation and year	Description
International Baby Food Action Network (IBFAN) http://www.ibfan.org/	IBFAN (1979)	Aims to protect, promote and support breastfeeding and optimal infant-feeding practices. Works towards universal and full implementation of the International Code and WHA Resolutions.
The International Code of Marketing of Breast-milk Substitutes https://www.who.int/publications/i/item/9241541601	WHO (1981)	Aim to contribute to the provision of safe and adequate nutrition for infants through the protection and promotion of breastfeeding, and by ensuring the proper use of breast milk substitutes, when necessary, on the basis of adequate information and through appropriate marketing and distribution.
International Code—World Health Assembly Resolutions https://www.who.int/teams/nutrition-and-food-safety/food-and-nutrition-actions-in-health-systems/netcode/code-and-subsequent-resolutions	WHA (1981 and every subsequent 2 years)	Updates the International Code to provide further clarification and guidance particularly regarding new marketing tactics and products.
Protecting, Promoting and Supporting Breastfeeding: The Special Role of Maternity Services https://apps.who.int/iris/handle/10665/39679	WHO/UNICEF 1989	Describes the critical role healthcare services play in the protection, promotion and support of breastfeeding.
The Innocenti Declaration https://waba.org.my/innocentideclaration.htm	WHO/UNICEF (1990, 2005)	Supports exclusive breastfeeding for all infants and recognises the significant infant, maternal, social and economic benefits that are associated with exclusive breastfeeding and longer breastfeeding duration.
The Baby Friendly Health Initiative https://bfhi.org.au/	WHO/UNICEF (1991)	BFHI launched globally following the adoption of the Innocenti Declaration and the Ten Steps to Successful Breastfeeding.
Ten Steps to Successful Breastfeeding https://www.who.int/teams/nutrition-and-food-safety/food-and-nutrition-actions-in-health-systems/ten-steps-to-successful-breastfeeding	WHO/UNICEF (1991, 2018)	Ten steps to increase support for breastfeeding in health facilities.
The Global Strategy for Infant and Young Child Feeding (GSIYCF) https://www.who.int/publications/i/item/9241562218	WHO (2003)	Aims to revitalise attention globally to the impact that feeding practices have on the nutritional status, growth and development, health, and survival of infants and young children.
The World Breastfeeding Trends Initiative (WBTi) https://worldbreastfeedingtrends.org/	WBTi (2004)	Aims to assist countries to assess the status of the implementation of the GSIYCF and is based on the WHO's tool for national assessment of policy and programs on infant and young child feeding.
Global Breastfeeding Collective https://www.globalbreastfeedingcollective.org/	WHO/UNICEF (2017)	Partnership of prominent international agencies calling on donors, policymakers, philanthropists and civil society to increase investment in breastfeeding worldwide.

- *WHO/UNICEF Baby Friendly Hospital Initiative/Ten Steps to Successful Breastfeeding*—baby-friendly maternity facilities aim to support all women to receive unbiased information and support regardless of their feeding method. The initiative incorporates the International Code of Marketing of Breast-milk Substitutes, and provides an audit tool to measure the quality of care provided to new mothers in relation to **breastfeeding protection**, promotion and support. The BFHI documents were reviewed in 2018 and updated guidelines released (WHO, 2018). The Ten Steps to Successful Breastfeeding were revised to reflect evidence-based guidelines and global public health policy (Box 32.1). BFHI Step 2 has moved from a focus on training for healthcare staff to competency verification with sixteen competencies identified as being necessary to implement the Ten Steps to Successful Breastfeeding (Chapin et al., 2021; WHO, 2020b). This change aims to place the responsibility on maternity facilities to ensure that staff have sufficient evidence-based knowledge, competence and skills to support breastfeeding and infant feeding practices (Chapin et al., 2021).

The BFHI in Australia and Aotearoa New Zealand

The BFHI was introduced into Australia in 1993 and has been governed by the Australian College of Midwives since 1995. In 2006 the name was changed to the Baby Friendly Health Initiative in order to better reflect the work of primary healthcare providers in both the hospital and community settings (BFHI Australia, 2020; Walsh et al., 2011).

The New Zealand Breastfeeding Alliance (NZBA) was formed as a non-profit, non-government organisation in 1999 with a primary role of establishing the BFHI in New Zealand. New Zealand legislation requires all maternity facilities to be BFHI-accredited and this is part of maternity service contract obligations. The uniqueness of the health system in Aotearoa New Zealand is reflected by the Treaty of Waitangi principles of protection, participation and partnership being incorporated as an integral part of BFHI, and including the Lead Maternity Carer (LMC) system where the majority of women choose a midwife for their antenatal, birth and postnatal care. The Aotearoa New Zealand documents and the Australian documents are aligned with the 2018 updated Ten Steps to Successful Breastfeeding.

Neo-BFHI

Neo-BFHI is the Baby Friendly Health Initiative for neonatal units and it is based on the Ten Steps to Successful Breastfeeding. There are three guiding principles for Neo-BFHI: 1) staff attitude to the mother must focus on the individual mother and her situation; 2) the facility must provide family-centred care supported by the environment; and 3) the healthcare system must ensure continuity of care—pre-,peri-, postnatal and discharge (Nyqvist, et al., 2012).

CRITICAL THINKING EXERCISE

- At a local maternity facility, determine when, or if, the facility has been BFHI accredited.
- Do the breastfeeding practices observed reflect the Ten Steps?

The International Code of Marketing of Breast-milk Substitutes

In recognition of declining breastfeeding rates globally, which in part are attributed to the unethical, misleading and aggressive marketing and advertising of breast milk substitutes (Kent, 2015; Palmer, 2009; WHO/UNICEF/IBFAN, 2016), the International Code of Marketing of Breast-milk Substitutes was adopted in 1981 (WHO, 1981). This Code is a set of recommendations from the collective membership of the World Health Assembly (WHA). The aim is to contribute to the provision of safe and adequate nutrition for infants through the protection and promotion of breastfeeding, and by ensuring the proper use of breast milk substitutes, when these are necessary, on the basis of adequate information and through appropriate marketing and distribution (WHO, 1981). Subsequent, relevant WHA resolutions ensure the Code stays current and up to date, and together with the 1981 Code their aim is to raise awareness of policy issues on infant and young child feeding at international and national levels. With reference to scope, the Code applies to all breast milk substitutes marketed or represented as either partial or total replacements for breast milk, which may include food and beverages such as infant, follow-on and other milk substitutes or products, cereals, fruit and vegetable mixes, and infant teas or juices (WHO, 1981, 2016b, 2017). It also includes the marketing of infant feeding bottles and teats. Ongoing issues with active and aggressive marketing of breast milk substitutes as a substantial barrier to breastfeeding has been highlighted (McFadden et al., 2016). A survey of 1360 mothers in the UK who were breastfeeding during the COVID-19 national lockdown found that 80% reported contact from formula companies (van Tulleken et al., 2020). Concerns have been expressed that the formula industry was violating the Code and actively exploiting COVID-19 concerns about breastfeeding to increase sales by inappropriately and unethically positioning themselves as sources of public health expertise (van Tulleken, 2020).

The Code calls upon governments to take action appropriate to their social and legislative framework to give effect to the Code's principles and aims. This includes enactment of legislation, regulations or other suitable measures (WHO, 1981). The World Health Organization publish reports about the legal status of Code implementation and the 2020 report highlighted the continued legal shortcomings of implementation in many countries, including Aotearoa New Zealand and Australia who have no legal measures in place (WHO, 2020a). Persistent challenges for countries included the absence of high-level political will, poor accountability, lack of monitoring and enforcement mechanisms, limited understanding of the Code, and insufficient human and financial resources (WHO, 2020a).

The International Code in Australia and Aotearoa New Zealand

Australia's response to the Code is the Marketing in Australia of Infant Formulas (MAIF) Agreement, operating since 1992 as a voluntary and self-regulatory code of conduct agreement between formula suppliers and importers, who agree to become signatories, and overseen by the Department of Health. After the closure of the Advisory Panel on the Marketing in Australia of Infant Formula (APMAIF) in November 2013, a new model was developed, an independent MAIF Complaints Committee was appointed, and since December 2014 this has been operational to review complaints and reported Code violations and to make determinations on potential breaches (Australian Government, 2021). It is important to note that the industry codes of conduct inadequately represent the International Code and ignore the World Health Assembly resolutions. The marketing activities of retailers including pharmacies and supermarkets are outside the scope of the MAIF Agreement as are milk products for toddlers over 12 months of age, baby foods, feeding bottles, teats and dummies (Australian Government, 2019).

Aotearoa New Zealand's initial response to the International Code was to set up a voluntary, self-regulatory implementation and monitoring process in 1997. The Code in New Zealand, a standard reference document, which includes the Code of Practice for Health Workers in New Zealand and the New Zealand Infant Formula Marketers' Association Code of Practice for the Marketing of Infant Formula, was developed later (Ministry of Health, 2007a). Four codes are now included in the New Zealand framework: the Health Workers' Code, the Marketers' Code of Practice (INC Code), and the Code for Advertising of Food and the Food Standards Code (MOH, 2007b). A compliance committee, appointed by the New Zealand Ministry of Health, meets four times a year to make decisions on complaints relating to a breach of either the Health Worker's Code or the INC Code (MOH, 2007c). The complaints-based process operating in Aotearoa New Zealand and Australia relies on public and health worker knowledge of the Code, adequate time to submit a complaint, and time to be actively involved with the industry responses to the report of violations. There is no formal, active or systematic monitoring of formula marketing in Aotearoa New Zealand or Australia. Targeted advertising of formula now dominates the marketing landscape on the internet and within social media platforms. Improved implementation and enforcement of the International Code in every country has been called for urgently (van Tulleken, 2020).

International Baby Food Action Network

The International Baby Food Action Network (IBFAN) was founded in 1979 and is made up of public interest groups working globally to reduce infant and young child morbidity and mortality. IBFAN provides information and guidance about key topics such as infant feeding in emergencies, conflicts of interest, human rights and maternity protection, and Code compliance is also monitored globally by IBFAN and partner organisations (IBFAN, 2018).

CRITICAL THINKING EXERCISE

Reflect on how breast milk substitutes are advertised in your local environment. When you visit the supermarket or see television, internet or magazine advertisements, consider the marketing strategies being used.

- How are formula ingredients promoted to make misleading health and nutrition claims?
- Are there any potential International Code violations and/or Australian and NZ Code violations? How can a violation be reported in Australia or Aotearoa New Zealand?

Breastfeeding policy in Australia and Aotearoa New Zealand

In response to the Innocenti Declaration, the National Health and Medical Research Council (NHMRC) in Australia developed guidelines for health workers to support breastfeeding (Commonwealth Departments of Health and Family Services, 2001). A national breastfeeding strategy was launched to provide a multifaceted primary healthcare approach to breastfeeding promotion, aimed at healthcare professionals, community agencies and the general public (Australian Government Department of Health, 2001). In 2009, the Australian Health Ministers endorsed the updated Australian National Breastfeeding Strategy for 2010–15 (Australian Government Department of Health, 2009), and in 2016 the Australian Health Ministries Advisory Council (AHMAC) set into motion the development of a new enduring strategy for 2017 onwards with a project team and a Breastfeeding Expert Reference Group (AHMAC, 2017). In 2019 an updated Australian Breastfeeding Strategy was launched with a vision statement focused on Australia providing an enabling and empowering environment to protect, promote, support and value breastfeeding as the biological and social norm for infant and young child feeding (Council of Australian Governments, 2019). The Strategy is described as enduring and without an end but reviews of the evidence underpinning the key priority/action areas and strategy evaluation will be undertaken periodically.

In 2002 the Ministry of Health in New Zealand published 'Breastfeeding: A Guide to Action', aimed at improving Māori and Pacific breastfeeding rates, and increasing the breastfeeding rates of all New Zealanders (MOH, 2002). In 2006 a National Transitional Breastfeeding Committee tasked with developing a strategic plan for breastfeeding was established. The Committee developed the National Strategic Plan of Action for Breastfeeding 2008–2012

(MOH, 2009) and then transitioned into the National Breastfeeding Committee, an advisory committee to the MOH. Due to the disestablishment of the committee in 2008 the strategic plan was not updated until late 2020 (Ministry of Health, 2020). 'The National Breastfeeding Strategy for New Zealand Aotearoa | Rautaki Whakamana Whāngote. A roadmap to action: 2020 and beyond', is also described as an enduring document that will be updated regularly. The breastfeeding strategies aim to address barriers to establishing and maintaining breastfeeding to increase population health and wellbeing.

Breastfeeding and infant feeding in emergencies

Climate change and disasters

Infant feeding in emergency plans are designed to safeguard the survival, health, growth and development of infants and young children in disaster situations. The International Confederation of Midwives (ICM) suggests that midwifery education should include knowledge and awareness of the health problems of women and families, both at the time of a disaster and in the mid- to long-term period afterwards (ICM, 2005). Australia and Aotearoa New Zealand both experience a high incidence of disasters and emergencies such as earthquakes, floods and fires. A midwifery consensus statement states that midwives are in a unique position to support breastfeeding and safe infant feeding during times of disaster (NZCOM, 2012). The New Zealand Ministry of Health (2015) produced guidelines for infant feeding in an emergency for emergency management staff which also outlines the roles and responsibilities of organisations and groups, and guidelines for parents and carers of infants have also been developed. Gribble et al. (2019) audited the content of Australian emergency management plans, polices and guidelines and found a lack of planning at all levels for the needs of infants and young children. They concluded that infant and young children were placed at severe health risk and that infant and young child feeding in emergency (IYCF-E) plans need developing. Breastfeeding is particularly critical during emergencies as it protects infants at a time when hygienic conditions are seriously threatened and water supplies are limited and/or unsafe. The circumstances that may have made formula feeding acceptable, feasible, affordable, sustainable and safe (AFASS) no longer exist, and bottle-fed/formula-fed infants are at a significantly increased risk of diarrhoeal diseases, morbidity and mortality (Gribble, 2011; Mother and Child Nutrition, 2016). Gribble & Berry (2011) developed information for emergency preparedness in a 'developed' country context that recognises the different needs of breastfed and formula-fed infants. If lactation needs to be re-established the infant requires alternative nutrition, and where powdered formula is used, care and support for parents should be provided to ensure that risks are reduced. Cups are easier to clean than bottles, and considered more appropriate in emergency situations where infants are not breastfed. It is recommended that donated or subsidised supplies of breast milk substitutes, bottles and teats be avoided in emergency situations, and that any supplies arriving in disaster zones should be placed under the control of a single designated agency (IFE Core Group et al., 2007). To protect breastfeeding, it is recommended that formula for use by non-breastfed infants should be purchased and distributed only to families who need it.

Pandemics: COVID-19 and infant feeding

On 11 March 2020, the Director General of the World Health Organization, Dr Tedros Adhanom Ghebreyesus, declared the coronavirus pandemic (COVID-19). The government and public health population responses, interventions and restrictions to contain the spread of the virus, resulted in some significant changes to health and maternity services globally. Countries made policy decisions to try and reduce transmission and to 'flatten the curve' of infections with varying effects on infection rates, inequity and population experiences. The International Confederation of Midwives expressed concerns that the human rights of women, their babies and their midwives were being violated by the introduction, in many countries, of inappropriate protocols for management of pregnancy, birth and postnatal care in response to the COVID-19 pandemic (ICM, 2020).

There have been no documented cases of vertical transmission of coronaviruses via human milk and, 'the ever accumulating evidence overwhelmingly indicates that human milk itself is safe and not a vector for viral transmission' (Spatz et al., 2021). Initial discussion about using the precautionary principle of separating mothers and infants, and avoiding breastfeeding, were rapidly challenged as being without sound evidence and ignoring the importance of breastfeeding (Davanzo et al., 2020). The World Health Organization recommended that infants and mothers with suspected or confirmed COVID-19 infections should not be separated, and should continue to have skin-to-skin contact after birth, breastfeed, and room-in within maternity facilities, while practising strict hygienic precautions (WHO, 2020c). Breastfeeding recommendations in some countries did not support breastfeeding and suggested separation of mothers and infants. Stuebe (2020) suggested that while the aim of recommendations to separate mothers and infants was to minimise the risk of viral transmission, the negative impacts of separation and potential loss of breastfeeding were 'additional considerations', and 'first do no harm' was a primary concern. The risk of maternal SARS-CoV-2 transmission needs to be weighed against undermining breastfeeding and the protection skin-to-skin contact, maternal proximity, and breastfeeding affords infants (Gribble et al., 2020). Tomori et al. (2020) highlighted the damage that can be caused by separation of mother and infant including disruption of breastfeeding and limiting its protection against infectious diseases.

The COVID-19 pandemic presented challenges for human milk banking. In terms of the use of donor human milk from a milk bank, research evidence from the COVID-19 pandemic has found that the virus is inactivated by pasteurisation (Shenker, 2020). The pandemic exposed a range of vulnerabilities in donor milk service provision and emergency preparedness. Milk banks faced the logistical challenges of adequate staffing, donor recruitment problems, safe handling and transportation of donor milk issues, alongside an increased demand for donor milk as a result of mothers and infants being separated (Shenker, 2020). Adapting milk bank operations to meet the needs of the pandemic and to sustain supply in the long term is necessary (Olonan-Jusi et al., 2021).

In terms of COVID-19 vaccinations for women who are breastfeeding, the vaccination is considered to be compatible with breastfeeding (Davanzo et al., 2021; RANZCOG et al., 2021) and there has been some research evidence showing SARS-CoV-2 antibodies have been detected in breast milk after vaccination (Baird et al., 2021; Perl et al., 2021).

Infant feeding, sustainability and climate change

The impact of infant-feeding decisions, not only on maternal and infant health, but also on the environment is a growing concern and formula usage adds to the existing climate change burden and increased carbon footprint (Dadhich et al., 2015). It is important to recognise that formula milk production is a source of greenhouse gas emissions, while breastfeeding generates no carbon footprint of its own (Dadhich et al., 2015). The environmental impact of formula production encompasses ingredient sourcing, processing, production, packaging, transportation, product use, disposal of feeding paraphernalia and environmental degradation. Intensification of dairy farming has a significant negative impact on the environment, causing degradation and water pollution (Foote & Joy, 2014). Smith (2019b) suggests that the environmental and health harms of increased formula use, combined with economic evidence, highlight the need for a strong public health response. Green Feeding is a term created to describe climate action from birth and it encompasses optimal and sustainable breastfeeding and complementary feeding for infants and young children (International Baby Food Action Network (IBFAN), GIFA, WBTi, 2019). Caution about the way breastfeeding and climate change messages are communicated is recommended to avoid directing messages at individual women (Shenker & Brown, 2019).

Conclusion

This chapter provides a broad overview of topics related to breastfeeding and reflects on ways that midwives can support breastfeeding. When midwives work with breastfeeding women and incorporate tailored, evidence-based, proactive, holistic care into practice, they are protecting, promoting and supporting breastfeeding. The science supporting breastfeeding is strong and evidence-based, but the key issues for the majority of women making decisions about infant feeding are related not to a misunderstanding or lack of knowledge about the importance of breastfeeding, but to the barriers to breastfeeding that they have to navigate. Support for breastfeeding requires not only a broad understanding of breastfeeding, but also recognition of the barriers to breastfeeding that many women may face, and an understanding of the need to provide accurate, contextual and unbiased information about breastfeeding and all aspects of infant feeding, including bottle-feeding and the safe usage and preparation of breast milk substitutes.

Review questions

1. In the context of health and emotional wellbeing, why is breastfeeding so important?
2. What are the main nutritional and immunological components of colostrum, transitional milk and mature milk?
3. Explain the different ways in which breast milk synthesis is regulated.
4. Describe the BFHI and the Ten Steps to Successful Breastfeeding.
5. How can midwives assist new mothers to initiate breastfeeding after birth?
6. What common clinical challenges might a breastfeeding woman experience and what can midwives recommend to support resolution?
7. How can mothers be supported to initiate and maintain lactation when separated from their infants?
8. What are the wider social, economic and environmental considerations associated with infant feeding?
9. What is the role of the midwife in protecting, promoting and supporting breastfeeding?
10. How can midwives support families who are bottle-feeding and using infant formula?

Acknowledgements

The authors would like to acknowledge the work of Erin Mandino, who contributed to the previous edition of this text.

Online resources

Australian Breastfeeding Association: http://www.breastfeeding.asn.au/.
Australian Breastfeeding Association. Breastfeeding, chest feeding and human milk feeding 2021: https://shop.breastfeeding.asn.au/.
Australian Government Department of Health. Australian National Breastfeeding Strategy collection: http://www.health.gov.au/breastfeeding.
Baby Friendly Health Initiative Australia: https://bfhi.org.au/.
BFHI Australia Maternity Facility Handbook: https://bfhi.org.au/wp-content/uploads/2020/03/BFHI-Handbook-Maternity-Facilities-2020.pdf.
Biological Nurturing: http://www.biologicalnurturing.com/.
Breastfeeding and Medication UK. https://breastfeeding-and-medication.co.uk/category/fact-sheet.
Breastfeeding Network Drug Factsheets: https://www.breastfeedingnetwork.org.uk/drugs-factsheets/.
First Steps Nutrition: https://www.firststepsnutrition.org/.
Hale Infant Risk Center: http://www.infantrisk.com/.
International Breastfeeding Journal: http://www.international-breastfeedingjournal.com/.
International Lactation Consultant Association: http://www.ilca.org/home.
LactMed, Drugs and Lactation database: https://www.ncbi.nlm.nih.gov/books/NBK501922/.
La Leche League (NZ): http://www.lalecheleague.org.nz/.
Ministry of Health (NZ): https://www.health.govt.nz/our-work/life-stages/breastfeeding.
Ministry of Health (NZ) National Breastfeeding Strategy: https://www.health.govt.nz/our-work/life-stages/breastfeeding/national-breastfeeding-strategy-new-zealand-aotearoa-rautaki-whakamana-whangote.
New Zealand Breastfeeding Alliance (Baby Friendly NZ): https://www.babyfriendly.org.nz/.
UNICEF UK Baby Friendly Initiative: https://www.unicef.org.uk/babyfriendly/.
World Alliance for Breastfeeding Action (WABA): http://waba.org.my/.
World Health Organization. Infant Nutrition: https://www.who.int/health-topics/infant-nutrition#tab=tab_1.

References

Academy of Breastfeeding Medicine Protocol Committee. Clinical protocol #9: Use of galactagogues in initiating or augmenting the rate of maternal milk secretion. *Breastfeed Med.* 2011;6(1):41–49.

Aghdas K, Talat K, Sepideh B. Effect of immediate and continuous mother-infant skin-to-skin contact on breastfeeding self-efficacy of primiparous women: a randomised control trial. *Women Birth.* 2014;27(1):37–40.

Akre JE, Gribble KD, Minchin M. Milk sharing: from private practice to public pursuit. *Int Breastfeed J.* 2011;6:8. doi:10.1186/1746-4358-6-8.

Allen LH, Hampel D. Water-soluble vitamins in human milk factors affecting their concentration and their physiological significance. In: Donovan S, German JB, Lonnerdal, B et al. *Human Milk: Composition, Clinical Benefits and Future Opportunities* (Vol. 90, pp. 69–81). Lausanne: Karger Publishers; 2019.

American Academy of Pediatrics. Section on breastfeeding. Breastfeeding and the use of human milk. *Pediatrics.* 2012;129(3): e827–e841.

Amir LH. Clinical protocol #4: Mastitis. *Breastfeed Med.* 2014;9(5): 239–243.

Amir LH, Donath SM, Garland SM, et al. Does Candida and/or Staphylococcus play a role in nipple and breast pain in lactation? A cohort study in Melbourne, Australia. *BMJ Open.* 2013;3(3):1–6.

Amir LH, Jones LE, Buck ML. Nipple pain associated with breastfeeding: incorporating current neurophysiology into clinical reasoning. *Aust Fam Physician.* 2015;44(3):127–132.

Anderson PO, Pochop SL, Manoguerra AS. Adverse drug reactions in breastfed infants: Less than imagined. *Clin Pediatr.* 2003; 42(4):325–340.

Appleton J, Laws R, Russell CG, et al. Infant formula feeding practices and the role of advice and support: an exploratory qualitative study. *BMC Pediatr.* 2018;18(12). doi:10.1186/s12887-017-0977-7.

Arbour M, Kessler J. Mammary hypoplasia: not every breast can produce sufficient milk. *J Midwifery Women's Health.* 2013; 58(4):457–461.

Assad M, Elliott MJ, Abraham JH. Decreased cost and improved feeding tolerance in VLBW infants fed an exclusive human milk diet. *J Perinatol.* 2016;36(3):216–220.

Australian Breastfeeding Association. *FeedSafe App.* 2021. Online: https://www.breastfeeding.asn.au/bf-info/safe-when-breastfeeding/alcohol-and-breastfeeding.

Australian College of Midwives (ACM). *ACM Position Statement—Use of Donor Human Milk.* 2014. Online: https://www.midwives.org.au/resources/acm-position-statement-use-donor-human-milk.

Australian Government. *Lodging complaints of alleged breaches of the MAIF Agreement.* 2019. Online: https://www1.health.gov.au/internet/main/publishing.nsf/Content/health-pubhlth-publicat-document-brfeed-complaints.htm.

Australian Government. *Marketing in Australia of Infant Formulas: Manufacturers and Importers Agreement 1992 (MAIF Agreement).* 2021. Online: https://www1.health.gov.au/internet/main/publishing.nsf/Content/health-pubhlth-strateg-foodpolicy-apmaif.htm.

Australian Government Department of Health. *National Breastfeeding Strategy Summary Report.* Canberra: Department of Health; 2001. Online: http://www.health.gov.au/internet/main/publishing.nsf/Content/health-pubhlth-publicat-document-brfeed-stratfeed-cnt.htm.

Australian Government Department of Health. *Australian National Breastfeeding Strategy.* Canberra: Australian Government Department of Health; 2009. Online: http://www.health.gov.au/internet/main/publishing.nsf/Content/6FD59347DD67ED8FCA257BF0001CFD1E/$File/Breastfeeding_strat1015.pdf.

Australian Government Department of Health. *Breastfeeding.* 2019. Online: https://www1.health.gov.au/internet/main/publishing.nsf/Content/health-pubhlth-strateg-brfeed-index.htm.

Australian Health Ministers Advisory Council (AHMAC). *Australian National Breastfeeding Strategy: 2017 and Beyond.* Fact Sheet 1. Updated May 2017.

Australian Institute of Health and Welfare (AIHW). *2010 Australian National Infant Feeding Survey: indicator results.* Canberra, AIHW; 2011.

Australian Institute of Health and Welfare (AIHW). *Australia's children.* Cat. no. CWS 69. Canberra: AIHW; 2020.

Ayton JE, Tesch L, Hansen E. Women's experiences of ceasing to breastfeed: Australian qualitative study. *BMJ Open.* 2019;9:e026234. doi: 10.1136/bmjopen-2018-026234.

Bagnoli F, Casucci M, Toti S, et al. Is vitamin D supplementation necessary in healthy full-term breastfed infants? A follow-up study of bone mineralization in healthy full-term infants with and without supplemental vitamin D. *Minerva Pediatr.* 2013; 65(3):253–260.

Baird JK, Jensen SM, Urba WJ, et al. SARS-CoV-2 antibodies detected in human breastmilk postvaccination. *MedRxiv.* preprint 2021. doi: https://doi.org/10.1101/2021.02.23.21252328.

Baker P, Smith J, Salmon L, et al. Global trends and patterns of commercial milk-based formula sales: Is an unprecedented infant and young child feeding transition underway? *Public Health Nutr.* 2016;19(14):2540–2550.

Baker P, Russ K, Kang M, et al. Globalization, first-food systems transformations and corporate power: a synthesis of literature and data on the market and political practices of the transnational baby food industry. *Global Health.* 2021;17(58). doi:10.1186/s12992-021-00708-1.

Ballard O, Morrow A. Human milk composition: nutrients and bioactive factors. *Pediatr Clin North Am.* 2013;60(1):49–74.

Balogun OO, O'Sullivan EJ, McFadden A, et al. Interventions for promoting the initiation of breastfeeding. *Cochrane Database Syst Rev.* 2016;(11):CD001688, doi:10.1002/14651858.CD001688.pub3.

Bartick MC, Schwarz EB, Green BD, et al. Suboptimal breastfeeding in the United States: Maternal and pediatric health outcomes and costs. *Matern Child Nutr.* 2017;13:e12366. doi:10.1111/mcn.12366.

Belfort MB, Anderson PJ, Nowak VA, et al. Breastmilk feeding, brain development, and neurocognitive outcomes: a 7-year longitudinal study in infants born at less than 30 weeks' gestation. *J Pediatr.* 2016;177:133–139.

Berens P, Brodribb W. ABM Clinical Protocol # 20: Engorgement. *Breastfeed Med.* 2016;11(4):159–163.

Bernt K, Walker WA. Human milk and the response of intestinal epithelium to infection. In: Newburg D, ed. *Bioactive Components of Human Milk.* New York: Springer; 2001:11–30.

Berry NJ, Jones S, Iverson D. It's all formula to me: women's understandings of toddler milk ads. *Breastfeed Rev.* 2010;18(1): 21–30.

Berry NJ, Gribble KD. Health and nutrition content claims on websites advertising infant formula available in Australia: A content analysis. *Matern Child Nutr.* 2017;13(4):e12383. doi:10.1111/mcn.12383

Betzold C. An update on recognition and management of lactational breast inflammation. *J Midwifery Womens Health.* 2007; 52(6):595–605.

BFHI Australia Baby Friendly Health Initiative. *Maternity Facility Handbook.* 2020. https://bfhi.org.au/maternity-facilities/

Blackburn S. *Maternal, Fetal and Neonatal Physiology.* 4th ed. Philadelphia: Saunders; 2007.

Blair A, Cadwell K, Turner-Maffei C, et al. The relationship between positioning, the breastfeeding dynamic, the latching process and pain in breastfeeding mothers with sore nipples. *Breastfeed Rev.* 2003;11(2):5–10.

Blyth R, Creedy D, Dennis C, et al. Effect of maternal confidence on breastfeeding duration: an application of breastfeeding self-efficacy theory. *Birth.* 2002;29(4):278–284.

Bode L. Human milk oligosaccharides: every baby needs a sugar mama. *Glycobiology.* 2012;22(9):1147–1162.

Borra C, Iacovou M, Sevilla A. New evidence on breastfeeding and postpartum depression: The importance of understanding women's intentions. *Matern Child Health J.* 2015;19(4):897–907.

Boyd CA, Quigley MA, Brocklehurst P. Donor breastmilk versus infant formula for preterm infants: systematic review and meta-analysis. *Arch Dis Child Fetal Neonatal Ed.* 2007;92(3): F169–F175.

Brimdyr K, Cadwell K, Widström A-M, et al. The association between common labor drugs and suckling when skin-to-skin during the first hour after birth. *Birth.* 2015;42(4):319–328.

Brimdyr K, Cadwell K, Svensson K, et al. The nine stages of skin-to-skin: practical guidelines and insights from four countries. *Matern Child Nutr.* 2020;e13042.

Brimdyr K, Cadwell K, Widström A-M, et al. The effect of labor medications on normal newborn behaviour in the first hour after birth: A prospective cohort study. *Early Hum Dev.* 2019;132:30–36.

Britton J, Britton H, Gronwaldt V. Breastfeeding, sensitivity, and attachment. *Pediatrics.* 2006;118(5):1436–1443.

Brodribb W. *Breastfeeding Management in Australia.* 5th ed. Melbourne: Australian Breastfeeding Association; 2019.

Brown A, Arnott B. Breastfeeding duration and early parenting behaviour: the importance of an infant-led, responsive style. *PLoS ONE.* 2014;9(2):e83893. doi:10.1371/journal.pone.0083893.

Brown A, Davies R. Fathers' experiences of supporting breastfeeding: challenges for breastfeeding promotion and education. *Matern Child Nutr.* 2014;10(4):510–526.

Brown A. Milk supply and breastfeeding decisions: the effects of new mothers' experiences. *NCT Perspective.* 2015;29:1–11.

Brown A. What do women really want? Lessons for breastfeeding promotion and education. *Breastfeeding Med.* 2016;11(3): 102–110.

Brown A. Midwifery Basics: Anatomy and Physiology 3. Understanding the impact of birth and the early postnatal environment on breastfeeding initiation and continuation. *Practicing Midwife.* 2018a; 21(10).

Brown A. What do women lose if they are prevented from meeting their breastfeeding goals? *Clin Lact.* 2018b; 9(4): 200–207.

Burkey B, Holmes A. Evaluating medication use in pregnancy and lactation: what every pharmacist should know. *J Pediatr Pharmacol Ther.* 2013;18(3):247–258.

Burns E, Fenwick J, Sheehan A, et al. Mining for liquid gold: Midwifery language and practices associated with early breastfeeding support. *Matern Child Nutr.* 2013;9(1):57–73.

Burns E, Fenwick J, Sheehan A, et al. 'This little piranha': A qualitative analysis of the language used by health professionals and mothers to describe infant behaviour during breastfeeding. *Matern Child Nutr.* 2016;12(1):111–124.

Buultjens M, Murphy G, Robinson P, et al. Women's experiences of, and attitudes to, maternity education across the perinatal period in Victoria, Australia: a mixed-methods approach. *Women Birth.* 2017;30(5):406–414.

Bystrova K, Widstrom AM, Ransjo-Arvidson AB, et al. Skin-to-skin contact may reduce negative consequences of "the stress of being born"—a study on temperature in newborn infants subjected to different ward routines in St Petersburg. *Acta Paediatr.* 2003;92:320–326.

Cacho NT, Harrison NA, Parker LA, et al. Personalization of the microbiota of donor human milk with mother's own milk. *Front Microbiol.* 2017;8(1470). doi: 10.3389/fmicb.2017.01470.

Cadwell K, Turner-Maffei C, Blair A, et al. Pain reduction and treatment of sore nipples in nursing mothers. *J Perinat Educ.* 2004;13(1):29–35.

Callen J, Pinelli J. A review of the literature examining the benefits and challenges, incidence and duration and barriers to breastfeeding in premature infants. *Adv Neonatal Care.* 2005; 5(2):72–88.

Campbell S. Recurrent plugged duct. *J Hum Lact.* 2006;22(3):340–343.

Cardwell CR, Stene LC, Ludvigsson J, et al. Breast-feeding and childhood-onset type 1 diabetes: a pooled analysis of individual participant data from 43 observational studies. *Diabetes Care.* 2012;35(11):2215–2225.

Castro T, Grant C, Wall C, et al. Breastfeeding indicators among a nationally representative multi-ethnic sample of New Zealand children. *N Z Med J.* 2017;130(1466):34–44.

Chapin EM, Chao-Huei C, Dumas L, et al. The paradigm shift in BFHI Step 2: From training to competency verification. *J Hum Lact.* 2021. doi:10.1177/0890334421995098.

Chow S, Chow R, Popovic M, et al. The use of nipple shields: a review. *Front Public Health.* 2015;3:236. doi:10.3389/fpubh.2015.00236.

Collaborative Group on Hormonal Factors in Breast Cancer. Breast cancer and breastfeeding: collaborative reanalysis of individual data from 47 epidemiological studies in 30 countries, including 50302 women with breast cancer and 96973 women without the disease. *Lancet.* 2002;360(9328):187–195.

Colson S. Maternal breastfeeding positions, have we got it right? Part 2. *Pract Midwife.* 2005;8(11):29–32.

Colson S, Meek J, Hawdon J. Optimal positions for the release of primitive neonatal reflexes stimulating breastfeeding. *Early Hum Dev.* 2008;84(7):441–449.

Commonwealth Departments of Health and Family Services. *National Breastfeeding Strategy.* Canberra, Australia: AGPS; 2001.

Cook EJ, Powell F, Ali N, et al. Improving support for breastfeeding mothers: a qualitative study on the experiences of breastfeeding among mothers who reside in a deprived and culturally diverse community. *Int J Equity Health.* 2021;20(92). doi:10.1186/s12939-021-01419-0.

Cotterman K. Reverse pressure softening: a simple tool to prepare areola for easier latching during engorgement. *J Hum Lact.* 2004;20(2):227–237.

Council of Australian Governments (COAG). *Australian National Breastfeeding Strategy: 2019 and Beyond.* Canberra: COAG; 2019.

Couread G, Moncombie A-S, Montigny D, et al. A pheromone that rapidly promotes learning in the newborn. *Curr Biol.* 2006;16:1956–1961.

Cox D, Owens R, Hartmann P. Blood and milk prolactin and the rate of milk synthesis in women. *Exp Physiol.* 1996;81(6):1007–1020.

Cramer R, McLachlan H, Shafiei T, et al. Women's experiences of infant feeding support: findings from a cross-sectional survey in Victoria, Australia. La Trobe. *Women Birth.* 2021. doi:10.26181/602b585b7b383.

Cregan M, Mitoulas L, Hartmann P. Milk prolactin, feed volume and duration between feeds in women breastfeeding their full-term infants over a 24 h period. *Exp Physiol.* 2002;87(1):207–214.

Cruz N, Korchin L. Breastfeeding after augmentation mammoplasty with saline implants. *Ann Plast Surg.* 2010;64(5):530–533.

Dadhich JP, Smith J, Iellamo A, et al. *Report on Carbon Footprints due to Milk Formula: A Study From Selected Countries of the Asia-Pacific Region.* IBFAN, BPNI; 2015.

Daly S, Owens R, & Hartmann P. The short-term synthesis and infant-regulated removal of milk in lactating women. *Exp Physiol.* 1993;78(2):209–220. doi:10.1113/expphysiol.1993.sp003681

Davanzo R, Moro G, Sandri F, et al. Breastfeeding and coronavirus disease-2019: Ad interim indications of the Italian Society of Neonatology endorsed by the Union of European Neonatal & Perinatal Societies. *Matern Child Nutr.* 2020; e13010. doi:10.1111/mcn.13010.

Davanzo R, Agosti, M, Cetin I, et al. Breastfeeding and COVID-19 vaccination: position statement of the Italian scientific societies. *Ital J Pediatr.* 2021;47(45) https://doi.org/10.1186/s13052-021-00998-.

den Hertog J, van Leengoed E, Kolk F, et al. The defecation pattern of healthy term infants up to the age of 3 months. *Arch Dis Child Fetal Neonatal Ed.* 2012;97(6):465–470.

Dener C, Inan A. Breast abscesses in lactating women. *World J Surg.* 2003;27(2):130–133.

Dennis CL, Jackson K, Watson J. Interventions for treating painful nipples among breastfeeding women (review). *Cochrane Database Syst Rev.* 2014;(12):CD007366, doi:10.1002/14651858.CD007366.pub2.

Department of Health (DOH). *Pregnancy Care Guidelines: Preparing for breastfeeding.* Online: https://www.health.gov.au/resources/pregnancy-care-guidelines/part-b-core-practices-in-pregnancy-care/preparing-for-breastfeeding. 2021.

do Carmo França-Botelho A, Ferreira MFJ, França E, et al. Breastfeeding and its relationship with reduction of breast cancer: a review. *Asian Pac J Cancer Prev.* 2012;13(11):327–332.

Doucet S, Soussignan R, Sagot P, et al. The smellscape of mother's breast: effects of odor masking and selective unmasking on neonatal arousal, oral and visual responses. *Dev Psychobiol.* 2007;49(2):129–138.

Doucet S, Soussignan R, Sagot P, et al. An overlooked aspect of the human breast: areolar glands in relation with breastfeeding pattern, neonatal weight gain, and the dynamics of lactation. *Early Hum Dev.* 2012;88(2):119–128.

Drugs and Lactation Database (LactMed) [Internet]. Bethesda (MD): National Library of Medicine (US); 2006. Online: https://www.ncbi.nlm.nih.gov/books/NBK501922/.

Duma L, Lepage M, Bystrova K, et al. Influence of skin-to-skin contact and rooming-in on early mother–infant interaction: a randomized controlled trial. *Clin Nurs Resid.* 2013;22(3):310–336.

Edmond K, Kirkwood B, Amenga-Etego S, et al. Effect of early infant feeding practices on infection-specific neonatal mortality: an investigation of the causal links with observational data from rural Ghana. *Am J Clin Nutr.* 2007;86(4):1126–1131.

Edmunds J, Miles S, Fulbrook P. Tongue-tie and breastfeeding: a review of the literature. *Breastfeed Rev.* 2011;19(1):19–26.

Emmott EH, Mace R. Practical support from fathers and grandmothers is associated with lower levels of breastfeeding in the UK Millennium Cohort Study. *PLoS ONE.* 2015;10(7):e0133547.

European Food Safety Authority (EFSA). Opinion of the Scientific Panel on Biological Hazards (BIOHAZ) Related to the Microbiological Risks in Infant Formulae and Follow-on Formulae. 2004.

Ewaschuk JB, Unger S, O'Connor DL, et al. Effect of pasteurization on selected immune components of donated human breastmilk. *J Perinatol.* 2011;31:593–598.

Feist N, Berger D, Speer C. Anti-endotoxin antibodies in human milk: Correlation with infection of the newborn. *Acta Paediatr.* 2000;89(9):1087–1092.

Feng LP, Chen HL, Shen MY. Breastfeeding and the risk of ovarian cancer: a meta-analysis. *J Midwifery Womens Health.* 2014;59(4):428–437.

Ferri RL, Rosen-Carole CB, Jackson J, et al. ABM Clinical Protocol #33: Lactation care for lesbian, gay, bisexual, transgender, queer, questioning, plus patients. *Breastfeeding Med.* 2020;15(5):284–293.

Fielder C. Determining the influencing factors of a caesarean section birth on breastfeeding. *Evid Based Midwifery.* 2016;14(2):57–63.

Flidel-Rimon O, Shinwell E. Breast feeding twins and high multiples. *Arch Dis Child Fetal Neonatal Ed.* 2006;91(5):F377–F380.

Foote K, Joy M. The true cost of milk: environmental deterioration vs. profit in the New Zealand dairy industry. NZ Agricultural and Resource Economics Society Inc. Conference, Nelson, August 28–29, 2014.

Frederick A. C, Busen NH, Engebretson JC, et al. Exploring the skin-to-skin contact experience during cesarean section. *J Am Assoc Nurse Pract.* 2016;28(1):31–38.

French CA, Cong X, Chung KS. Labor epidural analgesia and breastfeeding: a systematic review. *J Hum Lact.* 2016;32(3):507–20.

Furber C, Thompson A. Breastfeeding practice in the UK: midwives' perspectives. *Matern Child Nutr.* 2008,41(1):44–54.

Galante L, Milan AM, Reynolds CM, et al. Sex-specific human milk composition: The role of infant sex in determining early life nutrition. *Nutrients.* 2018;10(9). doi:10.3390/nu10091194.

Galipeau R, Dumas L, Lepage M. Perception of not having enough milk and actual milk production of first-time breastfeeding mothers: is there a difference? *Breastfeed Med.* 2017;12(4): 210–217.

Galipeau R, Baillot A, Trottier A, & Lemire L. Effectiveness of interventions on breastfeeding self-efficacy and perceived insufficient milk supply: A systematic review and meta-analysis. *Matern Child Nutr.* 2018;14(3):e12607.

Gatti L. Maternal perceptions of insufficient milk supply in breastfeeding. *J Nurs Scholarsh.* 2008;40(4):355–363.

Geddes D. Inside the lactating breast: the latest anatomy research. *J Midwifery Womens Health.* 2007;52(6):556–563.

Genuneit J, Boyle RJ. Hydrolysed formula and allergy prevention. *Pediatr Allergy Immunol.* 2021;32(4):667–669. doi:10.1111/pai.13470.

Gibson R, Makrides M. Long-chain polyunsaturated fatty acids in breastmilk: are they essential? *Adv Exp Med Biol.* 2001;501:375–383.

Girard LC, Côté SM, de Lauzon-Guillain B, et al. Factors associated with breastfeeding initiation: a comparison between France and French-speaking Canada. *PLoS ONE.* 2016;11(11): e0166946.

Gomez-Gallego C, Garcia-Mantrana I, Salminen S, et al. The human milk microbiome and factors influencing its composition and activity. Paper presented at the Seminars in Fetal and Neonatal Medicine. 2016.

Gonzalez-Viana E, Dworzynski K, Murphy MS, et al. Guideline Committee. Faltering growth in children: summary of NICE guidance. *BMJ.* 2017;358:j4219. doi:10.1136/bmj.j4219.

Graffy J, Taylor J. What information, advice and support do women want with breastfeeding? *Birth.* 2005;179–186.

Greer FR. Are breastfed infants iron deficient? The question that won't go away. *J Pediatr.* 2021; 231:34–35. doi:10.1016/j.jpeds.2020.12.01.

Gribble KD. Mechanisms behind breastmilk's protection against, and artificial baby milk's facilitation of, diarrhoeal illness. *Breastfeed Rev.* 2011;19(2):19–26.

Gribble KD. Summary of peer-to-peer milk donors and recipients' experiences and perceptions of donor milk banks. *J Obstet Gynecol Neonatal Nurs.* 2013;42(4):451–461.

Gribble KD, Berry NJ. Emergency preparedness for those who care for infants in developed country contexts. *Int Breastfeed J.* 2011;6(1):16. doi:10.1186/1746-4358-6-16.

Gribble K, Peterson M, & Brown D. Emergency preparedness for infant and young child feeding in emergencies (IYCF-E): an Australian audit of emergency plans and guidance. *BMC Public Health.* 2019;19(1):1278. doi:10.1186/s12889-019-7528-0.

Gribble K, Mathisen R, Ververs M, & Coutsoudis A. Mistakes from the HIV pandemic should inform the COVID-19 response for maternal and newborn care. *Int Breastfeed J.* 2020;15(67). Online: https://internationalbreastfeedingjournal.biomedcentral.com/articles/10.1186/s13006-020-00306-8.

Gribble KD, Bewley S, Bartick MC, Mathisen R, Walker S, Gamble J, Bergman NJ, Gupta A, Hocking JJ, Dahlen HG. Effective communication about pregnancy, birth, lactation, breastfeeding and newborn care: the importance of sexed language. *Front Glob Womens Health.* 2022. doi:10.3389/fgwh.2022.818856.

Groleau D, Sigouin C, D'Souza NA. Power to negotiate spatial barriers to breastfeeding in a western context: when motherhood meets poverty. *Health* Place. 2013;24:250–259.

Gunderson EP, Hurston SR, Ning X, et al. Study of women, infant feeding and type 2 diabetes after GDM pregnancy investigators. Lactation and progression to type 2 diabetes mellitus after gestational diabetes mellitus: a prospective cohort study. *Ann Intern Med.* 2015;163(12):889–898.

Gupta A, Suri S, Dadhich JP, Trejos M, et al. The World Breastfeeding Trends Initiative: Implementation of the Global Strategy for Infant and Young Child Feeding in 84 Countries. *J Public Health Pol.* 2019;40:35–65.

Hale TW, Rowe HE. *Medications and Mothers' Milk: A Manual of Lactational Physiology.* 17th ed. New York: Springer; 2017.

Hale TW. *Hale's Medications and Mothers' Milk: A Manual of Lactational Physiology.* New York: Springer; 2021

Hale TW, Kristensen JH, Ilett KF. The transfer of medications into human milk. In: Hale T, Hartmann P, eds. *Textbook of Human Lactation.* Amarillo: Hale; 2007.

Han Y, Chang E, Kim J, et al. Association of infant feeding practices in the general population with infant growth and stool characteristics. *Nutr Res Pract.* 2011;5(4):308–312.

Hanna S, Wilson M, Norwood S. A description of breast-feeding outcomes among U.S. mothers using nipple shields. *Midwifery.* 2013;29(6):616–621.

Hartmann PE. Lactation and reproduction in Western Australian women. *J Reprod Med.*1987; 32(7):543–547.

Hartmann BT. Ensuring safety in donor human milk banking in neonatal intensive care. *Clin Perinatol.* 2017;44(1): 131–149.

Hartmann BT, Pang WW, Keil AD, et al. Best practice guidelines for the operation of a donor human milk bank in an Australian NICU. *Early Hum Dev.* 2007;83:667–673.

Hassiotou F, Geddes D. Anatomy of the human mammary gland: Current status of knowledge. *Clin Anat.* 2013;26(1):29–48.

Hastings G, Angus K, Eadie D, et al. Selling second best: how infant formula marketing works. *Global Health.* 2020;16(77). doi:10.1186/s12992-020-00597-w.

Hauck FR, Thompson JMD, Tanabe KO, et al. Breastfeeding and reduced risk of sudden infant death syndrome: a meta-analysis. *Pediatrics.* 2011;128(1):103–110.

Henderson A. Understanding the breast crawl: implications for nursing practice. *Nurs Womens Health.* 2011;15(4):296–307.

Herrmann K, Carroll K. An exclusively human milk diet reduces necrotising enterocolitis. *Breastfeeding Med.* 2014;9(4):184–190.

Hillan R. Division of tongue tie: wicked and barbaric? *Pract Midwife.* 2008;11(10):22–25.

Hobbs AJ, Mannion CA, McDonald SW, et al. The impact of caesarean section on breastfeeding initiation, duration and difficulties in the first four months postpartum. *BMC Pregnancy Childbirth.* 2016;16(90). doi:10.1186/s12884-016-0876-1.

Hocking J, Hull N, & Smith J. Creating change for breastfeeding: the world breastfeeding trends initiative in Australia. *Women Birth.* 2019;32(1):S31.

Hoover K, Barbalinardo L, Platia M. Delayed lactogenesis II secondary to gestation ovarian theca lutein cysts in two normal singleton pregnancies. *J Hum Lact.* 2002;18(3):264–268.

Hoover K, Bentley S, Walters J. Perinatal and intrapartum care. In: Wambach K, Spencer B, eds. *Breastfeeding and Human Lactation.* Jones & Bartlett Learning; 2021:177–213.

Horta BL, Bahl R, Martines J, et al. *Evidence on the Long-Term Effects of Breastfeeding.* Geneva, Switzerland: World Health Organization; 2007.

Horta BL, Loret de Mola C, Victora CG. Long-term consequences of breastfeeding on cholesterol, obesity, systolic blood pressure and type 2 diabetes: a systematic review and meta-analysis. *Acta Paediatr.* 2015;104:30–37.

Hotham N, Hotham E. Drugs in breastfeeding. *Aust Prescr.* 2015;38(5):156–9. doi:10.18773/austprescr.2015.056. Epub 2015 Oct 1. Erratum in: *Aust Prescr.* 2016;39(1):27.

Huang Y, Lee J, Huang C, et al. Factors related to maternal perception of milk supply while in the hospital. *J Nurs Res.* 2009;17(3):179–188.

Huffman S, Harika R, Eilander A, et al. Essential fats: how do they affect growth and development of infants and young children in developing countries? A literature review. *Matern Child Nutr.* 2011;7(3):44–65.

Human Milk Banking Association of North America (HMBANA). *Guidelines for the Establishment and Operation of a Donor Human Milk Bank*. Fort Worth, TX: HMBANA; 2009.

Hunt F. The importance of kangaroo care on infant oxygenation levels and bonding. *J Neonatal Nurs*. 2008;14:47–51.

Hunter L, Magill-Cuerden J, & McCourt C. 'Oh no, no, no, we haven't got time to be doing that': Challenges encountered introducing a breast-feeding support intervention on a postnatal ward. *Midwifery*. 2015;31(8):798–804.

Hurst N. Recognising and treating delayed or failed lactogenesis II. *J Midwifery Womens Health*. 2007;52(6):588–646.

IFE Core Group (WHO, UNICEF, UNHCR, WFP, IBFAN-GIFA, CARE USA, Foundation Terre des hommes and the Emergency Nutrition Network (ENN)). *Infant and Young Child Feeding in Emergencies: Operational Guidance for Emergency Relief Staff and Programme Managers*. Version 2.1. Oxford: IFE Core Group; 2007.

Ingram J, Woolridge M, Greenwood R. Breastfeeding: it is worth trying with the second baby. *Lancet*. 2001;358(9286):986–7.

International Baby Food Action Network (IBFAN), GIFA, WBTi. *Green Feeding—climate action from birth*. 2019. Online: https://www.gifa.org/wp-content/uploads/2019/12/2019-Green-Feeding-Key-Messages-Dec2.pdf.

International Baby Food Action Network (IBFAN). *Monitoring of the International Code of Marketing of Breastmilk Substitutes*. 2018. Online: https://www.ibfan.org/code-monitoring.

International Confederation of Midwives (ICM). Health of Women and Children in Disasters: Position Statement. 2005, reviewed 2011.

International Confederation of Midwives (ICM). *Position Statement: Breastfeeding*. Adopted 2005, updated 2017.

International Confederation of Midwives (ICM). *Position Statement: Human Rights of Lesbian, Gay, Bisexual, Transgender and Intersex (LGBTI) People*. 2017.

International Confederation of Midwives (ICM). Women's rights in childbirth must be upheld during the Coronavirus Pandemic. 29 Mar 2020.

Jaafar SH, Ho JJ, Jahanfar S, et al. Effect of restricted pacifier use in breastfeeding term infants for increasing duration of breastfeeding. *Cochrane Database Sys Rev*. 2016;(8):CD007202. doi:10.1002/14651858.CD007202.pub4.

Jacobson LT, Hade EM, Collins, TC, et al. Breastfeeding history and risk of stroke among parous postmenopausal women in the women's health initiative. *J Am Heart Assoc*. 2018;7(17): e008739.

Jahanfar S, Ng C, Teng C. Antibiotics for mastitis in breastfeeding women. *Cochrane Database Syst Rev*. 2013;(2):CD005458. doi:10.1002/14651858.CD005458.pub3.

James L, Sweet L, Donnellan-Fernandez R. Breastfeeding initiation and support: A literature review of what women value and the impact of early discharge. *Women Birth*. 2017;30(2):87–99.

Jasani B, Simmer K, Patole SK, et al. Long chain polyunsaturated fatty acid supplementation in infants born at term. *Cochrane Database Syst Rev*. 2017;(3):CD000376. doi:10.1002/14651858.CD000376.pub4.

Jones W. *Breastfeeding and Medication*. London: Routledge; 2013.

Kelly NM, Smilowitz JT, Cagney O, et al. Delayed onset of lactogenesis and reduced breastfeeding frequency in mothers who give birth by caesarean section. The Proceedings of the Nutrition Society Cambridge. 2020;79. doi:10.1017/S0029665120003936.

Kendall-Tackett KM. A new paradigm for depression in new mothers: the central role of inflammation and how breastfeeding and anti-inflammatory treatments protect maternal mental health. *Int Breastfeed J*. 2007;2:2–41.

Kent G. Regulating fatty acids in infant formula: critical assessment of U.S. policies and practices. *Int Breastfeed J*. 2014;9:2. doi:10.1186/1746-4358-9-2.

Kent G. Global infant formula: monitoring and regulating the impacts to protect human health. *Int Breastfeed J*. 2015;10:6. doi:10.1186/s13006-014-0020-7.

Kent J. How breastfeeding works. *J Midwifery Women's Health*. 2007;52(6):564–570.

Kent J, Mitoulas L, Cregan M, et al. Volume and frequency of breastfeedings and fat content of breastmilk throughout the day. *Pediatrics*. 2006;117(3):e387–e395.

Kent JC, Ashton E, Hardwick CM, et al. Nipple pain in breastfeeding mothers: incidence, causes and treatments. *Int J Environ Res Public Health*. 2015;12:12247–12263.

Kent JC, Ashton E, Hardwick CM, et al. Causes of perception of insufficient milk supply in Western Australian mothers. *Matern Child Nutr*. 2021;17(1):e13080. doi:https://doi.org/10.1111/mcn.13080.

Kim J, Unger S. Human milk banking. *Pediatr Child Health*. 2010; 595:602.

Klaus M. Mother and infant: early emotional ties. *Paediatrics*. 1998;102(7):1244–1246.

Kornides M, Kitsantas P. Evaluation of breastfeeding promotion, support, and knowledge of benefits on breastfeeding outcomes. *J Child Health Care*. 2013;17(3):264–73.

Kramer M, Kakuma R. Optimal duration of exclusive breastfeeding. *Cochrane Database Syst Rev*. 2012;(8):CD003517. doi:10.1002/14651858.CD003517.pub2.

Kreemer F. Breastfeeding self-efficacy of women using second-line strategies for healthy term infants in the first week postpartum: an Australian observational study. *Int Breastfeed J*. 2013;8:1. doi:10.1186/1746-4358-8-18.

Laing I, Wong C. Hypernatraemia in the first few days: is the incidence rising? *Arch Dis Child Fetal Neonatal*. 2002;87(3): F158–F162.

Lapidaire W, Lucas A, Clayden JD, et al. Human milk feeding and cognitive outcome in preterm infants: the role of infection and NEC reduction. *Pediatr Res*. 2021. doi:10.1038/s41390-021-01367-z.

Lauwers J, Swisher A. *Counseling the Nursing Mother: A Lactation Consultant's Guide*. 5th ed. Sudbury, MA: Jones & Bartlett; 2011.

Lavigne V, Gleberzon B. Ultrasound as a treatment of mammary blocked duct among 25 postpartum lactating women: a retrospective case series. *J Chiropr Med*. 2012;11(3):170–178.

Lawrence R. Circumstances when breastfeeding is contraindicated. *Pediatr Clin North Am*. 2013;60(1):295–318.

Lawrence R, Lawrence R. *Breastfeeding: A Guide for Health Professionals*. 7th ed. St Louis: Mosby; 2011.

Leonard L. Breastfeeding triplets: the at-home experience. *Public Health Nurs*. 2000;17(3):211–221.

Leonard L. Breastfeeding higher order multiples: enhancing support during the postpartum hospitalisation period. *J Hum Lact*. 2002;4:386–392.

Li R, Fein SB, Chen J, et al. Why mothers stop breastfeeding: mothers' self-reported reasons for stopping during the first year. *Pediatrics*. 2008;122(suppl):S69–S76.

Lönnerdal B. Nutritional and physiologic significance of human milk proteins. *Am J Clin Nutr*. 2003;77(6):1537S–1543S.

Lubold, A.M. Historical-qualitative analysis of breastfeeding trends in three OECD countries. *Int Breastfeed J*. 2019; 14(36). doi:10.1186/s13006-019-0230-0.

Lucas A, Cole TJ. Breastmilk and neonatal necrotising enterocolitis. *Lancet*. 1990;336(8730):1519–1523.

Ludington-Hoe SM, Lewis T, Anderson L, et al. Breast-infant temperature with twins during shared kangaroo care. *J Obstet Gynaecol Neonatal Nurs*. 2006;35(2):223–231.

Ludington-Hoe SM, Morgan K. Infant assessment and reduction of sudden unexpected postnatal collapse risk during skin-to-skin contact. *Newborn Infant Nurs Rev*. 2014;14(1):28–33.

McBride GM, Stevenson R, Zizzo G, et al. Uses and experiences of galactagogues while breastfeeding among Australian women. *PLoS ONE*. 2021;16(7): e0254049.
McClellan H, Geddes D, Kent J, et al. Infants of mothers with persistent nipple pain exert strong sucking vacuums. *Acta Paediatr.* 2008;97(9):1205–1209.
McClellan L, Hepworth R, Garbin P, et al. Nipple pain during breastfeeding with or without visible trauma. *J Hum Lact.* 2012;28(3):511–521.
McFadden A, Mason F, Baker J, et al. Spotlight on infant formula: coordinated global action needed. *Lancet Breastfeed Series.* 2016;387(10033):413–415.
McFadden A, Gavine A, Renfrew MJ, et al. Support for healthy breastfeeding mothers with healthy term babies. *Cochrane Database Syst Rev.* 2017;(2):CD001141. doi:10.1002/14651858.CD001141.pub5.
McKechnie AC, Eglash A. Nipple shields: a review of the literature. *Breastfeed Med.* 2010;5(6):309–314.
Mangesi L, Dowswell T. Treatments for breast engorgement during lactation. *Cochrane Database Syst Rev.* 2010;(9):CD006946. doi:10.1002/14651858.CD006946.pub2.
Mangesi L, Zakarija-Grkovic I. Treatments for breast engorgement during lactation. *Cochrane Database Syst Rev.* 2016;(6): CD006946. doi:10.1002/14651858.CD006946.pub3.
Mass S. Breast pain: engorgement, nipple pain and mastitis. *Clin Obstet Gynecol.* 2004;47(3):676–682.
Matias S, Dewey K, Quesenberry C, et al. Maternal prepregnancy obesity and insulin treatment during pregnancy are independently associated with delayed lactogenesis in women with recent gestational diabetes. *Am J Clin Nutr.* 2014;115–121.
Medves JM. Three infant care interventions: reconsidering the evidence. *JOGNN.* 2002;31(5):563–569.
Meier P. Breastfeeding in the special care nursery. Premature and infants with medical problems. *Pediatr Clin North Am.* 2001;48(2):425–442.
Meier P, Furman L, Degenhardt M. Increased lactation risk for late preterm infants and mothers: evidence and management strategies to protect breastfeeding. *J Midwifery Womens Health.* 2007;52(4):579–587.
Mennella JA, Yourshaw LM, Morgan LK. Breastfeeding and smoking: short-term effects on infant feeding and sleep. *Pediatrics.* 2007;120(3):497–502.
Meyers D. Breastfeeding and health outcomes. *Breastfeed Med.* 2009;4(suppl 1):S13–S15.
Michaelsen K, Lauritzen L, Mortensen E. Effects of breast-feeding on cognitive function. *Adv Exp Med Biol.* 2009;639:199–215.
Michalopoulos K. The effects of breast augmentation surgery on future ability to lactate. *Breast J.* 2007;13(1):62–67.
Ministry of Health (MOH). *Breastfeeding: A Guide for Action.* Wellington, New Zealand; 2002.
Ministry of Health (MOH). *Implementing and Monitoring the International Code of Marketing of Breast-milk Substitutes in New Zealand: The Code in New Zealand.* Wellington, New Zealand; 2007a.
Ministry of Health (MOH). *Breast-milk Substitutes Complaints Procedure.* Wellington, New Zealand: MOH; 2007b.
Ministry of Health (MOH). *Compliance Panel.* Wellington, New Zealand: Wellington New Zealand; 2007c.
Ministry of Health (MOH). *National Strategic Plan of Action for Breastfeeding 2008–2012.* Wellington, New Zealand; 2009.
Ministry of Health (MOH). *Guidelines for Tuberculosis Control in New Zealand 2010. Chapter 5: Tuberculosis in children.* Wellington, New Zealand; 2010.
Ministry of Health (MOH). *Infant feeding in an emergency.* Wellington New Zealand; 2015.
Ministry of Health (MOH). *Breastfeeding by Women with HIV Infection.* Wellington New Zealand; 2016.
Ministry of Health (MOH). *Alcohol and breastfeeding.* Wellington New Zealand; 2018.
Ministry of Health (MOH). *National Breastfeeding Strategy for New Zealand Aotearoa Rautaki Whakamana Whāngote.* A roadmap to action: 2020 and beyond. Wellington New Zealand; 2020
Mirzaei-Aghsaghali A, Fathi H. Lactose in ruminants feeding. *Ann Biol Res.* 2012;3(1):645–650.
Mitchell-Box K, Braun K, Hurwitz E, et al. Breastfeeding attitudes: association between maternal and male partner attitudes and breastfeeding intent. *Breastfeed Med.* 2013;8(4):368–373.
Mizuno K., Nishida Y, Taki M. et al. Is increased fat content of hindmilk due to the size or the number of milk fat globules? *Int Breastfeed J.* 2009;4(7). doi:10.1186/1746-4358-4-7.
Mizuno K, Ueda A. Changes in sucking performance from nonnutritive sucking to nutritive sucking during breast- and bottle-feeding. *Pediatric Res.* 2006;59(5):728–731.
Mohammadi M, Bergh AM, Heidarzadeh M, et al. Implementation and effectiveness of continuous kangaroo mother care: a participatory action research protocol. *Int Breastfeed J.* 2021;16(24). doi:10.1186/s13006-021-00367-3.
Montgomery A, Hale TW, Academy Of Breastfeeding Medicine. ABM clinical protocol #15: analgesia and anesthesia for the breastfeeding mother, revised 2012. *Breastfeed Med.* 2012; 7(6):547–53.
Moore EAG, Bergman N, Dowsell T. Early skin-to-skin contact for mothers and their healthy newborn infants. *Cochrane Database Syst Rev.* 2012;(5):CD003519. doi:10.1002/14651858.CD003519.pub3.
Morland-Schultz K, Hill P. Prevention of and therapies for nipple pain: a systematic review. *J Obstet Gynecol Neonatal Nurs.* 2008;34(4):428–437.
Morns M, Steel A, McIntyre E, et al. 'It Makes My Skin Crawl': Women's experience of breastfeeding aversion response (BAR). *Women Birth.* 2022 in press.
Mortensen B, Diep LM, Lukasse M, et al. Women's satisfaction with midwife-led continuity of care: an observational study in Palestine. *BMJ Open.* 2019;9:e030324. doi: 10.1136/bmjopen-2019-030324
Morton J. *Maximising Milk Production.* 2009. Online: https://med.stanford.edu/newborns/professional-education/breastfeeding/maximizing-milk-production.html.
Morton J, Hall JY, Wong RJ, et al. Combining hand techniques with electric pumping increases milk production in mothers of preterm infants. *J Perinatol.* 2009;29:757–764.
Mother and Child Nutrition. *AFASS Principles.* 2016. Online: http://motherchildnutrition.org/info/afass-principles.html.
Much D, Beyerlein A, Kindt A, et al. Lactation is associated with altered metabolomic signatures in women with gestational diabetes. *Diabetologia.* 2016;59(10):2193–2202.
Murase M, Mizuno K, Nishida Y, et al. Comparison of creamatocrit and protein concentration in each mammary lobe of the same breast: does the milk composition of each mammary lobe differ in the same breast? *Breastfeed Med.* 2009;4(4):189–195.
Muresan M. Successful relactation—a case history. *Breastfeed Med.* 2011;6(4):233–239.
National Health and Medical Research Council (NHMRC). *Australian guidelines to reduce health risks from drinking alcohol.* Canberra Australia; 2020.
National Institute for Health and Care Excellence (NICE). *Donor Breastmilk Banks: The Operation of Donor Milk Bank Services. NICE Clinical Guidelines.* London: NICE; 2010:93.
National Institute for Health and Care Excellence (NICE). *Faltering Growth: Recognition and* Management of Faltering Growth in Children. London: NICE; 2017:24.
Netting MJ Moumin NA, Knight EJ, et al. The Australian Feeding Infants and Toddler Study (OzFITS 2021): Breastfeeding and

Early Feeding Practices. *Nutrients.* 2022;14:206. doi:10.3390/nu14010206.

Neville MC, Oliva-Rasbach J. Is maternal milk production limiting for infant growth during the first year of life in breast-fed infants? In: Goldman AS, Atkinson SA, Hanson LA, eds. *Human Lactation 3.* Boston, MA: Springer; 1987.

Neville M, Morton J, Umermura S. Lactogenesis. The transition from pregnancy to lactation. *Pediatr Clin North Am.* 2001;48(1):35–52.

Nevo N, Rubin L, Tamir A, et al. Infant feeding patterns in the first 6 months: an assessment in full-term infants. *J Pediatr Gastroenterol Nutr.* 2007;45(2):234–239.

New Zealand Breastfeeding Alliance (NZBA). *Baby Friendly Aotearoa National Infant Feeding Data at Discharge.* 2020a. Online: https://www.babyfriendly.org.nz/breastfeeding-data/.

New Zealand Breastfeeding Alliance (NZBA). *Protecting, supporting and promoting breastfeeding in New Zealand.* 2020b. Online: https://www.babyfriendly.org.nz/.

New Zealand College of Midwives (NZCOM). *Consensus Statement: Infant Feeding in Emergencies and Disasters.* Ratified 2012, updated 2016. Christchurch, New Zealand: NZCOM.

New Zealand College of Midwives (NZCOM). *Consensus Statement: Donor Human Milk and Milk Sharing.* Ratified 2019.

Newby RM, Davies PS. Why do women stop breast-feeding? Results from a contemporary prospective study in a cohort of Australian women. *Eur J Clin Nutr.* 2016;70(12):1428–1432.

Noel-Weiss J, Woodend K, Peterson W, et al. An observational study of associations among maternal fluids during parturition, neonatal output, and breastfeeding newborn weight loss. *Int Breastfeed J.* 2011;6:9. doi:10.1186/1746-4358-6-9.

Nommsen-Rivers L, Dolan L, Huange B. Timing and stage II lactogenesis is predicted by antenatal metabolic health in a cohort of primiparas. *Breastfeed Med.* 2012;7(1):43–49.

Noonan M. Breastfeeding; is my baby getting enough milk? *Br J Midwifery.* 2011;19(2):82–89.

Nye C. Transitioning premature infants from gavage to breast. *Neonatal Network.* 2008;27(1):7–13.

Nyqvist KH. Early attainment of breastfeeding competence in very preterm infants. *Acta Paediatr.* 2008;97(6):776–781.

Nyqvist KH. Lack of knowledge persists about early breastfeeding competence in preterm infants. *J Hum Lact.* 2013; 29(3):296–299.

Nyqvist KH, Häggkvist AP, Hansen MN, et al. Expansion of the ten steps to successful breastfeeding into neonatal intensive care: expert group recommendations for three guiding principles. *J Hum Lact.* 2012;28(3):289–296.

Nyqvist KH, Kylberg E, Hansen MN, et al. *Neo-BFHI: The Baby-friendly Hospital Initiative for Neonatal Wards. Three Guiding Principles and Ten Steps to Protect, Promote and Support Breastfeeding. Self-appraisal tool to assess standards and criteria.* Nordic and Quebec Working Group; 2015. Online: www.ilca.org/main/learning/resources/neo-bfhi/.

Obedin-Maliver J & Makadon HJ. Transgender men and pregnancy. *Obstetric Medicine.* 2016; 9(1):4–8.

Oddy W. Longer duration of exclusive breastfeeding associated with reduced risk of childhood asthma up to age six. *Evid Based Nurs.* 2013;16(1):18–19.

Odom E, Li R, Scanlon K, et al. Reasons for earlier than desired cessation of breastfeeding. *Pediatrics.* 2013;131(3):726–732.

Odom EC, Li R, Scanlon KS, et al. Association of family and health care provider opinion on infant feeding with mother's breastfeeding decision. *J Acad Nutr Diet,* 2014;114(8):1203–1207.

Olonan-Jusi, E., Zambrano, PG., Duong, et al. Human milk banks in the response to COVID-19: a statement of the regional human milk bank network for Southeast Asia and beyond. *Int Breastfeed J.* 2021;16(29). doi:10.1186/s13006-021-00376-2.

Otsuka K, Denis C, Tatsuoka H, et al. The relationship between breastfeeding self-efficacy and perceived insufficient milk among Japanese mothers. *J Obstet Neonatal Nurs.* 2008;5: 546–555.

Page-Goertz S, Chevreux E. The ill child: breastfeeding implications. In: Wambach K, Spencer B, eds. *Breastfeeding and Human Lactation.* Jones & Bartlett Learning; 2021:619–73.

Pak-Gorstein S, Haq A, Graham E. Cultural influences on infant feeding practices. *Pediatr Rev.* 2009;30(1):11–21.

Palmer G. *The Politics of Breastfeeding: When Breasts are Bad for Business.* London: Pinter & Martin; 2009.

Palmquist AEL, Holdren SM, Fair CD. 'It was all taken away': lactation, embodiment, and resistance among mothers caring for their very-low-birth-weight infants in the neonatal intensive care unit. *Soc Sci Med.* 2020;244:112648.

Pang WW, Hartmann PE. Initiation of human lactation: secretory differentiation and secretory activation. *J Mammary Gland Biol Neoplasia.* 2007; 12(4):211–21. doi: 10.1007/s10911-007-9054-4.

Paul IM, Schaefer E., Miller JR, et al. Weight change nomograms for the first month after birth. *Pediatrics.* 2016; 138(6):e20162625. doi:10.1542/peds.2016-2625.

Peila C, Moro GE, Bertino E, et al. The effect of Holder pasteurization on nutrients and biologically-active components in donor human milk: a review. *Nutrients.* 2016;8(8):477.

Perl SH, Uzan-Yulzari A, Klainer H, et al. SARS-CoV-2–specific antibodies in breastmilk after COVID-19 vaccination of breastfeeding women. *JAMA.* 2021. doi:10.1001/jama.2021.5782.

Pincombe J, Baghurst P, Antoniou G, et al. Baby Friendly Hospital Initiative practices and breastfeeding duration in a cohort of first-time mothers in Adelaide, Australia. *Midwifery.* 2008;24(1):55–61.

Pineda R, Dewey K, Jacobsen A, et al. Non-nutritive sucking in the preterm infant. *Am J Perinatol.* 2019;36(3):268–276.

Pokhrel S, Quigley MA, Fox-Rushby J, et al. Potential economic impacts from improving breastfeeding rates in the UK. *Arch Dis Child.* 2014;100(4):334–340. doi:10.1136/archdischild-2014-306701.

Prameela K, Vijaya L. The importance of breastfeeding in rotaviral diarrhoeas. *Malays J Nutr.* 2012;18(1):103–111.

Prime D, Geddes D, Hepworth A, et al. Comparison of the patterns of milk ejection during repeated breast expression sessions in women. *Breastfeed Med.* 2011;6(4):183–190.

Public Health Association Australia. *Breastfeeding background paper.* 2019. Online: https://www.phaa.net.au/documents/item/3820.

Raj S, Faridi M, Rusia U, Singh O. A prospective study of iron status in exclusively breastfed term infants up to 6 months of age. *Int Breastfeed J.* 2008;3(3). doi:10.1186/1746-4358-3-3.

Renfrew MJ, Dyson L, McCormick F, et al. Breastfeeding promotion for infants in neonatal units: a systematic review. *Child Care Health Dev.* 2010;36(2):165–178.

Renfrew MJ, Pokhrel S, Quigley M, et al. Preventing Disease and Saving Resources: The Potential Contribution of Increasing Breastfeeding Rates in the UK. UNICEF UK commissioned report. 2012a.

Renfrew MJ, McCormick F, Wade A, et al. Support for healthy breastfeeding mothers with healthy term babies. *Cochrane Database Syst Rev.* 2012b;(5):CD001141. doi:10.1002/14651858.CD001141.pub4.

Riordan J, Wambach K. *Breastfeeding and Human Lactation.* 4th ed. Boston: Jones & Bartlett; 2009.

Roll CL, & Cheater F. Expectant parents' views of factors influencing infant feeding decisions in the antenatal period: A systematic review. *Int J Nurs Stud.* 2016;60:145–155.

Rollins NC, Bhandari N, Hajeebhoy N, et al. Why invest, and what it will take to improve breastfeeding practices? *Lancet.* 2016;387(10017):491–504.

Royal Australian and New Zealand College of Obstetricians and Gynaecologists (RANZCOG). Covid-19 vaccine and breastfeeding infographic. Joint statement from RANZCOG, Australian Breastfeeding Association & the New Zealand Breastfeeding Alliance. April 2021.

Sabirov A, Casey J, Murphy J, et al. Breastfeeding is associated with a reduced frequency of acute otitis media and high serum antibody levels against NTHi and outer membrane protein vaccine antigen candidate P6. *Pediatr Res.* 2009;66(5): 565–570.

Schanler RJ. Human milk is the feeding strategy to prevent necrotizing enterocolitis. *Curr Pediatr Rep.* 2014;2(4):264–268.

Shenker, N. Maintaining safety and service provision in human milk banking: a call to action in response to the COVID-19 pandemic. *Lancet.* 2020. doi:10.1016/S2352-4642(20)30134-6.

Shenker N, Brown A. *Breastfeeding can help tackle climate change but it's on governments, not mums to save the world.* The Conversation; 2019;8 October. Online: https://theconversation.com/breastfeeding-can-help-tackle-climate-crisis-but-its-on-governments-not-mums-to-save-the-world-124676.

Schmied V, Beake S, Sheehan A, et al. Women's perceptions and experiences of breastfeeding support: a metasynthesis. *Birth.* 2011;38(1):49–60.

Schwarz EB. Infant feeding in America: enough to break a mother's heart? *Breastfeed Med.* 2013;8:454–457.

Schwarz EB, Ray RM, Stuebe AM, et al. Duration of lactation and risk factors for maternal cardiovascular disease. *Obstet Gynecol.* 2009;113(5):974–982.

Schwarz EB, Nothnagle M. The maternal health benefits of breastfeeding. *Am Fam Physician.* 2015;91(9):602–604.

Silano M, Paganin P, Davanzo R. Time for the 70 °C water precautionary option in the home dilution of powdered infant formula. *Ital J Pediatr.* 2016;42(17). doi:10.1186/s13052-016-0228-9.

Smith LJ. Postpartum care. In: Wambach K, Spencer B, eds. *Breastfeeding and Human Lactation.* Jones & Bartlett Learning; 2021:247–280.

Smith JP. Counting the cost of not breastfeeding is now easier, but women's unpaid health care work remains invisible. *Health Policy Plan.* 2019a;34(6):479–481.

Smith JP. A commentary on the carbon footprint of milk formula: Harms to planetary health and policy implications. *Int Breastfeed J.* 2019b;14(49):107.

Smriti A, Manju V, Vatsla D. A comparison of cabbage leaves vs. hot and cold compresses in the treatment of breast engorgement. *Indian J Community Med.* 2008;33(3):160–162.

Sobel H, Silvestre M, Mantaring JB 3rd, et al. Immediate newborn care practices delay thermoregulation and breastfeeding initiation. *Acta Paediatr.* 2011;100(8):1127–1133.

Spatz DL, Davanzo R, Müller JA, et al. Promoting and Protecting Human Milk and Breastfeeding in a COVID-19 World. *Front Pediatr.* 2021;8(633700). doi:10.3389 /fped.2020.633700.

Spencer B, Francis J. The composition and specificity of human milk. In: Wambach K, Spencer B, eds. *Breastfeeding and Human Lactation.* Jones & Bartlett Learning; 2021:85–126.

Stewart K, O'Reilly P. Exploring the attitudes, knowledge and beliefs of nurses and midwives of the healthcare needs of the LGBTQ population: An integrative review. *Nurse Educ Today.* 2017;53:76–77.

Stuebe AM. The risks of not breastfeeding for mothers and infants. *Rev Obstet Gynecol.* 2009;2(4):222–231.

Stuebe AM. Enabling women to achieve their breastfeeding goals. *Obstet Gynaecol.* 2014;123(2):643–652.

Stuebe AM, Rich-Edwards JW. The reset hypothesis: lactation and maternal metabolism. *Am J Perinatol.* 2009;26(1):81–88.

Stuebe, A. Should infants be separated from mothers with COVID-19? First, do no harm. *Breastfeed Med.* 2020;15(5):1–2.

Strong G. Provider management and support for breastfeeding. *J Obstet Gynaecol Neonatal Nurs.* 2011;40(6):753–764.

Su D, Pasalich M, Lee AH, et al. Ovarian cancer risk is reduced by prolonged lactation: a case-control study in southern China. *Am J Clin Nutr.* 2013;11(3):232–238.

Svensson KE, Velandia MI, Matthiesen A-S, et al. Effects of mother-infant skin-to-skin contact on severe latch-on problems in older infants: a randomized trial. *Int Breastfeed J.* 2013;8(1):1. doi:10.1186/1746-4358-8-1.

Sweet L. Expressed breastmilk as 'connection' and its influence on the construction of 'motherhood' for mothers of preterm infants: a qualitative study. *Int Breastfeed J.* 2008;3(30). doi:10.1186/1746-4358-3-30.

Swerts M, Westhof E, Bogaerts A, et al. Supporting breast-feeding women from the perspective of the midwife: A systematic review of the literature. *Midwifery.* 2016;37:32–40.

Szucs KA, Axline SE, Rosenman MB. Induced lactation and exclusive breastmilk feeding of adopted premature twins. *J Hum Lact.* 2010;26(3):309–313.

Taskforce on sudden infant death syndrome. SIDS and other sleep-related infant deaths: updated 2016 recommendations for a safe infant sleeping environment. *Pediatrics.* 2016;138(5):pii:e20162938.

Tomori C, Gribble K, Palmquist AEL, et al. When separation is not the answer: Breastfeeding mothers and infants affected by COVID-19. *Matern Child Nutr.* 2020;16(4):e13033. doi:10.1111/mcn.13033.

Tuc V, Camurdan A, Ilhan M, et al. Factors associated with defecation patterns in 0–24 month old children. *Eur J Pediatr.* 2008;167(12):1357–1362.

Tudehope D. Human milk and the nutritional needs of preterm infants. *J Pediatr.* 2013;162(3):S17–S25.

Underwood MA. Human milk for the premature infant. *Pediatr Clin North Am.* 2013; 60(1):189–207. doi:10.1016/j.pcl.2012.09.008.

United Nations International Children's Emergency Fund (UNICEF). Innocenti Declaration: On the Protection, Promotion and Support of Breastfeeding. 1990.

United Nations International Children's Emergency Fund (UNICEF). Innocenti Declaration 2005: On Infant and Young Child Feeding. 2005

United Nations International Children's Fund (UNICEF). *Breast Crawl, Initiation of Breastfeeding by Breastcrawl.* Mumbai, India: UNICEF; 2007.

United Nations International Children's Fund (UNICEF) UK Baby Friendly Initiative. *The Evidence and Rationale for the UNICEF UK Baby Friendly Initiative Standards.* London: UNICEF UK; 2013.

United Nations International Children's Fund (UNICEF) UK Baby Friendly Initiative. Responsive feeding: Supporting close and loving relationships. 2016.

United Nations International Children's Fund (UNICEF) UK Baby Friendly Initiative. Statement on Vitamin D Supplementation for Breastfed Babies (infosheet). 2017.

Uvnäs-Moberg K, Handlin L, Petersson M. Self-soothing behaviors with particular reference to oxytocin release induced by non-noxious sensory stimulation. *Front Psychol.* 2014;5:1529.

Van Tulleken C, Wright C, Brown A, et al. Marketing of breastmilk substitutes during the COVID-19 pandemic. *Lancet.* 2020;396:e58.

Victora CG, Bahl R, Barros AJD, et al. Breastfeeding in the 21st century: epidemiology, mechanisms, and lifelong effect. *Lancet.* 2016;387(10017):475–490.

Walker M. International breastfeeding initiatives and their relevance to the current state of breastfeeding in the United States. *J Midwifery Womens Health.* 2007;52(6):549–555.

Walker M. Maternal pathology: breast and nipple issues. In: Walker M, eds. *Breastfeeding Management for the Clinician using the Evidence.* 2nd ed. Sudbury, England: Jones & Bartlett; 2009:550–551. (Ch. 8).

Walker S, Armstrong M. The four pillars of safe breastmilk sharing. *Midwifery Today*. 2012;S101:34–36.
Walsh A, Pincombe J, Henderson A. An examination of maternity staff attitudes towards implementing Baby Friendly Health Initiative (BFHI) accreditation in Australia. *Matern Child Health J*. 2011;15(5):597–609.
Walters DD, Phan LTH, Mathisen R. The cost of not breastfeeding: global results from a new tool. *Health Policy Plan*. 2019;34(6): 407–417. doi:10.1093/heapol/czz050.
Wambach K. Breast-related problems. In: Wambach K, Spencer B, eds. *Breastfeeding and Human Lactation*. Jones & Bartlett Learning; 2021:281–312.
Wambach K, Watson Genna C. Anatomy and physiology of lactation. In: Wambach K, Spencer B, eds. *Breastfeeding and Human Lactation*. Jones & Bartlett Learning; 2021:49–83.
Wang Y, Zhao T, Zhang Y, Li S., Cong X. Positive effects of kangaroo mother care on long-term breastfeeding rates, growth, and neurodevelopment in preterm infants. *Breastfeed Med*. 2021;16(4):282–291.
Watt J, & Mead J. What paediatricians need to know about breastfeeding. *Paediatr Child Health*. 2013;23(8):362–366.
West D, Marasco L. *The Breastfeeding Mother's Guide to Making More Milk*. New York: McGraw Hill; 2009.
Whitford HM, Wallis SK, Dowswell T, et al. Breastfeeding education and support for women with twins or higher order multiples. *Cochrane Database Syst Rev*. 2017;2(2):CD012003. doi:10.1002/14651858.CD012003.pub2.
Widström A, Wahlberg V, Matthiesen A, et al. Short-term effects of early suckling and touch of the nipple of maternal behaviour. *Early Human Dev*. 1990;21(3):153–163.
Widström A, Lilja G, Aaltomaa-Michalias P, et al. Newborn behaviour to locate the breast when skin-to-skin: a possible method for enabling early self-regulation. *Acta Paediatr*. 2011;100(1): 79–85.
Widström A-M, Brimdyr K, Svensson K, et al. Skin-to-skin contact in the first hour after birth, underlying implications and clinical practice. *Acta Paediatrica*. 2019;108(7):1192–1204.
Widström A-M, Brimdyr K, Svensson K, et al. A plausible pathway of imprinted behaviours: Skin to skin actions of the newborn immediately after birth follow the order of fetal development and intrauterine training of movements. *Med Hypotheses*. 2020;134. doi:10.1016/j.mehy.2019.109432.
Wight NE, Morton KA, Kim JH. *Best Medicine: Human Milk in the NICU*. Amarillo: Hale; 2008.
Wilson-Clay B, Hoover K. *The Breastfeeding Atlas*. 4th ed. Manachaca, TX: Lactnet News Press; 2008.
World Breastfeeding Trends Initiative Australia. *Assessment Report Australia 2018*. 2018. Online: https://www.worldbreastfeedingtrends.org/uploads/country-data/country-report/WBTi-Australia-2018.pdf.
World Health Organization (WHO). *International Code of Marketing of Breastmilk Substitutes*. Geneva, Switzerland: WHO; 1981.
World Health Organization (WHO). *Global Strategy for Infant and Young Child Feeding*. Geneva, Switzerland: WHO; 2003.
World Health Organization (WHO). Infant and Young Child Feeding Counselling: An Integrated Course, p.19 (c) WHO; 2006.
World Health Organization (WHO). *Safe Preparation, Storage and Handling of Powdered Infant Formula: Guidelines*. Geneva, Switzerland: WHO; 2007.
World Health Organization (WHO). *Information Concerning the Use and Marketing of Follow-up Formula*. Geneva, Switzerland: WHO; 2013.
World Health Organization (WHO). *Infant Feeding in Areas of Zika Virus Transmission*. Geneva, Switzerland: WHO; 2016a
World Health Organization (WHO). *Guidance on Ending Inappropriate Promotion of Foods for Infants and Young Children*. Geneva, Switzerland: WHO; 2016b.
World Health Organization (WHO). *The International Code of Marketing of Breast-Milk Substitutes: Frequently Asked Questions*. Geneva, Switzerland: WHO; 2017.
World Health Organization (WHO). *Marketing of breastmilk substitutes: national implementation of the international code, status report*. Geneva, Switzerland: WHO/UNICEF/ IBFAN; 2020a.
World Health Organization (WHO). *Competency verification toolkit: Ensuring competency of direct care providers to implement the Baby-Friendly Hospital Initiative*. Geneva, Switzerland: WHO; 2020b. Online: https://www.who.int/publications/i/item/9789240008854.
World Health Organization (WHO). *Clinical management of severe acute respiratory infection (SARI) when COVID19 disease is suspected*. Geneva, Switzerland: WHO; 2020c.
World Health Organization (WHO). *Infant feeding for the prevention of mother-to-child transmission of HIV*. Geneva, Switzerland: WHO; 2021. Online: https://www.who.int/elena/titles/hiv_infant_feeding/en/.
World Health Organization (WHO)/UNICEF. *Protecting, Promoting and Supporting Breastfeeding: The Special Role of Maternity Services. A Joint WHO/UNICEF Statement*. Geneva, Switzerland: WHO; 1989.
World Health Organization (WHO)/UNICEF. *Acceptable Medical Reasons for Use of Breast-Milk Substitutes*. Geneva, Switzerland: WHO; 2009.
World Health Organization (WHO)/UNICEF. *Protecting, promoting, and supporting breastfeeding in facilities providing maternity and newborn services: the revised Baby-friendly Hospital Initiative 2018: Implementation guidance*. Geneva, Switzerland: WHO/UNICEF; 2018.
World Health Organization (WHO)/UNICEF. *Protecting, promoting and supporting breastfeeding: The Baby Friendly Hospital Initiative for Small, Sick and Preterm Newborns*. Geneva, Switzerland: WHO; 2020.
World Health Organization (WHO)/UNICEF/IBFAN. *Marketing of Breast-milk Substitutes: National Implementation of the International Code Status Report 2016*. Geneva, Switzerland: WHO; 2016.
Wright A, Elcombe E, Burns ES. 'Paper, face-to-face and on my mobile please': A survey of women's preferred methods of receiving antenatal education. *Women Birth*. 2020;S1871–5192(20) 30371-1. doi:10.1016/j.wombi.2020.10.014.
Xiao-Ming B. Nutritional management of newborn infants: practical guidelines. *World J Gastroenterol*. 2008;14(40): 6133–6139.
Young, C. 'Clickbait headlines as the media fails mothers (again)'. Analytical Armadillo blog post. 2018. Online: www.analyticalarmadillo.co.uk/search?q=RCM.
Zakarija-Grković, I., Cattaneo, A., Bettinelli, M.E. et al. Are our babies off to a healthy start? The state of implementation of the Global strategy for infant and young child feeding in Europe. *Int Breastfeed J*. 2020;15(51): https://doi.org/10.1186/s13006-020-00282-z
Zizzo G, Amir LH, Moore V, et al. The risk-risk trade-offs: Understanding factors that influence women's decision to use substances to boost breastmilk supply. *PLoS ONE*. 2021;16(5): e0249599.
Zuppa AA, Tornesello A, Papacci P, et al. Relationship between maternal parity, basal prolactin levels and neonatal breastmilk intake. *Neonatology*. 1988;53:144–147. doi:10.1159/000242775.

CHAPTER 33

Pharmacology and prescribing

Marion Hunter and Deborah Davis

LEARNING OUTCOMES

Learning outcomes for this chapter are:

1. To discuss the scope of midwifery practice in relation to prescribing medicines and the legislation associated with the prescription of medicines
2. To revise pharmacological concepts that inform the prescription of medicines and discuss the safety of medicines in pregnancy
3. To revise pharmaceutical medicines commonly used in maternity care
4. To review the use of antimicrobials in relation to maternity care and midwives' responsibility for minimising bacterial resistance
5. To examine the evidence in relation to accurate assessment, diagnosis and prescription of medicines related to the midwifery scope of prescribing
6. To be able to accurately prescribe appropriate medicines as part of autonomous midwifery practice.

CHAPTER OVERVIEW

In this chapter, the scope of midwifery practice is discussed with respect to independent prescribing. The authors assume that readers have current pharmacology knowledge and a comprehensive knowledge of normal and complicated childbirth. The discussion in this chapter is limited to pharmaceutical medicines and does not cover the use of complementary or non-pharmaceutical therapies. The authors acknowledge that prescription of medicines is always evolving according to evidence, availability of pharmaceuticals and cost. Midwife prescribers have an obligation to maintain a current knowledge of the safety of medicines in pregnancy and lactation, and of preferred pharmaceuticals for particular conditions.

KEY TERMS

dependent prescribing
independent or autonomous prescribing
over-the-counter (OTC)
pharmacodynamics
pharmacokinetics
therapeutic range

INTRODUCTION

Prescribing for women during pregnancy and lactation requires caution, as nearly all medicines transfer to the fetus or neonate. Knowledge and understanding of pharmacological concepts is essential for the administration or prescription of pharmaceuticals. Prescription of antimicrobials during childbirth should take account of increasing concerns over bacterial resistance. Common conditions in pregnancy are discussed, and research evidence is considered, in order to inform the prescription of medicines. In concluding this chapter, guidelines are given for midwife prescribers and for accurate prescription writing.

SCOPE OF MIDWIFERY PRESCRIBING

Dependent prescribing is prescribing according to standing orders or protocols where authority remains with the medical practitioner, whereas **independent or autonomous prescribing** occurs when the healthcare practitioner has the legal authority to issue prescription medicines. In Australia, midwives who meet the criteria set out by the Nursing and Midwifery Board of Australia (NMBA) (the Board) can apply to be endorsed for scheduled medicines. This endorsement means:

> *... that the midwife has met the requirements of the NMBA Registration Standard: Endorsement for scheduled medicines for midwives and is qualified to prescribe scheduled medicines and provide associated services required for midwifery practice in accordance with relevant state and territory legislation.*
> (NMBA, 2020)

The requirements include current general registration as a midwife, certain minimum clinical practice experiences and completion of a program of study focusing on prescribing that is approved by the Board. Endorsement relates to a context of care which includes across the continuum of care, antenatal, intrapartum, postnatal and lactation support. There are also a number of requirements that midwives must meet in order to maintain endorsement for scheduled medicines (NMBA, 2017). Endorsement enables midwives to prescribe Schedule 2, 3, 4 and 8 medicines as appropriate to the scope of midwifery practice. However, as the prescribing authority is conferred by Australian state and territory legislation the scope of midwifery prescribing varies depending on state and territory (NMBA, 2017). Midwives seeking endorsement in Australia, or those interested in more detail, should refer to the NMBA.

Midwives in Aotearoa New Zealand (NZ) undertake independent prescribing, and the Midwifery Council of New Zealand (MCNZ) expects all registered midwives to demonstrate competence in independent prescribing. Competency 2.13 (MCNZ, 2007) indicates that a midwife must demonstrate the ability to prescribe, supply and administer medicine, vaccines, and immunoglobulins safely and appropriately within the midwife's scope of practice and the relevant legislation.

Midwives in NZ gained lawful prescribing rights initially through the passage of the *Nurses Amendment Act 1990*, which included amendments to the *Misuse of Drugs Act 1975* and the *Medicines Act 1981*. The *Medicines Amendment Regulations (2011)* superseded the 1990 amendment to *Medicines Regulations (1984)*. There is no defined list of medicines that a NZ midwife may prescribe except for controlled drugs. The *Misuse of Drugs Amendment Regulations (2014)* specify that midwives can prescribe the controlled drugs pethidine, morphine and fentanyl. The Midwifery Council of New Zealand's statement on the scope of practice of the midwife in regard to the prescription of controlled drugs provides further information and restricts midwife prescribing of fentanyl to secondary or tertiary maternity facilities with available medical back-up services.

Shortly after legislation was amended in 1990 to allow for midwife prescribing, the Department of Health NZ circulated a guide to the *Nurses Amendment Act 1990* stating that midwifery prescribing would not include the treatment of underlying medical conditions such as asthma or hypertension, and that 'it would also not include the prescribing of medicines such as antibiotics or oral contraceptives' (Department of Health, 1990, p. 5). However, caseloading midwives found the latter restriction untenable. It imposed additional expense on women to consult a doctor in order to obtain medicines such as the progestogen-only contraceptive pill, or antibiotics for an uncomplicated urinary tract infection (UTI). The New Zealand College of Midwives (NZCOM) challenged the restrictions on prescribing and during 1995 the Ministry of Health (MOH) agreed that there was no legal basis for restricting the prescription of antibiotics and oral contraceptives and that it may indeed be appropriate for these to be prescribed by midwives during the course of providing antenatal, intrapartum and postnatal care (K Guilliland, personal communication, 1998).

The NZCOM Consensus Statement on Prescribing (NZCOM, 2014a) notes that midwives can prescribe for conditions commonly associated with uncomplicated pregnancy, labour and the postnatal period, up to 6 weeks after the birth of the baby. Midwives need to have knowledge of the effects, side effects and contraindications of medicines prescribed and prescribe within their knowledge and expertise. In relation to prescribing of opioid analgesia intrapartum, the NZCOM strongly discourages the use of opioids during labour at home and cautions that opioid analgesia administered intravenously can have immediate and significant respiratory depressant effects on the labouring woman (NZCOM, 2014b). The necessity for these types of medications is an indication for transfer to hospital. If an opioid is prescribed within a maternity setting, this must be discussed with the woman and the midwife must have the equipment and skills necessary to cope with the effects of this medication.

In the latter half of this chapter, specific conditions are discussed in relation to midwifery prescribing. The authors do not consider that all pregnancy-related conditions warrant treatment by midwives. Conditions such as severe morning sickness require careful assessment and consultation with an obstetrician; particular caution is required regarding safety of medication along with ensuring the woman maintains electrolyte balance.

Obstetric doctors need to prescribe adequate postoperative analgesia for women who have experienced caesarean birth. Independent prescribing of antidepressants, and medication for asthma or hypertension, are beyond the scope of midwifery practice. It is important that midwives do not issue prescriptions for medicines outside their scope of practice. Auditing processes can identify the practitioner who wrote the prescription and the types of medicines prescribed. Additional expertise is required for prescribing for unwell neonates owing to the immaturity of the neonate liver and renal system. In most cases medical practitioners prescribe any required systemic antibiotics (and paracetamol when indicated).

SAFETY OF MEDICINES DURING PREGNANCY AND LACTATION

Medication use during pregnancy should be restricted according to necessity, and to the use of medicines for which prior clinical evidence is available. The first trimester of pregnancy is considered the most critical period for teratogenic effects. After the first 11 weeks, exposure to teratogens will generally have an effect on the nervous system, gonadal tissue (due to slower development than other organs) or general growth restriction; however, little is known about ongoing effects of medication on neurological development and metabolic function (Al-Zidan, 2020). Vigilance is also necessary when midwives prescribe medicines during lactation. Resources should be utilised to ascertain the safety of medicines and midwives need to be aware of inconsistency in some web-based information.

The Swedish Catalogue of Approved Drugs, Australian Therapeutic Goods Administration (TGA) and US Federal Drug Administration (FDA) developed comprehensive systems for classifying drug safety. In 2015, the FDA created the 'Pregnancy and Lactation Labeling Rule' (PLLR) that abolished the letter-rating system for drug safety during pregnancy and lactation and replaced it with narrative-based labelling requirements. The letter-based system was considered oversimplified and erroneously implied that risk increases from A to X, with drugs in the same categories carrying the same risks (Al-Zidan, 2020).

The Therapeutic Goods Administration (TGA, n.d.) Australian Prescribing Medicines in Pregnancy Database provides additional narrative information to guide the prescriber noting where human data are lacking or inadequate for some medicines.

Prescribers are guided in addition by the Australian Quality Use of Medicines (http://www.health.gov.au/internet/main/publishing.nsf/Content/nmp-quality.htm), which refers to principles including selecting management options wisely, choosing a suitable medicine when indicated that a medicine is necessary and using medicines safely and effectively to achieve the best results. During pregnancy in particular, prescribers need to pose the questions of whether the drug is considered safe for this gestation and if the drug is necessary to treat the condition. Thalidomide is well known as the prototype for teratogens (Al-Zidan, 2020). Thalidomide prescribed to pregnant women in the late 1950s to relieve nausea and vomiting resulted in babies born with congenital anomalies particularly phocomelia, meaning short limbs, and this catastrophic effect shook the perception that the placenta provides a barrier to drugs. Drug licensing was less rigorous in the 1950s–1960s, and it was the compilation of case reports that established the link between thalidomide and infant deformities.

REFLECTIVE THINKING EXERCISE

Refer to the Australian Government TGA website Prescribing Medicines in Pregnancy Database (https://www.tga.gov.au/prescribing-medicines-pregnancy-database) and then answer the questions below.

1. Explain in your own words how medicines are classified during pregnancy in relation to safety.
2. List medicines commonly used during pregnancy and childbirth and the category or safety of each drug.
3. Review your personal habits regarding the use of pharmaceuticals in relation to pain, flu, or mild infections.
4. Discuss your personal biases with regard to medicine use during pregnancy and childbirth (e.g. women experiencing vomiting, women wishing to use antacids, or laxatives regularly).

Medication history

Studies show that many women use medicines prescribed during pregnancy as well as **over-the-counter (OTC)** and complementary and alternative medicines (CAM), which include, for example, herbal remedies. In a multinational study that included Australia, Lupattelli et al. (2014) found that over 80% of women reported use of at least one medication (prescribed or OTC) in pregnancy; these included analgesics, antacids, nasal decongestants/antiallergics and systemic antibiotics. It has also been found that a high proportion of pregnant women use CAM and that many do not disclose this to their caregiver. In one US-based study over 30% of pregnant women used CAM, with only half reporting this to their conventional caregiver (Holden et al., 2015).

From the data above, it appears there is a high prevalence of medicine and CAM use during pregnancy and therefore it is important that midwives establish a rapport with women regarding safety of medicines during pregnancy, particularly with the availability of OTC pharmaceuticals and CAM. It is also important that all caregivers are aware of the medications and other preparations (such as herbs) that women are taking as this may have implications for practice. Prescribers need to be aware of potential drug interactions (or interactions between herbal preparations and medicines like, for example, antidepressants and St John's wort). Prescribers need to be aware also when clinical signs might be masked by certain medicines (e.g. beta blockers and tachycardia), when symptoms might relate to the effects of medications or when results of investigations might be altered by the effect of medications. Understanding of the medicines the woman has taken previously and her response (including allergies) is helpful for planning future pharmacological treatment if it becomes necessary. Accurate and comprehensive documentation of the woman's medication history in her clinical notes is important in preventing avoidable errors such as medicine duplication (if, for example, the woman presents to a different caregiver for a health concern) or drug interactions.

Safe prescribing and good midwifery care are facilitated by a comprehensive medication history.

This includes: reviewing sources of available medicine information (e.g. medication containers), interviewing the woman about her medicines, verifying the history with one or more sources of information (e.g. community pharmacy, online systems) and recording the information in the woman's clinical record. The history should include all prescribed, OTC and CAM medicines and preparations (e.g. vitamins, minerals, herbs) taken in any form and by any route (e.g. tablets, pessaries, inhalers, patches, creams, injectables, eye/nose drops, sprays), with details of dose, route and frequency of each preparation and how well the woman is adhering to a prescribed medication (she may not be taking a medication as prescribed, for example). A comprehensive medication history is the first step in safe prescribing.

PRINCIPLES OF PHARMACOLOGY

Some key concepts are reviewed here. For a more extensive discussion, a pharmacology text should be consulted.

Pharmacokinetics

Pharmacokinetics is the term used to describe how drugs are absorbed, distributed, metabolised and eliminated by the body.

Absorption

In most cases, when a drug is administered to a person it has to be absorbed into the bloodstream before the molecules can be distributed around the body to the site of action. Absorption via the gastrointestinal tract is a complex process, as age, body mass, activity and fullness of the stomach can affect both the amount and the rate at which drugs are absorbed. Decreased gastrointestinal motility can increase or decrease drug absorption during pregnancy, and vomiting could mean that the drug is not absorbed at all (Bryant et al., 2019). Once the drug is dissolved in the gastrointestinal tract, the molecules can be absorbed. Because plasma membranes primarily consist of lipid substances, drug molecules generally need to be lipophilic (having an affinity with lipids) to pass through into the capillaries (Visovsky et al., 2019).

Distribution

Hepatic portal system

As with most other digested substances, drugs are absorbed from the intestine into the hepatic circulation via the portal vein. Therefore, before the drug molecules can reach the general circulation, they must pass through the liver. This is known as the *hepatic first pass*. At this point, a proportion of drug molecules can be metabolised and excreted by the liver. Drugs that have a significant proportion of molecules metabolised in this way are said to have a high hepatic first pass (Bryant et al., 2019).

Some of the metabolites from the liver are excreted into the small intestine via the bile duct. Bile salts are excreted in this way. The body uses intestinal bacteria to recycle bile salts. The bacteria deconjugate the bile salts, allowing them to be reabsorbed from the small intestine so that they can be conjugated again in the liver, excreted back into the small intestine and used once again in the normal digestion process. This is known as the *enterohepatic cycle*. A proportion of drug molecules metabolised in the liver on the hepatic first pass are excreted into the intestine, where they are also recycled by undergoing the process of deconjugation, reabsorption from the gut and then passing through the hepatic circulation a second time. Oestrogen (estrogen) in the combined oral contraceptive pill is an example of a drug that is affected in this way (Bryant et al., 2019).

General circulation

Once the molecules reach the general circulation, they are distributed to the site of action. Highly soluble drugs are carried in the plasma as free molecules in solution. Less-soluble drugs are carried partially bound to plasma protein molecules. Only drug molecules that are free in solution are pharmacologically active. They cannot bind to the receptor sites in the body while still bound to the serum protein. The levels of free and protein-bound drug molecules are in equilibrium. This means that drug molecules that are bound to protein molecules are released and become active as the free molecules are used. Therefore drugs that are distributed in the body partially bound to protein molecules take longer to be released to the receptor sites. The partially bound drug is pharmacologically active for longer than a highly soluble drug that has all its molecules available to the receptor sites and all its molecules available for metabolism by the liver at the same time. Drug distribution in the body may be affected by the physiological increase both in maternal plasma volume and in body fat during pregnancy (Bryant et al., 2019). This does not generally affect dosage regimens.

Decreased serum albumin can decrease protein binding of drugs and might be relevant for monitoring of drug concentrations such as phenytoin (Bryant et al., 2019). Phenytoin concentrations during pregnancy are extremely complicated and specialist interpretation of serum levels is necessary.

The blood–brain barrier and the placenta are barriers to distribution. For further information on this topic, see Bryant et al., 2019.

Metabolism and excretion

If the drug molecules remain lipophilic they will be reabsorbed at the nephron tubules or returned to the gut from the liver. Therefore, drugs are metabolised in the liver to make them water soluble (polar) so they can be excreted from the body. Two types of enzyme are involved in metabolism of drugs. The first type (sometimes called phase I) modifies the drug by chemical processes such as oxidation, reduction or hydrolysis to make water-soluble metabolites. The cytochrome P450 family of enzymes found in abundance in the hepatocytes is responsible for most of these reactions. Induction or inhibition of drug metabolism during pregnancy is dependent on the specific P450 enzymes involved. During pregnancy, metabolism of caffeine is decreased, whereas that of phenytoin is increased. Codeine is an example of a drug that is partially metabolised in the liver by a P450 enzyme. Genetic differences in the enzyme mean that some people metabolise codeine very rapidly (ultrarapid metabolisers), whereas others metabolise codeine at a slower rate than normal. Ultrarapid metabolism can result in very high blood levels and symptoms of overdose (see section on codeine in this chapter), whereas slow metabolism results in ineffective analgesia.

The second type of enzyme (phase II) conjugates the drug molecules, or a phase I metabolite, with a polar molecule such as glucuronic acid, rendering the molecule water soluble for excretion. Conjugation enzymes belong to the transferase family. Midwives will be familiar with the physiological process in neonates whereby excess lipophilic bilirubin molecules are conjugated to water-soluble molecules by the enzyme glucuronyl transferase in the liver (Bryant et al., 2019). Drugs are mainly excreted in the bile and urine; other routes include the lungs, sweat and saliva, and breast milk in lactating women (Visovsky et al., 2019). Drugs that are very water soluble are excreted virtually unchanged into the urine. This can be helpful when treating bacterial infections of the lower urinary tract.

Drug clearance and elimination may be increased during pregnancy owing to an increase in liver and renal blood flow. The glomerular filtration rate increases from early pregnancy and remains elevated throughout the pregnancy. Dosage adjustment may be required in some cases (Bryant et al., 2019).

Bioavailability

Bioavailability is the amount of drug that is available to the receptor sites. When injected intravenously, 100% of the drug is available, but when given orally some of the drug is lost during the absorption and hepatic-first-pass processes. Therefore, a smaller dose is usually required when the intravenous route is used (e.g. doses of opioids). Antibiotic therapy is the most common exception, as these drugs act directly on bacteria, not on body cells (Bryant et al., 2019).

Plasma concentration

Plasma concentration is the measure of a specific amount of drug in a specific volume of plasma (e.g. mmol/L). Measurement of plasma concentration is one of the ways that therapeutic levels of drugs can be monitored (Bryant et al., 2019). The time taken after a dose of a drug to reach maximum plasma concentration is affected by absorption, distribution, metabolism and elimination rates. Drugs given orally take longer than those administered intravenously to reach peak plasma concentration. The plasma concentration is related to the therapeutic effect.

Therapeutic range

In order to produce a clinical effect, a certain level of drug needs to be present in the general circulation. This level is called the *minimum effective concentration* (MEC) and is different for each drug. For all drugs there is also a level beyond which the drug will produce adverse effects on the person; this is known as the *maximum safe concentration* (MSC). The range between the MEC and the MSC that is associated with drug efficacy is known as the **therapeutic range**. Most drugs have a wide therapeutic range, which means that the serum levels will not normally rise to toxic levels when the usual size and frequency of dose is taken. However, a significant number of drugs, especially anticonvulsants and antibiotics from the aminoglycoside family (e.g. gentamicin), have a narrow therapeutic range. This means that it is possible for serum levels to rise to toxic levels even with normal dose and frequency regimens. People being treated with drugs that have a narrow therapeutic range need to have the serum levels of the drug regularly monitored so that, if necessary, the dose can be adjusted to maintain effectiveness without causing toxicity (Bryant et al., 2019).

Half-life

The length of time for which a drug is clinically effective in the body is called its *half-life*. Half-life is the length of time it takes to reduce the amount of drug in the circulation by half. For example, 500 mg of a drug that has a half-life of 4 hours will reduce to 250 mg 4 hours after administration, to 125 mg after another 4 hours, and so on. Although there are still active molecules of the drug in the body after 4 hours (in this example), the clinical effectiveness of the drug has been significantly reduced. This principle guides recommendations for the frequency of doses. Doses are given at the half-life interval (e.g. 4-hourly in the above example) (Bryant et al., 2019).

Steady-state concentration

The aim of dosing regimens is to achieve a steady-state concentration—that is, to maintain a constant concentration

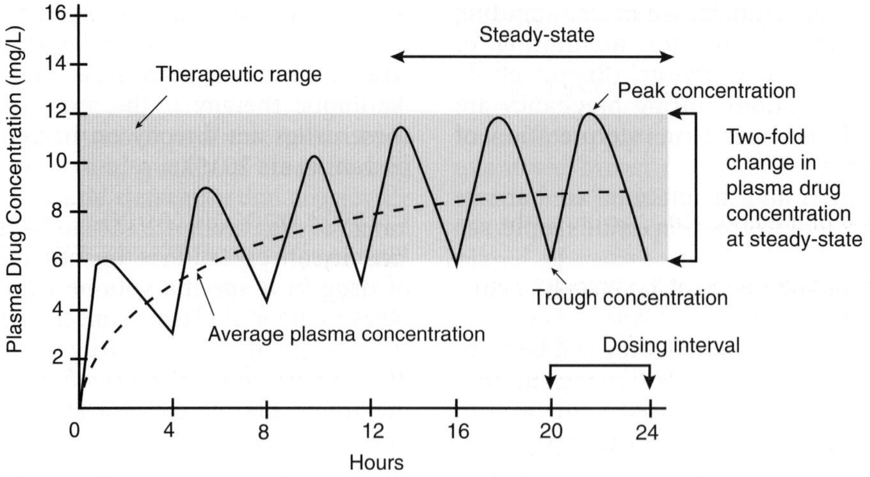

FIGURE 33.1 Achieving a steady state. The medicine in this example has a half-life of 4 hours.
(Source: Based on Bryant et al., 2019)

of the drug in the plasma that is consistent with a therapeutic response in the person (Fig. 33.1). In most cases, when a steady-state concentration is reached, the maintenance dose rate is equal to the elimination rate—that is, it is in equilibrium. Drugs are given at half-life intervals to reach a steady-state concentration. It takes several half-lives for an optimal steady state (Bryant et al., 2019). A *loading dose* is sometimes given when it is imperative to reach therapeutic plasma levels quickly (e.g. in severe infections). A loading dose is a larger dose than the maintenance dose. Loading doses are calculated by multiplying the volume of distribution and the target plasma concentration. While loading doses are often twice the ongoing dose, the desired plasma concentration and the apparent volume of distribution for individual drugs must be taken into account (Bryant et al., 2019). The initial dose is sometimes given parenterally, followed by oral administration of maintenance doses. Some antibiotics that are administered intravenously may have a loading dose prescribed. Women with infections severe enough to require a loading dose of antibiotics are generally hospitalised.

Pharmacodynamics

Pharmacodynamics is the term used to describe the action of a drug on the body. Nearly all drugs act on receptors in the body (antimicrobials act on microorganisms) by binding to a protein. Most drugs have some selectivity—that is, they 'see' or 'fit' particular receptors as targets. Generally, drugs act on four main types of regulatory proteins: carriers, enzymes, ion channels and transcription factors (Burchum & Rosenthan, 2019).

Carriers transport ions and small, poorly fat-soluble molecules across plasma membranes. Examples are carriers that uptake noradrenaline (norepinephrine) and serotonin at the nerve terminals. Drugs that target carriers usually inhibit carrier-mediated uptake of such transmitters (e.g. tricyclic antidepressants) (Bryant et al., 2019).

Enzymes are biological catalysts that control cellular biochemical reactions. Drugs that interact with enzymes inhibit or alter the biochemical reaction. The sulfonamide group of drugs, which includes the drug trimethoprim, is an example.

Ions are transported in and out of cells through specific channels in the plasma membrane so that the electrochemical gradient across the plasma membrane can be maintained. Drugs that interact with receptors to block the ion channels are widely used. These drugs generally have a high selectivity. Nifedipine, used for the control of hypertension, for example, is a calcium ion channel blocker that affects the arterioles, but has little effect on cardiac muscle and no effect on the transport of other ions such as sodium (Bryant et al., 2019).

Receptors are specific proteins usually found on or in the cell's plasma membrane. Drug molecules selectively bind with receptors in a 'lock-and-key' effect. Drugs that temporarily bind to receptors and stimulate the cell to carry out its normal biochemical actions are known as *agonists*, whereas those that bind to the receptors to temporarily block or inhibit the normal cell process are referred to as *antagonists*. Drugs called 'blockers' are antagonists. The beta-blocker labetalol is an example.

ANTIMICROBIALS

Midwives require a thorough understanding of antimicrobials, not only for prescribing and administration purposes, but also to encourage health-promoting activities in childbearing families. Opportunities to reinforce information about judicious use of antibiotics, recognising adverse effects and preventing the development of resistant bacteria, arise in the course of midwifery practice. Box 33.1 gives some prescription guidelines.

Midwives tend not to independently prescribe for infections that require intravenous antibiotics; guidance (from obstetric service/National Formulary) should be

Box 33.1 Prescription guidelines

To ensure accurate prescription of a pharmaceutical medicine:

- use accurate physical examination and diagnostic skills
- consider whether a pharmaceutical is appropriate for the condition
- have comprehensive knowledge of 'commonly' used drugs, including action/effect, and communicate this information to the woman
- ensure that the treatment is regarded as safe during pregnancy or during lactation
- consider the evidence in relation to the clinical scenario
- prescribe the appropriate drug, dose, frequency and duration of treatment
- monitor for any adverse reactions and refer accordingly
- do follow-up culture and sensitivity and alter drug if necessary
- be able to research information about drugs used less commonly
- have a low threshold for consultation with an obstetrician or general medical practitioner.

(Source: Adapted from Banning, 2004)

sought for conditions such as pyelonephritis or prophylactic antibiotics for cardiac conditions. Neonates with symptoms suggestive of systemic infection should be promptly referred to the paediatric service (or a medical practitioner in areas without a paediatric service). Neonates have immature liver enzymes and renal system, and therefore have limited ability to metabolise and excrete drugs. They can also become seriously ill very quickly. Referral should not be delayed.

Antimicrobials are groups of drugs that destroy or restrict the proliferation of infectious microorganisms. They work by inhibiting cell wall synthesis, disrupting plasma membrane permeability, interfering with the organism's metabolic processes, or by inhibiting protein synthesis in the organism.

Bacteriocidal antimicrobials destroy the organism and bacteriostatic drugs hinder bacterial growth, giving the body a longer period in which to mobilise its own defences. Antibiotics are used to treat bacterial infections. Other antimicrobials include antiviral, antifungal and antimycobacterial agents.

Antimicrobial stewardship

Midwives need to be cognisant of antimicrobial stewardship, alert to bacterial resistance and should base practice on research evidence. Comprehensive assessment, appropriate investigations and accurate diagnoses are essential to prevent either unnecessary exposure to antibiotics or, conversely, undertreatment.

Spectrum of activity

The number of types of organisms that are sensitive to a particular antibiotic is what determines its spectrum of activity. Antibiotics to which only a few groups of organisms are sensitive are said to have a narrow spectrum of activity, whereas those that are effective against a wide range of organisms are said to have a broad spectrum of activity.

Adverse reactions

It is important to take a careful history of hypersensitivity, adverse reaction, or an anaphylactic response in relation to exposure to antibiotics. There is clinical difference between adverse reactions such as diarrhoea, nausea and vomiting, candidiasis, sore mouth or tongue; fever and rash due to allergy; and an anaphylactic reaction. Clients do not always distinguish between types of adverse reaction. Persons who have a history of hypersensitivity to any antibiotic should have this recorded, so that it is not overlooked. In cases of hypersensitivity, medicines should be discontinued and consultation sought. Midwives need to be particularly cautious regarding women with a history of penicillin allergy. Approximately 7–15% of people have a history of allergy to penicillins; a proportion of these people will display cross-sensitivity to cephalosporins with rates varying from 1% to 15% (Burchum & Rosenthan, 2019). The tetracycline group of antibiotics cannot be used as an alternative, as they are contraindicated in pregnancy—there is risk to the fetus of teeth staining and inhibited bone growth. Midwives need to be aware of local policy for reporting adverse reactions of medicines and to refer women experiencing any adverse effects promptly to a medical practitioner.

Types of antimicrobials

Beta-lactam antibiotics

These drugs are bacteriocidal substances that contain a beta-lactam ring in their molecular structure. They include the penicillins, cephalosporins, monobactams, carbapenems and beta-lactamase inhibitors. Some bacteria have become resistant to antibiotics by developing the capacity to produce the enzyme beta-lactamase, which breaks the beta-lactam ring in the antibiotic molecule, rendering it ineffective (Burchum & Rosenthan, 2019).

Penicillins

The penicillins are a large group of antibiotics. They are grouped into several categories. Benzylpenicillin or penicillin G (parenteral) and phenoxymethylpenicillin or penicillin V (oral) are clinically comparable. Amoxicillin is considered a broad-spectrum penicillin in view of activity against some gram-negative bacilli. Amoxicillin is ineffective against beta-lactamase such as *S. aureus* (Burchum & Rosenthan, 2019).

Narrow-spectrum beta-lactamase-resistant penicillins

These penicillins are beta-lactamase resistant. Antibiotics effective against *S. aureus*, such as flucloxacillin, are used for lactating women when pharmacological treatment of mastitis is required. Flucloxacillin needs to be taken on an empty stomach (1 hour prior to food or 2 hours after food), which can be problematic.

Extended-spectrum penicillins

The spectrum of activity for amoxicillin/clavulanic acid, piperacillin/tazobactam and ticarcillin/clavulanic acid is extended with the addition of the beta-lactamase inhibitors clavulanic acid or tazobactam. This makes these antibiotics effective against otherwise-resistant strains of *S. aureus* and some anaerobes

Local patterns of bacterial resistance are an important consideration to prescribers. For example, when *Escherichia coli* resistance rates to amoxicillin are high, the prescriber needs to consider an antibiotic recommended for treating urinary tract infection during pregnancy or lactation.

Cephalosporins

Cephalosporins are a family of broad-spectrum antibiotics that are classified by their generation. The generation refers to the time frame over which each group was developed, rather than increasing improvement. Each generation has been designed to respond to a spectrum of antimicrobial activity. Community prescribing of cephalosporins is limited to the oral preparations.

Macrolide antibiotics

The macrolides are a group of primarily bacteriostatic antibiotics with some bacteriocidal effect that include erythromycin and azithromycin. They have a broad spectrum of activity against diverse organisms. Erythromycin might be considered for soft tissue infection (gram positive organism) when a person has a known allergy to penicillins and cephalosporins. Erythromycin estolate is contraindicated in pregnancy, because of drug-related hepatotoxicity due to estolate salt (Al-Zidan, 2020). Azithromycin is effective in the treatment of both Gram-positive and Gram-negative organisms; it is effective against infections by intracellular organisms such as *Chlamydia.*

Nitrofurantoin

Nitrofurantoin is frequently prescribed for pregnant women who have a history of, or suffer from, recurrent UTI. Nitrofurantoin is a broad-spectrum bacteriocide that inactivates or alters bacterial ribosomal proteins and other bacterial cell molecules. It is specific for the treatment of acute UTIs, as it is highly soluble and approximately 65% of the drug is excreted in the urine unchanged (Bryant et al., 2019). Nitrofurantoin is contraindicated when labour is imminent and during labour and birth because of the possibility of haemolytic anaemia in the neonate due to immature erythrocyte enzyme systems (glutathione instability). It is also contraindicated in women with glucose-6-phosphate dehydrogenase (G6PD) deficiency due to potential haemolytic anaemia and persons with renal impairment (Bryant et al., 2019).

The NZ MoH Centre for Adverse Reactions Monitoring (CARM) has received numerous reports of serious pulmonary reactions following the long-term use (greater than six months) of nitrofurantoin (Medsafe, 2020a). Long-term prophylaxis for recurrent UTIs in pregnancy requires referral to a medical practitioner.

Women should not take urine alkalinisers when taking nitrofurantoin, as the drug has more efficacy in an acidic environment. Antacid preparations containing magnesium trisilicate should be avoided when taking nitrofurantoin, to avoid the possibility of impaired absorption. Absorption is increased when taken with food.

CRITICAL THINKING EXERCISE

1. How do you make the decision as to which antibiotic is suitable for a woman at 24 weeks gestation who is symptomatic of UTI?
2. Discuss the rationale for prescribing more than one antibiotic in a particular circumstance, e.g. obstetrician prescribing of intravenous antibiotics to treat pyelonephritis or cardiac prophylaxis therapy.
3. Discuss the issue of 'caution' in relation to the prescription of antiemetics in the first trimester.

Trimethoprim

Trimethoprim, used to treat UTI, interferes with folate metabolism. Studies have shown that there may be an association between exposure to folate antagonists and birth defects in humans. Therefore, trimethoprim should be avoided in the first trimester owing to teratogenic risk.

Metronidazole

Metronidazole is a highly effective antimicrobial against anaerobic bacteria. It is used for the treatment of trichomonal infections and bacterial vaginitis. In relation to pregnancy and lactation, metronidazole is a category B2 pharmaceutical for both systemic and topical use and single-dose regimen is recommended for symptomatic trichomoniasis in pregnancy (New Zealand Sexual Health Society (NZSHS), 2017). In the *Trichomoniasis* guideline, the NZSHS (2017) recommends metronidazole for treatment of trichomonal infection in all trimesters in pregnancy, and notes that breast milk will carry an unpleasant taste. NZSHS indicates that treatment of all sexual contacts in past 2 months is required and the couple should use condoms or abstain from sex for 7 days after initiation of treatment. It is known that metronidazole crosses the placenta and is excreted in breast milk; the Lactmed website (see Online resources) shows concentrations in breastfed babies serum according to maternal dose and frequency. The New Zealand Formulary

(NZF, 2021a) refers to avoidance of high-single-dose use during breastfeeding.

Antivirals: aciclovir

Aciclovir is used as a topical or oral preparation to increase the healing rate and to decrease the pain of herpes lesions (NZF, 2021a). It acts by inhibiting viral DNA synthesis. The topical preparation is widely available as an OTC medicine, as it is primarily used for the treatment of herpes simplex I lesions. Although the topical preparation may also be prescribed by a medical practitioner, genital herpes requires systemic treatment (NZF, 2021a). Diagnosis of genital herpes, follow-up of partners and treatment regimens are generally beyond the scope of midwifery practice.

Aminoglycosides

Prescription of aminoglycosides is outside midwives' scope of practice. However, midwives do administer these drugs parenterally and monitor their effects. For example, gentamicin can be used to treat sensitive bacteria causing acute pyelonephritis in pregnancy.

The aminoglycosides are a group of potent bacteriocides that act by inhibiting protein synthesis. They are generally reserved for Gram-negative infections. They are: gentamicin, neomycin, netilmicin, streptomycin and tobramycin (Bryant et al., 2019). Adverse reactions include serious neurological and renal damage and ototoxicity, and therefore careful observation for signs of adverse reactions is required. Aminoglycosides have a narrow therapeutic range; therefore, if treatment is required for longer than 48 hours, plasma levels and renal function are monitored to determine dose regimens (Bryant et al., 2019).

Topical antibiotics in relation to neonates

Topical antibiotics are used for the treatment of conjunctivitis and occasionally superficial skin/umbilical cord infections in neonates. Care must be taken to use topical antibiotics only when there is an infection present. A significant proportion of neonatal 'sticky eyes' in the first week of life is related to an inflamed tear duct rather than to an infectious conjunctivitis. Regular cleansing of the eye, gentle massage of the tear duct and a few drops of expressed breast milk applied to the eye postfeed (when the mother wishes to do so) usually resolves 'sticky eyes'. If an infection is suspected, a swab should be taken for culture and sensitivities prior to starting treatment such as chloramphenicol eye drops. Antibiotic therapy can mask chlamydial eye infections. Midwives need to consider this condition if the eye is red and inflamed or an infection does not resolve quickly.

The use of topical antibiotics for minor neonatal skin infections is controversial. A mild antiseptic wash may be just as effective. The treatment of umbilical cord stumps with topical antibiotics should rarely be necessary. Most 'sticky cords' are the result of saprophytic action and require hygiene measures rather than antibiotics. Umbilical cord infections can rapidly spread to become serious systemic infections. Regular observation will assist early detection, and prompt referral is indicated for babies with umbilical infections.

> **RESEARCH ACTIVITY**
>
> **Antibiotic susceptibility**
>
> Compile a list of antibiotics that you see used in practice or referred to within this chapter. Write down the organisms that are susceptible to each antibiotic, and apply this knowledge by writing down which antibiotics are suitable for which conditions in relation to maternity prescribing.
>
> Resources such as an antibiotic susceptibility testing chart are available online.

An understanding of pharmacology and knowledge of commonly used antimicrobials is essential for safe prescribing practices. The following section refers to common conditions during pregnancy where midwives might need to consider prescription medicines in discussion with the woman.

COMMONLY ADMINISTERED PHARMACEUTICAL MEDICINES AND CONDITIONS ASSOCIATED WITH CHILDBIRTH

Selected pharmaceutical medicines other than antimicrobials that are commonly used, and conditions commonly prescribed for in the childbearing year, are described below.

Synthetic oxytocin

Synthetic oxytocin is used in labour to augment uterine contractions when they are absent or incoordinate, or during induction of labour. Synthetic oxytocin has an immediate onset and is rapidly inactivated in the liver. As it has a half-life of 1–6 minutes, synthetic oxytocin is administered in labour via an intravenous infusion in which the dose is incrementally titrated to achieve approximately three to four contractions every 10 minutes (Bryant et al., 2019). Caution is required if the woman has had prostaglandins (dinoprostone/Prostin E_2 gel) or inhalational anaesthetics, as the action of synthetic oxytocin may be enhanced; therefore concurrent use with other oxytocic agents is not recommended. If the woman requires augmentation with synthetic oxytocin, the manufacturer of dinoprostone recommends that synthetic oxytocin is not commenced within 6 hours following the administration of Prostin E_2 (Medsafe, 2019b).

Close monitoring of both maternal and fetal wellbeing is required. Adverse reactions include nausea, vomiting, hypotension, tachycardia and irregular heart rate. Occasional fetal bradycardia, dysrhythmias or neonatal jaundice have been reported (Bryant et al., 2019). Adverse effects include hypertonus, water intoxication and hyponatraemia. High doses and/or synthetic oxytocin administered for prolonged periods of time can cause fluid retention, placental abruption and amniotic fluid embolism.

Oxytocin is used as a uterotonic to prevent or control postpartum haemorrhage. A single-dose injection is used for the active management of the third stage of labour. Oxytocin alone is associated with significantly less nausea and vomiting as compared with combination ergometrine-oxytocin (5 IU oxytocin/0.5 mg ergometrine).

Synthetic oxytocin-ergometrine (Syntometrine) is contraindicated in hypertensive women, because it may exacerbate hypertension; it should be avoided in women who do not have their blood pressures measured during precipitate labours. The use of intramuscular synthetic oxytocin for active management of the third stage of labour is recommended in the NICE guidelines (NICE, 2021). The potential danger of ergometrine is its potent vasoconstrictor effect that can result in vasospasm.

RESEARCH ACTIVITY

Management of the third stage of labour

Review research evidence in relation to drugs used during the management of the third stage of labour. Compile a list of the drugs, contraindications, side effects, route of administration and strength used according to route of administration.

Local anaesthetic: lignocaine hydrochloride (lidocaine)

Lignocaine is a rapid-acting, stable, local anaesthetic used in perineal repair. A 0.5% w/v or 1% w/v solution without adrenaline (i.e. plain) is the usual strength employed. One percent concentration should not be exceeded. Injection should be given subcuticular with great care, undertaken slowly, with aspiration, to prevent intravascular injection, as this will produce systemic toxic effects (NZF, 2021a). The amount required for individual women will depend on the size of the woman, the extent of the perineal injury and whether the infiltration is into an intact perineum prior to birth or an injured perineum after the birth. The New Zealand Formulary advises that, for obese patients, the dose may need to be calculated on ideal body weight in order to avoid excessive dosage. The maximum dose is 200 mg in adults—i.e. 20mL of 1% w/v plain solution (NZF, 2021a). The usual dose is significantly less than the maximum. For perineal repair, a dose of 70–100 mg (7–10 mL of 1% plain solution) is often adequate. Midwives need to check the ampoule carefully with regard to strength of lidocaine.

Tocolytic drugs

Tocolytic drugs have been used in the management of pre-term labour to quieten uterine activity. The calcium ion channel blocker nifedipine is now the most commonly prescribed tocolytic agent in the management of pre-term labour in Australia, New Zealand and the UK (Bryant et al., 2019). This drug inhibits muscle contraction by interfering with the movement of calcium across the plasma membrane. In some larger centres, atosiban, an oxytocin antagonist, may be used in the management of pre-term labour (Bryant et al., 2019). Nifedipine has largely superseded the use of the β_2-adrenoceptor agonist salbutamol (Bryant et al., 2019).

RESEARCH ACTIVITY

Tocolytic drugs

Review research evidence in relation to the contraindications and side effects of nifedipine and other tocolytic drugs. State the rationale for nifedipine being used in preference to other tocolytics.

Non-steroidal anti-inflammatory drugs

Non-steroidal anti-inflammatory drugs (NSAIDs) act by inhibiting prostaglandin synthesis. They are prescribed or available as OTC medicines, for the relief of inflammation, pain and pyrexia. Medsafe (2019a) warned all NSAIDs (traditional and COX-2 selective NSAID) increased cardiovascular adverse events in otherwise healthy persons; risk entails both short-term and long-term use. NSAID use should be at the lowest effective dose for the shortest possible time (Medsafe, 2019a).

Bryant et al. (2019) similarly point to adverse reactions with use of NSAIDs including: acute myocardial infarction, gastric pain and / or ulceration bleeding, renal compromise and urticaria. Ibuprofen and NSAIDs should not be given to people with a history of aspirin or NSAID-induced asthma, rhinitis and urticaria, worsening of asthma, or previous reactions to NSAIDs. Contraindications to NSAIDs include the first and third trimesters of pregnancy; NSAIDs may cause constriction of the ductus arteriosus in utero during third trimester. Midwives should follow current medicine guidelines regarding NSAIDs.

RESEARCH ACTIVITY

Aspirin and preeclampsia

Research the evidence in relation to low-dose aspirin used for women at risk of preeclampsia.

Codeine

The use of codeine is not recommended in breastfeeding women owing to concerns over neonatal toxicity. Individual people can metabolise codeine at different rates, with some ultrarapid metabolisers (URM). Individuals who metabolise codeine quickly are at risk of severe opioid toxicity, given the high and uncontrolled conversion of codeine into morphine. While access to OTC codeine preparations is increasingly restricted, midwives need to remind breastfeeding women not to take analgesic medicines containing codeine. In April 2017, the FDA issued a strengthened warning to mothers that breastfeeding is not recommended when taking codeine or tramadol medicines owing to the risk of serious adverse reactions in breastfed infants. These can include excess sleepiness, difficulty in breastfeeding, or serious breathing problems that could result in death.

Topical treatment for haemorrhoids

Haemorrhoids are a common condition in pregnancy and after birth. Discomfort, swelling and itching can often be relieved by saline or witch hazel solution compresses. If these measures are ineffective, pharmaceutical preparations may be required.

Most pharmaceutical suppositories and ointments contain steroids. Topical steroids have anti-inflammatory, vasoconstrictor effects to relieve discomfort. Commonly available topical ointment/suppositories contain cinchocaine hydrochloride (a local anaesthetic), fluocortolone pivalate and fluocortolone hexanoate (Ultraproct). Topical products for the treatment of haemorrhoids that contain fluocortolones are contraindicated in the first trimester (Medsafe, 2020b).

An alternative preparation (Proctosedyl) contains hydrocortisone and cinchocaine hydrochloride. The NZ data sheet contains a caution that topical steroids should not be used extensively (in large amounts or for long duration) during pregnancy (Medsafe, 2018).

Lactulose

Lactulose is a semisynthetic disaccharide used for the treatment of constipation. It is not absorbed from the gut. It acts by increasing fluid accumulation in the intestinal lumen increasing peristalsis, thereby shortening the transit time of intestinal contents. It also promotes natural bowel flora rather than the proliferation of *E. coli.* Lactulose promotes bowel movement within 24–72 hours after oral administration (Bryant et al., 2019). Lactulose is probably compatible in pregnancy and lactation for the treatment of constipation, for postpartum women with haemorrhoids, operative birth or a third-degree perineal tear.

Antiemetic drugs

Full assessment of morning sickness and hyperemesis is covered in Chapter 37, and in severe cases the midwife is advised to refer the woman immediately for assessment by the obstetric team. Hyperemesis gravidarum requires regular antiemetic therapy, intravenous fluid and electrolyte replacement, and sometimes nutritional support. Supplementation with thiamine must be considered in order to reduce the risk of Wernicke's encephalopathy (NZF, 2021a).

First-line management of nausea and vomiting in pregnancy should include dietary and lifestyle interventions, with pharmacological treatment reserved for those cases where symptoms persist (NZF, 2021b). Medication(s) that may be considered vary according to safety during pregnancy (particularly first trimester), current guidelines and the severity of the person's symptoms / electrolyte status (Lowe et al., 2019; NZF, 2021b).

Folic acid

Supplementation with folic acid has been proven to decrease the incidence of neural tube defects and is recommended for primary prevention and for women with a previously affected pregnancy. Supplementation is recommended from the time of planning a pregnancy until 12 weeks of pregnancy (Table 33.1). At this point there is not enough evidence to determine whether folic acid prevents other birth defects.

The National Food Authority in Australia implemented mandatory fortification of breadmaking flour with folic acid in late 2009. The Australian Government recommends that women planning pregnancy take folic acid supplements (500 µg/day) from 12 weeks prior to conception and throughout the first 12 weeks of pregnancy (Health Direct, 2017).

Table 33.1 Folate recommendations for Australian and New Zealand women

Australia	New Zealand
Advise dietary supplementation of 400 µg of folic acid/day, ideally from 1 month before conception and throughout the first 3 months of pregnancy to reduce the risk of neural tube defects.	All women planning a pregnancy should supplement their diet with 800 µg (or 5 mg if risk factors) of folic acid/day beginning 1 month prior to conception until 12 weeks gestation.
Women at high risk of a neural tube defect (NTD) affected pregnancy are those who: • have previously had an NTD-affected pregnancy • have a family history of NTD, or whose partner has a family history • are affected by an NTD themselves, or whose partner is affected by an NTD • who are on insulin treatment for diabetes, or • women taking medications known to affect folate metabolism, such as anti-convulsants, infertility treatment, vitamin A analogues used to treat acne and some antitumour agents, e.g. carbemazepine, clomiphene, valproate, retinoids and etretinate.	

(Source: Ministry of Health NZ, n.d. From: http://www.health.govt.nz/our-work/preventative-health-wellness/nutrition/folate-folic-acid. https://creativecommons.org/licenses/by/4.0/)

In New Zealand, voluntary fortification of food has been permitted since 1996. The Ministry of Health NZ (n.d.) recommends that a folic acid 0.8 mg (800 µg) oral tablet be taken daily from 1 month pre-conception to the end of the 12th week of gestation. Women with risk factors require 5 mg tablet of folic acid daily as above.

Vitamin D

Vitamin D is necessary for healthy bones and muscle function. Neonatal vitamin D status is largely determined by maternal vitamin D status during pregnancy so it is important that women have sufficient vitamin D (Ekeroma et al., 2015). Vitamin D is formed mainly by the action of sunlight on the skin and also through dietary nutrients. Certain groups are more at risk of vitamin D deficiency including high body mass index, persons with dark or covered skin and those with minimal exposure to sunlight. Current guidelines in Australia and New Zealand do not recommend routine screening of pregnant women. Guidance regarding supplementation varies at time of writing; practitioners should consult national or regional guidance.

Iron supplementation (anaemia)

Prescribing supplements for women with iron deficiency and/or anaemia is relatively common when practising continuity of care throughout pregnancy and partum. Iron-deficiency anaemia (IDA) is the most common anaemia during pregnancy; however, midwives need to be aware of other types of anaemia, including folate, B_{12}, sickle cell, thalassaemia and autoimmune anaemia. Correct diagnosis is important to avoid inappropriate treatment that might be harmful to the woman and the fetus. Midwives need to consult with a haematologist or obstetrician when there is uncertainty with complex blood results.

Why iron is important

Iron is essential for the synthesis of haemoglobin, myoglobin and the function of iron-dependent enzymes. Compared with prepregnancy levels, iron requirements double during pregnancy; however, most pregnant women don't make substantial nutritional changes to increase iron intake (Milman 2020).

In developed countries, there is no consensus regarding routine versus need-based iron supplementation; nevertheless, Australia and New Zealand advocate a targeted need-based approach (RANZCOG, 2019). Anaemia in pregnancy guidelines are available online for various states and regions in Australasia. As pregnancy progresses, there is an increase in absorption of iron from the gut (hepcidin controls regulation and absorption of iron), yet iron depletion is common with increased demand for iron in the second half of pregnancy and increased fetal requirements in the third trimester (McLintock et al., 2010). Haem iron predominantly found in meat is readily absorbed and assists the absorption of non-haem iron, as discussed in Chapters 21 and 22.

Potential hazards of excess iron supplementation

Potential hazards of unnecessary iron supplementation include raised Hb with risk of placental insufficiency and secondary haemochromatosis in women with high iron. These risks can be avoided by assessing the complete blood count and ferritin within 2–4 weeks of commencing oral therapy to check diagnosis. Oxidant stress is linked with products of oxygen in contact with minerals such as iron resulting in free radicals. Free radicals can result from an excess of iron in tissue and potentially affect the placenta, which is susceptible to oxidative stress (McLintock et al., 2010).

Interpreting blood indices to diagnose iron deficiency and IDA

Haemoglobin (Hb)

Hb is a less reliable marker for assessment of iron status in pregnant women, in view of haemodilution and expanded volume. During iron depletion, haemoglobin levels are unlikely to change while serum ferritin is reduced. In IDA, there is reduction in Hb, serum ferritin and reduced transferrin saturation (Daru et al., 2016).

Mean cell volume (MCV) and mean cell haemoglobin (MCH)

MCV increases slightly in normal pregnancy (Percy et al., 2017) therefore is an unreliable marker until IDA is established. Low MCV (microcytic cells) alongside hypochromic cells (low MCH) are indicative of significant negative iron balance requiring urgent treatment to restore iron stores with relatively high-dose iron supplements (McLintock et al., 2010).

Serum ferritin

Serum ferritin is a stable glycoprotein that accurately reflects iron stores in the absence of active infection or inflammation. Ferritin is the first test to become abnormal as iron stores decrease and it is not affected by recent iron ingestion. Ferritin initially rises followed by a progressive fall by 32 weeks to about 50% of prepregnancy levels, owing to haemodilution and mobilisation of iron (Percy et al., 2017). The Royal College of Pathologists of Australia (RCPA, 2019) stated that serum ferritin concentration around 30 g/L or less is considered diagnostic of iron deficiency at any stage of pregnancy; however, there is some interassay variation (different laboratories) with ferritin levels around the 20–30 µg/L range. Serum ferritin levels fall in the last 4 weeks of normal pregnancy due to transfer of iron to the fetus, nevertheless, ferritin <30 µg / L remains indicative of iron deficiency (RCPA, 2019).

If ferritin level is above upper level, midwives are likely to question the woman about symptoms of infection and, with consent, repeat the serum ferritin. Serum C-reactive protein can be used to determine inflammation (Calje & Skinner, 2017). Milman (2020) stated that ferritin levels of approximately 60–70 µg/L are adequate reserves for the duration of pregnancy without the need for iron supplementation.

Iron studies or additional tests

Iron studies tend to be requested only when additional information is necessary to assist diagnosis. Low iron stores will reduce amount or saturation of iron bound to transferrin (iron transport protein), so that its capacity to bind iron is increased. A low transferrin saturation or increased total iron-binding capacity is often present in iron deficiency, but rapid fluctuations in levels make these tests on their own unhelpful in diagnosis of IDA (McLintock et al., 2010). Solubilised serum transferrin receptor increases in concentration when iron deficiency develops, but only when the storage compartment of iron is exhausted. Not all laboratories provide analysis of the serum transferrin receptor. Transferrin levels increase during pregnancy, thus total iron-binding capacity is unhelpful in diagnosis of iron deficiency during pregnancy (McLintock et al., 2010).

How much supplementation is required?

In Australia and New Zealand, usual daily doses of elemental iron vary between 60 and 105 mg elemental iron depending on individual need and the availability of subsidised supplements. Oral ferrous iron salt formulas are recommended because they have better intestinal iron absorption than do ferric iron salt preparations (Pavord et al., 2020). McLintock et al. (2010) noted there was little capacity for the gastrointestinal tract to absorb levels beyond 120–180 mg of elemental iron per day and that simultaneous calcium supplements can decrease absorption of iron.

The amount of supplementation required on an individual-needs basis is assessed according to the woman's blood results and the gestation of the pregnancy. Women with low Hb and absent iron stores in late pregnancy are likely to require higher-dose supplements and referral if there is no improvement. Midwives need to be cognisant of the fact that nutrition alone is unlikely to improve iron reserves. In consideration of accessibility and affordability, midwives should prescribe fully subsidised iron supplements with an adequate amount of elemental iron in order to treat IDA.

Recommended midwifery practice

- **Note:** Midwives need to ascertain the 'normal' serum ferritin values used at the laboratory where bloods are analysed in order to account for variance in normal range (RCPA, 2019).
- When undertaking first antenatal bloods, serum ferritin should be requested. Repeat serum ferritin with the second trimester bloods taken between 24–26 weeks gestation.
- If pregnant women present for care without serum ferritin undertaken at booking, review the complete blood count noting that MCV (and MCH) decrease only after IDA is established. Similarly, fatigue, pallor, weakness, headache, palpitations, dizziness, dyspnoea, irritability, restless leg and rarely pica might present after IDA is well established (McLintock et al., 2010; Pavord et al., 2020). If concerned that the woman is iron deficient, discuss the option of a further blood test for complete blood count and serum ferritin in partnership with the woman.
- New Zealand's National Women's Guideline (2015) recommendation is from 26 to 28 weeks gestation as follows: serum ferritin >50 µmol/L and Hb >100 g/L, no iron tablets likely to be necessary; ferritin <50 µmol/L and >15 alongside Hb >100 g/L, consider whether iron tablets are required later in pregnancy; ferritin <15 µmol/L and Hb >100 g/L, prescribe one low-dose iron tablet daily (approximately 65 mg elemental iron). Assess response after 4 weeks of iron therapy. See full guideline for further information.
- If the woman is a vegan or vegetarian, in addition to complete blood count (CBC) and serum ferritin, consider serum B_{12} and folate levels at booking. If results are abnormal for pregnancy range, discuss management with an obstetrician. Note that the 'development of macrocytic red cells that are induced by deficiencies of folate and/or cobalamin (B_{12}) may not occur in the presence of coexisting iron deficiency or the presence of thalassaemia or haemoglobinopathy' (McLintock et al., 2010, p. 52).
- If the haemoglobin level is <90 g/L, not responding to treatment, consultation with and/or referral to an obstetrician is indicated (MOH, 2012a).
- Check the amount of elemental iron (absorbable iron content) within iron supplements as this differs according to the type of iron preparation *and* the strength of the tablet or liquid preparation. This knowledge guides the safe dosage of supplemental iron. Therapeutic Guidelines Australia is a useful resource and the NZ Formulary online provides details regarding amount of elemental iron and fully subsidised supplements (see Online resources).
- Midwives need to be alert to vigorous marketing of some iron supplements that are costly yet contain very low levels of elemental iron. Midwives should research the amount of elemental (absorbable) iron in each product and share this information with women.
- Iron is absorbed best when administered separately, as opposed to multivitamin preparations where iron appears to be reduced by metal ions in zinc, copper, manganese, and selenium (Milman et al., 2016). Iron plus folic acid requires further studies to establish efficacy in developed countries (Peña-Rosas et al., 2015). Calcium inhibits absorption of haem and non-haem iron (McLintock et al., 2010); therefore antacids or other supplements containing calcium should be taken at a different time of day to iron supplements.
- Ensure that clients are advised to store iron supplements safely away from children.
- Assess full blood count and serum ferritin after 3–4 weeks of commencing iron therapy to check for improvement and to ensure that the diagnosis is IDA as opposed to another haemoglobinopathy or anaemia.

Hb concentrations should increase by approximately 10–20 g/L over 3–4 weeks (McLintock et al., 2010; Percy et al., 2017).

- When women report that iron supplements are not tolerated, options include: (a) recommending that the tablet be taken at bedtime; (b) recommending it be taken with food, although cereals, seeds, nuts, vegetables, fruit, tea, coffee and cocoa decrease iron absorption in a dose-dependent manner (Milman et al., 2016); (c) lowering the dose to improve compliance as fewer side effects occur with lower doses; or (d) suggesting iron supplements are taken on alternate days or three times per week (Peña-Rosas et al., 2015). Ingesting iron supplements with fruit juice improves absorption, but might increase gastrointestinal side effects, and additional vitamin C is not essential for the absorption of elemental iron in supplements.

Postpartum anaemia

Iron supplements can assist a woman's recovery with possible improvement in lactation and possible reduction in depressive illness. The CBC is used to assist decision making as ferritin level is unreliable postpartum owing to inflammatory processes. Postpartum iron deficit and IDA are undertreated resulting in poorer outcomes for women. Pavord et al. (2020) recommend haemoglobin testing within 48 hours of birth for women who experienced postpartum haemorrhage and those with symptoms of anaemia.

Medical prescribing of intramuscular and intravenous iron therapy

Medical prescribing of intravenous therapy is favoured above intramuscular iron therapy. Iron injections are painful and cause permanent staining of the skin with variable absorption (McLintock et al., 2010). Local guidelines should be adhered to during administration of intravenous iron preparation.

RESEARCH ACTIVITY

Iron supplementation

Research the emerging evidence that iron therapy in pregnancy improves neonatal iron status and development.

Antacids

Limited small studies suggested that heartburn in pregnancy could be completely relieved by pharmaceutical treatment; however, further research is needed to evaluate medications.

If dietary changes such as avoiding spicy or greasy food, acidic products and carbonated drinks do not solve reflux, calcium- or magnesium-based antacids, which neutralise stomach acids, can be used during pregnancy. High-dose aluminium-containing antacids are not generally recommended owing to common side effects of constipation and altered gastrointestinal (GI) motility. Combination antacids have been formulated to reduce the risk of diarrhoea or constipation. Alginic acid forms viscous cohesive foam, preventing reflux by increasing adherence of mucus. Simethicone disperses and prevents the formation of mucous gas pockets in the GI tract, relieving flatulence (Bryant et al., 2019). Antacids can bind with other medications and therefore should be taken at least an hour apart from iron preparations and other medicines. Histamine-2 receptor antagonists are also safe during pregnancy, and include cimetidine and ranitidine. The latter tend to be drugs used preoperatively and prescribed by a medical practitioner.

Recommended prescribing

- Ensure that there is no other pathology, and be aware that heartburn can mimic epigastric pain associated with preeclampsia. Always check the woman's blood pressure, urinalysis, fetal growth (according to customised growth chart), symptoms associated with preeclamptic toxaemia (PET) (after 20 weeks gestation) and undertake screening bloods where indicated prior to recommending or prescribing antacids.
- Encourage the woman to alter her dietary habits in the first instance before resorting to antacids.
- Oral magnesium salts (magnesium trisilicate) reduce absorption of oral iron and nitrofurantoin (NZF, 2021a)—antacids should not be taken at the same time as other drugs as they may impair absorption.
- If reflux continues to be troublesome, advise or prescribe antacid that is safe during pregnancy. Recommended dose depends on which preparation is given and prescribers should refer to a formulary to note maximum dose and refer to TGA for categorisation of safety during pregnancy.
- Aluminium-containing antacids: aluminium hydroxide dried.
- Calcium-containing antacids:
  - calcium with glycine (calcium carbonate + glycine—Titralac brand tablets)
  - calcium carbonate + magnesium hydroxide (Mylanta brand tablets).
- Simethicone-containing antacids:
  - aluminium + magnesium + simethicone (Mylanta brand liquid and tablet preparations)
  - alginate sodium + calcium carbonate + sodium bicarbonate (Gaviscon brand)
  - calcium carbonate + glycine (Titralac brand tablets).
- Medication prescribed by medical practitioners:
  - histamine H_2 blockers (prescribed by doctors or used according to hospital standing orders—e.g. ranitidine given to high-risk women intrapartum/prior to lower-segment caesarean section (LSCS))
  - medical prescribing only: proton pump inhibitors are rarely used during pregnancy (such as omeprazole).

Thrush (candidiasis or moniliasis)

Vaginal thrush

Vaginal thrush is a common complaint and increases in prevalence during pregnancy owing to changes in the vaginal flora. Predisposing factors include a recent course of antibiotics (which reduces the vaginal lactobacilli count, rendering a woman more susceptible to overgrowth of the yeast), diabetes, HIV infection, anaemia and urinary tract infection.

Young & Jewell (2001) in a Cochrane review revealed that topical imidazole drugs (clotrimazole, miconazole) are more effective than nystatin for treating vaginal candidiasis in pregnancy and recommend treatment for a longer period such as 7 days (clotrimazole 1% preparations are generally packaged for six nightly applications, and this should suffice) as curing 90% of cases versus a 4-day treatment, which cured about 50% of cases during pregnancy. The authors state that there are no reliable studies on complementary methods of treatment such as live yogurt. The primary mode of action of clotrimazole appears to be on the plasma membrane of the fungi, damaging the permeability barrier. Shorter courses of antifungal therapy are stronger: 10% cream preparation for a 1-night treatment compared with 1% for the 6-night course. Women are more likely to experience burning and irritation with the stronger preparations. It is possible that shorter-course treatments might contribute to non-*albicans* species such as *Candida glabrata* and *C. tropicalis*. Traditional imidazoles do not adequately treat non-*albicans* species, hence the rationale for culture of a vaginal swab. Oral antifungal agents (fluconazole preparations) are not recommended during pregnancy as fluconazole has a 'D' category by the TGA Australia drug safety in pregnancy. Education regarding careful insertion of the applicator should be discussed, as well as hygiene to decrease the risk of re-infection. There is no evidence that treating a male sexual partner makes any difference to this episode or any future episode unless the partner already has symptoms. Douching washes out lactobacilli as well as *Candida*; studies have shown increased pelvic infection rates after douching, so this is not a suitable treatment, particularly in pregnancy. Salt baths are helpful in reducing itching and swelling in the acute phase.

Recommended prescribing

- Treat only if the woman is symptomatic.
- Send vaginal swab for culture prior to commencing treatment to confirm organism/s.
- Prescribe clotrimazole 1% vaginal cream (35 g) or miconazole nitrate 2% vaginal cream (40 g) depending on subsidy. Advise the woman to insert applicator full of cream into vagina at bedtime for 6 (or 7) nights. There is sufficient cream to apply to the vulva twice daily—document succinct instructions for use on the prescription form.
- Occasionally women might prefer vaginal pessaries. If so, the midwife needs to offer a prescription for a cream for external use in addition to the pessaries.
- After checking HIV status and diabetes screening in partnership with a woman, it is best to consult with an obstetrician if a woman has symptomatic recurrent thrush during pregnancy.

Thrush on nipples

Thrush infection might occur after maternal antibiotic therapy or due to environmental factors. Nipple thrush can be over-diagnosed, therefore a swab is recommended to confirm thrush; however, it can be difficult to culture. Experienced clinicians might conclude a diagnosis using their assessment skills and the woman's symptoms. Women might complain of deep breast pain, stabbing pain or burning nipple pain that does not resolve after feeding. The midwife should inspect the nipple and areola for cracks indicative of poor positioning during breastfeeding; the nipple might appear pink and shiny. Conservative management re positioning and time may resolve pain. Pharmaceutical treatment includes topical antifungal cream (Amir et al., 2021), such as miconazole 2% cream applied after breastfeeding twice daily. The cream should be gently wiped off prior to breastfeeding.

Neonatal candidiasis

Thrush should be confirmed by swab or by recognition by an experienced practitioner prior to use of pharmaceuticals. If the baby has oral thrush, 1 mL of nystatin liquid 100,000 U/mL applied to the tongue four times daily after breastfeeding is recommended for a 6-day treatment. Gel products are not recommended for young babies because of the risk of choking. If the baby has thrush on the groin and buttocks, clotrimazole 1% cream or miconazole 2% cream should be applied sparingly twice daily and continued until 48 hours after the rash clears, which is usually around 5 days. A barrier cream can be applied over the antifungal cream. It is not necessary to use an antifungal cream with hydrocortisone.

Urinary tract infection

Urinary tract infection (UTI) is a common complication during pregnancy, and women can have asymptomatic or symptomatic UTI. Asymptomatic bacteriuria is prevalent in 2–10% of pregnant women; if not treated up to 30% will develop acute pyelonephritis that has an association with pre-term birth (Smaill & Vazquez, 2015). It is recommended that a clean midstream urine (MSU) sample be obtained from all pregnant women at approximately 12–16 weeks gestation to screen for bacteriuria (Australian Government Department of Health, 2019). The cost of screening MSU is likely to outweigh the cost of treatment for acute pyelonephritis and potential pre-term neonates.

Women who have had previous UTIs often recognise the symptoms associated with UTI and seek help early. Midwives should prescribe for lower tract infections only and refer to an obstetrician if there are any symptoms of pyelonephritis (pyrexia, loin pain) or if there are recurrent urinary infections during the pregnancy. An obstetrician might recommend prophylactic antibiotics for the continuation of the pregnancy and/or renal investigations.

Recommended assessment, diagnosis and prescribing

Asymptomatic bacteriuria

A Cochrane review has shown that antibiotic drug treatment substantially decreases the risk of pyelonephritis and pre-term delivery—Smaill & Vazquez (2015) concluded that a single-dose regimen of antibiotics may be less effective; women with asymptomatic bacteriuria in pregnancy should be treated by the standard regimen of antibiotics until more data become available testing 7-day treatment compared with shorter courses of 3- or 5-day regimens. Asymptomatic bacteriuria is diagnosed by the presence of a significant number of a single-organism bacteria in a clean MSU specimen. White cells might not be raised as the woman does not have an inflammatory process (she is asymptomatic). Prescribing should be 'directed' according to the culture results. The rule of prescribing the narrowest-spectrum antibiotic according to the culture results applies; for example, if *E. coli* cultures are susceptible to amoxicillin, then amoxicillin is a narrower-spectrum antibiotic and is preferred to the broader-spectrum antibiotics. Treat women with asymptomatic bacteriuria with a 7-day course (or follow local guideline) and screen monthly for UTI as there is a high recurrence rate.

Group B *Streptococcus* (GBS) significant in the urine culture (significant numbers) should be treated during the antenatal period. All women who have had GBS bacteriuria during the current pregnancy require GBS prophylaxis intrapartum, as this is indicative of heavy colonisation of vaginal GBS. GBS is known to be susceptible to penicillin in most instances, therefore either penicillin tablets or amoxicillin (which is without food restriction) could be used to treat GBS growth in urine.

Symptomatic UTI in pregnancy

For empirical prescribing while waiting for MSU culture results, antibiotic choice is dependent on: history of allergy, gestation of pregnancy alongside safety during pregnancy and bacterial resistance to antibiotics. In order to confirm clearance after antibiotic treatment, the woman needs to provide a clean MSU for culture not before 48 hours after completion of antibiotics. Vazquez & Abalos (2011) conducted a systematic review on treatment for symptomatic urinary tract infection during pregnancy. The authors noted there is a paucity of good quality data for pregnant women, however, cautioned use of data from non-pregnant women as pharmacodynamics of some drugs changed in pregnancy with increased renal excretion and greater presence of the antibiotic in urine. The authors found no significant difference between treatments, with all the antibiotics studied shown to be very effective with regard to cure rates, recurrent infection, incidence of pre-term birth and admissions to neonatal unit. The only exception in treatment outcome was cefuroxime compared with cephradine, where cefuroxime had better cure rates and fewer recurrences. Complications from treatments were very rare and the authors concluded that beta-lactams should be administered for 5 days (or longer), whereas 3-day treatment was adequate for trimethoprim. Adverse reactions increased in frequency when oral cephalosporins were used in treatment regimens for longer periods.

Diagnosis of symptomatic UTI involves assessment of history including dysuria (frequency alone is relatively common during pregnancy), cloudy or discoloured urine, assessment of the woman's temperature, pulse and respiratory rate, and assessment for loin pain and any uterine activity.

A clean MSU specimen must be obtained prior to the commencement of any antibiotics. Women should not 'pause' when undertaking MSU as bacteria can be trapped; the urine collected should be mid- or end-stream. MSU needs to be sent for laboratory analysis—microscopy, culture and sensitivity.

Empirical prescribing (prior to laboratory result being available) is undertaken in practice where UTI is diagnosed on symptoms. Women with history of UTI during or prior to pregnancy (particularly <15 years of age) are at high risk for recurrence (Schneeberger et al., 2015). Microscopy of urine can occur quickly (in 1–2 hours if indicated as urgent); however, culture of bacteria currently takes 36–48 hours. If laboratory service is unavailable, for example in a rural area of Australia or New Zealand, urine dipstick tests can detect white cells and nitrate associated with an established infection and Gram-negative organisms. However, dipstick analysis has limited value, as Gram-positive organisms or milder UTI are unlikely to be detected.

MSU culture showing a significantly high bacterial count (refer to local laboratory parameters) for either Gram-negative or Gram-positive organisms (the latter are slower growing), and usually a single organism is likely to indicate UTI (check that the bacteria cultured is an organism associated with UTI). A culture result of mixed bacterial species is frequently due to contaminants. Investigate the criteria used by your local laboratory, in order to interpret reports correctly. White cell count in urine is usually raised when a woman is symptomatic of UTI. A clean urine specimen should have only a small number or no epithelial cells from external contamination.

Beware of sterile pyuria where white cell count is raised but bacteria are absent; this result does not indicate a UTI. Screening for *Chlamydia* is recommended in the first instance (with consent), or consideration of other conditions, for example resolving UTI, woman on antibiotics, calculi, renal tuberculosis, and trauma.

If a prescription for antibiotics is indicated after careful assessment of symptoms (empiric prescribing):

- Assess the woman for allergies or adverse reactions prior to prescribing and document this assessment—note that allergy to penicillin is associated with co-allergy to cephalosporin drugs (cephalexin and cefaclor).
- Consider the resistance patterns for organisms associated with UTI and antibiotic susceptibility of common UTI pathogens, e.g. *E. coli*—the most prevalent organism; less prevalent organisms include: GBS, *Klebsiella*

pneumoniae, Proteus mirabilis, Staphylococcus saprophyticus, and *Enterococcus* species).
- Prescribe an antibiotic deemed appropriate for first-line treatment of UTI during pregnancy by local microbiologists.
- Refer the woman to the obstetric service if there are any symptoms associated with pyelonephritis.
- When prescribing empirically, perform a follow-up culture and sensitivity of the original MSU, and alter antibiotics where indicated according to the bacteria isolated and sensitivity.
- Ensure that the woman does a clean MSU 7–14 days after completing the last antibiotic, in order to ensure that the infection has cleared.

Antibiotics that can be used for UTI (these are not in order of preference)

Note: At the time of writing, shorter duration treatment is being studied; however, in a Cochrane review 7-day treatment was recommended for asymptomatic bacteriuria (Smaill & Vazquez, 2015).

- Amoxicillin 500 mg 8-hourly—suitable for asymptomatic bacteriuria when directed prescribing only (culture result is available showing sensitivity to Amoxicillin), as approximately 50% *E. coli* are resistant to amoxicillin.
- Nitrofurantoin—prescribers need to make clear distinction between formulations for safety: 50 mg 6-hourly (immediate release) for 5 days. Do not use urine alkalinisers during treatment, as this drug requires an acidic urinary pH to work effectively. Do not use in women with G6PD deficiency or when labour is imminent. Possible gastrointestinal side effects (long-acting nitrofurantoin 100 mg tablet 12 hourly is suitable also).
- Cefaclor or cephalexin (consult Formulary regarding strength/frequency). Oral cephalosporins should not be used where the woman has sensitivity to penicillin.
- Trimethoprim 300 mg at night for 3 days (3-day treatment adequate per Cochrane review)—contraindicated during the first trimester due to interference with folate metabolism.

CRITICAL THINKING EXERCISE

Jenner undertakes a routine MSU at 14 weeks gestation. She understands the need to provide a clean specimen as she had a UTI during her last pregnancy. Below are the results from Jenner's MSU. (Note that different laboratories might use different criteria for reporting results of microscopy and culture of MSU.)

- Protein: nil
- Glucose: nil
- Epithelial cells: $<10 \times 10^6$/L or small number
- Bacteria: heavy growth or large numbers
- Culture:
  - heavy growth of *E. coli* $>10^8$/L
  - sensitive to: amoxicillin, cefaclor, norfloxacin, amoxy-clavulanate
  - resistant to: trimethoprim.

State your rationale as to whether or not you would prescribe for Jenner, *and* which antibiotic is the *most* appropriate (remembering the rule of the narrowest-spectrum antibiotic to treat the organism, plus safety of medicines during pregnancy).

Sexually transmitted infections (STIs)

Midwives need to discuss the rationale for STI screening with women and partners and inform women that infections such as *Chlamydia* are usually silent or asymptomatic. Some STIs can be present but undetected for a number of years.

Before a woman is tested for a STI, a conversation needs to occur regarding the importance of treatment if it gives a positive result, along with simultaneous treatment of partner/s in the relationship. In the majority of cases, the midwife needs to refer the woman with a STI to a general practitioner or STI clinic for partner notification (see guidance re violence), contact tracing, potential notification of STIs and follow-up testing for cure.

Treatment for STIs

Treatment is usually prescribed by a specialist or doctor. Partners require treatment simultaneously for all STIs.

Chlamydia

The prescription is azithromycin 1 g orally stat (pregnancy category B1). Test for cure is recommended during pregnancy not before 5 weeks after treatment (NZSHS, 2017).

Trichomoniasis

Pregnancy (including first trimester)—metronidazole 2 g stat (category B2) *or* metronidazole 400 mg twice daily for 7 days (if intolerant to stat dose). Advise women not to have unprotected sex for 7 days or until sexual contacts have been treated. See full guidelines for advice regarding prescribing metronidazole during breastfeeding should this be required, as when metronidazole 2 g stat is prescribed, women need to refrain from breastfeeding for 12–24 hours. Breast milk during that time should be expressed and discarded (NZSHS, 2017).

Gonorrhoea

Current recommendations are to refer all women with gonorrhoea in pregnancy to an STI specialist in view of bacteria-resistant patterns associated with treating gonorrhoea. Women should be treated for *Chlamydia* simultaneously with gonorrhoea treatment. Resistance to penicillin, tetracycline and ciprofloxacin is widespread (NZSHS, 2017).

Human immunodeficiency virus (HIV)

HIV serology screening has been introduced antenatally to detect and treat women who are HIV positive. Treatment regimens continue to develop, and antenatal therapy clearly reduces the maternal–fetal transfer of HIV. This information should be shared with women when screening is discussed.

Mastitis

Antibiotic treatment should be reserved for infective mastitis. Management of problems associated with breastfeeding has been covered in Chapter 32; hence the focus of this discussion is assessment and correct diagnosis of infective mastitis. Complementary remedies lack formal evidence and are therefore to be used at the woman's discretion. Symptoms of mastitis include flu-like symptoms, episodes of shivering, muscle aching, extreme malaise and reluctance to breastfeed from a sore breast. A firm red wedge is usually confined to one lobe, often the upper outer quadrant of the breast. Redness of the breast might not be visible until 12 or more hours after the 'flu-like' symptoms (including 'chills') in a deep tissue breast infection. Mastitis frequently originates from a previous sore or cracked nipple. If rapid response to conservative management does not occur, or symptoms are severe or worsening, treatment with antibiotics is warranted in 12–24 hours (BPAC, 2021).

Recommended practice re assessment, diagnosis and prescribing

- Undertake a full physical assessment of the woman; it is important to exclude uterine infection and/or other pathology. Assess woman's temperature, pulse, respiratory rate, blood pressure, breasts, nipples, fundus, abdomen, lochia, perineum, bowel activity, micturition, venous thromboembolism (VTE) symptoms.
- Document the full assessment and history of symptoms. It can be useful to document the location of the affected breast lobe and measure size of the affected area (to exclude worsening signs and/or breast abscess).
- If the woman is systemically unwell and has symptoms of mastitis, exclude penicillin-related allergy prior to prescribing flucloxacillin 500 mg 6-hourly for 5–7 days (BPAC, 2021). Flucloxacillin is taken 1 hour prior to food or 2 hours after food. Flucloxacillin is recommended, as it is the narrowest-spectrum antibiotic and *Staphylococcus* are generally susceptible.
- Amoxicillin-clavulanate and cefaclor are broader-spectrum antibiotics and therefore have more side effects, such as diarrhoea and candidiasis. The use of these might encourage resistant organisms.
- If the woman is penicillin allergic, consultation with a general practitioner or obstetrician is warranted. It might be appropriate for the woman to take erythromycin ethylsuccinate 400 mg 6–8-hourly for 5–7 days. Side effects include gastrointestinal symptoms and poor tolerance.
- Advice to the woman should include starting a breastfeed from the affected breast, alternate cradle/football hold when breastfeeding to drain different ducts in the breast, and localised cold compress postfeed.
- Paracetamol may be used for temperature and analgesia; maximum dose of 4 grams in a 24-hour period.
- It is important to follow up seeing the woman within 24 hours of her commencing antibiotics to ensure improvement and no other underlying pathology. There should be notable improvement within 24 hours. If the woman is not improving, refer to a doctor for advice and/or admission to hospital. The woman might require intravenous antibiotics (medical prescribing) to combat severe infection, or might require an incision or aspiration to remove large amounts of pus when an abscess is present.
- Advise the woman about prevention of mastitis for the future. If the woman is expressing milk for storage (or during employment), the pattern of expressing and breastfeeding should remain consistent.

CRITICAL THINKING EXERCISE

Verity is 9 days postpartum with her second baby. She had attachment problems in the first few days of breastfeeding and had sore nipples. She telephones you (her midwife) to say that she felt cold last evening and was shivering through the night. This morning she has a sore breast and it hurts to breastfeed.

Discuss your full assessment of Verity and plan for management of this situation.

Postpartum sepsis/endometritis

Streptococcus pyogenes (community-acquired Group A β-haemolytic streptococcus (GAS)) is the most common organism causing maternal mortality from sepsis. GAS sepsis can present with non-specific symptoms such as fever, sore throat or vomiting and diarrhoea (Bowyer et al., 2017). Bowyer et al. state sepsis and immediate referral are needed (prior to laboratory assessments) when two or more of the following are present: systolic blood pressure of 90 mmHg or less; respiratory rate of 25 / minute or > (some literature state respiratory rate of 22 / minute or >); altered mental state. Midwives need to recognise signs of unwellness, assess for infection, including endometritis / sepsis and undertake prompt referral to obstetric services for investigations / intravenous antimicrobials.

Lower-segment caesarean-section wound infection

In view of rising caesarean rates and shorter postnatal stays, midwives are increasingly monitoring women in the community for wound infections and postpartum sepsis. If a wound infection is present, referral is needed to consider oral/intravenous antibiotics according to the risk for each individual woman and clinical presentation.

POSTPARTUM CONTRACEPTION

Contraceptive methods are covered in Chapter 34 thus the focus in this section is on pharmacological action of methods used postpartum, recent evidence of effects, and midwifery prescribing.

Progestogen-only pill (progestin-only oral contraception)

The progestogen-only pill (POP) has 96% to 97% efficacy, depending on compliance, and is often chosen as an oestrogen-free contraceptive method postpartum. POPs do not seem to reduce the milk volume for lactating women and minute amounts of the POP pass through the breast milk to the baby, less so with the highly bound levonorgestrel POP (Guillebaud, 2016). The POP, as with most other medicines, is metabolised by the liver. Midwives should not prescribe the POP to women with altered liver function. The POP is affected by enzyme-inducing drugs such as some anticonvulsants and rifampicin. Women taking medication should have a consultation with a medical practitioner, to assess drug interactions and safe prescribing. Other contraindications to midwifery prescribing (indication for medical assessment) include arterial disease, hypertension with either systolic or diastolic ≥140/90, abnormal lipids, any cancers, trophoblastic disease, pathological changes in nervous or muscle tissue, previous ectopic pregnancy, functional ovarian cysts (as these appear increasingly with use of the POP), acute porphyria, history of VTE, migraine with aura, strong family history of breast cancer and undiagnosed irregular menstrual bleeding (Guillebaud, 2016).

Assessment and prescribing recommendations

- Assess the woman's history (see Chs 23, 34), including ectopic pregnancy; document this discussion.
- Record the woman's blood pressure and document. If either systolic or diastolic pressure is elevated above or near 140/90, medical referral is warranted.
- Recommend options of starting POP at day 21 postpartum (Guillebaud, 2016), or the woman may elect to delay POP until 6 weeks or more postpartum—fertile ovulation has been documented at day 25 postpartum in non-lactating women. Younger women return to fertility more quickly than their older counterparts (Guillebaud, 2016).
- Provide education on the POP method. A pill needs to be taken every day of the month within 3 hours of the same time each day. There are no inactive/sugar pills in POP packages, unlike some combined oral contraceptives.
- If a POP is 'missed'—considered as >3 hours late (unless Cerazette is used)—then the woman should either abstain from sexual intercourse or use a barrier method of contraception for 48 hours until viscous cervical mucus is re-established.
- Antibiotics do not affect the POP unless they are enzyme-inducing drugs (oestrogen is recycled in the enterohepatic cycle, not progestogen) such as rifampicin for tuberculosis or meningitis prophylaxis, and griseofulvin used for fungal infections of the skin and nails (Guillebaud, 2016).
- Women should be informed regarding symptoms of ectopic pregnancy and to see a doctor urgently. Functional ovarian cysts and irregular bleeding should be discussed.
- Prescribers should not write 'mini-pill' on the prescription form, as the pharmacist might interpret this as a low-dose combined oral contraceptive pill.
- Brand names are acceptable on the prescription form. Check which brand/s are fully subsidised to minimise cost to the woman.

Combined hormonal contraceptive (CHC)

In general, midwives seldom prescribe CHC as this method is less suitable during lactation. Midwives can reference UK Faculty of Sexual and Reproductive Healthcare (FSRH, 2019) eligibility criteria for contraceptive use and similar guidelines. Prescribing of CHC requires careful assessment of the woman's personal and family history.

Although all CHCs carry a risk of VTE, this risk is greater in the postpartum period with an increase in concentration of clotting factors, which does not return to a prepregnancy state until 4 weeks postpartum for factors VIII and X, fibrinogen and plasminogen activator inhibitors 1 and 2 while factor VII and D-dimer may take 6 weeks or even 8 weeks for prothrombin fragments, protein S and activated protein C resistance (Jackson, 2011; Speroff & Mishell, 2008). Jackson (2011) quoted a systematic review that gave women in the first 6 weeks postpartum an increased risk 22–84-fold compared with similar-aged non-pregnant women without additional risk of combined contraception.

Historically, the 'third-generation-type' CHCs have been associated with an even higher incidence of VTE and fatal pulmonary embolism. Factor V Leiden mutation might also contribute to VTE and is reported as the most common genetic risk factor. Parkin et al. (2000) reviewed fatal pulmonary embolism in all NZ women of childbearing age from 1990 to 1998. Third-generation oral contraceptive pills containing the newer type progestogen, desogestrel and gestodene (purported to have less androgenic effects) were the most commonly used CHC by the women who died. Skegg (2000) concluded that women taking third-generation CHCs had approximately twice the risk of VTE in comparison with women using preparations containing levonorgestrel ('second-generation' CHC).

Assessment and prescribing recommendations

- Check thoroughly for history and risk factors that would preclude midwifery prescribing of CHCs; document informed choice. Ensure the woman is *not* breastfeeding.
- Record the woman's blood pressure. If either systolic or diastolic pressure elevated above or close to 140/90, medical referral is warranted.
- Educate the woman re symptoms of VTE.
- Earliest start date for CHC in a woman without risk factors is 3 weeks postpartum (FSRH, 2019).
- The midwife needs to have knowledge of appropriate CHC with regard to strength of ethinyloestradiol component combined with levonorgestrel or norethisterone.
- High-dose CHCs with 50 μg of synthetic oestrogen have an even greater risk of VTE and are prescribed by doctors only in certain circumstances, for example women medicated with enzyme-inducing drugs.

Injectable progestogen contraceptive (depot medroxyprogesterone acetate—DMPA)

There is a much higher dose of synthetic progestogen level initially with the injectable method, which then declines. It is essential that the injection site is deep intramuscular (thigh or outer area of buttock) and is not massaged, as this shortens the duration of action. FSRH (2019) placed DMPA as classification 2 for women without risk factors who are breastfeeding and <6 weeks postpartum. It is prudent practice to administer the injection in a setting where adult adrenaline (epinephrine) and resuscitation facilities are available and where the woman can be observed for 20–30 minutes after the injection.

RULES FOR WRITING PRESCRIPTIONS

Australian midwives have access to a formulary alongside the Australian Government Department of Health information for prescribers online (http://www.pbs.gov.au/info/healthpro/explanatory-notes/section1/Section_1_2_Explanatory_Notes). The Australian midwife can obtain personalised forms with name, qualifications, practice address/es, telephone number and prescriber number; non-personalised forms are distributed for emergency supply only. The following rules apply for Australian Pharmaceutical Benefits Scheme (PBS) prescriptions:

- They must be written in indelible form (i.e. ink or ball-point pen) in the prescriber's own handwriting (exceptions must be approved by Chief Executive Medicare) either on the standard PBS prescription, or on paper approximately 18 × 12 cm, or they can be generated by computer on a form approved by the Department of Human Services. For patient safety reasons, both the original and the duplicate must be legible.
- They must record the prescriber's name and address (and, in the case of dentists, optometrists, midwives and nurse practitioners, the prescriber number), the patient's name, address and entitlement status, and whether the prescription is under the PBS or Repatriation Pharmaceutical Benefits Scheme (RPBS).
- They should completely identify the pharmaceutical benefit by detailing the item, dose, form, strength, quantity and instructions for use.
- They should indicate where brand substitution is not permitted. PBS prescriptions must not be prepared using a computer prescribing program that contains a default which would result in all prescriptions being indicated as Brand Substitution Not Permitted.
- They must be signed by the prescriber and dated. Forward or back dating is not permitted.

There is no formulary list for New Zealand midwives. Midwives are expected to prescribe within their scope of practice. The following information covers changes to the *Medicines Regulations 1984/2012* under the *Medicines Act 1981*. The legislation referring to midwives prescribing for antenatal, intrapartum, and postpartum care has been revoked and replaced by the following legislation clause 39.

39 Conditions under which authorised NZ prescribers may prescribe prescription medicines

1. An authorised prescriber (including a designated prescriber) may only prescribe a prescription medicine if the authorised prescriber—
   (a) is prescribing the prescription medicine—
      (i) for the treatment of a patient under the authorised prescriber's care; and
      (ii) within, and in accordance with all conditions (if any) stated in, the authorised prescriber's scope of practice, as determined by an authorisation granted under section 21 of the *Health Practitioners Competence Assurance Act 2003* by the authority responsible for the registration of the authorised prescriber; and
   (b) is not prohibited by a notice under section 48(1) of the Act from prescribing that prescription medicine or any prescription medicines of a class or description that includes that prescription medicine.
2. An authorised prescriber who is a designated prescriber may only prescribe a prescription medicine if—
   (a) the prescription medicine is of a class or description that the designated prescriber is authorised to prescribe by regulations made under the Act; and
   (b) the requirements specified in or imposed under those regulations are satisfied.

Form of prescription NZ (*Medicines Regulations 1984*: reprint 28 May 2021 Part 7, 41)

- Every prescription given under these regulations shall—
  - (a) be legibly and indelibly printed; and
  - (b) be signed personally by the prescriber with his [sic] usual signature (not being a facsimile or other stamp), and dated; and
  - (c) set out the following information in relation to the prescriber:
    - (i) the prescriber's full name; and
    - (ii) the full street address of the prescriber's place of work or, in the absence of the prescriber having a place of work, the postal address of the prescriber; and
    - (iii) the prescriber's telephone number; and
  - (d) set out—
    - (i) the surname, each given name, and the address of the person for whose use the prescription is given; and
    - (ii) in the case of a child under the age of 13 years, the date of birth of the child; and
  - (e) indicate by name the medicine and, where appropriate, the strength that is required to be dispensed; and
  - (f) indicate the total amount of medicine that may be sold or dispensed, or the total period of supply; and
  - (g) if the medicine is to be administered by injection, or by insertion into any cavity of the body, or by swallowing, indicate the dose and frequency of dose; and
  - (h) if the medicine is for application externally, indicate the method and frequency of use.

Writing a prescription NZ (note that controlled drug prescription has additional requirements)

- Write your full name as the prescriber.
- Write 'Midwife Prescription' if you are not using an NZCOM prescription pad.
- Write the street address of your place of work (or the postal address if the prescriber does not have a fixed place of work).
- Write your phone number so that the Pharmacist can contact you urgently.
- Write your Midwifery Council Practising Certificate number (this might change to common person number in the future).
- Circle the code / s correctly on the prescription
- Write the given name(s) of the person for whose use the prescription is given (full name of client).
- Write the client NHI.
- Write date of birth if under 13 years of age—necessary for a prescription for a baby.
- The prescriber must specify the name of medicine (correct spelling), strength, route, dose and frequency of dose, and length of supply.
- Use generic prescribing (not brand or trade names) *except* for oral contraceptives.

Practicalities

- On the prescription form, use *one box per medicine* or pharmaceutical being prescribed—*never* write two different medicines or pharmaceuticals in one box.
- Use the first box on the left of the prescription to write the medicine name (correct spelling, and select a medicine that is fully subsidised from the NZ Formulary or current PHARMAC Schedule online).
- Write the strength of the drug where indicated in grams, milligrams, or micrograms.
- Write brief and professional instructions for use, which includes the 'route' and 'frequency' and supply. For example: Take one tablet orally daily. Supply 3 months.

Vaginal candidiasis prescription—clotrimazole cream 1%. Insert applicator filled with cream gently into the vagina at bedtime for 6 nights. Supply 35 grams (check the NZ Formulary or pharmaceutical schedule for amount of grams in the fully subsidised product).

- Strike out the unused boxes to prevent inappropriate 'tampering' of the prescription document.
- Write in the Period/Quantity box the Supply that matches the amount you wrote previously.
- Strike out any Period/Quantity boxes below that are not used.
- Prescriber must personally sign with usual signature and date the prescription; you cannot sign a prescription on behalf of another practitioner.
- The Prescriber must specify the total quantity of medicine or total period of supply, but no longer requires the prescriber to specify in what portions or at what intervals the medicine should be dispensed.
- The Prescriber's writing needs to be legibly and indelibly printed (black pen recommended).
- *Use Plain English* when writing prescriptions as abbreviations can cause errors.

What is the law regarding oral communication of a prescription in New Zealand?

Urgently required prescriptions of prescription medicines may be communicated orally, if later confirmed in writing. A written prescription must be forwarded to the pharmacist confirming the oral communication within 7 days.

Application to practice situation

On occasions midwives might need to fax a prescription to a Pharmacist. The original copy of a prescription that has been 'faxed' must be sent to the dispensing pharmacist *within 7 days.* The prescription must state that it has already been faxed by writing the word 'faxed' on it. This is to prevent fraud—cases have been reported where a client presented a faxed copy of a prescription to a number of different pharmacists.

Why was the legislation changed to include the telephone number of the prescriber and why is there a need for a postal address?

The pharmacist must be able to contact the prescriber by telephone, in order to clarify or amend prescriptions. If a prescription is incorrect, annotated changes are required by the prescriber. The Pharmacist will return the prescription to the prescriber via postal address. If midwives wish their home address to remain private, they can provide a clinic address or postal box number.

What is the period of supply for prescriptions?

Three months for all pharmaceuticals, *except* a 6-month supply is allowed for oral contraceptives prescriptions *only* (https://www.legislation.govt.nz/regulation/public/1984/0143/latest/DLM4189210.html).

CRITICAL THINKING EXERCISE

1. Explain the purpose of screening and treating asymptomatic bacteriuria during pregnancy.
2. Discuss the key clinical information that informs your decision making re managing mastitis conservatively or prescribing antibiotics immediately.
3. Explore research evidence in relation to contraceptive methods including efficacy of lactational amenorrhoea. Why do you think lactational amenorrhoea is 'underused' by Western postpartum women?
4. Discuss how you would explain to a woman the risk of venous thromboembolism in association with use of combined oral contraceptive pills <21 days postpartum.
5. Differentiate between the signs and symptoms associated with the following vaginal infections: candidiasis, trichomoniasis, *Chlamydia* and gonorrhoea.
6. Discuss the benefits versus side effects of injectable progestogen and the information that you would share with women considering this method of contraception postpartum.

Conclusion

In this chapter, an overview of pharmacology has been provided to assist readers with revision of pharmacology and the physiological changes during pregnancy. Medicines and antimicrobials commonly used during pregnancy and childbirth have been reviewed. Specific pregnancy-related conditions have been discussed in association with research evidence in relation to assessment, diagnosis and treatment. The authors stress the need for midwives to maintain a current knowledge base of pharmacology and pharmaceuticals. Midwives need to have a low threshold for referral, and to prescribe medicines only within the scope of midwifery practice and legislation. Midwives need to have particular concern for the wellbeing of the woman and baby, and consider the effects of pharmaceuticals upon the maternal–infant dyad. Midwives have a responsibility to encourage women and families to maintain optimal health and to minimise unnecessary use of antibiotics to prevent antimicrobial resistance. Finally, accuracy of prescription writing and follow-up of the client are essential for safe midwifery practice.

Review questions

1. How does the Australian Categorisation of Drugs and Safety during pregnancy assist midwives in safe prescribing practices?
2. List pre-existing conditions or pregnancy-related conditions that affect liver and renal function and therefore alter metabolism and/or excretion of medicines.
3. Explain the physiological changes that take place during normal pregnancy and how these might affect pharmacokinetics.
4. Explain bacterial resistance in relation to UTI and the implications this has upon prescribing practice.
5. List five principles that prescribers can employ to help minimise bacterial resistance.
6. Discuss differential diagnosis for a suspected UTI and whether or not you would treat prior to culture results.
7. Discuss differential diagnosis in relation to decision making (in partnership with the woman) regarding prescribing iron supplementation during pregnancy
8. State your response to a woman's partner who asks you to write a prescription for his/her own personal needs.
9. List all the assessments that you would undertake prior to prescribing a postpartum woman the progestogen-only pill.
10. Discuss how you will maintain current evidence-based knowledge to enable safe prescribing practice as a midwife.

Online resources

American College of Obstetricians and Gynaecologists: http://www.acog.org.
Australian Government, Department of Health and Ageing, Therapeutic Goods Administration, Prescribing medicines in pregnancy database: https://www.tga.gov.au/prescribing-medicines-pregnancy-database/.
Australian Government, Department of Health Prescribing Medicines—information for PBS prescribers: http://www.pbs.gov.au/info/healthpro/explanatory-notes/section1/Section_1_2_Explanatory_Notes.
Australian Quality Use of Medicines: http://www.health.gov.au/internet/main/publishing.nsf/Content/nmp-quality.htm.
Centers for Disease Control and Prevention (search for 'sexually transmitted infections and pregnancy'): https://www.cdc.gov.
Christchurch Medicines Information service: http://www.druginformation.co.nz/.
Infant Risk Center: https://www.infantrisk.com/.
- Breastfeeding and medication: https://www.infantrisk.com/categories/breastfeeding.
- Pregnancy and medication: https://www.infantrisk.com/categories/pregnancy.
- Drug entry into human milk reference: https://www.infantrisk.com/content/drug-entry-human-milk.

Lactmed: https://www.ncbi.nlm.nih.gov/books/NBK501922/?report=classic.
Medsafe (New Zealand Ministry of Health) information on medicines: http://www.medsafe.govt.nz.
Midwifery Council of New Zealand Midpoint Newsletters (see items under heading 'Newsletters'): http://www.midwiferycouncil.health.nz/publications/.
National Prescribing Service: Get It Right! Taking a Best Possible Medication History 2021: https://learn.nps.org.au/mod/page/view.php?id=5436.
New Zealand College of Midwives consensus statements and guidelines: http://www.midwife.org.nz/quality-practice/consensus-statements-and-guidelines/.
New Zealand Formulary: http://nzformulary.org/.
New Zealand referral guidelines for maternity services: http://www.health.govt.nz/publication/guidelines-consultation-obstetric-and-related-medical-services-referral-guidelines.
New Zealand Sexual Health Society (NZSHS) best practice guidelines: http://www.nzshs.org/.
NICE guidelines: http://www.nice.org.uk/guidance/index.jsp?action=byType&type=2&status=3.
NPS Medicine Wise: https://www.nps.org.au.
PHARMAC, Pharmaceutical Management Agency of New Zealand, online access to New Zealand Pharmaceutical Schedule detailing which pharmaceuticals attract subsidy: http://www.pharmac.govt.nz/.
Royal Australia New Zealand College of Obstetricians and Gynaecologists (RANZCOG): http://www.ranzcog.edu.au/.
Therapeutic Guidelines Australia: www.tg.org.au.

References

Al-Zidan, R. *Drugs in Pregnancy (online): A Handbook for Pharmacists and Physicians.* Apple Academic Press; 2020.
Amir L, Baeza C, Charlamb J, Jones W. Identifying the cause of breast and nipple pain during lactation. *BMJ.* 2021;374:n1628. doi:10.1136/bmj.n1628.
Australian Government Department of Health. *Asymptomatic bacteriuria symptomatic.* 2019. Online: https://www.health.gov.au/resources/pregnancy-care-guidelines/part-f-routine-maternal-health-tests/a38 -bacteriuria.
Banning M. Nurse prescribing, nurse education and related research in the United Kingdom: a review of the literature. *Nurse Educ Today.* 2004;24(6):420–427.
Best Practice Advocacy Centre NZ (BPAC). *Antibiotics: Choices for Common Infections.* Updated March 2021. Online: https://bpac.org.nz/antibiotics/guide.aspx.
Bowyer L, Robinson H, Barrett H, et al. SOMANZ Guidelines for sepsis in pregnancy, 2017. Society of Obstetric Medicine Australia and New Zealand. https://doi.org/10.1111/ajo.12646.
Burchum J, Rosenthal L. *Lehne's Pharmacology for Nursing Care.* 10th ed. St. Louis, Missouri: Elsevier; 2019.
Bryant B, Knights K, Darroch S, Rowland A. *Pharmacology for Health Professionals.* 5th ed. Chatswood, NSW: Elsevier; 2019.
Calje E, Skinner J. The challenge of defining and treating anemia and iron deficiency in pregnancy: a study of New Zealand midwives' management of iron status in pregnancy and the postpartum period. *Birth.* 2017;44(2):181–190. doi:10.1111/birt.12282.
Daru J, Cooper N, Khan K. Systematic review of randomized trials of the effect of iron supplementation on iron stores and oxygen carrying capacity in pregnancy. *Acta Obstet Gynecol Scand.* 2016;95(3):270–279. doi:10.1111/aogs.12812.
Department of Health NZ. *Nurses Amendment Act 1990: Information for Health Providers.* Wellington: Department of Health; 1990.
Ekeroma AJ, Camargo CA Jr, Scragg R, et al. Predictors of vitamin D status in pregnant women in New Zealand. *N Z Med J.* 2015; 128(1422):24–34.
Faculty of Sexual and Reproductive Health (FSRH). *UK Medical Eligibility Criteria for Contraceptive Use.* 2019. Online: http://ukmec.pagelizard.com/2016#.
Food and Drug Administration (FDA). *A strengthened warning to mothers that breastfeeding is not recommended when taking codeine or tramadol. 2017.* Online: https://www.fda.gov/Drugs/DrugSafety/ucm549679.htm.
Guillebaud J. *Contraception Today.* 8th ed. Atlanta, GA: CDC Press; 2016.
Health Direct. *Folate.* 2017. Online: https://www.healthdirect.gov.au/folate.
Holden SC, Gardiner P, Birdee G, et al. Complementary and alternative medicine use among women during pregnancy and childbearing years. *Birth.* 2015;42(3):261–269. doi:10.1111/birt.12177.
Jackson E. Controversies in postpartum contraception: when is it safe to start oral contraceptives after childbirth? *Thromb Res.* 2011;127:s35–s39. doi:10.1016/S0049-3848(11)70010-X.
Lowe SA, Bowyer L, Beech A, et al. *SOMANZ Guideline for the management of nausea and vomiting in pregnancy and hyperemesis gravidarum.* 2019. Online: https://www.somanz.org/content/uploads/2020/07/NVP-GUIDELINE-1.2.20-1.pdf.
Lupattelli A, Spigset O, Twigg M, et al. Medication use in pregnancy: a cross-sectional, multinational web-based study. *BMJ Open.* 2014;4(2):e004365. doi:10.1136/bmjopen-2013-004365.
McLintock C, Repke JT, Bucklin B. Haematological disease in pregnancy. In: Powrie R, Green M, Camann W, eds. *de Swiet's Medical Disorders in Obstetric Practice.* 5th ed. Singapore: Blackwell; 2010:48–81.
Medsafe. *New Zealand data sheet—proctosedyl.* 2018. Online: http://www.medsafe.govt.nz/profs/Datasheet/p/Proctosedylointsupp.pdf.
Medsafe. NSAIDs and cardiovascular risk. *Prescriber Update.* 2019a; 40(2). Online: https://www.medsafe.govt.nz/profs/PUArticles/June2019/NSAIDs-and-cardiovascular-risk..
Medsafe. *Data sheet—prostin E_2 1 mg and 2 mg vaginal gel.* 2019b. Online: www.medsafe.govt.nz/profs/datasheet/p/ProstinE2vaggel.pdf.
Medsafe. Spotlight on Nitrofurantoin. *Prescriber Update.* 2020a; 41(1). Online: https://www.medsafe.govt.nz/profs/PUArticles/March2020/Spotlight-nitrofurantoin.html.

Medsafe. *New Zealand data sheet*—ultraproct. Wellington: New Zealand Medicines and Medical Devices Safety Authority, Ministry of Health; 2020b. Online: http://www.medsafe.govt.nz/profs/Datasheet/u/ultraproctointsupp.pdf.

Midwifery Council of NZ (MCNZ). *Competencies for Entry to the Register of Midwives*. 2007. Online: http://www.midwiferycouncil.health.nz/midwifery-competence.

Milman N, Paszkowski T, Cetin I et al. Supplementation during pregnancy: beliefs and science. *Gynecol Endocrinol*. 2016; 32(7):509–516. doi:10.3109/09513590.2016.1129161.

Milman N. Dietary iron intake in pregnant women in Europe: a review of 24 studies from 14 countries in the period 1991–2014. *J Nutri Metab*. 2020. doi:10.1155/2020/7102190.

Ministry of Health NZ. *Folate/Folic Acid*. n.d. From: http://www.health.govt.nz/our-work/preventative-health-wellness/nutrition/folate-folic-acid. https://creativecommons.org/licenses/by/4.0/.

Ministry of Health (MOH). *Guidelines for Consultation with Obstetric and Related Medical Services (referral guidelines)*. Wellington, NZ: Ministry of Health; 2012a.

National Institute for Health and Care Excellence (NICE). *Intrapartum Care for Healthy Women and Babies. Clinical guideline*. London: NICE; 2021.

National Women's Guideline. *Pathway for Iron Supplementation for Pregnant Women*. 2015. Online: http://nationalwomenshealth.adhb.govt.nz/health-professionals/iron-in-pregnancy.

New Zealand College of Midwives (NZCOM). *Consensus Statement: Midwife Prescribing*. Christchurch: NZCOM; 2014a. Online: https://www.midwife.org.nz/quality-practice/nzcom-consensus-statements.

New Zealand College of Midwives (NZCOM) Consensus Statement. *Prescribing and Administration of Opioid Analgesia in Labour*. 2014b. Online: https://www.midwife.org.nz/quality-practice/nzcom-consensus-statements.

New Zealand Formulary (NZF). *Electronic edition*. 2021a. Online: http://nzf.org.nz/.

New Zealand Formulary (NZF). *Nausea and vomiting during Pregnancy*. Electronic edition, 2021b. Version 109; 1 July. Online: https://nzf.org.nz/nzf_2348?searchterm=vomiting%20 nausea%20and%20vomiting%20during%20pregnancy.

New Zealand Sexual Health Society (NZSHS). *Best Practice Guidelines*. 2017. Online: http://www.nzshs.org/docman/guidelines.

Nursing and Midwifery Board of Australia (NMBA). *2017 Registration standard: endorsement for scheduled medicines for midwives*. NMBA. Melbourne, Australia.

Nursing and Midwifery Board of Australia. *Safety and Quality Guidelines for Privately Practicing Midwives*. NMBA, Melbourne, Australia: NMBA; 2017.

Nursing and Midwifery Board of Australia. *FACT sheet: endorsement for scheduled medicines for midwives*. Melbourne, Australia: NMBA.

Parkin L, Skegg DC, Wilson M, et al. Oral contraceptives and fatal pulmonary embolism. *Lancet*. 2000;355(9221):2133–2134.

Pavord S, Daru J, Prasannan N, et al. UK guidelines on the management of iron deficiency in pregnancy on behalf of the BSH Committee. *Br J Haematol*. 2020;188:819–830. doi: 10.1111/bjh.16221.

Peña-Rosas JP, De-Regil LM, Garcia-Casal MN, et al. Daily oral iron supplementation during pregnancy. *Cochrane Database Sys Rev*. 2015;(7):CD004736, doi:10.1002/14651858.CD004736.pub5.

Percy L, Mansour D, Fraser I. Iron deficiency and iron deficiency anaemia in women. *Best Pract Res Clin Obstet Gynaecol*. 2017;40:55–67. doi:10.1016/j.bpobgyn.2016.09.007.

Royal Australian and New Zealand College of Obstetricians and Gynaecologists (RANZCOG). *Vitamin and Mineral Supplementation and Pregnancy*. 2019. Online: https://www.ranzcog.edu.au/RANZCOG_SITE/media/RANZCOG-MEDIA/Women%27s%20Health/Statement%20and%20guidelines/Clinical-Obstetrics/Vitamin-and-mineral-supplementation-in-pregnancy.

Royal College of Pathologists of Australia (RCPA). *Iron deficiency*. 2019. Online: https://www.rcpa.edu.au/Manuals/RCPA-Manual/Clinical-Problems/I/Iron-deficiency.

Schneeberger C, Geerlings SE, Middleton P, et al. Interventions for preventing recurrent urinary tract infection during pregnancy. *Cochrane Database Syst Rev*. 2015;(7):CD009279, doi:10.1002/14651858.CD009279.pub3.

Skegg D. Third generation oral contraceptives: caution is still justified. *BMJ*. 2000;321(7255):190–192.

Smaill F, Vazquez J. Antibiotics for asymptomatic bacteriuria in pregnancy. *Cochrane Database Syst Rev*. 2015;(8):CD000490, doi:10.1002/14651858.CD000490.pub3.

Speroff L, Mishell Jnr DR. The postpartum visit: it's time for a change in order to optimally initiate contraception. *Contraception*. 2008;78(2):90–98.

Therapeutic Goods Administration (TGA). *Prescribing medicines in pregnancy database*. n.d. Online: https://www.tga.gov.au/prescribing-medicines-pregnancy-database.

Vazquez JC, Abalos E. Treatments for symptomatic urinary tract infections during pregnancy. *Cochrane Database Syst Rev*. 2011;(1):CD002256, doi:10.1002/14651858.CD002256.pub2.

Visovsky C, Workman L, Edmunds M. *Introduction to Clinical Pharmacology*. 9th ed. St. Louis, Missouri: Elsevier; 2019.

Young G, Jewell D. Topical treatment for vaginal candidiasis (thrush) in pregnancy. *Cochrane Database Syst Rev*. 2001; (4):CD000225.

Statutes (NZ)

(see http://www.legislation.govt.nz).

Health Practitioners Competence Assurance Act 2003.

Medicines Act 1981.

Medicines Amendment Regulations 2011.

Medicines Regulations 1984.

Medicines Regulations 1984 Amendment No. 3 1990.

Misuse of Drugs Act 1975.

Misuse of Drugs Amendment Regulations 2014.

Nurses Amendment Act 1990.

Further reading

Spencer JP. Management of mastitis in breastfeeding women. *Am Fam Physician*. 2008;78(6):727-731.

Wulff M, Ekstrom EC. Iron supplementation during pregnancy in Sweden: to what extent is the national recommendation followed? *Acta Obstet Gynecol Scand*. 2003;82(7):628-635.

Student midwives should also access journals online and texts related to microbiology, pharmacology and prescribing practice.

CHAPTER 34

Contraception

Terri Foran

LEARNING OUTCOMES

Learning outcomes for this chapter are:

1. To be able to identify available contraceptive services in your local area
2. To describe the role of the midwife in providing contraception counselling
3. To identify the factors that influence the selection of a suitable method of contraception for a woman or couple
4. To discuss the influence of culture, disability, stage of reproductive life and pre-existing health problems on the choice of contraception
5. To explain the efficacy of various methods of contraception with typical and perfect use
6. To describe the way in which the following methods of contraception act, the reasons they may be selected as a method, and their suitability for use during lactation and the postpartum period: the lactational amenorrhoea method, fertility awareness-based methods, barrier methods, intrauterine devices, hormonal contraception, spermicides, coitus interruptus and sterilisation.

CHAPTER OVERVIEW

This chapter presents an overview of the methods of contraception available in Australia and New Zealand and will provide midwifery students with a basic knowledge in this area. It is not within the scope of this chapter to provide complete information about each method of contraception and midwives working with women in the antenatal and postnatal periods in particular are encouraged to read more extensively on this topic. Those seeking an even deeper understanding of this subject might consider enrolling in a course offered by their local sexual health clinic, family planning organisation or natural family planning centre. A list of the head offices across Australia and New Zealand is provided at the end of this chapter, as well as web addresses for other relevant organisations that provide reproductive health information (see Online resources).

KEY TERMS

barrier methods
combined hormonal methods
contraceptive implant
emergency contraception
fertility awareness methods
intrauterine devices (IUDs)
lactational amenorrhoea method (LAM)
long-acting reversible contraceptives (LARCs)
permanent contraception methods
progestogen-only contraceptive methods

INTRODUCTION

Attempts to control fertility have been documented throughout history (Varney, 1997). These have ranged from spells and amulets to postcoital douching and 'do-it-yourself' vaginal barriers made from half a lemon. However, it was not until the 20th century that we saw the advent of modern, more effective methods of birth control. In Australia and New Zealand, contraceptive services are provided in a variety of settings. These include sexual health and family planning clinics, general practice, women's health centres, community health centres, youth health centres, sexual health services and services provided within acute care hospitals.

REFLECTIVE THINKING EXERCISE

Many readers will come to any discussion of contraception with pre-existing opinions and experiences. Even before we start it might be useful to reflect on some of these. You might like to jot down some short notes as you consider the following questions.

1. Whose responsibility is contraception?
2. How do those in your particular community access contraceptive knowledge and services? Can you identify any potential barriers or problems?
3. If applicable you might also like at this point to reflect on your own experiences in seeking contraceptive advice and as a contraceptive user.

CONTRACEPTIVE COUNSELLING: THE ROLE OF THE MIDWIFE

It is estimated that approximately 50% of all pregnancies are unintended or mistimed, though not necessarily unwanted. Following delivery some women may wish to continue with their previous method of contraception, or alternatively they may lack confidence in their previous method and wish to consider a different method. Some women will decide that their family is now complete and seek to implement a more effective or even a permanent method of contraception. Midwives are therefore in a unique position to assist women during pregnancy, childbirth and the puerperium with their future contraception and safer-sex needs.

The most recent best-practice guidelines from the United Kingdom reinforce the message that the range of contraceptive options should be discussed with the woman in the postnatal ward before she leaves hospital and that appropriate staff be available to provide her with the option she feels may best suit her (Faculty of Sexual and Reproductive Healthcare (FSRH), 2017a). Initiation of contraception in the immediate postpartum period is a safe and cost-effective way of reducing the rates of both unintended pregnancy and early repeat deliveries (Teal, 2014). However, contraception is often neglected in the busy hospital setting, given the understandable immediate focus on pregnancy and delivery (Glasier et al., 1996). Traditionally, the discussion of contraception has often been deferred until the 6-week check, but this neglects the fact that ovulation can occur within 25 days of delivery in women who are not breastfeeding (Jackson & Glasier, 2011). The assumption that couples will not have resumed sexual activity by 6 weeks is also erroneous, as Australian research suggests that at least 41% have done so (McDonald & Brown, 2013). Ideally discussion about ongoing contraceptive needs should be initiated in the antenatal period and reinforced postnatally as this allows for a personalised dialogue between the woman and her health provider and builds on any written information made available to her (Saeed et al., 2008). An up-to-date list of local providers who have a special interest in contraception is an invaluable adjunct to initial counselling by the midwife.

A number of factors will influence the method of contraception selected by a woman or couple. These include:

- whether the individual or couple is seeking a permanent or temporary method of contraception
- their understanding of the effectiveness of the method—it is important to understand that for some methods there may be a significant difference between the theoretical failure rate seen in clinical trials and the typical failure rate likely to occur in a real-life setting (Table 34.1)
- health issues that may make some methods inappropriate
- the perceived or actual side effects of the method
- the woman's age and lifestyle
- previous positive or negative experience(s) of a method(s)
- the cost and convenience of the method
- the ease of use of particular methods
- the number of sexual partners
- the current popularity of a particular method
- the influence of the media, friends and family
- religious and/or cultural factors.

Contraceptive choices may vary greatly over a woman's lifespan depending on such factors as a desire for further children, stage of sexual relationship, medical history and the risks of sexually transmitted infection (STI) (Trussell & Guthrie, 2011). This variability of contraceptive use is exemplified in Tables 34.2–34.4. The effectiveness of the various contraceptive methods, both perfect and typical, should be discussed along with a conversation that no method, even sterilisation, is 100% effective (see Table 34.1). Also important is a discussion of how the various contraceptive methods work and their potential side effects. This should all be placed within the context of the benefits and risks of the method as they relate to the individual woman and her individual preferences and philosophy. The time it takes for fertility to return after cessation of the method is also important when couples indicate they want to have more children. Only

Table 34.1 Percentage of women experiencing an unintended pregnancy during the first year of use of a contraceptive method and the percentage continuing use at the end of the first year, USA

Method (1)	% of women experiencing an unintended pregnancy within the first year of use		% of women continuing use at 1 year[a]
	Typical use[b] (2)	Perfect use[c] (3)	(4)
No method[c,d]	85	85	
Spermicides[e]	29	18	42
Lactational amenorrhoea[f,g]		2	Only effective until 6 months postpartum
Fertility awareness-based methods	25	2–9	
Calendar method		9	
Ovulation (mucus) method		3	
Symptom—thermal		2	
Withdrawal	27	4	46
Barrier methods[h]			
Female condom (FC)	21	5	41
Male condom	15	2	43
Conventional diaphragm[i]	16	6	57
CAYA diaphragm with CAYA gel[g]	18	12	
Hormonal methods			
Combined pill and progestogen-only pill	8	0.3	67
NuvaRing[g]	8	0.3	67
DMPA	6	1	56
Intrauterine devices			
Copper T Load 375[g]	0.8	0.6	78
Mirena (LNG IUS)	0.1	0.1	80
Contraceptive implants			
Implanon NXT[g]	<0.1	<0.1	84
Jadelle	0.2–0.8	0.2–0.8	
Permanent contraception			
Female sterilisation	0.5	0.5	100
Male sterilisation	0.15	0.1	100

[a]Among typical couples who initiate a method (not necessarily for the first time), the percentage who experience an accidental pregnancy during the first year.
[b]Among couples who initiate use of a method (not necessarily for the first time), the percentage who experience an accidental pregnancy during the first year if they do not stop use for any other reason.
[c]Among couples who initiate use of a method (not necessarily for the first time) and who use it perfectly (both consistently and correctly), the percentage who experience an accidental pregnancy during the first year if they do not stop use for any other reason.
[d]Percentages becoming pregnant in columns (2) and (3) are based on data from populations where contraception is not used and from women who cease using contraception in order to become pregnant. Among such populations, about 89% become pregnant within 1 year. This estimate was lowered slightly (to 85%) to represent the percentage who would become pregnant within 1 year among women now relying on reversible methods of contraception if they abandoned contraception altogether.
[e]Foams, creams, gels, vaginal suppositories and vaginal film. Note: no spermicides are available in Australia and New Zealand.
[f]To maintain effective protection against pregnancy, another method of contraception must be used as soon as menstruation resumes, the frequency or duration of breastfeeds is reduced, bottle feeds are introduced or the baby reaches 6 months of age.
[g]Data not available for Trussell, so best alternative data provided (e.g. from manufacturers' studies).
[h]Without spermicides.
[i]With spermicides. Note: no spermicides are available in Australia and New Zealand.
DMPA = depot medroxyprogesterone acetate; LNG IUS = levonorgestrel-only intrauterine system.
(Adapted from Trussell & Guthrie, 2011)

Table 34.2 Contraceptive practices, Australia—primary contraceptive method reported by women who used any method[a]

Method	Total % use	% by age group (years)			
		16–19	20–29	30–39	40–49
Oral contraceptive	33.1	47.1	49.1	27.1	16
Condom	30.2	35	37.6	28.4	18.8
Partner has vasectomy	13.7	0	1.2	14.1	32.4
Intrauterine device (5.6% hormone-releasing IUD and 0.5% copper IUD)	6.1	1.2	2	10.4	7.6
Tubal ligation/occlusion	5.7	0	0.3	6	13.6
Implant	4.9	4.9	3.9	6.3	4.6
Breastfeeding	1.8				
Progestogen injection	1.5				
Safe period	1.4				
Withdrawal	1.3				
Other	0.5				

[a]No. of women surveyed= 4579.
IUD = intrauterine device.
(Adapted from Richters et al., 2016)

Table 34.3 Contraceptive practices, New Zealand 1999[a]

Method used[b]	% in each age group (years)					
	20–24	25–29	30–34	35–39	40–44	45–49
Non-Māori women (*n* = 1292)						
Sterilisation (male + female methods)	1	8	24	42	60	72
Pill, pill + other	47	45	29	17	11	5
Pill + condom	14	5	2	2	[0.4]	0
Condom, condom + other	21	20	20	16	8	7
IUD or injection or diaphragm or foam	9	4	7	7	8	3
Traditional methods	2	2	3	4	3	2
No method	6	16	15	11	10	11
Total %[c]	*100*	*100*	*100*	*100*	*100*	*100*
Māori women (*n* = 236)						
Sterilisation (male + female methods)	0	15	40	51	61	75
Pill, Pill + other	25	34	23	14	7	0
Pill + condom	9	0	5	0	3	0
Condom, condom + other	16	17	16	4	3	0
IUD or injection or diaphragm or foam[d]	18	9	7	6	7	0
Traditional methods	0	4	0	0	0	0
No method	32	21	9	25	19	25
Total %[c]	*100*	*100*	*100*	*100*	*100*	*100*

[a]Type of contraceptive method or methods used in the 4 weeks prior to the survey by women
[b]aged <50 years old, who were not pregnant and who had had intercourse in the previous 4 weeks, by age group at the time of survey and ethnicity.
[b]Excludes women who responded 'don't know' or 'refused'.
[c]Totals may not add to 100% due to rounding.
[d]Among Māori women, this category is mainly injection.
IUD = intrauterine device.
This appears to be the most recent comprehensive survey of contraceptive use in New Zealand women of all ages.
(Source: Pool et al., 1999)

Table 34.4 Current contraceptive usage in women in New Zealand aged 35–54 years[a]

	35–39 yrs	40–44 yrs	45–49 yrs	50–54 yrs	Total
	% using	% using	% using	% using	% using
Reversible methods					
OCPs	11	15	5		9
DMPA		3			1
Implant		2	2		1
IUD	7	14	10		8
Non-reversible methods					
Vasectomy	17	22	48	50	35
Tubal ligation		5	11	12	7
Hysterectomy		3	6	26	9
Oophorectomy			2	5	2
Period stopped[b]		5	15	60	20

[a]Data collected 2013–15. 'Ever-use' data was also collected but is not presented here.
[b]Includes natural menopause and surgically induced menopause.
DMPA = depot medroxyprogesterone acetate; IUD = intrauterine device; OCP = oral contraceptive pill.
This study is significantly limited by the age range of the people surveyed and the relatively poor response rate (47%). The authors compared their results with a similar earlier study and concluded that for 'ever-use' there had been a significant rise in ever-use of the OCP (75% to 89%) and a more than twofold increase in condom use (24% to 64%). There was a significant increase in ever-use of vasectomy (26% to 40%) and a fall in tubal ligation (22% to 8%). Only a slight increase in the use of DMPA and IUDs was observed.
(Adapted from Chesang et al., 2016)

condoms provide significant protection against STIs and raising the discussion of dual protection (i.e. condoms plus another more effective contraceptive method) may be useful for some women. Important too for midwives is an understanding of when particular methods can be commenced in the postpartum period, and their suitability during lactation. Some women have existing health problems that may affect the suitability of some methods. Both the World Health Organization (WHO) and the FSRH publish detailed medical eligibility criteria (MEC) for all contraceptive methods (FSRH, 2017b; WHO, 2015) and a link to these is provided in the Online resources section at the end of this chapter. These may assist in advising women with more complex medical problems.

Cultural and religious beliefs may also impact on contraceptive choice. It is not possible within the scope of this chapter to discuss each cultural group represented in Australia and New Zealand but it is important for midwives to be familiar with the cultural mores of the indigenous women and common groups of culturally and linguistically diverse (CALD) women in their care. Some women have a more restricted knowledge of contraceptive methods, particularly where virginity is highly prized and expected until marriage. In some cultures, information about contraception may have been withheld as being more appropriate to be discussed at the time of marriage. Other women may have been coerced to use methods of contraception without their informed consent and may be distrustful of all methods. Some may be refugees or have migrated from countries where access to contraceptive services was unavailable, limited or punitive, or may have experienced sexual assault or sexual exploitation in the past. Some may have come from countries with pronatalist policies, and others from countries where strict limitations are placed on family size. When discussing contraception with indigenous or CALD women, traditional values must be respected and dealt with sensitively. There must also be an acknowledgement that some women may want to move away from the traditional approaches to contraception countenanced by their partner and/or community (Srikanthan & Reid, 2008).

All advice and information provided should be non-judgmental and framed to complement the woman's own values and beliefs. Healthcare professionals should take care that their own values and preferences do not influence the advice they give to women. The midwife's counselling role also needs to extend beyond advice about contraception. Although the birth of a baby can strengthen a relationship and perhaps enhance sexual intimacy, resumption of sexual intercourse may take several months in some couples. Hormonal changes can result in a low libido, there can be physical discomfort from an episiotomy, perineal tear or caesarean, and there can be physical and emotional exhaustion from sleepless nights and the demanding role of parenting—all of which can be worse if the woman has postnatal depression (Guillebaud & MacGregor, 2017). Decreased lubrication due to low oestrogen levels may make intercourse uncomfortable even if artificial lubricants are used. Not only are there likely to be significant physical changes to the woman's body after childbirth, but also adjustment of the relationship to include a new family member can have a profound impact on erotic feelings and the opportunity to express these (Kennedy & Trussell, 2011).

RESEARCH ACTIVITY

Go to the website of your local sexual health and family planning organisation (see Box 34.12) and familiarise yourself with the services offered and the location of the clinics. Compile a resource list for use in your own clinical practice.

FERTILITY AWARENESS METHODS

Lactational amenorrhoea method

The lactational amenorrhoea method (LAM) is the informed use of breastfeeding as a contraceptive method. High levels of prolactin inhibit the pulsatile release of gonadotrophin- releasing hormone (GnRH) by the hypothalamus. This in turn reduces the production of follicle-stimulating hormone (FSH) and luteinising hormone (LH), which are required to initiate successful ovulation (Kennedy & Trussell, 2011). According to a 1988 consensus statement (Lancet, 1988) LAM provides 98% protection against pregnancy provided *all* three of the following criteria are met:

- The woman remains amenorrhoeic postpartum. The mean time for the return of menses in breastfeeding women is 28.4 weeks, with a range from 15 to 48 weeks.
- The woman is less than 6 months post-delivery.
- The baby is fully breastfed with no long intervals between feeds. Although no definitive guidance exists here, this interval is recommended to be no more than 4 hours during the day and 6 hours at night.

The key to the success of this method is frequent stimulation of the breast through suckling. Thus the effectiveness of LAM is compromised by any condition which affects attachment and suckling—such as prematurity or congenital abnormality. The method may also be less successful if there is routine use of expressed milk. One study looking at working women who regularly expressed suggested higher rates of pregnancy (5.2%) even on a background of good milk production and full breastfeeding (Valdes et al., 2000). If breastfeeding is supplemented only non-milk supplements are permitted (e.g. water/juice). These should be given infrequently (no more than and preferably less than 5%–15% of intake), and not via a bottle (Kennedy & Trussell, 2011).

Women should be advised to switch to another method of contraception once the infant reaches 6 months of age or should any of the other criteria fail to be met. LAM is not considered a suitable contraceptive option for women in Australia and New Zealand who are living with the human immunodeficiency virus (HIV) because of the potential for transmission of the virus in the breast milk (Panel on Treatment of HIV-Infected Pregnant Women and Prevention of Perinatal Transmission, 2021).

Other fertility awareness methods (FAMs)

These methods, sometimes called 'natural methods' or 'natural family planning', use recognition of the changes which occur during various times of the menstrual cycle in order to determine likely fertility. When used for contraception the aim is to avoid sexual intercourse during the fertile time but one of the advantages of this method is that it also provides the woman with the ability to optimise her chances of pregnancy when desired. Though the ovum is fertilisable for only up to 24 hours after ovulation, successful use of FAM must also take into account the length of time that sperm can survive in the upper female genital tract—an average of 3–4 days with a theoretical possibility of up to 7 days (Guillebaud & MacGregor, 2017).

To achieve maximum effectiveness such methods require the cooperation and commitment of both partners, as the couple must agree to abstain from intercourse throughout the potentially fertile period of the woman's menstrual cycle. Though the theoretical failure rate of this method is low, at 2%–9% per year, the typical failure rate is significantly higher with some studies reporting a failure rate of 25% in the first year of use (Smoley & Robinson, 2012). Some couples combine FAM with the use of a barrier method (condom/diaphragm) during the fertile time but unfortunately this strategy may compromise the effectiveness of both methods and there are no estimates of its likely efficacy. FAM could be considered when religious or cultural beliefs exclude the use of other contraceptive methods and also where there is a preference for a method that is completely free of physical and hormonal side effects.

A number of different methods follow by which the fertile time might be determined and some couples combine a number of these in an attempt to maximise efficacy. It is advisable that couples learn to use these methods correctly from expert practitioners, and Natural Fertility Australia/New Zealand provide a list of local accredited instructors. Their websites are listed in Box 34.12. Both these organisations also conduct courses for health professionals who are interested in becoming natural family planning instructors.

Implications for lactation and the postpartum period

FAMs may be even more difficult to use when cycles are irregular such as during breastfeeding and at perimenopause. Though signs of fertility may be apparent as early as 4 weeks in women who are not breastfeeding, previous experience in using the method is likely to make these easier to detect. The postpartum period is probably one of the more difficult times to implement FAM if it has not been used before.

Calendar-based methods

The calendar method, sometimes called the 'rhythm' method, is based on the dual premise that ovulation occurs

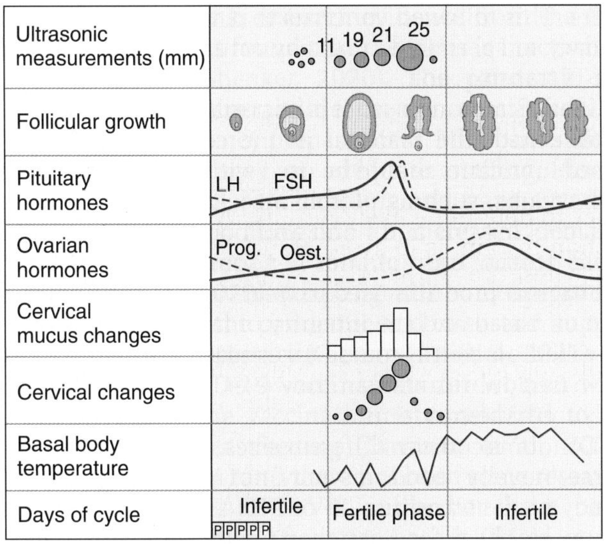

FIGURE 34.1 Fertility chart
(Based on Guillebaud, 2009)

11–16 days before the next menstrual period and that sperm can survive for up to 5 days (Fig. 34.1). The woman must chart at least three consecutive cycles in order to establish her usual cycle range and this calculation must be reviewed should she later experience a cycle which is outside the usual length. With day 1 being her first day of bleeding, the women should subtract 21 from her shortest cycle length in order to determine her first fertile day and 10 from her longest cycle for her last. For instance, in a women whose cycle length varied from 26 to 32 days, the first fertile day is calculated as day 5 (26 minus 21) and the last as day 22 (32 minus 10). The 'standard days' method is a relatively recent simplification of the calendar method and requires 12 days of abstinence per cycle from day 8 to day 19 (Nelson & Burke, 2011). It is not suitable for women who record more than two cycles per year outside the range 26–32 days. There are also a number of aids designed to assist calculation of fertile days using the calendar method. These range from the relatively low-tech 'cyclebeads' in which a bead is used to mark each day that passes, to smartphone applications of variable reliability. Calendar methods are considered the least effective FAM method (Wilcox et al., 2000) given that, even when strictly adhered to, life events may disrupt predictions and alter the fertile period unexpectedly.

Symptoms-based methods

Basal body temperature (BBT)

The BBT method relies on the detection of a 0.2–0.5°C rise in temperature following ovulation. This slight increase in temperature is caused by the secretion of progesterone from the corpus luteum and the temperature remains elevated until the onset of the next menstrual period. This sign is useful only in establishing when ovulation has already occurred and cannot be used to calculate the beginning of the fertile period. The temperature needs to be taken accurately each morning using the same (oral, vaginal or rectal) route each time and is then charted on a temperature chart. Couples using this method are advised not to have intercourse until there have been 3 consecutive days on which a higher temperature reading has been recorded when compared with the 6 previous days. One of the problems with this method is that there is significant individual variation in BBT, which can be affected by life events such as illness, emotional stress, irregular or disturbed sleep, smoking, some medications and travel (Barron & Fehring, 2005).

Mucus methods

These methods rely on the daily observation of the mucus discharge felt at the vaginal entrance. One variation of this method is the Billings' method, named after the two Australian doctors who first formalised a description of the differences in the mucus discharge from one part of the cycle to another. Three patterns of mucus are described:

- postmenstrual infertile mucus, which is described as thick, flaky and dry
- ovulatory or fertile mucus, which is watery and elastic, resembling egg white
- postovulatory infertile mucus, which is cloudy, sticky and dry.

This method dictates that intercourse should be avoided once the fertile mucus is detected and for 3 days after the last fertile mucus is seen. Some users combine an observation of the mucus pattern with daily temperature in order to provide additional confirmation that they are indeed postovulation.

Devices and personal fertility computers

There are an increasing numbers of apps and fertility computers designed to assist in determining fertile times and also some evidence that their use may increase the effectiveness of this method (Berglund et al., 2016). These utilise algorithms based on indicators such as cycle length and temperature and some are able to incorporate information from earlier cycles in an attempt to increase their accuracy further. The more accurate devices also incorporate testing for the presence of LH. This is detectable in the urine approximately 6 days before the ovum is released—conveniently at around the limit for sperm survival. One such device, the Persona, first marketed in 1996, claims a failure rate of around 6% in the first year of use.

BARRIER METHODS

Barrier methods include male and female condoms, diaphragms and cervical caps. Only one cervical cap—the FemCap—is presently manufactured and as it has never been marketed in Australia or New Zealand it must be accessed through a web supplier. It will not be covered in this chapter. Barrier methods have the advantage of being used only as required. Condoms are the only contraceptive method that also provide significant STI protection and for that reason they may be used in addition to the primary method of contraception when risk of infection is an issue. Such a practice is termed 'dual protection' or more colloquially 'double dutching'.

Male condom

This is a widely available and popular method of contraception (see Tables 34.2 and 34.3) in both Australia and New Zealand. Male condoms are single-use penile sheaths, most commonly made of latex (rubber). Polyurethane (plastic) and polyisoprene (synthetic non-allergenic rubber) condoms are also available, and provide a good alternative for individuals with allergies, sensitivities or personal preferences that might prevent the use of latex condoms (Gallo et al., 2006). They are both more expensive than the latex variety. In some countries, though not Australia or New Zealand, 'lambskin' condoms are also available. Made from lamb intestines, they are said to provide a more natural experience during intercourse than latex or polyurethane condoms. Though they provide adequate contraception the tiny pores present in lambskin condoms allow the passage of bacteria and viruses and so cannot be relied upon for STI protection. All male condoms provide high contraceptive efficacy if used correctly and consistently (Warner & Steiner, 2011), and have a perfect use failure rate of only 2%. Unfortunately the typical failure rate is significantly higher—up to 15%.

Condoms must be stored in a cool, dry place. Prior to their use the expiry date of the condom should be noted and a check made that there is no obvious damage to the packet. Care must be taken when handling condoms to minimise the risk of tearing during use. Each act of intercourse requires the use of a new condom and it should be placed onto the erect penis before any contact is made with the female partner. Many condoms come with a small teat at the end which is designed to collect semen after ejaculation. This should be squeezed between the thumb and forefinger, expelling any air, before the condom is rolled on. Failure to do this increases the chances of condom breakage. For condoms without a teat it is suggested that the very end of the condom be similarly compressed before rolling the rest down to the base of the erect penis. Following ejaculation, the condom should be held on at the base and the penis removed from the vagina before the erection is lost. This reduces the risk of the condom coming off accidentally during withdrawal and either being left within the vagina or spilling semen at the vaginal entrance. The condom should then be knotted at its open end and disposed of in the garbage. It is also important that the penis makes no contact with the vulva or vagina after ejaculation until the penis is cleansed as there may still be live sperm present in or around the male urethra. In some parts of the world, spermicides are used in conjunction with condoms; however, neither spermicides nor spermicide-lubricated condoms have been available in Australia or New Zealand for several years. This followed concerns that vaginal irritation secondary to spermicide use may actually increase the risk of STI transmission.

If lubricants are used it is important that they are compatible with the material in the condom. Only water-based lubricants should be used with latex condoms. Oils and creams, such as petroleum jelly, baby oil, massage oils, cooking oils and hand and body lotions, can cause rapid deterioration of latex condoms. Similarly many of the vaginal products used to treat vaginal candidiasis are also oil based and the integrity of latex condoms cannot be relied on if intercourse takes place during treatment. Oil-based lubricants can, however, be safely used with polyurethane condoms.

Condoms come in different sizes, colours and flavours. Some 'novelty' condoms may not protect against pregnancy or the transmission of STIs and so it is important that users check for Australian or New Zealand standards approval logo on the pack. Condoms are now available from many sources including supermarkets, pharmacies, vending machines, healthcare services and entertainment venues. They are reasonably cheap, particularly when bought in larger packets. Some manufacturers make wider, longer or tapered condoms for those who find standard condoms uncomfortable. It is important that condoms fit correctly to improve user acceptance and to optimise the prevention of STIs and unintended pregnancy (Cecil et al., 2010).

Condoms are most effective in preventing the transmission of STIs such HIV, gonorrhoea, chlamydia, trichomoniasis and hepatitis B. They are less effective against infections transmitted by skin-to-skin contact or contact with mucosal surfaces—such as genital herpes, human papilloma virus and syphilis. As the condom covers only the shaft of the penis it will not provide an effective barrier if lesions in either partner occur outside the area of coverage (Warner & Steiner, 2011).

If a condom is damaged or slips off during use then consideration should be given to the use of emergency contraception. Many authorities suggest that for those relying on barrier contraception it may be useful to have an 'in-date' pack of hormonal emergency contraception handy in case of non-use or accident. Box 34.1 gives emergency contraception advice.

Box 34.1 Emergency contraception alert—male condom

Women should be provided with information ahead of time about emergency contraception (see Emergency contraception section in this chapter), so they can prevent pregnancy if: the condom breaks, slips off or is damaged in any way; there is any semen leakage from the condom; there is contact of the penis with the female genital area before the condom is applied, or before it is removed and the penis cleansed.

Female condom (FC2)

The FC2 is the second-generation female condom. It is marketed in both Australia and New Zealand but it can be somewhat difficult to obtain as availability from local pharmacies is variable. Information on local access is best sought from the nearest family planning organisation (see Box 34.12). Female condoms cost approximately 10 times more than male condoms. The FC2 is a strong, thin, loose sheath (Fig. 34.2) which is 17 cm in length and is for single use only.

It is now made from nitrile rather than the previous polyurethane. Nitrile is a synthetic latex-like material which is safe to use with oil-based lubricants. It is also safe for use where either partner has a latex allergy. It has a 60 mm flexible ring at the closed end which assists its insertion high into the vagina. There is also a larger but thinner outer ring 70 mm in diameter that remains external to the vulva. This outer ring prevents the condom from being pushed into the vagina during intercourse. Female condoms have a perfect-use failure rate of 5% but a typical failure rate of 21% (Trussell, 2011). One perceived advantage is that they are under the control of the female partner, who can insert them several hours before they may be needed. Female condoms are prelubricated, although the use of a little additional lubricant can be useful in minimising the 'rustling sound' commonly described with their use during intercourse. As with male condoms, female condoms afford some protection against several STIs (Guillebaud & MacGregor, 2017).

Prompt access to emergency contraception provides a useful back-up in the event of non-use or slippage. Box 34.2 gives emergency contraception advice.

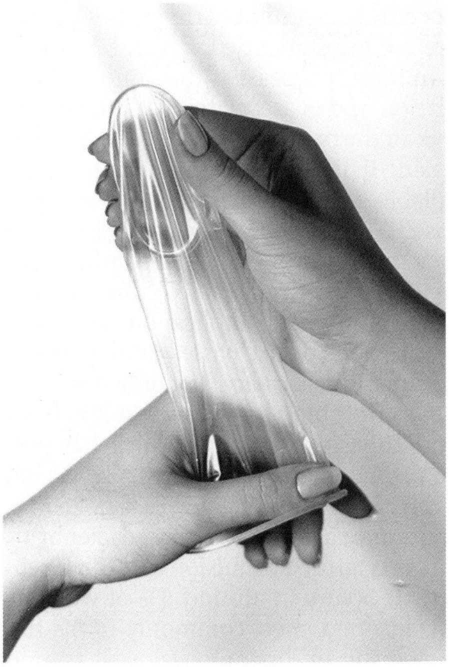

FIGURE 34.2 Female condom (Femidom)
(Source: Guillebaud, 2009)

Box 34.2 Emergency contraception alert—female condom

Women should be provided with information ahead of time about emergency contraception (see Emergency contraception section), so they can prevent pregnancy if: the penis is wrongly positioned (between the female condom and the vaginal wall); the female condom is damaged in any way; there is any semen leakage from the female condom; there is contact by the penis with the female genital area before the female condom is inserted, or before it is removed and the penis cleansed.

Implications for lactation and the postpartum period

Neither male nor female condoms interfere with lactation and can be used whenever the couple is ready to resume sexual intercourse. If vaginal dryness is a problem during lactation the addition of a suitable lubricant may make intercourse more comfortable.

Diaphragm

A traditional diaphragm comprises a soft dome of hypoallergenic, medical grade silicone with a firm, flexible rim and is designed to prevent sperm from reaching the upper genital tract. Conventional diaphragms have not been available in Australia and New Zealand for several years but can still be obtained from internet retailers if the woman's size is known. A 'one-size-fits-most' diaphragm known as a CAYA® is available in both Australia and New Zealand. It is advised that this device is used in conjunction with its companion CAYA GEL® to optimise efficacy. The manufacturer claims an effectiveness of 82% in real-life or 'typical' use when the device is used with the gel. The CAYA (Fig. 34.3) fits up to 90% of women (Schwartz et al., 2008). Though ostensibly 'one-size-fits-most' it is recommended that the size and

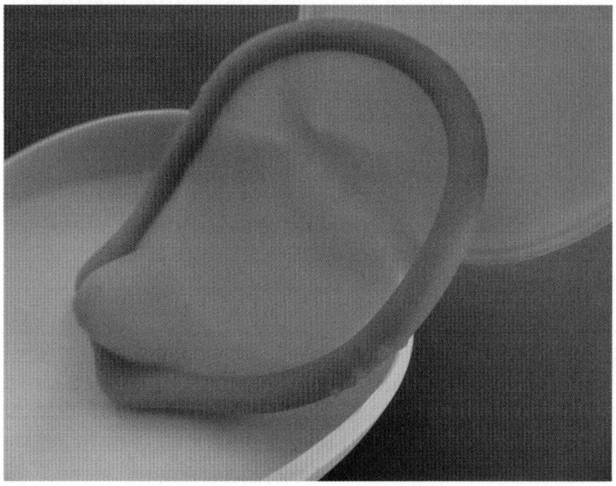

FIGURE 34.3 The CAYA
(Source: Terri Foran)

> **Box 34.3 Emergency contraception alert—barrier methods**
>
> Women should be provided with information ahead of time about emergency contraception (see Emergency contraception section), so they can prevent pregnancy if they become aware that the cervical barrier did not feel as though it fitted correctly, if it became dislodged, or if it was not used.

correct fit of the device be checked by a health provider before the intending user relies on it for contraception. CAYA is available without a prescription and is used in conjunction with the accompanying lactic acid buffer gel, which is applied to the inner surface of the dome prior to insertion.

The CAYA may not be suitable for those women with a shallow pubic ledge or poor pelvic floor muscle tone. Some women also find that the use of female barriers increases the incidence of urinary tract infection. Women who choose this method must feel comfortable with their bodies and confident in inserting and removing the device from their vagina. The CAYA can be inserted into the vagina several hours before intercourse but needs to be left in place for 6 hours afterwards. The device should be washed carefully after use with water and unperfumed soap, rinsed and dried well, and stored in the plastic box provided, away from light and heat. It should also be checked regularly for any holes or splitting, which would compromise its effectiveness as a barrier. CAYA has a recommended duration of use of 2 years and the gel used with it has a shelf-life of 3 months after opening. Box 34.3 gives emergency contraception advice.

Implications for lactation and the postpartum period

Like previous diaphragms, neither CAYA nor the cellulose gel used with it interferes with lactation. CAYA should not be used by women who are less than 6 weeks postpartum as pelvic laxity makes it less likely that it will ensure an adequate barrier to sperm.

LONG-ACTING REVERSIBLE CONTRACEPTIVES (LARCS)

This is a group of contraceptives gaining popularity as 'set-and-forget' forms of contraception that are highly effective and do not rely on daily or coitus-related use.

Intrauterine devices

Most intrauterine devices (IUDs) available worldwide have a plastic backbone around which is wrapped either copper or alternatively a hormone-releasing plastic sleeve. Hormonal IUDs are sometimes termed 'intrauterine systems' (IUSs). All IUDs require a minor surgical procedure to place them in the correct position inside the uterine cavity. Both copper and hormonal IUDs (Fig. 34.4) provide highly effective (see Table 34.1) and convenient contraception with prompt return of fertility on removal. IUDs fell out of favour in many parts of the world as a result of the litigation resulting from the use of the Dalkon Shield, an early IUD which was associated with high rates of pelvic infection in users. There is no doubt, however, that IUDs are an excellent contraceptive method for many women (Hubacher et al., 2011) and their use worldwide is increasing. It is now understood that the highest risk of infection occurs in the first 3 weeks after insertion. This is likely to be the result of asymptomatic cervical infection being introduced into the uterus during instrumentation and selective pre-insertion screening can greatly minimise this risk. Unfortunately the use of prophylactic antibiotics does not appear to alter this risk of infection at insertion (Grimes & Schultz, 2001) and is not therefore recommended. Beyond 3 weeks the risk of pelvic inflammatory disease is the same as that in the general population and is associated with the woman's risk of STI rather than the presence of the IUD. A smaller levonorgestrel-releasing IUD (Kyleena® in Australia, Jaydess® in NZ) is also available. Being smaller these devices may be a particularly useful LARC choice for younger women as trials suggest they may be easier and less painful to insert in this group. Box 34.4 gives emergency contraception advice.

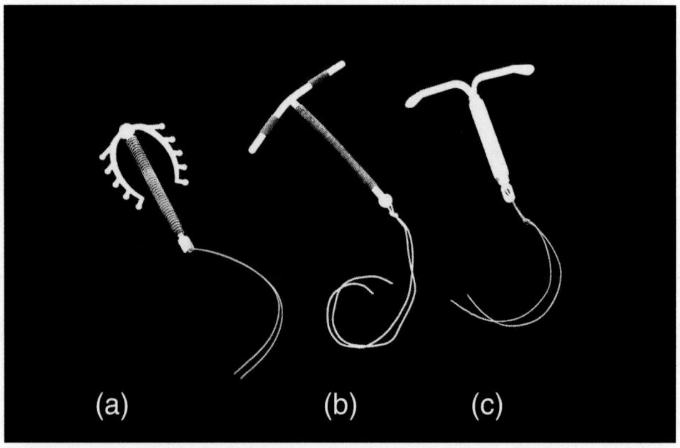

FIGURE 34.4 Intrauterine contraceptive devices: (a) Copper-T 380; (b) Multiload Cu 375; (c) Mirena
(Source: Contraceptive Flipchart—SHine SA; (c) SHINE SA)

Perforation is another complication of IUD insertion and this occurs when the device passes through the uterine wall and into the peritoneal cavity. Not only does this negate its contraceptive effect but also it may result in bowel/bladder injuries and adhesions. An IUD which has perforated requires prompt surgical retrieval usually via laparoscopy. Problems can also occur if the device is not correctly placed within the uterine cavity or is displaced later by uterine contractions. This is termed expulsion and can be either partial or complete. It occurs in around 5% of women who have had an IUD inserted, most commonly in the first year. Expulsion may result in discomfort as well as a potential reduction in the efficacy of the device. Women who regularly check their IUD strings may notice that they are longer than previously. Box 34.4 gives emergency contraception advice.

Box 34.4 Emergency contraception alert—intrauterine device

Women should be provided with information ahead of time about emergency contraception (see Emergency contraception section), so they can prevent pregnancy should the woman be unable to feel her IUD strings (when this had previously been possible) and sexual intercourse had occurred.

Copper IUDs

Copper IUDs do not have any hormonal side effects and do not disrupt the regularity of the menstrual cycle. Less than 1% of women with a copper IUD experience an unintended pregnancy and the typical failure rate is almost identical to the perfect rate (0.8% versus 0.6%) as user error is virtually eliminated (Trussell & Guthrie, 2011). In Australia and New Zealand, three copper IUDs are currently available:

- the TT-380 (licensed for up to 10 years use)
- the TT-380S (a smaller device and licensed for up to 5 years use)
- LOAD Cu-375 (licensed for up to 5 years use).

Copper is extremely toxic to sperm and the main action of a copper IUD is to impede the transport of sperm so as to block fertilisation (Guillebaud & MacGregor, 2017). Copper IUDs also have a secondary inflammatory effect on the endometrium making it unsuitable for implantation. This secondary effect is utilised when copper IUDs are inserted after unprotected intercourse for emergency contraception (see Emergency contraception section). The main disadvantage of copper IUDs is that they have a tendency to increase the amount of menstrual pain and bleeding, with one study indicating an average of about 50% more blood loss (Guillebaud et al., 1976).

Copper IUDs can be inserted up to 5 days after the day of estimated ovulation (which would be conservatively up to day 12 of the cycle) or no later than 5 days after a single act of unprotected intercourse in that cycle. They can, however, be inserted at any time if the woman is currently using an effective alternative contraceptive method. Most inserters require that nothing be placed in the vagina (avoid intercourse, use menstrual pads rather than tampons) for 3 days after insertion in order to minimise the risk of post-insertion infection. Each month, the woman should check for the IUD strings, which should be palpable at the cervical os, to confirm the presence and correct position of the device.

Hormonal IUDs

A variety of hormonal IUDs are available across the world. They provide convenient and very effective contraception, achieving both a perfect and a typical failure rate of 1 per 1000 (Trussell & Guthrie, 2011). The most widely used, the Mirena, releases 20 µg of the progestogen levonorgestrel per day into the uterine cavity at a constant rate over 5 years. Progestogen both thickens the cervical mucus plug and alters the composition of endometrial fluid so as to impede sperm transit to the fallopian tubes. It also thins the endometrium making it unsuitable for implantation. Unfortunately this effect on the endometrium takes up to a week to develop and therefore hormonal IUDs cannot be relied upon for emergency contraception.

Though irregular bleeding is very common in the first 3–5 months of use, almost all users report that bleeding is markedly reduced by 12 months. This makes hormonal IUDs an attractive option for women who experience heavy menstrual periods. Approximately 50% of women fitted with a Mirena report no menstrual bleeding after 6 months use and this too must be discussed prior to use as some women find the concept of amenorrhoea alarming (French et al., 2004). The hormonal IUD is a very useful option at perimenopause as not only does it reduce the heavier bleeding which is common at this time, but also it can act as the progestogen component of menopausal hormone therapy should this be required. Hormonal side effects are uncommon in those using hormonal IUDs as very little of the progestogen finds its way into the general circulation.

In Australia only one hormonal IUD, the Mirena, is presently available. This device is listed on the Australia Pharmaceutical Benefits Scheme (PBS) with specific indications and costs those with a Medicare card approximately $40. In New Zealand, women have access to both Mirena and a similar (but smaller) 3-year hormonal IUD called Jaydess. Jaydess has slightly lower rates of amenorrhoea than Mirena and its smaller size may make it a better choice in women with a smaller endometrial cavity or narrow cervical os. Neither of these hormonal IUDs is subsidised in New Zealand and the user must bear the entire cost of the device herself—around $350 for Mirena and $275 for Jaydess.

Implications for lactation and the postpartum period

Neither copper nor hormonal IUDs interfere with lactation. According to WHO (2015) guidelines a copper IUD can be inserted safely within 48 hours after delivery regardless of whether the woman plans to breastfeed, although such early insertion is associated with a slightly higher rate of expulsion (Lopez et al., 2015a). In the period from 48 hours to 4 weeks postpartum the expulsion rate may be as high as 70% (Eroğlu et al., 2006) and for that reason it is usually recommended that insertion of both copper and hormonal IUDs be avoided during this interval. A hormonal IUD can be safely inserted within the first 48 hours after delivery if the woman does not plan to breastfeed but should ideally be deferred to 4 weeks postpartum if she does. Both copper and hormonal IUDs can be safely inserted in suitable woman from 4 weeks postpartum, regardless of the method of delivery or whether the woman is breastfeeding.

The contraceptive implant

This is a highly effective and very convenient contraceptive method (see Table 34.1). There are a number of

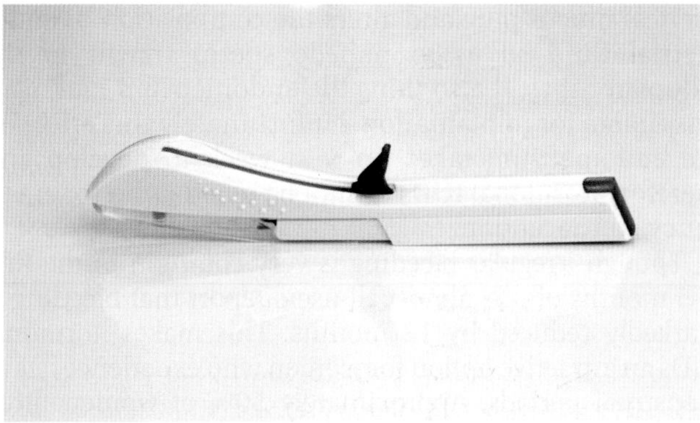

FIGURE 34.5 Contraceptive implant (Implanon)
(Source: Shutterstock/Akkalak Aiempradit)

contraceptive implants available worldwide in which one or more progestogen-releasing rods are inserted under local anaesthetic just under the skin of the upper arm (Fig. 34.5). Women using a contraceptive implant do not experience a predictable bleeding pattern. This can vary from no bleeding at all to troublesome frequent bleeding particularly in the first 6 months of use. Such unpredictable bleeding may be completely unacceptable to some women and their attitude to this should be canvassed before insertion. Other side effects, though uncommon, can include headache, acne, weight gain and mood changes (Trussell & Guthrie, 2011). Contraceptive implants are rapidly reversible, with a return to background fertility occurring within a few days of removal. The progestogens in a contraceptive implant are metabolised by the CYP3A4 system in the liver. Many antiepileptic medications, medications used to treat tuberculosis and HIV and even the herbal medication hypericum (St John's wort) act as enzyme inducers in this system and can significantly reduce the contraceptive efficacy of an implant. For a full list of medications which affect the CYP3A4 system see the Online resources section.

Implanon NXT is a single rod 40 mm long and 2 mm in diameter, containing 68 mg of the progestogen etonogestrel in total, which is released at around 60 µg per day over its 3-year lifespan. Implanon NXT is a very effective contraceptive method with a perfect and typical failure rate of less than 1 in 1000 (Trussell & Guthrie, 2011). The primary contraceptive action of Implanon NXT is to inhibit ovulation through suppression of the LH surge. It also makes cervical mucus impenetrable to sperm within 24–48 hours and thins the endometrium so that it is unsuitable for implantation. Provided that Implanon NXT is inserted within the first 5 of the woman's cycle (or replaces a previous implant) she will achieve immediate contraceptive cover. If the implant is inserted after day 5 she should be advised to use an additional non-hormonal barrier method (e.g. condoms) for 7 days after insertion or to avoid intercourse over that time. In addition, if the woman has been sexually active and the device is inserted after day 5, a pregnancy test should be performed 3 weeks after insertion to exclude an early pre-existing pregnancy. If the woman is currently using another effective method of contraception (e.g. pill, IUD, injection), implant insertion is permissible at any time. However, with a switch from another method the safest advice is for the woman to continue her current method of contraception for a further 7 days or, if she is keen to cease it, to use additional barrier contraception for that time (FSRH, 2017b).

Jadelle consists of two rods 43 mm in length and 2.5 mm in diameter. Each rod contains 75 mg of levonorgestrel. This releases a total of 100 µg of levonorgestrel per day in the month after insertion, which then falls to 30 µg per day by 2 years and beyond. It provides effective contraception for up to 5 years, though the failure rate appears to increase slightly after 4 years use particularly in heavier women. It does not inhibit ovulation as consistently as Implanon NXT and relies more on its effect on the cervical mucus and endometrium for its contraceptive efficacy. It has an annual pregnancy rate of 0.2%–0.8%.

Jadelle can be inserted within 7 days of the onset of the menstrual period but it is recommended that an additional non-hormonal barrier method (e.g. condoms) be used for 7 days after insertion. Similarly if the woman is changing from another contraceptive method to Jadelle she should be advised to continue that method for a further 7 days or to use an additional barrier contraception over that time (FSRH, 2017b).

In Australia, only Implanon NXT is available. It is subsidised by the PBS and costs a Medicare card holder around $40. In New Zealand, Jadelle is available on prescription at no cost to the consumer though there may be fees for insertion. Implanon NXT is also available in New Zealand but is unsubsidised.

Implications for lactation and postpartum

The evidence is unclear regarding effects of contraceptive implants on lactation and breastfeeding. However, minute amounts of the hormone are ingested by the infant through the breast milk and for some mothers this may be unacceptable. Both implants can be inserted immediately postpartum (FSRH, 2017a, 2017b). A Cochrane review found the quality of evidence for immediate versus delayed insertion after birth to be moderate to very low (Sothornwit et al., 2017).

COMBINED HORMONAL METHODS

Combined oral contraceptive pills (COCPs)

Combined oral contraception, commonly known as 'the Pill', is both an effective (see Table 34.1) and a popular (see Tables 34.2–34.4) method of contraception. The fact that the efficacy of the COCP relies greatly on consistent usage means that there is some disparity between perfect (0.3%) failure rate and that seen in typical use (8%). The type and dose of oestrogen and progestogen in the COCP varies from preparation to preparation. All tablets in the pack may contain the same hormone dose (monophasic) or differ in the dose of hormone from one part of the pack to another (bi-, tri- or multiphasic). The main action of COCPs is to block ovulation by suppressing FSH and LH production. They also impede sperm penetration by thickening the cervical mucus and thin the endometrium making it less suitable for implantation. If COCPs are commenced on days 1–5 of the menstrual cycle they provide immediate contraceptive cover even if the woman has had prior unprotected intercourse during that cycle.

Table 34.5 shows the currently available pill brands in Australia and New Zealand, along with the combination of hormones in each formulation. In Australia the COCP is currently only available on prescription from a medical practitioner. The Australian PBS subsidises some pills but not others. In New Zealand too some brands attract a

Table 34.5 Oral contraceptives available in Australia and New Zealand

Trade name	Oestrogen	Progestogen	Available in Australia—PBS listing	Available in New Zealand
Combined oral contraceptive pills				
Ava-20 Femme-Tab ED 20100 Lenest 20 ED Loette Microgynon 20 ED Microlevlen ED Micronelle 20 ED	20 µg ethinyloestradiol (EE)	100 µg levonorgestrel	Yes all but Ava-20 are available but only Femme-Tab 20100 is PBS listed	Ava-20, Loette, Microgynon 20 and Loette are available but only Ava-20 and Microgynon-20 ED are subsidised
Logynon ED Trifeme 28 Triphasil 28 Triquilar ED	6 × 30 µg EE 5 × 40 µg EE 10 × 30 µg EE	6 × 50 µg levonorgestrel 5 × 75 µg levonorgestrel 10 × 125 µg levonorgestrel	Ava-30 is not available in Australia but all other preparations are PBS listed	No
Ava-30 Eleanor 15030 ED Evelyn 15030 ED Femme-Tab ED 30150 Levlen ED Microgynon 30 ED Micronelle 30 ED Monofeme 28 Nordette 28	30 µg EE	150 µg levonorgestrel		Ava-30, Microgynon-30 and Monofeme are available but only Ava-30 and Levlen ED are subsidised
Microgynon 50 ED	50 µg EE	125 µg levonorgestrel		Yes and subsidised
Brevinor Norimin 28 day	35 µg EE	500 µg norethisterone		Yes and subsidised
Brevinor-1 Norimin-1 28 day	35 µg EE	1 mg norethisterone		Yes and subsidised
Norinyl-128	50 µg mestranol (equal to about 35 µg EE)	1 mg norethisterone		No
Improvil	35 µg EE	7 × 500 µg norethisterone 9 × 1 mg norethisterone 5 × 500 µg norethisterone	Neither Mercilon nor Ginet-35 is available in Australia; the remainder are available but are not PBS listed	No
Madeline Marvelon 28	30 µg EE	150 µg desogestrel		Madeline is not available. Mercilon is available but not subsidised
Mercilon	20 µg EE	150 µg desogestrel		Yes but not subsidised
Minulet	30 µg EE	75 µg gestodene		Yes but not subsidised

Continued

Table 34.5 Oral contraceptives available in Australia and New Zealand—cont'd

Trade name	Oestrogen	Progestogen	Available in Australia—PBS listing	Available in New Zealand
Brenda-35 ED Carolyn-35 ED Chelsea-35 ED Diane-35 ED Estelle-35 ED Ginet-35 Jene-35 ED Juliet-35 ED Laila-35 ED	35 μg EE	2 mg cyproterone acetate		Ginet-35, Estelle and Diane are available but are not subsidised for use as a contraceptive
Yasmin	30 μg EE	3 mg drospirenone		Yes—available but not subsidised
Yaz	20 μg EE	3 mg drospirenone		Yes—available but not subsidised
Valette	30 μg EE	2 mg dienogest		No
Oestradiol pills				
Qlaira	Oestradiol valerate 2 × 3 mg 5 × 2 mg 17 × 2 mg 2 × 1 mg	Dienogest 5 × 2 mg 17 × 3 mg	Yes but not PBS listed	Yes but not subsidised
Zoely	1.5 mg oestradiol	2.5 mg nomegestrol acetate	Yes but not PBS listed	Yes but not subsidised
Extended use pills				
Seasonique 84	30 μg EE (plus 7 × 10 μg EE every 4 packs)	150 μg levonorgestrel	Yes but not PBS listed	No
Yaz Flex	20 μg EE	3 mg drospirenone	Yes but not PBS listed	Yaz Flex is not available
Progestogen-only contraceptive pills				
Cerazette		75 μg desogestrel	No	Yes
Locilan		350 μg norethisterone	Yes and PBS listed	No
Micronor		350 μg norethisterone		
Microlut		30 μg levonorgestrel		Yes
Noriday		30 μg norethisterone		
Slinda®	(no oestrogen)	drospirenone	Yes	No

PBS = Pharmaceutical Benefits Scheme.

subsidy whereas others do not. In 2017 a number of the subsidised COCPs became available in New Zealand without a prescription. This requires a discussion with a trained pharmacist before the COCP is dispensed and is not open to first-time users or those under 16 years of age. If the supply is obtained from a pharmacist the cost is $45 for a 3-month supply compared with $5 per pack on prescription. Non-subsidised pills in New Zealand must be obtained on prescription and are more expensive.

Given the large number of COCPs available, it is usually possible to find a formulation that suits most women. Some pill packets have a total of 21 pills that are all active (hormone) pills, with the woman being instructed to take a 1-week break between packets. Others use placebo tablets (2–7 depending on the preparation) to mark the days in which active pills are not taken. The time off active pills is also called the 'pill-free interval' (PFI) and a withdrawal bleed, resembling a menstrual period, usually occurs during this time. Seven days off hormones is close to the time limit at which the COCP can reliably suppress ovulation in the next cycle. The most dangerous time, then, to miss an active pill is in the first and last weeks of the packet as this effectively extends the PFI, putting the woman at risk of pregnancy in the subsequent pill cycle. This is also the reason why some of the newer pills have reduced the number of placebo pills in the pack from 7 to only 2 or 4. Pills should be taken at the same time each day, though as long as it is taken within 24 hours of the usual time then contraceptive cover is maintained.

More recently some preparations have been marketed which extend the time between scheduled withdrawal bleeds by up to 120 days. It is also possible to achieve this with most standard monophasic pills by simply skipping the PFI. Numerous studies have demonstrated the safety of this practice but some women may require reassurance that there is no need to mimic the menstrual cycle with a monthly withdrawal bleed when using a COCP (Nelson, 2011). There is some limited evidence that scheduling less PFI may even increase the effectiveness of the COCP as the potential for a break-through ovulation should that interval be extended is also reduced (Howard et al., 2014).

Unscheduled bleeding is more common with such extended use than with conventional monthly cycling but most preparations can be continued for 3–4 months without significant 'break-through bleeding'. Another option is 'menstrually signalled' bleeding, which involves continuing active pills until more than 3 days of bleeding occurs. Then, provided the woman has taken more than seven pills since her last break, she should be advised to take a 4-day break from active pills allowing the endometrium to shed completely. She should then restart her active pills until the next time she has more than 3 days of bleeding.

In addition to its contraceptive effects, the other advantages of COCPs include regular, light and less painful periods, possible reduction in premenstrual symptoms, protection from pelvic infection and a decreased incidence of ectopic pregnancy. Longer-term benefits include a significant reduction in ovarian and endometrial cancer rates, which extends for up to 20 years after COCP use is ceased (Guillebaud & MacGregor, 2017).

Side effects and complications

Side effects experienced by those using the COCP include headaches, breast tenderness, nausea, weight increase, mood changes and loss of libido. These often diminish over time or may improve with a change of pill. One of the more severe side effects of COCPs is venous thromboembolism (VTE) and the COCP should never be used in those with a previous history of VTE. The risk of VTE is most clearly linked to the oestrogen content of the COCP and is significantly higher in 50 µg pills than in 20–35 µg pills. The presence of other risk factors such as a body mass index of greater than 30, immobility, long-haul travel, etc. may further increase the risk of VTE even with lower-dose COCPs. There remains some controversy as to whether the type of progestogen in the COCP may also affect the VTE risk—with the suggestion that preparations containing levonorgestrel or norethisterone may be safer in this respect.

The COCP also increases the risk of cerebrovascular accident (stroke) and ischaemic heart disease and should be avoided in women with risk factors for these conditions. Women who experience migraine with aura should be advised *never* to use combined contraception since this condition places them at an even higher risk of a cerebrovascular accident than the average user of the COCP (Nelson & Cwiak, 2011). Smoking potentiates most of the risks associated with COCP use (Nelson & Cwiak, 2011) and for this reason the COCP should not be used by those over 35 years of age who smoke more than 15 cigarettes per day.

The COCP should not be used by those with a personal history of breast cancer. A family history of breast cancer is not a contraindication to COCP use but it is not recommended in a woman with a known genetic mutation which is known to increase the risk of breast cancer (e.g. *BRCA1/BRCA2*) (FSRH, 2017b).

Precautions

In the section on contraceptive implants, medications which induce enzymes in the CYP3A4 system in the liver were discussed as they are known to significantly reduce the efficacy of what is otherwise a very effective contraceptive method. The same medications enhance the metabolism of both the oestrogen and progestogen in the COCP, leading to lower circulating levels of these hormones and reduced contraceptive efficacy. The COCP is generally, then, an unsuitable option for women taking these medications. Conversely the COCP may affect the efficacy of other medications. It is therefore important that a careful prescription and non-prescription medication history is taken from women who want to commence COCPs. Clear information about managing problems such as missed pills, vomiting, severe diarrhoea and interactions with other medications should also be provided to women who are taking COCPs. Box 34.5 gives emergency contraception advice.

Implications for lactation and the postpartum period

In a non-lactating woman with no identified risk factors for VTE it is preferable to wait for 3 weeks to commence COCPs (FSRH, 2017a, 2017b). Ovulation prior to that is unlikely and by this time the woman should have returned to her background risk of VTE (Guillebaud & MacGregor, 2017). For those who do not intend to breastfeed but who do have risk factors for VTE (e.g. immobility, transfusion at delivery, obesity, postpartum

Box 34.5 Emergency contraception alert—combined oral contraceptive

Women should be provided with information ahead of time about emergency contraception (see Emergency contraception section), so they can prevent pregnancy in the event that pills have been omitted (particularly those that extend the PFI), or when vomiting or severe diarrhoea has occurred.

haemorrhage, etc.) a non-oestrogen-containing method should be considered.

For the breastfeeding mother with no other risks it is suggested that commencement of the COCP be deferred until 6 weeks postpartum so that breastfeeding can be fully established. For breastfeeding women with no identified risk factors the COCP is considered broadly usable after 6 weeks and from 6 months on there are no restrictions at all to its use (FSRH, 2017a, 2017b). Obviously minute amounts of the hormones in the COCP will be ingested by the infant via the breast milk and the mother will need to make a personal decision about whether she is comfortable with this. She can, however, be reassured that to date no adverse effects on infant growth have been documented (Lopez et al., 2015b).

Hormonal vaginal ring (NuvaRing)

The hormonal vaginal contraceptive ring (Fig. 34.6) is a highly effective method of contraception (see Table 34.1) with failure rates comparable to the COCP. NuvaRing releases 120 μg etonorgestrel and 15 μg ethinyloestradiol from a soft flexible plastic ring (outer diameter of 54 mm) which is inserted into the vagina. It remains in place for 3 weeks before the device is removed for 1 week, at which time a withdrawal bleed occurs. The device is not reusable and a new ring is inserted 1 week later. In theory, as this method does not require daily commitment to maintain efficacy, it could lead to typical-use pregnancy rates lower than those with COCPs, though this has not been demonstrated in studies to date (Nanda, 2011). If the NuvaRing is inserted before day 5 of the menstrual cycle it provides immediate contraceptive cover even if the woman has had prior unprotected intercourse.

The mode of action of NuvaRing is exactly the same as the COCP—it suppresses ovulation, increases cervical mucus viscosity and thins the endometrium (Nanda, 2011). The contraindications and side effects are also the same though some women may find the contraceptive ring suits them better than the COCP because of the lower hormone doses and the more constant delivery system. The efficacy of the contraceptive ring is compromised by the same enzyme-inducing drugs which affect the COCP and contraceptive implants. However, as the contraceptive ring's efficacy is not dependent on absorption from the gut, its efficacy is unaffected by malabsorption syndromes, vomiting or diarrhoea. If the NuvaRing is removed from the vagina for more than 3 hours then contraceptive cover is lost for 1 week. For that reason it is recommended that the device be left in place during intercourse. In the uncommon event that its presence bothers a partner it can be removed but should be replaced within that 3-hour window. NuvaRing is available in Australia but is not subsidised by the PBS and costs the user approximately $30 per month. It was first marketed in New Zealand in 2013 but was withdrawn from sale there in 2017. Box 34.6 gives emergency contraception advice.

Box 34.6 Emergency contraception alert—hormonal vaginal ring

Women should be provided with information ahead of time about emergency contraception (see Emergency contraception section), so they can prevent pregnancy in the event that the ring is removed from the vagina for more than 3 hours and unprotected intercourse has occurred. Emergency contraception may also be appropriate in the first week of use if the woman has extended the length of her ring-free interval beyond 7 days.

Implications for lactation and the postpartum period

Considerations with regard to breastfeeding and postpartum use are identical to the COCP, although vaginal laxity and the presence of lochia may make it more difficult to use at less than 6 weeks postpartum.

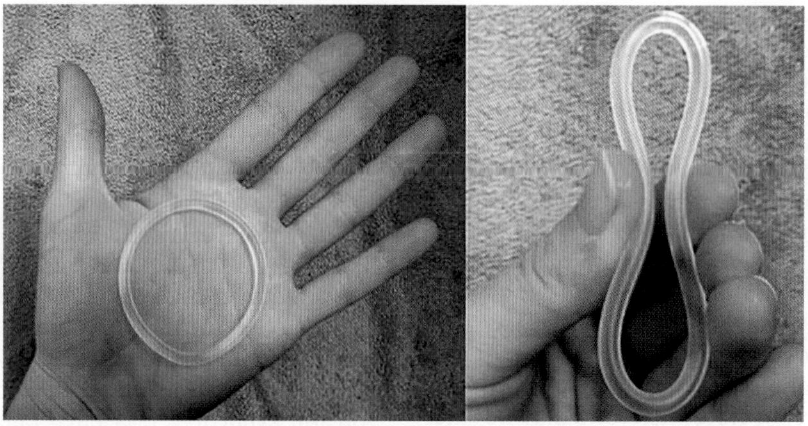

FIGURE 34.6 Hormonal vaginal contraceptive ring (NuvaRing)
(Source: WikimediaCommons/Sakky)

Progestogen-only contraceptive methods

The progestogen-only pill (POP)

The progestogen-only pill (POP), also known as the 'mini-pill', provides the same amount of one of four progestogens (levonorgestrel, norethisterone, drospirenone or desogestrel; see Table 34.5). It is suitable for women in whom oestrogen (and thus COCPs) is contraindicated. Efficacy is listed in Table 34.1, but it should be noted that in lactating women the efficacy of POPs is nearly 100% (Guillebaud & MacGregor, 2013). Most POPs are taken every day with no PFI and have to be taken within a 3-hour time to maintain efficacy, though the desorgestrel POP has a 12-hour window.

Slinda®, the drosprenone POP, has four placebo pills in addition to 24 active pills. It has the same 24-hour leeway for missed pills as the COCP. The action of most POPs is to block the passage of sperm by thickening the cervical mucus, reduce the ciliary action in the fallopian tubes, inhibit ovulation in a variable proportion of cycles and decrease endometrial receptivity (Raymond, 2011). Slinda® reliably suppresses ovulation and is therefore as effective as the COCP. As with the other progestin-only contraceptive methods, bleeding patterns may be altered during POP use, although amenorrhoea is likely during lactation. There are variable effects on ovulation inhibition. POPs containing levonorgestrel or norethisterone suppress ovulation only in perhaps up to 60% of cycles. By contrast, desogestrel POPs can be relied upon to suppress ovulation in a complex manner provided they are taken correctly and for that reason are more likely to be more effective than other POPs in typical use. As with all progestogen-only contraceptive methods, bleeding patterns are likely to be altered during POP use and these can range from amenorrhoea to persistent unpredictable light bleeding. If used during lactation most women experience either amenorrhoea or occasional light bleeding (Guillebaud & MacGregor, 2017).

Precautions

As most POPs are low-dose contraceptives, there is a very narrow margin of error for missed pills. If the pills are taken late, a back-up method of contraception should be used for 48 hours until the woman is back on schedule (Box 34.7). The exception is Slinda®, which, though it has a longer 24-hour leeway for missed pills, requires 7 days of additional contraception until full protection is achieved.

> **Box 34.7 Emergency contraception alert—progestogen-only pill**
>
> Women should be provided with information ahead of time about emergency contraception (see Emergency contraception section), so they can prevent pregnancy should a dose of POP be omitted or vomited.

In the event of vomiting, the usual pills should be taken and a back-up method (such as condoms) should be used for 48 hours. Provided POPs are commenced before day 5 of the cycle they provide immediate contraceptive cover. If the woman is not cycling, which will usually be the case during lactation or postpartum, the POP can be commenced at any time but additional cover will be required for a further 7 days. If the woman has had unprotected intercourse the POP can be commenced following a negative pregnancy test but this should be confirmed with a repeat test 3 weeks later. Like COCPs the efficacy of POPs is compromised by CYP3A4 inducers. Box 34.7 gives emergency contraception advice.

Implications for lactation and the postpartum period

POPs can be started at any time during the postpartum period; although small amounts of progestogen will be ingested by the infant in the breast milk there is no evidence that POPs affect either the quality or quantity of the milk and they have no known effect on infant health and growth (FSRH, 2017a, 2017b). Some women may find the narrow time frame of 3 hours in which to take POPs difficult to adhere to on a daily basis when they are experiencing erratic sleeping and waking patterns. A switch to a COCP/ring could be considered once the infant is 6 weeks old and breastfeeding is established. Alternatively the women may wish to look to the convenience of one of the longer-acting methods.

Injectable contraception

Depo-medroxyprogesterone acetate (DMPA) 150 mg, known as Depo-Provera or Depo-Ralovera, is a contraceptive injection that is effective for 12 weeks. It has a perfect failure rate of less than 1% but the typical failure rate is closer to 6% (see Table 34.1). Like the COCP its primary action is to suppress ovulation by inhibiting the LH and FSH surge. It also thickens the cervical mucus, slows tubal and endometrial motility, and thins the endometrium (Barz & Goldberg, 2011). The first injection should be administered before day 5 of the cycle, at which point it provides immediate contraceptive cover (FSRH, 2017b). If the injection is given later than day 5, or if the woman is not cycling (e.g. postpartum), it is recommended that pregnancy be reliably excluded before the injection is given. Additional precautions are then required for another 7 days (FSRH, 2017b).

DMPA may be a useful option in women with risk factors for the use of oestrogen-containing contraception or for those who experience oestrogenic side effects while using combined contraceptive methods. It is also unaffected by the liver enzyme-inducing medications that compromise the efficacy of methods such as implants, pills and rings, and may be a very useful option for women taking such medications. Irregular vaginal bleeding and spotting are common in the first few months of use though there is a trend to amenorrhoea over time (50% by 1 year). However, fertility may take up to a year to return after ceasing DMPA, making it unsuitable for

> **Box 34.8 Emergency contraception alert—hormonal injection**
>
> Women should be provided with information ahead of time about emergency contraception (see below), so they can prevent pregnancy in the event that the next DMPA injection is not given within the advised time limit and sexual intercourse has taken place.

women who want prompt reversibility of contraception. Some women on DMPA experience weight gain due to increased appetite (Barz & Goldberg, 2011). Other side effects such as headaches, dizziness, abdominal discomfort and fatigue have also been reported by some users (Guillebaud & MacGregor, 2017).

Another issue that has caused concern is the potential for reduced bone mineral density (BMD) in users of DMPA. The World Health Organization has concluded that, although there is some loss of bone density during DMPA use (on average 5%–7% in hip and spine over 4 years), this is regained quickly on cessation (WHO, 2007). Although not the first choice for adolescents or perimenopausal women, WHO stated that 'Women aged 18–45 should be able to use DMPA without any limitations' (WHO, 2007). A Cochrane review (Lopez et al., 2014) further concluded that the risk of subsequent fracture as a result of this transient decrease in BMD in DMPA users could not be determined from existing data.

DMPA is administered by deep intramuscular injection into the gluteus maximus or deltoid. The next injection is due 12 calendar weeks from that date, though there is a leeway of a further 2 weeks in which DMPA can be safely administered whilst maintaining contraceptive cover. Australasian family planning organisations suggest that ongoing contraceptive cover cannot be assured beyond 14 weeks from the last injection. This may require the use of emergency contraception and an alternative contraceptive method until pregnancy can be excluded and the next injection given. Box 34.8 gives emergency contraception advice.

Implications for lactation and the postpartum period

DMPA is broadly usable immediately following delivery whether the woman is breastfeeding or not, and from 6 weeks on there are no contraindications to its use at all. There is no evidence that DMPA affects the quality or quantity of the breast milk or that its use has any adverse effects on infant health and growth.

EMERGENCY CONTRACEPTION

Emergency contraception has been highlighted as a backup method throughout this chapter. It is an important and underused postcoital method of contraception that can be used:

- when the regular contraceptive method used is presumed to have failed—e.g. broken or slipped condom, missed pill(s), dislodged or damaged diaphragm, missing IUD strings
- after unprotected intercourse
- following sexual assault.

It is a method of contraception that should be included as part of counselling for most contraceptive methods and ideally there should be high community awareness of its safety, efficacy and availability (Calabretto, 2004). Unfortunately as late as 2011 around 50% of Australian women didn't know they could obtain hormonal emergency contraception from a pharmacist without a prescription (Hobbs et al., 2011).

Hormonal emergency contraception

Hormonal emergency contraception (EC) is the commonest emergency contraceptive method accessed in Australia and New Zealand. In the past, high-dose combined oral ethinyloestradiol and progestogen was used but this was superseded by levonorgestrel-only (LNG) emergency contraception. A single dose of 1500 µg of LNG is not only more effective than the previous combined method but is also safer and associated with fewer side effects. More recently another hormonal method of emergency contraception has become available in Australia, though not New Zealand, which contains 30 µg of the selective progesterone receptor modulator ulipristal acetate.

Hormonal EC is sometimes erroneously thought to be an abortifacient. It is important to understand that EC will not disrupt an already implanted pregnancy, nor will it cause any harm if inadvertently taken during early pregnancy (ACOG, 2010; Levy et al., 2014; Schwarz & Trussell, 2011; Zhang et al, 2009). The principal mechanism of action of hormonal EC is to inhibit or delay ovulation and it has no demonstrated effect on an already implanted ovum (International Consortium for Emergency Contraception/International Federation of Gynecology and Obstetrics (ICEC/FIGO), 2012).

In Australia, there are several brands of LNG EC available in a one-dose pill. These do not require a prescription but there is a requirement for the pharmacist to discuss the medication with the intending user prior to dispensing it. In New Zealand, the LNG EC can similarly be obtained from the pharmacy without the need for a prescription. Overall the percentage of expected pregnancies prevented is 85%—provided it is taken within the licensed 72 hours. However, LNG EC becomes less effective over time. If it is taken within 24 hours of intercourse the effectiveness is 95% compared with 58% on day 3 (Piaggio et al., 1999). This informs the advice that hormonal EC be commenced as soon as possible after unprotected intercourse and that those relying on less effective methods of contraception should preferably have a ready supply of EC on hand. LNG EC retains some effectiveness on day 4 but by 5 days after unprotected intercourse it is no more effective than placebo (Piaggio et al., 2011).

Ulipristal acetate is the newest hormonal EC, providing efficacy for up to 120 hours after unprotected sexual intercourse (Glasier et al., 2010). It is available in Australia, though not currently in New Zealand. It also more reliably prevents ovulation than does LNG EC, particularly if taken just before ovulation. Like LNG EC there is no evidence of any effect on implantation (Rosato et al., 2015). Pooled results from two trials (Creinin et al., 2006; Glasier et al., 2010) suggest that ulipristal acetate EC is generally a more effective method than LNG EC regardless of the time since unprotected intercourse. Ulipristal acetate is a slightly more expensive option than LNG EC.

One disadvantage associated with the use of ulipristal acetate is that it interacts with other hormonal contraception because of its direct action on progesterone receptors. The original concern was that it could reduce the efficacy of any hormonal contraceptive commenced shortly after its use. In fact the opposite appears to be the case: initiating hormonal contraception too soon reduces the efficacy of the ulipristal acetate EC. It is now recommended that users wait at least 5 days before initiating (or restarting) hormonal contraception and that additional contraception is then required for 2 days for a POP and 7 days for a COCP, ring or implant (FSRH, 2017c). Medications that affect the CYP3A4 system reduce the efficacy of both LNG EC and ulipristal acetate EC. The current advice is to double the dose of LNG EC in such cases, though this is an off-licence use of this medication. No similar recommendations exist for ulipristal acetate EC and its use should probably be avoided in women taking enzyme inducers (FSRH, 2017c).

Implications for lactation and the postpartum period

Hormonal EC is not required if unprotected intercourse occurs less than 3 weeks postpartum. Beyond that time both LNG EC and ulipristal acetate EC are safe to use. Although LNG EC can safely be used during lactation there are no long-term safety data on ulipristal acetate EC and it is currently recommended that women express but not breastfeed for 1 week after its use. Pragmatically then LNG EC is more commonly advised as the hormonal EC of choice in breastfeeding women.

The IUD as emergency contraception

A copper-bearing IUD (but not the LNG-IUD) can also be used as EC. It is more effective than either method of hormonal EC with a failure rate of 0.14% (Cleland et al., 2012).

It can be inserted up to 5 days after the most probable calculated date of ovulation, even if there have been multiple acts of unprotected intercourse up to that point. If there has been only a single act of intercourse it can be safely inserted within 5 days (Guillebaud & MacGregor, 2017). Use of the IUD for the purpose of EC is most appropriate for women who wish to use it as an ongoing method of contraception. A copper IUD does not interfere with breastfeeding and can be safely inserted from 4 weeks postpartum.

OTHER CONTRACEPTIVE METHODS

Spermicides

Spermicides are chemical agents that immobilise sperm, making them incapable of fertilising an ovum. Spermicides must be inserted prior to intercourse, and reapplied prior to any subsequent episodes of intercourse. They are generally not recommended as a stand-alone contraceptive method as their typical failure rate can be as high as 29% (see Table 34.1). They are more commonly used in conjunction with condoms and diaphragms in an attempt to boost the efficacy of these barrier methods. Nonoxynol-9 (chemically a detergent) is the active agent in most spermicides worldwide but there is good evidence that its potential to inflame the vaginal skin may actually increase the rate of STIs in users (Wilkinson et al., 2002). It is for this reason that conventional spermicides are no longer marketed in Australia or New Zealand although they can still be obtained through online suppliers. It is recommended that the CAYA diaphragm be used in conjunction with its companion cellulose gel. This is not actually a spermicide though it may assist in sperm immobilisation. CAYA gel should never be used alone for contraception.

Coitus interruptus (withdrawal)

This is a method that requires the man to withdraw his penis from the vagina before he ejaculates. The method may variously be described as 'withdrawal', 'being safe', 'being careful' and by numerous other euphemisms (Varney, 1997). It is important to be aware of the meaning behind such descriptions when a woman discusses her contraceptive method. Overall it must be conceded that withdrawal has a low rate of contraceptive efficacy as its failure rate in typical use is as high as 27% (see Table 34.1). However, when used consistently and correctly it approaches the efficacy of some barriers and spermicide alone and therefore is worth consideration when nothing else is available or acceptable. Some cultural groups use coitus interruptus as their main method of contraception when spacing families and, for some people, this is the only contraceptive method they will use throughout their reproductive lives.

One drawback with this method is that sperm from a previous ejaculation may still be present in the pre-ejaculate and therefore poses a pregnancy risk if intercourse occurs again within a short time. It is probably advisable

Box 34.9 Emergency contraception alert—withdrawal method

Women should be provided with information ahead of time about emergency contraception (see Emergency contraception section), so they can prevent pregnancy should ejaculation occur in the vagina or on the vulva.

Box 34.10 Emergency contraception alert—tubal ligation

Information about emergency contraception (see Emergency contraception section in this chapter) should be provided ahead of time so that pregnancy can be prevented should intercourse take place before an analysis has confirmed the tubes are blocked.

for the male to urinate if possible after ejaculation to remove any sperm from his urethra, and he should also cleanse the external surface of the penis before further contact with the woman's internal and external genitalia occurs (Kowal, 2011). Withdrawal is also more likely to fail if the man ejaculates on, or in the vicinity of, the female's external genitalia. The advantage of withdrawal is that it is free and is always available as a method or back-up method. It does, however, require good communication and cooperation between the couple and excellent control by the male. Box 34.9 gives emergency contraception advice.

PERMANENT CONTRACEPTION METHODS

These highly effective (see Table 34.1) surgical methods block the passage of the ova in women and sperm in men. Sterilisation should always be considered permanent as, although reversibility may be possible for some procedures, it can never be guaranteed. Appropriate counselling is critical for those considering permanent contraception so that expectations are accurate. Sterilisation procedures do not disrupt hormone levels and should not affect sexual functioning except in those individuals for whom fertility is an important aspect of their sexual identity. For many couples the procedure enhances sexual response because the fear of pregnancy is removed.

Tubal sterilisation

Female sterilisation, or tubal occlusion, is performed by a gynaecologist under conscious sedation or under general or local anaesthetic. Traditionally this required access to the tubes via laparotomy or more commonly laparoscopy. It is also possible to perform a sterilisation procedure after caesarean, though the failure rates are somewhat higher. Once the fallopian tubes have been accessed, they are sealed off with clips, rings or bands which are applied to the tubes. Alternatively diathermy may be used to heat and seal the tubes or a section of the tube may be surgically removed. Female sterilisation is immediately effective, and sexual intercourse may be resumed when the woman is ready to do so.

The failure rate after female sterilisation procedures in the first year is approximately 1 in 500. However, this rate rises to 1 in 54 by 10 years (Hillis et al., 1997), with one-third of failures occurring as ectopic pregnancies. Rates of female sterilisation have been falling in Australia from the mid 1990s, in part reflecting a greater uptake of the long-acting but reversible contraceptive methods once the desired family size is reached. New Zealand data also suggest a fall in the rates of female sterilisation over time (Chesang et al., 2016).

Box 34.10 gives emergency contraception advice.

Hysterectomy/salpingectomy

While obviously providing permanent contraception, hysterectomy is performed only where obstetric emergency or significant gynaecological problems indicate the need for such major surgery. A number of clinicians, however, are starting to recommend bilateral salpingectomy as a primary sterilisation procedure, rather than tubal occlusion. Salpingectomy is associated with a slightly higher risk of surgical complications than tubal occlusion but offers nearly 100% efficacy, which, unlike tubal occlusion, does not wane over time. It does not preclude the use of assisted conception techniques should the woman later regret her decision. Salpingectomy may even offer some protection against ovarian cancer as the most common ovarian cancer often originates in the fallopian tube rather than the ovary.

Vasectomy

This is a male method of permanent contraception in which the vas deferens are cut and the ends blocked to prevent the passage of sperm from the testes. After vasectomy, sperm are reabsorbed by the body. The procedure is usually performed under local anaesthesia by an urologist, surgeon or trained general practitioner. Men can expect some degree of local swelling and discomfort for a few days after the procedure. The failure rate of vasectomy is usually quoted as 1–2 in 1000. There are several techniques employed for vasectomy but the method chosen appears to have a minimal effect on efficacy, though there are limited data available (Cook et al., 2014). Following the procedure any sperm remaining in the seminal vesicles must be depleted before the procedure can be relied on for contraception. This takes up to about 16 ejaculations or 6 weeks—whichever comes first. At that point a semen analysis is performed to confirm the absence of sperm in the seminal fluid. The seminal fluid will not be noticeably different after vasectomy as sperm comprise only 2%–5% of semen with the remainder secreted by the seminal vesicles and prostate gland. The rate of vasectomy in Australia has been relatively steady at 23,000–30,000 procedures performed per year since 1994 (Medicare Australia, n.d.). New Zealand data from 2013–15 suggest that there has been a slight increase in the rate of vasectomy in that country, although the utility of the study is compromised by small numbers and its restriction to those over 35 years of age (Chesang, 2016).

Box 34.11 gives emergency contraception advice.

Box 34.11 Emergency contraception alert—vasectomy

Information about emergency contraception (see Emergency contraception section in this chapter) should be provided ahead of time so that pregnancy can be prevented should intercourse take place before a semen analysis has confirmed the absence of sperm.

CRITICAL THINKING EXERCISE

Complete a table using the model below, including commencement time and compatibility with breastfeeding.

Method of contraception	When can the method be commenced during the postpartum period?	Is the method compatible with breastfeeding?
COCs		
Condoms (female)		
Condoms (male)		
Diaphragm		
EC		
Fertility-awareness-based methods		
Implant		
Injectables		
IUDs		
LAM		
POPs		
Tubal ligation/ salpingectomy		
Vaginal contraceptive ring		

Conclusion

Midwives need to have a comprehensive understanding about the range of contraceptive options available to women. The need for contraception and contraceptive choice should be raised early in the postpartum period, and optimally in the antenatal period, because the return of fertility is variable, as is the resumption of sexual intercourse. The woman needs to be made aware that the return of fertility may precede her first period, so the timely initiation of a contraceptive method is vital if she does not wish to become pregnant at that time. All women need guidance in choosing a method that is best suited to their age, lifestyle, cultural values and health issues and one that will not affect the milk supply if she is breastfeeding. Where pregnancy has been unintended owing to non-use of contraception or a contraceptive failure, women may be sensitive about their future choice of contraception and this must be acknowledged as part of the discussion about contraceptive choice. Midwives should inform women that they can see their general practitioner for contraceptive advice and also provide them with the location of specialist contraceptive services in their area.

Contraceptive counselling is an important area of midwifery practice and it is important that it not be overlooked amongst the range of competing priorities in the postnatal period. The role of contraception in empowering women and their partners to plan their future pregnancies effectively and to optimise subsequent pregnancy outcomes should always be remembered.

Review questions

1. Are midwives adequately prepared to provide information about fertility control?
2. When is the best time to discuss fertility control with women?
3. Where would you refer women to for contraceptive counselling and services?
4. What resources should be available in clinics or units to assist midwives to discuss contraception with women?
5. How do midwives ensure that their own negative views about a particular method(s) of contraception are not imparted to women?
6. Do you always discuss emergency contraception when you talk to women about contraceptive methods? Think about strategies to ensure that this aspect is not omitted.
7. Think about why some women or couples may be ambivalent towards the use of contraception. How might you assist them?
8. Think about the reasons that a woman might stop using a method of contraception, and how you would counsel her in this situation.

9. Decreased bone mineral density is a potential problem for women who are long-term users of DMPA, and so these women should be taking adequate dietary calcium. How many milligrams of dietary calcium are adequate for a non-pregnant woman? Provide examples of common foods that would add up to this amount in a 24-hour period. Think about ways you could assess this aspect of nutrition with a woman you are counselling.

10. A woman in your care says that her partner does not want her to use any contraceptive method because of his cultural beliefs, although she would prefer to use a hormonal method, to space her family. Discuss the strategies you would use to assist your client to resolve this situation with her partner.

Acknowledgements

This is a revision of the chapter in an earlier edition of this text which was authored by Helen Calabretto. The present author, Dr Terri Foran, acknowledges the major contribution made by the previous author and also wishes to acknowledge the contribution of Dr Christine Roke, the National Medical Adviser, and Family Planning New Zealand, who assisted greatly with the collection of the New Zealand-specific information used in the earlier edition.

Online resources

Australasian Sexual Health and HIV Nurses Association. http://www.ashhna.org.au/.

Faculty of Sexual and Reproductive Healthcare (FSRH). CEU Clinical Guidance: Drug Interactions With Hormonal Contraception—Nov 2017. https://www.fsrh.org/standards-and-guidance/documents/ceu-clinical-guidance-drug-interactions-with-hormonal/.

Faculty of Sexual and Reproductive Healthcare (FSRH). MEC Eligibility Criteria for Contraceptive Use 2017; 2017. https://www.fsrh.org/ukmec/.

International Planned Parenthood Federation. http://www.ippf.org/.

World Health Organization (WHO). Medical Eligibility Criteria for Contraceptive Use. 5th ed. Geneva: WHO; 2015. http://www.who.int/reproductivehealth/publications/family_planning/MEC-5/en/.

National and regional sexual health and family planning organisations are listed in Box 34.12.

References

American College of Obstetricians (ACOG). Practice bulletin no. 112: emergency contraception. *Obstet Gynecol.* 2010;115(5):1100–1109.

Barron ML, Fehring RJ. Basal body temperature assessment. Is it useful to couples seeking pregnancy? *Am J Matern Child Nurs.* 2005;30(5):290–296.

Barz D, Goldberg AB. Injectable contraceptives. In: Hatcher RA, Trussell J, Nelson AL, et al., eds. *Contraceptive Technology.* 20th ed. NY: Ardent Media; 2011 [Ch. 9].

Berglund SE, Gemzell-Danielsson K, Sellberg JA, et al. Fertility awareness-based mobile application for contraception. *Eur J Contracept Reprod Health Care.* 2016;21(3):234–241.

Calabretto H. Emergency contraception—a qualitative study of young women's experiences. *Contemp Nurse.* 2004;18(12):152–163.

Cecil M, Nelson A, Trussell J, et al. If the condom doesn't fit, you must resize it. *Contraception.* 2010;82:489–490.

Chesang J, Richardson A, Potter J, et al. Prevalence of contraceptive use in New Zealand women. *N Z Med J.* 2016;129(1444):58–67.

Cleland K, Zhu H, Goldstuck N, et al. The efficacy of intrauterine devices for emergency contraception: a systematic review of 35 years of experience. *Hum Reprod.* 2012;27:1994–2000.

Cook LA, Van Vliet HAAM, Lopez LM, et al. Vasectomy occlusion techniques for male sterilization. *Cochrane Database Syst Rev.* 2014;(3):CD003991, doi:10.1002/14651858.CD003991.pub4.

Creinin MD, Schlaff W, Archer DF, et al. Progesterone receptor modulator for emergency contraception: a randomized controlled trial. *Obstet Gynecol.* 2006;108:1089–1097.

Eroğlu K, Akkuzu G, Vural G, et al. Comparison of efficacy and complications of IUD insertion in immediate postplacental/early postpartum period with interval period: 1 year follow-up. *Contraception.* 2006;74:376–381.

Faculty of Sexual and Reproductive Healthcare (FSRH). *Clinical Effectiveness Unit (CEU) Clinical Guidance: Contraception After Pregnancy—January 2017.* 2017a. Online: https://www.fsrh.org/documents/contraception-after-pregnancy-guideline-january-2017/.

Faculty of Sexual and Reproductive Healthcare (FSRH). *UK Medical Eligibility Criteria (MEC) for Contraceptive Use 2017.* 2017b. Online: https://www.fsrh.org/ukmec/.

Faculty of Sexual and Reproductive Healthcare (FSRH). *Clinical Effectiveness Unit (CEU) Clinical Guidance: Emergency Contraception—December 2017.* 2017c. Online: https://www.fsrh.org/standards-and-guidance/documents/ceu-clinical-guidance-emergency-contraception-march-2017/.

French R, Sorhaindo AM, Van Vliet HAAM, et al. Progestogen-releasing intrauterine systems versus other forms of reversible contraceptives for contraception. *Cochrane Database Syst Rev.* 2004;(3):CD001776, doi:10.1002/14651858.CD001776.pub2.

Gallo MF, Grimes DA, Lopez LM, et al. Nonlatex versus latex male condoms for contraception. *Cochrane Database Syst Rev.* 2006;(1):CD003550, doi:10.1002/14651858.CD003550.pub2.

Grimes DA, Schultz KF. Antibiotic prophylaxis for intrauterine contraceptive device insertion. *Cochrane Database Syst Rev.* 2001;(2):CD001327.

Glasier A, Logan J, McGlew TJ. Who gives advice about postpartum education? *Contraception.* 1996;53:217–220.

Glasier AF, Cameron ST, Fine PM, et al. Ulipristal acetate versus levonorgestrel for emergency contraception: a randomised non-inferiority trial and meta-analysis. *Lancet.* 2010;375(9714):555–562.

Guillebaud J. Contraception. *Your Questions Answered.* 5th ed. Edinburgh: Churchill Livingstone; 2009.

Guillebaud J, MacGregor A. *Contraception. Your Questions Answered.* 7th ed. Edinburgh: Churchill Livingstone Elsevier; 2017.

Guillebaud J, Bonnar J, Morehead J, et al. Menstrual blood-loss with intrauterine devices. *Lancet.* 1976;307(7596):387–390.

Hillis SD, Marchbanks PA, Tylor LR, et al.; for the U.S. Collaborative Review of Sterilization Working Group. Tubal sterilization and long-term risk of hysterectomy: findings from the U.S. Collaborative Review of Sterilization. *Obstet Gynecol.* 1997;89: 609–614.

Hobbs MK, Taft AJ, Amir LH, et al. Pharmacy access to the emergency contraceptive pill: a national survey of a random sample of Australian women. *Contraception.* 2011;83(2):151–158.

Howard B, Trussell J, Grubb E, et al. Comparison of pregnancy rates in users of extended and cyclic combined oral contraceptive (COC) regimens in the United States: a brief report. *Contraception.* 2014;89(1):25–27.

Hubacher D, Finer LB, Espey E. Renewed interest in intrauterine contraception in the United States: evidence and explanation. Contraception. 2011;83(4):291–294.

International Consortium for Emergency Contraception/International Federation of Gynecology and Obstetrics (ICEC/FIGO). *Statement on Mechanism of Action—How Do Levonorgestrel-only Emergency Contraceptive Pills (LNG ECPs) Prevent Pregnancy?* 2012. Online: https://www.gynmed.at/sites/default/files/statement_emergency_contraceptive_pills.pdf.

Jackson E, Glasier A. Return of ovulation and menses in postpartum nonlactating women: a systematic review. *Obstet Gynecol.* 2011;117(3):657–662.

Kennedy K, Trussell J. Postpartum contraception and lactation. In: Hatcher RA, Trussell J, Hatcher R, et al., eds. *Contraceptive Technology.* 20th ed. NY: Ardent Media; 2011 [Ch. 18].

Kowal D. Coitus interruptus (withdrawal). In: Hatcher RA, Trussell J, Nelson AL, et al., eds. *Contraceptive Technology.* 20th ed. NY: Ardent Media; 2011 [Ch. 15].

Lancet (n.a.). Breastfeeding as a family planning method. *Lancet.* 1988;2(8621):1204–1205. Online: http://www.sciencedirect.com/science/article/pii/S0140673688902796.

Levy DP, Jager M, Kapp N, et al. Ulipristal acetate for emergency contraception: postmarketing experience after use by more than 1 million women. *Contraception.* 2014;89(5):431–433.

Lopez LM, Grimes DA, Schultz KF, et al. Steroidal contraceptives: effect on bone fractures in women. *Cochrane Database Syst Rev.* 2014;(6):CD006033, doi:10.1002/14651858.CD006033.pub5.

Lopez LM, Bernholc A, Hubacher D, et al. Immediate postpartum insertion of intrauterine device for contraception. *Cochrane Database Syst Rev.* 2015a;(6):CD003036, doi:10.1002/14651858.CD003036.pub3.

Lopez LM, Grey TW, Stuebe AM, et al. Combined hormonal versus nonhormonal versus progestin-only contraception in lactation. *Cochrane Database Syst Rev.* 2015b;(3):CD003988, doi:10.1002/14651858.CD003988.pub2.

McDonald EA, Brown SJ. Does method of birth make a difference to when women resume sex after childbirth? *BJOG.* 2013;120(7): 823–830.

Medicare Australia. *Rates of Vasectomy.* n.d. Online: www.medicareaustralia.gov.au/statistics/mbs_item.shtml.

Nanda K. Contraceptive patch and vaginal contraceptive ring. In: Hatcher RA, Trussell J, Nelson AL, et al., eds. *Contraceptive Technology.* 20th ed. NY: Ardent Media; 2011 [Ch. 12].

Nelson AL. Communicating with patients about extended-cycle and continuous use of oral contraceptives. *J Womens Health.* 2011;16(4):463–470.

Nelson AL, Burke AE. Fertility awareness-based methods. In: Hatcher RA, Trussell J, Nelson AL, et al., eds. *Contraceptive Technology.* 20th ed. NY: Ardent Media; 2011 [Ch. 16].

Nelson AL, Cwiak C. Combined oral contraceptive. In: Hatcher RA, Trussell J, Nelson AL, et al., eds. *Contraceptive Technology.* 20th ed. NY: Ardent Media; 2011 [Ch. 11].

Panel on Treatment of HIV-infected Pregnant Women and Prevention of Perinatal Transmission. *Recommendations for Use of Antiretroviral Drugs in Pregnant HIV-1-Infected Women for Maternal Health and Interventions to Reduce Perinatal HIV Transmission in the United States.* 2021. Online: https://clinicalinfo.hiv.gov/sites/default/files/guidelines/documents/Perinatal_GL.pdf.

Piaggio G, von Hertzen H, Grimes DA, et al. Timing of emergency contraception with levonorgestrel or the Yuzpe regimen. Task Force on Postovulatory Methods of Fertility Regulation. *Lancet.* 1999;353(9154):721.

Piaggio G, Kapp N, von Hertzen H. Effect on pregnancy rates of the delay in the administration of levonorgestrel for emergency contraception: a combined analysis of four WHO trials. *Contraception.* 2011;84(1):35–39.

Pool I, Dickson J, Dharmalingam A, et al. *New Zealand's Contraceptive Revolutions. Social Science Monograph Series.* Waikato, NZ: University of Waikato Population Studies Centre; 1999:47–48.

Raymond E. Progestin-only pills. In: Hatcher RA, Trussell J, Nelson AL, et al., eds. *Contraceptive Technology.* 20th ed. NY: Ardent Media; 2011 [Ch. 10].

Richters J, Fitzadam S, Yeung A, et al. Contraceptive practices among women: the second Australian study of health and relationships. *Contraception.* 2016;94(5):548–555.

Rosato E, Farris M, Bastianelli C. Mechanism of action of ulipristal acetate for emergency contraception: a systematic review. *Front Pharmacol.* 2015;6:315.

Saeed G, Fakhar S, Rahim F, et al. Change in trend of contraceptive uptake—effect of educational leaflets and counseling. *Contraception.* 2008;77(5):377–381.

Schwarz EB, Trussell J. Emergency contraception. In: Hatcher RA, Trussell J, Nelson AL, et al., eds. *Contraceptive Technology.* 20th ed. New York: Ardent Media; 2011:113–145.

Schwartz JL, Ballagh SA, Creinin MD, et al. SILCS diaphragm: postcoital testing of a new single size contraceptive device. *Contraception.* 2008;78(3):237–244.

Schwartz JL, Warner DH, Lai JJ, et al. Contraceptive efficacy, safety, fit and acceptability of a single-size diaphragm developed with end-user input. *Obstet Gynecol.* 2015;125(4):895–903.

Smoley BA, Robinson CM. Natural family planning. *Am Fam Physician.* 2012;86(10):924–928.

Sothornwit J, Werawatakul Y, Kaewrudee S, et al. Immediate versus delayed postpartum insertion of contraceptive implant for contraception. *Cochrane Database Syst Rev.* 2017;(4):CD011913, doi: 10.1002/14651858.CD011913.pub2.

Srikanthan A, Reid RL. Religious and cultural influences on contraception. *J Obstet Gynaecol Can.* 2008;30(2):129–137.

Teal SB. Postpartum contraception: optimizing interpregnancy intervals. *Contraception.* 2014;89(6):487–488.

Trussell J. Contraceptive failure in the United States. *Contraception.* 2011;83(5):397–404.

Trussell J, Guthrie KA. Choosing a contraceptive. In: Hatcher RA, Trussell J, Nelson AL, et al., eds. *Contraceptive Technology.* 20th ed. NY: Ardent Media; 2011 [Ch. 3].

Valdes V, Labbock MH, Pugin E, et al. The efficacy of the lactational amenorrhea method (LAM) among working women. *Contraception.* 2000;62(5):217–219.

Varney H. *Varney's Midwifery.* 4th ed. London: Jones & Bartlett; 1997.

Warner L, Steiner MJ. Male condoms. In: Hatcher RA, Trussell J, Nelson AL, et al., eds. *Contraceptive Technology.* 20th ed. NY: Ardent Media; 2011 [Ch. 13].

Wilcox AJ, Dunson D, Baird DD. The timing of the 'fertile window' in the menstrual cycle: day-specific estimates from a prospective study. *BMJ.* 2000;321:1259–1262.

Wilkinson D, Ramjee G, Tholandi M, et al. Nonoxynol-9 for preventing vaginal acquisition of HIV infection by women from men. *Cochrane Database Syst Rev.* 2002;(3):CD003936, doi:10.1002/14651858.CD003936.

World Health Organization (WHO). *WHO Statement on Hormonal Contraception on Bone Health.* Geneva: WHO; 2007. Online: http://www.who.int/reproductivehealth/topics/family_planning/pbrief_bonehealth.pdf.

World Health Organization (WHO). *Medical Eligibility Criteria for Contraceptive Use.* 5th ed. Geneva: WHO; 2015. Online: http://www.who.int/reproductivehealth/publications/family_planning/MEC-5/en/.

Zhang L, Chen J, Wang Y, et al. Pregnancy outcome after levonorgestrel-only emergency contraception failure: a prospective cohort study. *Hum Reprod.* 2009;24(7):1605–1611.

Further reading

FPNSW/FPQ/FPV. *Contraception: An Australian Clinical Practice Handbook.* 4th ed. Sydney FPNSW/FPQ/FPV; 2017.

This is available for order through the websites of Family Planning NSW, Sexual Health Victoria and TRUE in Queensland (see Box 34.12).

Box 34.12 Additional resources: sexual health and family planning organisations

Useful information about clinic locations and services, and contraception is available from the sexual health and family planning organisations listed below. (See also the list of Online resources.)

ACT

Sexual Health & Family Planning ACT Inc.

Level 1, 28 University Ave, Canberra, ACT 2601

Phone: (02) 6247 3077

Website: http://www.shfpact.org.au

New South Wales

Family Planning New South Wales

Head Office, 10 Avenue of the Americas, Newington NSW 2127

Phone: (02) 8752 4316

Website: http://www.fpnsw.org.au/

Northern Territory

Family Planning Welfare Association of NT

Head Office, Unit 2, The Clock Tower, Dick Ward Drive, Coconut Grove, NT 0810

Phone: (08) 8948 0144

Website: www.fpwnt.com.au

Queensland

TRUE—Relationships and Reproductive Health

Building 1, 230 Lutwyche Road, Windsor, QLD 4030.

Phone: (07) 3250 0200

Website: www.true.org.au

South Australia

SHine SA

GP Plus Health Care Centre, 64c Woodville Road, Woodville, SA 5011

Phone: (08) 1300 794 584

Website: http://www.shinesa.org.au

Tasmania

Family Planning Tasmania

Head Office, 421 Main Road, Glenorchy, TAS 7010

Phone: (03) 6273 9117

Website: http://www.fpt.asn.au

Victoria

Sexual Health Victoria

Head Office, 901 Whitehorse Road, Box Hill, VIC 3128

Phone: (03) 9257 0100

Website: https://shvic.org.au/

Western Australia

Sexual Health Quarters

Head Office, 70 Roe St, Northbridge WA 6003

Phone: (08) 9227 6177

Website: http://shq.org.au

New Zealand

Family Planning Association Inc., New Zealand

National Office, Level 7, Southmark House, 203–209 Willis St, Wellington

Phone: (04) 384 4349

Website: http://www.familyplanning.org.nz/

Natural family planning organisations

Natural Fertility Australia

Website: http://naturalfertilityaustralia.com.au/

Natural Fertility New Zealand

Website: https://www.naturalfertility.co.nz/

CHAPTER 35

Women's psychosocial health and wellbeing

Virginia Schmied and Lesley Dixon

LEARNING OUTCOMES

The learning outcomes for this chapter are:

1. To discuss the risk and protective factors that influence maternal psychosocial health
2. To discuss the importance of optimal maternal psychosocial health and its influence on child development and health outcomes
3. To discuss the key elements of assessment and screening for psychosocial health
4. To discuss mental health problems (depression, anxiety, bipolar, schizophrenia, eating disorders) and their affect during pregnancy on the woman, her infant and family, and the potential consequences for the mother–infant relationship
5. To examine the impact of parental substance use on the health of women, infants and families
6. To examine the impact of domestic and family violence on the health of women, infants and families
7. To discuss the role of the midwife in caring for women and their infants with complex psychosocial needs.

CHAPTER OVERVIEW

This chapter provides an overview of psychological and social factors that influence maternal and newborn health including existing mental illness, antenatal depression and anxiety, eating disorders, substance use and domestic and family violence (DFV). We address the prevalence of mental health problems, the risk and protective factors for poor mental health, women's experiences and evidence-based interventions including approaches to screening and assessment. We also address the impact that maternal stress, situational or social difficulties and mental health problems have on the developing infant and child.

KEY TERMS

child development
domestic and family violence
parent–infant attachment
perinatal anxiety
perinatal depression
perinatal mental health
protective factors
psychosocial issues
psychosocial screening and assessment
risk factors
substance misuse

INTRODUCTION

Pregnancy and birth are usually times of celebration and excitement. They are also a time of increased emotional and social vulnerability, as a woman and her partner make a significant identity transition (Biaggi et al., 2016). Being a new mother or father can present unexpected challenges. Women with pre-existing physical or psychosocial needs, however, enter motherhood with additional challenges. Perinatal (defined here as from conception to 12 months post-birth) mental health problems such as anxiety and depression, stressful life events and poor social health are associated with adverse outcomes for women, their infant and family (Eastwood et al., 2021), in particular the mother's wellbeing and the relationship she has with her newborn baby (Fox et al., 2015).

Health and wellbeing are a combination of not just an individual's physical health but also their social and psychological health—with each influencing and having an impact on the other (Fig. 35.1). This is particularly relevant during the perinatal period when there are changes to family relationships, work and family circumstances as well as the physical changes and recovery for women following birth. Pregnancy changes and the return to physical health are discussed fully elsewhere in the textbook, so this chapter focuses on the psychological and social health of the woman and her baby.

Why maternal emotional and social health is important

Poor maternal mental health is now recognised as a significant public health problem and may be exacerbated by **substance misuse** and DFV (Thomson & Schmied, 2017).

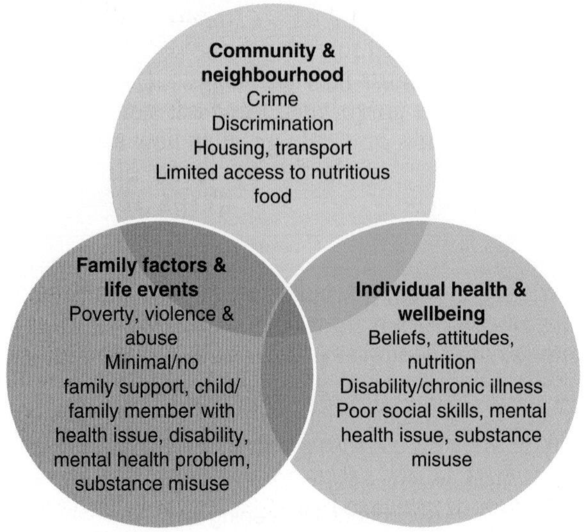

FIGURE 35.1 Diagram of the biopsychosocial determinants of maternal mental health
(Adapted from Lakhan, 2006. Online: http://www.medschool.lsuhsc.edu/medical_education/undergraduate/spm/SPM_100/documents/BiopsychosocialModel.pdf)

In Australia, Aotearoa New Zealand and other countries, mental health disorders are one of the leading causes of maternal morbidity and mortality (Humphrey, 2015; Perinatal and Maternal Mortality Review Committee (PMMRC), 2021). Suicide has been identified in the last decade as an alarming sequela of severe perinatal mental health problems (Humphrey, 2015) and continues to be a leading cause of maternal mortality in New Zealand, accounting for 23.8% of maternal deaths from 2006 to 2018, with Māori women over-represented in deaths from suicide (PMMRC, 2021). Globally, between 15% and 65% of women will experience depression in pregnancy (Dadi et al., 2020). The prevalence of self-reported anxiety symptoms fluctuates across pregnancy from approximately 18% in first trimester to 25% in the third trimester (Dennis et al., 2017).

MATERNAL SOCIAL AND EMOTIONAL HEALTH AND THE IMPACT ON THE INFANT

Studies in neuroscience and epidemiology emphasise that events during pregnancy and in the early years of life, and the quality of care received during these periods, strongly influence early infant development and adult life (Brockington et al., 2017). Maternal social and emotional distress in the perinatal period can have negative consequences for the infant and into childhood and adulthood (Glover et al., 2018). Depression and anxiety in pregnancy has been associated with prematurity and low birth weight (Ghimire et al., 2021), deficits in neurological development with impairments in physical and psychological development, language development and emotional and behavioural problems, decreased immune function with concomitant allergic reactions and an increased risk of depression in adulthood (Biaggi et al., 2016). An infant's risk increases if both parents experience mental health problems (Howard & Khalifeh, 2020).

Parental functioning can be compromised because of situational factors such as extreme poverty and homelessness, DFV or substance misuse, and this can impact on parenting capacity leading to physical, emotional or sexual abuse, or emotional or physical neglect, and will have a direct effect on infant wellbeing, possibly resulting in long-term negative trajectories (Eastwood et al., 2021; Howell et al., 2017).

The impact of these multiple factors on the developing brain is summarised in Box 35.1.

Other factors, outside of the family, also impact on child development. For example, the community that a child lives in and service availability can influence development.

The complexity of parental, family, community and societal factors that shape **child development** and outcomes are well represented in an ecological model. Bronfenbrenner's (1979) ecological model argues that the child's development is influenced not only by the more proximal, and relatively stronger influences, of the family, peers, school and neighbourhood, but also by the distal factors of the broader social context such as the media, parents' work arrangements and governmental policies.

Box 35.1 Summary: key points on brain development

- How the brain develops hinges on a complex interplay between the genes you are born with and the experiences you have.
- Early experiences have a decisive impact on the architecture of the brain and on the nature and extent of adult capacities.
- Early interactions don't just create a context; they directly affect the way the brain is 'wired'.
- Brain development is non-linear: there are prime times for acquiring different kinds of knowledge and skills.
- By the time children reach age three, their brains are twice as active as those of adults. Activity levels drop during adolescence.

(Shore, 1997; Moore et al., 2017)

CRITICAL THINKING EXERCISE

1. What are some of the difficulties that may be experienced by young children in families with high levels of unemployment or low levels of literacy or who live in disadvantaged neighbourhoods with higher rates of crime? Also consider the impact of social policies on mothers and young children—for example, government policies such as access / lack of access to paid parental leave and child care benefits.
2. What might be the impact for pregnant women and those with young babies of living through a natural disaster such as the Christchurch earthquakes and Queensland floods, or COVID-19? (See Moss et al., 2017.)

The physical, cognitive, social and emotional development of children undergoes rapid change in the first years of life. All of these aspects of growth and development are programmed by brain development, and all are interconnected. Development occurs in a strict hierarchical nature in the form of a 'bottom-up' sequence—this means that neural circuits that process basic information are wired earlier than those that process more complex information.

Newborns are born with millions of nerve cells, but these cells have minimal connections. These interconnections create circuits and highways for later use. They occur through 'synaptic density', where synapses are created with astonishing speed in the first three years of life. For the rest of the first decade of life, children's brains have twice as many synapses as adults' brains (Moore et al., 2017).

Attachment theory first articulated by John Bowlby was discussed in Chapter 30. Mary Ainsworth continued this work identifying the importance of maternal sensitivity for the developing child. The relationship that an infant has with their primary caregiver / s has a profound impact on the infant's future development. One of the earliest tasks of infancy is for the infant to be able to express and regulate emotions. They learn to do this with the help of a sensitive and responsive caregiver. Maternal sensitivity is defined as the mother's ability to be aware of and interpret the infant's behavioural cues and respond to the infant in a timely and appropriate manner (Ainsworth et al., 1978). Maternal sensitivity to infant cues and behaviours plays a strong role in secure attachment. Establishing a secure attachment relationship to a caregiver in infancy is an important basis for the development of lifelong mental health.

Epigenetics is an emerging area and refers to environmental influences that alter an individual's phenotype, the expressed characteristics of an individual's genetic code. The early caregiving environment may have a direct impact on an individual's phenotype with resultant positive or negative consequences (Glover et al., 2018). There is substantial evidence that maternal stress, depression, and anxiety in pregnancy can negatively influence the neurodevelopmental outcomes for the child (Howard & Khalifeh, 2020). Fetal programming refers to the capacity of the in-utero environment to modify the expression of genes and interact with the genetic substrate to determine disease susceptibility in the short- and long-term. High levels of stress and associated mental illnesses affect maternal and fetal outcomes, and also long-term offspring health into adulthood. If it is possible to minimise or eliminate negative events or exposures or replace them with positive factors, then outcomes for the mother and her infant can be improved (Dunkel Schetter & Tanner, 2012; Glover et al., 2018).

This increased knowledge of infant development and greater understanding of maternal distress has led to increased attention on the social and emotional needs of women and their families in the perinatal period. However, talking about or disclosing personal social or emotional health problems can be difficult for women and some choose not to disclose their concerns (Forder et al., 2020). There are interventions and services that can help women and families and it is important for both mother and baby that they receive the support needed. Midwives are in a privileged position to be able to support women through pregnancy, birth and the postnatal period. The first step is to understand the personal and situational risk and protective factors that make some women vulnerable to poor mental health outcomes and others not.

RISK AND PROTECTIVE FACTORS FOR POOR MATERNAL SOCIAL AND EMOTIONAL HEALTH

Risk factors are characteristics that increase the likelihood of poor mental health and include social and relationship issues relating to the individual, family circumstances, work, housing, friends, the neighbourhood, and broader community (See Box 35.2).

Previous or current birth experience, and health of the baby, can also be risk factors for maternal mental health

Box 35.2 Risk factors for poor maternal mental and social health

- *Individual maternal characteristics* including: poor nutrition, disability, low intelligence, chronic illness, difficult temperament, insecure or poor adult attachment style, poor social skills, poor problem solving, poor self-esteem, experiencing stigma, discrimination, alienation, being a single parent, young maternal age, tobacco smoking
- *Family factors and life events* including living in poverty, in a violent or abusive relationship, no family support, mental health problems in family, substance misuse in family
- *Community, neighbourhood factors* including living in an area of disadvantage, lack of access to health and support services, Housing - poor sewage, limited access to nutritious food, Neighbourhood violence and crime, social or cultural discrimination, community behaviour norms.

(Source: Fox et al., 2015; NSW Health, 2010)

Box 35.3 Protective factors

- Individual characteristics
  - optimism
  - good coping skills
  - self-confidence, high self-esteem
  - good physical health
  - preparedness to utilise services may also modify the relationship between risk factors and maternal and infant outcomes.
- Support from family, peers and boarder community
- Employment, sufficient financial resources
- Living in safe communities with access to good housing, transport

(Source: https://www.mindmatters.edu.au/docs/default-source/learning-module-documents/j4633_mm_module1-3-protectiveriskfactors_v2.pdf)

problems (Simpson, Schmied, Dickson, & Dahlen, 2018). Mothers of babies diagnosed with congenital problems in pregnancy are extremely anxious, as are those mothers who give birth prematurely (Feeley, 2017).

The presence of one or more risk factors does not mean that a woman or her child will develop a mental health problem; however, as the number of risk factors increases so does the likelihood of poorer psychosocial health (Eastwood et al., 2021; Thomson & Schmied, 2017). Some risk factors are particularly toxic (e.g. having experienced sexual or physical abuse).

Protective factors: Less is known about the protective factors for maternal mental health. Protective factors are characteristics that reduce the likelihood of poor mental health either on their own or when risk factors are present. They may be thought of as strengths or assets that help childbearing women and their families to maintain mental wellbeing and increase resilience (Box 35.3).

There are several situational factors that may increase risk for poor maternal mental health and outcomes for infants. Some women and families experiencing marginalisation are socially isolated and have less access to resources such as healthcare because of who they are or where they live (see Ch. 10). This includes families living in remote and rural areas of Australia and New Zealand; women living in poverty; Aboriginal and Torres Strait Islander, Māori and Pacific Islander women; migrants, particularly women who are refugees or asylum seekers; the LGBTI community; women with disabilities and young mothers. For example, many Indigenous families in Australia suffer ongoing trauma and mental health issues because of their separation from family and loss of culture and many women who are refugees have experienced significant pre-migration trauma, and loss and separation from family (Thomson & Schmied, 2017) (Box 35.4).

Box 35.4 Risk and protective factors scenario

Read the scenario below and identify the risk and protective factors that you think are present for Emily and her family.

You meet Emily in the antenatal clinic for her booking visit. In the course of your assessment Emily tells you about her family situation.

Emily is 32 years old and she lives in a three-bedroom housing department house with Steve and their three children Tom, Andrea and Samuel. Samuel is Emily's older son (9 years old) from her previous marriage who lives with them. He is a bright boy who sometimes gets into a bit of mischief at school. Tom is a quiet, easy-going four-year-old who attends preschool three days a week. Andrea is a lively two-year-old and needs a lot of Emily's time. Emily is 20 weeks pregnant when she first registers for maternity care because she hasn't had time to get herself organised. She explains that normally her mother comes to stay and help her two days a week, but she has been visiting Emily's sister for the last two months and will return home in two weeks' time.

Steve works as a truck driver and is often away from home for long periods. When Steve is away, Emily often runs out of money for food. When he is home, he is often quite short-tempered with the children, and sometimes he drinks, and occasionally really 'loses his cool'. Emily is so busy with the children she does not get out much and has no family or friends she can easily call on to give her a hand. She wishes they could afford a car so that she could get out a bit more.

PSYCHOSOCIAL ASSESSMENT AND SCREENING IN THE PERINATAL PERIOD

The early identification of potential risk factors in women who are currently unwell or at risk of developing mental health issues most often relies upon detection by the midwife or other maternity care provider. As most women attend antenatal care, this is an ideal time to enquire about and discuss their psychosocial health and wellbeing. As a result, most services in Australia and increasingly internationally have introduced *routine* psychosocial assessment and depression screening. Proponents of routine screening argue screening should be implemented because there are effective psycho-educational and pharmacological treatments (Dennis & Dowswell, 2013). However, there is debate about the implementation of *routine* psychosocial assessment and depression screening (Jomeen et al., 2017). Some authors argue that assessment and screening should not be implemented unless there are ongoing services, referral pathways and appropriate interventions to support women and families identified as distressed or being at risk.

Psychosocial health assessment in Australia

Australia has become a world leader in the development of national policy and clinical practice for routine screening of perinatal mental health. Guidelines such as the national Clinical Practice Guidelines for Depression and Related Disorders in the Perinatal Period (COPE, 2017) recommend routine psychosocial assessment and depression screening for all women in pregnancy and following birth using the Antenatal Risk Questionnaire (ANRQ) as it is a validated tool (Austin et al., 2013; Reilly et al., 2021) and the questions are acceptable to women (Mule et al., 2021). The questions / prompts used in ANRQ are in Table 35.1.

Table 35.1 Antenatal Risk Assessment Questionnaire (ANRQ)

*Please see link for more information and scoring of the ANRQ https://www.blackdoginstitute.org.au/wp-content/uploads/2020/04/anrqclinicians.pdf				Score
1. When you were growing up, did you feel your mother was emotionally supportive of you? (If you had no mother circle 6).	1 2 Very much	3 4 Somewhat	5 6 Not at all	
2. a) Have you ever had 2 weeks or more when you felt particularly worried, miserable or depressed?	Yes ☐	No ☐		
b) Do you have any other history of mental health problems? e.g eating disorders, psychosis, bipolar disorder, schizophrenia. Please specify: ______________	Yes ☐	No ☐		
If Yes to 2a or 2b, did this: c) Seriously interfere with your work and your relationships with friends and family?	1 2 Very much	3 4 Somewhat	5 6 Not at all	
d) Lead you to seek professional help?	Yes ☐	No ☐		
Did you see a: Psychiatrist ☐ Psychologist / Counsellor ☐ GP ☐ ______________ (Name of professional)				
e) Did you take tablets / herbal medicine? Please specify: ______________	Yes ☐	No ☐		
3. Is your relationship with your partner an emotionally supportive one? (If you have no partner circle 6)	1 2 Very much	3 4 Somewhat	5 6 Not at all	
4. a) Have you had any stresses, changes or losses in the last 12 months (e.g separation, domestic violence, unemployment, bereavement?) Please list: ______________	Yes ☐	No ☐		
b) How distressed were you by these stresses, changes or losses?	1 2 Very much	3 4 Somewhat	5 6 Not at all	

Continued

Table 35.1 Antenatal Risk Assessment Questionnaire (ANRQ)—cont'd

*Please see link for more information and scoring of the ANRQ https://www.blackdoginstitute.org.au/wp-content/uploads/2020/04/anrqclinicians.pdf				Score
5. Would you generally consider yourself a worrier?	1 2 Very much	3 4 Somewhat	5 6 Not at all	
6. In general, do you become upset if you do not have order in your life (e.g. regular timetable, a tidy house)?	1 2 Very much	3 4 Somewhat	5 6 Not at all	
7. Do you feel you have people you can depend on for support with your baby?	1 2 Very much	3 4 Somewhat	5 6 Not at all	
8. Were you emotionally abused when you were growing up?	Yes ☐	No ☐		
9. Have you ever been sexually ☐ or physically ☐ abused?				
If you would like to seek some help with any of these issues, please discuss this with your midwife or doctor.				
	Total score			

(Source: Austin et al., 2013)

In New South Wales, for example, SAFE START (NSW Health, 2010) is a framework guiding the practice of midwives, child and family health nurses and primary healthcare professionals in the promotion, prevention, early intervention and treatment of mothers, infants and their families. Similar frameworks are used in other states and territories. This model of care integrates psychosocial risk assessment and depression screening using the Edinburgh Postnatal Depression Scale (EPDS) with routine physical care during pregnancy and following birth. It endeavours to provide a coordinated network of support and health-related services in the perinatal period for mothers, infants and families. Psychosocial assessment occurs as part of history taking in the antenatal booking visit.

Following assessment, women's level of need is identified. For example, in the state of NSW, women are identified as having Level 1—no vulnerabilities detected; Level 2—predominantly social issues such as unstable housing, lack of social support, previous mental health problems including postnatal depression (PND) and Level 3—complex risk factors such as current maternal mental illness or substance use, presence of domestic violence and a history of involvement with child protection services. Women identified with multiple risk factors are referred to a multidisciplinary case review meeting where referral to more specialised services, for example, drug and alcohol services, is determined (NSW Health, 2010). Reassessment can occur at any time in pregnancy if a midwife is concerned about a woman's mental health and is routinely undertaken by child and family health nurses (CFHN) (maternal and child health nurses in Victoria and ACT) following birth. It is important to note that this routine assessment only occurs in public health antenatal services and, currently, most women accessing private maternity care are not screened.

These policies aim to increase collaboration and promote a seamless transition between primary (e.g. maternity, CFHN, Plunket services), secondary services (e.g. family care centres, social work) and tertiary services (e.g. drug and alcohol services), for women and their families. Some publicly funded health services offer specialist perinatal and infant mental health services where multidisciplinary teams provide case management and therapeutic models of care for women (Myors et al., 2014).

Psychosocial health assessment in New Zealand

In New Zealand (at the time of writing) there is no formal perinatal maternal mental health assessment or screening program, although the National Maternity Monitoring Group (2017) have recommended that district health boards develop referral pathways to guide assessment, screening and appropriate referral. It is recommended that midwives inquire about a woman's past and current mental health history and that of their family and offer appropriate referral as required. See Table 35.2 for recommended questions.

Mellor (2019) explored midwives' perceptions of maternal mental health through focus groups with 27 lead maternity carer midwives from urban and rural settings. These midwives acknowledged their pivotal role in assessment of maternal mental health and identified that they did assess women's mental health during antenatal care at booking and throughout the pregnancy in informal ways—through discussion of the woman's mental health history at booking and then continued observation of the woman, her partner and her home circumstances informally through the pregnancy. Most of the midwives used the EPDS selectively to validate any concerns and support referral. However, they also identified issues with the maternal mental health services in that only women with severe mental health issues were accepted following referral. Women with high levels of

Table 35.2 Screening for maternal mental health in New Zealand

Screening for maternal mental health in New Zealand
During the registration visit when discussing the woman's health, the midwife should ask:
• Are you currently receiving, or have you ever received treatment for a serious mental illness such as severe depression, bipolar disorder, schizophrenia or psychosis? • Have you ever had treatment from a psychiatrist or specialist mental health team in the past? • Is there anyone in your family who has (or has a history of) mental illness including being unwell when pregnant or following the birth (perinatal mental illness)?
If the women identifies a previous history of serious affective disorder or other psychoses she should be referred for psychiatric assessment and management even if she is currently well. This is because mental illness can deteriorate very rapidly in pregnancy and / or during the postnatal period. Regular monitoring and support is recommended during pregnancy and for at least three months following the birth.
During antenatal and postnatal care, depression can be identified through asking the following questions: • During the past month, have you often been bothered by feeling down, depressed or hopeless? • During the past month have you often been bothered by having little interest or pleasure in doing things?
If the answer is 'yes' to either question then the midwife should ask if this is something the woman would like help with so that referral to support services can be made.

anxiety and distress were unable to access support services leaving the midwife to fill the gap and resulted in additional responsibility as they sought to safeguard the woman's wellbeing. The disparity between women's needs and service provision was frustrating for the midwives and identified the major gap in service provision for women with mild to moderate mental health issues during the perinatal period.

In 2019 the government announced significant additional funding to improve access to mental health and addiction support services throughout Aotearoa New Zealand. This included a plan to expand access to and choice of primary mental health and addiction support over a period of five years along with the expansion of telehealth and digital supports for mental wellbeing (Budget, 2019). The PMMRC have recommended a stocktake of current mental health service across Aotearoa New Zealand to identify the strengths and gaps within the service. They also recommend that a funded maternal and infant mental health network be set up along with a national pathway for accessing maternal mental health services (PMMRC, 2021).

CRITICAL THINKING EXERCISE

You are undertaking a booking visit with Rosie. You explain that some of the questions you will ask her are about her emotional health and social wellbeing and may be sensitive questions. When you ask Rosie the question 'As a child, were you hurt or abused in any way (physically, emotionally, sexually)?', she tells you she was 'dreading this question coming up and can't you just look in my notes'. How would you respond to Rosie?

For midwives and women, the development of an ongoing and trusting relationship is necessary if women are to disclose the emotional and personal details of their lives—especially when these are potentially negative or stigmatising. This is where the benefits of having continuity of care and the building of trust within a relationship can make a difference for women and midwives. However, it is also imperative that there are a range of mental health and other social support services available and accessible to meet women's needs when mental health, addiction issues or domestic and family violence are disclosed.

PERINATAL MENTAL HEALTH ISSUES

Perinatal mental health disorders range from mild depression and anxiety, through to serious and chronic problems such as schizophrenia and bipolar affective disorder (Howard & Khalifeh, 2020; O'Hara & Wisner, 2014) and also include disorders like post-traumatic stress disorder and eating disorders. Perinatal depression and anxiety, however, are the more common mental health problems in the perinatal period. In this chapter we focus on depression and anxiety in pregnancy. Postnatal depression and other mental health problems in the postnatal period are examined in detail in Chapter 41.

Serious mental illness

Childbirth can trigger a bipolar episode with other psychotic disorders becoming more severe and developing more rapidly. Women who have a history of previous mental illness need to be referred to mental health services early in pregnancy. They experience poorer maternal and neonatal outcomes with higher rates of medical comorbidities, lifestyle and psychosocial risk factors that are known to contribute to poor obstetric outcomes, including premature birth (Frayne et al., 2019). They are at increased risk of suicide and more likely to have a recurrence of major depression or psychotic episodes in the first weeks following the birth (Howard & Khalifeh, 2020). Women who have had previous puerperal psychosis have a 50% (1 : 2) risk of this reoccurring.

Women with serious mental illness often delay seeking and attending antenatal care or may deny pregnancy, as they fear encountering stigma and judgmental attitudes of health professionals (McCauley et al., 2016). They may experience psychotic episodes postpartum or puerperal psychosis, and may have difficulty parenting with reduced responsiveness to their baby (Howard & Khalifeh, 2020).

Women with serious mental illness should be referred following antenatal booking and cared for by a multidisciplinary team who develop an integrated plan (NICE, 2014). One example of an integrated program for women with serious mental illness is the Childbirth and Mental Illness Antenatal Clinic (CAMI) in Western Australia (Hauck et al., 2013). This clinic uses a multidisciplinary team of obstetricians, midwives, social workers and psychiatrists to care for women with serious mental illness. Evaluation showed a reduction in depression and anxiety symptoms over the course of treatment at CAMI. Women in the study attended 90% of scheduled prenatal visits (Hauck et al., 2013). Women with serious mental health problems often struggle to parent effectively and will need family and professional support and advocacy (Megnin-Viggars et al., 2015).

Many women diagnosed with serious mental health problems discontinue their antipsychotic medications during pregnancy due to concerns related to the safety of the medications in pregnancy, which is currently largely unknown. Australian researchers have established the National Register of Antipsychotic Medications in Pregnancy. The analysis of the first 147 pregnancies reported 142 live births, with 18% of babies born preterm, and 43% of babies requiring special care nursery or intensive care after birth; 37% had a degree of respiratory distress and 15% of babies developed withdrawal symptoms (Kulkarni et al., 2014). However, if women cease their medications, they are more likely to experience a relapse of their mental illness, difficulties with parenting and an increased risk of losing custody of their children (McCauley et al., 2011).

Perinatal depression and anxiety

Perinatal depression is a mood disorder that encompasses antenatal depression arising during pregnancy, and PND, experienced for varying durations in the perinatal period. Perinatal depression is often defined symptomatically as exceeding a threshold on a screening measure, such as the EPDS when women score 13 or greater. Although in some instances a score of ≥ 10 is used, and women will be referred for further evaluation or treatment or for additional support. Following referral, more rigorous assessment occurs such as a clinical interview (O'Hara & Wisner, 2014).

Perinatal anxiety: A wide range of anxiety disorders are prevalent in the perinatal period. These include generalised anxiety, obsessive–compulsive disorder, panic and social anxiety disorders. O'Hara & Wisner (2014) note that, in many cases, the severity and effect of anxiety symptoms (e.g. worry, avoidance, and obsessions) do not rise to the level of an anxiety disorder diagnosis; nevertheless, they cause distress and some impairment. Similar to the case for perinatal depression, anxiety is detected using self-report measures.

The signs of antenatal depression and anxiety are listed in Box 35.5.

The prevalence of antenatal depression is estimated to be between 7 and 20% in high- income countries while rates of over 20% have been reported in low- and middle-income countries (Biaggi et al., 2016). Biaggi et al. (2016) reported that the prevalence of depression is 7.4% during the first trimester, increasing to 12.8% during the second, and 12% during the third trimester. In Australia, Eastwood et al. (2017) reported the prevalence of maternal depressive symptoms during pregnancy was 7.0% and Woolhouse et al. (2015) found 7.3% of pregnant women reported experiencing intense anxiety or panic attacks

Box 35.5 Signs of antenatal depression and anxiety

- Being nervous, 'on edge', or panicky
- Feeling constantly tired and lacking energy
- Having little or no interest in all the normal things that bring joy (like time with friends, exercise, eating, or sharing partner time)
- Sleeping too much or not sleeping very well at all
- Losing interest in sex or intimacy
- Withdrawing from friends and family
- Being easily annoyed or irritated
- Finding it difficult to focus, concentrate or remember (people with depression often describe this as a 'brain fog')
- Abrupt mood swings
- Feeling constantly sad, low, or crying for no obvious reason
- Panic attacks (a racing heart, palpitations, shortness of breath, shaking or feeling physically 'detached' from your surroundings)
- Persistent, generalised worry, often focused on fears for the health or wellbeing of the baby
- The development of obsessive or compulsive behaviours
- Engaging in more risk-taking behaviour (e.g. alcohol or drug use)
- Having thoughts of death or suicide

(Source: PANDA: https://www.panda.org.au/info-support/after-birth/symptoms-of-postnatal-anxiety-and-depression) either occasionally or often and 15.7% reported this in the first three months postpartum.

In Aotearoa New Zealand the Growing Up in New Zealand study found that 11.5% of the 5664 women in the study had symptoms of depression in their third trimester and 8% had symptoms for postnatal depression (Underwood et al., 2017).

Risk factors for the development of antenatal depression or anxiety

The most common risk factors associated with antenatal depression and anxiety are listed in Box 35.6. Notably, women with higher pregnancy anxiety tend to have lower personal resources (protective factors) such as self-esteem, optimism and perceived control over their pregnancies (Dunkel Schetter et al., 2016).

Recognising symptoms of anxiety and depression

The symptoms of depression and anxiety are listed in Box 35.5. However, anxiety can be more difficult to identify and may not be recognised by women and therefore not identified in assessment and screening. Women (talking on the COPE website) demonstrate their confusion or lack of knowledge about anxiety in pregnancy:

> *I didn't know you could get anxiety DURING pregnancy. It was only after the birth of my second child that I realised how unwell and how bad the anxiety was during my first pregnancy. It really surprises me that no one picked up on it.*
> (http://cope.org.au/pregnancy/mental-health-conditions-pregnancy/antenatal-anxiety/)

Impact on pregnancy outcomes

Women experiencing depression, anxiety and other mental health problems in pregnancy are more likely to have an induction of labour or assisted birth resulting in the infant being admitted into a special care nursery (Feeley, 2017). Some studies have shown an association between antenatal depression and preterm birth and low birth weight (Dadi et al., 2020) or small-for-gestational-age (SGA) babies (Szegda et al., 2014) and women may be less likely to initiate or maintain breastfeeding (Stuebe et al., 2014).

Women with mental ill-health are also more likely to perceive the birth as being traumatic (Boorman et al., 2014; Simpson et al., 2018) with possible subsequent post-traumatic stress disorder (PTSD). One review (Norhayati et al., 2015) and a recent Australian study (Eastwood et al., 2017) have shown that antenatal depression and anxiety are significant risk factors for PND. Around 40% of women who experience symptoms of depression during pregnancy will go on to experience PND if they do not receive treatment. In addition, depression may lead to negative health behaviours, such as increased smoking, alcohol consumption or inadequate nutrition, which, in turn, could increase risk (Szegda et al., 2014).

Box 35.6 Common factors associated with antenatal depression and anxiety

- Lack of partner or social support
- History of abuse or of domestic violence
- Personal history of mental illness
- Unplanned or unwanted pregnancy
- Adverse events in life and high perceived stress
- Unintended pregnancy
- Presence of domestic violence
- Present / past pregnancy complications
- Pregnancy loss

(Source: Biaggi et al., 2016; Dennis, et al., 2016; Dunkel Schetter et al., 2016; O'Hara & Wisner, 2014)

CRITICAL THINKING EXERCISE

Women experiencing depressive symptoms before or after birth may have difficulty responding sensitively to their baby's cues. How would you identify if a woman was not responding sensitively to her newborn baby and what might be the impact of this?

Management of antenatal depression and anxiety

The most important first step is to identify the depressive symptoms or anxiety and discuss with the woman what her needs are at that time and who you should refer her to. Many women describe a need to talk about how they are feeling and to receive reassurance about their pregnancy or baby. In addition, women may benefit from psychological counselling, antidepressant medication, or a combination of these treatments (COPE, 2017; O'Hara & Wisner, 2014).

Other antenatal interventions include support and education offered to all women through antenatal education, advice regarding physical activity in pregnancy, and interventions with a psychological focus (Wadephul et al., 2016). The interventions in Box 35.7 can be offered individually or in groups and increasingly women can access cognitive behavioural therapy (CBT) and other programs for depression online (Dennis & Dowswell, 2013; Howard & Khalifeh, 2020). The United Kingdom's (UK) National Institute for Health and Care Excellence guidelines provide recommendations for evidence-based psychological and pharmacological treatment for anxiety disorders and may be used in the postpartum period. In addition, women may be offered support through peer support programs (Dennis et al., 2016) and attachment-based programs to support women in developing a relationship with their baby in pregnancy as well as following birth (Myors et al., 2014).

Box 35.7 Interventions for antenatal depression and anxiety

- *Cognitive behavioural therapy* (CBT) is widely used to treat anxiety and depression, including in a perinatal context. It is based on the theory that thoughts, emotions and behaviours are interconnected and that distorted or negative thinking affects feelings and behaviours and can lead to negative patterns. The focus in CBT is on changing thoughts and behaviours in order to manage problems in a more positive, constructive way (Jomeen et al., 2017).
- *Interpersonal therapy* (IPT) is a structured form of therapy relating psychological distress to difficulties in interpersonal relationships. IPT focuses on both psychological symptoms and relationship conflict and on identifying and strengthening social support (Dennis et al., 2007).
- *Mindfulness-based** approaches are becoming increasingly popular and focus on cultivating 'a mental state of awareness and acceptance of present moment experiences, including one's current sensations, thoughts, bodily states and environment' (Wadephul et al., 2016). They use techniques such as progressive muscle relaxation, yoga and various forms of meditation and are often taught in groups.
- CBT and IPT are also offered as computer-assisted and internet-based treatments (e-interventions) and can provide support to those who do not otherwise have access (e.g. people who live in rural and remote locations) or prefer anonymity (Dennis et al., 2007).

*The evidence base for Mindfulness is not yet established but is promising.

EATING DISORDERS IN PREGNANCY AND AFTER BIRTH

Most attention to women's weight in pregnancy is on women who have a raised BMI (see Ch. 21). A number of women develop 'eating disorders' related to 'underweight' and 'undereating' either as adolescents or later in life. Midwives may encounter women who are still struggling with an eating disorder or for whom disordered eating may re-emerge with pregnancy or in the postpartum period (Fogarty et al., 2018).

The most common and well-recognised eating disorders are anorexia nervosa, bulimia nervosa, and binge eating disorder (Hudson et al., 2007). Bulimia nervosa and binge eating disorder both involve binge eating (uncontrolled episodes of overeating) and in bulimia nervosa these are followed by compensatory behaviours such as purging (self-induced vomiting, diuretics, or laxatives) or excessive exercise (Hudson et al., 2007).

Incidence

In a recent UK study, Bye et al. (2020) reported that 15.4% of their sample of pregnant women had experienced an eating disorder in their lifetime and that 1.47% of the women experienced an eating disorder during their pregnancy (Bye et al., 2020). This rate in pregnancy is lower than that reported in other studies. For example, Easter et al. (2013) reported that 7.5% of pregnant women met diagnostic criteria for an eating disorder. However, the high pre-pregnancy incidence suggests that a significant proportion of pregnant women have a history of eating disorders which may impact on pregnancy outcomes. A recent review (Fogarty et al., 2018) found that approximately one-quarter of women (23.4%) reported high weight and shape concern during pregnancy; 8.8% reported binge eating and 2.3% engaged in regular compensatory behaviours such as purging.

Some women with an eating disorder may be motivated to cease disordered eating behaviour during pregnancy, others may only manage a reduction of disordered eating and for some eating patterns stay the same or get worse (Fogarty et al., 2018). It is also important to recognise that some women may develop eating disorders during pregnancy or the postnatal period and that this is associated with mental health problems and other **psychosocial issues** (Baskin et al., 2021).

Impact on maternal and baby outcomes

Women who have a pre-existing or current eating disorder commonly report adverse childhood experiences such as sexual abuse (Fogarty et al., 2018) and have low self-esteem and poor body image leading to dangerous weight control methods such as misuse of insulin stimulant abuse (Hay et al., 2015). Women therefore need a thorough antenatal assessment to pinpoint problems early and provide a multidisciplinary approach to their care. Symptoms of depression and anxiety during pregnancy are common amongst women with eating disorders (Easter et al., 2013). Eating disorders are also associated with adverse pregnancy and birth outcomes, including: impaired fertility, unplanned pregnancy, low birth weight, premature birth, hypertension, pre-eclampsia and miscarriage, and delivering large-for-gestational-age babies (Bye et al., 2020). Following birth, some women report that their eating disorder symptoms either worsen or return to their pre-pregnancy levels, motivated by the desire to return to a pre-pregnancy weight and shape (Cardwell, 2013). Returning to eating disorder behaviours in the postpartum period may result in a shorter duration of breastfeeding and may impact on the interaction the mother has with her baby and her relationship with her partner (Fogarty et al., 2018). These women are also apprehensive about how they are perceived, and this has the potential to impact on the interaction with the baby, the method of infant feeding and relationship with the partner (Fogarty et al., 2018).

Managing eating disorders

Treatment of pregnant women with anorexia nervosa is the same as treatment of women who are not pregnant (Cardwell, 2013). Referrals for support should be made to local eating disorders services. Nutritional advice is important to ensure that women have an appropriate dietary intake and variety of food for fetal growth. Sensitive and thoughtful care is necessary to adequately address concerns unique to women who suffer from an eating disorder during the perinatal period (Cardwell, 2013).

CRITICAL THINKING EXERCISE

It can be difficult framing questions about women's weight in pregnancy and their eating patterns. How would you approach this in an antenatal visit? Consider also how you might phrase a question to identify if a woman had a previous or current eating disorder.

Alcohol and substance use during pregnancy

In Australia, the National Drug Strategy Household Survey (AIHW, 2020) estimated that at least 1 in 8 (15%) women continued to drink alcohol during pregnancy, which had reduced from 1 in 4 in 2016; 1 in 9 (11%) smoked, 2.3% used an illicit substance and 1.6% used prescription medications in non-medical ways. Overall, at least 1 in 2 pregnant women (150,000 women a year) report using legal (e.g. alcohol, prescription medications, nicotine) or illegal (e.g. cannabis, heroin, methamphetamines, cocaine, inhalants) substances during pregnancy (AIHW, 2020).

Pregnant women may use substances for many reasons that reflect individual or family situations or external pressures including financial stress and poor or no housing. For example, women with histories of familial substance use and / or who currently live with a partner who uses substances are more likely to be using substances and substance use is also common for women experiencing violence in relationships (Latuskie et al., 2019). Women may use alcohol or drugs as a way of managing stress or depression, or to deal with the fears / stresses from other aspects of their lives (Young-Wolff et al., 2020). Women may also have used substances during the first trimester because they were unaware of the pregnancy and women may experience guilt associated with this use (Latuskie et al., 2019). They do not deliberately choose to harm their baby but may be unaware of the harm the substance use is causing or unable to stop without addiction support.

For substance-dependent women, attempts to discontinue use can be a source of stress, due to withdrawal symptoms and the habitual nature of substance use, and women can also experience many barriers to seeking treatment including financial instability or no access to transport, all of which can act as barriers to accessing treatment (Latuskie et al., 2019).

Addiction to drugs or alcohol, whilst relatively uncommon, is important because any untreated addiction has the potential to have a major impact on both maternal mental and physical health as well as neonatal health.

Alcohol consumption during pregnancy

Whilst drinking alcohol is a widely accepted feature of both Australian and New Zealand societies, excessive consumption and misuse of alcohol is known to be harmful. Being exposed to alcohol during pregnancy can affect the development of the fetus leading to fetal alcohol spectrum disorder (FASD). FASD is an umbrella term that encompasses a range of physical, behavioural, cognitive and neurodevelopmental disorders that occur when a fetus is exposed to alcohol during pregnancy (MOH, 2020; Oei, 2020). A safe level of alcohol use is not known so women should be advised to abstain from drinking alcohol if they are planning pregnancy or as soon as they know they are pregnant and during breastfeeding (MOH, 2020; Oei, 2020).

Incidence

Many women do not plan pregnancy resulting in a high proportion consuming alcohol in the early weeks of pregnancy. However, once a woman finds out she is pregnant the majority will discontinue alcohol consumption. A systematic review of 14 studies found the most consistently reported predictors of alcohol use in pregnancy were pre-pregnancy alcohol use (quantity and frequency), smoking, and maternal exposure to violence and abuse (Skagerström et al., 2011). Smoking as a key predictor of alcohol consumption in pregnancy has been confirmed by a review of international cohort studies (O'Keefe et al., 2015). A New Zealand longitudinal, prospective study interviewed 6822 women during pregnancy and found that nearly 30% did not drink alcohol at all (Growing up in New Zealand, 2015). A further 71% reported drinking alcohol at some level before they were aware they were pregnant. This reduced to 23% in the first trimester after they became aware of the pregnancy and 13% after the first trimester. Some women continued to drink and there were different patterns of alcohol consumption during their pregnancy, with approximately 2% continuing to drink throughout the pregnancy. Most women responded to the public health message to abstain from drinking alcohol during pregnancy but if women had a high level of alcohol use prior to pregnancy, they were less likely to stop drinking alcohol during pregnancy. An Australian study examined the patterns of alcohol consumption in pregnancy and identified two distinct groups of women—those who stop drinking as soon as they know they are pregnant and those who continue to drink, either because they are unaware of, or despite, the recommendation of abstinence (Muggli et al., 2016). Interestingly, women who continued to consume alcohol in low and moderate levels had a higher education and income, smoked cigarettes and were in their early to mid-thirties.

Screening for alcohol consumption

Questions are best embedded in the usual antenatal history at initial assessment and repeated during each trimester if the woman indicates she has been drinking during pregnancy (Department of Health, 2020; MOH, 2020). This will help to identify the women who restart or continue to drink during pregnancy.

In New Zealand and Australia, midwives are required to ask about alcohol consumption and recommend that women stop drinking alcohol. Three steps are advised:

1. Ask if the woman is drinking alcohol.
2. Provide brief advice—that she should not drink alcohol and why.
3. Assist women to identify if they are having difficulty stopping or that drinking is a problem and refer them to specialist addiction services.

There are many different screening tools for alcohol misuse—some of which are more useful and context-specific than others. In New Zealand and in most states and territories in Australia, health professionals are advised to use three questions from the Audit C (MOH, 2010; NSW Department of Health, 2014) (see Table 35.3).

Consequences of alcohol consumption during pregnancy

There continues to be uncertainty about the relationship between alcohol and the effects on the fetus, specifically what level of alcohol consumption leads to FASD (FASD Working Group, 2016; Oei, 2020). Drinking during pregnancy can increase the risk of miscarriage, stillbirth, premature birth, physical abnormalities and a range of physical and neurodevelopment impairments (FASD Working Group, 2016; Leemaqz et al., 2016; Oei, 2020). An action plan has been developed in New Zealand and in Australia in an attempt to take 'a strategic and coordinated national approach to fetal alcohol spectrum disorder *(FASD)*' (FASD Working Group., 2016, p iii; Department of Health, 2018). The approach is to prioritise prevention and early identification to ensure that support can be provided to families / whanau.

Women with problems related to their use of alcohol have potentially high-risk pregnancies and are often less likely to access antenatal care than other women. Consequently, the potential to screen, provide advice and refer for treatment is lost, which can contribute to an increased risk of poor pregnancy outcomes for mother and baby (Breen et al., 2014).

Management of alcohol consumption in pregnancy

The first line of management is to ensure that women are screened using appropriate tools to assess alcohol use in pregnancy (Oei et al., 2021). Women who have drunk alcohol before they knew they were pregnant or during their pregnancy and have subsequently avoided alcohol should be reassured that most babies exposed to low levels of alcohol suffer no observable harm. Women who find it difficult to decrease their alcohol intake during pregnancy will require support and treatment.

A recent systematic 'evidence check' (Oei et al., 2021) concluded that there is some evidence for individual brief face-to-face interventions (e.g. motivational interviewing, self-interviewing with a self-help manual, supportive counselling, psychoeducational interventions) and case management reducing alcohol dependency and increasing engagement with services. These also decreased the risk of low birthweight, neonatal intensive care unit admissions, and child maltreatment risk. Similarly, group support interventions using informed consequences, social support, goal setting, and action planning strategies have demonstrated some efficacy in supporting abstinence (Oei et al., 2021).

Table 35.3 Screening for alcohol use

AUDIT-C is the first three questions of the longer AUDIT tool, which is a more comprehensive assessment of problem drinking

	0	1	2	3	4	Score
How often do you have a drink containing alcohol?	Never	Monthly	2–4 times a month	2–3 times a week	4 or more times a week	
How many drinks containing alcohol do you have on a typical day when you are drinking?	1–2	3 or 4	5 or 6	7 to 9	10 or more	
How often do you have six or more drinks on one occasion?	Never	Less than monthly	Monthly	Weekly	Daily or almost daily	
A score of 3 or less indicates a low-risk drinking pattern.						
A score of 4–7 indicates a risky pattern of drinking.						
A score of 8+ indicates a high–risk pattern of drinking.						
This may be useful information when referring women for support.						

(Source: Department of Health. Information for health professionals on assessing alcohol consumption in pregnancy using AUDIT-C I: http://www.alcohol.gov.au/internet/alcohol/publishing.nsf/Content/65598B7652DC1C5CCA257CD70019CF9A/$File/Women-want-to-know-AuditC-A4-flyer-2017.pdf)

It is important that women are referred to the appropriate services. In New Zealand this will often be a community alcohol and drug service (CADS). In the Australian context, substance use in pregnancy and parenting services (SUPPS) are specialist programs that provide support during and / or after pregnancy, aimed at improving better outcomes for women and their children. Some of these programs support mothers for up to two years after birth but there are no published reports on the outcomes of these programs. Coupland and colleagues (2021) recently outlined the key elements of a SUPPS model of care (see below). There are also several pilot services within New Zealand which are providing specialist pregnancy and parenting services to pregnant women and parents (with children under 3 years of age) who are experiencing issues with alcohol and drugs or prescribed medicines (MOH, 2020).

Substance misuse during pregnancy

Antenatal exposure to drug misuse mostly occurs in the presence of environmental and contextual risk factors that together can impede healthy outcomes. Pregnant women who are drug dependent require support to manage their addiction as well as pregnancy care; referral to a multidisciplinary team with integrated service delivery is crucial.

Table 35.4 identifies some of the illicit substances that may be used and the impact on the pregnancy and fetus/ infant. The detrimental effects of substance use during pregnancy are influenced by the type and amount of drug used, the mother's overall health (nutrition, comorbidities and lifestyle) and the gestational age of the fetus at the time of use.

A qualitative study exploring the experiences of 20 women attending a specialist service in Western Australia and who were using methamphetamine as their primary drug of choice identifies multiple layers of adversities. The participants identified that drug use was often part of their social environment and introduced by family members, partners or friends—often at an early age. Addiction often led to unemployment, homelessness and crime. The women describe mental health issues, and for some, the

Table 35.4 The most common illicit substances used and impact on pregnancy

Substance	Incidence	Impact on pregnancy	Impact on fetus / infant	References
Marijuana / cannabis Used to alter the mental state and contains more than 120 chemicals known as cannabinoids	• 15% of NZ population and 11.6% of Australian adult population • Relatively high incidence in pregnancy and increasing • Between 2% to 3% acknowledge use in pregnancy	Increased risk of miscarriage, congenital malformations, preterm birth, SGA, placental abruption and antepartum haemorrhage	• Affects fetal and infant neurodevelopment • Excreted into breast milk and may have an impact on the baby's nervous system development and endocannabinoid-related functions, with growth, motor skill development and intellectual development potentially affected	Carter et al., 2016; Leemaqz, et al., 2016; Young-Wolffe et al., 2019
Methamphetamine (P) meth, speed, ice or crystal meth A stimulant; increases the experience of pleasure, with chronic use leading to paranoia, delusions, hallucinations, insomnia and extreme weight loss	1% of adults in New Zealand and 1.3% of Australians	Increased risk of severe maternal morbidity, gestational hypertension, preeclampsia and fetal death, fetal anomalies such as heart defects, gastroschisis, cleft lip and palate and preterm birth and SGA	Children exposed to meth during pregnancy have been reported to have poorer developmental functioning at 1 year of age, increased stress, decreased arousal, decreased school achievements and behavioural problems	Forray & Foster, 2015; MOH, 2016a; AIHW, 2020; Gabrhelik et al., 2016; O'Connor et al., 2020
Cocaine Stimulant effects include euphoria, agitation, loss of contact with reality	Estimated 1.1% use in pregnant population	Increased risk of premature rupture of the membranes, placental abruption, preterm birth and SGA	Affects ability to focus, impairs language and executive function, negative effects on perceptual reasoning, IQ and visual motor skills	Dos Santos et al., 2018; Forray & Foster, 2015; Singer et al., 2015

Continued

Table 35.4 The most common illicit substances used and impact on pregnancy—cont'd

Substance	Incidence	Impact on pregnancy	Impact on fetus / infant	References
Opioids Includes diamorphine and heroin; treated with methadone		• Increases the risk of miscarriage, fetal growth restriction, prematurity, placental abruption, oligohydramnios • Sudden withdrawal during pregnancy increases risk of stillbirth • Effects can last into adulthood	• Risk of neonatal abstinence syndrome (NAS) and sudden infant death (SIDS) • NAS is due to the sudden withdrawal of opiates with symptoms including irritability, hypertonia, tremors, feeding intolerance, emesis, watery stools, seizures and respiratory distress	MOH, 2014; Jumah, 2016; Oei, 2018; Yeoh et al., 2019

use of drugs to block the pain of childhood sexual abuse, with many also describing intergenerational trauma. Many of the women had attempted suicide and had self-harmed, many had also experienced family violence and had children removed from their care by child protection services (O'Connor et al., 2021).

CRITICAL THINKING EXERCISE

What is the public view of women who are using substances during pregnancy? How do you think these women may feel about themselves? What can midwives do to support women in the perinatal period?

Irrespective of threats or actual sanctions, most drug-dependent women cannot simply stop 'using' and threats of arrest and interventions by child protection or welfare authorities may deter women from seeking antenatal care or enrolling in treatment programs. Unplanned pregnancy in drug-dependent women is common and often complicated by late presentation for antenatal care and poly drug use. It is important to remember that these women want and hope to be 'good mothers' but experience stigma, shame and guilt (Nichols et al., 2020).

Management of substance use in pregnancy

Management of substance use in pregnancy varies depending upon the substance. For example, maternal opioid substitution programs can improve outcomes for pregnant women by supporting the woman with opiate substitutes. Buprenorphine is the preferred treatment over methadone for opioid use disorder resulting in improvements in maternal and neonatal outcomes; however, there is also good evidence that methadone is an effective treatment for opioid use disorder and it is currently the most commonly used treatment worldwide (Oei et al., 2021; Stover & Davis, 2015).

As identified above, psychoeducation and counselling delivered as parental education and leaflets show evidence of improving the mother's and the child's overall social-emotional functioning for any type of substance use. Interventions that focus on mother and child interaction are recommended to reduce maternal hostility and intrusiveness, and improve the quality of mother–infant interaction. They also succeed in sustaining high maternal abstinence, treatment retention, and alleviating depressive symptoms (Oei et al., 2021). In general, stopping the substance use will improve outcomes, however, for women using opiates, it is important that they don't try to suddenly withdraw from opiate use but are enrolled into a maintenance program until after the pregnancy. In contrast to abstinence programs, many advocate harm reduction approaches to reduce stigma for women and increase engagement with services, particularly child protection, with the potential to reduce placement of children into out-of-home care (O'Connor et al., 2021).

Working with pregnant women who use substances is complex and challenging. Drug use needs to be considered along with other factors such as homelessness, poverty, family violence, trauma and mental health issues. Drug-dependent women may be difficult to engage in antenatal care, but pregnancy is often a time when women want to change their behavior (Nichols et al., 2020).

Most importantly, women who are receiving support for substance use in the perinatal period must be approached in a sensitive and non-judgmental way. It is critical that services and clinicians take a trauma-informed approach to care, which includes being woman-centred, limiting the number of staff clients must interact with and avoiding multiple psychosocial assessments where clients have to re-tell their trauma history. Services need to be flexible and reflect the social determinants of health and promoting engagement in a context where they perceive more may be lost than gained (O'Connor et al., 2021). There needs to be good communication across service providers, achieved best in integrated models of care (Coupland et al., 2021; O'Connor et al., 2021). Community Alcohol and Drugs Services (CADS) or Substance Use in Pregnancy Programs (SUPPS) are available in many areas of New Zealand and Australia where specialised drugs in pregnancy clinics are either linked to antenatal services or established as outreach clinics (Coupland et al., 2021; O'Connor et al., 2021). These services provide specialist support and management for women with substance addiction. Increasingly there is a move to extend integrated models of care beyond antenatal and maternity services, to child and adolescent health (Coupland et al., 2021).

CRITICAL THINKING EXERCISE

Women who are taking substances during pregnancy or are on a methadone program often have many competing priorities and challenges in their lives. Following birth, it is possible that without support, they will have difficulty meeting their baby's emotional needs. What might be the consequences for mother and baby if the situation for the mother remains chaotic? How can you best support this mother?

Drawing on the concepts of **parent–infant attachment** discussed previously, it is likely that the baby in the situation above may become insecure. An insecure child is not confident that the caregiver will meet his or her emotional needs. If a child cannot rely on the caregiver to respond to his / her distress, he / she may intensify his / her display of emotion by being very fussy or demanding to ensure he / she is not ignored. As the child is often angry that he / she cannot rely on the caregiver, he / she may also refuse to accept the caregiver's attempts to provide comfort. This can be very confusing to the caregiver, who cannot distinguish when the child is experiencing true distress or needs to be held and comforted, thereby continuing disharmony and dissatisfaction in the relationship.

Another way children respond to insensitive or unresponsive care is by downplaying their distress and suppressing emotion in order to not provoke the anger of the caregiver. This is termed avoidant attachment. Although the child may seem independent and self-sufficient, insecurity and distress lie beneath this exterior. When upset, a child may retreat to the use of objects such as toys to make contact with the caregiver in order to keep him / her physically near. Infants who have not developed secure relationship are more likely to experience social and biological dysregulation.

DOMESTIC AND FAMILY VIOLENCE

Domestic and family violence (DFV) is a health issue that occurs globally and is not limited to any gender, religion, culture or income group with multi-factorial causes (MOH, 2016b). Women and girls are more likely to be subjected to physical and sexual violence than men, and in most cases the perpetrator is known to their victims. Worldwide, almost one-third (30%) of all women who have been in a relationship have experienced physical and / or sexual violence by their intimate partner (WHO, 2013). Strong associations exist between abuse in childhood and the occurrence of mental health problems later in life and between DFV and mental health problems in adult women.

Indigenous women experience a higher level of DFV as do those women living outside metropolitan centres (Dillon, et al., 2013) and younger women are also at high risk (ABS, 2013). Indigenous women are 35 times more likely to be hospitalised due to DFV than non-Indigenous Australians (COAG, 2016).

Definitions

Many terms are used to describe violence against women. In this chapter the term **domestic and family violence** (DFV) is used as a term that captures the multiplicity of terms and experiences. In New Zealand, family violence is defined as: violence or abuse of any type, perpetrated by one family member against another family member, including child abuse, partner abuse and elder abuse (MOH, 2016b). The term *intimate partner violence* (IPV) is used in much of the literature and therefore IPV may be used depending on the source. Campo (2015) provides a clear overview of the common terms used (Box 35.8).

While there is no single definition, the central element of DFV is an ongoing pattern of behaviour aimed at controlling a partner through fear, for example by using behaviour which is violent and threatening. In most cases, the violent behaviour is part of a range of tactics to exercise power and control over women and their children and can be both criminal and non-criminal (COAG, 2016).

Prevalence of DFV in the perinatal period

Pregnancy is a risk factor for the commencement of violence, however women who are abused during pregnancy have most commonly been abused beforehand (Taft & Hooker, 2017). Pregnant and postpartum women may experience higher risk of partner violence than non-pregnant women, with estimates varying from 4–24% (Devries et al., 2014; Feder et al., 2009; James et al., 2013). A study of pregnant women in Australia suggests up to 17% of nulliparous women experienced physical or emotional abuse in the first year postpartum (Gartland et al., 2011) and 29% reported experiencing IPV by the time their child turned four (Gartland et al., 2014).

Risk factors for DFV

Factors associated with DFV occur at individual, family, community and wider society levels. Some women are more at risk of violence than others, for example those

Box 35.8 Definitions of violence

The United Nations defines violence against women as: any act of gender-based violence that causes 'physical or psychological harm or suffering to women, including threats of such acts, coercion or arbitrary deprivation of liberty' (United Nations, 1993). This can include a host of specific forms of violence experienced by women and girls including sexual violence, intimate partner violence, and domestic and family violence as well as practices that are harmful to women and girls such as female genital mutilation and forced marriage (WHO, 2010a).

Intimate partner violence or domestic violence generally, describes violence perpetrated by a current or previous partner and is the most common form of violence against women (Phillips & Vandenbroek, 2014; WHO., 2010b). 'Domestic violence' or 'family violence' are the terms commonly used to describe violence perpetrated against women in the home.

Family violence is a broader term encapsulating violence between family members as well as intimate partners (Phillips & Vandenbroek, 2014). Family violence is the preferred term in Indigenous populations as it better captures kinship and extended family relationships in Indigenous communities (COAG, 2016).

Intimate partner violence, domestic violence and family violence include behaviours that are coercive and controlling and include physical abuse, emotional / psychological abuse, sexual abuse, financial deprivation and social and cultural isolation (COAG, 2016). Sexual violence includes sexual harassment, sexual bullying, sexual coercion, unwanted touching or kissing, as well as sexual assault (Tarczon & Quadara, 2012). Sexual violence can occur in intimate relationships and / or family contexts as well as in community or work contexts.

Box 35.9 Risk factors for DFV

- Lower levels of education (both for perpetrators of sexual violence and those experiencing sexual violence)
- Exposure to child maltreatment (both perpetrators and those experiencing violence)
- Witnessing family violence (both perpetrators and those experiencing violence)
- Antisocial personality disorder (perpetrators)
- Harmful use of alcohol (both perpetrators and those experiencing violence)
- Having multiple partners or suspected by their partners of infidelity (perpetrators)
- Attitudes that are accepting of violence and gender inequality (both perpetrators and those experiencing violence)

Factors specifically associated with IPV include:

- past history of violence
- marital discord and dissatisfaction
- difficulties in communicating between partners.

Factors specifically associated with sexual violence perpetration include:

- beliefs in family honour and sexual purity
- ideologies of male sexual entitlement
- weak legal sanctions for sexual violence.

The unequal position of women relative to men and the normative use of violence to resolve conflict are strongly associated with both intimate partner violence and non-partner sexual violence.

(Source: Capaldi et al., 2012; Hahn et al., 2018; WHO, 2013)

with young children, sex workers and the homeless, refugees and asylum seekers. An extensive multi-country review by the WHO identified multiple factors associated with DFV (Capaldi et al., 2012; Hahn et al., 2018; WHO, 2013) (Box 35.9).

Impact of DFV

Severe physical violence can end in loss of life (Alhusen et al., 2015). In Australia, over a 10-year period (2002–12), 41% of homicides were domestic / family homicides. Sixty percent of these domestic homicides (654) were related to those in intimate partner relationships, with 75% of all homicide victims being women (Cussen & Bryant, 2015).

Depression is the most common mental health consequence of DFV. Women experiencing partner violence during pregnancy have a threefold likelihood of experiencing PND and a greater prevalence of anxiety and PTSD symptoms in the ante- and the postnatal period (Oliveira et al., 2017). Alhusen et al. (2015) report that around 40% of abused women report depressive symptomatology, and between 19% and 84% experience PTSD. Women experiencing violence are also more likely to have suicidal ideation and commit suicide (Devries et al., 2014). Australian research demonstrated depression can continue years after the birth (Woolhouse et al., 2015).

DFV may also lead to poorer physical health in pregnancy with a higher proportion of abused women reporting urinary incontinence, faecal incontinence and vaginal bleeding, high blood pressure, severe nausea, and kidney and urinary tract infections (Howell et al., 2017). Living with DFV also impacts on women's health behaviours. Women who are experiencing DFV during pregnancy are more likely to miss antenatal care appointments or initiate care late and are more likely to miss three or more antenatal visits (Alhusen et al., 2015). Women are also more likely to engage in unhealthy practices such as smoking and higher alcohol consumption, have poor nutrition and inadequate gestational weight gain (Alhusen et al., 2015).

Insufficient antenatal care, together with events related to physical abuse during pregnancy lead to higher rates of miscarriage, preterm delivery and low birth weight (Donovan et al., 2016). Neurobiological research suggests that newborns exposed to DFV in utero are born with high levels of stress-related hormones (De Bellis & Zisk, 2014) and a US study found exposure to DFV in utero predicted externalising and internalising problems at age 10 years (Martinez-Torteya et al., 2015). Living with abuse, high levels of stress and potentially depression and anxiety, can be disruptive to the development of the maternal–infant relationship and damage attachment at this vulnerable time (Taft & Hooker, 2017).

Women reporting DFV are less likely to breastfeed or to cease breastfeeding early (Howell et al., 2017). Unsurprisingly, a recent Australian study found that women who have experienced DFV have a worse experience of motherhood than women who have not experienced violence (Hooker et al., 2016).

Women's experiences of DFV

It is important to understand women's experiences of DFV. Women's words are a powerful illustration of the experience of violence during the perinatal period (Box 35.10).

Women experiencing violence are also impacted by their individual circumstances (e.g. education level, race / ethnicity, religion, ability / disability), and their environment (e.g. poverty, isolation, disconnection from culture) as well as historical trauma and discriminating public policy (WHO, 2013).

Historical trauma is central to the experience of Australian Indigenous women and as such places additional burden upon individuals and communities. Historical trauma refers to psychosocial and emotional distress that has been experienced over generations (Bowen & Murshid, 2016). Within healthcare, a trauma-informed care approach also recognises the micro (service provider) and macro (public policy) level of healthcare.

Box 35.10 Women's experience of DFV

Torchalla and colleagues captured the trajectory of childhood abuse to abusive intimate relationships:

> *I was heavily abused as a child. Mentally and physically by my mother. And, sexually by her boyfriends. And I watched her getting raped. And I watched her get the crap beat out of her, I walked in on her slitting her wrists. (...) I had, uh, a traumatic childhood (White woman, 36 years)*
>
> (Torchalla et al., 2015, p. 4)

Pregnancy may be something that women hope will change things. Torchalla found several participants were hoping for a new beginning in their lives and their relationship.

> *We moved to Vancouver because we wanted to, raise this baby and, get away from the drugs and alcohol. This is where we came to start fresh and I thought maybe he would be better. And then, he was getting worse, physical, verbal abuse, you know, emotional, everything (Aboriginal woman, 29)*
>
> (Torchalla et al., 2015, p. 6)

The most heartbreaking thing for women experiencing DFV was to be criticised as a mother, to feel unappreciated and unworthy:

> *I can say that I have felt like the bearer of his child. I have not felt that I was important to him at all. He has never allowed me to feel as if I was a nice mum, that I was important to him, never, he has never, he has pushed that away all the time.*
>
> (Wood & Barter, 2015, p. 193)

Women also help us to understand why they stay with their partner:

> *There's no support to do it on your own, I clung to him, 'cos I had no other support, if like benefits they muck you up, one time it took 3 months to get a penny from anybody, where was I to turn, where was I to get money, food, I clung to him*
>
> (Wood & Barter, 2015, p. 196)

Working with women experiencing DFV

Women experiencing violence tend to be under recognised in healthcare settings often due to reluctance to identify the issue but also due to misconceptions that the main effects are physical injury (MOH, 2016b). Taft & Hooker (2017) stress there are two premises that a midwife or health professional must commence with when interacting with women experiencing DFV.

1. *DFV is a serious public health issue, rather than a private problem, which falls within the purview of health professional care.*
2. *No woman, under any circumstances, deserves to be physically, sexually or emotionally abused.*

(Taft & Hooker, 2017, p. 97)

All health professionals must be very sensitive when working with women in cases of suspected DFV including sexual violence—being empathetic, non-judgmental, compassionate and caring. In recent Australian research, the key factor influencing disclosure was that the person was caring (Spangaro, Koziol-McLain et al., 2016). Understanding the influences and complexities of any relationship is important as often over-simplified solutions are suggested for what is a complex issue. Professionals should never therefore prescribe that women leave an abuser; but provide support to the woman. When the woman judges she is sufficiently resourced, safe and confident enough to leave, she will herself know best when she can do so (Taft & Hooker, 2017). Rather than exploring details, it may be more helpful for a midwife to offer suspected DFV or rape survivors general trauma counselling, and allow any sexual assault issues to emerge as trust develops in a confidential setting.

Addressing DFV: prevention and early intervention

Both the New Zealand and Australian governments have made preventing and reducing DFV a priority and have developed cross-agency responses to ensure a country-wide commitment to reduce further violence (Department of Social Services, 2010; MOH, 2016b). In New Zealand for example, a coordinated community response is in place, involving local government, social services, the justice system, education, religion, media and health services. Health providers are supported to ensure increased identification and active responses to DFV and child abuse. This has resulted in greater cross-agency collaboration and information sharing to provide more effective responses for victims of family violence.

Routine enquiry for DFV

Universal or routine enquiry usually involves a set of questions asked by the midwife or other health professionals to detect DFV (e.g. the questions in Table 35.1) (NSW Health, 2010). The Australian Government Clinical Practice Guidelines recommend that all women are asked about DFV at their first antenatal visit (Australian Health Ministers' Advisory Council, 2012). In New Zealand, midwives are expected to routinely ask all pregnant women about DFV as part of a comprehensive health assessment which includes routinely asking about child abuse if abuse is disclosed or there are concerns identified (NZCOM, 2015).

It is important to understand how women feel about being asked about DFV. Salmon and colleagues (2015) found that 94.4% of women surveyed in their study in England indicated they were comfortable with a midwife asking about previous or current experience of violence or abuse. Over 96% of the participants also believed it was appropriate for a midwife to ask and that midwives should be able to respond to positive disclosure. Interviewees subject to abuse during pregnancy were happy to be questioned, even though they did not always feel able to disclose immediately.

Australian research (Spangaro, Koziol-McLain et al., 2016) reported that direct asking was an important trigger which prompted women to consider whether they were safe from the abuser finding out they had disclosed, as well as from shame and institutional control. But most importantly direct asking had to occur in the context of 'care'. The other important trigger for pregnant women is concern about the baby's wellbeing (Spangaro, Koziol-McLain et al., 2016). One study participant stated:

> *If she hadn't have asked I wouldn't have trusted her enough. If she's got the balls to ask, then, yeah, I will give her an answer.*
> (Spangaro, Koziol-McLain et al., 2016, p. 49)

and another,

> *If she didn't ask me about it, I wouldn't have said anything to her. So, it was definitely a good thing they asked.*
> (Spangaro, Koziol-McLain et al., 2016, p. 49)

Disclosure of current or previous violence including childhood sexual abuse is not easy:

> *So, questions like the rape and things like that are always confronting [...] because sometimes you can get through days without having to relive things. And then when you're stopped and asked to think about those things, then you have to, yeah, bring up things from the past. And it can be very daunting.*
> (Spangaro, Koziol-McLain et al., 2016, p. 51)

Spangaro, Herring and colleagues (2016) also investigated Aboriginal women's experience of screening for DFV finding similar experiences; however, unique to Aboriginal women's decisions to disclose abuse, was cultural safety. Cultural safety included trust, building the relationship first, coming at it slowly. One study participant emphasized the importance of attending a service in a trusted place with trusted professionals, in this case the midwife who was providing care through the Aboriginal Medical Service. Spangaro and colleagues (2020) later identified the different impact that routine inquiry may have on women depending on their readiness to disclose and the approach taken by the midwife. Benefits of screening for IPV included naming the abuse, connection with services and knowing others may experience the same, unburdening and having the chance to talk, taking steps to safety, and enabling informed care. For example, some women choose not to disclose but are receptive to receiving information about IPV and can benefit from screening:

> *I think it's just the fact that when she gave me that purple card at the end, and then I realized that there's so many other people out there who can help us in relation to our past experience. (Bridget)*
> (Spangaro et al., 2020, p. 344)

These authors found that key conditions for positive impact of IPV enquiry were care in asking, and support and validation from the midwife. If the midwife did not take this approach and there was no continuity of care then it was most likely there was no positive impact from screening as reflected in the following quote:

> *Cause you get one lady that asks you about that type of stuff and then you talk to that person and you go to your next visit but THAT lady has no idea and then you go to your NEXT visit and then THAT person has no idea. Yeah. It kind of loses track of why the lady asked the first time.*
> (Spangaro et al., 2020, p. 346)

There is debate about the effectiveness of DFV enquiry. The Cochrane systematic review on the impact of routine screening for DFV in the perinatal period (O'Doherty et al., 2015) showed that routine screening or enquiry increases the identification of women experiencing DFV in healthcare settings. Overall, however, rates of disclosure are low (often between 4 to 8%), much lower than the prevalence of DFV in women in the community. The authors did not find that routine enquiry resulted in outcomes such as increased referral, uptake of services, or improved health outcomes (O'Doherty et al., 2015).

Proponents argue that routine enquiry provides the opportunity for women to talk about their concerns and understand there is support, even if she decides not to leave the relationship. Research suggests that women tend not to disclose their experience of DFV unless they are directly asked about it (Alhusen et al., 2015). When asked, women may choose not to disclose about the abuse at the initial time of asking, for fear of their own safety but asking signifies that she can disclose about at a later contact (Salmon et al., 2015).

As a result of this debate there is inconsistent and at times poor uptake of screening in antenatal services in Australia (Baird & Mitchell, 2014). The New Zealand College of Midwives (NZCOM) have developed a Consensus Statement about the responsibility of midwives in relation to family violence (NZCOM, 2015). Similarly, the Australian Clinical Practice Guidelines for Pregnancy Care recommend routine inquiry for domestic violence (DOH, 2020).

There have been several legislative changes designed to reduce family and child abuse which are discussed in more detail in Ch. 14. The introduction of the Vulnerable Children's Act requires all children's workers (which includes midwives) to undergo a safety check to ensure they do not pose a danger to children. It also requires that all midwives adopt a child protection policy. The New Zealand College of Midwives have set out a Child Protection Policy to provide guidance to midwives and assist them to identify and respond to child abuse and neglect (NZCOM, 2016).

CRITICAL THINKING EXERCISE

Think about situations where you have asked about domestic violence—what was your approach? Reflect on the key issues that come to your mind.

The *New Zealand Family Violence Assessment and Intervention Guideline* (MOH, 2016b) and the Australian Department of Health (2020) have set out information to support health practitioners undertaking routine enquiry, as shown in Box 35.11.

Box 35.11 Key principles for conducting routine inquiry for DFV

- Enquire about family violence when alone with the woman.
- Explain that the woman's responses will be kept confidential (subject to legal requirements).
- Actively listen to what the woman tells you.
- Do not blame or judge the woman or her partner.
- Inform the woman that she is not alone, there are other women experiencing family violence.
- Affirm that the woman has made an important step by discussing her experiences.
- Reinforce that family violence is against the law.
- Reinforce that the woman should not self-blame.
- Affirm that the decision to discuss family violence is a major step to enhance her safety.
- Assist the woman to assess her safety and that of children in her care.
- Discuss options for safe temporary accommodation if needed and available (e.g. safe house, family or friends, hospital, women's refuge).
- Encourage the woman to access specialist support services (e.g. woman's health centre, social worker, counsellor, mental health service, family violence and sexual assault service)
- Inform the woman of her legal right to protection and provide information on legal support services.
- Inform the woman that disclosure of family violence may require further discussion and possible reporting in relation to child protection issues.
- Be aware of security supports that can be used to protect the woman and yourself if needed.
- Document a woman's responses (ensuring that records are kept confidential and secure).
- Report any incidents of violence according to organisational policy and jurisdictional legislation.

(Source: DOH, 2020; MOH, 2016b)

Setting up the framing statement is important as it explains the relevance of the question and can facilitate disclosure. An example of a framing question is: '"Because violence affects people's health, I routinely ask all my clients about any violence they have experienced"' (MOH, 2016b, p. 54). Routine enquiry involves asking direct questions about specific behaviours, and includes physical violence, sexual violence, physiological / emotional abuse and controlling behaviour. An example is: 'Within the past year did anyone scare you or threaten you, or someone you care about?'

Confidentiality is important but practices differ as to when this is introduced to women. For example, in New Zealand making a statement about confidentiality before the routine enquiry is not recommended. If information is disclosed that raises concerns it is important to identify the limits of confidentiality and discuss the need to talk to others to support safety. In Australia the practice varies, with many services recommending the following introduction to enquiry about DFV:

> *In this health service we routinely ask all women the same questions about violence at home. This is because violence in the home is very common and can be serious and we want to improve our response to women experiencing family violence. You don't have to answer the questions if you don't want to. All answers to the questions will remain confidential to the health service except where you give us information that indicates that you or your children are at immediate risk of serious harm. We would discuss this with you.*
>
> (NSW Health, 2010)

The response of the healthcare provider to disclosure is important with women needing validation of their experience and affirmation that the perpetrator's behaviour is unacceptable (Hooker et al., 2016). This should be followed by a safety and risk assessment.

Safety plans

A thorough safety assessment for both women and children is required, with a subsequent safety plan to be discussed, along with counselling and referral to specialist DFV services (Valpied & Hegarty, 2015). Safety planning may be one of the most important and meaningful aspects of care and a key outcome to measure when assessing intervention efficacy (O'Doherty et al., 2015). Safety planning has been shown to increase women's safety. Safety assessment involves asking women about their immediate safety (including children) and ability to return home.

CRITICAL THINKING EXERCISE

In a recent antenatal visit with Sarah, she disclosed that she was frightened of her partner. How would you assess Sarah's safety at that time and what information would you provide to Sarah? (Check your response in Box 35.12.)

The most dangerous time for an abused woman is after she ends the relationship; leaving the home, asking the perpetrator to leave and / or reporting the abuse are significant factors that place a woman at 'higher risk' of becoming a victim of homicide (Valpied & Hegarty, 2015).

Box 35.12 Safety planning when a woman discloses DFV

- Provide the woman with resources including hotline numbers to call (police and local refuges).
- Recommend that she packs a safety bag that includes anything she and her children might need including money, keys and important documents that can either be taken quickly if the woman needs to leave the house or can be left with someone she trusts.
- Encourage her to memorise important phone numbers or web addresses.
- Care must be taken to ensure that providing this information will not put the woman at greater risk of violence by always respecting the woman's choice of what she wants to do.
- Other useful strategies include the removal of dangerous weapons and the use of code words that family, friends and / or neighbours are aware of when in danger and urgent assistance is needed.

(Adapted from Women's Aid, Making a Safety Plan: https://www.womensaid.org.uk/the-survivors-handbook/making-a-safety-plan/)

It is therefore very important for a woman to make her own decision to leave a relationship because she is in the best position to assess the potential danger. When there is evidence of escalating violence or 'lethality' (i.e. the woman's life is at risk) the midwife must immediately refer her to the appropriate tertiary services.

Women exposed to DFV need comprehensive support

Ideally healthcare should weave together different components of support depending on the individual's needs. For example, mental health needs (resilience) should be supported along with relational (e.g. DFV), parental (e.g. antenatal health, parenting skills) and systemic (e.g. social and instrumental support, community resources) supports. See Box 35.13.

In general, interventions focused on problem solving / solution seeking / enhanced choice making and the alteration in distorted self-thinking and perception are promising in facilitating and maintaining positive physical and mental health changes for women who experience violence (Trabold et al., 2020). Counselling interventions such as IPT are beneficial in that they directly address known mental health consequences associated with IPV-exposure (Howell et al., 2017).

Therapeutic responses that focus on fostering mother–infant bonding and attachment, based on relational trauma and attachment theory, are an emerging, promising approach to responding to women in the perinatal period. Parent–infant psychotherapy can begin during pregnancy as it is thought mothers begin to develop internal representations of themselves as mothers during this time (Myors et al., 2014). Home visitation interventions up to two years after birth (Kemp et al., 2011) and community-based mentorship programs (Taft et al., 2011) offer unique opportunities to join with women in addressing multifaceted and systemic needs. A recent review suggests some benefits from both face-to-face and remote delivery of interventions, offering the opportunity to improve access for vulnerable women who might

Box 35.13 Comprehensive care for women experiencing DFV

Comprehensive care is needed to:

- Improve access to and utilisation of antenatal and medical care
- Address negative mental health outcomes
- Rebuild compromised social support networks
- Reduce exposure to violence
- Enhance the woman's conceptualisation of her child
- Improve parenting practices

(Source: Howell et al., 2017)

be unable to or are unwilling to access care at hospitals and registered clinics (Ogbe et al., 2020). Finally, community connections can be particularly important for women with low social support. Ogbe et al. (2020) examined the impact of social support interventions for women experiencing DFV; in their systematic review they found most interventions that use advocacy with strong community linkages and a focus on community networks showed significant effects on mental health outcomes and access to social support, highlighting the benefits of community connectedness for women.

Service system response to support maternal and infant social and emotional health

The complexity of the perinatal period warrants systems and services that are well networked. Poor communication and cooperation between services only widens the gap between what is needed and what is available to support women and families experiencing mental ill-health. Women with a history of mental illness—particularly serious mental illness and / or complex psychosocial issues—require a well-planned, coordinated approach to care that involves case management and the maintenance of support networks (Eastwood et al., 2021). To achieve this, there needs to be effective collaboration between services and professionals.

CRITICAL THINKING EXERCISE

Certain conditions or factors are needed to ensure effective interprofessional collaboration. From your experience in practice, what do you think are the key characteristics of effective collaboration and teamwork?

In collaborative practice, midwives need an awareness of their own and others' roles, interpersonal relationship skills and organisational support. Researchers have identified several key characteristics of effective collaboration. A summary of these is presented in Box 35.14.

See Chapter 18 for more on collaboration.

Box 35.14 Key characteristics of successful collaboration

- Shared vision and values
- Agreement on common goals and clearly stated aims
- Inspirational and energetic leadership
- Built on the enthusiasm and commitment of others
- Sound governance, clarity of leadership and assessment of risks
- Recognition of and valuing diverse professional contributions
- Capacity to address issues of power and achieve an equitable distribution of resources
- A willingness to share risks and problems as well as any positive outcomes
- Mechanisms in place to deal with conflict
- Recognising all contributions
- Public recognition of worth
- Evaluations to assess effectiveness and cost-effectiveness
- The need for frequent and effective communication
- Time and resources, particularly time to spend in building relationships with other professionals
- Mechanisms to facilitate sharing of information and administrative data as appropriate
- Understanding participants' practice, philosophy, culture, ideas and beliefs

(Source: Psaila & Schmied, 2017)

Conclusion

In this chapter we have examined a range of mental health and social situations that impact on health outcomes for women and their babies. A small proportion of women experience significant pre-existing mental health concerns including eating disorders, however a higher proportion experience mood disorders—antenatal depression and anxiety. These feelings may also be associated with PTSD following birth. Drug and alcohol issues and DFV also pose significant difficulties for women during pregnancy. Midwives are in a key position to support women. Risk factors associated with poor mental health are well known and this has informed tools and approaches to early identification. Women's response to **psychosocial screening and assessment** varies and it is important that midwives undertake assessment in a non-judgmental, respectful way. It is also important that effective interventions are available, and women have access to appropriate referral pathways and secondary-level services. Midwives, particularly when working in continuity models, have the potential to influence positive outcomes for women and their babies.

Review questions

1. What are the key risk and protective factors associated with maternal mental health in the perinatal period?
2. What are the main components of psychosocial assessment? When should a midwife assess a woman's mental health and social wellbeing?
3. What are the benefits and / or negative aspects of routine psychosocial assessment in pregnancy?
4. Why might maternal anxiety be increasing and how might be this affect child development?
5. What are the signs and symptoms of perinatal depression and anxiety?
6. What are the key psychological and psycho-educational interventions for maternal depression and anxiety?
7. What advice would you give to a woman about alcohol consumption in pregnancy?
8. What is the midwife's role in assessing alcohol consumption in pregnancy?
9. What are the known adverse effects of substance misuse in pregnancy?
10. What are the main forms of domestic and family violence and what are the known risk factors for DFV?
11. What are the key elements of safety planning?
12. What are the key characteristics of working in partnership with women who have complex needs?

Online resources

Depression and anxiety

Australia

BeyondBlue—provides support, advice and action for mental health problems including perinatal mental health: https://www.beyondblue.org.au/about-us/about-our-work/perinatal-mental-health.

COPE (Centre for Perinatal Excellence)—aims to prevent and improve the quality of life of those living with emotional and mental health problems that occur in the perinatal period. COPE informs and educates through providing high-quality, evidence-based information to empower people and guide them to care; also equips health professionals with knowledge, skills and confidence to provide safe and effective care: http://cope.org.au/.

PANDA (Perinatal Anxiety and Depression Australia)—a specialist not-for-profit organisation that has helped tens of thousands of Australian women get vital information and support: https://www.panda.org.au/.

New Zealand

Mental Health Foundation of New Zealand—provides information, advice and support about depression and postnatal depression: https://www.mentalhealth.org.nz/get-help/a-z/resource/26/postnatal-depression.

Depression and anxiety—provides information, self-tests and self-help. Helpline – 0800 111 757 or free text 4202: https://depression.org.nz/.

Postnatal depression—overview and information by the Ministry of Health https://www.health.govt.nz/your-health/pregnancy-and-kids/first-year/helpful-advice-during-first-year/postnatal-depression.

Mothers matter—aims to provide up-to-date information to women, families and healthcare providers. Includes PND, anxiety and bipolar disorders, contains information on local supports available: https://www.mothersmatter.nz/.

Perinatal Anxiety & Depression Aotearoa (PADA): https://pada.nz/.

Anxiety New Zealand—helpline 0800 269 4389: https://www.anxiety.org.nz/.

Healthline—0800 611 116: https://www.health.govt.nz/your-health/services-and-support/health-care-services/healthline.

Suicide Crisis Helpline—0508 828 865: https://www.lifeline.org.nz/services/suicide-crisis-helpline.

Domestic and family violence

Australia

1800RESPECT: https://www.1800respect.org.au/.

ANROWS (Australia's National Research Organisation for Women's Safety Limited)—an independent, not-for-profit company established as an initiative under Australia's National Plan to Reduce Violence against Women and their Children 2010–2022. Delivers relevant and translatable research evidence which drives policy and practice leading to a reduction in the levels of violence against women and their children: https://anrows.org.au/.

Services Australia—Family and Domestic Violence: https://www.servicesaustralia.gov.au/family-and-domestic-violence.

ECAV (NSW Education Centre Against Violence)—a state-wide unit responsible for workforce development and training programs in the areas of adult and child sexual assault, domestic and Aboriginal family violence and physical and emotional abuse and neglect of children: http://www.ecav.health.nsw.gov.au/.

New Zealand

Shine—provides information, resources and support for victims of domestic abuse, including a free national Helpline, crisis advocacy, women's refuge / transition housing along with help for children exposed to domestic abuse: http://www.2shine.org.nz/how-shine-helps/shine-services.

National Campaign: Family Violence – It's not Ok: It is OK to ask for help: http://www.areyouok.org.nz/

NZ Police, Help for Family violence—provides a legal perspective and information about police safety orders: http://www.police.govt.nz/advice/family-violence/help.

Small Steps—mental health support: https://www.smallsteps.org.nz/.

Drugs and alcohol

Australia

Drug and Alcohol Foundation: https://adf.org.au/drug.

National Drug and Alcohol Research Centre (UNSW)—Australia's leading research centre into drugs and alcohol; has undertaken relevant research related to pregnancy: https://ndarc.med.unsw.edu.au/search/node/pregnancy.

New Zealand

NZ Drug Foundation—provides advice and advocacy aimed at reducing drug harm: https://www.drugfoundation.org.nz/.

Alcohol Drug Helpline service directory—lists services in different locations through NZ: http://www.addictionshelp.org.nz/Services/Home.

Community Alcohol and Drug Services, Auckland (these services are also available in other regions): http://www.cads.org.nz/.

New Zealand Alcohol Drug Helpline: 0800 787 797

Pot Help—an online support resource for those struggling with cannabis use: https://www.pothelp.org.nz/.

Ministry of Health—Help with mental health and addiction: https://www.govt.nz/browse/health/help-with-mental-health-and-addiction/.

References

Ainsworth MDS, Blehar MC, Waters E, et al. *Patterns of Attachment: A Psychological Study of the Strange Situation*. Hillsdale, NJ: Erlbaum; 1978.

Alhusen JL, Ray E, Sharps P, Bullock L. Intimate partner violence during pregnancy: maternal and neonatal outcomes. *J Womens Health*. 2015;*24*(1):100–106. doi:10.1089/jwh.2014.4872.

Australian Bureau of Statistics. Personal Safety Survey. *Australia (cat. No. 4906.0)*; 2013. Online: http://www.abs.gov.au/ausstats/abs@.nsf/mf/4906.0.

Australian Health Ministers' Advisory Council. Clinical Practice Guidelines Antenatal care – Module I; 2012. Online: http://www.health.gov.au/internet/publications/publishing.nsf/Content/clinical-practice-guidelines-ac-mod1.

Australian Institute of Health and Welfare. National Drug Strategy Household Survey *Drug Statistics series no. 32. PHE 270;* 2020. Online https://www.aihw.gov.au/getmedia/77dbea6e-f071-495c-b71e-3a632237269d/aihw-phe-270.pdf.aspx?inline5true.

Austin MP, Colton J, Priest S, Reilly N, Hadzi-Pavlovic D. The antenatal risk questionnaire (ANRQ): acceptability and use for psychosocial risk assessment in the maternity setting. *Women Birth*. 2013;*26*(1):17–25. doi:10.1016/j.wombi.2011.06.002.

Baird KM, Mitchell T. Using feminist phenomenology to explore women's experiences of domestic violence in pregnancy. *Br J Midwifery*. 2014;*22*(6):418–426. doi:10.12968/bjom.2014.22.6.409.

Baskin R, Meyer D, Galligan R. Predicting the change in perinatal disordered eating symptoms: An examination of psychosocial factors. *Body Image*. 2021;*37*:162–171.

Biaggi A, Conroy S, Pawlby S, Pariante CM. Identifying the women at risk of antenatal anxiety and depression: a systematic review. *J Affect Disord*. 2016;*191*:62–77. doi:10.1016/j.jad.2015.11.014.

Boorman RJ, Devilly GJ, Gamble J, et al. Childbirth and criteria for traumatic events. *Midwifery*. 2014;30(2):255–261.

Bowen EA, Murshid NS. Trauma-informed social policy: a conceptual framework for policy analysis and advocacy. *Am J Public Health*. 2016;*106*(2):223–229. doi:10.2105/AJPH.2015.302970.

Breen C, Awbery E, Burns L. Supporting Pregnant Women Who Use Alcohol or Other Drugs: A Review of the Evidence; 2014. Online https://ndarc.med.unsw.edu.au/sites/default/files/ndarc/resources/Supporting%20Pregnant%20Women%20who%20use%20Alcohol%20or%20Other%20Drugs%20-%20A%20review%20of%20the%20evidence.pdf.

Brockington I, Butterworth R, Glangeaud-Freudenthal N. An international position paper on mother-infant (perinatal) mental health, with guidelines for clinical practice. *Arch Womens Ment Health*. 2017;20(1):113–120.

Bronfenbrenner U. *The Ecology of Human Development*. Cambridge, MA: Harvard University Press; 1979.

Budget 2019: Mental Health, Wellbeing and Addiction Initiatives. Online: https://www.health.govt.nz/our-work/mental-health-and-addiction/he-ara-oranga-response/budget-2019-mental-health-wellbeing-and-addiction-initiatives#primarycare.

Bye A, Nath S, Ryan EG, et al. Prevalence and clinical characterisation of pregnant women with eating disorders. *Eur Eat Disord Rev*. 2020;*28*(2):141–155.

Campo M. *Children's Exposure to Domestic and Family Violence (CFCA Paper 36)*. Melbourne: CFCA; 2015. Online: https://aifs.gov.au/cfca/publications/childrens-exposure-domestic-and-family-violence.

Capaldi DM, Knoble NB, Shortt JW, Kim HK. A systematic review of risk factors for intimate partner violence. *Partner Abuse*. 2012;*3*(2):231–280. doi:10.1891/1946-6560.3.2.231.

Cardwell MS. Eating disorders during pregnancy. *Obstet Gynecol Surv*. 2013;*68*(4):312–323. doi:10.1097/OGX.0b013e31828736.

Carter R, Wainwright H, Molteno C, et al. Alcohol, methamphetamine and marijuana exposure have distinct effects on the human placenta. *Alcohol Clin Exp Res*. 2016;*40*(4):753–764.

Centre of Perinatal Excellence (COPE). Mental Health Care in the Perinatal Period: Australian Clinical Practice Guideline; 2017. Online: https://www.cope.org.au/wp-content/uploads/2018/05/COPE-Perinatal-MH-Guideline_Final-2018.pdf.

COAG. COAG Advisory Panel on Reducing Violence against Women and their Children – Final Report; 2016. Online: http://www.coag.gov.au/sites/default/files/communique/COAGAdvisoryPanelonReducingViolenceagainstWomenandtheirChildren-FinalReport.pdf.

Coupland H, Moensted ML, Reid S, et al. Developing a model of care for substance use in pregnancy and parenting services, Sydney, Australia: Service provider perspectives. *J Subst Abuse Treat*. 2021;*131*:108420. doi:10.1016/j.jsat.2021.108420.

Cussen T, Bryant W. Domestic/Family Homicide in Australia; 2015. Online http://www.aic.gov.au/publications/current%20series/rip/21-40/rip38.html.

Dadi AF, Akalu TY, Baraki AG, Wolde HF. Epidemiology of postnatal depression and its associated factors in Africa: a systematic review and meta-analysis. *PLoS ONE*. 2020;15(4):e0231940. doi:10.1371/journal.pone.0231940.

De Bellis MD, Zisk A. The biological effects of childhood trauma. *Child Adolesc Psychiatr Clin N Am*. 2014;*23*(2):185–222. doi:10.1016/j.chc.2014.01.002.

Dennis C-L, Ross S, Grigoriadis S. Psychosocial and psychological interventions for treating antenatal depression. *Cochrane Database Syst Rev*. 2007;(3):CD006309.

Dennis C, Brown HK, Morrell J. Interventions (other than psychosocial, psychological and pharmacological) for preventing postpartum depression. *Cochrane Database Syst Rev*. 2016;(5). doi:10.1002/14651858.CD012201.

Dennis CL, Dowswell T. Psychosocial and psychological interventions for preventing postpartum depression. *Cochrane Database Syst Rev (Online)*. 2013;*2*.

Dennis CL, Falah-Hassani K, Brown HK, Vigod SN. Identifying women at risk for postpartum anxiety: a prospective population-based study. *Acta Psychiatr Scand*. 2016;*134*(6):485–493. doi:10.1111/acps.12648.

Dennis CL, Falah-Hassani K, Shiri R. Prevalence of antenatal and postnatal anxiety: systematic review and meta-analysis. *Br J Psychiatry*. 2017;*210*(5):315–323. doi:10.1192/bjp.bp.116.187179.

Department of Health. National Fetal Alcohol Spectrum Disorder Strategic Action Plan; 2018. Online: https://www.health.gov.au/sites/default/files/national-fasd-strategic-action-plan-2018-2028.pdf.

Department of Health. (2020) *Clinical Practice Guidelines: Pregnancy Care*. Canberra: Australian Government Department of Health; 2020. Online: https://www.health.gov.au/resources/pregnancy-care-guidelines.

Department of Social Services. The National Plan to Reduce Violence against Women and their Children 2010 – 2022; 2010. Online: https://www.dss.gov.au/sites/default/files/documents/08_2014/national_plan1.pdf.

Devries KM, Child JC, Bacchus LJ, et al. Intimate partner violence victimization and alcohol consumption in women: a systematic review and meta-analysis. *Addiction.* 2014;*109*(3):379–391. doi:10.1111/add.12393.

Dillon G, Hussain R, Loxton D, Rahman S. Mental and physical health and intimate partner violence against women: a review of the literature. *Int J Family Med.* 2013;*2013*:313909. doi:10.1155/2013/313909.

Donovan BM, Spracklen CN, Schweizer ML, Ryckman KK, Saftlas AF. Intimate partner violence during pregnancy and the risk for adverse infant outcomes: a systematic review and meta-analysis. *BJOG.* 2016;*123*(8):1289–1299. doi:10.1111/1471-0528.13928.

dos Santos JF, de Melo Bastos Cavalcante C, Barbosa FT, et al. Maternal, fetal and neonatal consequences associated with the use of crack cocaine during the gestational period: a systematic review and meta-analysis. *Arch Gynecol Obstet.* 2018;*298*(3): 487–503. doi:10.1007/s00404-018-4833-2.

Dunkel Schetter C, Niles AN, Guardino CM, Khaled M, Kramer MS. Demographic, medical, and psychosocial predictors of pregnancy anxiety. *Paediatr Perinat Epidemiol.* 2016;*30*(5):421–429. doi:10.1111/ppe.12300.

Dunkel Schetter C, Tanner L. Anxiety, depression and stress in pregnancy: implications for mothers, children, research, and practice. *Curr Opin Psychiatry.* 2012;*25*(2):141–148. doi:10.1097/YCO.0b013e3283503680.

Easter A, Bye A, Taborelli E, et al. Recognising the symptoms: how common are eating disorders in pregnancy? *Eur Eat Disord Rev.* 2013;*21*(4):340–344. doi:10.1002/erv.2229.

Eastwood J, Ogbo FA, Hendry A, Noble J, Page A. The impact of antenatal depression on perinatal outcomes in Australian women. *PloS ONE.* 2017;*12*(1). doi:10.1371/journal.pone.0169907.

Eastwood J, Wang A, Khanlari S, Montgomery A, Yang J. Psychosocial stratification of antenatal indicators to guide population-based programs in perinatal depression. *BMC Pregnancy Childbirth.* 2021;21:277. doi:10.1186/s12884-021-03722-8.

FASD Working Group. *Taking Action on Fetal Alcohol Spectrum Disorder:* 2016–2019: An Action Plan. Wellington: Ministry of Health; 2016. Online: https://www.health.govt.nz/system/files/documents/publications/taking-action-on-fetal-alcohol-spectrum-disorder-2016-to-2019.pdf.

Feder G, Ramsay J, Dunne D, Rose M, Arsene C. How far does screening women for domestic (partner) violence in different health-care settings meet criteria for a screening programme? Systematic reviews of nine UK National Screening Committee criteria. *Health Technol Assess.* 2009;*13(16).*

Feeley N. Giving birth earlier than expected. Mothers whose newborn requires neonatal *intensive care. In: Thomson G, Schmied V, eds. Psychosocial Resilience and Risk in the Perinatal Period: Guidance for Professionals.* London: Routledge; 2017:140-153.

Fogarty S, Elmir R, Hay P, Schmied V. The experience of women with an eating disorder in the perinatal period: a meta-ethnographic study. *BMC Pregnancy Childbirth.* 2018;*18*(1):121.

Forder PM, Rich J, Harris S, et al. Honesty and comfort levels in mothers when screened for perinatal depression and anxiety. *Women Birth.* 2020;*33*(2):e142–e150. doi:10.1016/j.wombi.2019.04.001.

Forray A, Foster D. Substance use in the perinatal period. *Curr Psychiatry Rep.* 2015;*17*(11):91. doi:10.1007/s11920-015-0626-5.

Fox S, Southwell A, Stafford N, Goodhue R, Jackson D, Smith C. *Better Systems, Better Chances: A Review of Research and Practice for Prevention and Early Intervention.* Canberra; 2015. Online: https://www.aracy.org.au/shop/publications/better-systems-better-chances.

Frayne J, Nguyen T, Allen S, Hauck Y, Liira H, Vickery A. Obstetric outcomes for women with severe mental illness: 10 years of experience in a tertiary multidisciplinary antenatal clinic. *Arch Gynecol Obstet.* 2019;*300*(4):889–896. doi:10.1007/s00404-019-05258-x.

Friedrich J, Khatib D, Parsa K, Santopietro A, Gallicano GI. The grass isn't always greener: the effects of cannabis on embryological development. *BMC Pharmacol Toxicol.* 2016;*17*(1):45. doi:10.1186/s40360-016-0085-6.

Gabrhelik R, Nechanska B, Mravcik V, Skurtveit S, Lund IO, Handal M. A unique opportunity to study short and long term consequences in children prenatally exposed to illicit drugs and opioid maintenance treatment using Czech and Scandinavian registers. *Cent Eur J Public Health.* 2016;*24*(3):248–251. doi:10.21101/cejph.a4474.

Gartland D, Hemphill SA, Hegarty K, Brown SJ. Intimate partner violence during pregnancy and the first year postpartum in an Australian pregnancy cohort study. *Matern Child Health J.* 2011;*15*(5):570–578. doi:10.1007/s10995-010-0638-z.

Gartland D, Woolhouse H, Mensah FK, Hegarty K, Hiscock H, Brown SJ. The case for early intervention to reduce the impact of intimate partner abuse on child outcomes: results of an Australian Cohort of First-Time Mothers. *Birth.* 2014;*41*(4): 374–383. doi:10.1111/birt.12123.

Ghimire U, Papabathini SS, Kawuki J, Obore N, Musa TH. Depression during pregnancy and the risk of low birth weight, preterm birth and intrauterine growth restriction- an updated meta-analysis. *Early Human Development.* 2021;*152*:105243. doi:10.1016/j.earlhumdev.2020.105243.

Glover V, O'Donnell KJ, O'Connor TG, Fisher J. Prenatal maternal stress, fetal programming, and mechanisms underlying later psychopathology—a global perspective. *Dev Psychopathol.* 2018;*30*(3):843–854.

Growing up in New Zealand. *Patterns and Dynamics of Alcohol Consumption during Pregnancy in a recent New Zealand Cohort of Expectant Mothers.* Wellington: Social policy Evaluation and Research Unit (Superu); 2015.

Hahn CK, Gilmore AK, Aguayo RO, Rheingold AA. Perinatal Intimate partner violence. *Obstet Gynecol Clin North Am.* 2018;*45*(3):535–547. doi:10.1016/j.ogc.2018.04.008.

Hauck Y, Allen S, Ronchi F, Faulkner D, Frayne J, Nguyen T. Pregnancy experiences of western australian women attending a specialist childbirth and mental illness antenatal clinic. *Health Care Women Int.* 2013;*34*(5):380–394. doi:10.1080/07399332.2012.736577.

Hay P, Chinn D, Forbes D, et al. Royal Australian and New Zealand College of Psychiatrists clinical practice guidelines for the treatment of eating disorders. *Aust N Z J Psychiatry.* 2014;*48*(11): 977–1008.

Hooker L, Samaraweera NY, Agius PA, Taft A. Intimate partner violence and the experience of early motherhood: a cross-sectional analysis of factors associated with a poor experience of motherhood. *Midwifery.* 2016;*34*:88–94. doi:10.1016/j.midw.2015.12.011.

Howard LM, Khalifeh H. Perinatal mental health: a review of progress and challenges. *World Psychiarty.* 2020;*19*(3):313–327.

Howell KH, Miller-Graff LE, Hasselle AJ, Scrafford KE. The unique needs of pregnant, violence-exposed women: a systematic review of current interventions and directions for translational research. *Aggress Violent Behav.* 2017. doi:10.1016/j.avb.2017.01.021.

Hudson JI, Hiripi E, Pope Jr HG, Kessler RC. The prevalence and correlates of eating disorders in the National Comorbidity Survey replication. *Biol Psychiatry.* 2007;*61*(3):348–358. doi:10.1016/j.biopsych.2006.03.040.

Humphrey MD. Maternal mortality trends in Australia. *Med J Aust.* 2015;*205*(8):344-346.

James L, Brody D, Hamilton Z. Risk factors for domestic violence during pregnancy: a meta-analytic review. *Violence Vict.* 2013;*28*(3):359–380. doi:10.1891/0886-6708.28.3.359.

Jomeen J, Fleming S, Martin CR. Women with a diagnosed mental health problem. In: Thomson G, Schmied V, eds. *Psychosocial Risk and Resilience in the Perinatal Period: Guidance for Professionals.* London: Routlege; 2017.

Jumah NA. Rural, pregnant, and opioid dependent: a systematic review. *Subst Abuse.* 2016;*10*(suppl 1):35–41. doi:10.4137/SART.S34547.
Kemp L, Harris E, McMahon C, et al. Child and family outcomes of a long-term nurse home visitation programme: a randomised controlled trial. *Arch Dis Child.* 2011;*96*(6):533–540.
Kulkarni J, Worsley R, Gilbert H, et al. A prospective cohort study of antipsychotic medications in pregnancy: the first 147 pregnancies and 100 one year old babies. *PloS ONE.* 2014;9(5). doi:10.1371/journal.pone.0094788.
Latuskie KA, Andrews NCZ, Motz M, et al. Reasons for substance use continuation and discontinuation during pregnancy: a qualitative study. *Women Birth.* 2019;*32*(1):e57–e64. doi:10.1016/j.wombi.2018.04.001.
Leemaqz SY, Dekker GA, McCowan LM, et al. Maternal marijuana use has independent effects on risk for spontaneous preterm birth but not other common late pregnancy complications. *Reprod Toxicol.* 2016;*62*:77–86. doi:10.1016/j.reprotox.2016.04.021.
Martinez-Torteya C, Bogat GA, Levendosky AA, Von Eye A. The influence of prenatal intimate partner violence exposure on hypothalamic-pituitary-adrenal axis reactivity and childhood internalizing and externalizing symptoms. *Dev Psychopathol.* 2015;*28*(1):55–72. doi:10.1017/S0954579415000280.
McCauley K, Elsom S, Muir-Cochrane E, Lyneham J. Midwives and assessment of perinatal mental health. *J Psychiatr Ment Health Nurs.* 2011;*18*(9):786–795. doi:10.1111/j.1365-2850.2011.01727.x.
McCauley KM, Cross W, Kulkarni J. Mental health: outcomes of 10 babies of mothers with a history of serious mental illness. *J Psychiatr Ment Health Nurs.* 2016;*21*(7):580–586. doi:10.1111/jpm.12111.
Megnin-Viggars O, Symington I, Howard LM, Pilling S. Experience of care for mental health problems in the antenatal or postnatal period for women in the UK: a systematic review and meta-synthesis of qualitative research. *Arch Womens Ment Health.* 2015;*18*(6):745–759.
Ministry of Health (MOH). *Alcohol and Pregnancy: A Practical Guide for Health Professionals.* Wellington, NZ: Ministry of Health; 2010.
Ministry of Health. *New Zealand Practice Guidelines for Opioid Substitution Treatment.* Wellington: Ministry of Health; 2014.
Ministry of Health. *Amphetamine use 2015/16. New Zealand Health Survey.* Wellington: Ministry of Health; 2016a.
Ministry of Health. Family Violence Assessment and Intervention Guidelines; 2016b. Online: http://www.health.govt.nz/publication/family-violence-intervention-guidelines-child-and-partner-abuse.
Ministry of Health. Fetal Alcohol Spectrum Disorder; 2020. Online: https://www.health.govt.nz/our-work/diseases-and-conditions/fetal-alcohol-spectrum-disorder.
Moore TG, Arefadib N, Deery A, West S. *The First Thousand Days: An Evidence Paper.* Parkville, Victoria: Centre for Community Child Health, Murdoch Children's Research Institute; 2017. Online: https://apo.org.au/sites/default/files/resource-files/2017-09/apo-nid108431_1.pdf.
Moss KM, Simcock G, Cobham V, et al. A potential psychological mechanism linking disaster-related prenatal maternal stress with child cognitive and motor development at 16 months: the QF2011 Queensland flood study. *Dev Psychol.* 2017;*53*(4):629–641. doi:10.1037/dev0000272.
Muggli E, O'Leary C, Donath S, et al. "Did you ever drink more?" A detailed description of pregnant women's drinking patterns. *BMC Public Health.* 2016;*16*(1):683.
Mule V, Reilly NM, Schmied V, Kingston D, Austin MP. Why do some pregnant women not fully disclose at comprehensive psychosocial assessment with their midwife? *Women Birth.* 2021. doi:10.1016/j.wombi.2021.03.001.
Myors KA, Schmied V, Johnson M, Cleary M. Therapeutic interventions in perinatal and infant mental health services: a mixed methods inquiry. *Issues Ment Health Nurs.* 2014;*35*(5):372–385.
New Zealand College of Midwives (NZCOM). *Consensus Statement: Family Violence.* Christchurch: New Zealand College of Midwives; 2015.
New Zealand College of Midwives (NZCOM). *New Zealand College of Midwives Child Protection Policy.* Christchurch: New Zealand College of Midwives; 2016.
NICE. Antenatal and postnatal mental health: clinical management and service guidance. Clinical guidelines; 2014. Online: nice.org.uk/guidance/cg192.
Nichols TR, Welborn A, Gringle MR, Lee A. Social stigma and perinatal substance use services: recognizing the power of the good mother ideal. *Contemp Drug Probl.* 2020. doi:10.1177/0091450920969200.
Norhayati MN, Nik Hazlina NH, Asrenee AR, Wan Emilin WM. Magnitude and risk factors for postpartum symptoms: a literature review. *J Affect Disord.* 2015;*175*:34–52. doi:10.1016/j.jad.2014.12.041.
NSW Department of Health. NSW Clinical Guidelines for the Management of Substance Use during Pregnancy, Birth and the Postnatal Period; 2014.
NSW Health. *Families NSW: Supporting Families Early Package.* North Sydney, NSW: NSW Department of Health; 2009.
O'Connor A, Harris E, Hamilton D, Fisher C, Sachmann M. The experiences of pregnant women attending a specialist service and using methamphetamine. *Women Birth.* 2021;*34*(2):170–179. doi:10.1016/j.wombi.2020.01.011.
O'Doherty L, Hegarty K, Ramsay J, Davidson LL, Feder G, Taft A. Screening women for intimate partner violence in healthcare settings. *Cochrane Database Syst Rev.* 2015;7:CD007007. doi:10.1002/14651858.CD007007.pub3.
Oei JL. Adult consequences of prenatal drug exposure. *Intern Med J.* 2018;*48*(1):25–31. doi:10.1111/imj.13658.
Oei JL. Alcohol use in pregnancy and its impact on the mother and child. *Addiction.* 2020;*115*(11):2148–2163. doi:10.1111/add.15036.
Oei JL, Azim SI, Lee E, et al. Substance use during pregnancy, birth and the postnatal period: an evidence check rapid review brokered by the Sax Institute (www.saxinstitute.org.au) NSW Ministry of Health, January 2021.
Ogbe E, Harmon S, Van den Bergh R, Degomme O. A systematic review of intimate partner violence interventions focused on improving social support and/ mental health outcomes of survivors. *PloS ONE.* 2020;*15*(6):e0235177. doi:10.1371/journal.pone.0235177.
O'Hara MW, Wisner KL. Perinatal mental illness: definition, description and aetiology. *Best Pract Res Clin Obstet Gynaecol.* 2014;*28*(1):3–12. doi:10.1016/j.bpobgyn.2013.09.002.
O'Keeffe LM, Kearney PM, McCarthy FP, *et al.* Prevalence and predictors of alcohol use during pregnancy: findings from international multicentre cohort studies. *BMJ Open.* 2015;**5:e006323. doi:10.1136/bmjopen**-2014-006323.
Oliveira AGS, Reichenheim ME, Moraes CL, Howard LM, Lobato G. Childhood sexual abuse, intimate partner violence during pregnancy, and posttraumatic stress symptoms following childbirth: a path analysis. *Arch Womens Ment Health.* 2017;*20*(2):297–309. doi:10.1007/s00737-016-0705-6.
Perinatal and Maternal Mortality Review Committee. Fourteenth Annual report of the Perinatal and Maternal Mortality Review Committee: Reporting Mortality and Morbidity 2020; 2021. Online: https://www.hqsc.govt.nz/our-programmes/mrc/pmmrc/publications-and-resources/publication/4210/.
Phillips J, Vandenbroek P. *Domestic, Family and Sexual Violence in Australia: An Overview of the Issues. Parliamentary Library Research Paper;* 2014. Online: http://www.aph.gov.au/About_Parliament/Parliamentary_Departments/Parliamentary_Library/pubs/rp/rp1415/ViolenceAust.

Psaila K, Schmied V. Interprofessional collaboration: a crucial component of support for women and families in the perinatal period. In: Thomson G, Schmied V, eds. *Psychosocial Risk and Resilience in the Perinatal Period: Guidance for Professionals.* London: Routlege; 2017.

Reilly N, Loxton D, Black E, Austin MP. The antenatal risk questionnaire-revised: development, use and test-retest reliability in a community sample of pregnant women in Australia. *J Affect Disord.* 2021;*293*:43–50. doi:10.1016/j.jad.2021.05.081.

Salmon D, Baird KM, White P. Women's views and experiences of antenatal enquiry for domestic abuse during pregnancy. *Health Expect.* 2015;*18*(5):867–878. doi:10.1111/hex.12060.

Shore R. *Rethinking the Brain: New Insights into Early Development.* NY: Families and Work Institute; 1997. Online: https://eric.ed.gov/?id5ED418770from.

Simpson M, Schmied V, Dickson C, Dahlen HG. Postnatal post-traumatic stress: an integrative review. *Women Birth.* 2018;*31*(5):367–379. doi:10.1016/j.wombi.2017.12.003.

Singer LT, Minnes S, Min MO, Lewis BA, Short EJ. Prenatal cocaine exposure and child outcomes: a conference report based on a prospective study from Cleveland. *Hum Psychopharmacol.* 2015;*30*(4):285–289. doi:10.1002/hup.2454.

Skagerstr√≥m J, Chang G, Nilsen P. Predictors of drinking during pregnancy: a systematic review. *J Womens Health.* 2011;*20*(6):901–913. doi:10.1089/jwh.2010.2216.

Spangaro J, Herring S, Koziol-Mclain J, Rutherford A, Frail MA, Zwi AB. 'They aren't really black fellas but they are easy to talk to': factors which influence Australian Aboriginal women's decision to disclose intimate partner violence during pregnancy. *Midwifery.* 2016;*41*:79–88. doi:10.1016/j.midw.2016.08.004.

Spangaro J, Koziol-McLain J, Zwi A, Rutherford A, Frail MA, Ruane J. Deciding to tell: qualitative configurational analysis of decisions to disclose experience of intimate partner violence in antenatal care. *Soc Sci Med.* 2016;*154*:45–53. doi:10.1016/j.socscimed.2016.02.032.

Spangaro J, Koziol-McLain J, Rutherford A, Zwi AB. "Made Me Feel Connected": a qualitative comparative analysis of intimate partner violence routine screening pathways to impact. *Violence Against Women.* 2020;*26*(3–4):334–358. doi:10.1177/1077801219830250.

Stover MW, Davis JM. Opioids in pregnancy and neonatal abstinence syndrome. *Semin Perinatol.* 2015;*39*(7):561–565. doi:10.1053/j.semperi.2015.08.013.

Stuebe AM, Horton BJ, Chetwynd E, Watkins S, Grewen K, Meltzer-Brody S. Prevalence and risk factors for early, undesired weaning attributed to lactation dysfunction. *J Womens Health.* 2014;*23*(5):404–412. doi:10.1089/jwh.2013.4506.

Szegda K, Markenson G, Bertone-Johnson ER, Chasan-Taber L. Depression during pregnancy: a risk factor for adverse neonatal outcomes? A critical review of the literature. *J Matern Fetal Neonatal Med.* 2014;*27*(9):960–967. doi:10.3109/14767058.2013.845157.

Taft A, Hooker L. Domestic and family violence. In: Thomson G, Schmied V, eds. *Psychosocial Risk and Resilience in the Perinatal Period: Guidance for Professionals.* London: Routlege; 2017.

Taft A, Small R, Hegarty KL, Watson LF, Gold L, Lumley JA. Mothers' AdvocateS In The Community (MOSAIC)-non-professional mentor support to reduce intimate partner violence and depression in mothers: a cluster randomised trial in primary care. *BMC Public Health.* 2011;*11*:178. doi:10.1186/1471-2458-11-178.

Tarczon C, Quadara A. The Nature and Extent of Sexual Assault and Abuse in Australia. *ACSSA Resource Sheet No. 5;* 2012. Online: https://aifs.gov.au/publications/nature-and-extent-sexual-assault-and-abuse-australia.

Thomson G, Schmied V. *Psychosocial Risk and Resilience in the Perinatal Period: Guidance for Professionals.* London: Routlege; 2017.

Torchalla I, Linden IA, Strehlau V, Neilson EK, Krausz M. "Like a lots happened with my whole childhood": violence, trauma, and addiction in pregnant and postpartum women from Vancouver's Downtown Eastside. *Harm Reduct J.* 2015;*11*(1). doi:10.1186/1477-7517-11-34.

Trabold N, McMahon J, Alsobrooks S, Whitney S, Mittal M. A systematic review of intimate partner violence interventions: state of the field and implications for practitioners. *Trauma Violence Abuse.* 2020;*21*(2):311–325.

Underwood L, Waldie KE, D'Souza S, Peterson ER, Morton SM. A Longitudinal study of pre-pregnancy and pregnancy risk factors associated with antenatal and postnatal symptoms of depression: evidence from growing up in New Zealand. *Matern Child Health J.* 2017;*21*(4):915–931. doi:10.1007/s10995-016-2191-x.

United Nations. *Declaration on the Elimination of Violence Against Women.* Geneva; 1993. Online: https://eeas.europa.eu/delegations/un-geneva_en/36191/Statement%20on%20the%20International%20Day%20for%20the%20Elimination%20of%20Violence%20against%20Wome.

Valpied J, Hegarty K. Intimate partner abuse: identifying, caring for and helping women in healthcare settings. *Womens Health.* 2015;*11*(1):51–63. doi:10.2217/WHE.14.59.

Wadephul F, Jones C, Jomeen J. The impact of Antenatal Psychological Group Interventions on psychological well-being: a systematic review of the qualitative and quantitative evidence. *Healthcare.* 2016;*4*(2):32. doi:10.3390/healthcare4020032.

WHO. A 2013 analysis conduct by WHO with the London School of Hygiene and Tropical Medicine and the Medical Research Council; 2013. Online: http://www.who.int/reproductive-health/publications/violence/9789241564625/en/.

Wood M, Barter C. Hopes and fears: teenage mothers' experiences of intimate partner violence. *Child Soc.* 2015;*29*(6):558–568. doi:10.1111/chso.12100.

Woolhouse H, Gartland D, Mensah F, Brown SJ. Maternal depression from early pregnancy to 4 years postpartum in a prospective pregnancy cohort study: implications for primary health care. *BJOG.* 2015;*122*(3):312–321. doi:10.1111/1471-0528.12837.

World Health Organization. *A Conceptual Framework for Action on the Social Determinants of Health.* Geneva: World Health Organization; 2010a.

World Health Organization. *Preventing Intimate Partner and Sexual Violence Against Women: Taking Action and Generating Evidence.* Geneva: WHO; 2010b.

Yeoh SL, Eastwood J, Wright IM, et al. Cognitive and motor outcomes of children with prenatal opioid exposure: a systematic review and meta-analysis. *JAMA Netw Open.* 2019;*2*(7):e197025. doi:10.1001/jamanetworkopen.2019.7025.

Young-Wolff KC, Sarovar V, Tucker L-Y, et al. Self-reported daily, weekly, and monthly cannabis use among women before and during pregnancy. *JAMA Netw Open.* 2019;*2*(7):e196471. doi:10.1001/jamanetworkopen.2019.6471.

Young-Wolff KC, Sarovar V, Tucker L-Y, et al. Association of depression, anxiety, and trauma with cannabis use during pregnancy. *JAMA Netw Open.* 2020;*3*(2):e1921333. doi:10.1001/jamanetworkopen.2019.21333.

Further reading

Austin M-P, Highet N, Expert Working Group. *Mental Health Care in the Perinatal Period: Australian Clinical Practice Guideline.* Melbourne: Centre of Perinatal Excellence; 2017. Online: File://ad.uws.edu.au/dfshare/HomesPTA$/30020148/ Downloads/Final-COPE-Perinatal-Mental-Health- Guideline%20(1).pdf.

Thomson G, Schmied V. *Psychosocial Risk and Resilience in the Perinatal Period: Guidance for Professionals.* London: Routlege; 2017.

SECTION 2

Collaborative practice

CHAPTER 36

Variations in normal

Sally K Tracy

LEARNING OUTCOMES

Learning outcomes for this chapter are:

1. To describe the ways in which midwives work to keep birth emotionally and physically safe when variations in presentation occur
2. To explore the known benefits and harms of vaginal breech birth
3. To outline the underlying physiology and aetiology of multiple pregnancy
4. To discuss the use of various manoeuvres to facilitate the birth of the shoulders and the head of a breech baby
5. To describe the indications and contraindications of external cephalic version
6. To outline the current evidence and best practice around breech birth.

CHAPTER OVERVIEW

This chapter discusses the variations from normal in pregnancy and labour, with an emphasis on multiple pregnancy, occipitoposterior (OP) presentation and breech birth. It provides a broad overview of the issues and considers some of the core technical components of clinical practice incorporating and promoting evidence-informed midwifery practice. The chapter establishes a framework for understanding the way of doing things, with reference to the guiding principles which are fundamental for midwives working within the midwifery model.

KEY TERMS

amnionicity
anteroposterior diameters of a newborn head
breech birth
breech presentation
chorionicity
external cephalic version (ECV)
moxibustion
multiple pregnancy
occiput posterior position
zygosity

INTRODUCTION

Occipitoposterior position of the fetus

> *The fetal occiput posterior position poses clinical challenges in every aspect of intrapartum care—prevention, diagnosis, correction, supportive care, labor management, and delivery of the fetus ... Although the occiput posterior fetus usually rotates to occiput anterior eventually, it often occurs after many hours and efforts to deal with a painful, exhausting, and non-progressing labour.*
>
> (Simkin, 2010, p. 61)

Occiput posterior position occurs in about 10%–25% of pregnancies during the early stage of labour and in 10%–15% during the active phase. The occiput posterior position of the fetal head in the pelvis during the first and second stage of labour is diagnosed by palpating the fontanelles and sutures of the fetal skull (Fig. 36.1). If you find the larger, diamond-shaped fontanelle is anterior in the pelvis, the fetus is in an OP position. Although about 2%–10% of singleton term cephalic fetuses will be born in an OP position, some of these may have been in an occiput anterior (OA) position in labour but rotated during labour to the OP position. One of the most significant predisposing factors includes epidural anaesthesia (Lieberman et al., 2005), although the exact mechanism for this is not clearly understood.

The OP fetal position in particular has been reported as a cause of back pain in labour possibly because there is usually some degree of deflexion of the fetal skull, presenting the larger diameter as it enters and progresses through the maternal pelvis. This results in delayed descent and reduced contact between the fetal skull and maternal cervix, with less-effective contractions. Through this mechanism women are often predisposed to labour dystocia, characterised by slow progress in the first and second stages of labour, and increased pain (Lee et al., 2015).

In the OP position, in about 10%–25% of pregnancies the fetal head enters the maternal pelvis with the occiput lying in the posterior segments of the pelvis. In most cases the architecture of the pelvis is normal, but in others the pelvic diameters may be reduced. OP positions are more common in the presence of long, narrow pelvic walls (oval-shaped pelvis) or with convergent pelvic side walls and prominent ischial spines. For the baby lying in a right occipitoposterior (ROP) position, to rotate to a right occipitoanterior (ROA) the head must rotate 135° from an ROP to a right occipitolateral (ROL), then to ROA and then, as the head begins to birth, to a direct OA (DOA). Thus, lengthy labours are associated with an OP position. In nearly two-thirds of cases, the fetal head spontaneously achieves this rotation.

In about 15% of cases the fetal attitude is one of deflexion, and the sinciput becomes anterior. If this happens, the sinciput, not the occiput, rotates to the front of the pelvis so that the fetal head completes a short rotation of 45° and the head is born 'face-to-pubes'. With a deflexed fetal head, the presenting diameter is 12.5 cm—much larger than the 9.5 cm of the suboccipitobregmatic diameter of the well-flexed head, and so as the head births there is a much higher chance of perineal lacerations. In 20% of cases the fetal head attempts the 'long rotation' but arrests at the level of the ischial spines—known as deep transverse arrest.

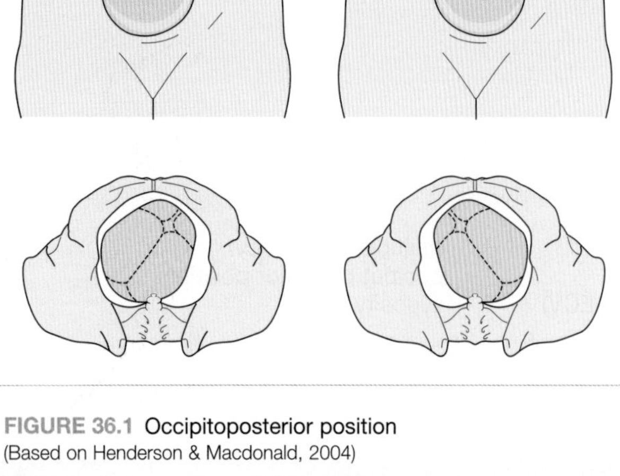

FIGURE 36.1 Occipitoposterior position
(Based on Henderson & Macdonald, 2004)

CLINICAL POINT

Outline the four potentially different posterior positions of a baby's head during labour.

Working with a woman experiencing an OP labour

Woman usually experience a long, discouraging and trying labour with intense pain in the small of the back. Others will have an uncontrollable urge to push before the cervix is completely dilated. Many require pharmaceutical analgesia, including epidurals, to cope with intolerable pain and exhaustion. However, encouraging the woman to ambulate, assume positions such as the all-fours position and squat in the first and second stages, as well as offering massage or labouring in water, helps the pain and may aid the fetus to rotate anteriorly. Stremler et al. (2005) identified that the all-fours position significantly reduced back pain and suggested that adopting this position assisted fetal rotation to the OA position. This was supported by a review by Hunter et al. (2007).

Prevention

To date, there is no strong evidence that the OP position can be prevented and sustained through to birth (Simkin, 2010). A trial undertaken in Australia in 2004 examined the use of a hands-and-knees position with slow pelvic rocking exercises for 10 minutes twice daily, beginning in the 37th week of gestation and continuing until the time of labour, and found no difference between those randomised to either arm of the trial (Kariminia et al., 2004). Once in labour, however, many women find staying upright and frequently changing position more comfortable than assuming a supine or semirecumbent position in bed. The UK National Institute for Health and Care Excellence guidelines (NICE, 2017) on intrapartum care actively encourage women to mobilise during labour and not to give birth in a supine position on a bed, but this is still often the position many women adopt especially in the hospital setting, though rarely at home (Westbury, 2014).

A randomised controlled trial undertaken in the US to determine whether a lateral asymmetric decubitus posture could facilitate the rotation of fetal occiput posterior into occiput anterior positions showed that lying on the side opposite that of the fetal spine did not facilitate rotation of fetal head (Le Ray et al., 2016).

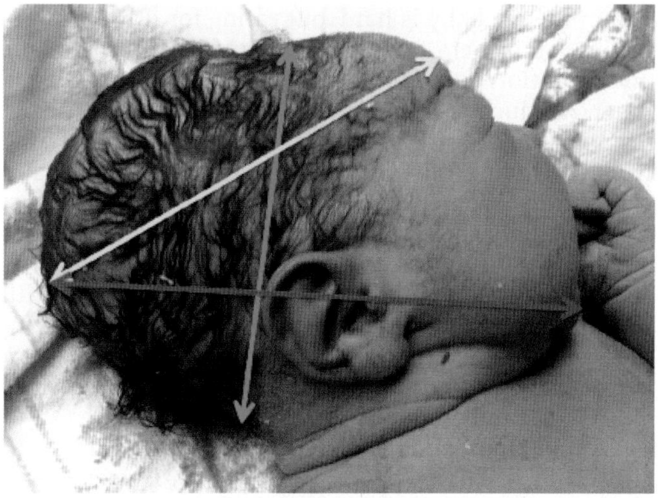

FIGURE 36.2 Anteroposterior diameters of a newborn head: for occiput anterior delivery, the suboccipitobregmatic diameter (green) typically passes through the outlet and over the perineal body. For occiput posterior deliveries, the larger occipitofrontal (yellow) or occipitomental (red) diameters typically pass through the outlet as a result of extension of the fetal head.
(Source: Barth, 2015)

Diagnosis

On abdominal palpation, the fetal back is often felt on the far side of the mother's flanks or not at all. There is a sensation of 'limbs everywhere', and the fetal head is deflexed and slow to engage in the pelvis. A saucer-shaped depression may be seen at, or just below, the umbilicus because the shoulder is lying posteriorly (see Fig. 36.1). On vaginal examination, the anterior fontanelle can be felt in the anterior quadrant of the mother's pelvis and the posterior fontanelle at the back. Palpation using Leopold's manoeuvres may be helpful in determining fetal presentation, weight and other characteristics (Lydon-Rochelle et al., 1993). (Palpation is described in Ch. 23. For details on the Sharma technique, a more recent modification of the Leopold manoeuvres, see Sharma (2009).)

The use of intrapartum scanning is possibly the most reliable means to determine the fetal position when OP is suspected (Simkin, 2010). It is always important, however, to consider the mother's views and the potential but unknown risks of frequent ultrasound exposure.

Deep transverse arrest (where the widest part of the fetal head is blocked at the level of the ischial spines) must always be considered if, during second stage on vaginal examination:

- sagittal suture remains in the transverse diameter of the pelvis
- in a primigravida the uterine contractions become hypotonic or irregular
- there is increasing and extensive moulding of the fetal head
- there is increasing caput succedaneum
- the fetal head does not descend past the maternal ischial spines.

Potential problems for mother and baby from an OP position include:

- slow engagement of the fetal head
- false labour and incoordinate uterine action
- early and severe backache
- possibility of deep transverse arrest
- increased incidence of operative delivery
- persistent OP position ('face-to-pubes'), which may result in a higher incidence of perineal trauma.

Complications

Because the deflexed fetal head presents a wider diameter and more irregular presentation (Fig. 36.2), progress in cervical dilation and fetal descent tends to be slow with an OP baby. The labour is often prolonged and painful. If an OP persists, it greatly increases the likelihood of an operative delivery (caesarean or instrumental delivery), especially for the first birth.

Operative birth carries with it the inherent risks of major surgery: severe perineal trauma, infection, haemorrhage, wound infection, urinary retention and infection, pulmonary embolism and anaesthesia-related complications. As in all instances of dystocia with an OP position, there is a higher incidence of early rupture of membranes, chorioamnionitis, fetal infection, fetal compromise and asphyxia. Infection may occur because the membranes are ruptured for a longer period of time and from multiple vaginal examinations.

MULTIPLE PREGNANCY

A diagnosis of a **multiple pregnancy** is one that often brings both surprise and anxiety for parents and midwives.

Parenting one baby is hard, but caring for two (or more) babies can be very taxing. Parents try to split their time and attention equitably between the siblings and each other. As much as they try, parents of multiples may not feel they can devote the quality and quantity of care they would wish and this may lead to feelings of failure and exhaustion. Women will require considerable support from not only their family but also midwives, obstetric and neonatal services during pregnancy, birth and well into the postnatal period. Complications associated with multiple pregnancies have resulted in a significant increase in the proportion of pre-term births and the number of babies admitted to neonatal intensive care units (NICUs) (Chamberlain et al., 2017).

Overall, approximately 50–60% of multiple pregnancies result in babies being born before 37 weeks, with about 9–12% of those being born before 32 weeks gestation (Liem et al., 2013).

In Australia in 2019 around 64% of twins and all other multiples (triplets and higher) were born pre-term (AIHW, 2021). The majority of multiple births, given that they are pre-term, were more likely to be admitted to NICUs than singletons (68% for twins, 99% for other multiples) and more than half or these babies had hospital stays of 6 days or more (AIHW, 2021).

Incidence of multiple pregnancies

The number of multiple births in Australia each year is small and has remained relatively stable at around 2–3% of all births (from 9285 (3.1%) of births in 2009 to 8915 (2.9%) of births in 2019). In 2019, of this small proportion, almost all multiple births (98%) were twins, while the remaining 2% were other multiples (that is, triplets, quadruplets or higher). The proportion of multiple pregnancies was lowest among mothers aged less than 20 (0.8%) and increased to 2.8% among mothers aged 40 and over (AIHW, 2021). In Aotearoa New Zealand the proportion of twin or multiple births has not changed much over the last decade, ranging from 1.3% to 1.6% of all women giving birth. Amongst NZ women giving birth to twins, 64% were more likely to have a caesarean section (MOH, 2021). (See Table 36.1; see also NICE, 2013).

Classification

Zygosity

There are two major types of twin gestations: *dizygotic (DZ)* and *monozygotic (MZ)* (Box 36.1, Fig. 36.3). MZ twins (uniovular and identical) occur sporadically. In contrast, the incidence of DZ twins (binovular and fraternal) increases with advancing maternal age and parity. In some families, DZ twinning is probably inherited. DZ twins are more common than MZ twins. In Caucasians, about 30% of twin pregnancies are MZ and about 70% DZ (Rankin, 2017).

DZ twins develop from two ova fertilised by different spermatozoa. They have separate gestational sacs with separate placentas, chorion, amnion and umbilical cords (Fig. 36.4). The developing fetuses may be of the same or different sex and are no more alike than non-twin siblings. In contrast, MZ twins develop from a single ovum, which splits within a few days of embryogenesis into two identical halves, each developing into one twin with a separate amnion and umbilical cord but usually sharing one placenta and chorion (Fig. 36.5). These babies are of the same sex, have the same blood group and share very similar physical and psychological characteristics.

Chorionicity

Chorionicity refers to the type of placentation caused by the number of chorionic (outer) membranes that surround the fetuses in a multiple pregnancy. If there is only one membrane the pregnancy is described as monochorionic; if there are two it is described as dichorionic, and a triplet pregnancy with three membranes is described as trichorionic. Monochorionic twin pregnancies and dichorionic and monochorionic triplet pregnancies carry higher risks because fetuses share a placenta (NICE, 2021).

All dizygotic twins have DC (dichorionic/diamniotic) placentas. The placentas may be fused or separate but,

Table 36.1 The percentage of women giving birth, by plurality and type of birth, New Zealand, 2017

Type of birth	Singleton (N= 58,481) %	Twin (N=767) %	Multiple (N=16) %
Spontaneous vaginal	63.1	23.4	0
Assisted birth	9.5	12.4	0
Emergency caesarean	15.1	24.9	50
Elective caesarean	12.3	39.3	50
Unknown	–	–	–
Total	**100.0**	**100.0**	**100.0**

(Source: NZMOH, *Report on Maternity*, 2019 p. 58)

Box 36.1 What is zygosity?

Dizygotic (DZ) (fraternal) twins occur when two eggs are released at a single ovulation and are fertilised by two different sperm. These two fertilised eggs then implant independently in the uterus. DZ twins share around 50% of their genes, which is the same type of genetic relationship as non-twin siblings, hence the term fraternal, and:

- approximately half are the same-sex and half, different sex
- each has its own placenta, which is continuous with the chorion (outer membrane), with rare exceptions
- each is as genetically similar as any same-sex or different-sex siblings.

Monozygotic (MZ) (identical) twins develop when one egg is fertilised by a single sperm and during the first 2 weeks after conception the developing embryo splits into two. As a result, two, genetically identical babies develop:

- approximately one-third have separate placentas
- approximately two-thirds share a single placenta despite maintaining their own inner sac (amnion), umbilical cord and share of the placental mass
- all MZ twins are the same sex with rare exceptions
- all are genetically identical, or almost 100% identical.

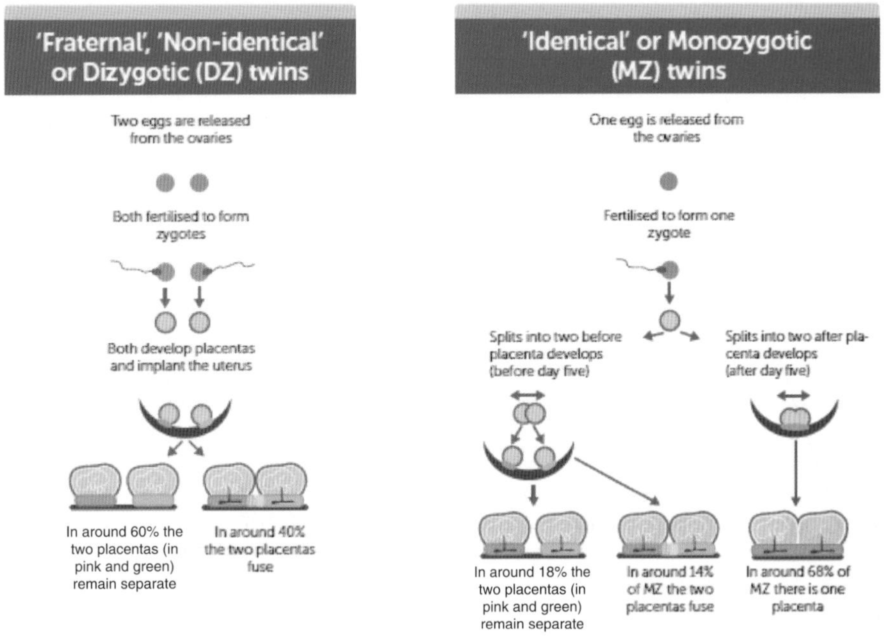

FIGURE 36.3 What is zygosity?

(Source: Twins Research Australia: https://www.twins.org.au/how-to-determine-zygosity)

when examined after birth, blood vessel anastomoses between the two vascular beds are seldom discovered (Rankin, 2017).

Amnionicity

Amnionicity refers to the number of amnions (inner membranes) that surround fetuses in a multiple pregnancy. Pregnancies with one amnion (so that all fetuses share one amniotic sac) are described as monoamniotic; twin or triplet pregnancies with two amnions are diamniotic; triplet pregnancies with three amnions are triamniotic (NICE, 2021).

Box 36.2 summarises chorionicity and amnionicity.

Mortality/morbidity

Multiple pregnancies are considered to be 'high risk' because the mortality rate is about four times that for singletons. Based on current research, approximately 10–20% of women with a confirmed pregnancy will experience early pregnancy loss. However, after 12 weeks of pregnancy this rate is reduced to about 3–4% (Cohain et al., 2017; Vasak et al., 2017; Stirrat 1990). In many cases the loss is due to congenital abnormalities, which are more common in monozygotic and monochorionic twins (Khalil & O'Brien, 2007). In the so-called 'vanishing twin' syndrome, the 'lost' twin is reabsorbed into the

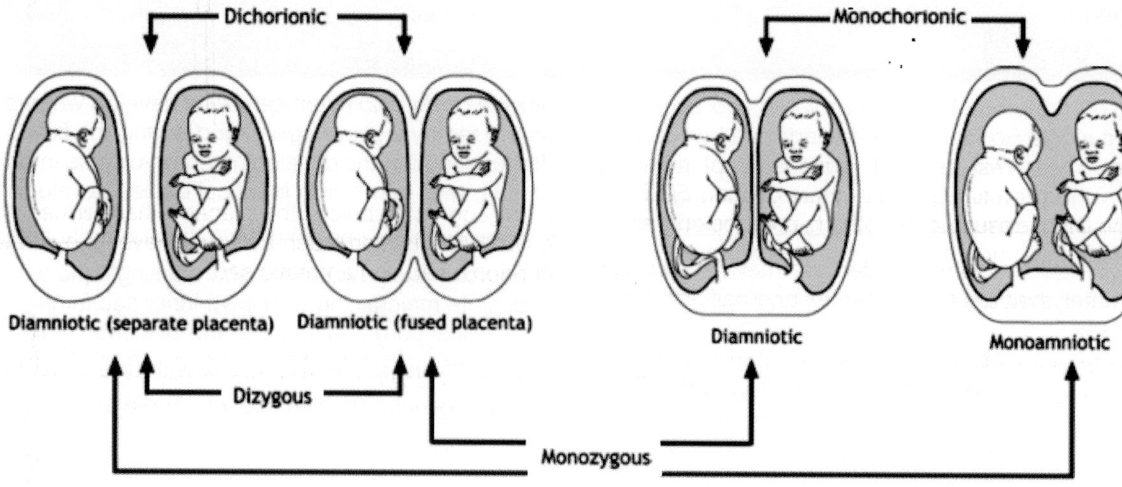

FIGURE 36.4 Zygosity, chorionicity and amnionicity: different patterns of placentation for twins.
(Source: Shetty A, Smith AP. The sonographic diagnosis of chorionicity. *Prenatal Diagn*. 2005;25(9):735–739)

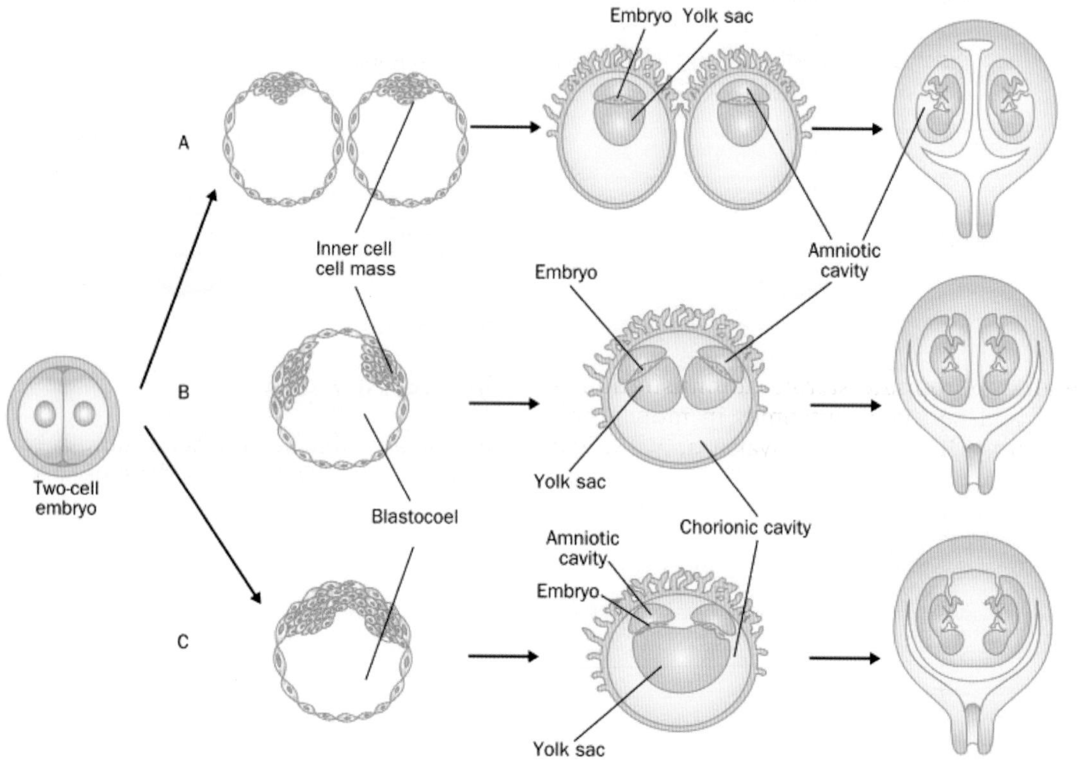

FIGURE 36.5 Three types of monozygotic placenta and membrane: A: dichorionic diamniotic; B: monochorionic diamniotic; C: monochorionic monoamniotic.
(Source: Hall JG. Twinning. *Lancet* 2003;362(9385):735–743)

mother's body or miscarried with few or no symptoms. Occasionally one fetus dies early in the pregnancy and is retained in the uterus until term, becoming flattened and mummified. This is known as a fetus papyraceus ('paper-like'). Depending on local regulations, the fetus may require birth and death certificates.

Higher-order multiple births have even higher mortality and morbidity rates compared with twins and singletons. This is mostly due to the increased proportion of infants with low birth weight and pre-term delivery and the complications associated with these. Several authors dispute this, however, arguing that regular fetal

Box 36.2 Understanding chorionicity and amnionicity

Identical twins

Identical or monochorionic twins occur in 25% of twin pregnancies. The latest research indicates that identical twins have a very similar genetic makeup (sharing about 88% of their DNA), resulting in both children looking alike.

Identical twins are the same gender, and may have similar fingerprints, ear shapes, eye colour, hair colour and teeth imprints. They will often develop at similar rates and experience developmental stages simultaneously—for example, when they learn to walk, and grow their first teeth. They may also have similar brain wave patterns. Mirror image identical twins have mirror image features, such as left and right hair crown swirl, left- or right-handedness and similar moles or body marks, but on different sides of the body.

What causes a fertilised egg to divide and create identical twins is still unknown.

Identical twins and chorionicity

Identical twins are categorised by chorionicity—depending on when the fertilised egg splits and how it splits, such as top/bottom or right side/left side. After an egg is fertilised it will develop a yolk sac (important for nourishing the forming embryo) and around the same time the embryo's placenta and chorionic sac begin to form. Finally, an amniotic sac surrounds the developing baby. There are different types of chorionicity for identical twins, depending on the timing of the above-mentioned events.

Diamniotic dichorionic twins

If the egg splits before the placenta has formed, within 3 days of fertilisation, each baby will have its own placenta, chorionic sac and amniotic sac.

Diamniotic monochorionic twins

If the egg splits after the placenta has formed, after the third day following fertilisation, then the babies will share a placenta and chorionic sac, but may have their own amniotic sac.

Monoamniotic monochorionic twins

Monoamniotic twins occur when the egg splits after the amniotic sac has begun to form, around 9 days after conception. As a result, both babies share an amniotic sac. Monochorionic twin pregnancy is more common where assisted reproductive technology has been used. Many monoamniotic twins lie very close to, or on top of, each other and early ultrasounds cannot tell that they are separate babies.

Conjoined twins

If the egg splits later than 12 days after fertilisation, and does not split completely, then conjoined twins occur.

(Source: Reinhard J, Reichenbach L, Ernst T, et al. Delayed interval delivery in twin and triplet pregnancies: 6 years of experience in one perinatal center. *J Perinatal Med*. 2012;40:551–555)

surveillance and appropriate steroid administration is necessary for good perinatal outcomes in monoamniotic twin gestations (Imaizumi & Hayakawa, 2013; Van Mieghem et al., 2014; Vasak et al., 2017). Twin-to-twin transfusion syndrome, in which blood from one twin is transfused to the other twin via blood vessels in their shared placenta, is a rare but serious and potentially life-threatening condition affecting 15% of MZ twins (Johnson, 2015).

Other complications include:

- pre-term labour and birth
- low birth weight
- placenta praevia
- placental abruption, particularly after the birth of the first twin
- intrauterine growth restriction (IUGR)
- preeclampsia
- increased frequency of birth asphyxia, again for twin B
- malpresentation
- prelabour and pre-term rupture of the membranes and group B *Streptococcus* (GBS) infection
- anaemia
- umbilical cord accidents
- operative delivery
- postpartum haemorrhage.

Goals of care

Care of the woman and her multiple baby pregnancy should be designed to assess, diagnose and treat the complications that may occur in order to optimise physical and psychosocial outcomes for the mother, babies and family. Supporting the parents of twins is not just about obstetric management of the pregnancy; it is also about helping the woman and her family to adapt to a rapid increase in their family (NICE, 2021). Maternal adaptations to pregnancy are exaggerated with twins. Plasma volume increases an additional 10%–20% in twin over singleton pregnancies. Nutritional requirements rise and carbohydrate metabolism may differ, but the most marked changes arise because of the increase in maternal blood volume and consequently maternal cardiac output. Red blood cell mass increases to a lesser degree than plasma volume, and so there is a relative anaemia because of this haemodilution. Both iron and folate requirements are higher in twin pregnancies; thus, iron and vitamin supplementation is common practice. Because of the complications associated with multiple pregnancies, most women are referred to an obstetrician and advised to prepare for hospital births and, increasingly often, an operative birth. However, many of the complications associated with multiple pregnancy occur irrespective of the place of birth and, indeed, hospitalisation cannot prevent their occurrence (NICE, 2021).

Diagnosis of multiple pregnancy

Generally, the diagnosis of twins is not difficult for the midwife. By the end of the first trimester the uterine size is larger than expected, upon abdominal palpation, for gestational age by last menstrual period and/or earlier examinations (Dodd et al., 2011). The woman may report excessive nausea and vomiting or that she 'feels as if she is having twins'. In the second trimester, abdominal palpation of multiple fetal parts may suggest the presence of more than a single fetus, and occasionally, two sets of fetal heart rates may be detected. Ultrasound early in the first trimester usually confirms any suspicion the woman has that she is having twins. During abdominal ultrasonography, two gestational sacs can be visualised after 6 weeks gestation; vaginal ultrasound allows for an even earlier diagnosis. If the initial diagnosis is made very early in pregnancy, a repeat ultrasound several weeks later will be advised to confirm the presence of twins, rule out anomalies and determine chorionicity. Because of the increased rate of congenital abnormalities, women should be offered both biochemical genetic and nuchal translucency tests (Dodd et al., 2011). Many practitioners recommend serial scans every 4–6 weeks to evaluate fetal growth and for concordance, especially if the twins are MZ. Cardiotocography (CTG), Doppler flow studies and combined CTG/Doppler flow studies all play an important role in the ongoing assessment of fetal wellbeing, especially IUGR and growth discrepancies (Giles et al., 2003).

In the event that one of the twins dies, the parents will be caught in a difficult dichotomy of grieving for the dead baby while at the same time celebrating the life of the other baby.

A WOMAN'S STORY

We were thrilled to find that at last I was having twins, after so many unsuccessful cycles of IVF. And then one day they told me one of my precious babies had died. Knowing that I was carrying a dead baby and a live one was very strange. Every time I went for a scan I was terrified that they would tell me that the second baby was going to die. I used to wonder if the one who was left knew that her sister was dead. I wanted to grieve for my dead baby and I felt guilty if I felt happy for the one who was still alive, but I was. When Linda was born, so beautiful and so healthy, we were so grateful and wanted to celebrate her birth, but I mourned for my second baby girl all over again. I wasn't sure what I was supposed to feel and I alternated between relief, guilt, sorrow and intense joy. Linda is too young to talk about it yet but I often wonder if she misses her identical sister. One day we will talk about it, but not today.

Preparation for birth

The type of birth for twins is usually determined by the presentations of both babies. Where they are cephalic presentations and if twin B is a breech presentation, vaginal birth is the usual mode of delivery (Khalil & O'Brien, 2007). There is the potential for 'locked twins' for a leading breech and then cephalic presentation, so a caesarean section is advisable in this case. The mechanisms involved in vaginal birth of the first twin are similar to those for singleton pregnancies; however, malpresentation, fetal compromise, maternal and placental bleeding and the need for abdominal delivery are increased in twin pregnancies. Therefore, intensive and continuous monitoring of maternal and fetal wellbeing and the progress of labour is advised. Induction of labour, augmentation with synthetic oxytocin and artificial rupture of membranes for one or both babies are used if necessary (Khalil & O'Brien, 2007). Blood is cross-matched and intravenous access obtained because of the increased risk of postpartum haemorrhage (PPH) owing to overdistension of the uterus. Epidural analgesia is recommended if the woman has hypertension, or if the labour is pre-term or complicated by the possibility that there may be a malpresentation of the second twin.

Equipment is prepared for the births of two babies, keeping in mind that the babies may be small for dates or pre-term and that the birth of the second twin may not be straightforward. Each twin is monitored simultaneously. Depending on the gestation of the twins and the fetal wellbeing, the midwife will need to decide how much paediatric or anaesthetic support will be required. In the event of a healthy pregnancy that has progressed to term, there is less urgent need for support from paediatricians and an anaesthetist.

Birth of the second twin

The birth of the second twin engenders significant controversy in the intrapartum management of twins (Fox et al., 2010). There is general agreement that vaginal birth is safe in twins who both present as vertex, and caesarean delivery is indicated only in the presence of the usual obstetric and fetal indications (Easter et al., 2016; Rzyska et al., 2017) (Box 36.3).

Management of vertex–non-vertex twins is perhaps the most controversial. The options are caesarean delivery, **external cephalic version (ECV)** and assisted vaginal **breech birth**. The most important factor in this decision is the skill and experience of the personnel available. If the decision is made to proceed with a vaginal birth, as long as the fetal heartbeat of the second twin is reassuring, the time interval until the baby's birth is not critical. What is critical, however, is that the labour is progressing. As soon as the first baby is born, the second baby's heart tones are monitored continuously (Easter et al., 2016; Vogel et al., 2014), and the baby's position, lie and presentation determined by palpation and vaginal examination or, as is increasingly common, with real-time ultrasound.

Box 36.3 Asynchronous birth of a twin

One of the mysteries surrounding the birth of twins relates to whether it is safe to await asynchronous delivery in twin and triplet pregnancies. A German study published in 2012 (Reinhard et al., 2012) aimed to assess the outcome of delayed interval delivery for twin and triplet pregnancies at 22 + 0 to 25 + 0 weeks of gestation. The study, involving five twin pregnancies and two triplet pregnancies, found the interval between delivery of the first baby and the remaining twin/triplets was 1–18 days (mean, 9.7 days). In all cases, the first baby was born vaginally. Survival of the first twin/triplet was 14.3%, whereas 57.1% of the second born twin/triplets survived. The amount of weight gained due to delayed delivery was 131 g on average with no signs of severe maternal complications.

The first time a delay was described between a first and second twin was in 1880 when it was reported that the second twin was delayed by 44 days.

(Source: Reinhard et al., 2012)

If the lie is longitudinal, whether the vertex or the breech is presenting, a short period of time is left to elapse to see whether contractions establish (Easter et al., 2016; Vogel et al., 2014). If they do not, augmentation with oxytocin is warranted. The birth of the second twin usually occurs quite quickly as the cervix has already been fully dilated.

The midwife should always be aware of the increased risk of PPH in multiple births. Oxytocin is given only after the birth of the second baby and after confirming that there is not a third baby waiting to be born. Many clinicians recommend that an intravenous infusion of Hartmann's solution or normal saline containing 40 mIU of Syntocinon is commenced to ensure that the uterus remains well contracted in the immediate postpartum period, thereby avoiding a PPH. The placenta and membranes are examined to determine whether they are complete and whether the twins are MZ or DZ, although this can be confirmed by placental histology.

Postpartum care of the family

Care of the postpartum woman proceeds as for a singleton pregnancy, though the woman will require extra practical support and assistance to establish feeding and organise the care of two babies. Contact with local support groups such as the local multiple birth association is encouraged from early in pregnancy. Lack of professional and family support can be a serious problem for mothers of multiples, and caring for two or more babies is physically and emotionally draining. Multiple birth associations are well placed to offer support and guidance about coping in the early days at home. (See Ch. 32 for breastfeeding of twins.)

Mothers of multiples are most at risk of postnatal depression (see Ch. 35). As they try to cope with exhaustion exacerbated by sleep deprivation, it is not surprising that mothers of multiples often experience isolation.

BREECH PRESENTATION

Epidemiology of breech presentation

Breech presentation occurs in 3%–4% of all births (Evans, 2012a). The proportion of breech presentations decreases with advancing gestational age, from about 25% of births before 28 weeks gestation, to less than 10% at 32 weeks gestation, and to 1%–3% of births at term (Impey et al., 2017b).

Predisposing factors for breech presentation include prematurity, uterine malformations or fibroids, polyhydramnios, placenta praevia, fetal abnormalities (e.g. central nervous system (CNS) malformations, neck masses, aneuploidy), and multiple gestations. Fetal abnormalities are observed in 17% of pre-term breech births and in 9% of term breech births (Fischer, 2016). Perinatal mortality is increased two- to fourfold with breech presentation, regardless of the mode of birth. Deaths are most often associated with malformations, prematurity and intrauterine fetal demise.

Current midwifery and obstetric practice is heavily informed by the Term Breech Trial (TBT) (Hannah et al., 2000). The trial included 2083 women who had a frank or complete breech presentation, 1041 of whom were randomly assigned to undergo a planned caesarean birth and 1042 randomised to planned vaginal birth. In the planned-vaginal-birth group, a little more than half the women (57%) actually achieved a vaginal birth. The trial found that planned caesarean delivery was associated with a lower risk of perinatal mortality compared with planned vaginal birth—3 per 1000 versus 13 per 1000. Caesarean delivery was also associated with a lower risk of 'serious' neonatal morbidity—1.4% versus 3.8% (relative risk (RR) 0.33; 95% confidence interval (CI) 0.19–0.59; $p < 0.0001$).

CRITICAL THINKING EXERCISE

How would you explain the risks and benefits of having a vaginal breech baby to prospective anxious parents?

Make a table of the arguments for and against the findings of the TBT (Hannah et al., 2000, 2004; Whyte et al., 2004). For this you will need to research the response from professional colleges and papers from New Zealand, Australia, the Netherlands and Canada.

It is important to remember that the morbidity and mortality in relation to breech birth may be caused by factors such as prematurity and congenital abnormality and may have little to do with the breech birth technique itself.

Fahy (2011) and Evans (2012b) acknowledge that the single most important factor relating to safe breech birth outcomes is the skill of the birth attendant. The TBT has had a profound impact over nearly one and a half decades resulting in an almost complete loss of confidence and erosion of skills in supporting women to give birth to a breech baby, in both the obstetric and the midwifery communities (Evans, 2012a; Lawson, 2012; Walker et al., 2018a, 2018b). The findings of the TBT, which was never fully completed, deduced that caesarean section was the safest mode of birth for breech babies (Hannah et al., 2000; Whyte et al., 2004). The findings of this research were so seriously flawed that even one of the trial's collaborators, Glezerman's (2006) review of the TBT, concluded that the recommendation that all breech babies should be born by caesarean should be rescinded, as in some cases neonatal death and morbidity should not have been attributed to the mode of birth. Re-analysis of the data (Su et al., 2004) demonstrated no significant differences between vaginal and abdominal birth outcomes for breech babies but continued to argue that caesarean birth was the safest option for breech birth. As Lawson (2012) highlighted, in his review of the TBT 10 years on, five maternal deaths have since been reported in women who underwent caesarean section for a breech presentation. He suggests that these statistics are most likely an underrepresentation of the true incidence of maternal mortality following a caesarean for breech presentation. As this author and others wisely state, vaginal breech births will continue to occur regardless, for the following reasons: maternal choice, women booked for an elective caesarean who labour and who give birth spontaneously, and undiagnosed breech presentations prior to labour. In part, these practice realities and current recent research findings (Bjellmo et al., 2017; Goffinet et al., 2006) led both the American College of Obstetricians and Gynecologists Committee on Obstetric Practice (ACOG, 2006) and the Royal College of Obstetricians and Gynaecologists (RCOG) in the United Kingdom (Impey et al., 2017b) to modify their guidelines on planned vaginal breech birth to include recommendations that the woman's choice and clinical judgment should be taken into account when decisions about the mode of birth are made (Kotaska, 2007). Australia's and New Zealand's professional obstetric body, the Royal Australian and New Zealand College of Obstetricians and Gynaecologists (RANZCOG), states in the current guideline (2016) that:

> *Almost 90 per cent of fetuses presenting by the breech at term are now delivered by caesarean section. However, with careful case selection and intrapartum management, in an institution with adequate experience and infrastructure, it is possible to plan for attempted vaginal delivery in some cases. This will depend upon the experience of the clinical team, and the infrastructure available.*
>
> (RANZCOG, 2016)

The New Zealand Guidelines Group (NZGG) was a multidisciplinary team that produced guidelines for clinicians. It has since been dissolved and the breech guideline not updated; however, it provides a good example of a woman-centred approach to care when breech occurs at term. While recognising the potential complications associated with breech presentations and vaginal breech birth, the guideline recommended that women be given evidence-based information about the risks and benefits of both vaginal breech birth and caesarean section *prior to* (our emphasis) birth so that they can make informed decisions and choices about their care (NZGG, 2004). Few breech babies are currently born vaginally in Australia and New Zealand. Less than 1 in 10 (4.1%) mothers had a baby in the breech position (buttocks or feet first) in Australia 2019 and only 0.7% of mothers who had a baby in the breech position had a non-instrumental vaginal birth, compared with 10.4% of mothers who had a caesarean section (AIHW, 2021).

The number of breech presentations in New Zealand is not recorded; however, in the most recent report on Maternity a total of 222 women had a vaginal breech birth, with 133 having a spontaneous breech birth, 57 an assisted breech birth and 32 by breech extraction. The proportion of vaginal breech births ranged from 0.4% to 0.5% of all births between 2008 and 2017 (MOH, 2021).

The NZGG stressed that maintaining skills for facilitating vaginal breech birth remains an important goal for all clinicians. Although these guidelines have been developed specifically for the care of women undergoing a breech birth, they hold true for all women with any complication in labour.

Perinatal morbidity and mortality

Breech presentation is associated with increased mortality and morbidity, largely due to:

- pre-term gestation
- congenital malformations
- birth asphyxia or trauma.

However, not all babies presenting by the breech should be birthed vaginally. There are risks associated with all births and breech births are no different. Other factors increasing perinatal morbidity and mortality are: cord prolapse, intracranial haemorrhage, low Apgar scores, asphyxia, cervical spine injury, fractures of the long bones (humerus and femur) and fracture of the clavicle. Although it is true that a few babies presenting by the breech are born at home, it is generally accepted that because a breech is generally classified as a 'malpresentation' all babies diagnosed as a breech should ideally, except in an emergency situation, be referred to a medical consultant for collaborative care in a hospital with facilities for caesarean section and ready access to a team of midwives, obstetrician, paediatrician and anaesthetist if needed. In the New Zealand Referral Guidelines (MOH, 2012), breech at >36 weeks or in labour is an indication for consultation with an obstetrician, but not necessarily for handing over care. The LMC midwife, the woman and the obstetrician have a three-way conversation to plan for birth, including roles and responsibilities. Midwives supporting women giving birth to an unexpected breech baby are part of New Zealand's Midwifery *Scope of Practice*, as the midwife 'identifies complications and implements emergency measures as necessary' (Midwifery Council of New Zealand (MCNZ), 2010). While the Australian Nursing and Midwifery Accreditation Council (ANMAC, 2014) Midwife Accreditation Standards do not specifically refer to the expertise required to assist in the birth of breech babies, they too expect midwives to 'recognise and respond effectively in emergency or urgent situations'. In Australia, breech birth at home would be considered to fall outside the scope of the midwife's practice. (See also the *National Midwifery Guidelines for Consultation and Referral*, 3rd ed. (ACM, 2013).)

Contributing factors to breech presentation include:

- nulliparity
- previous breech birth
- uterine (anatomical) anomaly
- oligohydramnios
- polyhydramnios
- extended fetal legs
- multiple pregnancy
- short umbilical cord
- early gestation
- fetal abnormality
- poor fetal growth (ACOG, 2017).

REFLECTIVE THINKING EXERCISE

Do you think a breech baby is a variant of the 'normal' or a 'high-risk complication'? Why do you think this is so?

How do different belief systems about the 'normality' of a breech impact on the way birth is 'managed'?

Diagnosis

Many clinicians 'miss' diagnosing a breech presentation because, in late pregnancy or during labour, the breech may be well engaged in the pelvis and the fetal head positioned under the diaphragm, making it very difficult to diagnose a breech on abdominal palpation and even during vaginal examination when the membranes are intact. A vaginal examination should always be performed if there are indications in labour suggesting that the baby is presenting breech so as to enable midwifery decision making and the development of a plan of action.

The four key landmarks of breech presentation are the fetal sacrum, the deep depression of the anal cleft between the fetal buttock, and the two ischial tuberosities. The type of breech can be determined by the presence or absence and positioning of feet (and, seldomly, knees). Real-time ultrasonography will confirm the diagnosis and may rule out contraindications for a vaginal breech birth.

Types of breech presentation

There are four types of breech presentation: legs flexed at the hips and extended at the knees (frank or incomplete), 65%; both legs flexed at the hips and knees (complete), 10%; a single or double footling breech—one or both feet tucked underneath the buttocks, 25% (Fig. 36.6) or a kneeling breech where the leg is flexed at the knee (rare). Both these two last presentations are also incomplete breeches.

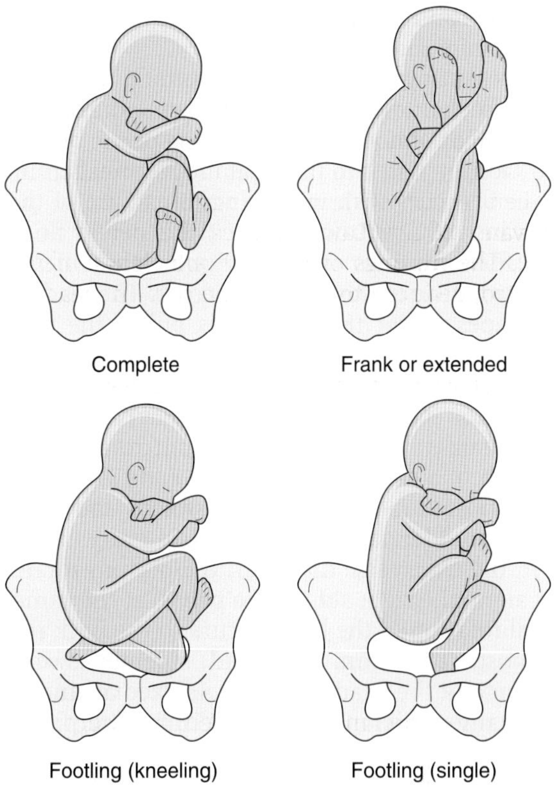

FIGURE 36.6 Breech presentations
(Based on Henderson & Macdonald, 2004)

- *Frank breech*: the fetus is in a pike position with the buttocks presenting and the hips flexed, but knees extended.
- *Complete breech*: the fetus has both knees and hips flexed so the feet are near the buttocks, but the buttocks are presenting.
- *Incomplete breech*: the fetus has either one or both knees flexed and one or both hips flexed resulting in either the feet or the knee below the buttock.
- *Footling breech*: a type of incomplete breech wherein the fetus has one or both feet presenting.

Breech positions—mechanisms of labour

There are three main mechanisms of labour in a breech birth: first the bottom and legs, then the shoulders and arms, and finally the head.

The mechanisms of a right sacroanterior (RSA) position are as follows:

- the lie is longitudinal
- the attitude is complete flexion
- the presentation is breech

- the position is RSA
- the denominator is the sacrum
- the presenting part is the right buttock
- the bitrochanteric diameter of 10 cm enters the pelvis in the right oblique diameter of the pelvic brim
- the sacrum points to the right iliopectineal eminence.

Descent occurs with increasing impaction of the buttocks. The right buttock reaches the pelvic floor and rotates forwards into the pelvis one-eighth of a circle; internal rotation of the buttocks occurs. The leading buttock escapes under the symphysis pubis; the posterior buttock sweeps the perineum and the buttocks are born by lateral flexion. Restitution of the buttocks now occurs. The anterior shoulder enters the pelvis in the same oblique diameter as the buttocks and rotates forwards one-eighth of a circle, escaping under the symphysis pubis. The posterior shoulder now sweeps the perineum and the shoulders are born. The head enters the pelvic brim in the transverse diameter; the occiput rotates forwards along the right side of the pelvis; at the same time external rotation of the body occurs so the back remains uppermost. The chin, face and sinciput sweep the perineum and the head is born in a flexed attitude.

For many clinicians and women, a baby presenting by the breech is not considered an abnormality but a variant of the normal. Spontaneous labour and birth are in many instances possible and in most cases a better option for the mother in terms of recovery from the birth, ability to care for her newborn and, most importantly, for her future pregnancies. The risks associated with caesarean section tend to be overlooked, as do the longer-term impacts on the mother's psychological wellbeing. Given the most recent research on the benefit of being born vaginally, vaginal breech birth should always be considered an option for women where there are no mitigating circumstances and the midwife or obstetrician is confident in their skills for vaginal birth. All women and their partners should receive counselling about the process of breech births and possible associated procedures where risks are discussed, along with the safeguards that are in place where risks are encountered.

Labour and breech birth

Before proceeding to a spontaneous vaginal breech birth it is important:

- to exclude IUGR or other signs of fetal compromise
- to ensure a clinically adequate pelvis
- to ascertain that presentation should be complete or frank breech
- to ascertain that the estimated fetal weight is 2500–4000 g
- to exclude hyperextended head
- to aim for spontaneous onset of labour
- to group and save blood in case a caesarean section is required
- to ensure that caregivers are appropriately experienced, available and prepared to proceed to caesarean section if complications occur.

With a few exceptions, midwifery support and care during labour is no different from that for a cephalic presentation. According to the Canadian Consensus Statement (Kotaska et al., 2009), there is no evidence that epidural analgesia is an essential component of vaginal breech birth. The RCOG (Impey et al., 2017a) also recommends epidural analgesia should not be routinely advised; offer women a choice of analgesia during breech labour and birth. Induction or augmentation of labour is also not recommended (Impey et al., 2017a; Kotaska, 2007). According to the Society of Obstetricians and Gynaecologists of Canada (SOGC) (Kotaska, 2007), continuous electronic fetal heart monitoring (EFM) is preferable in the first stage and mandatory in the second stage of labour. Unless telemetry is in use, continuous EFM means that the woman is restricted to a semisupine position in bed, which may restrict descent of the buttocks.

Vaginal examination ideally should be performed whenever a breech presentation is suspected, not only to establish that labour has commenced but also to exclude cord presentation and cord prolapse, as well as a foot, knee or compound presentation. It is important not to break the membranes during the examination.

When labour is well established, asking the woman to remain upright and mobile will aid descent of the buttocks and dilation of the cervix. There is as yet no consensus from those with experience of breech births with regards to the 'best' position for women to adopt when birthing a breech baby, beyond women-led positioning (Banks, 1998; Evans, 2012a; Walker et al., 2016). There is no evidence to suggest continuous EFM is more beneficial than intermittent auscultation of the fetal heart beyond a reduction in neonatal seizures, but it is associated with an increase in caesarean sections and instrumental births (Alfirevic et al., 2017; Impey et al., 2017a). Many institutions have protocols in place for continuous EFM. Overt cord prolapse occurs in more than 1% of breech births (RCOG, 2014):

- 0.5% of cephalic and frank breech presentations
- 5% of complete breech
- 15% of footling breech.

The membranes should be left intact to help prevent cord or foot prolapse. If the membranes spontaneously rupture, meconium is often apparent. In breech births, as the baby comes down the birth canal the gut is squeezed causing the fetus to pass meconium. As soon as the membranes break, the fetal heart rate should be recorded (unless EFM is in situ when the trace is assessed) and a vaginal examination performed to again exclude cord or limb prolapse.

Consideration of the birthing environment is essential prior to the baby's birth. The room should be kept warm and neonatal resuscitation equipment prepared in advance. Once the woman wants to bear down in the second stage, a vaginal examination will ensure that the cervix is completely dilated. The buttocks or legs may descend through the cervix (especially if the fetus is small) even if it is not completely dilated. Banks (1998, p. 70) writes that 'the premature urge to push before full dilation that is often mentioned to women as being problematic in breech births is unlikely to be noticeable in a term infant who will have a hip size in a flexed or extended legs position equal to head size'.

An upright position during the second stage will aid gravity and descent of the baby once pushing begins, but active pushing should not commence until the buttocks distend the vulva. As the buttocks are born, it is possible to see the buttocks move 'up and down' just before crowning—this is known as 'rumping'.

Physiological birth of a breech baby

Many clinicians recommend that the 'best' way to birth by the breech is to facilitate spontaneous birth with a 'hands-off' approach. This is most likely to occur if the woman is standing, on all-fours or squatting rather than lying in a supine position (Banks, 2014). Louwen et al. (2017) studied a large cohort of women with breech-presenting babies who gave birth vaginally in upright positions—leaning over the back of the hospital bed, on the knees, on all fours, or occasionally standing up—compared with those in a dorsal position (on their back) or who planned a caesarean birth. The researchers found that vaginal breech birth in an upright position was associated with a significantly reduced length of the second stage, caesarean rate and frequency of neonatal injuries and manipulations to extract the neonate, compared with vaginal breech birth in a dorsal position. More than half the upright births required no manoeuvres at all (Louwen et al., 2017). Physiological birth relies on a non-interventionist approach by the midwife in the presence of continuing and timely descent of the baby who is responding well to labour. The key principles to remember with a vaginal breech birth are:

- Never be in haste.
- 'Hands off the breech' when birth is proceeding normally.
- Always keep the fetus with the back anterior.

When the breech meets the resistance of the perineum the anterior buttock climbs up the fourchette; the anus is then visible and the posterior buttock then distends the perineum (see Fig. 36.7). Both the onset and progress in labour should be spontaneous, enabling the baby, as Evans (2012a, p. 18) describes, to 'adopt his/her optimal position and to progress at his/her own pace through the

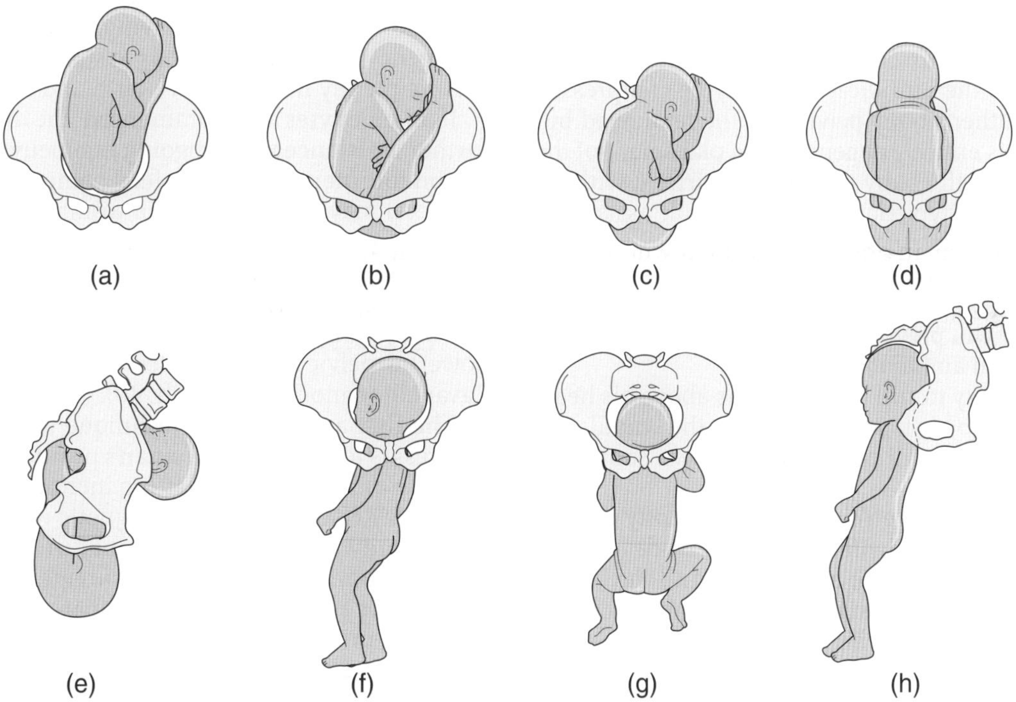

FIGURE 36.7 Mechanism of standing breech birth: (a) The bitrochanteric diameter (10 cm) enters the widest diameter of the pelvis (oblique or transverse). (b) The buttocks (anterior buttock leading) descend through the pelvis while rotating clockwise. (c) The baby then rotates anticlockwise so the sacrum now lies in the direct sacrum anterior (DSA) position. (d) The shoulders now move into the oblique/transverse diameter of the pelvic brim. (e) The buttocks are born by lateral spinal flexion (wiggling from side to side), followed by the baby's legs. Once the legs and pelvis are born the baby arches its spine so its torso rounds the mother's symphysis pubis and the head moves around the maternal sacral prominence. (f) Still rotating anticlockwise, the head enters the brim of the pelvis, freeing the arms and shoulders from under the pubic arch. (g) The baby then rotates clockwise. Flexion of the legs and arms causes the head to flex which brings the chin down onto the chest, pivoting the occiput. (h) The mother often changes to a position that promotes flexion of the head and it births spontaneously.
(Based on Evans, 2012a)

various planes of the pelvis'. Following rumping the legs of a flexed legs breech will be born while those of an extended legs breech may not be released until the baby is born to the nipple line. Watchful patience will usually see the legs birth without intervention.

Evans's observations of breech birth suggest that baby arches its spine and the head moves backwards by extending its pelvis along its journey past the maternal sacral prominence, and the baby's rotation also brings the arms down with assistance from the mother's pelvic floor muscles, ideally with the baby in the right sacral anterior position. She also observes that many women will drop forwards to a more horizontal position from an upright position as the baby is birthed. Banks (2014, 2017) notes the intuitive movement to increase spinal curvature helps rotate the fetal head under the pubic arch or, when done earlier, tips the pelvic brim forwards to enable movement of the head into the pelvis. Maternal movements must be led by the birthing mother, not forced or suggested by the midwife as otherwise the baby's head might deflex and result in damage to the baby. Midwives identify that the babies of non-medicated women actively participate in birth through pedalling, lurching, twisting, pulling their arms down and 'tummy scrunching' (lifting legs and often arms to flex the chin towards their chest). This later movement internally makes the baby's head roll onto the internal aspect of the mother's symphysis pubis (Evans, 2012a).

As the baby's head first enters the pelvis, the fetal heart rate may drop as the umbilical cord may be compressed between the mother's bony pelvis and the fetal head but this occurrence is entirely dependent on placement of the cord. If this occurs the baby needs to be birthed without delay to minimise hypoxia; the woman will assist this with her pushing to facilitate a timely birth.

The tone, colour and energy of the baby can also be observed at this point. Wrapping a warm towel around the baby's body will prevent hypothermia in an environment that lacks an ambient temperature.

The baby is likely to still have his arms above his head, which helps to keep his head flexed. Once the scapula appears the active baby will pull his arms down spontaneously.

The baby 'hangs' while the midwife patiently continues to honour the midwifery adage—'hands off the breech'. Once the nape of the baby's neck and the baby's hairline is visible, the woman may lean forwards from the waist to tilt her pelvis or she may tilt her buttocks, increasing the spinal curvature, to aid clearance of the nose and mouth from the perineum while the rest of the head is born slowly. Birth of the head will be by flexion, which ensures the same favourable diameters for birth as with a cephalic presentation.

The baby's head should be birthed slowly, because rapid birth of the head can cause sudden decompression of the head and tearing of tentorium cerebelli with intracranial haemorrhage and perinatal death. The midwife may need to remind the woman to 'release' the baby's head rather than pushing if she is having expulsive urges that may bring the baby's head too quickly. Aspiration of the oropharynx should be avoided to prevent activation of the Moro reflex, gasping and possibly inhalation of meconium.

Once born the baby should be placed in the mother's arms with the midwife calmly assessing his transition to extrauterine life.

Sometimes the midwife may find herself attending a woman who finds it more comfortable to remain supine. Fig. 36.8 shows the birth of a baby when the mother is supine.

Boxes 36.4, 36.5, 36.6 and Fig. 36.9 illustrate techniques to achieve the physiological birth of a breech baby.

Manoeuvres to assist vaginal breech birth

Various manoeuvres are designed to correct any deviation from the normal mechanism of spontaneous birth or to expedite birth in the event of a problem. These techniques are rarely required if the woman maintains an upright position, is not sedated and has patient birth attendants. Should delay occur prior to rumping, consultation with an obstetric specialist is warranted and delivery by caesarean section should be considered, as 'adequate' progress in labour is the major forerunner to an uncomplicated breech birth.

Practising the following manoeuvres using a doll and pelvis or mannequins is an effective way to learn manoeuvres and to reduce fear of having to perform them in an emergency. The midwife needs to simulate these manoeuvres frequently in both active birth and supine positions.

If manoeuvres are commenced the baby may need further assistance with ongoing manoeuvres because the reason for intervention (e.g. fetal compromise or delay in progress) may still persist. The woman continues to participate fully in the birth with her pushing efforts, albeit directed by the midwife. She may also assist with repositioning; for example, the woman may be able to 'suck up her baby' and reposition him slightly using the same powerful pelvic floor muscles that are activated in the Zavanelli manoeuvre (see Ch. 40).

The first and foremost technique to correct a lack of progress is to change the woman's position to increase the capacity of her pelvis; squatting increases the pelvic outlet by 28% (Banks, 2017). A magnetic resonance imaging (MRI) study undertaken in Frankfurt showed how the maternal transverse pelvic measurements widen significantly in a kneeling crouch compared with the supine position, providing anatomical rationale for getting a woman up and moving in second stage (Reitter, 2014) (Fig. 36.10). The kneeling squat position significantly increases the bony transverse and anteroposterior dimension in the mid-pelvic plane and the pelvic outlet. The study showed a striking and significant increase in the transverse diameters of the mid-pelvis and the pelvic outlet (0.9–1.9 cm) when women changed from the supine dorsal position to a kneeling squat position; this increase is larger than the increase in the corresponding anteroposterior measurements. The increase is even more pronounced in pregnant women. The modern imaging in

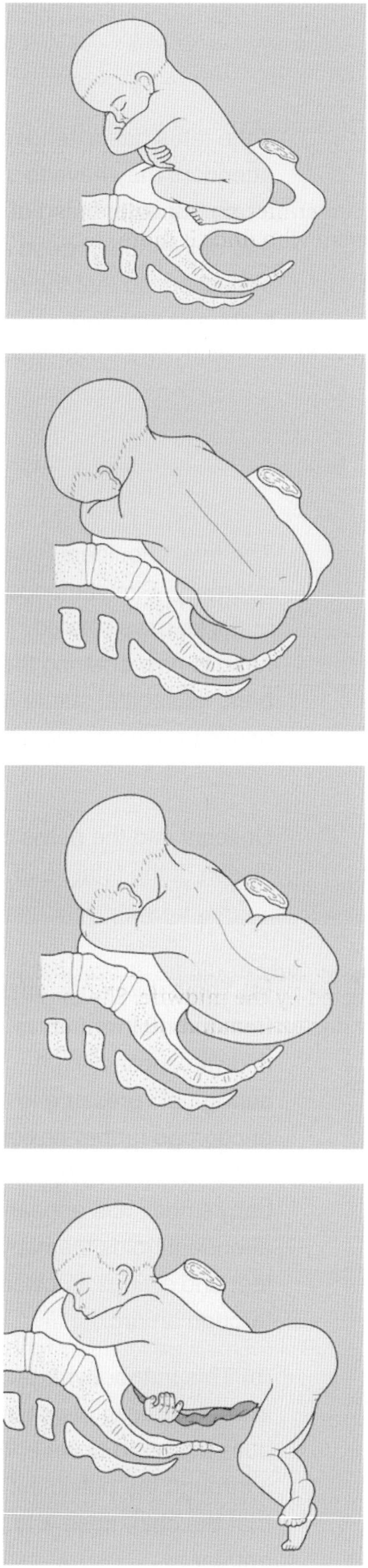

The breech is presenting in the right sacral anterior position.
With full dilation of the cervix, the buttocks descend deeply into the pelvis.

When the buttocks reach the pelvic floor, the shape of the pelvis causes the buttocks to rotate internally.

The anterior buttock appears at the vulva. With further uterine contractions the buttocks distend the vaginal outlet.

Lateral flexion of the fetal trunk takes place and the shoulders rotate so that they may enter the pelvis.

The buttocks have been born and the shoulders have entered the pelvis in its transverse diameter.

This causes the external rotation of the buttocks so that the fetal back becomes uppermost.

FIGURE 36.8 Birth of the breech with mother supine

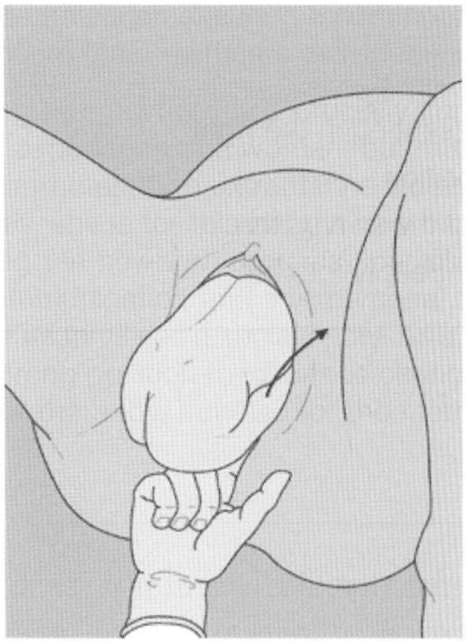

If the fetus has extended legs, the attendant may have to slip a hand along the anterior leg of the fetus and deliver it by flexion and abduction, so that the rest of the birth may proceed.

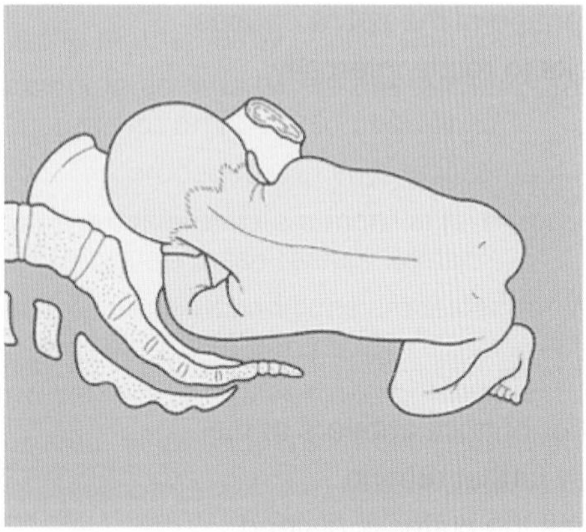

The fetal shoulders have rotated internally. Simultaneously, the buttocks have rotated. The fetal head is now entering the pelvic brim, its sagittal suture lying in the brim's transverse diameter.

Descent into the pelvis occurs with flexion of the fetal head.

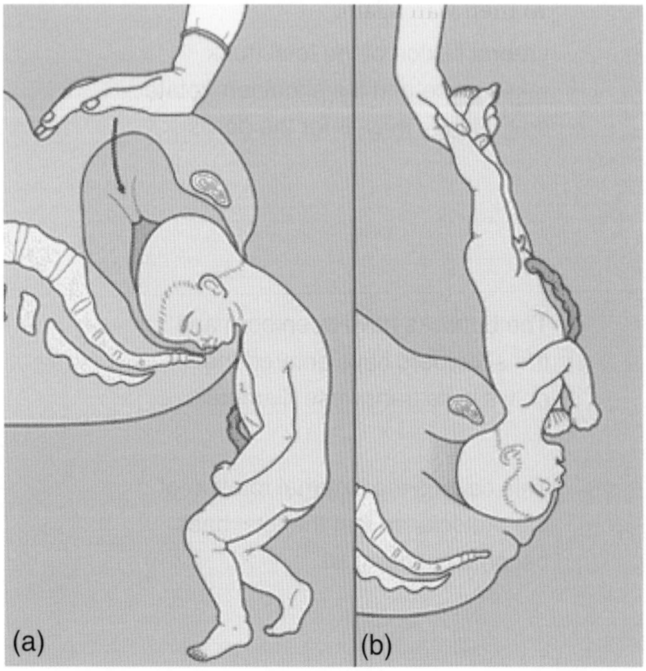

(a) The baby hangs unsupported from the mother's vulva. The midwife applies slight suprapubic pressure to encourage further flexion of the head. When the nape of the baby's neck has appeared, the attendant holds the baby by the feet and swings it upwards through an arc.

(b) This manoeuvre, by using the lower border of the sacrum, pulls the head down and rotates it through the pelvic outlet so that the chin, nose and forehead appear

FIGURE 36.8, cont'd

Box 36.4 Hands off the breech—the Bracht manoeuvre

Erich Bracht, a German gynaecologist, described in 1935 the manoeuvre named after him for delivering the frank breech with minimal interference.

'Hands off the Breech' is the phrase derived from the writings of Dr Eric Bracht who in 1938 first described the obstetrician's role in spontaneous breech birth as one that involved minimal handling. Although his technique was adopted and subjected to extensive trials in Germany, France, Spain, Holland and South America, with fetal mortality figures suggesting its considerable superiority over more active management, the procedure seems to have been overlooked in the United Kingdom and the United States.

(Source: Dunn P. 'Erich Bracht (1882–1969) of Berlin and his "breech" manoeuvre'. *Arch Dis Child Fetal Neonatal Ed.* 2003;88:F76–F77)

Box 36.5 The Bracht manoeuvre

1. The force applied is derived solely from contractions of uterine and abdominal muscles. The element of pull is absent.
2. The breech appears in transverse position.
3. The breech rotates slowly to SA position as the buttocks and trunk are delivered.
4. The forces applied from above produce a lordotic curvature of the baby's back around the mother's symphysis.
5. The rotation around the symphysis continues upwards. Head and shoulders remain at right angles to each other.
6. Elbows, arms and hands are delivered spontaneously; they are forced out by the aftercoming head.
7. The neck is in extreme extension, the head in AP position in the mid pelvis with the face appearing at the outlet.
8. The head is delivered spontaneously in direct AP position.

AP = anteroposterior; SA = sacroanterior.

(Source: Plentl AA, Stone RE. The Bracht maneuver. *Obstet Gynecol Surv.* 1953;8:313–325)

this study provides anatomical justification for the long-held obstetric and midwifery opinions regarding the advantage of an upright position during birth for both cephalic and breech presentations (Reitter, 2014).

Fetal rotation back into a sacroanterior position following rumping usually occurs over one contraction and with maternal expulsive effort. However, if the woman is in a supine position the baby's back may instead begin to rotate to a sacroposterior position following rumping. If the back starts to rotate posteriorly the midwife gently rotates it back with two hands circling the pelvic girdle so that the back remains anterior. At this point the baby is again left to 'hang' and to descend through maternal effort.

Freeing extended legs

If the legs are extended and there is delay in their release it is necessary to abduct the thigh and flex the fetal knee to bring the legs down. The midwife does so by placing a thumb and applying pressure in the popliteal fossa with two fingers of the same hand over the baby's shin. Abducting the knee in this manner will free it from the perineum.

Louwen's manoeuvre to free nuchal arms

Louwen's manoeuvre (Louwen, 2017), performed with the woman in a hands-and-knees position, is used when the baby's descent is halted prior to the nipple line being visible (Fig. 36.11). Louwen calls this the first sign of dystocia. The baby does not rotate to a sacroanterior position (as in Louwen's top-left diagram) but rather remains in a sacro-oblique position (as in Louwen's top-right diagram) with shoulders transverse to the pelvic inlet. The midwife's hands circle the baby's body with pressure supporting the hips and fingers embraced over the ribs and spine. The thumbs will be placed within the vagina as the baby is also braced laterally over the chest (as in Louwen's middle row illustrations).

The baby's shoulder is turned back 180° to the direction in which it came, then 90° back. This manoeuvre turns the shoulders transverse to the inlet and the baby will be in a sacroanterior position.

Louwen notes that the arms might still be above the head following this. But the manoeuvre will have brought the baby's arms forward past his / her ear and will be in a position to draw down the arms. He cautions the midwife to then wait again.

Løvset manoeuvre

The Løvset manoeuvre (Fig. 36.12) is another method to free fetal arms which are extended, or in the presence of one but more commonly both arms being nuchal. One or both arms may be fully extended along the side of the head or behind the neck. This usually results from inappropriate earlier traction placed on the fetus. The diagnosis is made by noticing the winging of scapula and absence of flexed limbs in front of the chest. Løvset's manoeuvre is a very effective way of dealing with this complication (Mukhopadhyay & Arulkumaran, 2002). It is primarily used when the woman is in a supine position and progress is halted at the umbilicus. It is based on the principle that when the anterior shoulder remains above the symphysis pubis, the posterior shoulder will be below the sacral promontory. Therefore, if the fetal trunk is rotated keeping the back anterior and maintaining gentle downward traction, the posterior shoulder will appear below the symphysis pubis. The Løvset manoeuvre involves a series of rotations combined with downward traction. Lateral flexion of the fetus is exaggerated to enable descent of the posterior shoulder below the sacral promontory. The midwife rotates the body 180°, always

Box 36.6 The art of vaginal breech

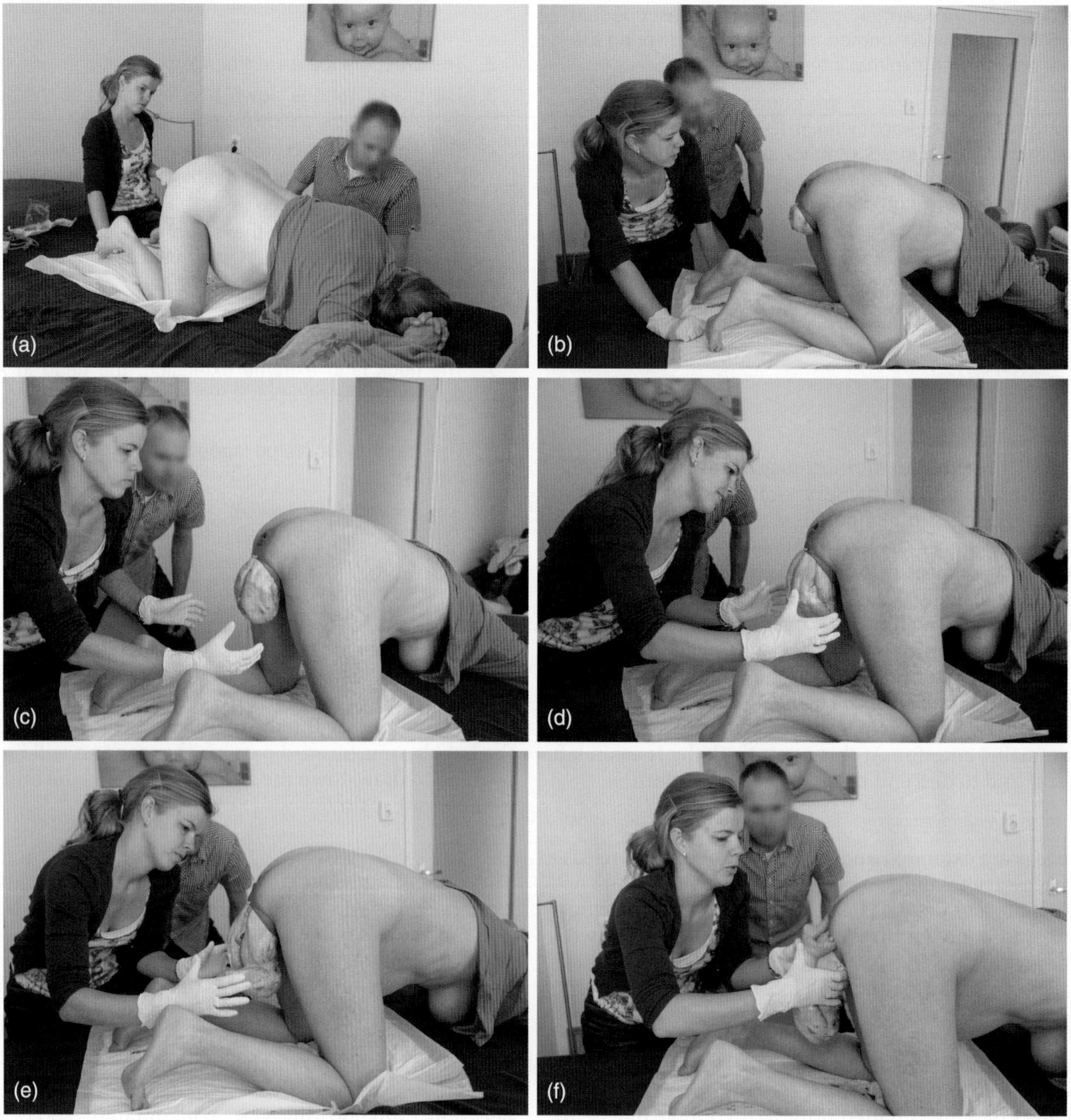

FIGURE 36.9 The art of vaginal breech: (a) 7.45 a.m.: the mother-to-be is on all fours talking to her husband while the attending midwife (vB-S) calmly awaits further events. (b) The hips progressively descend with the sacrum in the anterior position. (c) The lower part of the body in the frank breech position progressively distends the perineum. The mother is encouraged to continue to push. (d) Watchful waiting. At this stage of birth, the hands of the attending midwife do not touch the lower part of the body of the baby. (e) The left leg of the baby has now been born spontaneously, while the right leg remains in flexion, with extension at the knee. The cord is clearly visible. (f) The attending midwife applies both hands at the trunk and both legs of the baby while the mother is encouraged to push.

Box 36.6 The art of vaginal breech—cont'd

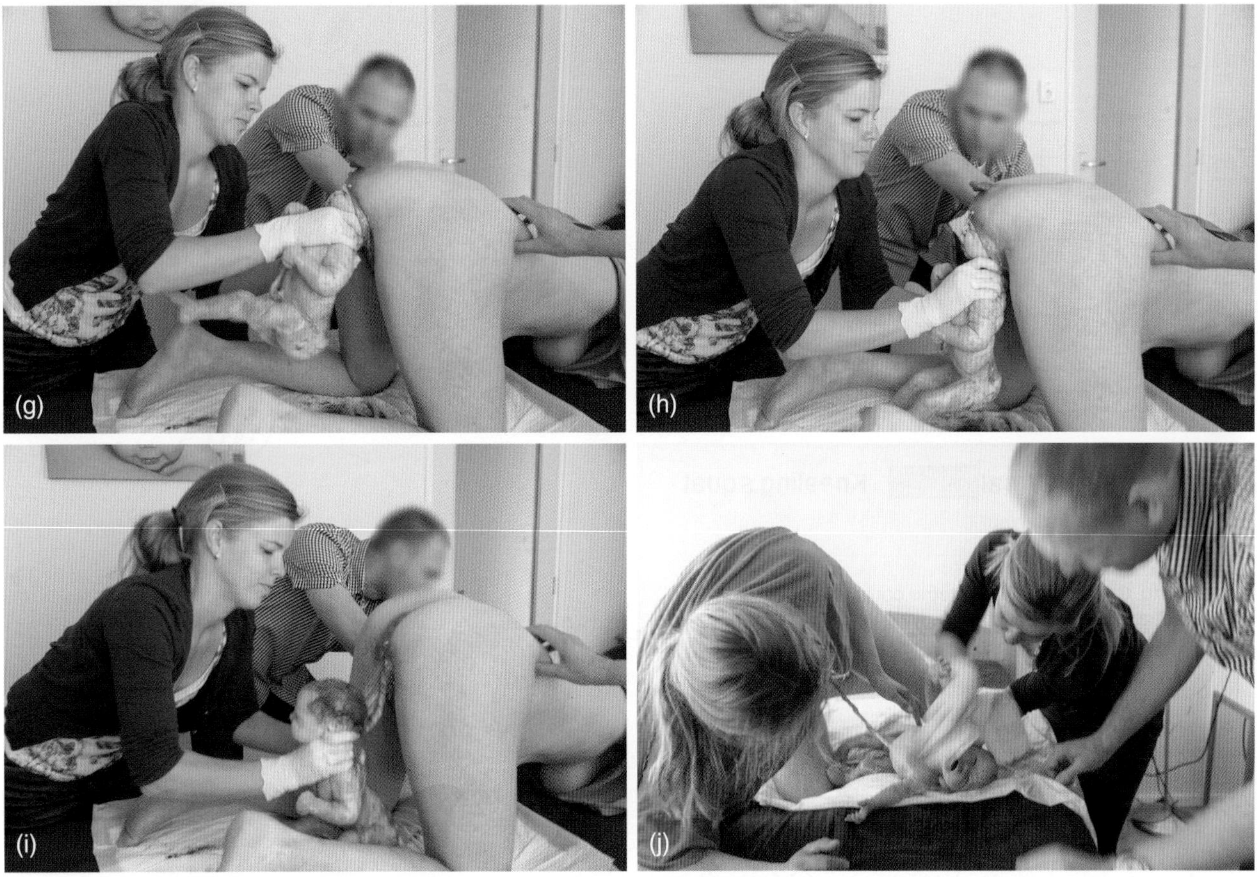

FIGURE 36.9, cont'd (g) Following the spontaneous release of both arms, the midwife ushers the body of the baby with gentle anterior and downward traction. (h) The body continues to descend until the head becomes visible. (i) 8.04 a.m.: the baby is born. (j) The first gasps of the baby while she is shown to her parents

(Reproduced from Wildschut HIJ, van Belzen-Slappendel H, Jans S. The art of vaginal breech birth at term on all fours. *Clin Case Rep*. 2017;5(2):182–186, with permission of Hinke van Belzen-Slappendel, Midwife, Independent Midwifery Practice)

keeping the back anterior; the posterior shoulder rotates anteriorly, and then lies beneath the symphysis pubis. The midwife then brings the arm downwards, then rotates the body back 180° in the opposite direction to deliver the second shoulder anteriorly once it too rotates to below the symphysis pubis. The other arm can now be delivered in the same way. The fetus should then be left to hang from the vulva again until the nape of the neck (hairline) is visible at the anterior vulva though maternal pushing continues. This affords descent of the head into the pelvis. As the baby who has needed this assistance may continue to be compromised, assistance with the birth of the head may be needed.

The Frank nudge

This manoeuvre flexes the head by pushing the baby's head up slightly and towards the pubic bone (Fig. 36.13). The midwife's fingers support the scapulae and the thumbs press over the clavicles while the palms help to round the shoulders over. This will enable the head to emerge.

It is important to continue to avoid traction on the cervical spine during birth of the head. Arms can be swept across the chest and out of the birth canal.

For example, a flexed fetal arm can be brought down across the chest by use of the index and middle fingers splinting the baby's arm and bringing the arm down across its face 'like a cat washing its face' (Banks, 1998, p. 88). As the head begins to birth, it is crucial not to apply traction on the body because this may deflex or extend the head, causing entrapment of the head behind the symphysis.

Assisted vaginal breech birth

In an *assisted* vaginal breech birth, the baby still births spontaneously by uterine action and maternal effort

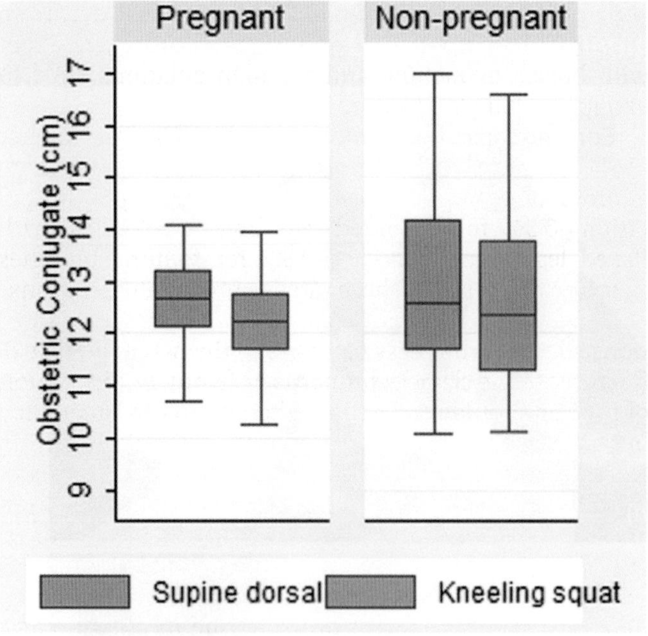

FIGURE 36.10 Changes in the obstetric conjugate of the women in a pregnant and non-pregnant state, lying and squatting
(Source: Reitter et al., 2014)

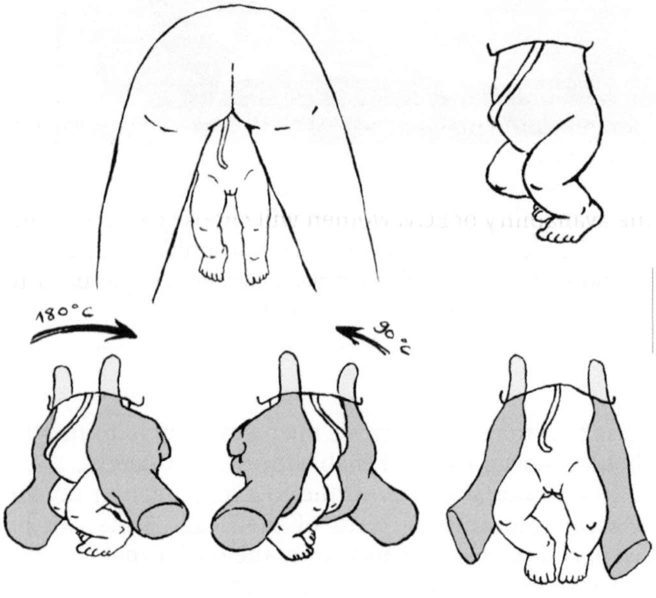

FIGURE 36.11 Louwen manoeuvre: Professor Frank Louwen's manoeuvre to free nuchal arms
(Source: Louwen et al. *Int J Gynecol Obstet*. 2017;136:151–161)

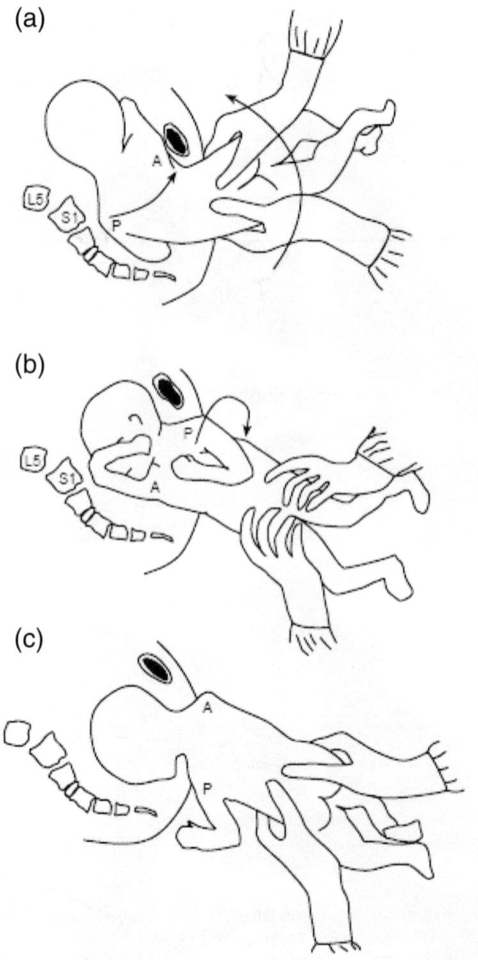

FIGURE 36.12 The Løvset manoeuvre to release the extended arms: (a) The fetus is grasped using both hands by a femoropelvic grip, keeping the thumbs parallel to the vertebral column. The body is lifted anteriorly to cause lateral flexion and promote descent of the posterior shoulder below the sacral promontory. (b) The fetal trunk is rotated through 180°, keeping the back anterior and maintaining gentle downward traction. This will bring the posterior arm to emerge under the pubic arch, which is then hooked out. (c) The body is then rotated through 180° in reverse direction to deliver the anterior shoulder under the symphysis pubis
(Source: Mukhopadhyay & Arulkumaran, 2002)

until he is born to the umbilicus. Once the legs and abdomen have emerged, the fetus should be allowed to hang from the vulva until the tip of the scapula appears. Once the legs and abdomen are born the woman is encouraged to push again with contractions and the shoulders should present in the anterior–posterior plane and birth spontaneously, one at a time, along with the arms, which are usually crossed in front of the chest. Birth of the rest of the body, up to delivery of the mouth, should be achieved over the next one or two contractions (Frye, 2004).

Kristellir manoeuvre

Others, working with women in a supine position, recommend that an assistant may apply suprapubic pressure to maintain flexion of the occiput.

Mauriceau–Smellie–Veit manoeuvre

A modified Mauriceau–Smellie–Veit (MSV, Fig. 36.14) manoeuvre can be used to maintain flexion of the baby's head as it births. It is best to do this from a position below and in front of the baby, probably kneeling. One hand

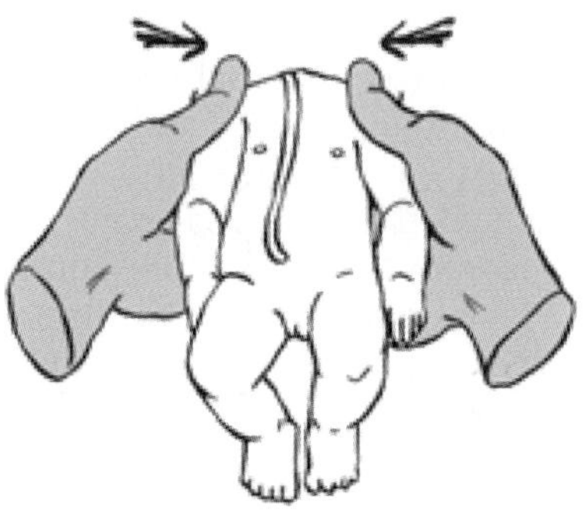

FIGURE 36.13 The Frank nudge
(Source: Louwen et al. *Int J Gynecol Obstet*. 2017;136:151–161)

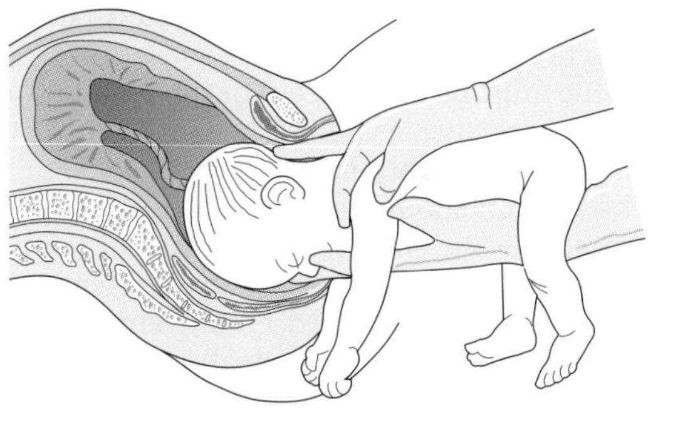

FIGURE 36.14 Birth of the after-coming head using the Mauriceau–Smellie–Veit manoeuvre
(Source: Baskett TF, Calder AA, Arulkumaran S. *Munro Kerr's Operative Obstetrics*. 12th ed. Philadelphia: Saunders; 2014; © 2014 Saunders Elsevier, reproduced with permission)

and forearm supports the baby's body, which straddles the arm, with the ring and index finger on the maxillae and the middle finger being placed under the chin (not the mouth). The other hand is placed on the baby's back with a finger pushing down on the occiput to keep the head flexed. The head is delivered by drawing the baby downwards. Some traction on the shoulders by the upper hand may be required. As the head is birthed very slowly, the baby's body is kept in a neutral position with respect to the head and then gently raised in a large arc so that the child rests on the mother's abdomen. An assistant may also apply suprapubic pressure to encourage head flexion and descent.

Breech extraction

Total breech extraction is inappropriate for term singleton breech delivery (Kotaska et al., 2009).

Complications of a breech birth

The main aetiologies for the mortality and morbidity for breech babies are due to pre-term birth, anoxia due to cord compression, mechanical trauma which occurs to the baby's non-moulded after-coming head, particularly with breech extraction, and the manipulations done to extract the baby's hands or shoulders.

Cord prolapse is commonly cited at 10 times higher (3.7%) than with cephalic presentation (0.3%). It is more appropriate to apply the incidence to a particular presentation—0.5% for extended legs breech; 5%–10% with flexed legs breech; and 8%–18% for footling breeches (Confino et al., 1985); these rates apply for all gestations.

The breech baby can be at risk of birthing complications such as Erb's palsy (damage to the brachial plexus), fractures of the clavicle, humerus or femur, or dislocation of hips or shoulders. The last often occurs in pregnancy but may be exacerbated during birth, particularly during extracted breech birth, which is associated with 25% of birth injury and up to 20% of breech mortality (Ekeus et al., 2017). This includes trauma to the adrenal glands or gut and rupture of the spleen or liver if the baby's abdomen rather than the fetal pelvis is grasped during manoeuvres. Some degree of bruising due to pressure and prolonged congestion is to be expected, especially of the male genitalia, and so the parents should be informed about this before the birth.

External cephalic version (ECV)

Approximately 3%–4% of all pregnant women at term will have a fetus presenting by the breech. The procedure of turning the baby from a breech position to a cephalic presentation is useful and recommended in cases where women would prefer a vaginal birth. However, an Australian study found that the majority of women with a breech presentation did not receive ECV. Regardless of the availability of ECV, women will choose caesarean section if there is a medical indication (Gamble et al., 2007). Version or turning of the breech is a technique used to change a fetal presentation by abdominal or intrauterine manipulation. The latter, usually an 'internal podalic version', is rarely performed. It is used in second stage to convert a second twin from a transverse lie by grasping the feet and bringing them through the woman's cervix for a breech extraction. In contrast, ECV is increasingly common and effectively reduces the incidence of breech presentation. A Cochrane review on ECV in term pregnancies showed this procedure to be effective in the reduction of non-cephalic birth (RR 0.46; 95% CI 0.31–0.66) and caesarean delivery (RR 0.63; 95% CI 0.44–0.90) (Hofmeyr et al., 2015). They concluded that ECV at term reduces the incidence of both non-cephalic presentation and caesarean section. International guidelines recommend an ECV for all women with an uncomplicated breech presentation at term (de Hundt et al., 2014; Impey et al., 2017b).

If ECV is performed very early in the third trimester (32–4 weeks), it does not affect how the baby is lying at full term; nor does it seem to change the number of babies born by caesarean delivery. However, there are insufficient data to say whether beginning ECV between 34

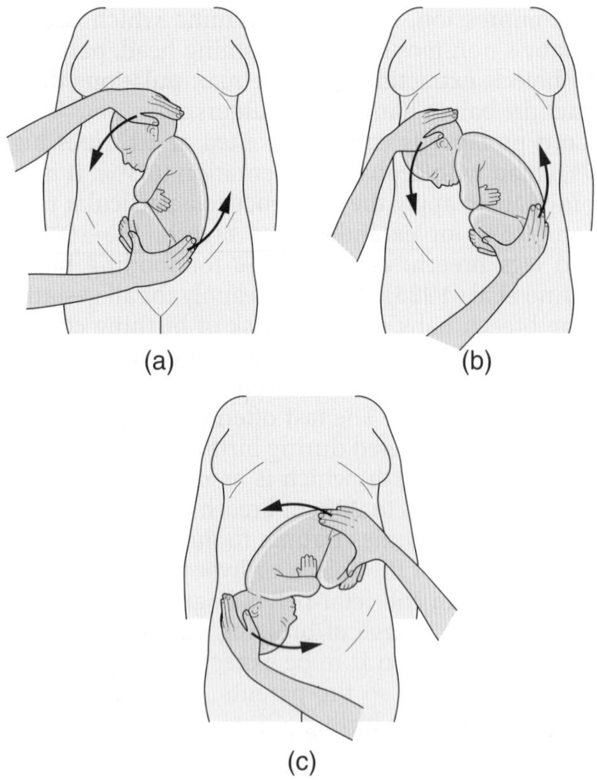

FIGURE 36.15 External cephalic version: (a) The right hand lifts the breech out of the pelvis. The left hand makes the head follow the nose. Flexion of head and back is maintained throughout. (b) Flexion is continued. The left hand brings the head downwards. The right hand pushes the breech upwards. (c) Pressure is exerted on head and breech simultaneously until the head is lying at the pelvic brim
(Based on Fraser & Cooper, 2003)

and 36 weeks compared with beginning it after 37 weeks results in fewer breech babies at birth and fewer caesarean sections.

This section focuses on the use of ECV to turn a breech presentation to a cephalic one (Fig. 36.15).

Spontaneous version of a breech presentation occurs in about 20% of cases. For the remaining percentage of women, an ECV is a useful technique to 'turn a breech', and has been practised since the time of Hippocrates. Most versions are performed at about 37 weeks, because at this stage most babies still in a breech position will not spontaneously revert to a cephalic presentation. In addition, if complications occur as a result of the ECV, the risk of pre-term birth is eliminated.

Factors associated with a successful ECV

ECV is best carried out with the woman awake and facilities for emergency caesarean birth nearby. A paper presenting some of the findings of the Canadian Early External Cephalic Version Trial (Hutton et al., 2008) described the factors associated with a successful ECV procedure. The authors stated that multiparity and a non-engaged presenting part were the only significant preprocedural predictors of ECV success. Procedural factors predictive of ECV success included lower reported maternal pain scores during the procedure, a single attempt at ECV, and a more mobile fetus (that is before engagement of the fetus in the pelvis). The authors commented that maternal pain may have been because more vigorous (and thus more painful) attempts at ECV are made when a fetus is not turning readily, or because when pain is reported the ECV attempt is abandoned (Hutton et al., 2008).

Criteria for ECV

According to the Cochrane review (Hofmeyr et al., 2015), before an ECV is attempted the following criteria should be met:

- The fetus must be a singleton.
- The breech must not be engaged.
- There must be adequate amniotic liquor.
- A reactive non-stress test (NST) should be obtained prior to the procedure.
- The fetus must be 36–7 weeks or more gestation.
- Other authors, such as Edelstone (2000), make the following recommendations:
  - The woman should give informed consent for the procedure. She should be informed of the benefits and risks of ECV—failed version, reversion (2%), fetal stress related to cord entanglement or abruption, ruptured uterus and abruption and unexplained fetal death. Benefits of a successful ECV (more than 50%) include decreased caesarean section rate. The woman and her support people also need information about alternatives to an ECV—postural exercises, moxibustion and visualisation.
  - The ECV should be performed only in a maternity unit that can proceed to an immediate caesarean section.
  - A real-time ultrasound should be performed prior to beginning the procedure to rule out placenta praevia and to confirm fetal presentation and position.
  - A subcutaneous injection of a tocolytic drug such as terbutaline (Bricanyl) is administered to achieve uterine relaxation.

Contraindications for ECV

Apart from maternal refusal, there are a few absolute contraindications to ECV. These include any factors that may prevent successful vaginal birth, such as maternal or fetal compromise (including significant IUGR) and placenta praevia, or where ECV is not possible such as in multiple gestation. Oligohydramnios is also a contraindication owing to the need for adequate amniotic fluid to enable version (Burgos et al., 2014). Although a perception exists that a previous caesarean section is a contraindication for ECV, there is little evidence that caesarean section should be considered an absolute contraindication (Rosman et al., 2013). There is some evidence that the associated risks of ECV in women with one previous caesarean section are similar to those in women without a previous caesarean section. Nevertheless an Australian population-based study found that previous caesarean section was the most common reason for excluding women from ECV, with only 2.6% of women with ECV having a history of caesarean section compared with 16.6% in women with breech presentation overall (Bin et al., 2017).

ECV procedure

The woman is admitted to a day-only unit or delivery suite in case an immediate caesarean section is necessary. Before the procedure begins, the obstetrician checks that the woman has given consent for the version, understands the risks and benefits of the procedure and has had all her questions answered. An ultrasound confirms that the baby is still in a breech position and that there is no evidence of congenital anomalies that preclude vaginal birth. A CTG is performed for 20 minutes or until it is reactive. Maternal and fetal vital signs are recorded and documented. A tocolytic is sometimes administered according to the unit's protocols. The woman assumes a recumbent position (with a wedge under her buttocks); once she is relaxed, the obstetrician gently turns the baby by pushing the presenting part upwards, and the fetal head is pushed in the opposite direction towards the pelvis (ACOG, 2017; Hofmeyr et al. 2015). This procedure should not be painful. After the version has been completed, the CTG is reconnected and the fetal heart rate (FHR) observed for signs of fetal compromise and the occurrence of uterine contractions that may herald the onset of labour. Because of the risk of alloimmunisation, anti-D prophylaxis is recommended for non-sensitised D-negative women following ECV attempts (McBain et al., 2015). Before she goes home, the woman should be asked to contact her lead carer if there are signs of vaginal bleeding, if the membranes rupture, if contractions begin or if she is worried about her own or the baby's wellbeing. Women are sometimes asked to complete a kick chart for 24 hours after the version. If the ECV is unsuccessful or if the fetus reverts to a breech, the version may be repeated in 1 week (ACOG, 2017).

Reinhard et al. (2012) studied the use of hypnosis for ECV and found that it helped during ECV on several levels. First they found women were more comfortable during the ECV procedure with the help of hypnosis; secondly they found that hypnosis appeared to help relax the uterine muscles. This study found that, when women were offered clinical hypnosis and a relaxation technique (to visualise Lorenz-Wallacher's 'smiling child' (Reinhard et al., 2012, p. 187)) versus standard medical care, of the 78 women who received a hypnosis intervention prior to ECV, 41.6% ($n = 32$) had successful ECV, whereas the control group of 122, who had similar baseline characteristics, had a 27.3% ($n = 33$) successful ECV procedure ($p < 0.05$). The study was designed to test whether hypnosis could improve the success rate of ECV.

Complications of ECV

Very low complication rates have been reported following ECV (Hofmeyr et al., 2015). The most frequently reported complication is a transient abnormal baby's heart rate pattern (5.7%). Less-frequent complications were persisting pathological baby's heart rate patterns (0.37%), vaginal bleeding (0.47%), placental abruption (0.12%), emergency caesarean section (0.43%) and perinatal mortality (0.16%) (Hofmeyr et al., 2015).

Alternative techniques to reduce the incidence of breech presentation

There is no evidence that postural management—'breech exercises'—are effective in converting a breech to a cephalic presentation (Hofmeyr et al., 2015). Similarly, although there is anecdotal evidence that moxibustion is effective in converting a breech into a cephalic presentation, there is as yet limited evidence to support its use (Coyle et al., 2012). On the other hand, there is no evidence that moxibustion is harmful.

Moxibustion involves the application of a heated mixture made from the dried leaves of a herb, mugwort (*Artemisia vulgaris*), directly to the designated meridian point (Bladder-67), located beside the outer corner of the fifth toenail. It is applied close to the skin until it produces hyperaemia from local vasodilation. Treatment may take from 2 to 7 weeks. Alternatively, the heat from a burning moxa stick is used to warm acupuncture needles that have already been inserted in the appropriate meridian point. The heat and aroma of the mugwort is believed to stimulate the meridian point, so that energy moves through it, increasing fetal activity and encouraging the fetus to move to a cephalic presentation (Coyle et al., 2012).

Moxa is an emerging therapy used by women in Western settings to promote cephalic version. Researchers in Australia examined the views of acupuncturists and researchers to identify key aspects of treatment to promote cephalic version for women with a breech presentation, and to establish a research treatment protocol to guide effective and safe self-administration of moxa; further work is being undertaken in this area with larger sample sizes (Smith et al., 2014).

CLINICAL POINT

It is important that those who birth babies arriving by breech are skilled, confident and share a trusting relationship with the woman. The fundamentals of best practice—astute, accurate clinical assessments, an excellent grasp of the physiology of breech labour, experience of attending breech births, considerable patience and skilful techniques—hold true for breech births. It is also important for midwives to have established and effective collaborative support frameworks with efficient lines of communication.

Conclusion

Importantly, women, midwives and obstetricians recognise the importance of listening to the woman's body, and to work with it not against it to preserve the normal physiology of birth. Internationally and within Australia and New Zealand, maternity guidelines and policies have been revised to reflect a new understanding of breech birth. In 2017, NSW Health issued a statement in their breech birth policy stating:

> *Local and international guidelines support the provision of vaginal breech birth in selected circumstances. For women with a singleton breech presentation at term, research has demonstrated that in maternity units with policies and guidelines to direct clinical care, there is no significant excess additional risk associated with planned vaginal birth compared with planned caesarean section ... Access to a supportive vaginal breech birth service within NSW is limited. It is an obligation of NSW Health to provide women with birthing options that offer appropriate safety controls and processes within a tiered network of maternity services. Consultation, referral and transfer processes should be in place to ensure all women are provided with the option of vaginal breech birth. To ensure the best outcomes for mothers and babies, vaginal breech birth should be managed in services with expertise in this birth option, including support for informed decision making. Information should be provided on the benefits and risks, both for current and future pregnancies, of planned caesarean section versus planned vaginal birth for breech presentation at term.*
>
> (NSW Health Guideline: *Maternity—Supporting Women Planning a Vaginal Breech Birth.* GL2017_008, May 2017; © State of New South Wales NSW Ministry of Health. For current information go to www.health.nsw.gov.au.)

Review questions

1. When is the breech baby likely to turn to a vaginal position for birth?
2. Why is this so?
3. What are the predisposing factors that influence a baby remaining in the breech position for birth?
4. What is moxibustion? What ancient science does it adhere to?

Acknowledgements

I wish to acknowledge the major contribution made by authors Carol Thorogood and Catherine Donaldson in previous editions of the text; and I also wish to acknowledge the contribution of Dr Maggie Banks and the generous photographic contribution of the independently practising midwife from the Netherlands, Hinke van Belzen-Slappendel.

Online resources

Association of Radical Midwives UK. https://www.midwifery.org.uk/articles/breech-birth/.

Birthspirit. Breech birth: monitoring in labour. Dr Maggie Banks. http://www.birthspirit.co.nz/.

Birthwell birthright. Everything you wanted to know about breech birth, but were afraid to ask. Tanya Strusberg. http://birthwell-birthright.com/everything-wanted-know-breech-birth-afraid-ask/.

Breech Birth Network. https://breechbirth.org.uk/about/.

Mary Cronk midwifery services breech birth workshops. http://www.homebirth.org.uk/marycronk/.

Midwifery Today. *Breech Birth* e-book. https://www.smashwords.com/books/view/172532.

References

Alfirevic Z, Devane D, Gyte GM, et al. Continuous cardiotocography (CTG) as a form of electronic fetal monitoring (EFM) for fetal assessment during labour. *Cochrane Database Syst Rev.* 2017;(2):CD006066.

American College of Obstetricians and Gynecologists Committee on Obstetric Practice (ACOG). ACOG Committee Opinion No. 340. Mode of term singleton breech delivery. *Obstet Gynecol.* 2006;108:235–237.

American College of Obstetricians and Gynecologists Committee on Obstetric Practice (ACOG). Practice Bulletin No. 184 Summary: vaginal birth after cesarean delivery. *Obstet Gynecol.* 2017;130:1167–1169.

Australian College of Midwives (ACM). *National Midwifery Guidelines for Consultation and Referral.* 3rd ed.; 2013. Online: http://midwives.rentsoft.biz/lib/pdf/documents/National/Guidelines2013.pdf.

Australian Institute of Health and Welfare (AIHW). *Australia's Mothers and Babies.* 2021. Online: https://www.aihw.gov.au/reports/mothers-babies/australias-mothers-babies/contents/about

Australian Nursing and Midwifery Accreditation Council (ANMAC). *Midwife Accreditation Standards 2014.* Canberra: ANMAC; 2014.

Banks M. *Breech Birth Woman-Wise.* Hamilton: Birthspirit Books; 1998.

Banks M. *The obstetric bed: resistance in action.* 2014. Online: https://www.birthspirit.co.nz/the-obstetric-bed-resistance-in-action/.

Banks M. *Breech birth: optimal maternal positioning.* 2017. Online: https://www.birthspirit.co.nz/breech-birth-optimal-maternal-positioning/.

Barth WH Jr. Persistent occiput posterior. I. *Obstet Gynecol.* 2015;125(3):695–709. doi:10.1097/AOG.0000000000000647.

Baskett TF, Calder AA, Arulkumaran S. *Munro Kerr's Operative Obstetrics.* 12th ed. Philadelphia: Saunders; 2014.

Bin YS, Roberts CL, Nicholl MC, et al. Uptake of external cephalic version for term breech presentation: an Australian population study, 2002–2012. *BMC Pregnancy Childbirth.* 2017;17:244.

Bjellmo S, Andersen GL, Martinussen MP, et al. Is vaginal breech delivery associated with higher risk for perinatal death and cerebral palsy compared with vaginal cephalic birth? Registry-based cohort study in Norway. *BMJ Open.* 2017;7:e014979.
Burgos J, Cobos P, Rodriguez L, et al. Is external cephalic version at term contraindicated in previous caesarean section? A prospective comparative cohort study. *BJOG.* 2014;121:230–235, discussion 235.
Chamberlain C, O'Mara-Eves A, Porter J, et al. Psychosocial interventions for supporting women to stop smoking in pregnancy. *Cochrane Database Syst Rev.* 2017;(2):CD001055.
Cohain JS, Buxbaum RE, Mankuta D. Spontaneous first trimester miscarriage rates per woman among parous women with 1 or more pregnancies of 24 weeks or more. *BMC Pregnancy Childbirth.* 2017;17(1):437. doi:10.1186/s12884-017-1620-1.
Confino E, Gleicher N, Elrad H, et al. The breech dilemma. A review. *Obstet Gynecol Surv.* 1985;40:330–337.
Coyle ME, Smith CA, Peat B. Cephalic version by moxibustion for breech presentation. *Cochrane Database Syst Rev.* 2012;(5):CD003928, doi:10.1002/14651858.CD003928.pub3.
de Hundt M, Velzel J, de Groot CJ, et al. Mode of delivery after successful external cephalic version: a systematic review and meta-analysis. *Obstet Gynecol.* 2014;123:1327–1334.
Dodd JMG, Grivell RM, Crowther CA. Multiple pregnancy. In: James D, Steer P, et al., eds. *High-Risk Pregnancy: Management Options.* St Louis: Saunders; 2011:1053–1064.
Dunn P. Erich Bracht (1882–1969) of Berlin and his "breech" manoeuvre. *Arch Dis Child Fetal Neonatal Ed.* 2003;88:F76–F77.
Easter SR, Lieberman E, Carusi D. Fetal presentation and successful twin vaginal delivery. *Am J Obstet Gynecol.* 2016;214:116. e1–116.e10. doi:10.1016/j.ajog.2015.08.017.
Edelstone DI. Breech presentation. In: Kean LHB, Baker PN, Edelstone DI, eds. *Best Practice Labour Ward Management.* London: WB Saunders; 2000:142–165.
Ekeus C, Norman M, Aberg K, et al. Vaginal breech delivery at term and neonatal morbidity and mortality – a population-based cohort study in Sweden. *J Matern Fetal Neonatal Med.* 2017;1–6. doi:10.1080/14767058.2017.1378328.
Evans J. Focus on understanding physiological breech birth. *Essentially MIDIRS.* 2012a;3:17–21.
Evans J. Joining-up knowing. The final piece of the breech birth jigsaw. *Essentially MIDIRS.* 2012b;3:46–49.
Fahy K. Is breech birth really unsafe? Treatment validity in the Term Breech Trial. *Essentially MIDIRS.* 2011;2:17–21.
Fischer R. *Breech delivery.* e-Medicine; 2016. Online: http://emedicine.medscape.com/article/262159-overview.
Fox NS, Silverstein M, Bender S, et al. Active second-stage management in twin pregnancies undergoing planned vaginal delivery in a U.S. population. *Obstet Gynecol.* 2010;115: 229–233.
Fraser D, Cooper M. *Myles' Textbook for Midwives.* 14th ed. London: Churchill Livingstone; 2003.
Frye A. *Holistic Midwifery: A Comprehensive Textbook for Midwives in a Homebirth Practice, Vol. II: Care from Onset of Labor through the First Hours after Birth.* Portland, OR: Labrys Press; 2004.
Gamble J, Creedy DK, McCourt C, et al. A critique of the literature on women's request for cesarean section. *Birth.* 2007;34: 331–340.
Giles W, Bisits A, O'Callaghan S, et al. The Doppler assessment in multiple pregnancy randomised controlled trial of ultrasound biometry versus umbilical artery Doppler ultrasound and biometry in twin pregnancy. *BJOG.* 2003;110:593–597.
Glezerman M. Five years to the term breech trial: the rise and fall of a randomized controlled trial. *Am J Obstet Gynecol.* 2006;194:20–25.
Goffinet F, Carayol M, Foidart JM, et al. Is planned vaginal delivery for breech presentation at term still an option? Results of an observational prospective survey in France and Belgium. *Am J Obstet Gynecol.* 2006;194:1002–1011.
Hall JG. Twinning. *Lancet.* 2003;362(9385):735–743.
Hannah ME, Hannah WJ, Hewson SA, et al. Planned caesarean section versus planned vaginal birth for breech presentation at term: a randomised multicentre trial. Term Breech Trial Collaborative Group. *Lancet.* 2000;356:1375–1383.
Hannah ME, Whyte H, Hannah WJ, et al. Maternal outcomes at 2 years after planned cesarean section versus planned vaginal birth for breech presentation at term: the international randomized Term Breech Trial. *Am J Obstet Gynecol.* 2004;191:917–927.
Henderson C, Macdonald S. *Mayes' Midwifery.* 13th ed. London: Baillière Tindall; 2004.
Hofmeyr GJ, Kulier R, West HM. External cephalic version for breech presentation at term. *Cochrane Database Syst Rev.* 2015;(4):CD000083, doi:10.1002/14651858.CD000083.pub3.
Hunter S, Hofmeyr GJ, Kulier R. Hands and knees posture in late pregnancy or labour for fetal malposition (lateral or posterior). *Cochrane Database Syst Rev.* 2007;(4):CD001063.
Hutton EK, Saunders CA, Tu M, Early External Cephalic Version Trial Collaborators, et al. Factors associated with a successful external cephalic version in the early ECV trial. *J Obstet Gynaecol Can.* 2008;30:23–28.
Imaizumi Y, Hayakawa K. Infant mortality among singletons and twins in Japan during 1999–2008 on the basis of risk factors. *Twin Res Hum Genet.* 2013;16:639–644.
Impey LWM, Murphy DJ, Griffiths M, et al. Management of breech presentation. *BJOG.* 2017a;124:e151–e177.
Impey LWM, Murphy DJ, Griffiths M, Royal College of Obstetricians and Gynaecologists, et al. External cephalic version and reducing the incidence of term breech presentation. *BJOG.* 2017b;124:e178–e192.
Johnson A. Diagnosis and management of twin–twin transfusion syndrome. *Clin Obstet Gynecol.* 2015;58:611–631.
Kariminia A, Chamberlain ME, Keogh J, et al. Randomised controlled trial of effect of hands and knees posturing on incidence of occiput posterior position at birth. *BMJ.* 2004;328:490.
Khalil A, O'Brien P. Challenges of twin pregnancy. *Br J Midwifery.* 2007;15:266–272.
Kotaska A. In the literature: combating coercion: breech birth, parturient choice, and the evolution of evidence-based maternity care. *Birth.* 2007;34:176–180.
Kotaska A, Menticoglou S, Gagnon R. Vaginal delivery of breech presentation. *J Obstet Gynaecol Can.* 2009;31:557–566.
Lawson GW. The term breech trial ten years on: primum non nocere? *Birth.* 2012;39:3–9.
Le Ray C, Lepleux F, De La Calle A, et al. Lateral asymmetric decubitus position for the rotation of occipito-posterior positions: multicenter randomized controlled trial EVADELA. *Am J Obstet Gynecol.* 2016;215:511.e1–7.
Lee N, Kildea S, Stapleton H. 'Facing the wrong way': exploring the Occipito Posterior position / back pain discourse from women's and midwives perspectives. *Midwifery.* 2015;31:1008–1014.
Lieberman E, Davidson K, Lee-Parritz A, et al. Changes in fetal position during labor and their association with epidural analgesia. *Obstet Gynecol.* 2005;105:974–982
Liem, S., Shuit E,. Hegeman M et al Cervical pessaries for prevention of preterm birth in women with a multiple pregnancy (ProTWIN): a multicentre, open-label randomized controlled trial. *Lancet.* 2013; 382: 1341–49
Louwen F, Daviss BA, Johnson KC, et al. Does breech delivery in an upright position instead of on the back improve outcomes and avoid cesareans? *Int J Gynaecol Obstet.* 2017;136:151–161.
Lydon-Rochelle M, Albers L, Gorwoda J, et al. Accuracy of Leopold maneuvers in screening for malpresentation: a prospective study. *Birth.* 1993;20:132–135.

McBain RD, Crowther CA, Middleton P. Anti-D administration in pregnancy for preventing Rhesus alloimmunisation. *Cochrane Database Syst Rev.* 2015;(9):CD000020, doi:10.1002/14651858.CD000020.pub3.

Midwifery Council of New Zealand (MCNZ). *Scope of Practice.* Wellington, NZ: MCNZ; 2010.

Ministry of Health (MOH). *Guidelines for Consultation with Obstetric and Related Medical Services (Referral Guidelines).* Wellington, NZ: Ministry of Health; 2012. Online: https://www.health.govt.nz/system/files/documents/publications/referral-glines-jan12.pdf.

Ministry of Health (MOH). *Report on Maternity web tool;* 2021. Online: https://www.health.govt.nz/publication/report-maternity-web-tool.

Mukhopadhyay S, Arulkumaran S. Breech delivery. *Best Pract Res Clin Obstet Gynaecol.* 2002;16:31–42.

National Institute for Health and Care Excellence (NICE). *Multiple pregnancy: twin and triplet pregnancies.* 2013. Online: https://www.nice.org.uk/guidance/qs46/resources/multiple-pregnancy-twin-and-triplet-pregnancies-2098670068933?.

National Institute for Health and Care Excellence (NICE). *CG190 Intrapartum Care for Healthy Women and Babies.* London: NICE; 2017, updated 2021. Online: https://www.nice.org.uk/guidance/cg190/resources/intrapartum-care-for-healthy-women-and-babies-pdf-35109866447557.

National Institute for Health and Care Excellence (NICE). *Twin and triplet pregnancy.* London: NICE; 2021. Online: www.nice.org.uk/guidance/ng137.

New South Wales Health. *Guideline: Maternity—Supporting Women Planning a Vaginal Breech Birth.* GL2017_008. May 2017.

New Zealand Guidelines Group (NZGG). *Care of Women with Breech Presentation or Previous Caesarean Birth.* Wellington: NZ NZGG; 2004.

Plentl AA, Stone RE. The Bracht maneuver. *Obstet Gynecol Surv.* 1953;8:313–325.

Rankin J. *Physiology in Childbearing: With Anatomy and Related Biosciences.* 4th ed. London: Elsevier; 2017.

Reinhard J, Reichenbach L, Ernst T, et al. Delayed interval delivery in twin and triplet pregnancies: 6 years of experience in one perinatal center. *J Perinat Med.* 2012;40:551–555.

Reitter A, Daviss BA, Bisits A, et al. Does pregnancy and/or shifting positions create more room in a woman's pelvis? *Am J Obstet Gynecol.* 2014;211:662.e1–662.e9.

Rosman AN, Guijt A, Vlemmix F, et al. Contraindications for external cephalic version in breech position at term: a systematic review. Acta Obstet Gynecol Scand. 2013;92:137–142.

Royal Australian and New Zealand College of Obstetricians and Gynaecologists (RANZCOG). *Management of Breech Presentation at Term.* 2016. Online: https://www.ranzcog.edu.au/RANZCOG_SITE/media/RANZCOG-MEDIA/Women%27s%20Health/Statement%20and%20guidelines/Clinical-Obstetrics/Management-of-breech-presentation-at-term-(C-Obs-11)-Review-July-2016.pdf?ext=.pdf.

Royal College of Obstetricians and Gynaecologists (RCOG). *Umbilical Cord Prolapse. Green-top Guideline no. 50.* London: RCOG; 2014. Online: https://www.rcog.org.uk/globalassets/documents/guidelines/gtg-50-umbilicalcordprolapse-2014.pdf.

Rzyska E, Ajay B, Chandraharan E. Safety of vaginal delivery among dichorionic diamniotic twins over 10 years in a UK teaching hospital. *Int J Gynaecol Obstet.* 2017;136:98–101.

Sharma JB. Evaluation of Sharma's modified Leopold's maneuvers: a new method for fetal palpation in late pregnancy. *Arch Gynecol Obstet.* 2009;279:481–487.

Shetty A, Smith AP. The sonographic diagnosis of chorionicity. *Prenat Diagn.* 2005;25(9):735–739.

Simkin P. The fetal occiput posterior position: state of the science and a new perspective. *Birth.* 2010;37:61–71.

Smith CA, Betts D. The practice of acupuncture and moxibustion to promote cephalic version for women with a breech presentation: implications for clinical practice and research. *Complement Ther Med.* 2014;22:75–80.

Stirrat GM. Recurrent miscarriage I: definition and epidemiology. *Lancet.* 1990. 336:673–75.

Stremler R, Hodnett E, Petryshen P, et al. Randomized controlled trial of hands-and-knees positioning for occipitoposterior position in labor. *Birth.* 2005;32:243–251.

Su M, Hannah WJ, Willan A, et al. Planned caesarean section decreases the risk of adverse perinatal outcome due to both labour and delivery complications in the Term Breech Trial. *BJOG.* 2004;111:1065–1074.

Van Mieghem T, De Heus R, Lewi L, et al. Prenatal management of monoamniotic twin pregnancies. *Obstet Gynecol.* 2014;124:498–506.

Vasak B, Verhagen JJ, Koenen SV, et al. Lower perinatal mortality in preterm born twins than in singletons: a nationwide study from The Netherlands. *Am J Obstet Gynecol.* 2017;216:e161–e169.

Vogel JP, Holloway E, Cuesta C, et al. Outcomes of non-vertex second twins, following vertex vaginal delivery of first twin: a secondary analysis of the WHO Global Survey on maternal and perinatal health. *BMC Pregnancy Childbirth.* 2014;14:55.

Walker S, Scamell M, Parker P. Principles of physiological breech birth practice: a Delphi study. *Midwifery.* 2016;43:1–6.

Walker S, Scamell M, Parker P. Deliberate acquisition of competence in physiological breech birth: a grounded theory study. *Women Birth.* 2018a;31(3):e170–e177. doi:10.1016/j.wombi.2017.09.008.

Walker S, Parker P, Scamell M. Expertise in physiological breech birth: a mixed-methods study. *Birth.* 2018b;45(2):202–209. doi:10.1111/birt.12326.

Westbury B. Mobility and upright positioning in labour. *Pract Midwife.* 2014;17:24–26.

Whyte H, Hannah ME, Saigal S, et al. Outcomes of children at 2 years after planned cesarean birth versus planned vaginal birth for breech presentation at term: the International Randomized Term Breech Trial. *Am J Obstet Gynecol.* 2004;191:864–871.

Wildschut HIJ, van Belzen-Slappendel H, Jans S. The art of vaginal breech birth at term on all fours. *Clin Case Rep.* 2017;5(2):182–186.

Further reading

Catling C, Petrovska K, Watts N, et al. Barriers and facilitators for vaginal breech births in Australia: clinician's experiences. *Women Birth.* 2015;29:138–143.

Daviss BA, Johnson KC, Lalonde AB. Evolving evidence since the term breech trial: Canadian response, European dissent, and potential solutions. *J Obstet Gynaecol Can.* 2010;32:217–224.

Evans J. *Breech Birth—What Are my Options?* Camberley, Surrey: AIMS UK; 2005.

King TL, Brucker MC, Kriebs JM, et al. *Varney's Midwifery.* Burlington, MA: Jones & Bartlett Learning; 2013.

Louwen F, Daviss B, Johnson KC, et al. Does breech delivery in an upright position instead of on the back improve outcomes and avoid cesareans? *Int J Gynaecol Obstet.* 2017;136:151–161.

Petrovska K, Watts NP, Catling C, et al. Supporting women planning a vaginal breech birth: an international survey. *Birth.* 2016;43:353–357.

Petrovska K, Watts NP, Catling C, et al. "Stress, anger, fear and injustice": an international qualitative survey of women's experiences planning a vaginal breech birth. *Midwifery.* 2017;44:41–47.

Pilliod RA, Caughey AB. Fetal malpresentation and malposition: diagnosis and management. *Obstet Gynecol Clin North Am.* 2017;44:631–643. doi:10.1016/j.ogc.2017.08.003.

CHAPTER 37

Challenges in pregnancy

Catherine Donaldson and Lesley Dixon

LEARNING OUTCOMES

Learning outcomes for this chapter are:

1. To describe the effects that complications in pregnancy have on the woman, her family, the pregnancy and the unborn baby
2. To discuss the diagnosis, evidence for, treatment of and expected outcomes associated with common complications in childbearing
3. To identify strategies to support women as they are challenged by and deal with the physical and psychological complications of 'high-risk' birthing.

CHAPTER OVERVIEW

For most women the expectation is that pregnancy is a time of wellness for herself and her unborn baby regardless of their socioeconomic and cultural contexts (Downe et al., 2016). For some, however, complications that arise during the pregnancy and/or pre-existing health problems may put the woman and her baby at risk of adverse outcomes. These complications can lead to serious illness, trauma, and even the death of the woman, her baby or both. Irrespective of the final outcomes, challenges in pregnancy place tremendous stress on the woman and her family from a physical, social and sometimes economic perspective. It is essential that midwives have the knowledge and skills to recognise the physical signs that a pregnancy is not progressing as it should and can identify psychosocial and environmental stressors that may create or exacerbate complications in pregnancy. Midwives have a professional, legal and ethical responsibility to act on their findings irrespective of the practice setting and the woman should remain the primary focus of maternity care.

The midwife, working in partnership with the woman, initially manages many of these pregnancy challenges in the primary health setting. When complications fall outside the scope of midwifery practice, midwives, still working in partnership with the woman, consult colleagues in a timely manner and work collaboratively with them to jointly manage secondary and tertiary levels of care.

KEY TERMS

deep vein thrombosis
gestational diabetes
gestational hypertension
hyperemesis gravidarum
molar pregnancy (hydatidiform mole)
placenta praevia
placental abruption
preeclampsia
miscarriage
thromboembolic disease

INTRODUCTION

This chapter focuses on an exploration of the most common complications arising in pregnancy and those that pre-exist pregnancy (cardiac disease, renal disease, rheumatic heart disease, thyroid disease, tuberculosis, diabetes type 1 and 2 (T1DM and T2DM), venous thromboembolic disease). Usually, these conditions are exacerbated by pregnancy and a few occur anew such as hyperemesis gravidarum (HEG), bleeding in early and late pregnancy including ectopic pregnancy, gestational diabetes mellitus (GDM) and preeclampsia (PE). For convenience, the chapter commences with a description of conditions that occur early in pregnancy (hyperemesis) and then moves on to bleeding in early and late pregnancy including Rhesus (Rh) sensitisation. All pose challenges for the parents and their unborn baby, and the clinicians' role is to support optimal care and outcomes. This chapter builds on the philosophy, principles and actions described in previous chapters because if a midwife is to understand the parameters outside the normal she must first know the 'normal'.

Complex and high-risk childbearing

'High-risk' maternity care is not just about assessments, investigations, diagnoses, conditions and medical treatment. It is also about women from different ethnic, socioeconomic and cultural backgrounds who, while pregnant, must still face common life stressors while they deal with pregnancy complications as well as their anxieties and fears about their own and their baby's health and the wellbeing of their family (Downe et al., 2016). Thus, midwifery care is also about supporting women as they make the uncertain journey towards birth, one sometimes complicated by obstacles that result in actual or potentially life-threatening situations.

High-risk pregnancies are those complicated by one or more factors that threaten the wellbeing of the woman and her developing baby. The term 'high risk' may have different meanings to women. Mobbs et al. (2018) pose the question 'does the language we use matter?' and suggest that midwives develop a style of language that respectfully supports and empowers women. Midwives should therefore take the time to reflect on what the terms 'high risk', 'complex' and 'clinical complexity' mean for them and their practice. How women perceive their risk status or the complexity of their pregnancies affects how they think about themselves and the choices they make. For example, consider the two phrases describing so-called 'breech babies'—'a breech presentation is high risk' and 'a breech presentation is a variant of the normal'—and how this language impacts on women's emotions and choices. It is important that midwives work with women as they reflect on their perceptions of 'risk'.

VOMITING IN PREGNANCY AND HYPEREMESIS GRAVIDARUM

Nausea and vomiting of pregnancy

Nausea and vomiting of pregnancy (NVP) is a common complication of pregnancy. As many as 85%–90% of women experience nausea and/or vomiting during their pregnancies, which ranges from mild to moderate to the more severe and debilitating hyperemesis gravidarum (HEG) (Argenbright, 2017). NVP is termed a minor disorder of pregnancy, although it can have a major impact on the woman's life as they juggle caring for children, cooking nutritious meals and working while feeling nauseated (Heitmann et al., 2016). Women with NVP, and the more severe HEG, are expected to accomplish all these tasks and endure nausea and vomiting sometimes for months.

For some women NVP can be a very distressing condition that has considerable impact upon a woman's social, physical and psychological wellbeing (Argenbright, 2017). NVP usually begins between the fourth and seventh week and resolves by the 20th week of pregnancy with or without treatment. It can last for a longer period of time and occur at any time of the day, and affects each individual quite differently.

Hyperemesis gravidarum

Hyperemesis gravidarum (HEG) occurs in 0.3%–3% of pregnancies (McParlin et al., 2016). As well as its effects on women's quality of life, HEG can lead to severe medical complications. It is a debilitating illness; symptoms usually begin at about the sixth week of pregnancy and are improving by the 20th week in 90% of women, although some women continue to have recurring bouts throughout the whole pregnancy (Heitmann et al., 2016; Royal College of Obstetricians and Gynaecologists (RCOG), 2016). It is characterised by persistent and intractable vomiting leading to fluid and electrolyte depletion and imbalance, marked ketonuria, and nutritional deficiency and rapid weight loss. Severe HEG requires hospital admission and is the commonest indication for early admission to hospital during a pregnancy (Heitmann et al., 2016; RCOG, 2016).

Pathophysiology

There are a range of aetiological theories about the cause of both nausea and vomiting in pregnancy and HEG; the most common is that it is due to fluctuations in hormonal levels (Argenbright, 2017). RCOG's (2016) guideline suggests that these theories range from genetic and biochemical to feto-protective. There is scant evidence to suggest that any particular socioeconomic, racial or ethnic group is at increased risk of either NVP or HEG.

HEG is characterised by persistent, severe nausea and vomiting. Serum hCG levels peak during the first trimester, and changes in its concentration mirror the clinical course of NVP and HEG. The possible role of hCG is also supported by the observation that women with multiple gestations and molar pregnancies—conditions with higher hCG levels—are at higher risk (RCOG, 2016) (Box 37.1).

Assessment

Midwives should take a detailed history of all physical symptoms, including asking about emotional wellbeing, to identify which factors make NVP / HEG better or worse for each woman. This enquiry needs to include a detailed personal and family medical history, the times of the day when she vomits, what exactly is vomited and whether or not vomiting is associated with food intake. Accompanying symptoms to NVP may include hypersalivation, an odd metallic taste in the mouth, neck and backache, abdominal distension and discomfort, flatulence, constipation or diarrhoea. A full account of all associated symptoms is key, both to determine any other potential causes and to enable informed decision making of appropriate self-help strategies or medical treatment, if required (Argenbright, 2017).

One validated assessment tool used to try to determine the severity of NVP is the Motherisk Pregnancy Unique Quantification of Emesis and Nausea PUQE-24 scoring index (SOMANZ, 2019). This tool (Table 37.1) can be used to assist the diagnosis of HG but can also help midwives and women gauge the degree of their particular experience.

Box 37.1 Theories related to physiological factors for HEG

- Elevated pregnancy hormones (e.g. hCG, oestrogen and progesterone)—hCG levels are higher than usual in some conditions associated with hyperemesis, nausea and vomiting in pregnancy (molar pregnancy and multiple pregnancy); hCG has been associated with HEG because its peak concentration in pregnancy coincides with the peak of nausea and vomiting, especially in cases of hydatidiform molar pregnancies (see Molar pregnancy later in this chapter)
- Gastric dysrhythmias—displacement of the gastrointestinal tract, delayed gastric emptying, lower oesophageal sphincter pressure and increased levels of gastric hydrochloric acid, hyperacuity of the olfactory system, and altered hormone levels. Many pregnant women report that the smell of cooking food, particularly meat, triggers nausea. Striking similarities between HEG and motion sickness suggest that subclinical vestibular disorders may account for some cases of HEG
- Autonomic nervous system changes—in blood volume, temperature, heart rate and vascular resistance
- Nutritional deficits (e.g. trace elements—zinc, copper and pyridoxine)
- Liver enzyme abnormalities—though elevated serum bilirubin, aminotransferase and alkaline phosphatase may be secondary to HEG rather than a cause of it
- A slow adaptation of the liver to the increased levels of hormones in pregnancy, which may result in abnormal levels of serum lipids and lipoproteins
- Chronic infection with *Helicobacter pylori*
- Psychogenic factors, for example ambivalence or rejection of the pregnancy, and depression
- High thyroxine (T_4) levels

Table 37.1 PUQE-24 scoring system

☐ **Mild = 4–6**
☐ **Moderate = 7–12**
☐ **Severe ≥ 13**

1. In the last 24 hours, for how long have you felt nauseated or sick to your stomach?				
Not at all (1)	1 hour or less (2)	2–3 hours (3)	4 to 6 hours (4)	More than 6 hours (5)
2. In the last 24 hours, have you vomited or thrown up?				
I did not throw up (1)	1 to 2 (2)	3 to 4 (3)	5 to 6 (4)	7 or more times (5)
3. In the last 24 hours, how many times have you had retching or dry heaves without throwing up?				
None (1)	1 to 2 (2)	3 to 4 (3)	5 to 6 (4)	7 or more times (5)

Management

Women who develop NVP are offered a combination of behaviour and dietary interventions, complementary therapies and pharmacological treatments (Argenbright, 2017). A Norwegian study investigated the attitudes of both women and GPs about nausea in pregnancy. Women felt ignored by their GPs due to the GPs trivialising and normalising NVP (Heitmann et al., 2016). The researchers concluded that pregnant women suffering from NVP do need reassuring and comprehensive information about all treatment options before any medical treatment.

HEG can have an adverse impact upon a woman's mental health which includes social isolation, anxiety, depression, guilt, loss of self, a sense of death, suicide or termination of pregnancy. Dean et al. (2018) suggests a thorough holistic biopsychosocial assessment and treatment plan. Midwives and doctors need to encourage women to express their feelings about NVP and then feel validated by her experiences.

Collaborative support for a woman with hyperemesis

The goals of care include alleviation of nausea and vomiting, correction of dehydration and electrolyte abnormalities, prevention of extreme maternal weight loss and complications, and provision of emotional support for the woman as she deals with the stress related to the hyperemesis (Box 37.2.). Early treatment of NVP *may* prevent progression to HEG. First-line treatment involves rest and avoidance of the sensory stimuli that seem to act as triggers. Frequent small meals with avoidance of spicy or fatty foods and increasing high-protein snacks may reduce the frequency and severity of the vomiting.

Given the high risk of recurrence in a subsequent pregnancy, many women ask about preventive measures as soon as they contact their midwife. When a pregnant woman contacts her midwife with a history of persistent vomiting for most of the day, is unable to tolerate fluids and voids only small amounts of concentrated urine, an immediate midwifery assessment is warranted. In severe cases the woman will be dehydrated and will show signs of electrolyte imbalance—initially alkalosis from the loss of hydrochloric acid and then, as her condition worsens, she will become acidotic and ketonuric, hypovolaemic, hypotensive and tachycardic. If any of these signs are observed, medical referral and hospital admission are essential.

It is important to rule out other pregnancy- and non-pregnancy-related causes such as pyelonephritis, drug toxicity, biliary tract and liver disease and a molar pregnancy. Traditionally the treatment of hyperemesis has been supportive, with reassurance, dietary modifications and lifestyle changes, but there is no clear evidence of the benefits of any of these interventions (RCOG, 2016).

Hospitalisation is often required for HEG (McParlin et al., 2016; RCOG, 2016). The digestive tract is rested and intravenous fluids and electrolytes are used to replace fluids and correct electrolyte imbalances. A few women will require enteral or short-term total parenteral nutrition (TPN) via a peripherally inserted catheter (PIC) line, but these should be last-resort treatments reserved for those who continue to vomit and lose weight despite less-interventionist strategies. However, an advantage is that these can be managed at home (McParlin et al., 2016).

Box 37.2 Support for women with hyperemesis

Clinical support

Most sufferers with hyperemesis gravidarum (HEG) require multiple hospital admissions for each pregnancy. Intravenous fluids may be warmed before administration to avoid discomfort and calorie loss due to shivering. Warmed blankets will also help. If multiple intravenous sites are required, it is important to use local anaesthetics and to use the most skilled personnel to site them, to avoid undue pain and scarring. A peripherally inserted central catheter (PICC or PIC) line is useful if total parenteral nutrition is required.

Multiple intramuscular injections should be avoided because of muscle atrophy and general discomfort. It is important to minimise stimuli (light, noise and odours), as well as interruptions to the woman's rest. Occupational or physiotherapy consultations can be used to develop progressive exercise regimens that minimise muscle atrophy. Women with HEG need the chance to express their feelings in an atmosphere of compassion and empathy. These feelings should be taken seriously, and the woman with HEG needs to know that her midwife will do all she can to help her cope with the misery, stress and discomfort of HEG.

HER Foundation

The Hyperemesis Education and Research (HER) Foundation is dedicated to those suffering from HEG and those who have survived it. HER can be contacted at: http://www.hyperemesis.org.

CRITICAL THINKING EXERCISE

Francesca is 12 weeks pregnant. She comes to your clinic for her first antenatal check, and tells you that she vomits all day and 'can't keep anything down'.

Formulate questions for Francesca that will help you determine the severity of her nausea and vomiting, and the potential for HEG. Your questions should focus on:

- the frequency and severity of vomiting
- risk factors
- other symptoms such as pain or pyrexia
- tolerance of food and fluid.

Medications for HEG

A number of published reviews, including a systematic review in 2016 by McParlin et al., examined a range of pharmaceutical and non-pharmaceutical treatments for nausea and vomiting in pregnancy. In summary, they concluded that ginger, antihistamines, pyridoxine and anti-emetics for mild nausea and emesis of pregnancy were of more benefit than a placebo. When symptoms were moderate then metoclopramide (anti-emetic) or promethazine (antihistamine) or the combination of pyridoxine (vitamin B6, because a lack of pyridoxine may be a factor in NVP) with doxylamine (antihistamine) were found to be more effective than a placebo. The drug ondansetron, which has the added advantage of being given orally as a wafer, has, however, resulted in improvement in a range of symptoms for HEG. Concern has been raised over use of this drug in the first trimester so it is recommended for use only if other antiemetics are not effective (RCOG, 2016). Finally, corticosteroids may have benefit for severe cases or, as the RCOG (2016) suggests, when other therapies have failed.

Non-pharmaceutical treatments

There are a number of non-pharmacological therapies that have been used for the treatment of nausea and vomiting in pregnancy and HEG (Argenbright, 2017). Acupressure and electrical stimulation wristbands have been associated with benefit for nausea/vomiting of early pregnancy, although the evidence is mixed and limited. Ginger is another commonly recommended non-pharmacological intervention for the treatment of nausea and vomiting in pregnancy (Argenbright, 2017).

Practitioners of Traditional Chinese Medicine maintain that stimulation of acupuncture point Pericardium 6 (P6) can relieve nausea and possibly the symptoms of HEG. Acupressure can be used as an alternative or complement to Western medications. However, the data about acupressure for nausea are equivocal. 'Sea Bands' are an easy over-the-counter product that stimulates the P6 site.

Ongoing treatments

Left untreated, the woman with HEG may develop renal, neurological or hepatic damage. In severe cases, splenic avulsion, oesophageal rupture, peripheral neuropathy and preeclampsia as well as fetal intrauterine growth restriction (IUGR) and increased mortality can occur (Dean, 2018; RCOG, 2016). Termination of pregnancy may be the woman's final choice, especially if severe renal, neurological or hepatic involvement is apparent.

CLINICAL POINT

The following clinical pointers suggesting how midwives can support women with HEG are adapted from Argenbright (2017) and Dean (2018).

- Reduce stimuli and triggers as far as possible—e.g. lighting (low level lights) and noise levels (use of earplugs or headphones), odours (ventilation), motion and interruptions to rest.
- Listen: loneliness and isolation may well have featured heavily during the course of the illness.
- Watch for signs of psychological illness (repeat EDPS) and refer for assessment as appropriate if possible.
- Refer to a physiotherapist to minimise the effects of muscle atrophy.
- Ask for permission to discuss food and before mentioning food names.
- Ascertain the level of sickness by asking what foods and drinks have been tried, what has helped/what has not.
- Be careful about recommending 'cures' to an HEG sufferer; she will have been told innumerable times to try crackers and ginger.
- Do not challenge what she is or is not eating/drinking; anything is better than nothing.
- Refer to the Hyperemesis Education and Research (HER) website (http://www.hyperemesis.org) for a list of foods, drinks and vitamins that may work.
- Suggest use of the new HEG app for smartphones, details to be found on the HER site. The app will enable the woman to keep many of the details you ask for.
- Watch for signs of dehydration.
- Refer for medical assessment as appropriate.
- Alleviate any guilt and reassure her if she has been unable to take antenatal supplements.
- Remind her to take the pregnancy a day at a time and that the HEG will usually improve by the second trimester.
- Remember that pregnancy sickness is not always a 'good sign'. There are cases of women whose HEG has continued despite later discovering that the fetus died weeks earlier.
- Encourage the woman to take appropriate medication. If she cannot tolerate oral medications these may be administered intramuscularly or intravenously.
- Those with prolonged illness and inadequate medical care—e.g. those with greater than 10% loss of pre-pregnancy body weight or those who fail to gain weight for consecutive trimesters—are at increased risk of serious maternal and/or fetal complications. A referral should be made to an obstetrician or assessment unit to check for signs of IUGR.
- Remember that recovering from HEG takes time and that there may be a long-term impact on both mother and baby.

BLEEDING IN EARLY PREGNANCY

Bleeding in early pregnancy is a very distressing symptom, which leads a woman to seek reassurance that she has an ongoing pregnancy from her healthcare provider, often her GP or lead maternity carer (LMC) (Breeze, 2016). About 20%–40% of women with a clinically diagnosed pregnancy will experience bleeding during the first trimester

(Breeze, 2016) and approximately 20% of all pregnancies are thought to end in a **miscarriage** (Sheerin et al., 2019).

Miscarriage

Any bleeding in early pregnancy—that is, the first or second trimester—is considered a threatened or an actual miscarriage (abortion) until proved otherwise. Diagnosis of a miscarriage is not always possible at the first consultation and there might be a need for further investigations and referral to a gynaecologist or early pregnancy assessment service. Most miscarriages occur during the first trimester and are called 'early miscarriages'. Those occurring between 13 and 20 weeks are 'late miscarriages'. The first imperative is to establish the location of the pregnancy to exclude an ectopic pregnancy (see section on ectopic pregnancy below). Less common causes of bleeding are cervical and vaginal lesions, for example infection, cervical malignancy, cervical ectropion, polyps or a uterine infection (Breeze, 2016).

Definition and classification

Miscarriage in Australia and Aotearoa New Zealand (NZ) is defined as a pregnancy that ends spontaneously before 20 weeks' gestation or a fetal weight of less than 400 g (Breeze, 2016). This definition is *medical* and can impact on the way a miscarriage is perceived both socially and politically. However, women's grief and loss over the death of 'their baby' frequently does not fit medical terminology and its definitions. Ultrasonography and over-the-counter pregnancy tests mean that as never before women have been able to 'see and know' their baby and to bond with the child early in pregnancy. A wide range of emotions may be experienced after a miscarriage, some of which may be intense and long lasting. Grief counselling may assist and women should be asked to let their GP or midwife know if they are experiencing profound sadness verging on depression (Sumarno et al., 2020) (Box 37.3).

A miscarriage can be an intensely sad and frightening experience for everyone. A pregnancy that seemed normal suddenly ends, leaving the expectant parents devastated. For most women, pregnancy loss is associated with fear, grief, guilt and sorrow. Medical terminology such as 'spontaneous abortion', 'habitual abortion' and 'pregnancy failure' or 'abnormal pregnancy' may exacerbate the negative self-perceptions that women may already have—bringing a sense of failure, shame, guilt and insecurity (Bellhouse et al., 2019). Women-centred care is paramount to enable and support informed decision making, taking fully into account women's needs and preferences about all options for treatment in partnership with health professionals (NICE, 2019a). Midwives also need to ensure that the language they use is acceptable to the woman and other clinicians. When unsure, it is preferable to adopt the words the woman uses. The use of a common language is a step towards offering positive support for women. While there are many terms used to describe a miscarriage, it is best considered a process rather than an event. For ease of understanding in medical and hospital circles, the different 'types' of miscarriage are presented here as separate entities although they rarely occur as distinct steps.

> **Box 37.3 Miscarriage support**
>
> Miscarriage Support (http://www.miscarriagesupport.org.nz/) is a team of New Zealand volunteers who have all experienced the loss of a baby. Sharing their experience with others has assisted many women with the grieving progress and set them on the road to recovery.
>
> In Australia, an online resource provides a directory of grief and child loss counselling support groups, miscarriage support and child bereavement support groups: https://www.pregnancybirthbaby.org.au/emotional-support-after-miscarriage.

Threatened miscarriage (abortion)

Vaginal bleeding (spotting) before the 20th week of pregnancy, possibly accompanied by low back or abdominal pain, is usually the first sign of a threatened miscarriage. The bleeding is usually self-limiting, and is sometimes attributed to trophoblastic implantation within the endometrium rather than a miscarriage per se. On examination, the cervix remains closed, and the uterus is soft and non-tender and of appropriate size for gestational age. Breeze (2016) suggests that there is an increased risk (2.6 times) of miscarriage later in this pregnancy and that some women, about 17%, may go on to experience complications in pregnancy including IUGR and preterm labour.

Inevitable (imminent) miscarriage

When vaginal bleeding persists, and is accompanied by dilation of the internal cervical os or rupture of the fetal membranes, a miscarriage is usually inevitable. Bleeding is usually more severe than with a threatened miscarriage and often associated with uterine contractions. An early-pregnancy ultrasound can usually detect pregnancies that are destined to miscarry inevitably, including those that are already non-viable. Non-viable pregnancies are either a 'missed miscarriage' if an embryo or fetus is still present but is dead, or an 'anembryonic pregnancy' if no embryo has developed within the gestation sac.

Complete miscarriage

In a complete miscarriage, the products of conception have been expelled. Women report a history of vaginal bleeding, abdominal pain and perhaps passing the products of conception. Once miscarriage is completed, the bleeding and pain usually subside, the uterus contracts and the cervix closes. A completed miscarriage can be confirmed by ultrasound, which shows an empty uterus with close apposition of relatively thin and regular endometrial interfaces.

Urine or serum β-hCG values will gradually fall below discriminatory threshold levels.

Incomplete miscarriage

Not all miscarriages will be complete, however, and surgical intervention may be required to perform an ERPC (evacuation of the retained products of conception), commonly referred to as a 'dilatation and curettage' (D&C). Recent evidence suggests that expectant management (i.e. waiting for a miscarriage to finish), having medical treatment and having surgery are safe, acceptable and effective (Kim et al., 2017). The choice should be the woman's after oral and written information is given (NICE, 2019a). An incomplete miscarriage is more likely to occur between 6 and 14 weeks of pregnancy. Bleeding and pain may persist if the miscarriage is not completed, and this increases the risk of infection. Vaginal bleeding is usually heavy and accompanied by increasingly severe uterine contractions. The cervical os is open. The woman may say that she has passed fetal or placental fragments. Ultrasonography may reveal some fragments are still present in the uterus.

Silent or delayed miscarriage (missed abortion, blood mole, carneous mole or stony/fleshy mole)

Women can experience a miscarriage without knowing it. In a silent (missed) miscarriage, the fetus has died but is retained in the uterus. Uterine and breast growth cease and the woman may report vaginal 'spotting' or a brown, sometimes offensive, vaginal discharge. With widespread use of transvaginal ultrasonography, a silent miscarriage (presence of a non-viable fetus) or an anembryonic pregnancy (blighted ovum, delayed miscarriage) reflects different aspects or stages of the same clinical process. An anembryonic pregnancy occurs when a fertilised egg implants into the uterine wall but fetal development does not begin. Most are caused by chromosomal abnormalities. The woman may report that her pregnancy symptoms have stopped and there is dark-brown vaginal bleeding. Diagnosis is confirmed by the woman's story, physical examination, laboratory tests and ultrasonography. Blood and urine tests will show a drop in β-hCG levels. An ultrasound examination shows early evidence of an intrauterine pregnancy but only an empty pregnancy sac.

Septic (infected) miscarriage

In a septic miscarriage, retained products of conception become infected (Box 37.4). Septic abortion remains a leading cause of maternal death across the world, especially in countries where termination of pregnancy is illegal (WHO, 2016a). If not treated, the infection may spread into the myometrium and parametrium and cause peritonitis. In this case the woman may develop generalised septicaemia and will require aggressive antibiotic therapy. Pelvic inflammatory disease (PID) and infertility are common long-term complications of this life-threatening disorder.

Box 37.4 Signs of infected miscarriage

Any woman of childbearing age presenting with fever, tachycardia, abdominal pain, vaginal discharge or bleeding should be evaluated for a possible septic miscarriage. Immediate referral to a medical practitioner is warranted.

Warning signs include:

- history of recent pregnancy
- pyrexia and general malaise
- abdominal pain
- vaginal discharge, which may be purulent
- vaginal bleeding.

Management

Initial assessment

The first step is to consider the woman's degree of pain, bleeding and most importantly her haemodynamic stability (shock). Young women may experience a significant amount of blood loss before showing signs of being in shock so this must be considered at all times. Transfer to an emergency department for treatment is then imperative. The most common causes of shock are a massive haemorrhage after a miscarriage, a ruptured ectopic pregnancy or cervical shock due to parasympathetic nerve stimulation from retained products of conception following an incomplete miscarriage (Breeze, 2016). If this happens then a speculum examination is performed in hospital with rapid transfer to theatre for a suction curettage, laparoscopy or laparotomy.

If no signs of shock are present, then a more detailed assessment can continue in a community setting, firstly taking a detailed history, noting relevant risk factors such as previous pelvic infection or a sexually transmitted infection (STI) such as chlamydia or an intrauterine device (IUCD) as these are significant in a suspected ectopic pregnancy (Breeze, 2016).

Early-pregnancy assessment units

Sometimes the medicalisation of miscarriage means that it is viewed as a singular medical event, its 'outcome' measured in terms of subsequent complications such as infection or haemorrhage. Miscarrying women may, however, view the miscarriage holistically as an event with emotional, psychological, practical and social aspects. The woman grieves for the death of her baby and a person. In a medicalised model the 'baby' is reduced to an 'outcome' (or conceptus), which can easily be replicated. The need for formal and informal support and sensitive care for those who have experienced a miscarriage has been conclusively shown to improve outcomes. Researchers such as Bellhouse et al. (2019) and Sumarno et al. (2020) have suggested that perceptions of unsatisfactory care contribute to women's distress after the experience of a miscarriage. Some (but not enough) Australian and

New Zealand health services offer women the option of an early-pregnancy assessment service with direct access for women, midwives and medical personnel. A dedicated early-pregnancy assessment unit/clinic (EPAU/C) can streamline the management of women with early-pregnancy bleeding or pain and thus improve the quality of care in the presence of a supportive, multidisciplinary team who are educated in delivery of sensitive communication (NICE, 2019a).

To be effective, EPAU/Cs should have:

- an appointment system and be open every day, ideally for 24 hours
- a discrete waiting area and quiet and private consulting rooms
- onsite ultrasound equipment (including transvaginal probes) and/or access to ultrasound evaluation
- convenient access to laboratory facilities for Rh antibody screening as well as facilities for β-hCG and serum progesterone testing.

CLINICAL POINT

Women often report that they were not informed about the physical processes of miscarriage or that it may involve significant pain or differing levels of bleeding, the passing of tissue and clots and sometimes a discernible fetus; also that they wished they had been informed that sometimes after a miscarriage, they would require surgery.

Collaborative care

In many cases, and if the bleeding is not severe, women often prefer to wait at home, supported by their midwife, 'to see what happens' rather than attend the local hospital or EPAU/C. In most cases, the woman spontaneously passes the products of conception. Nevertheless, any bleeding in pregnancy requires medical referral because it may result in a potential risk to fetal growth and wellbeing (New Zealand College of Midwives (NZCOM), 2021).

There are three different management options for women with an incomplete miscarriage: surgical evacuation, medical therapy and expectant treatment. Management options depend largely on the woman's preferences NICE (2019a).

Investigations

In a woman bleeding in early pregnancy, a combination of measurement of serum hCG and ultrasound assessment is used. Serum hCG levels measured at intervals of 48–72 hours and that are falling usually indicate a non-viable pregnancy but do not indicate a failed uterine or an involuting ectopic pregnancy (Breeze, 2016). A non-viable pregnancy is usually seen on ultrasound; if there is any doubt a repeat scan should be done 1 week later. A pregnancy of unknown origin should be suspected if there are no signs of an intra- or extrauterine pregnancy. Magnetic resonance imaging (MRI) can be used if locally available to diagnose a caesarean scar pregnancy, the definition of which is 'implantation into the myometrium defect occurring at the previous uterine incision' (Elson et al., 2016). This may be when there is bleeding in early pregnancy, either an ongoing possibly viable pregnancy or a miscarriage within the scar. The prevalence of a caesarean scar pregnancy is thought to be 1 in 2000 pregnancies (Elson et al., 2016), but it may be higher with the increasing number of caesareans being performed worldwide.

Until the late 1980s, D&C was the 'gold standard' for management of miscarriage because it was quickly performed and it was possible to remove any remaining retained products of conception (Kim et al., 2017). Histological examination of the removed tissues also allowed exclusion of trophoblastic disease. With the advent of transvaginal sonography (TVS), clinicians have adopted a more conservative approach to management (Breeze, 2016; NICE, 2019a). Conservative or expectant approaches usually involve making the diagnosis of an incomplete miscarriage with ultrasound followed by a dose of misoprostol on its own or in combination with Mifepristone vaginally (PV) or orally depending upon the woman's choice (Kim et al., 2017; Sheerin et al., 2019; NICE, 2019a). This should be given with analgesics, an antiemetic and, importantly, information shared with women about what to expect and any potential side effects of this treatment, for example diarrhoea, vomiting and pain (NICE, 2019a). Women who miscarry should:

- be advised what to expect in the recovery period including postoperative care if they have had surgery, what to do if they become pregnant again and when to start sexual activity
- be given information on the potential impact of any treatment upon future fertility
- be guided that they can expect a grief reaction and be advised about where and how to access counselling and support services including helpline services; this should include leaflets and web-based information
- be offered the opportunity of a follow-up appointment with a health professional of their choice (NICE, 2019a)
- have their plans for follow-up clearly recorded in the discharge letter from the EPAU/C to the lead carer.

CLINICAL POINT

Retained products of conception

Hospital personnel often refer to 'products of conception' but the woman may perceive these 'products' differently. During an incomplete miscarriage, such products may be caught in the cervix, causing profound vagal stimulation, bradycardia and shock. If this is suspected, urgent hospital admission is needed. Removal of retained products leads to rapid clinical improvement and reduction in bleeding. Any tissue passed should accompany the woman to hospital.

Emotional recovery from early pregnancy loss

Cesare et al. (2020) have investigated how social media provides a support system for women who have experienced a miscarriage. Their findings showed that when 'celebrities' tell their stories, this leads to an increase of discussion about miscarriage and provides information on the public's level of understanding of miscarriage.

For some couples, miscarriage causes severe, protracted distress at a level not always appreciated by healthcare providers (Sumarno et al., 2020).

The purpose of follow-up support and counselling is to provide:

- open discussion about the loss, monitoring of progress and counselling for the woman and her partner about future pregnancies
- an opportunity for the woman and her partner to discuss their loss and have their mourning acknowledged
- the family with information about the normal grief process
- facilitation of the mourning process by enabling expression of their feelings of ambivalence, guilt and self-blame, particularly when there is no medical explanation for the miscarriage
- acknowledgement that pregnancy loss among gender-diverse couples can also be devastating
- an opportunity for the woman and her family to discuss their care and identify any issues or dissatisfaction

Before the midwife–woman relationship ends, it is important to ensure that the woman has access to physical and psychological support services for miscarriage.

A woman's story

I experienced intense grief and loss following an early miscarriage. It didn't occur to me that my body would 'fail' and I was profoundly shocked when I began to bleed at 14 weeks. My feelings, wants and hopes see-sawed—from wanting to 'get it over with' to hoping it 'wouldn't happen'. After several weeks of 'spotting' and 'not knowing' I miscarried in the toilet. I am a midwife and should have known that sometimes the miscarriage hurts but was shocked that it did! Even though I knew the baby (and it was a baby to me) was dead I immediately went to hospital for a D&C. At no time did a nurse or doctor talk to me about our loss. It was all very clinical and our conversations were limited to 'sign here', 'have you taken your wedding ring off' and 'come and see me in my rooms in 2 weeks'. I went home the next day, numb and very sad but reluctant to cry about something I knew was probably for the best. My family and friends were little different. Apart from the usual 'you can have another pregnancy' there was little acknowledgement about my 'baby'. I went back to work 2 days later and told no one. My husband didn't know what to say so he said nothing and went back to work. In retrospect we both grieved but in silence. A few weeks later a friend had a stillbirth and I felt so guilty because her loss was so much greater than mine. I can remember thinking that I had no right to be sad when my friend was suffering so much. Twelve months later I gave birth again. My pregnancy and birth were 'physiologically normal' but this time I knew my body could fail me again and experienced considerable anxiety throughout the pregnancy. My midwives did not refer to the miscarriage and neither did I—probably because it seemed 'unworthy'.

Recurrent miscarriage (habitual abortion)

The occurrence of miscarriage in healthy women is around 15%–20% and it can reoccur in 2%–3% of these women. Recurrent miscarriage is defined as the loss of three or more pregnancies before 20 weeks gestation, but experts now suggest that two or more miscarriages is enough for a diagnosis of recurrent miscarriage and that each loss requires appropriate referral and assessment (Garrido-Gimenez & Alijotas-Reig, 2015). Any miscarriage is distressing for the parents but recurrent miscarriages are devastating, especially if it is not possible to identify a cause and therefore a 'cure'. Potential parents need to know that, despite the battery of tests usually ordered during investigation of recurrent miscarriage, only 50% of couples will be given an answer for their inability to carry a live baby beyond two trimesters (Garrido-Gimenez & Alijotas-Reig, 2015). An interviewee in the study by Bellhouse et al. (2019) remarked:

> *...after my third miscarriage, like you start facing infertility at that point. So like, 'Am I not going to have a child? Am I not going to have any babies?', like that all becomes a real possibility at that point. And it can be really all consuming.*

Causes of miscarriage

The causes of miscarriage are becoming more clearly understood but clinicians are frequently unable to give grieving parents a precise response to questions about why the miscarriage occurred. Usually no treatable cause is found for a miscarriage.

In summary, when it can be determined, recurrent miscarriage may be caused by one or more of the following according to Garrido-Gimenez & Alijotas-Reig (2015):

- reproductive history—women who have had a recent live birth are less likely to have a miscarriage next pregnancy

- gestational age—miscarriages tend to occur at the same gestation
- genetic factors—in around 2%–4% of couples one of them, more often the woman, will have genetically balanced structural chromosome rearrangement
- chromosomal abnormalities—occur more frequently, in around 50%, and account for the increased risk of fetal aneuploidy
- endocrine abnormalities—occur in 15%–20% of all recurrent miscarriages, including thyroid autoimmunity, poorly controlled type 1 diabetes, coeliac disease, antiphospholipid antibodies and antiphospholipid syndrome
- inherited thrombophilic disorders
- infectious disease—but these are rare
- environmental factors—cigarette smoke, alcohol, cocaine use, moderate to heavy caffeine use and obesity are all poorly supported by current evidence.

There is emerging evidence about circulating microparticles, glycoproteins and leptin.

Rhesus sensitisation and miscarriage

Rhesus (Rh) sensitisation and disease is caused by a specific mix of blood types between a pregnant mother and her unborn baby. Rh sensitisation and disease can occur only if the mother has an RhD-negative blood type, the baby has an RhD-positive blood type, and the mother has previously been exposed to RhD-positive blood and has developed an immune response to it (known as sensitisation). Rh sensitisation can occur after a transplacental haemorrhage of <0.1 mL, and so there is a potential for sensitisation in pregnancies of less than 12 weeks gestation (Breeze, 2016). Since the late 1960s, anti-D immunoglobulin has been used successfully for Rh prophylaxis.

In Australia and New Zealand, non-sensitised Rh-negative women should be offered anti-D immunoglobulin for any sensitising event; these include: ectopic pregnancy, all threatened or diagnosed miscarriages over 12 weeks, all miscarriages, and when the uterus has been surgically evacuated (Royal Australian and New Zealand College of Obstetricians and Gynaecologists (RANZCOG), 2019).

RhD immunoglobulin should be administered as soon as possible after the sensitising event, but always within 72 hours for successful immunoprophylaxis. If RhD immunoglobulin has not been administered within 72 hours, a dose offered within 10 days may provide protection (Breeze, 2016). Administration of 250 international units (IU) RhD-Ig is sufficient to cover a fetomaternal haemorrhage (FMH) of 2.5 mL of packed fetal red blood cells (Breeze, 2016). To ensure adequate protection against immunisation this dose should be offered to every RhD-negative woman who has an indication for RhD-Ig and who has no pre-existing immune anti-D. For recurrent bleeds in an ongoing pregnancy, this dose will be effective for a period of 6 weeks up to and including 12 weeks gestation. However, a subsequent miscarriage or a procedure requiring instrumentation of the uterus requires an additional dose of RhD-Ig irrespective of when the first dose was administered (RANZCOG, 2019). Administration of 625 IU of RhD-Ig is required in multiple pregnancy. Discharge documentation should always clearly state whether or not anti-D immunoglobulin was offered, given and by whom.

Local causes of vaginal bleeding in early pregnancy

Vaginal bleeding may occur at any time in pregnancy, from benign conditions such as implantation, cervicitis or polyps, or after coitus, or from more serious conditions such as carcinoma, miscarriage, ectopic pregnancy or placenta praevia and abruption and domestic assault (domestic violence). Pregnancy can be a time of heightened risk for women with abusive partners. Violence against pregnant women can result in breast and genital injury, miscarriage, premature birth or miscarriage, later-trimester bleeding and infection, blunt or penetrating abdominal trauma, and death and so it is important that the midwife looks for signs of trauma and sexual assault. Box 37.5 summarises the causes of bleeding in early pregnancy.

Implantation bleeding

Some healthcare professionals still believe that, as the trophoblast implants into the endometrial layer of the uterus, bleeding can sometimes occur and escape from the uterine cavity into the vagina—hence the term 'implantation bleeding'. However, there is no evidence that implantation causes vaginal bleeding.

Decidual bleeding

During pregnancy, menstruation ceases. Occasionally, however, there is a slight blood loss from the decidua in the first 10 weeks of pregnancy, often at a time the period would be due. Decidual bleeding may be mistaken for a menstrual period and affect the accuracy of estimations of the expected birth date. Most pregnancies proceed without further complication.

Cervical pathology

In pregnancy the increased vascularity of the cervix may result in slight bleeding from cervical ectropion (previously called erosion). A cervical polyp may also be the cause of minimal, irregular bleeding in pregnancy. These are seen as bright-red, fleshy protrusions that extend out from the cervical canal. Treatment, if required, is left until after pregnancy has been completed

Carcinoma

Malignancy complicates as many as 1 in 1000 pregnancies. In industrialised countries such as New Zealand and Australia, carcinoma of the cervix is a serious but rare occurrence in pregnancy. Cancer of the cervix is usually detected by a Papanicolaou smear. On examination the cervix is hard and irregular and bleeds when touched. Treatment will depend on the stage of the cancer and the stage of the pregnancy. For cervical cancer found to be at

Box 37.5 Causes of bleeding in early pregnancy

- Decidual bleeding
- Miscarriage
- Ectopic pregnancy
- Termination of pregnancy
- General maternal causes:
  - chronic maternal disease
  - infection (bacterial vaginosis)
  - hormonal deficiencies
  - nutritional deficiency
  - poorly controlled diabetes
  - thyroid disease
  - autoimmune disease—systemic lupus erythematosus
- Local maternal causes:
  - weakened cervix
  - abnormally shaped uterus
  - rarely a retroverted gravid uterus
  - polycystic ovary syndrome
- Other maternal causes:
  - lifestyle factors (smoking, illicit and licit drug and alcohol abuse)
  - environmental and workplace hazards
  - increased maternal age
- Hydatidiform mole
- Cervical pathology:
  - dysplasia
  - polyp
  - carcinoma
- Vaginal bleeding from non-pregnant horn of a bicornuate uterus
- Urinary tract infection
- Haemorrhoids
- Ruptured vulval varicosities

a very early stage, or for cancer found during the last trimester of pregnancy, it may be possible to delay treatment until after the baby is born.

Cervicitis and/or vaginitis

An increased vaginal discharge is normal in pregnancy. Normal pregnancy discharge, known as leucorrhoea, is non-irritating and has no odour. Vaginal discharge may also be a symptom of genital infection. Vaginitis and cervicitis are usually due to STIs, or trichomoniasis or candidiasis (thrush) infection. Microscopic examination of the discharge isolates the cause of the infection, which is then treated with antibiotics.

Haemorrhoids/vulval varicosities/urinary tract infection

While not strictly pregnancy-related bleeding, a urinary tract infection (UTI) presenting as haematuria can be the cause of a woman presenting with bleeding in pregnancy. Similarly, bleeding from haemorrhoids or vulval varicosities needs to be excluded in any assessment of bleeding in pregnancy.

Molar pregnancy (gestational trophoblastic disease)

Following a silent miscarriage, a few women develop gestational trophoblastic disease. This term covers a spectrum of disorders characterised by abnormal and rapid growth of trophoblastic tissue, ranging from a **molar pregnancy (hydatidiform mole)** to a malignant choriocarcinoma. Trophoblastic disease is rare, occurring in 1 out of every 1000 pregnancies in Europe and north America, but in Asia can be around 2 out of every 1000 pregnancies (Lurain, 2019). The condition varies between regions and age groups. The reasons for these geographic and age differences are unknown but may be related to poor nutrition, particularly a low intake of carotene (vitamin A precursor).

The main risk factor for a molar pregnancy is advanced maternal age—women over 40 having greater chance of a molar pregnancy (Lurain, 2019). In addition, women who have had a prior molar pregnancy have a 1 in 100 chance of having another in a subsequent pregnancy.

Complete and partial molar pregnancies (hydatidiform moles)

Molar pregnancies are the result of a genetic error during fertilisation and comprise two distinct entities (Lurain, 2019). Irrespective of whether they are complete or partial, a molar pregnancy poses a threat to the woman not only because it produces an abnormal pregnancy, but also because it may cause life-threatening complications.

Hydatidiform mole can be subdivided into complete and partial moles based on genetic and histopathological features. Complete moles are diploid and androgenetic in origin, with no evidence of fetal tissue (Lurain, 2019). They arise from the fertilisation of an 'empty egg'—one that has lost its maternal genetic material. There is no embryo and no normal placental tissue. However, the placenta continues to grow and produces β-hCG, so the woman thinks and feels that she is pregnant. A complete mole demonstrates a characteristic vesicular pattern (resembling a bunch of grapes).

Partial moles are triploid in origin with two sets of paternal haploid genes and one set of maternal haploid genes (Lurain, 2019). They occur, in almost all cases, following dispermic fertilisation of an ovum. Thus a partial mole has duplicate paternal genetic material while the maternal chromosomal complement is intact, so the genetic material is in triplicate. The embryo has 69 chromosomes instead of the normal 46. The fetus nearly always dies in utero.

Signs

The typical clinical presentation of complete molar pregnancies has changed with the advent of high-resolution ultrasonography. Most are now diagnosed in the first trimester before the onset of the classic signs and symptoms (Lurain, 2019). Women with a 'partial mole' usually report signs and symptoms consistent with an incomplete or late miscarriage abortion (e.g. vaginal bleeding and absence of fetal heart tones).

A molar pregnancy begins 'normally' and may entail common signs and symptoms of pregnancy: a missed period, positive pregnancy test and nausea. From about the 10th week, most women report dark-brown vaginal bleeding and perhaps pass vesicular tissue. These symptoms usually mimic those of a miscarriage, although about 50% of women with a complete mole have uterine enlargement that is too advanced for the expected gestational age. Rarely, PE may develop before the 20th week of pregnancy. A few women have signs of hyperthyroidism.

Women with partial molar pregnancies usually have fewer symptoms, and so the condition is often confirmed only on histological examination following treatment for a silent or inevitable miscarriage. They rarely have abnormally excessive uterine enlargement, hyperthyroidism or PE. Occasionally the fetus survives beyond 16 weeks and diagnosis is confirmed on ultrasound.

Medical diagnosis

The widespread use of ultrasound has led to earlier diagnosis of pregnancy and has changed the pattern of molar pregnancy (Lurain, 2019). The 'gold standard' of diagnosis remains the characteristic vesicular appearance of the placenta on ultrasound scan, typically a 'cluster of grapes' or a 'snowstorm' appearance (Fig. 37.1). Initially, levels of β-hCG—although not diagnostic—are often higher than normal with a complete mole but lower than normal with a partial mole (Lurain, 2019).

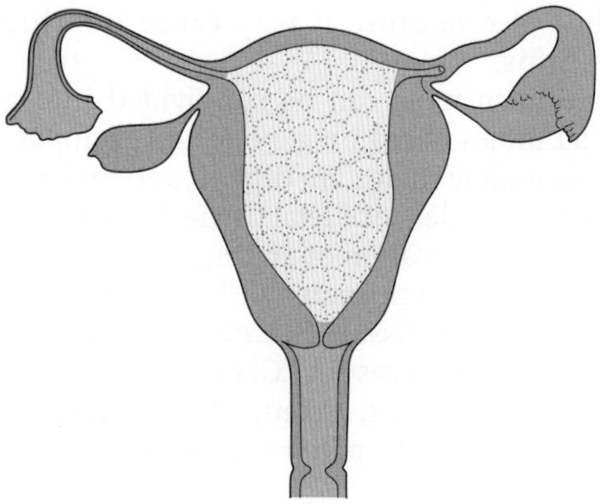

FIGURE 37.1 Molar pregnancy. A grape-like cluster of tissue (called a hydatidiform mole) forms around the area that normally would become the placenta, and may cause life-threatening complications

In a twin pregnancy, where there is one viable fetus and the other pregnancy is molar, the pregnancy should be allowed to proceed if the mother wishes. The probability of achieving a viable baby is around 40% without a significant risk of gestational trophoblastic neoplasia (GTN) (Lurain, 2019) but there is an increased risk of maternal complications such as pulmonary embolism and PE.

Collaborative management

A molar pregnancy is a very frightening experience. Not only does the woman lose a pregnancy, but she also learns that she has a risk, albeit a slight one, of developing trophoblastic disease and perhaps GTN, a fast-growing but rare malignant growth of the chorion (Lurain, 2019). In order to protect the woman from these complications, all molar tissue is removed from the uterus (Lurain, 2019). In the first trimester this is usually done with suction curettage, sometimes followed by surgical curettage, under general anaesthesia. In the second trimester, uterine stimulation with prostaglandin E_2 and an oxytocin infusion followed by surgical evacuation helps to avoid the risk of uterine perforation and haemorrhage (Lurain, 2019). If the mole is extensive and the woman has decided against future pregnancies, she may be advised to have a hysterectomy.

Follow-up

All women who have had a molar pregnancy are advised to have regular β-hCG urine tests, because molar pregnancies can recur, and to ensure that no chorionic tissue remains in the uterus because of the risk of choriocarcinoma. Follow-up may include chest X-ray, review of pathology specimens and regular physical examinations of the uterus until it returns to normal size (Lurain, 2019). Women should be advised not to conceive until β-hCG levels have been normal for 6 months.

Ectopic pregnancy

As a midwife may be the first point of contact for a pregnant woman in early pregnancy, it is vital that midwives have knowledge and understanding about ectopic pregnancy. A prompt diagnosis is vital and may even save the woman's life (Montgomery et al., 2017). An ectopic pregnancy occurs if a fertilised ovum implants at a site other than the endometrial lining of the uterus; in 95% of cases this is in a fallopian tube, although ovarian, cervical and abdominal pregnancies are also possible. The incidence of ectopic pregnancy is estimated to be 1%–3% of all pregnancies, with associated causation of maternal mortality and morbidity in the first trimester (Montgomery et al., 2017).

The diagnosis of ectopic pregnancy can be made by non-invasive methods, primarily by high-resolution transvaginal scan (TVS). Improvements and greater efficiency in diagnosis have resulted in a range of both conservative and radical treatment options.

Tubal ectopic pregnancy

In a tubal ectopic pregnancy, the blastocyst embeds in the epithelium of the fallopian tube, burrowing into blood vessels in the same way that it does in a normal implantation, and continues to develop and increase in size.

Abdominal ectopic pregnancy

In an intra-abdominal ectopic pregnancy, implantation occurs within the intraperitoneal cavity. The placenta attaches to an abdominal structure, usually the surface of the uterus, broad ligaments or ovaries. Because the invading trophoblastic tissue is not held in check, it can erode major blood vessels because they are not cushioned by the myometrium.

Low-lying implantation ectopic pregnancy

This term is used to include both cervical ectopic pregnancy and caesarean scar pregnancy. In cervical ectopic pregnancy the fertilised ovum bypasses the uterine endometrium and implants itself in the cervical mucus. In a caesarean scar pregnancy (CSP) the ovum embeds within myometrium and fibrous tissue of the caesarean scar and can occur following multiple caesarean births; it has an incidence of 1/1800, and can cause life-threatening haemorrhage (Knat-Petkas et al., 2016).

Risk factors for ectopic pregnancy

Montgomery et al. (2017) point out that, although there are identifiable risk factors for an ectopic pregnancy, about one-third of women will not have any of these. The prime risk factors are a previous ectopic pregnancy, a history of infertility, IVF (in vitro fertilisation), smoking, tubal blockage or damage following surgery or following chlamydia trachomatis infection (Montgomery et al., 2017). Lesser-known risk factors are advancing maternal age, previous spontaneous miscarriages and a partner who smokes—all of these offer the opportunity for lifestyle information sharing by the midwife.

Clinical presentation

In the Western world it is rare for women with an ectopic pregnancy to present to a maternity setting with collapse and shock. Most are diagnosed before they rupture—women often report non-specific vague symptoms that can be confused with signs of miscarriage, an ovarian cyst or pelvic inflammatory disease (PID). In the initial stages of an ectopic pregnancy, although the fertilised ovum embeds into the fallopian tube the uterus still undergoes the normal changes of early pregnancy, and so the woman experiences the normal symptoms of pregnancy. Women who present to hospital in severe shock usually report warning signs that have been overlooked. While the woman typically has experienced non-specific signs similar to those of a threatened miscarriage, she may complain of lower abdominal pain that precedes bleeding. Immediately prior to rupture, increasing abdominal pain is felt and rigidity and rebound tenderness are palpable. These signs, especially if they are accompanied by vaginal bleeding, may initially be minimal but may quickly become torrential, together with signs of haemodynamic compromise / shock—hypotension, tachycardia, pallor, cold clammy skin, faintness and vomiting—and should always alert the lead carer to the possibility of a ruptured ectopic pregnancy. In addition, shoulder-tip pain may be present, or pain may be referred to an iliac fossa. A mass may be felt to one side of the uterus. Any woman presenting with these signs requires immediate transfer to hospital and specialist consultation. If the clinical diagnosis is still unclear, an ultrasound scan will confirm or exclude the presence of an extrauterine gestational sac and, occasionally, a viable fetus.

CLINICAL POINT

Always consider the possibility of ectopic pregnancy in women of childbearing age with abdominal pain (NICE, 2019a). A sexually active woman with abdominal pain and vaginal bleeding after an interval of amenorrhoea has an ectopic pregnancy until proved otherwise! If there is no history of a missed period, check whether the last period was normal in duration and blood loss. The index of suspicion rises if the woman reports a history of infertility, has missed a period while using an IUCD, or has been sterilised. Always ask about contraception use and remember that not all women will disclose being sexually active. Others may not be aware that they are pregnant.

Diagnosis

Imaging studies

Transvaginal ultrasound is used to diagnose an ectopic pregnancy (Elson et al., 2016; Montgomery, 2017). If there are concerns or a pregnancy is not identified within the uterus, serum β-hCG levels can help to confirm pregnancy when used in conjunction with transvaginal ultrasonography.

Laboratory studies

In a pregnancy of unknown location, a diagnosis can't be made based upon a single serum β-hCG analysis. The recommendation is that two serum β-hCG are done over a period of 48 hours (NICE, 2019a).

Collaborative management of a woman with an ectopic pregnancy

A woman with classic signs of a ruptured ectopic pregnancy plus signs of haemodynamic compromise needs rapid transfer to a healthcare facility with the resources to support a critically ill woman. Venous access is obtained before transport or en route for cross-matching of blood and so as to administer intravenous (IV) fluids to maintain blood pressure. The receiving unit is alerted before arrival. On arrival at the medical facility, treatment consists of resuscitation (according to local or national guidelines) followed by immediate surgery, possibly with laparotomy to remove the blood and blood clot and to stop the bleeding. It is often necessary to remove the fallopian tube.

CLINICAL POINT

The ABCs are the mainstay of all primary resuscitative efforts for a woman in shock from a ruptured ectopic pregnancy. If the radial pulse is palpable, the blood pressure can be assumed to be adequate. If it is not palpable, restore circulation volume by giving IV fluids until the radial pulse is palpable again. It is crucial that lines of communication between care providers, the woman and her family are accurate and timely.

Options for management of ectopic pregnancy

Three options for ongoing management are most commonly used: (i) expectant or conservative, (ii) surgical management (salpingectomy or salpingostomy) and (iii) medical management (methotrexate).

Expectant management

Expectant management is used for women with declining β-hCG levels, minimal or no pain and who are able to attend a follow-up appointment, ideally at an early pregnancy assessment unit (Montgomery et al., 2017).

Surgical management of an ectopic pregnancy

Most women with an ectopic pregnancy undergo surgical management. The two options are a salpingectomy (removal of the fallopian tube) or a salpingotomy (removal of the ectopic pregnancy and preservation of the fallopian tube). Women choosing to have a salpingotomy should be informed that there is a need to monitor their β-hCG levels. Laparoscopy is the common surgical method used and women can be discharged the same day, with a supportive psychological support plan, and pain control as long as they are haemodynamically stable (Montgomery et al., 2017; NICE, 2019a).

Medical management of an ectopic pregnancy

Medical therapy of ectopic pregnancy is appealing over surgical options for a number of reasons, including eliminating morbidity from surgery and general anaesthesia, potentially less tubal damage, and less cost and need for hospitalisation. Methotrexate is used in the treatment of ectopic pregnancy directly using ultrasound or as single or multiple intramuscular injections.

Treatment with methotrexate requires follow up including serum β-hCG levels on days 4 and 7. Importantly, the woman is advised not to become pregnant again for at least 3 months, and her liver function tests need to be normal. All of this is because methotrexate is a chemotherapeutic treatment with adverse side effects.

Woman-focused information about their postoperative care (for women undergoing surgery) and follow-up care includes:

- information about resuming normal activity and the emotional impact of the loss of a baby on the family's life
- potential future complications and what to do next time if the woman becomes pregnant again (advice about how long to wait before trying to conceive)
- what follow-up support is available from within the hospital and formal and informal support groups
- how the woman can contact a healthcare professional for postoperative advice, and who this will be
- how to find further information—for example, on when to return to work.

Fertility after treatment

The prognosis for women with an ectopic pregnancy is good, provided there is early diagnosis and prompt, effective treatment. Fertility may be preserved, especially if there is early diagnosis followed by conservative management.

BLEEDING IN THE SECOND AND THIRD TRIMESTERS OF PREGNANCY

Antepartum haemorrhage

Antepartum haemorrhage (APH) is defined as any bleeding from the genital tract after the 24th week of pregnancy and before the onset of labour (Varouxaki et al., 2018) (Box 37.6).

Decisions about the management of an APH depend on:

- whether the bleeding has settled or stopped
- whether the bleeding continues but is not life threatening
- whether the bleeding continues and is life threatening
- the condition of the fetus
- the gestational age of the pregnancy.

CLINICAL POINT

Placenta praevia and placental abruption can produce massive obstetric haemorrhage without any warning. With placental abruption, the clinician may not be aware of the full extent of the blood loss because a proportion of the blood may be concealed behind the placenta. Pregnant women may remain haemodynamically stable until they lose between a third and a half of their circulating blood volume.

Box 37.6 Causes of antepartum haemorrhage

- Bleeding from a normally situated placenta (accidental haemorrhage)
- Placental abruption (concealed, revealed, combined)
- Bleeding from an abnormally situated placenta (unavoidable or inevitable haemorrhage):
  - placenta praevia
  - placenta percreta/accreta/increta
- Extraplacental/incidental causes:
  - ruptured uterus/dehiscence of uterine scar (complete or incomplete)
  - ruptured vasa praevia
  - excessive bloody show
  - cervical erosion, polyp, carcinoma
  - vaginitis
  - urinary tract infection
  - haemorrhoids
  - bleeding from the non-pregnant horn of a bicornuate uterus
  - ruptured vulval varicosities.

Placental abruption

Placental abruption is defined as bleeding caused by premature separation of a normally situated placenta from the myometrium in the uterus. If bleeding occurs in the decidua basalis under the placenta, a haematoma is formed, which eventually leads to separation in various degrees of the placenta from the maternal vascular system (Giordano et al., 2010, Varouxaki et al., 2018). Placental separation may be partial or complete.

The precise aetiology is uncertain but documented associations are (RCOG, 2011a):

- factors predisposing to an abruption, including bleeding prior to 20 weeks of pregnancy, chronic hypertension, PE, thrombophilia, previous placental abruption, IVF, fetal growth restriction, advanced maternal age, low body mass index, non-vertex presentations, domestic violence, smoking, cocaine and amphetamine use
- sudden reduction in size of an overdistended uterus, e.g. rupture of the membranes in association with polyhydramnios, between births of multiple pregnancies
- trauma, e.g. motor vehicle accident.

Classification of placental abruption

Placental abruption is described as the separation of a normally situated placenta; the diagnosis is based upon findings during an abdominal ultrasound, or if an emergency through clinical presentation and placental examination at birth (Kasai et al., 2014). See Fig. 37.2:

- *Concealed*—the separation occurs near the centre of the site of the placental attachment; blood cannot escape so it is retained between the uterine wall and the placenta as a large retroplacental haematoma. In severe cases, the blood infiltrates the myometrium until the uterus becomes swollen and engorged with blood; this is known as a Couvelaire uterus, and increases the woman's risk of postpartum haemorrhage (PPH) because the uterus loses its ability to contract and retract postpartum.

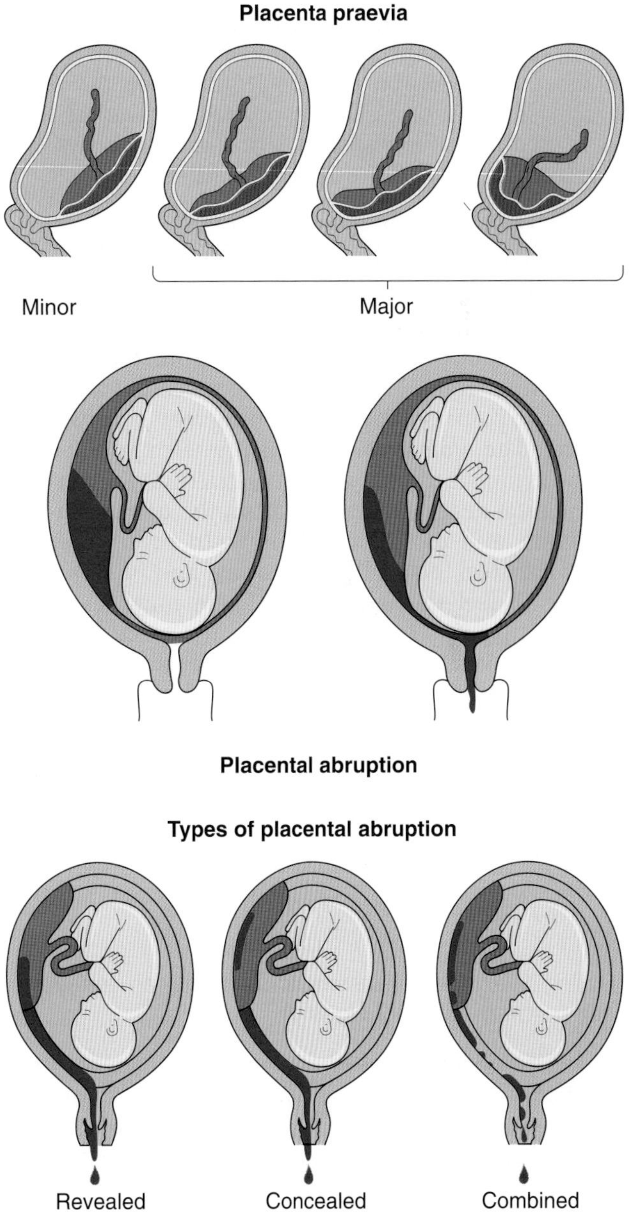

FIGURE 37.2 Placenta praevia and placental abruption (Based on Oats & Abraham, 2004)

- *Revealed*—the separation occurs near the edge of the placenta and blood tracks down between the membranes and the decidua, through the cervix and into the vagina and is seen at the vulva. The woman's condition is relative to the amount of blood loss.
- *Partially separated*—this is a combination of concealed and revealed bleeding, where some of the blood escapes into the vagina, the rest remaining trapped in the uterus.

Incidence

Placental abruption complicates around 3%–5% of pregnancies (RCOG, 2011a) and it is associated with a high perinatal mortality rate of over 300 per 1000 diagnosed, with greater than half of perinatal demises occurring before admission to hospital. A history of an abruption in a previous pregnancy increases the risk, as does hypertension and preeclampsia, smoking, bleeding in the first trimester and cocaine use (Varouxaki et al., 2018). Regardless of these associations and risk factors many placental abruptions can occur in a pregnancy with no obvious complexity (Varouxaki et al., 2018).

Clinical presentation and diagnosis

A placental abruption most commonly presents with vaginal bleeding associated with a variable degree of abdominal pain. This is in contrast to the painless bleeding of placenta praevia or bleeding from the cervix or lower genital tract. However, some placental abruption can also be painless. Vaginal bleeding may occur without warning. The woman may be in pre-term labour; there may be evidence of fetal growth restriction or even intrauterine fetal death. On examination the uterus is tender to palpate, and pain is continuous. In severe cases the uterus may feel 'board like or woody' and it is often impossible to feel the fetal parts. There may be referred shoulder-tip pain.

However, it is important to remember there may be no evidence of vaginal bleeding (in completely or partially concealed APH); or the blood may be bright, dark or intermixed with amniotic fluid. A chronic form of abruption may manifest as recurrent vaginal bleeding with episodic pain and uterine contractions.

CLINICAL POINT

During the initial assessment following an antepartum haemorrhage, look for signs of:

- cardiovascular collapse
- shock
- sepsis
- rigid abdomen
- heavy vaginal bleeding
- complications of labour
- fetal compromise.

No vaginal examinations should be performed until the cause of the bleeding is found in case the examining fingers rupture a placental blood vessel.

The vaginal bleeding may be:

- *mild*—with some abdominal pain, a non-tender uterus and a live fetus; the woman shows no signs of haemodynamic compromise
- *moderate*—with stronger abdominal or back pain, perhaps uterine contractions, a firm, tender uterus and signs of fetal distress; cardiotocography (CTG) and Doppler sonography reveal ominous features and the woman will exhibit some degree of hypovolaemic shock
- *profuse*—with severe abdominal pain, a 'board-like', enlarging, tender uterus that fails to relax. Usually no fetal heart tones are heard on auscultation and an ultrasound scan shows fetal demise. The woman will be severely shocked, to a degree often out of proportion to the amount of visible blood loss. In severe cases, significant amounts of thromboplastin are released into the circulation, making the woman at risk of disseminated intravascular coagulation (DIC) (see also Ch. 40).

CLINICAL POINT

Midwives should remember that if they observe vaginal bleeding it is also likely that there is a significant concealed quantity of blood in the uterus. Revealed loss is invariably underestimation of the total blood loss. In the presence of a typical severe abruption (with fetal death), the woman will probably require at least 4–6 units of blood owing to the concealed haemorrhage. Considerable further blood loss should be anticipated around the time of birth. There are degrees of abruption that will reflect the range of maternal and fetal compromise.

Management

Immediate management

Community-based midwives should ask women to immediately contact them if they experience blood loss during their pregnancy. Management of APH depends on the nature and severity of clinical signs and symptoms. An initial assessment at home by the midwife may be indicated, if the bleeding is minimal or occurred some days prior, to assess the woman's and baby's wellbeing. However, it is important to remember that the observed blood loss may not give an accurate picture of the extent of the bleeding. Midwives should consult a medical practitioner following signs of vaginal bleeding. If the bleeding is moderate, the woman is advised to seek immediate midwifery/medical advice followed usually by timely admission to a maternity unit to confirm the cause of the bleeding as well as assessment of wellbeing. If bleeding is severe, after initial maternal resuscitation and stabilisation at home, prompt admission to a maternity unit is essential (Box 37.7). After 20 weeks of pregnancy all cases of vaginal bleeding are treated as if the cause was a placenta praevia until proven otherwise by an ultrasound scan or clinical diagnosis. The woman and her family/whānau should be treated respectfully and kept fully informed of all procedures to enable mutual trust and confidence to develop (RCOG, 2011a). Ongoing effective communication between the collaborative healthcare team assists with this process (RCOG, 2011a).

Assessment

A thorough assessment of maternal and fetal wellbeing allows clinicians to implement an action plan based on the degree of maternal and fetal compromise and the quantity and type of blood loss. It includes:

- *history*—risk factors (i.e. trauma, hypertension, drug use), estimated birth date, gestation, parity
- *vaginal loss*—volume, old or new blood, clots, tissue, products of conception and liquor. All pads and linen are saved for inspection and weighing; the quantity of revealed blood loss should be estimated and clinical signs (blood pressure, pulse, respiration rate)
- *general signs*—blood pressure, pulse, colour, respiration rate, oxygen saturation levels, urinary output, anxiety (i.e. signs and symptoms of hypovolaemic shock), signs of DIC, fetal heart sounds (or heart beat on ultrasound or CTG)
- *urine output*—should be at least 30 mL/h; an indwelling urinary catheter with a urometer will assist with accurate measuring of output.

Box 37.7 Emergency treatment of abruption

- Call for help and arrange escorted transfer to obstetric unit for further assessment even if bleeding seems to settle, as the fetus may still be compromised or the blood loss concealed.
- Treat shock beginning with the ABCs.
- Keep talking to the woman and her support people.
- Give oxygen via facemask at 6–8 L/min.
- Insert IV lines (two wide-bore cannulae); consider the use of CVP/arterial monitoring.
- Cross-match 6 units of blood, FBC, coagulation profile, including platelets and Kleihauer–Betke tests.
- Ongoing and accurate evaluation of blood loss.
- Restore blood loss quickly with IV fluids—replace estimated losses plus 2 L of IV fluid. Give isotonic solutions followed by colloids until packed cells are available
- Urinary catheterisation to monitor output and keep output at >30 mL/h.
- Ultrasound examination if the placenta is unsighted or if history or clinical features suggest placenta praevia.
- Continuous monitoring of fetus, mother and labour (vital signs, fluid balance intake and output) in a high-dependency unit.

(See also Ch. 40)

ABC = airway, breathing and circulation; CVP = central venous pressure; FBC = full blood count; IV = intravenous.

Initial assessment and management

Maternal assessments include:

- *gentle abdominal palpation*—to assess tenseness of uterus and measurement of uterine size/abdominal girth and to observe for signs of labour; a hard 'woody' uterus is pathognomonic of placental abruption; an engaged vertex almost always excludes a major degree of placenta praevia
- *CTG (EFM)*—(dependent on gestation) to assess fetal status and contraction pattern; contractions are often frequent with a short resting period between the contractions
- *haemoglobin, coagulation studies*—to exclude disseminated intravascular coagulopathy as a consequence of large blood loss; fibrinogen levels increase in pregnancy, therefore 'normal' or low fibrinogen levels and a prolonged prothrombin time are suggestive of DIC
- *Kleihauer–Betke test or flow cytometry*—to measure the degree of fetomaternal haemorrhage
- *ultrasound*—to look for evidence of a retroplacental haematoma, increased placental thickness or echogenicity
- *woman's emotional status*—including ability to cope
- *gentle vaginal examination with a sterile speculum only*—to assess the site of bleeding, cervical changes and evidence of liquor.

Fetal assessments: all pregnancies that have had a placental abruption require increased fetal surveillance. The woman should be carefully advised with respect to the observation of fetal movements and the reporting of any decrease in fetal activity. Regular and ongoing CTG and serial ultrasound scans are appropriate and should be tailored according to the woman's and fetal wellbeing.

Once the maternal condition has stabilised, an ultrasound will exclude placenta praevia, determine the site and degree of placental separation and confirm fetal position and presentation. If necessary, the woman is referred to a specialist team and ongoing management of midwifery and obstetric care is transferred to the hospital collaborative team. Ultrasound is not advised as a diagnostic tool due to decreased sensitivity; instead, the initial diagnosis should be based upon presentation and observation (Varouxaki et al., 2018).

Ongoing management

Ongoing management depends on the diagnosis, gestation, viability and condition of the fetus, the amount of bleeding and the degree of maternal haemodynamic compromise. Corticosteroids should be administered (if necessary and if no contraindications) for fetal lung maturation in pregnancies of less than 34 weeks gestation. For women who are bleeding from an abruption and experiencing uterine contractions, the use of tocolysis is controversial and should be used only with caution by experienced clinicians (RCOG, 2011a). Intravenous magnesium sulfate may be considered for neuroprotection in pregnancies where birth is planned at less than 30 weeks gestation, especially if the woman is to be transferred to a tertiary hospital (Doyle et al., 2009). Similarly, the administration of narcotic analgesia requires careful consideration because of the risks to the pre-term infant. The woman should be asked to consent to have 625 IU anti-D, as an intramuscular injection, if she is Rhesus D negative. Additional doses of anti-D immunoglobulin may be required if the Kleihauer–Betke test indicates a large fetomaternal haemorrhage.

Even after a 'minor' APH, bed rest and close monitoring in hospital for at least 24 hours is recommended. If the bleeding ceases and maternal and fetal condition remain stable, discharge home to care of the community-based midwife may be indicated. Serial ultrasonography and antepartum surveillance in the third trimester are appropriate for women with chronic (repeated) abruption because of the potential for uteroplacental insufficiency. Women who smoke cigarettes or engage in recreational drug use should be advised of the strong association with placental abruption.

Expediting the birth of the fetus and placenta are the definitive treatments following an APH. Some women will begin labour spontaneously; if not, induction of labour and artificial rupture of membranes (ARM) may facilitate a vaginal birth—the decision is determined by the degree of blood loss and gestation. A caesarean section may be the safest option, especially if the haemorrhage is severe. If the fetus is dead, vaginal birth is then the preferable option because the effects of serious coagulation defects are less dangerous than with a caesarean section. There is, however, a significant danger that consumptive DIC may develop with hypofibrinogenaemia. Persistent haemorrhage after birth may be due to coagulopathy, a Couvelaire uterus, an atonic uterus or trauma.

The Australian 3 Centres Collaboration (2010) and RCOG (2011a) guidelines state that, if the baby has died, conservative management of the birth in consultation with the woman is an option in the presence of an abruption. However, this does not apply if there is a major abruption. In these instances birth should be expedited and managed by an experienced multidisciplinary team. For women at or near term, even if the current abruption appears to be minimal, birth is recommended owing to the risk of further, possibly catastrophic placental abruption. Between 32 and 37 weeks, conservative management can be considered for what appears to be only a minor placental abruption. However, if there is substantive revealed blood loss together with significant uterine tenderness, evidence of coagulopathy or fetal compromise, birth should be expedited. Between 28 and 32 weeks gestation and in cases of extreme prematurity (less than 28 weeks), conservative management may be considered even in the presence of substantive revealed bleeding and significant uterine tenderness—provided both maternal and fetal conditions are stable and the mother is fully informed of the risks and benefits of each mode of birth. Decisions on birth timing must weigh the risks of the maternal condition and prematurity against those of continuing the pregnancy.

Place of birth

In all cases, women will be referred to an obstetrician, many are admitted to hospital and many will remain as inpatients until birth. There is, however, minimal robust evidence that the policy of 'routine admission' is efficacious. After a period of assessment, some women may be discharged home to their primary care midwife or GP and monitored at home provided that if bleeding restarts they have ready access to hospital, collaborative care and:

- the initial bleeding has completely abated and there is no further evidence of haemorrhage
- clinical features were those of a minor placental abruption (low volume revealed blood loss and minimal uterine tenderness)
- tests of fetal and maternal wellbeing are reassuring.

Women who have experienced bleeding are at risk of having a PPH. Chapter 40 discusses its management in more detail.

Complications of abruption

Postpartum haemorrhage is relatively common following a placental abruption and may occur as a consequence of both a bleeding disorder (thrombocytopenia +/− DIC) and uterine atony. The latter may occur in association with a Couvelaire uterus—where blood has suffused into the myometrium, giving the serosal surface a mottled black appearance. Uterotonic agents such as oxytocin, ergometrine and prostaglandin analogues may be administered according to the local policy and keeping in mind contraindications and possible adverse effects. Platelets and clotting factors should be replaced.

Rare and ongoing complications

Sheehan's syndrome (anterior pituitary necrosis) is a rare complication following massive haemorrhage. Women with this condition demonstrate the symptoms of amenorrhoea, failure to lactate, coarsening of the hair and skin, feeling cold and, later, genital atrophy and premature sterility.

Placenta praevia

Placenta praevia occurs when the placenta is inserted wholly or partly into the lower segment of the uterus in the third trimester of pregnancy (see Fig. 37.2). Placental pathology may identify the aetiology and pathophysiology of an abruption. Abnormalities such as placental thrombosis, perivillous fibrin deposition, infarction and decidual abnormalities may be observed. The diagnosis is made by transvaginal ultrasound, where the distance between the inferior edge of the placenta and the internal cervical os is measured. If the placenta lies over the cervical os, it is considered a major placenta praevia; otherwise it is considered a minor placenta praevia. TVS or translabial ultrasound is the preferred method for localisation of a low-lying placenta (RCOG, 2011b). Both have been shown to be significantly more accurate than transabdominal sonography and are safe to perform even in the presence of bleeding. TVS makes it easier to identify an anterior than a posteriorly located placenta praevia. This is because the fetus often obscures the leading edge of a posterior placenta. However, many women find TVS invasive and prefer transabdominal sonography.

The low-lying placenta

A low-lying placenta occurs in 28% of pregnancies found at the 20-week anomaly scan but most will have moved higher by a subsequent scan at 32–34 weeks with an incidence of around 3% at term (Varouxaki et al., 2018). The change of placental position results from the formation of the lower uterine segment, which moves the placenta upwards with the expanding uterus. If there is still evidence of a low-lying placenta then women should be forewarned by their primary community-based midwife that they may be at risk of placenta praevia, advised that this increases the risk of vaginal bleeding and informed about the urgent need for midwifery / medical attention if they have any vaginal bleeding until the diagnosis has been confirmed.

The maternal mortality rate secondary to placenta praevia is approximately 0.03%. Babies born to women with placenta praevia tend to have a higher incidence of intrauterine growth restriction according to a systematic review and meta-analysis by Balayla et al. (2019).

Incidence

The incidence of placenta praevia is on the rise, primarily resulting from an increase in caesarean sections, along with a growing number of complications from this operation such as placenta accreta; it is also associated with increasing maternal age (RCOG, 2011b; Varouxaki et al., 2018).

Causes

There is no known 'cause' of placenta praevia, it is thought to be primarily due to prepregnancy factors (Varouxaki et al., 2018). The predisposing factors include:

- uterine scarring (especially following repeated caesarean sections, myomectomy, etc.) is a major risk factor for placenta praevia; as the number of caesareans increases, so too will the prevalence of placenta praevia and placenta accreta
- past history of placenta praevia
- a large placenta (e.g. with fetal erythroblastosis or multiple pregnancy)
- high parity
- an abnormally shaped uterus (e.g. fibroids, bicornuate uterus)
- artificial reproductive technology (in vitro fertilisation, gamete intrafallopian transfer)
- advancing maternal age.

Clinical presentation and diagnosis

Women with a placenta praevia generally present in the following ways:

- with an antepartum haemorrhage
- as a finding on ultrasound in an asymptomatic woman
- with a fetal malpresentation or a high mobile presenting part in late pregnancy
- with vaginal bleeding in labour.

Symptomatic placenta praevia usually manifests as bright-red, painless vaginal bleeding, although it is not uncommon for women to experience some painful uterine contractions after the bleed (RCOG, 2011b) in the late second or third trimesters, often after sexual intercourse (Table 37.2). The bleeding is typically painless unless labour begins or if placental abruption occurs. The most common pregnancy complication arising from a placenta praevia is intermittent vaginal bleeding and this should be managed individually depending upon the woman's needs (RCOG, 2011b). Even small 'bleeds' may lead to

Table 37.2 Comparison between an abruption and a placenta praevia

	Abruption	Placenta praevia
Pain	Constant	Painless
Haemodynamic compromise	The actual amount of bleeding may be far in excess of observed vaginal blood loss.	The degree of shock is in proportion to the amount of vaginal blood loss.
Uterus	Uterus is tender and tense.	Uterus is non-tender.
Fetus	Normal presentation and lie.	May have abnormal presentation and / or lie.
Fetal condition	Fetal heart trace non-reassuring / absent.	In general, fetal heart trace is reassuring.
Associated problems	May be a complication of PE; may cause DIC.	Small APH may occur before larger bleed.

These comparisons are generalisations and specific cases may vary in their clinical features.
APH = antepartum haemorrhage; DIC = disseminated intravascular coagulopathy; PE = preeclampsia.

maternal anaemia and so it is important to ensure and maintain adequate maternal haemoglobin levels and iron stores with diet and, if necessary, supplements. Bleeding is more likely to occur in the third trimester when the lower uterine segment is developing or during contractions with cervical dilation, which is thought to cause shearing forces, leading to disruption of the placental attachment. Bleeding can also be provoked by a digital examination or intercourse.

CLINICAL POINT

In the presence of vaginal bleeding, do not perform a vaginal examination until placenta praevia is ruled out. This is in case there are blood vessels lying across the cervical os which may be damaged and cause severe haemorrhage

The amount of blood lost can be highly variable—from a few spots to several litres. The initial bleed usually ceases spontaneously as soon as the blood clots. This initial sentinel bleed usually is not sufficient to produce haemodynamic instability or to threaten the fetus. Unlike an abruption, gentle abdominal palpation does not cause the woman pain and fetal parts are easily palpable. The presenting part usually does not engage in the pelvis and remains high, because the placenta occupies the lower uterine segment, preventing it from descending into the pelvis.

Diagnosis is confirmed by ultrasonographic imaging techniques revealing the relationship of the leading edge of the placenta to the cervical os and the leading fetal pole. When the placental edge lies between 20 mm away from the internal os and 20 mm overlap after 26 weeks gestation, ultrasound should be repeated at regular intervals depending on the gestational age, distance from the internal os, and clinical features such as bleeding. If the placental edge overlaps the internal os by 20 mm or more at any time in the third trimester it is highly likely that the woman will require a caesarean section.

Management

The goal of management is to obtain the maximum fetal maturation while minimising the risk to both fetus and mother. Management and place of birth are determined by the degree of placenta praevia present, the gestational age of the fetus and the presence and amount of vaginal bleeding. Following any episode of vaginal bleeding, it is important that the woman be referred and transferred to the nearest hospital for immediate assessment. In the presence of significant haemorrhage it may be necessary to summon an ambulance and initiate resuscitative measures.

On admission to hospital and depending on her haemodynamic status:

- The ABCs are always the first priority.
- The woman's general condition and vital signs are assessed and her records are reviewed.
- An accurate history is taken including details of the bleeding onset, volume and precipitating factors.
- For a diagnosis of placenta praevia to be confirmed, the location of the placenta must be determined. A transabdominal ultrasound facilitates this process and should be performed as quickly as possible.
- Unless bleeding is such that the woman's haemodynamic status is compromised, following a gentle abdominal palpation the fetal condition is assessed through a CTG and / or Doppler ultrasonography of the fetal heart rate.
- A speculum or vaginal examination shouldn't be performed until localisation of the placenta is known.
- Give corticosteroids (to support fetal lung maturation) if gestation is less than 34 weeks.
- Handheld Doppler and / or Pinards can be used to assess presence of fetal heart rate.
- Administer 625 IU anti-D, as an intramuscular (IM) injection, if the woman is RhD negative; additional doses of anti-D immunoglobulin may be required.
- If the diagnosis cannot be confirmed by ultrasound, a vaginal examination using a speculum may be required. This should be performed in an operating theatre as a 'double set-up'—so the team can proceed to an immediate caesarean section should the haemorrhage become torrential.

Emergency management

Optimal outcomes depend on prompt diagnosis and appropriate, timely intervention to prevent further complications by:

- maternal resuscitation using the ABCs (see Ch. 40)
- continuous assessment of blood loss and maternal response to treatment
- rapid blood product replacement
- confirmation of the position of the placenta
- determination of gestational age
- administration of corticosteroids if the fetus is between 23 and 34 weeks gestation
- ruling out other causes of bleeding.

Continuous fetal monitoring is recommended. Decelerations or loss of variability may resolve with adequate maternal resuscitation; however, a persistently non-reassuring fetal heart rate tracing may require urgent caesarean delivery before the aetiology of the haemorrhage is established. Tocolytic therapy *may* be used to inhibit labour if this commences, and only after bleeding has resolved and for neuroprotection in pre-term infants for 48 hours.

Once the diagnosis is established, the clinical team must decide whether the woman is a suitable candidate for expectant management, or whether an immediate caesarean section is needed to save the life of the mother and her baby.

Ongoing care

Once the initial haemorrhage is controlled, decisions about ongoing care depend on the mother's haemodynamic status, fetal gestational age and extent / frequency of bleeding. If risks of pre-term birth outweigh those of another potentially catastrophic bleed, expectant management is preferred as it allows more time for the fetal lungs to mature. The mother remains in hospital for at least 48 hours and a caesarean section is planned for about 38 weeks gestation or sooner if the maternal or fetal condition deteriorates (RCOG, 2011b, Varouxaki et al., 2018).

Inpatient or outpatient care?

Traditionally women with an asymptomatic placenta praevia (that is, without vaginal bleeding) have been admitted to hospital at 34 weeks gestation or earlier. There is limited evidence to support women who are asymptomatic staying at home rather than being in hospital (RCOG, 2011b). Some clinicians make decisions regarding inpatient versus outpatient management on a variety of individualised factors including:

- gestational age
- the woman's preferences
- bleeding history including: severity, frequency, how recent
- home issues such as:
  - likelihood of obtaining rest
  - carer continuously in attendance
  - absence of sexual intercourse and trauma
  - ability to obtain timely treatment in the event of catastrophic haemorrhage
- hospital proximity with respect to:
  - ability to transport immediately to hospital
  - resuscitation and massive transfusion capability
  - immediate caesarean section if needed.

The woman is closely monitored for signs of another bleed, the onset of labour, and evidence of fetal wellbeing and/or compromise. In addition:

- blood samples for cross-match are always available at the blood bank
- an IV cannula is inserted but it may be luered
- fetal wellbeing is monitored (CTG and Doppler flow ultrasonography)
- corticosteroids are administered if the mother is <34 weeks pregnant
- preparations for an immediate caesarean section are always in place
- women with bleeding in late pregnancy who are Rh negative should receive Rh_0(D) immunoglobulin after performance of a Kleihauer–Betke test to determine the appropriate dose.

Measures are put in place to support the family as they deal with fear and anxiety related to the threats to the woman's life and that of her baby. These measures include:

- sharing information and education about placenta praevia and treatment plans
- diversional and supportive activities to help with the boredom and anxiety associated with prolonged hospitalisation as well as the difficulties associated with being away from the family
- education about the signs of bleeding and the onset of labour.

Ongoing management

The woman usually stays in hospital until there has been no further evidence of bleeding for about 24–72 hours. Outpatient collaborative management of placenta praevia may be appropriate for haemodynamically stable women with home support, close proximity to a hospital, readily available transportation and telephone communication. Before going home, the woman and her family are advised about the steps they can take to reduce the likelihood of another bleed (avoid sexual intercourse or any activity that may trigger labour). However, if they are to go home it is crucial that the woman always has access to transportation and can, if necessary, return to hospital at the start of another episode of bleeding. If significant bleeding occurs in the third trimester, the only management option is admission to hospital until birth by caesarean section can be undertaken.

Mode of birth

Planning for complicated birthing and control of haemorrhage is critical in cases of placenta praevia. Where the placenta is not overlying the internal os, recommendations should consider:

- likelihood of a placenta accreta (e.g. in cases of previous caesarean section)
- considerations with respect to immediate caesarean section (birth within 15 minutes)
- presence of a vasa praevia
- placental edge proximity to the internal os
- availability of high-volume blood transfusion; this may be limited by local factors or the presence of anti-red-cell antibodies
- individual considerations such as acceptability of blood transfusion, and of an elective caesarean section.

Caesarean section

When the placental edge is more than 20 mm away from the internal cervical os (low-lying placenta rather than a placenta praevia) women may choose to labour and birth vaginally. Although a distance of 0–20 mm from the cervical os does not absolutely preclude a vaginal birth, it is associated with a likelihood of significant intrapartum bleeding; an elective caesarean section is often recommended. Whenever possible, the timing of a caesarean section should be deferred until after 39 weeks to improve neonatal morbidity. However, in a major placenta praevia, planning for a caesarean section at 37–8 weeks may avoid the possibility that an emergency caesarean may be needed owing to the onset of labour before the scheduled caesarean section at 39+ weeks (RCOG, 2011b).

It is imperative that the woman and her family are supported in their decision making and are counselled regarding the risks associated with having a placenta praevia, including the potential need for a blood transfusion and/or hysterectomy.

About 50% of babies will be born pre-term and so the place of birth may be dictated by the need for neonatal intensive care post birth. Expectant management is terminated as soon as the fetus is mature, in the presence of excessive bleeding, if active labour begins or if signs of other complications such as chorioamnionitis occur. When there is a definite ultrasound diagnosis of major placenta praevia, an elective caesarean section is performed at about 38 weeks gestation. The choice of regional or general anaesthesia will depend on the grade of placenta praevia and position—anterior or posterior—and the risk of haemorrhage at delivery. If there has been a previous caesarean section there is a significant risk of placenta accreta. In this situation there is a significant risk of major haemorrhage and DIC (see Ch. 40).

CLINICAL POINT

Maternal health risks

- Hypovolaemic shock
- Postpartum haemorrhage
- Anaemia
- Sepsis
- Invasive placenta (accreta, increta and percreta following severe haemorrhage due to major placenta praevia)
- Rhesus isoimmunisation
- Disseminated coagulopathy

Perinatal health risks

- Malpresentation
- Prematurity and intrauterine growth restriction
- Fetal anaemia from fetomaternal haemorrhage

Before they are discharged from hospital, it is important to counsel women with placenta praevia about the risk of recurrence, so that they can plan for their next pregnancy.

Complications

Complications of placenta praevia include:

- placenta accreta, percreta and increta and vasa praevia
- PPH (secondary to the poor contractibility of the lower uterine segment)—a frequent complication
- coagulation disorders
- acute renal failure
- anaemia
- infection—prophylactic antibiotics should therefore be used for emergency caesarean section and considered for elective procedures
- manual removal of the placenta
- thromboembolism.

CRITICAL THINKING EXERCISE

When a woman presents with vaginal bleeding, the history should also include the following questions. Role-play asking these questions, and the woman's responses. Reflect on the different responses a woman with an abruption or with a placenta praevia may give you:

- When did the bleeding start, how much bleeding, and did the bleeding stop?
- Was this the first episode of bleeding?
- What was the colour of the blood (dark or bright red), were any clots present, and what was their size?
- What were you doing at the time of the bleed?
- Has anyone hurt you?
- Did you bleed with any of your other pregnancies?
- Have you felt the baby move?
- When did you last have sexual intercourse?
- Are you feeling any contractions?
- How is your general health?
- Do you have any abdominal pain?

Vasa praevia

Vasa praevia is a condition in which the umbilical vessels, unsupported by either the umbilical cord or placental tissue, traverse the fetal membranes of the lower segment above the cervix. Although vasa praevia is rare, it is important for midwives to be familiar with this condition because rapid intervention is essential for fetal survival (Varouxaki et al., 2018).

Incidence

The reported incidence varies from 1 in 2000 births to 1 in 6000 births and can result in neonatal mortality (Varouxaki et al., 2018). Vasa praevia usually occurs in association with velamentous insertion of the umbilical cord, bipartite placenta or succenturiate lobe. It typically manifests as onset of profuse haemorrhage at the time of vaginal examination, amniotomy and spontaneous breaking of the membranes. Sudden severe abnormalities of the fetal heart rate in labour can often be the first sign. The haemorrhage is from fetal blood, and exsanguination can occur rapidly because the average blood volume of a term fetus is approximately 250 mL. When performing a third-trimester ultrasound for a woman with a suspected placenta praevia, some clinicians include colour Doppler imaging specifically to detect the presence of fetal vessels.

Diagnosis of vasa praevia can be made from Doppler flow studies or ultrasound scan or, in rare cases, palpation of a pulsating vessel during a vaginal examination. Sudden onset of vaginal bleeding that is accompanied by acute fetal distress immediately after an ARM should alert the midwife to the possibility of a ruptured vasa praevia. In the event of vaginal bleeding with a known vasa praevia, if time permits, a rapid biochemical test for fetal haemoglobin could be conducted, followed by an urgent caesarean section if a confirmed result is returned. However, performing a CTG or listening to the fetal heart rate may be a quicker way, in many situations, to infer the diagnosis and institute appropriate management. There is typically an initial tachycardia as the fetus first becomes hypovolaemic, soon followed by a sustained bradycardia, a sinusoidal trace and then fetal demise if delivery by caesarean section is not immediate. An emergency caesarean birth is the only option to birth a live baby, who then will require blood transfusion to restore the blood circulating volume. Reported survival rates of 97% can occur when a vasa praevia is detected antenatally (RCOG, 2011b).

MATERNAL MEDICAL CONDITIONS DIAGNOSED BEFORE AND DURING PREGNANCY

Various medical diseases may preclude women from achieving a successful pregnancy and birth, although many women will go on to birth safely. Sometimes these conditions are diagnosed before pregnancy and others occur as a result of the pregnancy. Often, medical complications affect the mother's pregnancy, her illness and her fetus's wellbeing. It is not possible to cover all the medical disorders in a textbook of this nature, and so only the most common have been selected: diabetes, thyroid disease, heart disease, respiratory disease, renal disease, obstetric cholestasis, epilepsy, thromboembolic disease, genital infections and hypertension in pregnancy.

Diabetes mellitus

Pregnancy presents particular challenges for women with diabetes, irrespective of whether they have just been diagnosed with **gestational diabetes** or have been living with diabetes since childhood. However, advances in medical, midwifery, obstetric and intensive care of the diabetic woman and her baby have resulted in significantly better outcomes. Most women with diabetes can and do have healthy pregnancies. Nevertheless, a diagnosis of diabetes requires urgent modifications in lifestyle and close surveillance by a multidisciplinary team.

Diabetes mellitus is a heterogeneous group of diseases characterised by impaired carbohydrate metabolism and elevation of glucose in the blood because the body is unable to produce enough insulin for its own needs, because of either impaired insulin secretion, impaired insulin action, or both. These diseases all pose significant threats to maternal and perinatal health.

In its chronic forms, diabetes is coupled with long-term vascular complications, including retinopathy, nephropathy, neuropathy and vascular disease. Diabetes in pregnancy is negatively linked to the health and wellbeing of the woman and to the developing fetus. Miscarriage, PE and pre-term labours are more common in women with pre-existing diabetes. Women with diabetes have a two- to threefold greater risk of having a baby with a major congenital malformation compared with the general population. In addition, diabetic retinopathy can deteriorate quickly during pregnancy. Stillbirth, congenital malformations, macrosomia, birth injury, perinatal morbidity and mortality and neonatal adaptation problems (such as hypoglycaemia) are widespread in babies born to women with pre-existing diabetes.

Epidemiology

Australia and New Zealand, like many other countries, are facing a challenge in health provision and the inevitable resulting economics owing to a rising tide of people with diabetes. A global report from the World Health Organization (WHO) in 2016 revealed that the incidence of diabetes in adults is believed to have quadrupled since 1980 to that of 422 million currently. This striking increase is understood to be due to type 2 diabetes and some of the factors causing this escalation are from adults being overweight and obese.

The consequence of this explosive rise in the number of people with diabetes may be that 21st-century Australian and New Zealand children will be the first for many centuries to have a shorter life expectancy than their parents or grandparents. In 2016, diabetes was thought to have been the direct cause of 1.6 million deaths worldwide and linked to strokes, heart attacks, blindness, lower limb amputation and kidney failure (WHO, 2020). The outlook for indigenous peoples is even grimmer. In many rural and remote communities such as in Australia's Northern Territory, diabetes is the norm and many families have at least one person on dialysis due to end-stage diabetes-related kidney disease. The incidence of diabetic retinopathy leading to blindness is much higher in indigenous communities. Increasingly, type 2 diabetes, once a disease with a 'mature onset', is seen in children and young adults—meaning that the development of serious complications of diabetes occurs when adults are at their peak working age. The Australian Institute of Health and Welfare (AIHW, 2020b) health services report identified that 4.9% of the total population had diabetes in 2017–18 with 7.9% of Indigenous Australians having diabetes, a rate of almost three times that of the non-Indigenous peoples.

In developed countries, approximately 1 in 20 pregnancies are complicated by diabetes, of which 90% is attributed to gestational diabetes and 8% to pre-existing insulin-resistant (i.e. adult-onset) diabetes. In New Zealand a large, ongoing longitudinal cohort study, the Growing up in New Zealand study, identified a diagnostic rate of 6.2% in 2010 (Lawrence et al., 2019). Diabetes that is poorly controlled can lead to an increase of complications for both the mother and her baby (WHO, 2020).

Overview of carbohydrate metabolism in pregnancy

Glucose homeostasis and carbohydrate metabolism are complex processes and so, before proceeding with this section, you are advised to refresh your knowledge of these topics by referring to a text such as Coad et al. (2020), Blackburn (2017) or Rankin (2017). In addition, Chapters 20 and 21 provide an overview of carbohydrate metabolism. Boxes 37.8 and 37.9 summarise the roles of insulin and glucagon respectively.

Pregnancy is a diabetogenic state

Pregnant women are normally in a diabetogenic state, which ensures that the fetus has an adequate and continuous supply of glucose. It is characterised by insulin resistance with compensatory hyperinsulinaemia, beginning in the second trimester and remaining throughout the pregnancy, to levels that resemble the levels in type 2 diabetes. The insulin resistance seen in pregnancy may be the consequence of increased maternal adiposity combined with the insulin-desensitising effects of placental hormones.

All pregnant women experience mild fasting hypoglycaemia and after-meal hyperglycaemia. Increased secretion of insulin between meals and during sleep enables the fetus to continue to draw glucose across the placenta from the maternal bloodstream, even during periods of maternal fasting. In the second and third trimesters, increased placental steroids and peptide hormones exacerbate tissue insulin resistance. However, if the maternal pancreatic insulin response to food intake is inadequate, first maternal and then fetal hyperglycaemia occurs.

Box 37.8 Role of insulin

Insulin:

- facilitates the uptake of glucose by facilitating its movement from the blood into target cells (liver, skeletal and muscle)
- stimulates formation and storage of lipids and glycogen
- lowers circulating blood glucose.

It does this by:

- increasing glucose transport by target cells
- accelerating glucose utilisation (target cells) and enhanced ATP production
- stimulating glycogen synthesis (skeletal, muscle and liver cells)
- decreasing glucogenesis.

ATP = adenosine triphosphate.

Box 37.9 Role of glucagon

Glucagon:

- mobilises energy reserves and promotes glucose synthesis and glycogen breakdown
- elevates blood glucose concentrations.

It does this by:

- stimulating the breakdown of glycogen in skeletal, muscle and liver cells
- stimulating the breakdown of triglycerides in adipose tissues
- stimulating the production of glucose in the liver.

Causes of diabetes mellitus

In diabetes mellitus there is an absolute or relative deficiency of the insulin produced by the pancreas. Glucose cannot be converted to glycogen or released as energy, so it accumulates in the bloodstream, causing hyperglycaemia, some of which is excreted in the urine. Glucose is osmotically active and draws water after it, causing polyuria and thirst. Faced with a lack of glucose, the body tries to mobilise energy from fats and proteins, which leads to the production of ketones by the liver, and ketosis. Glucose crosses the placenta and stimulates fetal glucose production; maternal or exogenous insulin does not.

Classification of diabetes

Diabetes is classified into three major types (see below) that are different disease entities but share the symptoms and complications of hyperglycaemia. In addition, people with 'pre-diabetes' or 'borderline diabetes' have a degree of glucose intolerance and hyperglycaemia that precedes the onset of type 2 diabetes. The three major types of diabetes that affect pregnancy are as follows:

- *Type 1 diabetes* (T1DM, or 'insulin-dependent diabetes mellitus' (IDDM), formerly called 'juvenile diabetes')—T1DM develops as a result of an autoimmune response directed against insulin-producing β-cells, located in the pancreas. It is usually characterised by progressive β-cell destruction, usually leading to absolute insulin deficiency. Evidence suggests that both a genetic predisposition and environmental factors, such as a viral infection, are involved.
- *Type 2 diabetes mellitus* (T2DM, formerly called 'non-insulin-dependent diabetes mellitus', NIDDM, 'type II' or 'adult-onset')—is the most common form of diabetes (80%–90%) and its incidence is increasing worldwide. It comprises a group of disorders characterised by hyperglycaemia and is associated with microvascular (i.e. retinal, renal, possibly neuropathic), macrovascular (i.e. coronary, peripheral vascular) and neuropathic (i.e. autonomic, peripheral) complications, along with insulin resistance in peripheral tissues and an insulin secretory defect of the β-cells. Recently a new, rare form of type 2 diabetes known as 'maturity-onset diabetes of the young' (MODY) has been identified. MODY is caused by an autosomal dominant gene. Sufferers are usually women of normal weight and under 25 years old. During pregnancy, women with MODY do not require insulin.
- *Gestational diabetes mellitus* (GDM)—is defined as diabetes with onset or first recognition during pregnancy. It encompasses any type of diabetes first diagnosed in pregnancy. For example, it includes type 2 diabetes

recognised for the first time in pregnancy. GDM is often diagnosed following routine glucose tolerance screening. As with other forms of hyperglycaemia, GDM is characterised by pancreatic β-cell function that is insufficient to meet the body's needs. Most women classified with GDM have normal glucose homeostasis during the first half of the pregnancy and develop only a relative insulin deficiency (and hyperglycaemia) during the second half of the pregnancy. The hyperglycaemia resolves in most cases after birth but places such women at significant risk of developing type 2 diabetes in later life.

Effects of diabetes on the woman and her pregnancy

Whatever its causation, diabetes can result in a range of complications for the mother, her baby and the progress of her disease. In women with either type 1 or type 2 diabetes, glycaemic control worsens and insulin requirements change as the pregnancy progresses. Poorly controlled type 1 diabetes causes life-threatening metabolic reactions, such as ketoacidosis and diabetic coma. Hyperglycaemia is the prime determinant of the following microvascular and metabolic complications:

- diabetic ketoacidosis
- cardiovascular disease
- peripheral vascular disease
- diabetic retinopathy
- diabetic nephropathy and end-stage renal disease
- peripheral nerve disease
- cancer of the pancreas
- liver disease
- depression.

Metabolic complications associated with diabetes

During pregnancy, lack of knowledge about the effects of pregnancy on diabetes, as well as the effects of pregnancy on glycaemic control, increases the risks of hypoglycaemic episodes as well as diabetic ketoacidosis. Women and their partners need ongoing, evidence-based information and education about the management of these conditions, including the use of glucagon to alleviate hypoglycaemia and how to recognise and prevent ketoacidosis. Midwives are well placed to work with the family to develop an emergency plan that they know works and is kept in an accessible place. This plan should contain a list of local emergency contacts.

Microvascular complications for the woman

Retinal and renal disease associated with diabetes can worsen during pregnancy:

- *Retinopathy*—first-trimester poor glycaemic control, PE and chronic hypertension are all independently associated with the progression of retinopathy. Diabetic retinopathy may develop or worsen during pregnancy. Women should consult an ophthalmologist before conception and to plan further follow-up consultations during the course of the pregnancy.
- *Nephropathy*—there is an association between pre-existing nephropathy and adverse maternal and perinatal outcomes. Complications associated with nephropathy and PE, especially if the latter is superimposed on chronic hypertension, are strongly associated with pre-term birth.

Effects of diabetes on the fetus

Ornoy et al. (2015) investigated the impact of prepregnancy diabetes and gestational diabetes upon the developing fetus in pregnancy. They found that cardiovascular and neural tube defects were the most commonly occurring fetal abnormities. Neural tube defects occur 13–20 times more frequently in diabetic pregnancies. About a third of fetuses of women with diabetes mellitus in pregnancy are large for gestational age (LGA). The fetus has a larger shoulder and extremity circumference, a decreased head-to-shoulder ratio, significantly higher body fat and thicker upper-extremity skinfolds.

Parrettini et al. (2020) considered the prepregnancy metabolic challenges of women with obesity and diabetes. They describe the effects that the nutritional status may have on the developing fetus as well as the risks of premature birth and fetal mortality. For these reasons women with type 1 diabetes are advised to maintain good blood glucose control pre-conceptually and throughout pregnancy to reduce the potential of congenital malformations, miscarriage, premature birth, stillbirth and neonatal death (NICE, 2020; Parrettini, 2020).

Other risks to perinatal health include:

- unexplained stillbirth in the third trimester
- prematurity due to a higher incidence of spontaneous pre-term labour and of elective premature birth to prevent stillbirth
- low birth weight due to intrauterine growth restriction, resulting from metabolic dysfunction (Castillo-Castrejon et al., 2017)
- congenital malformations
- birth trauma often caused by macrosomia.

Because it is the most frequently diagnosed form of diabetes, this chapter focuses on the collaborative management of type 2 diabetes. Interventions specifically designed for women with type 1 diabetes are also described in the following sections.

Aetiology of type 2 diabetes

Type 2 diabetes is a condition in which the body either makes too little insulin or is unable to use the insulin it makes (i.e. insulin resistance) and is the most common of the three 'types'. Often, type 2 diabetes can be controlled through dietary modifications and exercising regularly. The aetiology of type 2 diabetes mellitus is multifactorial and, like T1DM, probably genetically based, but there are also strong behavioural components. In Australia and New Zealand (Box 37.10), it is more common in women:

- of advancing age
- who are obese
- with a sedentary lifestyle
- with a family history of type 2 diabetes

Box 37.10 Diabetes (GDM and T2DM) in New Zealand and Australia

New Zealand

Māori and Pacific populations are among the highest risk groups for diabetes and for cardiovascular disease and related conditions. The prevalence of diabetes is three times higher in Māori and Pasifika populations compared with other ethnic groups (MOH, 2014b). This increase reflects changing demographic factors (including increased population size and changes in population age structure) and epidemiological factors (such as obesity and physical inactivity).

Effective primary prevention programs for type 2 diabetes are largely based on programs to reduce diabetes risk factors, such as reducing overweight/obesity, stopping smoking and increasing physical activity. Such programs extend beyond the health sector, involving local government, employers, education and community groups, amongst others.

Māori and Pacific populations traditionally have strong community links, which are important to the success of health programs targeting the above risk factors.

Australia

Diabetes is more common in men (4.9%) than in women (3.8%) and is most prevalent in the Northern Territory (10.6%) and least prevalent in the Australian Capital Territory (3.0%). The high prevalence of diabetes in the Northern Territory mainly reflects the high burden of type 2 diabetes in Aboriginal Australians.

GDM = gestational diabetes mellitus; T2DM = type 2 diabetes mellitus.

(Sources: AIHW, 2017a; MOH, 2014b, https://www.health.govt.nz/our-work/diseases-and-conditions/diabetes/about-diabetes)

- with impaired glucose tolerance
- with a genetic predisposition
- with a history of gestational diabetes
- with an 'apple-shaped figure'
- who are Chinese, Indian, Māori, Pacific Islanders, or Australian Indigenous people
- with socioeconomic disparity and health and education inequities.

CLINICAL POINT

Some studies suggest that an in-utero environment leading to low birth weight may predispose some individuals to type 2 diabetes mellitus in later life. Intrauterine exposures including diabetes in pregnancy can modify the expression of genes in the fetus related to carbohydrate metabolism (Ornoy et al., 2015; Parrettini et al., 2020).

Pathophysiology

Type 1 diabetes (T1DM)

Type 1 diabetes mellitus (T1DM) accounts for 5%–10% of diagnosed diabetes. The exact cause of T1DM still eludes scientists, but it is known that a general inflammatory state, termed insulitis, precedes overt diabetes. Due to the destruction of β-cells, people with T1DM require insulin replacement to achieve euglycaemia. Onset of the disease generally occurs before age 30, and it thus can affect women during their reproductive years. Fluctuations in insulin sensitivity occur during pregnancy, mostly due to changes with diabetes. Women with T1DM are at increased risk for complications such as infertility, stillbirth, hypoglycaemia, diabetic ketoacidosis, retinopathy, nephropathy, PE, and pre-term labour and birth.

Type 2 diabetes (T2DM)

People develop type 2 diabetes at any age—even during childhood, although usually when older. A relative lack of endogenous insulin plus pancreatic β-cell dysfunction reduces glucose uptake by cells, resulting in hyperglycaemia. Insulin deficiency usually occurs because of resistance to the actions of insulin in muscle, fat and the liver, and an inadequate response by the pancreatic β-cells. Evidence supports inherited components for both pancreatic β-cell failure and insulin resistance.

CLINICAL POINT

The midwife is a crucial member of a multidisciplinary team (MDT) and the guardian of 'normality' within a high-risk pregnancy. This role is crucial for women with all forms of diabetes so that normal pregnancy information and planning is not pushed to the back of care priorities within a medical model of care. The midwife's role includes ensuring that the woman's 'voice' is central in all decisions and that she is provided with evidence-based care. The midwife is also often the best placed to coordinate a collaborative midwifery, obstetric, medical, allied health approach to care.

Collaborative management of type 1 and type 2 diabetes during pregnancy

The management of type 1 and frequently type 2 diabetes involves daily administration of exogenous insulin by injection or an insulin pump, combined with carefully designed meal plans and exercise regimen of walking or swimming. This, however, assumes that the insulin regimen is the guiding component of therapy and this may not be the case in T2DM. In reality, the individual's typical eating pattern and lifestyle should be the key factors and the determinants of the best insulin regimen. Antenatal care involves teamwork. Healthcare professionals working collaboratively and in partnership with the woman plan her care before conception, and during pregnancy and labour. The woman should always be referred to a consultant unit attached to a neonatal nursery. Diabetes specialist midwives and nurses have an important role in educating women about the need for home blood glucose monitoring, urine testing, intensive insulin regimens, dietary management and regular exercise.

Prepregnancy care

Statistically, the level of risk for a woman with T1DM or T2DM and for the baby is determined largely by the woman's health just before conception and during the first trimester. Attendance at a multidisciplinary prepregnancy clinic is associated with a reduction in the rate of spontaneous miscarriage, in the risk of congenital malformations and in complications of pregnancy. The aim of prepregnancy care is to achieve optimal glycaemic control (e.g. diet, insulin) (Box 37.11). Care will often involve regular HbA_{1c} testing as well as consultations with eye specialists and podiatrists to identify / treat any existing issues. The midwife works with the woman to discuss how to optimise her health within her context, and is provided with information about health promotion—such as smoking cessation, stopping alcohol consumption and folic acid supplementation. At these meetings the woman is able to make realistic plans about the best time to stop contraception.

Antenatal care

Pregnant women with diabetes require immediate referral to a multidisciplinary team (MDT) as soon as the pregnancy is confirmed. Ideally the members of the MDT are all in the same setting at the same time to make it easier for the women to consult each one. Communication is an integral component of effective care. Following referral a plan of care should be identified with the woman continuing to have care from her primary care provider in collaboration with the MDT.

The key components of antenatal care specifically for pregnant women with diabetes are:

- history taking—current and past contraception, menstrual history
- screening for existing diabetic complications (retinal and renal complications)
- documentation and management of comorbidities
- review of medications—especially ACE inhibitors and anticonvulsants, etc.
- high-dose (5-mg) folic acid supplementation pre-conception and during the first trimester
- documentation of smoking, alcohol intake; cessation programs
- measurement of weight, height and body mass index, and referral to dietitian
- encouragement for women to monitor their blood glucose levels regularly before and after meals and adjust insulin accordingly
- negotiation of individual targets for blood glucose levels and glycated haemoglobin (HbA_{1c}); generic targets to aim for are: blood glucose <5.6 mmol / L before meals and <7.8 mmol / L after meals
- discussion about risks of hypoglycaemia / ketoacidosis during pregnancy
- education about driving and glucagon kit
- early booking and need for regular ongoing multidisciplinary care.

Because of the increased risk of congenital anomalies, women with diabetes should be offered combined first trimester screening for aneuploidy, with β-hCG and a pregnancy-associated plasma protein test (PAPP-A) measured at 10 weeks gestation, followed by an ultrasound examination for dating, nuchal transparency, gross morphology and plurality. Because of the higher incidence of complications, women with type 1 diabetes are referred for ultrasonography at least three times in pregnancy: early or at first booking to recognise possible early growth delay or congenital malformations, later at about 28 weeks to determine fetal size and hydramnios, and finally at about 36 weeks to identify the possible presence of macrosomia.

Insulin

Not all type 2 diabetics require exogenous insulin. People with type 1 diabetes, because they experience absolute insulin deficiency, in the vast majority of cases must use insulin to control their blood sugar levels. Requirements change during pregnancy because of the effects of insulin-antagonistic placental hormones. Regimens vary, but the consensus seems to be that a 'tight control' plan (Box 37.12) with frequent administration of insulin (up

Box 37.11 Reducing insulin resistance

Insulin resistance may be decreased with dietary modification, weight loss, and perhaps antidiabetic agents such as the biguanide metformin. There is some evidence that infants exposed to maternal diabetes in utero may have an increased incidence of childhood obesity and diabetes and become insulin resistant.

Box 37.12 'Tight control' plan

Working with pregnant women with diabetes

The type of diabetes treatment program that aims to normalise blood glucose levels is referred to as a 'tight control' plan. Cornerstones of tight glycaemic control are:

- administering insulin and adjusting the doses, depending on results of self-monitoring of blood glucose (SMBG)
- frequent SMBG
- following an appropriate meal plan
- adding or maintaining an appropriate level of physical activity
- controlling / treating hypoglycaemia.

to four times daily) and the use of different insulin types (e.g. rapid- and long-acting insulin analogues), as well as more frequent blood glucose measurements, is better able to achieve normal blood glucose levels.

CLINICAL POINT

Metformin therapy is more frequently used for women with pregnancies complicated by T2DM (Frier et al., 2017) as well as in pregnancies complicated by gestational diabetes following the findings of the Metformin in Gestational Diabetes (MIG) Trial (Rowan et al., 2008). If a woman with T2DM and taking metformin presents to the antenatal clinic already pregnant, she should be reassured that there is no evidence of teratogenesis with its use. There is data suggesting a small increase in childhood body mass index for children exposed to metformin during pregnancy but further larger studies are needed to explore this further (ADIPS, 2020). The woman should continue taking the medication until ongoing treatment options are discussed with her and clinicians in her team.

Blood glucose monitoring

Monitoring blood glucose levels is fundamental to achieving 'tight' diabetic metabolic control. Self-monitoring of blood glucose levels (SMBG) empowers women who have diabetes, enabling them to achieve their goals actively. In addition, the instant feedback that SMBG provides enables women to learn more about portion sizes, foods that cause hyperglycaemia, maintenance of stable temporal patterns of elevated blood glucose levels, and when exercise is most likely to help keep blood glucose in the targeted range. With this information, women are better able to make choices about their diet and exercise activities on an individual basis and to see the effects of these in a timely manner.

Women should aim to maintain blood glucose levels as near to their non-diabetic range as possible without increasing the risk of hypoglycaemia. This usually means targeting levels between 4 and 7 mmol/L. The glycated haemoglobin (HbA_{1c}) should be measured at the first antenatal visit and repeated monthly, with a target level of <6.5%.

CLINICAL POINT

Women with type 1 diabetes may be using continuous glucose monitoring (CGM), which provides a detailed view of glucose levels over 24 hours. CGM measures interstitial glucose and can be linked to a mobile phone, reading device and/or continuous subcutaneous insulin infusion pump (ADIP, 2020).

Lifestyle and dietary advice

Lifestyle advice, including diet and weight management (Box 37.13), is the cornerstone of management of all forms of diabetes (MOH, 2014). Expert nutritional advice should be available in all diabetic antenatal clinics in order to encourage the entire family to have a diet low in saturated fat, with high levels of complex carbohydrates, soluble fibre and vitamins. Women with diabetes are encouraged to take folic acid 2.5–5 mg daily from 3 months prior to conception until 12 weeks of gestation (Rudland et al., 2020).

Box 37.13 Type 2 diabetes and weight management

An unhealthy lifestyle featuring a lack of physical activity and excessive eating initiates and propagates the majority of T2DM. A woman's weight influences her body image. Women with type 2 diabetes or gestational diabetes mellitus are often overweight. Obesity makes it more difficult to maintain tight glycaemic control and this is especially true for the woman with type 2 diabetes. Women with diabetes are often advised to 'maintain a healthy weight' but this is easier said than done. It may be helpful to separate the issue of how much the woman weighs from the behaviours required for the woman to maintain a healthy weight.

Type 1 and type 2 diabetes are both risk factors for the development of preeclampsia and women should be provided with low-dose aspirin (100–150 mg daily) from 12 weeks gestation until 36 weeks gestation. Calcium intake (1.5 g daily) should also be supplemented (Rudland et al., 2020).

Exercise. The benefits of exercise include cardiovascular fitness and psychological wellbeing. In contrast to women with T2DM, women with T1DM are rarely overweight but exercise is still beneficial especially when they use a continuous glucose monitoring device (Jaklevic, 2021). For women with T2DM or gestational diabetes, the benefits of regular exercise also include a decrease in body fat, better weight control and improvements in insulin sensitivity.

Maternal and fetal monitoring

Diabetic pregnancies are 'high risk' and therefore regular monitoring is appropriate. It is recommended that women with all forms of diabetes are assessed more frequently than usual. This may be in the form of serial ultrasound every 2–4 weeks from 28 weeks gestation to examine fetal growth and identify fetal growth restriction (ADIP, 2020). Other monitoring of fetal wellbeing includes CTG and ultrasound/Doppler flow studies commencing at 34 weeks (ADIP, 2020; NICE, 2020).

Ongoing laboratory tests

Ongoing evaluation of glycaemic control and the assessment of diabetic complications are essential components of any management plan for women with all forms of diabetes. Tests include:

- HbA_{1c}—as red blood cells are made, they combine with glucose in the blood to make HbA_{1c}. How much HbA_{1c} is produced depends on the blood glucose level

at the time each red blood cell is made. HbA_{1c} levels of 7% or less are associated with a reduced risk of microvascular complications, whereas levels >9% are associated with increased risks. It is advisable therefore to aim for levels of 7% or less.
- urinary PCR—a one-off positive of ≥30 mg/mmol PCR result confirms proteinuria and does not need to be repeated. Additionally, rising serum creatinine alongside falling serum albumin would be of concern, as would deranged liver function tests.
- random plasma glucose and SMBG
- in the third trimester, ultrasound examination at 30 weeks for assessment of fetal growth—this should be repeated as clinically indicated, or at 36 weeks to identify growth discordance.

Self-management skills

Practical self-management skills for good glycaemic control include:
- counselling and education about the risks and prevention of congenital anomalies, maternal and perinatal complications, the effects of pregnancy on diabetes and the effects of diabetes on pregnancy, the need for effective contraception and pre-conceptual care, the importance of tight glycaemic control and its relationship to maternal and perinatal complications
- selection of appropriate antihyperglycaemic therapy
- development of a workable and acceptable plan to achieve low-risk glycaemia—<1% above the normal range
- an appropriate diet and meal plan
- self-monitoring of blood glucose levels
- self-administering of insulin and self-adjustment of insulin dose
- treatment of hypoglycaemia (woman and her family members)
- development of an emergency plan to deal with hypoglycaemia
- incorporation of daily physical activity—at least 30 minutes a day
- development of techniques to reduce stress and help cope with the condition and its potential complications.

Labour and birth

During labour, a collaborative team approach is essential to regulate diabetic control. As yet there is no clear evidence to inform decisions about the optimal timing for birth with significant disagreement between international guideline recommendations (MOH, 2019). In Australia guidelines regarding timing of IOL may vary from state to state and obstetricians' practice preferences. There is an increased risk of stillbirth in women with prepregnancy diabetes. The New Zealand IOL guidelines recommend that if the prepregnancy diabetes is well controlled then there is no need to offer induction of labour unless there are other obstetric or fetal indications for induction. In addition:
- For women with gestational diabetes, expectant management can continue to at least 40 weeks gestation if there is good glycaemic control, normal fetal growth and no other complications.
- For women with type 2 diabetes, expectant management to 39 weeks can continue unless there are obstetric or fetal indication or diabetes complications indicating earlier birth is indicated.
- Women with type 1 diabetes should be managed on a case-by-case basis.

If there is a risk of pre-term birth, antenatal corticosteroids should be administered in line with local protocols. Even after controlling for confounding factors, women with diabetes have a high rate of caesarean section. This is possibly because of clinicians' concerns about the relationship between macrosomia and shoulder dystocia.

During labour and birth, blood glucose levels should be monitored hourly and adjusted as per local guidance—the aim is to maintain maternal plasma glucose levels usually between 4 and 7 mmol/L. Titration of plasma glucose levels during labour can be achieved using IV infusions of regular insulin and 5% dextrose according to institutional protocols. If the woman is using an insulin pump then this may be continued but may require adjustment of basal rates because insulin requirements fall during labour (Rutland et al., 2020). In this situation a written plan of care should be provided for all involved.

Postpartum period

After birth, insulin sensitivity increases greatly owing to the rapid decline of hormonal influences. Women quickly return to their prepregnancy insulin requirements. Frequent blood sugar estimations are recommended. Usually the same meal plan used during the pregnancy is adequate to meet the needs of the breastfeeding mother with diabetes. Adjustments are made in consultation with the woman's endocrinologist and dietitian. Early breastfeeding is important and adjustment of the mother's food intake to accommodate this must be recognised. There are well-documented health benefits for diabetic women in breastfeeding their babies. For some women with type 1 diabetes, breastfeeding may complicate their glycaemic control—they may have erratic blood glucose levels and an increase in insulin reactions. For others, it is easier to maintain tight glycaemic control; some women can eat more and take less insulin. Others find that symptoms of hypoglycaemia are different while they are breastfeeding; perhaps these symptoms appear more quickly or without any warning. Such women may need to take extra precautions and have some form of glucose (non-diet soft drink, or glucose tablets) nearby so that they do not have to interrupt breastfeeding if a hypoglycaemic episode occurs.

Postnatal follow-up

Postnatal follow-up is a good opportunity for the team to begin prepregnancy care for any subsequent pregnancy, to support the woman as she works to attain good glycaemic control, and to assist the family to develop lifelong good health habits. Effective ongoing communication between the woman, hospital-based team, family doctor and diabetes clinic is essential. It is at this stage that a carefully documented outcome assessment for both mother and baby must take place.

Gestational diabetes mellitus

GDM is defined as 'any degree of glucose intolerance with onset or first recognition during pregnancy' and is now one of the most frequently seen complications in pregnancy and brings challenges for midwives and obstetricians. Worldwide, GDM affects between 2% and 17% of pregnancies and in New Zealand over 3000 women are diagnosed with GDM annually (Lawrence et al., 2017). GDM includes previously unrecognised T2DM and, rarely, T1DM arising in pregnancy. In most women, GDM is asymptomatic and diagnosed on routine testing between 8 and 24 weeks gestation.

Changes to screening and diagnosis criteria for GDM have been adopted in both Australia and New Zealand and have resulted in an increased number of pregnant women being diagnosed with GDM. Simmons (2020) argues that this has led to an escalating medicalisation of pregnancy and a loss of confidence for women, as well as an increased workload for health professionals. Simmonds (2020) suggests that the adoption of the International Association of Diabetes in Pregnancy Study Groups Guidelines (IADPSG) for GDM would be of more benefit.

In New Zealand a national guideline for screening, diagnosis and treatment of diabetes was developed to improve consistency in the identification and treatment of GDM (MOH, 2014). Many, but not all, women have recognised risk factors for GDM but, using the recommended diagnostic criteria, clinicians can determine if women with GDM will also develop T2DM later in life and the risk to their children (Simmons, 2020).

GDM generally resolves once the pregnancy is completed, although 50% will develop T2DM in later life. About 50% of women diagnosed with GDM will require insulin during pregnancy. Women with GDM are more likely to experience repeated miscarriage and develop hypertensive disorders, although some of this additional risk may be associated with the underlying risk factors for GDM (e.g. increased maternal age or obesity). They are also more at risk of caesarean birth. Clinicians' fears about perceived associations between fetal macrosomia, shoulder dystocia and GDM may account for this finding. Other potential complications for the woman include polyhydramnios, pre-term labour and birth, as well as genital tract infections from *Candida albicans* and UTIs.

There is a greater risk of congenital abnormalities, particularly neural tube defects (Lawrence et al., 2017; Simmonds, 2020). Episodes of fetal hyperglycaemia and hyperinsulinaemia may lead to fetal macrosomia, and possibly traumatic birth. Many babies are born pre-term even if they are macrosomic and thus prone to neonatal hypoglycaemia, hypocalcaemia, hyperbilirubinaemia and polycythaemia.

Risk factors for GDM

Risk factors for GDM include obesity, family history of diabetes and being of Aboriginal or Torres Strait Islander background, or of Māori, Pacific Island, Middle-Eastern or Asian ethnicity.

Other risk factors include:

- previous unexplained stillbirth
- poor obstetric or social history
- polycystic ovarian syndrome
- obesity
- previous diagnosis of GDM
- having a previous baby with a birth weight over 4500 g
- maternal age >25 years.

In a current pregnancy, accelerated weight gain, polyhydramnios, newly detected glycosuria and multiple pregnancies are all associated with GDM.

Diagnosis of GDM

Australia. The Australian Diabetes in Pregnancy Society (ADIPS) and the International Association of the Diabetes and Pregnancy Study Groups (IADPSG) criteria for the diagnosis of GDM are shown in Table 37.3. ADIPS recommend that all women should be tested for GDM with the offer of an oral glucose tolerance test (OGTT) at 24–28 weeks. Women with risk factors should have tests offered earlier in pregnancy and the method of testing should be based on clinical judgement, local health care policy and risk stratification. Women considered higher risk can be offered an oral glucose tolerance test (OGTT) or an HbA_{1c} test.

Table 37.3 Criteria for diagnosis of gestational diabetes mellitus and diabetes mellitus in pregnancy with a 2-hour pregnancy OGTT (2015)

Diagnosis	Fasting plasma glucose (mmol/L)	1-h glucose (mmol/L) following 75-g oral glucose load	2-h glucose (mmol/L) following 75-g oral glucose load
Normal	<5.1	<10.0	<8.5
GDM	5.1–6.9	>10.0	8.5–11.0
Diabetes mellitus in pregnancy	>7.0	—[a]	>11.1

[a]There are no established criteria for the diagnosis of diabetes based on the 1-hour post-load value.
GDM = gestational diabetes mellitus; OGTT = oral glucose tolerance test.
(Source: WHO, 2013)

New Zealand. In New Zealand, national guidelines recommend that all pregnant women should be offered a glycated haemoglobin test as part of their first routine antenatal blood test (generally in the first trimester and ideally prior to 20 weeks gestation) (MOH, 2014).

- If the HbA_{1c} result is ≥50 mmol / L the woman should be advised of the need to be referred to diabetes specialists because the results indicate prepregnancy diabetes.
- If the HbA_{1c} result is 41–9 mmol / L, the woman should be offered the 75 mg load 2-hour oral glucose tolerance test (OGTT) when she is between 24 and 28 weeks gestation. She is considered to be at increased risk of developing gestational diabetes.
- If the HbA_{1c} result is <40 mmol / L, a 50 g oral glucose, or as it is often called a 'Polycose', test should be offered between 24 and 28 weeks gestation. If the result of the Polycose test is >11.1 mmol / L the woman is referred directly to specialist diabetic services; if the result is 7.8–11.0 mmol / L then a further 75 g load 2-hour OGTT is recommended.

Collaborative management in GDM

The keystones of therapy—control of blood glucose levels, monitoring, diet and exercise—have already been discussed, and this section explores only material that is of direct relevance to GDM. Women at significant risk of, or with, GDM require an interdisciplinary team approach. If the woman has been diagnosed with GDM in earlier pregnancies, it may be possible to begin her care before conception so that she and her team can develop evidence-based strategies aimed at maintaining the maternal blood sugar levels as near to normal as possible. It is possible to stabilise the GDM by diet alone, but 50% of women require metformin, insulin or a combination of both as the pregnancy progresses. Each woman requires regular antenatal assessment, including a management plan. This is usually achieved through a combination of hospital and home visits, with hospital admission if the woman's diabetes becomes unstable or if she presents with any infection or other complication.

After the initial visit and once she becomes pregnant (or once the condition is diagnosed), the woman is seen by the team at 4- to 8-week intervals, depending on her ability to keep to her management plan and pre-existing complications, if any.

Treatment for GDM

Medical treatment for GDM used to be varying sliding scale doses of insulin given in subcuticular injections, in response to the mother's blood glucose levels. More recently, following on from the results of the MIG trial (Rowan et al., 2008), this has changed to treatment with an oral hypoglycaemic, metformin, used in combination with insulin if required (MOH, 2014). Metformin has not been found to be linked with a rise in perinatal complications compared with insulin and is preferred by women (Rowan et al., 2008). Not all women with GDM require treatment but those that have poor glycaemic control, including a poor response to lifestyle and dietary changes, are offered pharmacological treatment. Decisions about treatment will be made collaboratively with the woman, her obstetric specialist and importantly her midwifery LMC. Ultrasound is recommended at the time of a diagnosis of GDM, when clinically required and at 36–7 weeks gestation but should not be the sole reason for initiation of treatment, as there is no evidence to indicate this is of benefit to either mother or baby (MOH, 2014).

REFLECTIVE THINKING EXERCISE

What would you say to a woman who says, 'My doctor says my ultrasound shows that my baby is much larger than expected. He says he thinks this is because I have diabetes and that I will need a caesarean section'?

Dietary modification and exercise

Dietary management, with or without metformin and / or insulin, causes a modest but consistent reduction in neonatal birth weight (Frier et al., 2017). Unfortunately, the optimal distribution of calories as carbohydrates, fats and protein for women with GDM is unknown, and there is little consensus and wide variability in clinical practice. Working in partnership, the mother and midwife aim to meet the following goals for nutrition: (i) optimal nutrition for both the developing fetus and the pregnant woman / mother, (ii) maternal euglycaemia without distortion of dietary patterns, (iii) good nutrition for all the family, and (iv) nutritional patterns that prevent or forestall recurrence of GDM and the onset of T2DM in later pregnancies. Exercise can be helpful in lowering blood glucose (BG) levels; the most acceptable form of exercise for most women is to introduce daily walks into their normal routine.

Frequency of visits

If gestational diabetes is well controlled, the pregnancy is treated as 'normal' and proceeds to term. It is, however, most likely to proceed to term if the woman's GDM is well controlled by diet alone. As the third trimester begins, a woman with GDM is more at risk of complications and so the schedule of antenatal visits should increase. Women receiving insulin should be seen weekly from 34 weeks. The frequency of consultations is increased if there are other complications, such as: pre-existing or pregnancy-induced hypertension, fetal macrosomia, IUGR, poor glycaemic control and inability to stop smoking.

CLINICAL POINT

Community-based care

Telephone /email management can be a financially and time-effective way for the midwife to maintain close contact with a woman with GDM during the intervals between face-to-face consultations with the diabetic team. Women are asked to call or email their records weekly. A midwife skilled in working with women with GDM can use these records to assess the woman's health and to reinforce health education, answer questions and monitor records to identify those in need of extra support. Self-maintenance of these records is empowering for the woman and also reinforces their importance. This type of monitoring also identifies the high blood glucose levels that are not necessarily brought to the attention of the diabetic team, perhaps from fear or denial of their significance. Telephone calls, rather than the more impersonal email or fax management, are probably more likely to lead to the formation of a trusting relationship between the woman and the midwife.

Labour and birth

In women with good glycaemic control and no complicating factors, there is no need to induce labour before term (MOH, 2014). A vaginal birth is the suggested approach for women with gestational diabetes but this would also depend upon any obstetric factors or complications that may have arisen. The woman's need for exogenous insulin by itself is not an indication for earlier birth or a caesarean section. During labour, blood sugar levels are monitored depending upon local guidelines. The 2015 NICE guidelines recommend hourly recordings of blood sugar levels, which should be maintained at 4–7 mmol / L. The woman's condition and that of her fetus are observed and monitored as in any normal labour, although the fetal heart rate is usually continuously electronically monitored once labour commences.

Postnatal care and follow-up

A management plan should be made by the multidisciplinary team prior to birth. During the early postnatal period this includes blood sugar estimations to detect hypoglycaemia, as the postpartum woman's insulin requirements will fall rapidly after the birth for 24 hours (MOH, 2014). If she is on metformin this will be stopped after the birth and doses of insulin are reduced, depending on the blood sugar levels. Early breastfeeding is recommended and encouraged; although it does alter the woman's blood glucose levels, it is associated with better neonatal outcomes and maternal weight loss postpartum. Breastfeeding also improves fasting blood glucose levels, glucose tolerance and lipid levels. The baby should be observed, have an early breastfeed and regular recording of blood sugar levels from 2 hours following birth to detect hypoglycaemia (MOH, 2014).

Before going home, the woman should be counselled about the risk of having GDM in another pregnancy as well as the increased likelihood of getting type 2 diabetes in her lifetime. She should be given advice on healthy eating and lifestyle modifications for her own wellbeing, which can often improve the eating and regular exercise habits of her family at the same time. Women are advised to have HbA_{1c} measurement 3 months after the birth postpartum and annually thereafter with their GP (MOH, 2014).

Thyroid disease

Numerous hormonal changes occur during pregnancy, resulting in complex metabolic adaptations in maternal thyroid function. Despite this, a normal pregnancy is considered to be a euthyroid state. If not treated during pregnancy, hyperthyroidism and hypothyroid disease can be harmful to both mother and baby (Gorringe, 2019; ACOG, 2020). There is insufficient evidence at present to support routine screening for thyroid disease (Gorringe, 2019; ACOG, 2020).

The following women have an increased risk of thyroid disease in pregnancy and thyroid level testing should be considered (Gorringe, 2019):

- family history of thyroid dysfunction / goitre
- history of thyroid dysfunction and / or thyroid surgery
- women with anti-thyroid antibodies with symptoms or clinical signs of hypothyroidism
- infertility
- history of miscarriage or pre-term birth
- morbid obesity, or prepregnancy BMI >30
- type 1 diabetes or other autoimmune disorders
- from an area of known moderate to severe iodine deficiency
- previous birth of an infant with thyroid disease
- prior head or neck irradiation.

During pregnancy, thyroid-stimulating hormone (TSH) and free thyroxine (FT_4) levels can be used to diagnose thyroid disease

- During the first trimester of pregnancy, TSH levels should be <2.5 mU / L.
- Second and third trimester TSH levels should be <3.0 mU / L (Gorringe, 2019; ACOG, 2020).

In Australia and New Zealand, all women are advised to take a 0.150 mg / 150 µg iodine-only tablet daily throughout pregnancy and whilst breastfeeding. This can be prescribed by their midwife.

Hyperthyroidism

Hyperthyroidism, also known as thyrotoxicosis, occurs in 0.2%–0.7% of pregnancies and is primarily due to Graves' disease, which accounts for more than 95% of hyperthyroid cases (ACOG, 2020). Signs of this disease are excessive perspiration, fatigue, disturbed sleep, heat intolerance, raised metabolic rate, weight loss where there is good calorific intake, rapid irregular heart rate, palpitations, hypertension and nervousness (ACOG, 2020). It is not easy to diagnose in pregnancy because of normal thyroid changes; there is often slight palpable enlargement of the thyroid gland (a goitre) at this time. If left untreated, severe thyrotoxicosis, a life-threatening thyrotoxic crisis (i.e. thyroid storm), can occur (ACOG, 2020). Predominant tri-iodothyronine (T_3) thyrotoxicosis, commonly seen in patients with toxic nodules and some patients with Graves' disease, is a management dilemma. Treatment to normalise T_3 may result in hypothyroxinaemia and potentially compromise the fetus. Treatment of hyperthyroidism during pregnancy is different from that in non-pregnant women, because radioactive iodine cannot be given and surgery should not be performed because of an increased risk of miscarriage. Propylthiouracil (PTU) is the treatment of choice in any woman with Graves' disease planning pregnancy or in the first trimester because carbimazole is associated with a rare embryopathy. In the second and third trimesters, changing to carbimazole is advised because of the risk of fulminant hepatitis with PTU (ACOG, 2020).

Hypothyroidism

Overt hypothyroidism is defined as an elevated TSH associated with a low free T_4 and is thought to be associated with significant adverse pregnancy outcomes, gestational diabetes, PE and pre-term birth (ACOG, 2020). Hypothyroidism can be caused by defects in the thyroid gland, or TSH release, or in the control pathways of thyrotrophin-releasing hormone (TRH). Untreated hypothyroidism is associated with infertility and, if pregnancy does occur, there is an increased risk of miscarriage or prolonged pregnancy. Symptoms include constipation, low basal metabolic rate (BMR), thick and dry skin, feeling cold, oedema, puffy eyes, lethargy and mental sluggishness (ACOG, 2020). Overt maternal hypothyroidism requires urgent treatment with thyroxine. T_4 is also secreted in breast milk, but, provided the dosage in the mother is maintained in the physiological range, it appears to be quite safe for the mother on T_4 to breastfeed. After birth, the dose of T_4 is gradually returned to prepregnancy levels. There is an association between postnatal depression, failure to lactate and hypothyroidism, so thyroid levels should be checked in these situations. Subclinical hypothyroidism (SCH) is associated with adverse pregnancy outcomes, particularly miscarriage, but not impaired cognitive function. Drug therapy is controversial. Some clinicians consider low-dose T_4 replacement, aiming for TSH values falling within the trimester-specific reference ranges for euthyroid pregnant women. Postpartum thyroiditis (tPPT) affects one in 20 women. Its onset is usually about 3–6 months after birth. Generally the condition is self-limiting—beta-blockers can be used for symptomatic thyrotoxicosis (ACOG, 2020).

CRITICAL THINKING EXERCISE

An Australian woman asks you whether she should take an iodine supplement during pregnancy and when she is breastfeeding because she has heard that many Australian women are iodine deficient. What will you say? Which foods in Australia have been iodine fortified?

Heart disease

Fifty years ago, women with heart disease were advised to avoid pregnancy. Now it is not unusual for women with heart disease to have a normal (albeit carefully monitored) pregnancy. Heart disease in pregnancy has the potential to cause significant maternal morbidity or death and has been identified as a prime cause of maternal death in both the UK and the US (Knight, 2020). Women who die from acquired heart conditions are frequently not known to have a cardiac problem before pregnancy. Heart disease may be congenital or related to illness, ischemic heart disease and most commonly rheumatic heart disease. This is more common in indigenous populations in both Australia and New Zealand, resulting in major cardiac and perinatal morbidity (Sullivan et al., 2020). In Australia, cardiac disease was the leading cause of deaths classed as indirect maternal mortality in 2018 (AIHW, 2020c). Contraindications for women with heart disease to become pregnant include severe pulmonary hypertension or Eisenmenger's syndrome, cardiomyopathy with severe symptoms, severe uncorrected valvular disease and unrepaired congenital heart disease (CHD).

The mechanical stress placed upon the heart begins at conception; there is an increase in blood volume, compensatory lowering of systemic vascular resistance and an increase in heart rate and cardiac output. For women with cardiac disease the usual pregnancy changes in both anatomy and physiology, normally well tolerated, can become life threatening (Sullivan et al., 2020).

There are two reasons why a rise in the number of women with heart disease is occurring:

- Better medical care and technologies mean that women with congenital cardiac disease are surviving to reproductive age.
- Demographic changes have also resulted in an increase in incidence in areas where there are large immigrant communities (Bortnick, 2020).

Risk factors for heart disease in pregnancy include a positive family history of inherited cardiac disease, hypertension and obesity, and increased maternal age. The last is increasingly important as more women in older age groups delay childbearing or seek assisted conception.

Pre-conceptual maternity care

Ideally all women with known cardiac disease should be offered pre-conceptual counselling by a multidisciplinary team in ways that enable them to choose their best options. Pre-conceptual information sharing will often explore sensitive issues such as maternal life expectancy so that the woman and her partner are able to make informed decisions about whether they want to have children. Women with congenital heart defects will often want to know about the statistical likelihood of their children inheriting their condition. Pre-counselling enables the team to offer advice regarding healthy behaviours, smoking cessation, diet and exercise and to optimise medications and cease drugs that are contraindicated in pregnancy. Pre-conceptual clinical assessment should include a thorough clinical assessment (physical and psychosocial), relevant cardiac imaging, chest X-ray and/or cardiac catheterisation and exercise testing. Whenever possible, symptomatic or severe valvular lesions should be repaired prior to conception.

CLINICAL POINT

Healthy pregnancies are often associated with fatigue, dyspnoea and decreased exercise capacity. Pregnant women often have dependent oedema and jugular venous distension. Indeed, most have audible physiological systolic murmurs, created by augmented blood flow. A physiological third heart sound (S3), reflecting the volume-overloaded state, can often be auscultated. Thus normal haemodynamic changes in pregnancy may alter the presentation of a variety of cardiac conditions.

History taking

Given the increased prevalence of cardiac disease in pregnant women the following should be elucidated at the booking clinic:

- past history of congenital or acquired heart disease
- family or personal history of congenital heart disease
- history of hypertension
- history of dyspnoea, fatigue or oedema.

Signs of cardiac disease. Signs of cardiac compromise depend on the nature of the disease, and may include hypertension, dyspnoea, fatigue and ankle oedema. Other signs are: new regurgitant heart murmurs, pulmonary crackles, elevated jugular venous pressure and hepatomegaly. Occasionally pregnant women may present with atypical features of cardiac ischaemia, such as dyspnoea, vomiting or dizziness.

CLINICAL POINT

Heart murmurs

One study of 199 healthy pregnant women found that 93.2% had a systolic murmur at some time during their pregnancy. They are invariably systolic, may be early, mid or late and there may be a diastolic component. They are located predominantly at the second left intercostal space or along the left sternal border, although they may radiate widely. They may occur at any stage in pregnancy and may come and go.

Congenital heart disease

Most but not all pregnant women with CHD are aware of their condition and are already receiving cardiologist care. History taking at the first antenatal contact and questions about a past history of rheumatic fever plus auscultation of abnormal heart sounds may be the woman's first inkling that she has heart disease.

Specialist care, a multidisciplinary approach and all clinicians working as a team leads to better outcomes for both mother and baby. Individual counselling should ideally include information regarding contraception, maternal and fetal risks of pregnancy, and expected long-term outcomes.

Measures designed to optimise intravascular volume and systemic loading conditions enable many women with CHD to have successful outcomes. Pregnant women with mechanical valve prostheses have a need for anticoagulation. Unfortunately, there are significant risks for both the mother and fetus from either haemorrhage or thrombosis with the use of either warfarin or heparin.

Ischaemic heart disease

Atherosclerotic coronary artery disease was rarely seen among pregnant women until several decades ago. It is now becoming a relatively common cause of indirect maternal death. The increased incidence of myocardial infarction has occurred because of increased maternal age and less-healthy lifestyles leading to obesity, smoking, hypertension, hypercholesterolaemia and diabetes. Women with known risk factors should be screened preconceptually and should be treated before they embark on pregnancy (Nallapati & Park, 2021).

Rheumatic heart disease

Rheumatic heart disease (RHD) continues to decline as a major cause of maternal mortality in the Western world. However, it remains a major cause of morbidity and mortality in developing countries and for Aboriginal Australians and Torres Strait Islander young people (AIHW, 2020a). In New Zealand, acute rheumatic fever is now almost exclusively a disease affecting Māori and Pacific children, aged 4–19 years, living in low socioeconomic communities in the northern and central North Island and in pockets around the Wellington region (MOH, 2017a). In 2011, the New Zealand MOH Rheumatic Fever Prevention Programme began, with the intention of reducing the number of cases of group B streptococcal sore throat infections, which can lead to acute rheumatic fever (ARF) (MOH, 2017a). Recurrent episodes of ARF frequently lead to RHD, which can damage heart valves with associated morbidity. ARF/RHD is a neglected public health problem and is associated with poverty and neglect (AIHW, 2020a).

Management plans

Women with more than mild RHD should be identified as having a higher than normal risk of complications in pregnancy, and should receive antenatal care at an appropriate referral centre with an experienced obstetrician, in collaboration with an obstetric physician and/or cardiologist. The most severe cases should be seen at a referral centre with cardiology and intensive care facilities. Discussions with the woman regarding timing, nature and site of planned delivery should occur before or early in pregnancy.

During pregnancy, women with valvular heart disease should be reviewed regularly by a cardiac specialist, and cardiac status should be reviewed whenever there is a change in symptoms (Bortnick, 2020). A multidisciplinary approach to management is an important principle for care of the pregnant patient with rheumatic valvular disease. It is often necessary to advise women with heart disease to cease work earlier in pregnancy for medical reasons, as cardiac demands increase significantly as pregnancy proceeds. Most women with valvular heart disease become more symptomatic in the third trimester.

Rheumatic heart disease in Northern Australia

Australia's Aboriginal and Torres Strait Islander peoples living in remote areas have one of the highest rates of RHD in the world. Data on ARF (acute rheumatic fever) and RHD in Australia is reported in a national data collection set from all the states in the Commonwealth. The incidence of ARF is the greatest in 5–14-year-olds, with 60% of Indigenous Australians under 25 years of age when diagnosed with RHD (AIHW, 2020a). In the Northern Territory, prevalence rates of RHD have risen steadily to 141 per 100,00 (AIHW, 2020a). For these reasons this section on cardiac disease is primarily focused on the effects of RHD with special emphasis on the effects of valvular disease on pregnancy and its management.

The predictors of increased maternal and fetal risk in the pregnant patient with rheumatic valvular disease are:

- reduced left ventricle (LV) systolic function
- significant aortic or mitral stenosis
- moderate or severe pulmonary hypertension
- a history of heart failure
- symptomatic valvular disease before pregnancy
- atrial fibrillation, especially when anticoagulation is required
- pregnant women with mechanical valves are a very high-risk group, in whom all anticoagulation options carry maternal and/or fetal risks.

Valvular heart disease

Valvular heart disease is often first recognised in pregnancy when the profound haemodynamic changes that normally occur during pregnancy put additional strain on the heart, sometimes precipitating heart failure.

Clinical presentation

Mitral stenosis is the most common rheumatic valvular lesion encountered during pregnancy. Depending on the severity and duration of the disease, pregnant women with mitral stenosis frequently present clinically with symptoms of both left-sided heart failure and right ventricular failure. However, left-sided heart failure is more common and symptoms include orthopnoea, paroxysmal nocturnal dyspnoea and dyspnoea on exertion.

> **CLINICAL POINT**
>
> Symptoms of normal pregnancy can mimic those of valvular heart disease. The presence of a loud fourth heart sound, a diastolic murmur, a grade 3/6 or greater systolic murmur, a fixed split of the second heart sound and an opening snap should raise suspicion of cardiac abnormalities. The presence of one or more of these signs should signal the need for referral to specialist care and echocardiographic evaluation.

Diagnostic assessment

Invasive diagnostic testing is rarely indicated in pregnant women with mitral stenosis. Echocardiography is the diagnostic test of choice because it both confirms the diagnosis and helps to determine the severity of the condition. In addition, it is used to determine pulmonary pressures, right ventricular function and mitral regurgitation.

Management in pregnancy

Generally, the onset of RHD occurs in childhood and adolescence; it affects more women than men. Potentially RHD can complicate pregnancy and labour. There are a number of factors that are important in ensuring a good outcome for both mother and child.

Important factors in the early detection and management of RHD in women who are planning to become pregnant, or who are pregnant, include the following:

- Detect early and exclude RHD.
- In populations at high risk of RHD, all women who have a heart murmur require an early echocardiogram. Echocardiography is an essential tool in the diagnosis, assessment of severity and management of RHD.
- If there is a history of ARF, the result of a recent echocardiogram should be reviewed.
- Assess and treat before pregnancy occurs.
- Refer women with known RHD for specialist physician/cardiologist review.
- Discuss options for fertility planning and contraception with women with RHD.
- Once pregnancy occurs it is important that the woman is involved in all decisions about the planned model of care including place and mode of birth.
- Ensure a coordinated and multidisciplinary care team is in place early—pregnant women with RHD require a team approach linking primary healthcare, obstetric services, anaesthetics and specialist physicians/cardiologists.

In addition to the measures designed to manage symptoms, rest is encouraged and dietary advice given to aid weight control. Iron and folic acid are prescribed to prevent anaemia (common in Indigenous Australians) and haemoglobin estimation is undertaken frequently. To prevent bacterial endocarditis (see below), a dental referral is made early in pregnancy. If the woman presents with any signs of infection, she is commenced on antibiotics. Any deterioration in her condition, such as dyspnoea and a cough, requires hospital admission. Rarely, women require mitral valvotomy during pregnancy to increase the size of a narrowed mitral valve. A cardiologist may restrict salt and fluid intake. However, diuretics are used with caution to avoid hypotension and tachycardia as well as fetal compromise caused by maternal hypotension and hypoxaemia. Beta-blocking drugs to slow the heart rate can dramatically improve the woman's symptoms.

Labour and birth

In view of the increased cardiac output during labour and after giving birth, it is important to plan management carefully. With very few exceptions, vaginal birth is preferable in most women with cardiac disease. Pre-term induction is rarely indicated, but planned induction of labour and birth for women with increased risk can ensure availability of appropriate staff and equipment. Heparin anticoagulation is discontinued at least 12 hours before induction of labour, or reversed with protamine sulfate if spontaneous labour develops, and can usually be resumed 6–12 hours postpartum.

Optimal management may also require invasive haemodynamic studies in women with moderate to severe mitral stenosis. Continuous oxygen via facial mask may be helpful to reduce pulmonary pressures and fluid restriction, and use of diuretics and epidural anaesthesia with adequate volume preloading is the technique of choice. Epidural fentanyl is particularly advantageous in women with cyanotic heart disease because it does not lower peripheral vascular resistance. Instrumental birth will shorten the second stage of labour and reduce the need for maternal expulsive efforts. Active management of the third stage of labour can reduce the incidence of PPH and its complications.

Antibiotic prophylaxis against endocarditis

The incidence of endocarditis is no different in pregnant women with valvular heart disease to that in non-pregnant women with the same condition. Streptococcal organisms are the most common cause of subacute bacterial endocarditis, but acute endocarditis is usually due to more virulent organisms such as *Staphylococcus aureus*, *Streptococcus pneumoniae* and *Neisseria gonorrhoeae*. The 2007 American Heart Association guidelines for the prevention of infective endocarditis do not recommend antibiotic prophylaxis for prevention of infective endocarditis in pregnant women.

Anticoagulation

Pregnancy involves a state of hypercoagulability caused by increased levels of various clotting factors and increased blood viscosity. Systemic anticoagulation poses major problems during pregnancy in women with prosthetic heart valves, venous or arterial thromboembolism, or atrial fibrillation with valvular heart disease.

Anticoagulation therapy during pregnancy

The three most common agents considered for use during pregnancy are unfractionated heparin (UH), low-molecular-weight heparin (LMWH) and warfarin. All three medications are useful in the management of cardiac disease in pregnancy and the puerperium. Before embarking on a treatment plan, the healthcare team and the woman need to carefully discuss the risks and benefits of warfarin, UH and LMWH.

Postnatal care and follow-up

Maternal haemodynamics do not return to baseline for many days after giving birth, so women may require ongoing monitoring for up to 72 hours postpartum. They should be encouraged to rest to support their recovery. Breastfeeding is not contraindicated

Prior to discharge contraception and future pregnancies should be discussed. The woman should be followed up at the cardiology clinic, in addition to the midwife and GP follow-up.

CRITICAL THINKING EXERCISE

- How will you respond to a woman with mitral valve stenosis who asks whether it is safe to take warfarin in early pregnancy?
- Women who have had valve replacements are often on oral anticoagulation therapy. Then, as the anticipated birth date draws near, this is changed to subcutaneous heparin. Why is this change of therapy necessary and what are the evidence-based advantages and disadvantages of LMWH versus UH in pregnancy and the postpartum period?

Respiratory disease

Pregnancy induces profound changes in the mother, resulting in significant alterations in normal physiology. The anatomical and functional changes of pregnancy affect the respiratory and cardiovascular systems. Management of respiratory problems in pregnancy requires an understanding of these changes for interpretation of clinical and laboratory manifestations of respiratory diseases.

Asthma

Asthma is a commonly occurring medical condition with increasing incidence in the general population and has been found to often get worse during pregnancy (Hindley, 2018). Severe and / or poorly controlled asthma has been associated with numerous adverse perinatal outcomes, including congenital malformations, placenta praevia, pre-term birth, gestational diabetes, PE, small for gestational age (SGA), low birth weight, caesarean section, neonatal hospitalisation and death (Hindley, 2018; Cusack & Gauvreau, 2020).

In pregnancy, asthma can be triggered by: allergies, upper respiratory tract infection, sinusitis, exercise, aspirin, non-steroidal anti-inflammatory drugs (NSAIDs), environmental toxins (e.g. tobacco smoke, chemical fumes), humidity, anxiety and emotional distress (Hindley, 2018). In these circumstances, it is vital that midwives are aware of the potential impact of asthma to ensure optimal health for both mother and baby (Hindley, 2018). A critical issue for pregnant women with asthma is cigarette smoking and being around others who smoke, as data indicate that if they do so they are more at risk of episodes of acute exacerbation with more severe symptoms (Clifton, 2019; Cusack & Gauvreau, 2020). Smoking cessation programs and one-to-one advice can be effective during pregnancy and therefore should be promoted to women with asthma.

Asthma medications during pregnancy

The aim of effective asthma control in pregnancy is to enable the best achievable asthma control and prevent acute exacerbations. These goals are accomplished by the prevention of day- and night-time symptoms, and the maintenance of lung function and normal activity (Cusack & Gauvreau, 2020). Although care providers have a natural reluctance to prescribe drug therapy in pregnancy, poorly controlled asthma is potentially more dangerous for the fetus than medication (Cusack & Gauvreau, 2020). Women with asthma should therefore be advised to continue with their prepregnancy medication in consultation with a multidisciplinary team, working with asthma in pregnancy guidelines and an achievable management plan (Hindley, 2018).

Diagnostic testing for asthma in pregnant women

Asthma is assumed in the presence of typical symptoms, such as chest tightness, wheezing, associated shortness of breath with a cough. A diagnosis of asthma is ideally established by the evidence of reversible airway obstruction, which usually takes the form of an increase in forced expiratory volume in 1 second (FEV_1) by $\geq$12% and at least 200 mL after an inhaled short-acting bronchodilator. The partial pressure of oxygen in arterial blood (P_aO_2) is higher in pregnant women than in non-pregnant women, ranging from 102 mmHg to 116 mmHg). In addition, the normal physiological increase in minute ventilation results in a lower P_aCO_2 range of 28 mmHg to 30 mmHg. Therefore, a low P_aO_2 or a high P_aCO_2 associated with an acute episode of asthma may represent significantly more severe respiratory compromise than similar blood gas values in a non-pregnant woman.

Management of asthma (Box 37.14)

Asthma education programs tailored to pregnant women and delivered by an asthma educator / midwife can contribute to significant improvements in all aspects of asthma self-management including inhaler technique, knowledge of and adherence to prescribed medications. There is extensive evidence for the safety of major drug classes used to treat asthma during pregnancy, including short-acting beta-2 agonists, some inhaled corticosteroids (ICSs) and theophylline. The safety of oral corticosteroids is less clear.

As with non-pregnant women, beta-2 agonists are used for symptomatic benefit during acute asthma. ICSs remain the mainstay of therapy for asthma control. Occasionally corticosteroids are necessary but should be used for only short periods. An increased risk of cleft palate and placental abnormalities is reported in animals given oral steroids in the first trimester, but not in humans. Nevertheless, the benefits of oral steroids may outweigh the risks if they are used to manage severe asthma or during life-threatening exacerbations because the steroid- to oral-cleft-palate relationship is irrelevant after the first trimester.

Updates on asthma management guidelines are available online from the Asthma + Respiratory Foundation NZ (see Online resources).

Box 37.14 Asthma management

Environmental control, pharmacological treatment and specific allergen immunotherapy are the cornerstones of asthma management for all patients. Of these, institution of environmental control measures to lessen exposure to triggers is even more vital during pregnancy. Helping women to learn how to watch for and avoid these triggers will probably improve symptom control, and may possibly result in pregnant women needing less medication. Gastro-oesophageal reflux is a common problem in late pregnancy and is a documented asthma trigger. Advising the woman to eat small meals and to raise the head of her bed by several centimetres may help alleviate this problem. Some women may require antacids or H_2-receptor-blocking medications.

CLINICAL POINT

Medications for asthma have been shown to be safe for both the mother and the developing baby (Clifton, 2019; Cusack & Gauvreau, 2020). It is more dangerous to have untreated asthma during pregnancy than to continue with prescribed asthma therapy. Asthma reduces the amount of oxygen available to the fetus. To maintain optimal asthma control it is important for women to follow their asthma action plan very carefully.

Breastfeeding

Breastfeeding should be encouraged in women with asthma, because breast milk confers some immunity to infection to the baby, especially to respiratory and gastrointestinal infections. Breast milk contains very small amounts of the usual medications used to prevent and treat asthma, but there is no evidence that this is harmful to the infant.

Women should be reassured that, although asthma medications do enter breast milk, their concentrations are extremely small and do not have any adverse effects on their babies.

Acute asthma exacerbation

Acute exacerbations that necessitate emergency department visits typically require a course of systemic corticosteroids. In addition, oxygen therapy is used to maintain oxygen saturation levels at or above 95% to ensure both maternal and fetal wellbeing. There is no evidence of teratogenic effects associated with bronchospasm relaxants such as the beta-2 agonists (category A)—salbutamol, terbutaline and fenoterol.

Client education

Most complications of asthma during pregnancy are from undermedication; thus, the goal is to emphasise the importance and safety of therapy. Education should cover the following aspects of asthma and pregnancy:

- signs and symptoms of asthma
- the effect of pregnancy on asthma
- importance and safety of the medication to the fetus and to the mother
- warning signs that indicate the woman should seek urgent help
- potential harm to their fetus and increased risk to themselves with poor compliance with treatment or unnecessary delays in seeking medical assistance
- prevention, minimising known triggers
- correct use of metered-dose inhalers and peak flow meters
- adverse effects of therapies
- use of written diaries to record peak expiratory flow rate (PEFR)
- use of action plans for managing an exacerbation of the disease.

Tuberculosis

In contrast with many countries, Australia and New Zealand are fortunate in having a low but relatively constant pattern of tuberculosis (TB). This is due predominantly to the reactivation of latent infection in people who were previously infected in their countries of birth or during their childhood. The incidence of TB in Australia averages around 1000 new cases per year (in Victoria, 250–320 per year). If a woman receiving medication for active TB becomes pregnant, she continues with her medications. If the disease is diagnosed for the first time during pregnancy, antituberculoid medication is still commenced and this protects the fetus from the disease. Labour is managed normally and, in the presence of active disease, an elective vacuum extraction or forceps delivery may be recommended to shorten the second stage of labour.

The risk of disease developing in a tuberculin-positive pregnant woman with a normal chest X-ray is the same as that for a non-pregnant woman.

The disease may reactivate in the postnatal period. Breastfeeding is contraindicated if the woman has active TB while treatment is established; antituberculoid drug therapy crosses into the breast milk. To minimise the level of antituberculoid drugs in the newborn, the woman is advised to take her antituberculoid drugs immediately after breastfeeding and then use formula until the next day.

Vaccination is always recommended in high-risk groups, such as people from Asian or Pacific Island backgrounds and Aboriginal Australians, or if other members of the household have or have had a history of pulmonary TB, or if they are likely to come into contact with people at high risk of infection. In Australia and New Zealand, parents are encouraged to immunise their babies with BCG (bacille Calmette–Guérin) vaccine.

Untreated TB represents a far greater hazard to a pregnant woman and her fetus than does the treatment of the disease. Isoniazid and ethambutol are both category A drugs, and considered safe in pregnancy. Drug companies recommend that rifampicin (category C) be avoided in pregnancy although evidence regarding the teratogenicity of rifampicin is inconclusive.

Renal disease

The renal system undergoes major physiological and anatomical changes during a normal pregnancy (see Ch. 20). An understanding of these changes is necessary in order to understand how they may lead to or worsen pre-existing or new renal disease. Only the most common conditions are dealt with in this section. Others, such as glomerular nephritis, chronic renal disease and renal transplantation, are not included here and the reader should refer to the appropriate specialist texts.

Urinary tract infection

Urinary tract infections (UTIs), especially asymptomatic bacteriuria and cystitis, are common pregnancy complications. Pyelonephritis is less common but has the potential to cause significant morbidity and adverse outcomes. Early identification and treatment of UTIs in pregnancy and postpartum are crucial because of their close association with maternal hypertension, anaemia and pre-term labour, putting the fetus at risk of all the complications associated with low birth weight. The fetus is also at risk of IUGR. It seems that the bacterium that causes the UTI has the potential to infect fetal membranes, leading to chorioamnionitis. Finally, inadequately treated UTIs and upper tract infections such as pyelonephritis have a high incidence of later chronic renal pathology.

Contrary to popular belief, non-culture methods such as dipsticks are not generally reliable for the identification of bacteriuria in asymptomatic populations, including pregnant women.

Traditionally, and still current in practice today, screening pregnant women's urine for glucose, ketones and protein at every antenatal visit was 'routine'. In addition to laboratory screening tests, as a key aspect of the initial or, as it's often referred to, booking visit, it is important that the midwife gathers data about the woman's history of infections and existing renal pathology, renal function studies and family or personal history of renal disease, hypertension or connective tissue disorders.

Asymptomatic bacteriuria and cystitis

As identified in a recent systematic review (Wingert et al., 2019), there is no reliable evidence to recommend routine screening in early pregnancy or in the third trimester for asymptomatic bacteriuria, as was the traditional practice for many years. Many of the studies supporting this practice were done in the 1950s–80s, and as such application of these studies to current practice was questioned and found to be limited by today's research standards. Therefore, the practice has largely been discontinued. The rationale for screening was that there was an association between adverse pregnancy outcomes, primarily SGA babies and premature birth, with infections of the urinary tract, which can occur quite frequently for some women owing to physiological changes that occur in pregnancy. The Wingert et al. (2019) review determined that for women with significant bacteriuria, having antibiotic treatment probably reduces the incidence of pyelonephritis and low birth weight. A Cochrane review by Schneeberger et al. (2015) considered various therapeutic interventions, both pharmacological using antibiotics and non-pharmacological such as cranberry, acupuncture or probiotics, and found these to be ineffective to prevent reoccurring UTIs in pregnancy.

Normal anatomical and physiological changes in pregnancy

The normal anatomical and physiological changes in pregnancy predispose the pregnant woman to UTIs (see also Ch. 20). In brief, starting in the first weeks of pregnancy, most pregnant women develop hydronephrosis of pregnancy. Under the influence of pregnancy hormones, increased bladder volume and decreased bladder tone, along with decreased ureteral tone, contribute to increased urinary stasis and ureterovesical reflux. This urine becomes a good growth medium for bacteria. Also, an increase in the plasma volume during pregnancy decreases urine concentration. More than two-thirds of pregnant women develop glycosuria, which encourages bacterial growth in the urine. Increases in urinary progestins and oestrogens reduce the ability of the lower urinary tract to resist pathogens. Midwives are ideally placed to work with women to prevent the initial occurrence of UTIs and ongoing problems (Box 37.15).

In a urinary tract infection, the choice of antibiotic should address the most common infecting organisms (i.e. Gram-negative gastrointestinal organisms such as *E. coli*). Historically, ampicillin has been the drug of choice, but in recent years *E. coli* has become increasingly resistant to ampicillin. Other antibiotics include nitrofurantoin, the cephalosporins, and Fosfomycin (Monurol), which is taken as a single dose. Sulfonamides can be taken during the first and second trimesters, but during the third trimester their use carries a risk of kernicterus of the newborn, especially pre-term infants. Tetracyclines are contraindicated for use in pregnancy because of rare maternal acute fatty liver necrosis. In addition, they cause permanent staining of the fetal dentition. A 5- to 10-day course of antibiotic treatment is usually sufficient to eradicate the infecting organism(s). Some authorities have advocated shorter courses of treatment—even single-day therapy.

Box 37.15 Preventing urinary tract infections (UTIs)

Measures include the following:

- Drink 6–8 glasses of water each day, to flush out bacteria. Unsweetened cranberry juice may prevent UTIs.
- Avoid refined foods, fruit juices, caffeine, alcohol and sugar.
- Develop a habit of urinating as soon as the need is felt, emptying the bladder completely.
- Wipe the perineum from front to back after voiding or defecation.
- Avoid using strong soaps, douches, antiseptic creams, feminine hygiene sprays and powder.
- Urinate before and after sexual intercourse.
- Wear cotton underwear and avoid tight-fitting pants.
- Use lubricating jelly if needed during sexual intercourse.
- Report early signs of UTI or genital infection.
- Always complete a course of antibiotics.

Symptomatic cystitis

A woman with symptomatic cystitis often complains of urgency and frequency of micturition and dysuria. She may have some lower abdominal discomfort and a slightly raised temperature and pulse rate. In general, treatment is initiated before the results of the culture are available. A midstream urine sample (MSU) is sent to the laboratory for a bacterial count, the leucocyte (pus) cell count and the identification of the organisms present and their sensitivity to several antibiotics. If the bacterial count is over 10^5 organisms per mL of urine, the woman is commenced on a broad-spectrum antibiotic (see above).

A repeat MSU should be obtained 1–2 weeks later and a further course of antibiotics prescribed if infection is still present. Women who present with more than three UTIs in the antenatal period require referral to a renal physician.

Pyelonephritis

Acute pyelonephritis during pregnancy is a serious systemic illness that can progress to maternal sepsis and pre-term birth. Pyelonephritis occurs in 2% of pregnant women and almost 25% will have another episode of the disease in the same pregnancy. The diagnosis is made when the presence of bacteriuria is accompanied by systemic symptoms or signs such as pyrexia, rigors, nausea and vomiting, and flank pain. Symptoms of lower tract infection (i.e. frequency of micturition and dysuria) may or may not be present.

Collaborative management of UTIs

Treatment varies according to the nature of the renal infection. Aggressive treatment is important in preventing complications from pyelonephritis. Hospitalisation is indicated for women who are exhibiting signs of sepsis, who are vomiting, perhaps dehydrated and who may be having uterine contractions. The woman is observed for any signs of the onset of labour, and fetal wellbeing is assessed through CTG and/or Doppler ultrasonography. Intravenous rehydration and IV antibiotic therapy may be initiated before obtaining the results of urine culture and sensitivity. Follow-up and repeat MSUs are undertaken to ensure the infection has been adequately treated. Other diagnostic tests may include renal ultrasonography or, if indicated, an abbreviated IV pyelogram.

CLINICAL POINT

The most common reason for treatment failure in pyelonephritis is antibiotic resistance.

'Natural' remedies for the prevention of UTIs

There are a number of non-pharmacological, 'natural' remedies for the prevention of UTIs. There is some evidence that undiluted cranberry juice may decrease the number of symptomatic UTIs in non-pregnant women. However, to date, there has been little research examining the effectiveness of complementary remedies. Any complementary therapy should be prescribed and administered by a suitably-qualified health practitioner and avoided in the 1st trimester.

Obstetric cholestasis (intrahepatic cholestasis)

Obstetric cholestasis is a rare liver disease and multifactorial condition of pregnancy characterised by intense pruritus in the absence of a skin rash, with abnormal liver function tests (LFTs) and/or raised bile acids (Lee et al., 2021), neither of which has an alternative cause and both of which resolve following birth of the baby. Influences upon the prevalence of this rare condition of pregnancy are thought to be possibly environmental and genetic but vary between populations worldwide (Lee et al., 2021). The wide-ranging definitions applied to obstetric cholestasis, along with the lack of agreed diagnostic criteria, make comparisons between published literature a challenge and result in limitations to provide detailed recommendations for specific aspects of care for women affected by this condition (Lee et al., 2021).

The clinical importance of obstetric cholestasis lies in the potential fetal risks to the baby; these are iatrogenic pre-term birth, premature birth and still birth. The risk of stillbirth is considered to be comparable to whole population figures, except for women with bile acids of 100 μmol/L or more, where an association with increased stillbirth has been found (Ovadia, 2019) After birth, meconium is often found to have been passed. There can also be significant maternal morbidity in association with the intense pruritus and consequent sleep deprivation (Lee et al., 2021).

The cause of obstetric cholestasis is still unknown it has been suggested it is caused by the higher levels of circulating oestrogen in pregnancy along with genetic factors. It can reoccur in subsequent pregnancies (Lee et al., 2021).

Once a diagnosis has been confirmed, women will need care, support and surveillance from the obstetric team. If a woman has severe pruritus without alteration in her LFTs then these should be repeated every 1–2 weeks. Other indicators of cholestasis are dark urine, pale stools and possibly jaundice. These should be noted and investigated. Any other potential risk indicators should be explored, such as a personal or family history of obstetric cholestasis, the presence of gallstones, a multiple pregnancy or a carrier of hepatitis C (Lee et al., 2021).

There is no clear evidence that any specific treatment improves maternal symptoms or neonatal outcomes. The woman with obstetric cholestasis requires close monitoring of her and her fetus. This includes regular ultrasound assessment for growth, and weekly LFTs, CTG recordings and/or Doppler ultrasonography, (RCOG, 2011c). Rest and a good diet are encouraged. Frequent cool baths, the use of skin lotions to soothe the itch and the wearing of loose-fitting cotton clothing may be helpful. Ursodeoxycholic acid (Urso) improves the itching and normalises biochemistry. Dexamethasone and vitamin K administration are also helpful. In New Zealand the IOL guidelines advise expectant management unless the bile acid concentration is equal or more than 100 μmol/L or if the woman is experiencing problematic symptoms (MOH, 2019). Current practice in many places is induction of labour at about 37 weeks to avoid the potential risk of stillbirth (Lee et al., 2021).

Postpartum LFTs return to normal but their measurement should be delayed until a postnatal follow-up appointment or after the first 10 days owing to a usual rise in LFTs following birth; the associated pruritus quickly resolves. Before the primary care provider terminates her relationship with the woman, it is important to ensure that the woman is reassured about the lack of long-term sequelae for her and her baby, informed about the high recurrence rate during pregnancy, as well as the increased incidence of obstetric cholestasis in other family members, and discusses contraceptive choices (usually avoiding oestrogen-containing methods).

Epilepsy

Epilepsy is a term used to describe a neurological disorder that results in unprovoked seizures. It is a commonly seen medical disorder, affecting 50 million people all over the world (Doyle et al., 2016). Epilepsy has been described as 'abnormal discharges of cerebral neurons [that] result in the alteration or impairment of consciousness, sensation or motor function' (Doyle et al., 2016, p. 830). Although most women with seizure disorders find that pregnancy has no effect on their disease, about one-third will have an increase in seizure activity. The causes of epilepsy are hard to identify and can be complex owing to many unknown reasons. The following are identified by the UK's Epilepsy Society (2017):

- a genetic tendency that can be either inherited from one or both parents or not inherited
- a structural or symptomatic change in the brain from a birth injury, infection, stroke or a tumour
- genetic conditions resulting in structural changes, for example neurofibromatosis or tuberous sclerosis.

Epileptic seizures can be stimulated by lack of sleep, increase in temperature, hypoglycaemia, water intoxication, drugs, emotional and physical stress, hyperventilation, strobe lights, some music and constipation.

Pre-conceptual care and planning with a multidisciplinary team of healthcare professionals is aimed at reducing risks to both mother and her unborn child, with a heightened awareness of potential complications from pregnancy (Morley, 2018).

Risks during pregnancy

Women with sub-optimal levels of anticonvulsants are at risk of sudden unexpected death in epilepsy (SUDEP). This risk is exacerbated when there are difficult social circumstances or there is delayed referral or barriers to access for specialist services (PMMRC, 2015). The effectiveness of the anti-epileptic drugs (AED) can be disrupted during pregnancy which may lead to lack of seizure control. Some women experience an increase in seizure frequency because they have changed or reduced the amount of anticonvulsant medication they take. Therefore, whenever possible, the anticonvulsant medication the woman has been prescribed prior to becoming pregnant should be maintained, although the dosage may require adjusting later in the pregnancy.

Risks to the fetus

Antiepileptic medications pose significant risks for the fetus with reports of congenital malformations associated with many of the commonly prescribed AEDs: phenytoin, phenobarbitone, primidone, valproate, carbamazepine and trimethadione. In addition, children born to women with epilepsy are, on average, smaller in size and weight than those born to women who do not have epilepsy. The reasons for this discrepancy are not clear. However, such disparities and congenital malformations occur even without AED use. Just as importantly, maternal seizures increase the risk of injury, miscarriage, epilepsy in the offspring and children's developmental delay.

Therefore the goal during pregnancy should be to prevent all seizures. In general, as the risk from the drugs is very small, having a seizure during pregnancy is much more dangerous to the fetus than the dangers associated with antiepileptic medications. Therefore, if the risk for recurrent seizures is high, then medication should still be used. However, in women at low risk of seizure, before becoming pregnant it may be possible for these women to decrease pharmacotherapy or to taper the dosages of AEDs.

Collaborative management

All women diagnosed with epilepsy require referral to a multidisciplinary team who will work collaboratively with the woman to provide her and the baby with quality care. Women with epilepsy should be encouraged to register in the Australian Pregnancy Register (APR) of AEDs.

A major component to healthy pregnancy for sufferers of epilepsy is multivitamin therapy with folate. Research shows the use of folate can help to minimise the risk of some of the major congenital anomalies, especially those involving the spinal cord. The vast majority of women will have a good outcome and so it is important to reassure them of this. The mainstays of treatments are: preconception counselling, focusing on optimisation of AEDs, folic acid supplementation and reliable contraception to prevent unplanned pregnancy and reduce the risk of complications.

Pre-conceptual care

All women who are epileptic should be offered genetic counselling. Prepregnancy discussions should enable shared decision making and include information about the risks to mother and fetus as well as the need for modification of her AED regimen to reduce the number of drugs and total dose (Morley, 2018).

CRITICAL THINKING EXERCISE

Below is a checklist for pre-conceptual discussion with a woman with epilepsy. Using it as a guide, assess what the woman knows, wants to know and what information you should share with her.

- Discuss the diagnosis and its implications for childbearing.
- Review seizure frequency and severity.
- Consider use of a seizure diary.
- Discuss drugs—benefits, disadvantages, modifications and side effects.
- Discuss the impact of pregnancy on the woman and her family's lifestyle.
- Provide contact information of support organisations.
- Discuss contraception and pregnancy.

Pregnancy

Adjustment of the anticonvulsant regimen during pregnancy may be necessary dependent on the medications being used. Lamotrigine and levetiracetam should be increased in the second and third trimesters under the supervision of the physician (PMMRC, 2015). Excessive weight gain due to fluid retention during pregnancy may exacerbate seizure activity and so the woman will need advice about optimal weight gain.

CLINICAL POINT

Epilepsy in pregnancy

The PMMRC recommends that:

1. All pregnant women with epilepsy on medication be referred to a physician. Women with a new diagnosis of epilepsy or a change in seizure frequency should be referred urgently.
2. The dose of anti-epileptic drugs may need to proactively increase. In particular, lamotrigine and levetiracetam should be increased in the second and third trimesters.
3. Labour and birth care for women with epilepsy should be provided in a secondary or tertiary obstetric hospital (NICE, 2012).
4. Communicate and document the plan of care for the woman, her family/whānau, and all practitioners involved in her care.

(PMMRC, 2017)

Intrapartum care

Women should be advised to plan birth in a secondary or tertiary unit due to an increased risk of seizures during labour. The woman's usual anticonvulsant regimen is maintained during labour with usual labour care provided. If seizures occur, intravenous benzodiazepine (e.g. lorazepam or diazepam) is the medication of choice. Where possible, a paediatrician should review the baby to exclude the possibility of rare congenital malformations secondary to the teratogenic effects of anticonvulsants.

Postpartum care

There remains an increased risk of seizures into the postpartum, so women should be advised to consider how to modify that risk (PMMRC, 2015). The woman's family / whānau should be aware of first aid procedures during a seizure. Discussion during the postpartum should consider how to minimise risks and include topics such as sleeping, bathing and the care of young children, and who is available to provide support. Women should be advised not to drive if they have had a recent seizure.

Management of seizures

Seizures can occur at any time and any place, and can be especially tricky to manage if they occur in water or in a confined space. In the community or in hospital, for women with generalised tonic–clonic seizures, the following general guidelines should be followed:

- Secure the airway (the priority is always the DRABC).
- Call for help—midwives, anaesthetist, obstetrician, physician and paediatrician.
- Give oxygen.
- Assess cardiac and respiratory function.
- Secure IV access in large veins.
- Seizures will usually be managed with IV medications such as diazepam and phenytoin. If there is a delay in IV access diazepam can be given rectally.
- Assess the fetal heart rate or fetal status.
- Rule out eclampsia.

Following a seizure, hospital care may include the following:

- Collect blood for full blood count, urea and electrolytes, LFTs, calcium, glucose, clotting, AED levels and storage for later analysis.
- Check fetal status. A non-reassuring heart rate trace may indicate an emergency caesarean section.
- Measure blood gases to assess extent of acidosis.
- Establish aetiology and treat as necessary.

If the seizures persist (status epilepticus), the woman is:

- admitted to an intensive care unit and administered general anaesthesia
- monitored using EEG to assess seizure control
- referred for specialist advice.

Thromboembolic disease

Pulmonary embolism and **deep vein thrombosis** (DVT) are the two components of venous thromboembolism (VTE). Pregnant women have an increased risk (four- to fivefold) over that of non-pregnant women of developing a VTE owing to hypercoagulability, increased venous stasis, decreased venous outflow and compression of the inferior vena cava and pelvic veins by the enlarging uterus (Middleton et al., 2021). VTE used to be one of the leading causes of maternal deaths worldwide but has become less so owing to improved prevention and treatment.

Pathology

During pregnancy a woman's body is in a prothrombolic state (Alshawabkeh et al., 2016). The development of VTE requires the compounding effect of three factors, often referred to as Virchow's triad. The triad consists of stasis, vessel trauma and hypercoagulability. Progesterone-mediated changes in the blood vessels during pregnancy cause stasis of the venous blood flow, resulting in pooling of blood. Compression of the pelvic blood vessels compounds this physiological change. Second, damaged endothelium may be caused by direct trauma, such as during birth via caesarean section, infections of surrounding soft tissue, and IV catheters or prolonged use of these. The trauma releases platelet-activating factors, initiating the coagulation cascade, which results in platelet adhesion to the blood vessel wall and the beginning of thrombus formation. Third, clotting factors alter during pregnancy. There are increased levels of factors V and VIII and fibrinogen, acquired resistance to activated protein C (an endogenous anticoagulant) and a reduction of its cofactor, protein S. Increased inhibitors of plasminogen activator result in impaired fibrinolysis. In addition, hypercoagulability of blood may be caused by other haematological conditions such as anaemia or infectious disease (pneumonia) or as a secondary complication to renal disease or hypercoagulable medications. VTE is more common in the postnatal period as blood viscosity is altered because of the diuresis that occurs in the first 24 hours after birth and remains to up to 12 weeks after birth (Alshawabkeh et al., 2016). This is of significance currently owing to the increasing operative birth rate.

Risks for venous thromboembolism

The incidence of VTE is estimated at 1 per 1000 pregnancies (RCOG, 2015). Almost 80% of VTE events are caused by DVT and 20%–25% by a pulmonary embolus, of which 1 in 40 will lead to maternal death. Pregnancy is a risk factor for VTE with a 10-fold increase in risk when compared to non-pregnant women (Alshawabkeh et al., 2016). The risk is increased if the birth is by caesarean section, especially if it is an emergency procedure. VTE during pregnancy is rare unless the woman develops a pulmonary embolism but is associated with increased morbidity and mortality. Pregnancies affected by COVID-19 may also increase coagulopathy and thromboembolism (Servante et al., 2021).

Diagnosis

A venous thromboembolism happens when a blood clot forms in a deep vein, commonly in the leg, resulting usually in swelling and pain. Diagnosis is confirmed by compression duplex ultrasound when there is a clinical suspicion and indication of a DVT (RCOG, 2015). Once a DVT is diagnosed then the recommendation is that anticoagulant treatment is commenced. A number of anticoagulants are considered safe to use in pregnancy but should be balanced by possible risk or harm and benefit to the fetus and mother (Middleton et al., 2021). The drugs most commonly used are low molecular weight heparin (LMWH) and low dose aspirin. The RCOG guidelines (2015) advise that blood should be taken for a full blood count, coagulation screen, urea and electrolytes, and LFTs prior to starting anticoagulation treatment during pregnancy.

Superficial thrombophlebitis

Women at an increased risk of VTE tend to be older, obese and of higher parity. The superficial leg veins (most commonly the left) are usually affected but vulval varicosities are not uncommon. Use of supportive leg stockings, elevation of the lower limbs and rest may be helpful. There is, however, limited risk of pulmonary embolism unless there is associated deep vein thrombosis.

Management

Following diagnosis and commencement of anticoagulant treatment, the woman needs to be taught how to self-inject heparin with safe disposal of all equipment, about the wearing of compression stockings on the affected leg and that she will be having these injections daily for the rest of her pregnancy and for at least 6 weeks postnatally. She also needs to be advised that when she is going into labour, or thinks she is, she needs to cease injecting the anticoagulant. Warfarin is not used in pregnancy because it is a vitamin K antagonist and can have an adverse effect upon the baby in utero (RCOG, 2015). An adjunct to anticoagulant treatment, commonly used in hospitals in both Australia and New Zealand, is mechanical thromboprophylaxis. These come in the form of pneumatic compression devices and thromboembolic stockings even though there is limited evidence as to their effectiveness in pregnant or postpartum women (O'Shaughnessy et al., 2020).

Pulmonary thromboembolism

Pulmonary thromboembolism (PTE) is more common in the postnatal period than in pregnancy. The signs and symptoms of PTE are non-specific, and so the clinical recognition of PTE is notoriously inaccurate. The lack of sensitivity of the clinical diagnosis of PTE is evident from postmortem studies demonstrating that most cases of PTE detected postmortem were not diagnosed (or treated) prior to death. Shortness of breath and rapid respirations accompanied by leg or chest pain with cyanosis are the most common symptoms, although a cardiac arrest may also be the first indication. Frothy, blood-stained sputum may also be apparent. To confirm the diagnosis, the woman requires blood gases, a chest X-ray, electrocardiogram and a ventilation–perfusion (V/Q) scan of the lungs. If the scan shows low or intermediate probability of a PTE, a pulmonary angiography is indicated. In non-pregnant people a d-dimer assay is often used to diagnose PTE. Because of the intrinsic prothrombotic state inherent in pregnancy, the assay elevates and becomes progressively more positive during the second and third trimester and for some time after birth.

CLINICAL POINT

Signs of pulmonary embolism

These include dyspnoea, pleuritic chest pain, haemoptysis, faintness and collapse. The woman may have focal signs in the chest, tachypnoea, a raised jugular venous pressure and there may be ECG changes (S1, Q3, T3). Arterial blood gases with the woman in a seated position may show respiratory alkalosis and hypoxaemia. There may also be symptoms or signs of a DVT.

Any woman with a suspected PTE requires hospitalisation, anticoagulation and supportive care in consultation with an obstetrician and a physician. Supplemental oxygen should be provided to reverse hypoxia and maintain a P_aO_2 of more than 60 mmHg. Intubation may be required to maintain adequate fetal oxygenation (i.e. P_aO_2 of <60 mmHg) or for uncontrolled rising maternal P_aCO_2. Fluid resuscitation and pressors such as dopamine may be used to maintain adequate blood pressure (systolic pressure >80 mmHg), but there is a significant risk that uterine blood flow may be compromised. Narcotic analgesics should not be withheld. Only women with life-threatening manifestations of PTE should be treated with a fibrinolytic agent such as tissue plasminogen activator, since as yet there are currently no data on the risk of placental abruption or potential injury to the fetus. These agents are contraindicated postpartum. Emergency thoracotomy and embolectomy may be beneficial as a last-ditch effort for critically ill patients.

Once the woman's condition has been stabilised, anticoagulation treatment to prevent further clot formation is commenced with heparin (RCOG, 2015).

Hypertension in pregnancy

Hypertension is the most common medical problem encountered during pregnancy, complicating 5%–10% of pregnancies worldwide (Sheehan et al., 2019) and associated with significant maternal and perinatal morbidity and mortality. In healthy pregnant women there is little alteration in systolic pressure but a marked fall in the diastolic pressure mid-pregnancy with a rise to non-pregnant levels at term (Rankin, 2017).

Hypertension is classified as:

- chronic / pre-existing hypertension
- gestational hypertension
- preeclampsia
- eclampsia
- HELLP syndrome.

Eclampsia and HELPP syndrome are discussed in Chapter 40; this section discusses chronic and gestational hypertension and preeclampsia.

Identifying risk factors for hypertension in early pregnancy

At the initial pregnancy assessment a comprehensive risk assessment for hypertensive disorders should be undertaken (MOH, 2022). This involves identifying any major risk factors (MRF) for hypertension (Table 37.4). Baseline laboratory evaluations should be performed early in pregnancy for all women known to be at high risk of PE.

Women with pre-existing major risk factors should be referred to a multidisciplinary team, with low dose aspirin (100 mg daily taken in the evening) commenced from 12 weeks gestation and calcium supplementation considered during the pregnancy.

Blood pressure monitoring during pregnancy

All women should have a blood pressure assessment at each antenatal consultation during pregnancy. Women with pre-existing hypertension may require more frequent monitoring during pregnancy. When undertaking blood pressure monitoring a liquid crystal sphygmomanometer should be used. If this is unavailable, use a validated and appropriately calibrated automated device.

Table 37.4 Major pre-existing risk factors for hypertension in pregnancy

Pre-existing risk factor	Relative risk/ odds ratio	95% CI
Antiphospholipid antibodies/SLE	9.72[b]	4.3–21.7
Previous history of pre-eclampsia	7.2[b]	5.9–8.8
ART (oocyte donation)	4.3[a]	3.1–6.1
Renal disease	4.1[a]	2.2–7.7
Chronic hypertension	3.6[a]	2.0–6.6
Previous history of HELLP	3.7[a]	0.9–16.1
Pre-existing diabetes	3.6[b]	2.5–5.0
Family history of pre-eclampsia in mother or sister	3.3	1.5–7.4

[a]Adjusted odds ratio
[b]Relative risk
ART = assisted reproductive technology
(Source: MOH, 2022)

Identifying hypertension during pregnancy

During assessment, hypertension is identified if the blood pressure is raised (a systolic BP ≥140 or diastolic BP ≥90 mmHg), as measured on two or more consecutive occasions at least four hours apart (Box 37.16).

CLINICAL POINT

Women should be advised of the symptoms of preeclampsia (MOH, 2022). These symptoms include:

- severe headaches
- visual disturbances
- severe epigastric pain
- shortness of breath
- retrosternal pressure / pain
- nausea, vomiting
- sudden swelling of face, hands or feet
- hyperflexia

Pre-existing / chronic hypertension

For women with pre-existing / chronic hypertension there is an increased likelihood of developing preeclampsia (PE) and so they require close clinical surveillance (Lovell et al., 2019).

Complications of chronic hypertension are: an exacerbation of maternal hypertension, superimposed PE and uteroplacental insufficiency, IUGR and placental abruption.

Box 37.16 Identifying hypertension

- Defined as systolic BP ≥140 and/or diastolic BP ≥90 mmHg.
- Blood pressure should be repeated to confirm true hypertension
  - if blood pressure is severe (SBP ≥160 and/or DBP ≥110 mmHg) then the blood pressure should be confirmed within 15 min;
  - for less severe blood pressure, repeated readings should be taken over a few hours.

(Source: Brown et al., 2018, p. 291)

Pre-existing/chronic hypertension (BP >140/90) is apparent pre-conceptually or before the 20th week of pregnancy. This type of hypertension is more likely to occur in pregnancy when there is a family history of hypertension, and if the woman is obese or overweight. Secondary hypertension, seen less frequently in pregnancy, is caused by an underlying medical condition such as:

- chronic kidney disease (e.g. glomerulonephritis, reflux nephropathy and adult polycystic kidney disease)
- renal artery stenosis, systemic disease with renal involvement (e.g. diabetes mellitus, systemic lupus erythematosus)
- endocrine disorders (e.g. phaeochromocytoma, Cushing syndrome and primary hyperaldosteronism)
- coarctation of the aorta (Brown et al., 2018; Lovell et al., 2019).

Management includes antihypertensive agents with the aim to achieve a diastolic blood pressure of less than 90 mmHg during pregnancy. Appropriate baseline assessment is preferable prior to pregnancy and includes an evaluation of pre-existing target organ damage, cardiomegaly, renal insufficiency and retinopathy.

CLINICAL POINT

Chronic hypertension in pregnancy is associated with serious maternal and fetal complications, including superimposed preeclampsia, fetal growth restriction, pre-term birth, placental abruption and stillbirth.

Prepregnancy counselling and management of pre-existing/chronic hypertension is essential to good management. It is important that the woman knows that some commonly prescribed antihypertensive drugs are contraindicated or best avoided before conception and during pregnancy, such as the ACE inhibitors, diuretics and beta-blockers. Women with chronic hypertension should continue taking antihypertensive medication but it is recommended that they switch from ACE inhibitors to different hypertensive medications, such as nifedipine, labetalol or methyldopa, during pregnancy (Lovell et al., 2019; MOH, 2022). Other recommendations are as follows:

- Initiate calcium supplementation and low-dose aspirin after 12 weeks gestation.
- The woman needs to be informed of the signs and symptoms and made aware of the risk of developing preeclampsia (Box 37.17).
- Refer to the obstetric team.

The aim of management is to ensure that the woman's blood pressure stays at prepregnancy levels or if possible lower. If the baby's wellbeing and, in particular, fetal growth is of concern, this is an indication for more-frequent scans in combination with umbilical artery Doppler and CTGs. If a small-for-gestational-age (SGA) baby is diagnosed then SGA guidelines should be followed.

Birth is not usually anticipated before 37 weeks gestation and if the woman has a low chance of adverse outcomes, she can anticipate going into labour spontaneously and having a normal birth with more-frequent assessment of her wellbeing in the last few weeks of pregnancy. During the birth the blood pressure should be monitored every hour and she should continue to take her usual antihypertensive medication.

Following the birth the woman may re-commence her prepregnancy antihypertensive medication such as ACE inhibitors. She will need to have a daily BP assessment while in hospital, at 24 hours following discharge, then at one week and weekly up to 6 weeks, before being referred back to her usual GP with a detailed discharge summary.

Gestational hypertension

In contrast to chronic hypertension, **gestational hypertension** is a provisional diagnosis made when, after 20 weeks gestation, there is a rise in the diastolic BP to greater than or equal to 90 mmHg or systolic BP >140 mmHg, with no associated signs of PE such as proteinuria (but not limited to) or alterations in renal or hepatic status. This condition resolves usually within 3 months postpartum. The BP increase more commonly occurs at 36 weeks gestation if not before, but about 25% of women may go on to develop proteinuria (PE), whereas others may have pre-existing hypertension that has been masked by the physiological drop in BP in the early part of pregnancy. A diagnosis of gestational hypertension is confirmed if PE does not develop and the BP returns to normal by 12 weeks postpartum. There is an indication that gestational hypertension is a marker for hypertension and cardiovascular disease later in life, so women should be informed about this and advised as to the maintenance of a healthy lifestyle (Brown et al., 2018). Having gestational hypertension also puts women (and their babies) at increased risk for other pregnancy complications, including IUGR, pre-term birth, placental abruption and stillbirth.

Upon diagnosis, a blood screen for PE and a spot urine protein creatinine ratio (PCR) should be done along with referral to the specialist team. Assessment of fetal wellbeing may include more-frequent scans to identify intrauterine growth restriction and/or evidence of placental dysfunction. Scans should evaluate umbilical artery Doppler studies and fetal growth discordance via biometry which should be plotted on a growth chart. CTG monitoring may also be indicated. Antihypertensive medications may be started and importantly the woman is informed about the signs of PE (Box 37.17). A plan for ongoing monitoring will be made enabling shared decision making with the team, the woman and her LMC.

A blood screen for PE consists of taking a full blood count, creatinine levels, LFTs including AST and ALT, electrolytes and coagulation if AST and ALT levels are not normal or if platelet levels are low. Unless warranted, women can stay at home rather than in hospital with weekly blood pressure assessment and urinalysis to detect for the development of proteinuria along with ongoing assessment of fetal wellbeing, and in particular fetal growth. Again, if there are concerns then umbilical artery Doppler and CTGs can be done, according to need, following assessment.

Birth may be advised prior to 40 weeks gestation and following a shared, informed decision process (involving the woman and her LMC). During labour the woman's BP should be assessed hourly and her antihypertensive medications taken but adjusted if she has an epidural. Postpartum care should include a daily BP assessment while in hospital, within 24 hours of discharge, then weekly for 6 weeks, before being referred back to her usual GP with a detailed discharge summary (Bick, 2020; NICE, 2019b).

Preeclampsia

Preeclampsia (PE) complicates about 8% of pregnancies. It is defined as the development of hypertension after 20 weeks gestation and with one or more of the following complications:

- abnormalities of the coagulation system
- disturbed liver function
- renal failure
- cerebral ischaemia
- fetal growth restriction (Brown et al., 2018).

It is known as a multifactorial disease of pregnancy. The exact mechanisms that lead to PE are still unclear. What is known is that some women have predisposing factors and are more at risk of the disease than others (Box 37.17). Table 37.5 lists the effects of PE and the primary body systems affected.

Box 37.17 Risk factors for preeclampsia (PE)

Any one of the following factors predisposes women in a given pregnancy to PE:

- first pregnancy
- previous PE
- ≥10 years since last baby
- age ≥40 years
- body mass index ≥35
- family history of PE (mother or sister)
- booking diastolic blood pressure ≥80 mmHg
- proteinuria at booking (≥0.3 protein:creatinine on more than one occasion or 300 mg/24 h)
- multiple pregnancy
- underlying medical conditions: pre-existing hypertension, renal disease, or diabetes.

Diagnosis

Preeclampsia is diagnosed when there is:

- hypertension after the 20th week of gestation, and rarely earlier than this (perhaps when there are extensive hydatidiform changes in the chorionic villi)

Table 37.5 Effects of preeclampsia

System	Effects
Maternal	
CVS	Widespread vasoconstriction Normal or increased systemic vascular resistance Left ventricular failure Increased vascular permeability and oedema Decreased circulating blood volume
CNS	Headaches Visual disturbance Hyper-reflexia Cerebral haemorrhage Convulsions
Renal	Reduced glomerular filtration rate Reduced urea clearance and increased uric acid concentration Proteinuria and hypoproteinaemia Oliguria Acute renal failure
Respiratory	Pulmonary oedema Facial and laryngeal oedema Adult respiratory distress syndrome
Liver	Abnormal liver function tests Subcapsular haemorrhage and epigastric pain Liver rupture
Coagulation	Increased turnover of fibrinogen, fibrin and platelets Thrombocytopenia Impaired platelet function Disseminated intravascular coagulation HELLP syndrome
Fetal	
	Decreased placental circulation Placental ischaemia and infarction Intrauterine growth restriction Placental abruption Pre-term labour

CNS = central nervous system; CVS = cardiovascular system; HELLP = haemolysis, elevated liver enzymes, low platelet count.
(Source: Hart & Coley, 2003, p. 39)

- a diastolic blood pressure of at least 90 mmHg and a systolic blood pressure of at least 140 mmHg; these blood pressures must be manifested on at least two occasions 4 hours or more apart
- spot urine protein:creatinine ratio ≥30 mg/mmol established by a protein creatinine ratio; proteinuria using a 2+ reaction on a standard urine dipstick is no longer considered mandatory for the diagnosis of PE but should be investigated through spot urine creatinine
- evidence of two of the following: renal insufficiency, liver disease, neurological problems, haematological disturbance or fetal growth restriction.

Oedema is now considered to be of little clinical importance because it occurs equally in women experiencing normal pregnancy and in PE. However, the rapid onset of oedema is usually abnormal. Pathological oedema is defined as a generalised accumulation of fluid of greater than 1+, pitting oedema after 12 hours of bed rest or weight gain of 2 kg or more in 1 week, or both.

In addition, many women with PE will have abnormal LFTs (Brown et al., 2018):

- aspartate aminotransferase (SGOT) level higher than 72 IU/L, and lactate dehydrogenase (LDH) levels >600 IU/L
- alanine transaminase (ALT) levels >40 IU/L
- alkaline phosphatase levels >60 IU/L in first trimester, >80 IU/L in second trimester and >140 IU/L in third trimester
- total albumin level 34 g/L decreasing to 28 g/L at term; there is a strong relationship between low serum albumin levels and adverse maternal and fetal outcomes
- total bilirubin levels >17 µmol/L.

Although transaminase levels rise as a result of hepatocellular necrosis, prothrombin time remains within the reference range. As PE worsens there may be evidence of haematological abnormalities: haemolysis (haemoglobin <110 g/L, with reticulocytosis) or thrombocytopenia (<150 × 10^9 g/L platelets).

Renal function tests (plasma creatinine, creatinine clearance, blood urea and total urea protein and uric acid) are often abnormal. A total urinary protein of >500 mg/L in 24 hours is associated with severe PE. A serum creatinine level ≥0.10 mmol/L also indicates significant renal impairment. Current evidence suggests that serum uric acid levels could help distinguish those women that have gestational hypertension from those developing PE but this evidence is weak and insufficient to be used in diagnosis or to determine disease progression (Brown et al., 2018; MOH, 2022; NICE 2019b).

CRITICAL THINKING EXERCISE

You find that a woman who books into your antenatal clinic for the first time at 25 weeks pregnant has a blood pressure of 150/95. There is no proteinuria. What is the most likely cause of her hypertension and what are you going to do about it?

Classification

Brown et al. (2018) and the NZ MOH practice guidelines (2022) also describes PE as severe if the following features are present.

- *Severe hypertension (dBP ≥110 mmHg or sBP ≥160 mmHg)*
- *Worsening of* ***thrombocytopenia*** *(platelet count less than 100 × 109/L)*
- ***Impaired liver function*** *not responding to treatment and not accounted for by alternative diagnosis—elevated transaminases (AST, ALT)—at least twice upper limit of normal ± right upper quadrant or epigastric abdominal pain)*
- ***Progressive renal insufficiency*** *(serum creatinine >90 µmol/L or doubling of serum creatinine concentration in the absence of other renal disease, urine output of <80 mL/4h)*
- *Pulmonary oedema*
- *New onset of headaches and visual disturbances*
- *HELLP syndrome*
- *Eclampsia.*

HELLP and eclampsia are discussed in Chapter 40.

Management

The diagnosis of PE requires urgent review by the obstetric team and transfer of care from primary care. Clinical deterioration can be rapid (MOH, 2022). A multidisciplinary team approach (obstetrician, midwife, neonatologist, anaesthetist and physician) is usually required. Because PE is a multiorgan disease that compromises maternal and fetal health, women should be advised to birth in a secondary /tertiary hospital. Management of PE depends on several factors:

- gestational age of the pregnancy
- severity of the disease
- presence of complicating factors
- evidence of maternal or fetal compromise.

The multi-disciplinary team will make a management plan for ongoing care and monitoring. This will generally involve hospital in-patient care.

The definitive treatment for PE is birth of the fetus and placenta (Brown et al., 2018; MOH, 2022; NICE 2019b). Birth may be expedited if the fetus is viable and if the mother's health is significantly compromised with concerns related to:

- impending eclampsia
- pulmonary oedema
- compromised renal function
- placental abruption
- a platelet count <100,000/µL
- a ratio of serum alanine aminotransferase to serum aspartate aminotransferase that is twice the reference range with concomitant epigastric and right upper quadrant tenderness
- persistent severe headache or visual changes
- uncontrolled severe hypertension.

Antihypertensive therapy

The first aim of treatment is to stabilise the woman's blood pressure. Antihypertensive therapy will be commenced usually with what are known as first-line hypertensives—nifedipine, methyldopa or hydralazine—depending upon the woman's condition upon admission.

Antihypertensive therapy for PE is indicated once the BP is persistently >160/100 mmHg, with the aim of achieving a diastolic BP of 90–100 mmHg. This is to avoid 'overcorrection' and the risk of exacerbating placental hypoperfusion. Antihypertensive drugs used to control hypertension include methyldopa, atenolol and labetalol. Angiotensin-converting enzyme (ACE) inhibitors are contraindicated in pregnancy due to the possibility of congenital abnormalities (Lovell, 2019; NICE, 2019b).

Antihypertensive treatment should be commenced in all women with a systolic blood pressure of ≥110 mmHg because of the risk of intracerebral haemorrhage and eclampsia (Brown et al., 2018; NICE, 2019b).

Monitoring disease progression

Further assessment of rapidly increasing, generalised oedema or maternal facial and periorbital oedema combined with rapid weight gain is warranted because marked fluid retention may be associated with the onset of severe PE. It is crucial that an accurate fluid balance chart is maintained and reviewed daily to ensure that renal impairment is detected quickly.

Once hypertension is suspected, laboratory tests to confirm the diagnosis and to track its progression include hepatic enzyme levels, platelet counts, serum creatinine levels and a 12- to 24-hour urine collection (or spot creatinine tests) for total protein measurement. Blood tests include a full blood count, urea and electrolytes and coagulation profiles (APTT, PT and fibrinogen) (Brown et al., 2018; NICE, 2019b).

Impact on fetus

Intrauterine growth restriction and oligohydramnios are associated with PE (Brown et al., 2018), with evidence suggesting that these may be occurring long before the diagnostic criteria for PE is apparent. Daily CTG and/or Doppler flow studies are used to monitor fetal growth and to ascertain the most appropriate and safest time to expedite the birth.

Education for the woman and her family begins as soon as the diagnosis is confirmed, and should include information about the disease process, signs and symptoms of worsening disease, proposed course of treatment including physical and laboratory assessment, medications, potential complications for the woman and her baby and the plan for birthing (NICE, 2019b).

Table 37.6 lists the systemic complications of eclampsia/PE. Management options will depend on the level of services available at each facility, the woman and baby's health and also distance to a tertiary hospital with an intensive care unit, availability of 24-hour operating theatres and a NICU. Consultation with and/or transfer to a higher level service may be indicated for:

- pre-term pregnancies (24–32 weeks gestation) with PE, severe PE, eclampsia or HELLP syndrome
- term pregnancies complicated by eclampsia or HELLP syndrome
- any pregnancy in which the healthcare provider believes the healthcare facility will be unable to manage the complications of hypertension of pregnancy.

Table 37.6 Systemic complications of eclampsia/preeclampsia

System	Complication
Cardiovascular	Cardiogenic and non-cardiogenic pulmonary oedema
Neurological	Cerebral oedema Cerebral haemorrhage, a direct consequence of hypertension Convulsions, coma
Hepatic	Subcapsular haematoma (epigastric or right upper quadrant pain) Hepatic rupture
Renal	Renal failure Proteinuria
Haematological	Thrombocytopenia Disseminated intravascular coagulopathy Haemolysis
Fetal	Fetal growth restriction Placental abruption

(Source: Lew & Klonis, 2003, p. 362)

Timing of birth

Expediting the birth of the baby and placenta is the only 'cure' for clinically diagnosed PE and should be accomplished as soon as the fetus is mature, or earlier if the mother's condition deteriorates or there is evidence of significant fetal compromise. The timing and management of birth require close collaboration between the woman and her obstetric, midwifery, paediatric and anaesthetic team members. If the fetus is between 24 and 34 weeks gestation corticosteroids are administered to the mother to stimulate fetal lung maturation and the production of surfactant (Brown et al., 2018; NICE, 2019b).

Vaginal birth is preferable and epidural analgesia is the preferred choice of analgesia for labour. Epidurals reduce the maternal stress response and release of catecholamines, which occur in labour when pain cannot be controlled. Epidural analgesia and anaesthesia are contraindicated if there is evidence of coagulopathy (platelet count $<50{,}000 \times 10^9/L$) (Brown et al., 2018; NICE, 2019b).

Indications for expediting the birth immediately are as follows.

- *Fetal indications are:* IUGR, non-reassuring CTG, oligohydramnios.
- *Maternal indications are:* progressive deterioration of liver function, progressive deterioration of renal function, suspected placental abruption, persistent severe headache or visual changes, and persistent severe epigastric pain, nausea or vomiting.

CLINICAL POINT

Up to 40% of eclamptic seizures occur before birth; approximately 16% occur more than 48 hours after birth (see Ch. 40 for the management of HELLP syndrome and eclampsia).

Preeclampsia superimposed on chronic hypertension

Preeclampsia superimposed on chronic hypertension is characterised by new-onset proteinuria (or by a sudden increase in the protein level if proteinuria is already present), a rapid increase in blood pressure (assuming hypertension already exists) or development of the HELLP (haemolysis, elevated liver enzymes, low platelet count) syndrome. Recognising PE superimposed on chronic hypertension can be very challenging (Brown et al., 2018; NICE, 2019b).

The condition should be suspected when any one of the following is present: blood pressure >160/110 mmHg, heavy proteinuria (more than 2 g per day) or existing proteinuria that abruptly worsens, blood pressure suddenly increasing after a period of good control, or serum creatinine levels rising to more than 110 mmol/L. Immediate management is similar to that described for PE. Once the baby is born, further assessment and treatment of ongoing hypertension is required (Brown et al., 2018; NICE, 2019b). The blood pressure should be monitored daily while in hospital. Once stable the woman can be discharged home with BP monitored within 24 hours of discharge, then at one week and weekly until 6 weeks.

CRITICAL THINKING EXERCISE

Your client says: 'I'm 35 weeks pregnant and yesterday my doctor admitted me to hospital for bed rest because he thinks I have PE. He sent my urine to the lab for testing. I have high blood pressure, high heart rate and my ankles are swollen. If it turns out I have it, at what point do they induce labour? He said 35 weeks is still too early to bring the labour on ...'.

What will you say? Support your answer with research.

Conclusion

This chapter has identified a range of challenges and complexity that can affect a woman, her baby and her family during pregnancy. Midwives need to understand these often complex challenges, recognise and identify the signs and symptoms of pathology, and support referral to a multidisciplinary team. Women experiencing the issues identified within this chapter will need emotional and psychological as well as physical support and assistance. Midwives along with other members of the multidisciplinary team need to listen with compassion and understanding to the woman's fears and anxiety. She may well need to be away from her home following referral and transfer to a tertiary hospital, leaving other children and family members behind. The midwife's involvement in each individual woman's pregnancy journey is fundamental to ensure that she receives the best care possible, in accordance with up-to-date current best practice evidence and guidelines.

Review questions

1. At 10 weeks pregnant, Neve is unable to eat any food without vomiting and feels nauseated all day. What actions will you take?
2. Beth is 8 weeks pregnant and rings you to say she has had some fresh vaginal bleeding. What advice will you give her?
3. Lydia is 32 weeks pregnant. She tells you she has had some fresh vaginal bleeding. What are possible causes for the bleeding? What information will you need to help you make a diagnosis? Describe the advice you will give Lydia.
4. Victoria is 22 weeks pregnant. She comes to your clinic complaining of feeling unwell and with lower abdominal crampy pain. What other information do you require? What will you do?
5. Isabella's first pregnancy has progressed normally. However, at her 36-week antenatal check, she has a blood pressure recording of 140/98 mmHg and + protein on dipstick. What actions do you take?
6. At 32 weeks pregnant, Joanna rings you, saying that her skin feels very itchy, especially on her palms. She tells you that she has no rash. What do you advise?
7. The results of Kelly's 28-week gestational diabetes challenge test (50-g glucose polymer load) at 1-hour post-glucose dose is 9 mmol/L. What are your obligations as the midwife providing Kelly's care?

Online resources

Asthma +Respiratory Foundation NZ. A national foundation representing the interests of people living with respiratory disease: https://www.asthmafoundation.org.nz/health-professionals.

Diabetes Australia. National body for people affected by all types of diabetes: https://www.diabetesaustralia.com.au/about-us/.

Diabetes New Zealand.Charitable organisation providing support for women with diabetes: https://www.diabetes.org.nz/.

Epilepsy New Zealand. The national epilepsy association of NZ: http://epilepsy.org.nz/.

Health Navigator NZ. What you need to know about pregnancy if you have diabetes: https://www.healthnavigator.org.nz/health-a-z/d/diabetes-pre-existing-and-pregnancy/.

Hyperemesis Education and Research (HER) Foundation: http://www.hyperemesis.org.

Ministry of Health guidelines for hypertension during pregnancy: https://www.health.govt.nz/search/results/hypertension%20in%20pregnancy.

Miscarriage Support Auckland: http://www.miscarriagesupport.org.nz/.

National Asthma Council Australia. Australian Asthma Handbook. Version 1.3. Melbourne: National Asthma Council; 2017. http://www.asthmahandbook.org.au.

The Perinatal Loss Centre: https://www.theperinatallosscentre.com.au/.

RHD Australia. Supports the prevention, diagnosis and management of acute rheumatic fever and rheumatic hear disease in Australia: https://www.rhdaustralia.org.au/.

Society of Obstetric Medicine of Australia and New Zealand (SOMANZ). Guidelines for medical disorders related to pregnancy: https://www.somanz.org/.

References

Argenbright C. Complementary approaches to pregnancy induced nausea and vomiting. *Int J Childbirth Educ.* 2017;32(1):6–9.

Alshawabkeh L, Economy K, Valence A-M. Anticoagulation during pregnancy, evolving strategies with a focus upon mechanical values. *J Am Coll Cardiol.* 2016;68(16):1804–1813.

American College of Obstetricians & Gynecologists. Thyroid disease in pregnancy. ACOG Practice Bulletin No. 223. *Obstet Gynecol.* 2020;135:e261–74.

Australian Institute of Health and Welfare (AIHW). *Acute rheumatic fever and rheumatic heart disease in Australia 2014–2018.* 2020a. Online: https://www.aihw.gov.au/reports/heart-stroke-vascular-diseases/acute-rheumatic-fever/contents/rheumatic-heart-disease.

Australian Institute of Health and Welfare (AIHW). *Diabetes 2017–2018 data tables.* 2020b. Online: https://www.aihw.gov.au/reports/diabetes/diabetes/contents/what-is-diabetes.

Australian Institute of Health and Welfare (AIHW). *Maternal Deaths in Australia 2009–2018.* Canberra: AIHW; 2020c. Online: https://www.aihw.gov.au/reports/mothers-babies/maternal-deaths-in-australia-2008-2012/.

Balayla J, Desilets J, Shrem G. Placenta previa and the risk of intrauterine growth restriction (IUGR): a systematic review and meta-analysis. *J Perinat Med.* 2019;47(6):577–584. doi: 10.1515/jpm-2019-0116.

Bellhouse C, Temple-Smith MJ, Watson S, et al. "The loss was traumatic... some healthcare providers added to that": women's experiences of miscarriage. *Women Birth.* 2019;32:137–146.

Blackburn ST. *Maternal, Fetal and Neonatal Physiology: A Clinical Perspective.* 5th ed. St Louis, MO: Saunders; 2017.

Bick D, Silverio SA, Bye A, et al. Postnatal care following hypertensive disorders of pregnancy: a qualitative study of views and experiences of primary and secondary care clinicians. *BMJ Open.* 2020;10: e034382. doi:10.1136/bmjopen-2019-034382.

Bortnick A. Valvular Heart Disease in Pregnancy. *Clin Obstet Gynecol.* 2020;63(4):910–922.

Breeze C. Early pregnancy bleeding. *Aust Fam Physician.* 2016;45(5): 283–286.

Brown M, Magee L, Kenny L, et al. Hypertensive disorders of pregnancy: ISSHP classification, diagnosis and management recommendations for international practice. *Hypertension.* 2018; 72 (1). Online: https://www.ahajournals.org/doi/full/10.1161/HYPERTENSIONAHA.117.10803.

Castillo-Castrejon M, Powell TL. Placental nutrient transport in gestational diabetic pregnancies. *Front Endocrinol (Lausanne).* 2017;8:306. doi:10.3389/fendo.2017.00306.

Cesare N, Oladeji O, Ferryman K, et al. Discussions of miscarriage and preterm births on Twitter. *Paediatr Perinat Epidemio..* 2020. doi:10.1111/Ppe.12622.

Clifton V. Managing asthma in pregnancy: effects on future child health. *Lancet Respir Med.* 2019;7(6):485–486.

Coad J, Pedley K, Dunstall M. *Anatomy and Physiology for Midwives.* 4th ed. Sydney: Elsevier; 2020.

Cusack R. Gauvreau G. Pharmacotherapeutic management of asthma in pregnancy and the effect of sex hormones. *Expert Opin Pharmacother.* 2020;22:339–349.

Dean C, Bannigan K, Marsden J. Reviewing the effect off hyperemesis gravidarum on woman's lives and mental health. *Br J Midwifery.* 2018;26(2):109–119.

Downe S, Finlayson K, Tuncalp Ö, et al. What matters to women: a systematic scoping review to identify the processes and outcomes of antenatal care provision that are important to healthy pregnant women. *BJOG.* 2016;123:529–539.

Doyle L, Geraghty S, Folan M. Epilepsy in pregnancy: pharmacodynamics and pharmacokinetics. *Br J Midwifery.* 2016;24(12): 830–835.

Doyle LW, Crowther CA, Middleton P, et al. Magnesium sulphate for women at risk of preterm birth for neuroprotection of the fetus. *Cochrane Database Syst Rev.* 2009;(1):CD004661, doi:10.1002/14651858.CD004661.pub3.

Duckitt K, Harrington D. Risk factors for pre-eclampsia at antenatal booking: systematic review of controlled studies. *BMJ.* 2005;330(7491):565. doi:10.1136/bmj.38380.674340.E0.

Frier E, McKay G, Carty D. Metformin in pregnancy. *Pract Diabetes.* 2017;34(5):178–179.

Gorringe C. Thyroid disease in pregnancy. *Aust J Med Sci.* 2019; 40(1 & 2):2–12.

Heitmann K, Svendsen HC, Sporsheim IH, et al. Nausea in pregnancy: attitudes among pregnant women and general practitioners on treatment and pregnancy care. *Scand J Prim Health Care.* 2016;34(1):13–20. doi:10.3109/02813432.2015.1132894.

Hindley C. Asthma in pregnancy: Physiology, management and recommendations for midwives. *Br J Midwifery.* 2018;26(7): 446–450.

Kasai M, Eoki S, Ogawa M, et al. Prediction of perinatal outcomes based on primary symptoms in women with placental abruption. *J Obstetrics Gynaecol.* 2014;41(6):850–856. doi:10.1111/jog.12637.

Kim C, Barnard S, Neilson JP, et al. Medical treatments for incomplete miscarriage. *Cochrane Database Syst Rev.* 2017;(1):CD007223, doi:10.1002/14651858.CD007223.pub4.

Knat-Petkas M, Bodur S, Dundar O, et al. Systematic review: what is the best first-line approach for caesarean section ectopic pregnancy? *Taiwan J Obstet Gynecol.* 2016;55:263–269.

Knight M. Acquired heart disease in pregnancy—need for a greater focus. *BJOG.* 2020;127:57.

Lawrence L, Wall R, Bloomfield F. Prevalence of gestational diabetes according to commonly used data sources: an observational study. *BMC Pregnancy Childbirth.* 2019. Online: https://bmcpregnancychildbirth.biomedcentral.com/articles/10.1186/s12884-019-2521-2.

Lawrence L, Wall R, Bloomfield F, et al. Dietetic management of gestational diabetes in pregnancy in New Zealand: A cross-sectional survey. *Nutr Diet.* 2017;74(95):1–4.

Lee R. Grenburg M. Metz. Pettker C. Intrahepatic cholestasis of pregnancy. *Am J Obstet Gynecol.* 2021;224(2):B2–B9.

Lovell H, Wilson HM, Whybrow R, et al. Caring for women with chronic hypertension. *Br J Midwifery.* 2019;2(6):343–351.

Lurain R. *Hydatifiorm mole: Recognition and management.* Contemporary OB/GYN; 2019;64(3). Online: https://www.contemporaryobgyn.net/view/hydatidiform-mole-recognition-and-management.

McParlin C, O'Donnell A, Robson S. Treatments for hyperemesis gravidarum and nausea and vomiting in pregnancy: a systematic review. *JAMA.* 2016;316(13):1392–1401. doi:10.1001/jama.2016.14337.

Middleton P, Shepherd E, Gomersall JC. Venous thromboembolism prophylaxis for women at risk during pregnancy and the early postnatal period. *Cochrane Database Syst Rev.* 2021;3:CD001689. doi:10.1002/14651858.CD001689.pub4.

Ministry of Health (MOH). *Diabetes in Pregnancy: Quick Reference Guide for Health Professionals on the Screening, Diagnosis and Treatment of Gestational Diabetes in New Zealand.* Wellington, NZ: Ministry of Health; 2014a. Online: https://www.health.govt.nz/system/files/documents/publications/diabetes-in-pregnancy-quick-reference-guide-dec14-v4.pdf.

Ministry of Health (MOH). *About Diabetes.* Wellington, NZ: Ministry of Health; 2014b. Online: https://www.health.govt.nz/our-work/diseases-and-conditions/diabetes/about-diabetes.

Ministry of Health (MOH). *Rheumatic Fever.* Wellington, NZ: Ministry of Health; 2017a. Online: http://www.health.govt.nz/our-work/diseases-and-conditions/rheumatic-fever.

Ministry of Health (MOH). *Induction of Labour in Aotearoa New Zealand. A Clinical Practice Guideline.* Wellington, NZ: Ministry of Health; 2019. Online: https://www.health.govt.nz/publication/induction-labour-aotearoa-new-zealand-clinical-practice-guideline-2019.

Ministry of Health (MOH). *Diagnosis and Treatment of Hypertension and Pre-eclampsia in Pregnancy. A Clinical Practice Guideline.* Wellington, NZ: Ministry of Health; 2022.

Mobbs N, Williams C, Weeks AD. *Humanizing birth: does the language we use matter?* The bmj opinion; 2018. Online: https://blogs.bmj.com/bmj/2018/02/08/humanising-birth-does-the-language-we-use-matter/.

Morley K. Epilepsy in pregnancy: The role of the midwife in risk management. *Br J Midwifery.* 2018;26(9):564–573.

Montgomery A, Hannon G, Muhammad S, et al. *Br J Midwifery.* 2017;25(11):700–705.

Nallapati C. Park K. Ischemic heart disease in pregnancy. *Cardiology Clinics.* 2021;39:91–108.

National Institute for Health and Clinical Excellence (NICE). *Ectopic Pregnancy and Miscarriage: Diagnosis and Initial Management. Clinical guideline (CG154).* London: NICE; 2019a. Online: https://.www.nice.org.uk/guidance/ng126.

National Institute for Health and Clinical Excellence (NICE). *Hypertension in Pregnancy: Diagnosis and Management. Clinical Guideline 133*; 2019b. Online: https://www.nice.org.uk/guidance/ng133.

National Institute for Health and Clinical Excellence (NICE). *Diabetes in Pregnancy: Management From Preconception to the Postnatal Period.* London: NICE; 2020. Online: https://www.nice.org.uk/guidance/ng3.

New Zealand College of Midwives (NZCOM). *Practice Guidance. Assessment and Promotion of Fetal Wellbeing During Pregnancy.* Christchurch: NZCOM; 2021.

Oats J, Abraham S. Llewellyn-Jones *Fundamentals of Obstetrics and Gynaecology.* 8th ed. Sydney: Elsevier; 2004.

Ornoy A, Albert Reece E, Pavlinkova G, et al. Effect of maternal diabetes on the embryo, fetus, and children: congenital anomalies, genetic and epigenetic changes and development outcomes. *Birth Defects Res C Embryo Today.* 2015;105:53–72.

O'Shaughnessy E, O'Reilly D, Ainle F. Current opinion and emerging trends on the treatment, diagnosis, and prevention of pregnancy-associated venous thromboembolic disease: a review. *Transl Res.* 2020;225:20–32.

Ovadia C, Seed PT, Sklavounos A, et al.. Association of adverse perinatal outcomes of intrahepatic cholestasis of pregnancy with biochemical markers: results of aggregate and individual patient data meta-analyses. *Lancet.* 2019;393: 899–909. doi:10.1016/S0140-6736(18)31877-4.

Parrettini S, Carroli A, Torone E. Nutritional and metabolic adaptions in physiological and complicated pregnancy: Focus on Obesity and Gestational Diabetes. *Front Endocrinol.* 2020. doi:10.3389/fendo.2020.611929.

Perinatal and Maternal Mortality Review Committee (PMMRC). *Eleventh Annual Report of the Perinatal and Maternal Mortality Review Committee: Reporting Mortality and Morbidity 2015.* Wellington, NZ: Health Quality and Safety Commission; 2017. Online: https://www.hqsc.govt.nz/our-programmes/mrc/pmmrc/publications-and-resources/publication/2929/.

Rankin J. *Physiology in Childbearing: With Anatomy and Related Biosciences.* 4th ed. Edinburgh: Elsevier; 2017.

Rowan JA, Hague WM, Gao W, et al. MiG Trial Investigators. Metformin versus insulin for the treatment of gestational diabetes. *N Engl J Med.* 2008;358(19):2003–2015. doi:10.1056/NEJMoa0707193.

Royal College of Obstetricians and Gynaecologists (RCOG). *The Management of Nausea and Vomiting and Hyperemesis Gravidarum. Green-top Guideline no. 69.* London: RCOG; 2016. Online: https://www.rcog.org.uk/globalassets/documents/guidelines/green-top-guidelines/gtg69-hyperemesis.pdf.

Rudland V, Price S, Hughes, et al. ADIPS 2020 guideline on pre-existing diabetes and pregnancy. *Aust NZ J Obstet Gunaecol.* 2020;60:E18–E52.

Schneeberger C, Geerlings SE, Middleton P, et al. Interventions for preventing recurrent urinary tract infection during pregnancy. *Cochrane Database Syst Rev.* 2015;(7):CD009279. doi:10.1002/14651858.CD009279.pub3.

Servante J, Swallow G, Thornton J, et al., Haemostatic and thromboembolic complications in pregnant women with Covid-19: a systematic review and critical analysis. *BMC Pregnancy Childbirth.* 2021;108. doi:10.1186/s12884-021-03568-0.

Sheehan E, Khalil A, Kay L. Using a smartphone app to identify signs of pre-eclampsia and/or worsening blood pressure. *Br J Midwifery.* 2019;2(2):92–99.

Sheerin M, McDonald E. Management of first trimester pregnancy loss: mifepristone plus misoprostol. *Br J Midwifery.* 2019: 27(11)711–714.

Simmons D. The benefits of the use of the new International Association of Diabetes in Pregnancy Study Groups guidelines for gestational diabetes mellitus. *Aust N Z J Obstet Gynaecol.* 2020;60:486–488. doi:10.1111/ajo.13167.

SOMANZ. *Guideline for the Management of Nausea and Vomiting in pregnancy and Hyperemesis Gravidarum.* 2019. Online: https://www.somanz.org/content/uploads/2020/07/NVP-EXEC-SUMMARY-1.2.20.pdf.

Sullivan E, Vaughan G, Carapetic J, et al. The high prevalence and impact of rheumatic heart disease in pregnancy in First Nations populations in a high-income setting: a prospective cohort study. *BJOG.* 2020;127:47–56.

Sumarno V, Temple- Smith M, Bilardi J. Whose role is it? Primary care and the provision of emotional support for women experiencing miscarriage: a pilot qualitative Australian study. *Aust J Prim Health.* 2020;26:388–395. doi:10.1071/PY20042.

Varouxaki N, Gnanasambanthan S, Datta S, et al. Antepartum haemorrhage. *Obstet Gynaecol Reprod Med.* 2018;28(8):237–242. doi:10.1016/j.ogrm.2018.07.001.

Wingert A, Pillay J, Sebastianski M. et al. Asymptomatic bacteriuria in pregnancy: systematic reviews of screening and treatment effectiveness and patient preferences. *BMJ Open.* 2019;9: e021347. doi:10.1136/bmjopen-2017-021347.

World Health Organization (WHO). *Diagnostic Criteria and Classification of Hyperglycaemia First Detected in Pregnancy.* Geneva: WHO; 2013. Online: http://apps.who.int/iris/bitstream/handle/10665/85975/WHO_NMH_MND_13.2_eng.pdf?sequence=1.

World Health Organization (WHO). *Preventing Unsafe Abortion Fact Sheet.* Geneva: World Health Organization; 2016a. Online: http://www.who.int/mediacentre/factsheets/fs388/en/.

World Health Organization (WHO). *Diabetes–Key facts.* Geneva: World Health Organization; 2020. Online: https://www.who.int/news-room/fact-sheets/detail/diabetes.

Further reading

Ministry of Health (MOH). *Guidelines for Consultation With Obstetric and Related Medical Services (Referral Guidelines).* Wellington, NZ: Ministry of Health; 2012. Online: https://www.health.govt.nz/system/files/documents/publications/referral-glines-jan12.pdf.

Ministry of Health (MOH). *Induction of Labour in Aotearoa New Zealand: A Clinical Practice Guideline 2019.* Wellington, NZ: Ministry of Health 2021. Online https://www.health.govt.nz/publication/induction-labour-aotearoa-new-zealand-clinical-practice-guideline-2019.

Ministry of Health (MOH). *National Maternity Clinical Guidance.* Wellington NZ. Online: https://www.health.govt.nz/our-work/life-stages/maternity-services/national-maternity-clinical-guidance.

Queensland Clinical Guidelines, Translating evidence into best clinical practice. Maternity and Neonatal Clinical Guideline. Health. Queensland Maternity and Neonatal Clinical Guidelines Program. Hypertensive and Pregnancy. Brisbane: Queensland Health; 2021. Online: https://www.health.qld.gov.au/__data/assets/pdf_file/0034/139948/g-hdp.pdf.

Rankin J, ed. *Physiology in Childbearing: with Anatomy and Related Biosciences.* 4th ed. Sydney: Elsevier; 2017.

CHAPTER 38

Disturbances in the rhythm of labour

Nigel Lee

LEARNING OUTCOMES

Learning outcomes for this chapter are to:

1. Analyse the causes, identification, effects and management of disturbances in the rhythms of labour and birth
2. Critically discuss the evidence that supports common obstetric interventions in birth
3. Describe the ways in which midwives work to keep birth culturally, emotionally and physically safe for women when disturbances in the rhythms of labour occur.

CHAPTER OVERVIEW

Maternity care in most developed countries including Australia and, until recently, Aotearoa New Zealand is dominated by a medicalised, technologically orientated, interventionist model of maternity service provision. Soaring intervention rates suggest two things: that Western women's bodies are no longer able to cope with labour and birth without medical intervention, and that intervention is occurring in many 'normal' labours and births. Whatever the cause, increased intervention in birth, including inductions of labour, caesarean sections, the use of regional anaesthesia and analgesia, and operative births, has not made substantial differences in improving maternal and neonatal outcomes for women living in resource-rich nations.

Despite the very best of care and support, not all labours proceed as planned and an exploration of the causes, associations and management of these deviations from the usual birthing journey is the overall aim of this chapter. The chapter is lengthy and deals with complex topics. The chapter has been written so that you can 'dip into' the sections that are of most interest to you. This is why headings are used to signpost each topic. The chapter begins by reflecting on what a 'normal' journey is and what it is not. It describes the factors that disturb the rhythms of labour, leading to what is commonly called **dystocia** (difficult labour)—such as prolonged labour and pre-term labour, as well as the interventions used to manage these, such as augmentation and induction of labour. It draws on woman-focused and empowering language—disturbance in the rhythms of birth—to describe some of the causes of dystocia, rather than mechanistic and disempowering idioms such as the oft-used but ill-defined 'failure to progress' or 'trial of labour' and 'trial of scar', because the former is more woman-centred and does not ascribe notions of failure and inadequacy or blame to the birthing woman. However, because the latter terms are part of the everyday language found in the literature and in most birthing units, they are included here as well.

The anatomical structures, physiology and biosciences underpinning disturbances in the rhythms of labour are covered only briefly in this chapter. Therefore it is important that readers who may be unfamiliar with these concepts refer to a specialised text such as Blackburn (2017, 5th edn) and/or Rankin (2017, 4th edn) to enable them to apply this material to the content of this chapter. In addition, Chapter 24 in this text provides an excellent overview of physiological changes during labour.

KEY TERMS

augmentation of labour
dystocia
Friedman's curve
incoordinate uterine action
induction of labour
latent and active phases of labour
partogram
pre-term labour
prolonged labour
tocolysis

INTRODUCTION

Many midwives do not subscribe to an interventionist model of maternity care. For example, in New Zealand, the Midwifery Council's Scope of Practice statement (Midwifery Council of New Zealand (MCNZ), 2010) clearly places emphasis on the midwife supporting the physiological processes of normal birthing, and this is evident throughout the Council's competency requirements for registration as a midwife (MCNZ, 2007) and the New Zealand College of Midwives' (NZCOM, 2006) consensus statement on normal birth.

As Powell-Kennedy & Shannon (2004) reported in a qualitative study, the support of normalcy is fundamental to a midwifery model of care, one that is prefaced by a view that birth for most women should be a normal process (even though some labours are more difficult than others) and that women's bodies are physiologically prepared for labour and birth. Research by Dixon et al. (2013) examined women's perceptions of labour progress; importantly women in this study considered labour as a continuum rather than as stages. Descriptions of stages and phases as well as criteria for 'normalcy' serve to meet organisational and professional requirements rather than the needs of women. These researchers challenge practitioners to re-evaluate the more common midwifery and obstetric discourses and understanding of labour, and reconsider them in light of women's experiences, in particular to review labour progress based in time and measurement of cervical dilation. Midwives who work with women throughout pregnancy, and attend the entire labour and birth, are best placed to know what is normal and not normal for this woman. Unfortunately, this is not the case for the majority of birthing women. Therefore, maternity carers need systematic ways of judging and documenting labour in ways that the team understands—hence documents such as the **partogram** (partograph), which enables each carer to determine the progress of labour and when dystocia begins.

A review of the literature concerned with labour and birth reveals that, since the 17th century, clinicians have endeavoured to differentiate between a 'normal' and an 'abnormal' labour and birth. Certainly, the history of midwifery and obstetrics suggests that, across time and place, clinicians have created, eliminated and reworked descriptions of 'normal' labour (Gould, 2000). Many of these are still in use, although they are not supported by scientific or research-based evidence, and more often than not have been created according to the authors' hunches, opinions, cultural beliefs or convenience. Gross and colleagues (2005) comment on the difficulties associated with determining the precise onset of labour and the duration of each of its phases and stages. As yet there is no consensus about the appropriate length of each stage of labour, or how to differentiate between a 'normal' and an 'abnormal' labour with its identified risk factors. Neal et al. (2015) identified only six national midwifery and obstetric college statements and guidelines amongst United Nations member nations and international organisations that provided a non-ambiguous definition of normal first-stage labour progress, and within these descriptions the stated normal parameters still differed.

In practice, medical and midwifery students are often introduced to notions of specific time intervals expected from each phase of labour, and this knowledge is reinforced by what they see in the hospital environment—even though these are arbitrarily timed. However, although they are frequently the lead decision makers in these circumstances, there remains a lack of consensus amongst obstetricians regarding a definition of normal progress in the first stage of labour and how to manage abnormal progress (White et al., 2017). It has been suggested that a lack of agreement on what constitutes normal progress amongst clinicians and extraneous factors, such as a woman-unfriendly birth environment combined with a medical model of practice premised on pathology, and an institutional requirement to keep the birthing assembly line moving (Walsh, 2005, 2012), have led to the overdiagnosis of labour 'dystocia'.

The Greek word for 'difficult' or abnormal labour is 'dystocia', and this topic is the focus of this chapter. Irrespective of where they practise, every midwife will at some time be confronted with complications in labour or deviations from a normal labour. Midwives should know how to recognise these variations and instigate appropriate action until they are resolved, or make a referral and transfer care to a specialist lead carer. Irrespective of the place of birth, the composition of the healthcare team or planned interventions, midwives always work in partnership with each woman to create a space for birth that is culturally, emotionally and physically safe (MirzaeeRabor et al., 2016).

Midwives who are evidence-informed and reflective practitioners often find that obstetric interventions such as the induction of labour (IOL), especially if there are no accepted medical indications for the procedure, pose ethical and professional dilemmas that need to be addressed. The New Zealand College of Midwives consensus statement (2006, updated 2009) on normal birth recognises that 'each action the midwife makes, from their first interaction with the woman, needs to support keeping birth normal thereby supporting the normal cascade that occurs when labour and birth happen physiologically. Any and every interaction/decision affects this natural cascade in a positive or negative way.'

A clearly defined midwifery philosophy, along with the relevant standards for practice and codes of ethics, enables midwives to determine their own boundaries in regards to decision making about their participation in interventions in the labour and birth processes.

REFLECTIVE THINKING EXERCISE

If they are to provide quality midwifery care, midwives need to consider how knowledge is generated, where it comes from, and how their own value and belief systems affect their understanding of 'normal' birth, its duration, the role of pain in labour and complications such as cephalopelvic disproportion.

As you work through this chapter, reflect on the 'facts' about labour, especially those taken for granted, by asking the kinds of questions posed by Walsh (2003):

- Whose purpose does knowledge serve?
- Where does knowledge come from?
- Who created it and why?
- Who benefits?
- How has knowledge of birth been influenced by a technological–mechanistic view of birth that is readily apparent in 21st-century popular and medical culture?

RESEARCH ACTIVITY

Understanding the physiology and the mechanisms or cardinal movements of labour, including how the shape of the maternal pelvis influences the passage of the fetus through the birth canal, aids recognition of deviations from the usual pattern and rhythm of labour. Before you embark on an exploration of disturbances in the rhythms of labour, make sure that you refresh your understandings about what is known about the causes of the onset of labour and its processes (see Rankin, 2017 and/or Blackburn, 2017).

WHEN DOES LABOUR BEGIN?

McDonald & Magill-Cuerden (2013), in a review of the latent phase of labour, make an important point that the childbirth continuum results in a multitude of calculations used to divide the labour into timed stages and phases. These parameters often dictate what is a 'normal' and an 'abnormal' labour. During the latent phase of labour, uterine contractions become more regular and increase in intensity; there is slow but gradual cervical dilation and effacement, often referred to as prelabour. The so-called latent phase of labour is both challenging to understand and difficult to define. So probably the best option is to ask the woman when her labour began, and believe her (Greulich & Tarrant, 2007) because there is no 'objective' or 'scientific' way of measuring when labour actually begins. Research by Gross et al. (2003, 2006) into the 'latent' phase of labour radically challenges the accepted textbook descriptions of how labour begins. Their work established that, for less than 60% of nulliparous women, contractions are the starting point of labour. The remaining women experienced a variety of signs from vaginal loss to gastrointestinal and sleep disturbances. Objectively, the presence of cervical changes is the most accurate means of determining the onset of labour. Work by Burvill (2002) suggests that there are multiple factors that influence midwives' decisions about determining when labour starts—workloads, guidelines and protocols, risk-management strategies, the need to justify actions to others, institutional constraints and the desire to provide a degree of continuity of care—all of which interfere with the woman's validation of her lived experience. Women empowered to take control of their birth experience will alert the midwife to changes in their labour and are best placed to determine whether they are 'in' or 'not in' labour. Indeed, Walsh (2003, 2012) makes the point that, in a partnership of reciprocal respect and trust, women's fear of intervention during the usual ebb-and-flow patterns of labour can be minimised. NICE (2014) guidelines suggested the following definition of the latent phase of labour: (i) a period of time, not necessarily continuous, when there are painful contractions; and (ii) some cervical change, including cervical effacement and dilation up to 4 cm. However, work by Zhang et al. (2010) indicates that labouring women may take up to 6 hours to progress from 4 cm to 5 cm and over 3 hours to progress from 5 cm to 6 cm. A systematic review of cervical dilation patterns of low-risk women with spontaneous labour also concluded that the progress of labour did not naturally start to accelerate until the cervix had dilated to 5–6 cm (Oladapo et al., 2017). This suggests that many women may still be in the latent phase of labour until 6 cm of cervical dilation. Also both nulliparous and multiparous women progress at a similar rate until 6 cm. Given that the current obstetric opinion dictates the average length of a latent phase, ending at 4 cm dilation, for a spontaneous labour at term, with a fetal vertex position, in a well woman and fetus to be an estimated 12 hours for nulliparous women (but could be as long as 20 hours) and 6 hours for multiparous women, these new parameters will require a more patient approach to the estimation of a normal duration of latent stage. The American College of Obstetricians and Gynecologists (ACOG, 2014) has published guidelines that reflect this approach. The World Health Organization (WHO) recommends using cervical dilation of 5 cm for the end of latent phase, however they also acknowledge the limitations of having a defined threshold and advise that varying definitions of latent phase should not impact on birth outcomes (WHO, 2018).

ACTIVE MANAGEMENT OF LABOUR

Midwives' and women's perceptions of the expected length of labour have been seriously undermined by dominant medical hegemony (Bates 2004; Walsh, 2012). This has culminated in the overuse of protocols such as the 'active management of labour' (Box 38.1) and guidelines focused on a predetermined timeline. Even though authors such as Thornton as early as 1996 argued there was (and still is) scant evidence to support active management of labour, this practice is still used in many maternity units. Possibly midwives are not challenged by 'managing' the differing labour rhythms that women experience but more by hospital guidelines and protocols, which aim to restructure labours in a linear fashion not entirely congruent with labour physiology (Neal & Lowe, 2012).

Box 38.1 Active management of labour

In the early 1970s, O'Driscoll et al. (1973) introduced to maternity units in Dublin a 'package' of care that they termed 'active management', which, they argued, resulted in a reduced incidence of prolonged labour and a caesarean section rate of less than 7%. The package included: antenatal education; one-to-one midwifery care; precise criteria for the diagnosis of the onset of labour; 2-hourly timed vaginal examinations; and early use of high doses of synthetic oxytocin (e.g. Syntocinon) that achieved a rate of cervical dilation of at least 1 cm/h.

The active management of labour approach gained worldwide popularity through the 1980s and 1990s and continues to influence labour management. A Cochrane review of active management versus delayed augmentation found no statistically significant differences in rates of caesarean section but women were more likely to have a shorter labour (2.7 hours) (Brown et al., 2013). These findings were supported by another Cochrane review that compared early oxytocin with no or delayed treatment of slow progress in labour (Bugg et al., 2013). In fact, the only component of the package that has been demonstrated to reduce the caesarean section rate is continuous support from a midwife during labour (Bohren et al., 2017).

CRITICAL THINKING EXERCISE

The following list identifies the assessments a midwife often makes and records during labour care. Make sure that you can define each of these.

- fetal heart rate—by intermittent auscultation, or continuous electronic fetal heart rate monitoring
- labour progress—rate of cervical dilation and descent of the fetus through the pelvis
- uterine contractions—quantification of frequency, duration and strength
- amniotic fluid (if the membranes have broken)—state of fluid, presence of meconium
- maternal urine production—presence of ketones and protein
- maternal adaptation to labour—blood pressure, pulse rate and temperature
- hydration and nutrition—fluid and dietary intake and output
- maternal wellbeing—behaviour and response to labour, levels of fatigue, pain and coping ability
- family support—level, type and effect.

Using the above headings as a guide, determine how frequently clinicians (medical practitioners; midwives working in the community, birth centres or in tertiary hospitals) assess these variables and the range they use to establish whether labour is progressing normally.

Rate of cervical dilation using 'objective' means

The first clinician to provide a definitive instrument, a cervicograph, for the assessment of individual labours was US obstetrician Emanuel Friedman. Friedman (1955) plotted the labours of 500 women and depicted labour as a sigmoid curve, with the first stage of labour divided into two distinct phases: the **latent and active phases of labour** (Fig. 38.1). In **Friedman's curve** the active stage begins at 2–3 cm of cervical dilation (you will note how this parameter continues to change) and can be further subdivided into three sequential phases: acceleration, maximum slope and deceleration. Friedman set the slowest normal progress of labour as a cervical dilation rate of 1.2 cm/h for primigravidas and 1.5 cm/h for multigravidas during the maximal slope phase. This has remained the basis for defining the normal progress of active first-stage labour until research by Albers (1999), Zhang et al. (2001, 2002, 2010) and Neal et al. (2010a), amongst others, challenged Friedman's theories.

Partogram

In an attempt to improve maternity outcomes in Rhodesia (now Zimbabwe), Philpott & Castle (1972) refined Friedman's work. They described the active phase of labour as progressing in a straight line with a cervical dilation rate of 1 cm/h, with no distinction for parity. They also placed an alert line on a cervicograph. The alert line, unlike the sigmoid curve described by Friedman, was a straight line, commenced at 4 cm of cervical dilation and was drawn at an angle equal to a rate of cervical dilation of 1 cm/h irrespective of parity. A second parallel line, known as the 'action line', was later drawn on the cervicograph (partogram), 4 hours to the right of the alert line. The partograph with alert and action lines (Fig. 38.2) was originally designed for use in countries with developing health systems to promote timely transfer of women

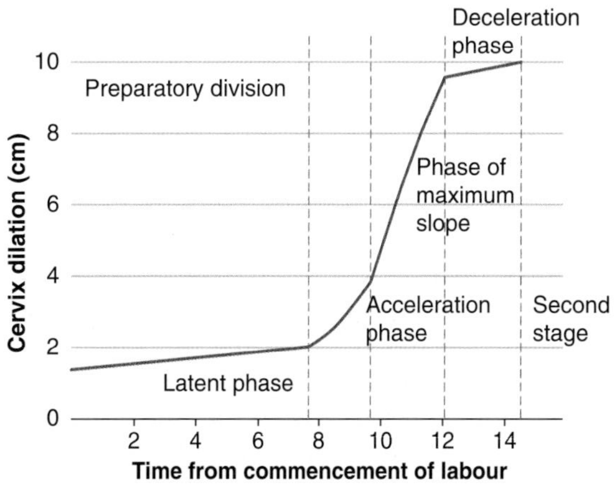

FIGURE 38.1 The Friedman curve
(Based on Friedman, 1955)

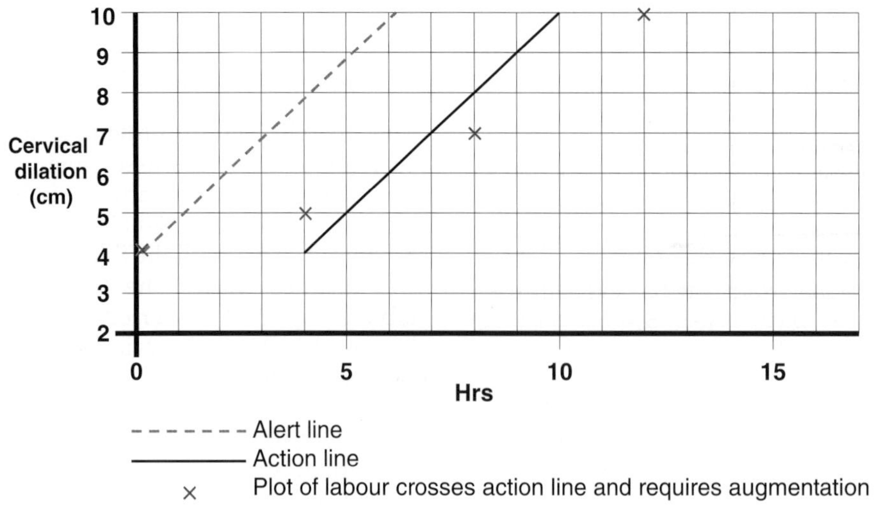

FIGURE 38.2 Partogram plotting the alert and action lines
(Adapted from Lee et al., 2018, p. 357. Reprinted with permission from Springer Nature. Lee NJ, Neal J, Lowe NK, et al. Comparing different partograph designs for use in standard labor care: a pilot randomized trial. *Matern Child Health J.* 2018;22:355–363. https://doi.org/10.1007/s10995-017-2366-0)

from regional 'clinics' to hospitals where suspected obstructed labour could be medically managed. For example, if the plot of the woman's labour crossed the alert line she was transferred to a hospital and if she then crossed the action line her labour was managed as being abnormally slow. The use of the partograph has been demonstrated to improve maternal and infant outcomes in developing countries (WHO, 1994); however, there is little evidence regarding their use in developed countries. It was estimated that 10% of labouring women would cross the alert line; however, in a number of studies more than 30% crossed the line (Lavender et al., 1998, 2006). Some evidence suggests that partograms with alert and action lines remain in use in countries such as Australia and New Zealand; however, they are often misinterpreted with interventions being introduced after the alert line is crossed (White et al., 2017). A 2018 Cochrane review of the effect of partogram use on outcomes for women in spontaneous labour at term concluded that there was insufficient evidence to recommend its routine use (Lavender et al., 2018) and suggested that the use of partograms in labour is so widespread that until further research indicates otherwise its use should be determined locally.

More realistic estimations of a normal rate of cervical dilation

As we have previously discussed, evidence from research which informs our practice indicates that the prime influence that results in high intervention rates in labour may be the commonly held beliefs around the rate of cervical dilation. Following a literature review, Neal et al. (2010b) found that the slowest-yet-normal linear dilation rate for low-risk nulliparous in spontaneous labour was approximately 0.5 cm / h. The authors highlight the issue of an overdiagnosis of labour dystocia in practice, using the premise of 1 cm / h cervical dilation, resulting in an overuse of interventions such as artificial rupture of membranes and **augmentation of labour** with titrated doses of exogenous oxytocin to accelerate labour progress. Based on the work by Zhang et al. (2010), the American College of Obstetricians and Gynecologists (ACOG, 2014) produced guidelines that recommended that (i) 6 cm should be considered the start of active-phase labour; (ii) prior to 6-cm progress, standards of active-phased labour progress should not apply; (iii) slow but progressive labour should not be an indication for intervention. Whilst the management principles presented by the ACOG guidelines have not been widely implemented across Australia and New Zealand, they do present a more physiologically based approach to labour management. However, they may present challenges to midwives confronted with hospital policies that enforce a more aggressive approach with early use of high doses of synthetic oxytocin.

Although the use of oxytocin may be advantageous in some circumstances, inappropriate use of oxytocin to augment labour has been shown to have both adverse maternal and perinatal effects (Clark et al., 2009). A recent study indicated that in women exposed to synthetic oxytocin in labour, serum levels remained abnormally high for 2 months post birth (Prevost et al., 2014). Whilst the long-term health implications of this are largely unknown, other studies have reported associations between fetal exposure to synthetic oxytocin and decreased sucking behaviours, breastfeeding duration (Olza Fernández et al., 2012) and increased risk of abnormal cognitive development, bipolar disorder (Freedman et al., 2015) and autism spectrum disorder (Kenkel et al., 2014). Synthetic oxytocin has been classed by the Institute for Safe Medical Practice as a high-alert medication. Such drugs may have a 'heightened risk of harm when they are used in

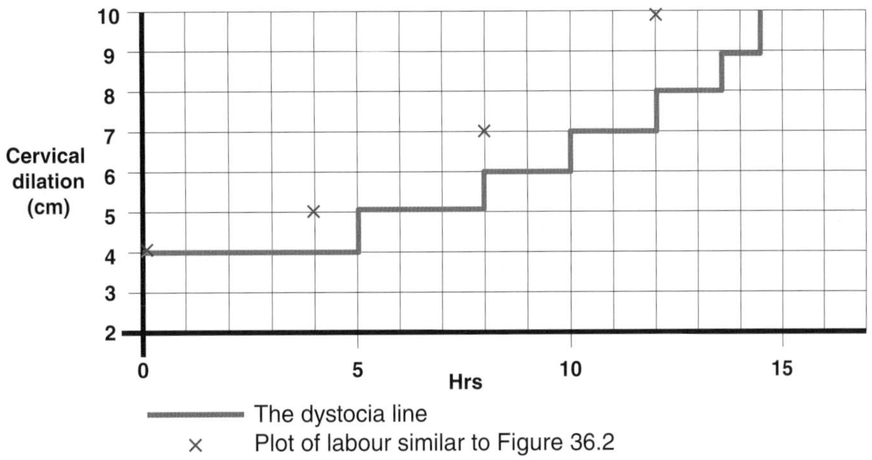

FIGURE 38.3, A dystocia line partograph
(Source: Lee et al., 2018, p. 357. Reprinted with permission from Springer Nature. Lee NJ, Neal J, Lowe, NK, et al. Comparing different partograph designs for use in standard labor care: a pilot randomized trial. *Matern Child Health J.* 2018;22:355–363. https://doi.org/10.1007/s10995-017-2366-0)

error' and 'require special safeguards to reduce the risk of error' (Institute for Safe Medical Practices, 2015). A Cochrane review comparing early oxytocin with no treatment or placebo and early compared with delayed treatment found no difference in mode of birth, but early oxytocin resulted in increased uterine hyperstimulation with fetal heart changes (Bugg et al., 2013).

It would seem reasonable then to develop documentation and guidelines to safely limit the use of oxytocin to women who are diagnosed with an abnormally slow labour. American midwifery researchers Neal & Lowe (2012) designed a physiological partograph that incorporates a stepwise 'dystocia' line. The dystocia line (Fig. 38.3) follows the curve of labour described by Zhang et al. (2010), and used in the ACOG guidelines, and functions much the same as the action line we previously discussed (i.e. intervention is considered only once the plot of labour crosses the line). The Neal & Lowe partograph allows for greater variation in labour progress and limits the use of oxytocin to labouring women with abnormally slow progress. A pilot randomised controlled trial of the Neal & Lowe partograph suggested its use could result in a significant reduction (40%) in synthetic oxytocin augmentation (Lee et al., 2018). A large multi-centre trial (LaPS trial) comparing the action line partograph with labour progression guidelines based on the work by Zhang et al. (2010) reported only a small reduction (47% vs 41%) in synthetic oxytocin use in nulliparous women when the parameters described by Zhang et al. were used to determine labour dystocia (Bernitz et al., 2019). It is alarming that in both groups over 40% of the spontaneously labouring women had their labours augmented and that 19% of women in the Zhang group and 23% in the action line group received synthetic oxytocin without a diagnosis of labour dystocia (Bernitz et al., 2019; Dalbye et al., 2019). These outcomes suggest that decisions regarding labour progress and the use of synthetic oxytocin to augment labour are being made without reference to partograph. It is interesting to note that there is no reference in the trial publication to the level of consultation between the attending obstetrician (decision maker), the midwife and the labouring woman regarding how, if at all, this may have been a consideration in the decision to intervene and augment the labour. Future studies may be needed to explore the decision-making process around labour augmentation and how varying the design of partographs may influence this.

REFLECTIVE THINKING EXERCISE

Do midwives sometimes refute women's descriptions of early labour or their explanation of when it started? How do you think women feel when their perceptions about what they are experiencing are not believed? Imagine how you would react if you told the dentist that she was hurting you, only to be told that you couldn't be in pain and it was all in your imagination! Reflect on how the environment and the dentist's behaviours would affect your perceptions and behaviours.

CRITICAL THINKING EXERCISE

Friedman described three stages in the active phase of labour: acceleration, maximal slope and deceleration. Make your own partogram and draw the typical curve. As you support women in labour, plot their labours on a 'personal' partogram. Later, reflect on the 'normal' labours that actually fitted this pattern compared with those that did not, and the birth outcomes for each.

DISTURBANCES IN THE RHYTHM OF LABOUR—DYSTOCIA

As we have demonstrated, the overdiagnosis of the poorly defined entity 'dystocia' (abnormally slow labour) leads to interventions that have been overused in healthy labours. However, there remains a need for sentinel indicators to identify when the wellbeing of mother and fetus may become compromised. We now know that the clinical phenomenon of labour dystocia is complex and multifactorial (Lowe, 2007) and more often than not it is not possible to determine its cause. The reasons for the observed increased incidence of dystocia in industrialised countries are only partly known. Poor application of the fetal head-to-cervix may be associated with dystocia caused by slow progress of labour (Allman et al., 1996), as is slow engagement of fetal head at onset of labour (Roshanfekr et al., 1999). Malposition and malpresentations are associated with both these problems. Iatrogenic factors have also been used to explain the increase of augmentation of labour and caesarean birth. An increased need for augmentation has been reported in affluent countries and some studies show augmentation is now used in up to 50% of nulliparas (Lavender et al., 2013; Neal et al., 2010a).

Even though we do not know much about its causes and associations, labour 'dystocia' remains the most common reason for performing a caesarean section in nulliparous women (ACOG, 2014). Interestingly, Zhang et al. (2002) suggest that maternal obesity and increasing fetal weight might result in a slower labour (dystocia). Thus fetal macrosomia may increase the risk of dystocia and possibly the increased incidence of caesareans (Scott-Pillai et al., 2013). Other studies show that BMI >35 (referred to as 'morbid obesity') in pregnancy is associated with longer gestation and significantly higher risk of post-term birth, which contributes to the greater need for IOL for prolonged pregnancy. As gestation progresses beyond term, perinatal morbidity and mortality increase, as do maternal complications such as preeclampsia, postpartum haemorrhage and caesarean birth (Arrowsmith et al., 2011). However, these authors also show that following induction of labour there is little difference in outcomes between women with BMI >35 and those with BMI <25. The authors conclude that induction of labour followed by spontaneous birth is a safe option for women classed as 'morbidly obese'. In other words, these women do not require a caesarean section.

Slow progress in the latent phase of labour

It is difficult to determine whether a period of slow progress in the latent phase of labour is pathological and therefore requires treatment, or is a normal variation in the physiological process of the cervix becoming more responsive to the uterine contractions and commencing to dilate. Hence, evidence-informed midwives are aware that slow progress in this phase of labour is not necessarily indicative of dystocia in the later stages of labour. Further, active interventions to accelerate labour in the latent phase are not associated with improvements in outcomes, and may be harmful (Bugg et al., 2011; Clark et al., 2009). In most cases the treatment of choice for a lengthy latent labour phase is rest, simple analgesia and sleep—none of which are easily achieved in hospital. Numerous studies have demonstrated that women who are admitted to hospital in the latent phase of labour are more likely to receive interventions and less likely to have a vaginal birth compared with those admitted in the active phase (McNiven et al., 1998; Neal et al., 2014). This does require midwives to act as 'gatekeepers' to 'protect' women from the time-based expectations of hospital labour management (Cheyne et al., 2007). However, when a woman has made the decision to come to hospital, such advice may be viewed as impacting on the woman's sense of autonomy and seem at odds with a woman-centred approach (Carlsson et al., 2012). Therefore an appropriate midwifery response to a woman presenting in latent phase needs to emphasise the normality of the process and positively reinforce her progress whilst responding effectively to her immediate needs (Ängeby, 2018).

Slow progress in the active phase of labour

The diagnosis of the active phase of labour has been identified as one of the most problematic yet significant aspects of intrapartum care (McDonald & Magill-Cuerden, 2013). According to the traditional obstetric approach based upon Friedman's research and the active management of labour, the active phase of labour is characterised by increasing frequency and intensity of contractions, progressive descent of the presenting part and dilation of the cervix of 1 cm/h. It covers the period from the end of the latent phase (3–4 cm of cervical dilation) to complete dilation of the cervix (10 cm of cervical dilation). Fig. 38.2 shows how a partogram is used to plot the expected progress of labour and the typical pattern of **prolonged labour** based on Friedman's 'ideal' of normal labour and the action lines devised by Philpott & Castle (1972). On the other hand, using work by Zhang et al. (2010) and Neal & Lowe (2012) that allows for greater variation of progress in the early active stage, we can see the same progress of labour plotted on Fig. 38.3 and how this is now considered normal. It has also been noted that, even in the presence of seemingly effective contractions, cervical dilation may pause for up to 4 hours prior to 8 cm and still be considered normal (Zhang et al., 2010). Effective midwifery responses to slow progress in the active phase should be aimed at addressing the underlying cause, which is not always obvious and may be multifactorial. These are discussed in greater detail later in this chapter.

Slow progress in the second stage of labour

It is often observed that the second stage of labour has its own latent stage where the contractions may slow or stop as the woman's mind and body prepare for the work of birth. This period may last for up to an hour. In many cases this is 'normal'; however, after the very strong and frequent contractions associated with the 'transition' at the end of the first stage this can often be misdiagnosed as abnormal and augmentation inadvertently commenced. Slow progress in second stage may result from analgesia such as epidurals, malposition, fetal size or pelvic shape.

Assessing progress in labour

As we have discussed, a misdiagnosis of slower than expected labour progress in the active phase can lead to unnecessary obstetric intervention, such as augmentation of labour using oxytocic drugs and artificial rupture of the membranes (ARM) (NICE, 2014). On the other hand, failure to diagnose complications related to dystocia may have catastrophic consequences. Prolonged labour can lead to increased maternal and neonatal mortality and morbidity owing to increased risks of maternal exhaustion, postpartum haemorrhage and sepsis, fetal distress and asphyxia, and it requires early detection and appropriate clinical responses including referral (Rohwer et al., 2013). Empowered, knowledgeable women will alert the midwife to an apparent slowing down in the pattern of contractions once labour has established. As we work in partnership with women we should also consider that our understanding of labour progress has primarily not been developed with input from women and may not equate with their experience (Dixon & Foureur, 2010). If a woman states that *she* feels that something is wrong with her labour or progress, this should be sufficient reason to assess her further.

Midwives may not need to perform vaginal examinations, particularly on a routine 2–4-hourly basis to assess the progress of labour, unless there is good reason to suspect that progress has halted. However, many hospitals have protocols or guidelines that require the use of partograms and assessment criteria so midwives may be required to follow these. Women may also decline vaginal assessment, or this may be inappropriate in certain cultures or for women with histories of sexual abuse. Less-invasive methods to determine the progress of labour include the evaluation of contraction patterns by gentle abdominal palpation to track the descent of the fetus through the birth passage, combined with careful assessment of the strength, regularity and duration of contractions, and are effective techniques. However, these assessments are also subjective, and should always be considered along with the patterns in the woman's behaviour and her reactions to each contraction.

The pattern of contractions can be altered by factors that include fear, anxiety and uncontrolled pain rather than problems in what are often called the 'passages—disproportion between the pelvis and the fetus'. Maternal fears about transfer to hospital will often slow labour down. Similarly, labour often slows just before the commencement of the second stage of labour, probably to give the mother a much-needed rest before the work of the birth begins.

Although a longer than expected, albeit normal, duration of labour is not uncommon in primigravidas, there are other potentially problematic reasons for observed changes in contraction rhythms and these are now explored. Apart from the factors associated with dystocia described in earlier sections they are:

- maternal dehydration or ketosis
- anxiety and fear
- ineffective pattern of contractions
- malposition (a persistent occipitoposterior position)
- malpresentation (face, shoulder, brow)
- relative or absolute cephalopelvic disproportion.

MATERNAL DEHYDRATION, KETOSIS AND THE PROGRESS OF LABOUR

Labour is hard work, and the body needs energy to work effectively. However, in developed countries, the costs and benefits of restricting fluids and food in labour remain controversial issues. Restricting women's oral intake to fluids or ice chips during labour is a widely accepted obstetric tradition, which began about 50 years ago when women frequently gave birth under general anaesthesia and were therefore at risk of aspiration pneumonia (Mendelson's syndrome). However, modern anaesthesia has improved, and in any case general anaesthesia is rare in 21st-century obstetrics. Moreover, no period of fasting guarantees an empty stomach, and clear liquids leave the stomach almost immediately. Some authors argue, with limited evidence to support their hypothesis, that fasting increases ketosis and dehydration, which leads to more painful contractions, slower labours and fatigue (Nahaee et al., 2020; Singata et al., 2013). However, preventing the woman from meeting her body's calorific requirements and consequent suboptimal functioning of vital organs caused by fasting may slow the progress of labour. In addition, the effect of malnourishment on the woman's psyche needs to be addressed (Nahaee et al., 2020). A woman in active labour requires up to 47 kCal/h (197 kJ/h) to prevent ketosis (Hall et al., 2006) (see Chs 21 and 24). Routine administration of intravenous fluids to reduce ketosis is not supported by evidence (Hall et al., 2006). Neither does administering intravenous fluids to low-risk women reduce the duration of labour (Dawood et al., 2013; Fong et al., 2017). Administration of intravenous glucose to women in labour risks fluid overload and lactic acidosis in the mother and hyponatraemia and decreased PO_2 in the fetus (Ames et al., 1975; Mauad-Filho et al., 1982). For these reasons, restrictions placed on eating and drinking during normal labour are no longer justified. The woman should be supported to eat and drink according to her own preferences. Unrestricted eating in low-risk labours has also been shown to reduce the duration of labour (Ciardulli et al., 2017). A Cochrane review (of five studies) (Singata et al., 2013) concluded that the evidence shows no benefits or harms; there is no justification for the restriction of fluids and food in labour for women at low risk of complications. No studies reviewed by the authors looked specifically at women at increased risk of complications, hence there is as yet no evidence to support restrictions in this group of women either.

Sports medicine isotonic calorific drinks (e.g. Gatorade 105 kJ / 100 mL) administered in labour reduce the incidence of ketosis without increasing gastric volume (Kubli et al., 2002). However, Singata et al. (2013) found conflicting evidence on the effect of carbohydrate solutions on labour. One study reported a significant increase in caesarean sections for women taking carbohydrate drinks in labour compared with water only, but the reviewers caution the interpretation of these results because the sample size was small. The authors state that further studies are needed and it is critical that any future studies assess women's views of their usefulness.

THE EFFECT OF ANXIETY AND FEAR ON LABOUR PROGRESS

Various factors shape the physiological and psychological processes of birth; the ways women experience the pain as well as their reactions to it. Prior experience of birthing, culture and ethnicity, educational attainment, support from a partner and her ability to cope with the pain of labour are significant mediating variables on the experience of labour pain (Lowe, 2002). The relationships between continuous support in labour, fear, anxiety and the progress of labour are described elsewhere in this text. In brief, anxiety, excessive pain and fear increase the amount of catecholamines ('fight-or-flight' hormones) released into the maternal circulation, and these influence the effectiveness of uterine contractions. It has long been considered that uncontrollable anxiety and fear increase the pain of labour and inhibit its progress. A notable proponent of this explanation was Grantly Dick-Read, an English obstetrician (1890–1959). Dick-Read developed his ideas about a possible relationship between fear and pain in childbirth after attending a birth in the slums of Whitechapel (London) in the 1930s. The birthing woman refused to allow him to administer chloroform and, following her infant's birth, remarked, 'It didn't hurt. It wasn't meant to, was it, doctor?' (Dick-Read, 1946). From this remark, and his observations of birth practices in other countries, Dick-Read proposed two questions:

> *Is labour easy because she is calm, or is she calm because her labour is easy? And conversely, is a woman pained and frightened because her labour is difficult, or is her labour difficult and painful because she is frightened?*
>
> (Dick-Read, 1946, p. 55)

Dick-Read theorised that fear had a physiological effect on the uterus which gave rise to pain and that when a woman (and her birth attendants) were calm, confident and relaxed, labour would not be painful and progress more easily. To this end, Dick-Read insisted that women be instructed in the facts of natural childbirth and relaxation and breathing techniques; he subsequently devised the first program of antenatal classes. Moreover, we now know that women who feel in control of their bodies, their labour and what is happening to them are less likely to experience uncontrollable pain (Neerland, 2018). Women who experienced sexual abuse in childhood or have had prior traumatic birth experiences, or have strong 'control' issues, may sometimes have difficulty surrendering to the power of their labour (Leeners et al., 2016). When the fear of labour and birth (tocophobia) becomes so intense a woman may avoid pregnancy and vaginal birth. Indeed, maternal fear of childbirth is the most common reason for nulliparous women's request for caesarean birth (Handelzalts et al., 2017). Women with extreme fear of labour (tocophobia) may develop post-traumatic stress disorder if they feel 'forced' to go through vaginal birth, but may benefit from counselling or psychiatric consultation (Striebich et al., 2018) (see also Ch. 41).

CLINICAL POINT

Strategies to prevent, or support women in dealing with, anxiety and fear in labour are:

- one-to-one midwifery care in which a trusting relationship has been established
- eating and drinking to avoid fatigue and dehydration, which may slow labour
- massage, acupressure, sterile water injections or showers to ease pain and induce relaxation, which may enhance progress
- warm-water immersion, which has been called the 'midwives' epidural'
- talk, which provides comfort, reassurance and encouragement, and aims to relieve anxiety and explore the psychological or emotional issues or adverse environmental elements that might be causing the 'slow' labour.

INEFFECTIVE CONTRACTION PATTERNS

As already shown, dystocia encompasses various complications in labour, the most common being incoordinate uterine contractions that result in an extremely painful and prolonged / slow labour. Other contraction patterns include coordinate hypotonic and hypertonic uterine activity. Research by Wuntakai et al. (2013) has postulated that leptin—a protein synthesised in the adipose tissues in humans—opposes the effect of oxytocin on myometrium, which may result in a 'dysfunctional' slow labour caused by ineffective uterine action in women with a BMI >35. These authors recommend early and incremental use of synthetic oxytocin in labour may stimulate effective contractions in women whose BMI is >35. However, as noted previously, labour progress may vary with each individual woman and such interventions should be implemented only after careful assessment. Many women with a high BMI will labour normally.

Incoordinate uterine action

Incoordinate uterine action is characterised by asynchronous, hypotonic or hypertonic uterine contractions. There is a loss of fundal polarity, and in hypertonic incoordinate uterine action there is an increased uterine resting tone (see Rankin, 2017 or Blackburn, 2017). Consequently, placental blood flow is reduced and fetal compromise may occur (Murray, 2020). Two variations of hypertonic incoordinate uterine activity are the so-called 'colicky uterus' and 'constriction ring dystocia'. In the former, various parts of the uterus contract independently and this is combined with generalised and severe pain. An extreme form of incoordinate uterine action occurs with a localised spasm of one part of the uterus. In association with ineffectual uterine contractions it occurs when an annular spasm arises at the junction between the upper and lower uterine segment, usually in late first stage or early in the second stage of labour. Unlike Bandl's pathological retraction ring, constriction rings are not associated with obstructed labour and cannot be palpated abdominally (Table 38.1). Constriction rings may also arise from injudicious use of oxytocin or during intrauterine manipulation such as an internal podalic version. Relaxants, terbutaline or on rare occasions deep anaesthesia with a drug such as halothane may eliminate the localised myometrial spasms, but as a last resort caesarean section with a vertical incision may be required (Rohwer et al., 2013).

Table 38.1 Patterns of incoordinate uterine action

Bandl's pathological retraction ring	Constriction ring
Primarily occurs in second stage	Occurs in the first, second or third stage
Always occurs at the junction of the thinned lower uterine segment and the thick retracted upper uterine	Occurs at any level of the uterus
Rises up anteriorly	Does not change its position
Felt and seen abdominally	Felt only vaginally
Uterine pain is constant and the fetal parts cannot be felt	The uterus is not tonically retracted and the fetal parts can be felt
Maternal distress and evidence of fetal compromise or death	Maternal and fetal compromise may not be present
Relieved only by birth of the fetus (caesarean section)	May be relieved by anaesthetics or antispasmodics

Hypotonic uterine contractions

Ineffective contractions are commonly associated with a poorly fitting presenting part on the cervix. Hypotonic uterine action (contractions are short in duration and of weak intensity) result in a slower than expected rate of cervical dilation and in prolonged labour. The pattern may occur in early labour (primary), or later after a normal contraction pattern has been established (secondary). Typically, this pattern is briefly observed after the administration of epidural or narcotic analgesia, but is more frequently associated with a degree of malposition or cephalopelvic disproportion. There is also evidence that women are genetically predisposed to hypotonic uterine action (Algovik et al., 2010).Once the presence of factors that preclude the use of oxytocics is eliminated, many obstetric clinicians advocate augmentation of labour with an artificial rupture of membranes and synthetic oxytocin infusion. However, studies of the effectiveness of amniotomy have not demonstrated that it significantly improves outcomes or reduces the duration of labour (Smyth et al., 2013). Epidurals may also impact on the duration of labour, with a Cochrane review reporting that women who used epidurals were more likely to require oxytocin augmentation and have a longer second stage (Anim-Somuah et al., 2011), whereas another Cochrane review concluded that women with continuous labour support (e.g. midwives, doulas) were more likely to have shorter labours, spontaneous vaginal births and require less pain medication than women without such support (Bohren et al., 2017).

Hypertonic uterine contractions

A precipitate labour is defined as one with a total duration of less than 2 hours (Janga & Bickerton, 2015). For some women this may be their normal pattern, but the most common cause of hypertonic uterine action is the injudicious use of oxytocic drugs. Fetal welfare may be compromised when the intensity of uterine contractions is increased, resting intervals are shortened and the duration of the contractions is increased. Hypertonic contractions may also cause maternal trauma—including uterine rupture or perineal damage—or increase risk of postpartum haemorrhage. A combination of excessively forceful uterine contractions and minimal soft-tissue resistance can give rise to precipitate labour, fetal anoxia and cerebral trauma, maternal lacerations, and postpartum haemorrhage caused by uterine atony. Early recognition of the problem, and timely preparation for birth under controlled conditions, may minimise these risks. If oxytocin administration is the cause of the hypertonic contractions, the infusion should immediately be stopped. The problem typically resolves in less than 15 minutes. If excessive uterine activity is associated with fetal heart rate abnormalities, and this pattern persists despite discontinuation of oxytocin, a beta-mimetic such as terbutaline can be given.

Working with women experiencing ineffective contraction patterns

Walsh (2012) suggests that a greater understanding of labour physiology and hormonal control, referred to as the 'dance of labour' (Buckley, 2004), enables midwives to appreciate the purpose of an apparent imbalance in endogenous oxytocin release during labour. A longer-than-expected labour for the woman and her birth supporters can affect her ability to cope, leading to an increased release of catecholamines (stress hormones), which causes the labour to slow. The midwife will need to use all their skills in supporting women in a long labour, in particular taking care to avoid maternal dehydration and moderate ketosis, which is best determined by documentation of fluid input and output and urinalysis. Ketosis and dehydration may exacerbate ineffective contraction patterns and dysfunctional labour (Toohill et al., 2008). However, gastric emptying (increasing the risk of aspiration) is delayed in women receiving an epidural during labour (Desgranges et al., 2019).

It is important for the woman to avoid a full bladder because this may inhibit descent of the presenting part into the pelvis and delay the second stage of labour, and potentially contribute to a postpartum haemorrhage. Observation and assessment of the rhythms of normal labour are useful to detect the onset of complications. Simple measures such as midwives undertaking regular abdominal assessment to determine the position of the baby during labour, encouraging the woman to ambulate, frequent changes of position, creating a restful birthing environment and the presence of supportive birth companions assist the birth process (Deakin, 2001; Walsh, 2012). Research by Cluett et al. (2004) demonstrated that labouring in water may alleviate the effects of labour dystocia rather than invasive and potentially harmful interventions such as ARM and intravenous oxytocin. Moreover, fasting, enforced bed rest, intravenous therapy and continuous electronic fetal monitoring imply notions of loss of control, sickness and helplessness, which may also interfere with the progress of labour and necessitate intervention such as augmentation of labour, epidural analgesia and operative birth (Nahaee et al., 2020).

Women experiencing ineffective contraction patterns and prolonged labour are more at risk of postpartum haemorrhage (PPH). Therefore, a discussion of the management of the third stage of labour should occur early enough for the woman to be able to make informed decisions about the need for an active management of the third stage of labour.

REFLECTIVE THINKING EXERCISE

The woman, as the final decision maker, is asking you as the midwife to explain the doctor's advice that her labour requires augmentation. What information, alternatives and support can you offer to support her to make an informed decision?

Collaborative interventions

The primary goal of all clinicians working with women as they labour is to provide the safest outcome for both mother and infant. It is crucial that midwives have the skills and knowledge required to assess labour and contraction patterns that pose risks for the mother and fetus. Once dystocia is recognised, it is important to identify and, if possible, to treat the cause in partnership with the woman, minimising any potentially harmful outcomes. Often, dystocia can be relieved by simple measures such as alleviating intolerable pain or rehydration, although in some cases management will include transferring primary care to a multidisciplinary team. The lead midwife should avail themselves of support from the back-up midwife in primary settings or support from the midwifery staff in secondary/tertiary hospitals, so that the lead carer can take regular breaks and have adequate rest (Australian College of Midwives (ACM), 2013; NZCOM, 2012).

Delay in the active phase of labour—one example of diagnosis and management

The active phase of labour has been described in various ways. Frequently, it is described as when there are painful, regular contractions (3 in 10 minutes) and progressive cervical dilation from 4 cm (NICE, 2014).

Diagnosis of delay in the active phase should consider all aspects of labour progress and include (NICE, 2014):

- cervical dilation of less than 2 cm in 4 hours for first labours
- cervical dilation of less than 2 cm in 4 hours or slowing of progress for second or subsequent labours
- moulding of the fetal head (>2+); marked caput succedaneum; malpresentation
- slow/absent descent and rotation of the fetal head; asynclitism
- reduced changes in the strength, duration and frequency of uterine contractions
- signs of fetal and maternal compromise.

Collaborative interventions may include ARM (see next section), augmentation of labour with oxytocin and possibly pharmaceutical analgesia (epidural or intramuscular narcotics). Operative birth (instrumental or caesarean section) may be the preferred option.

Amniotomy (artificial rupture of membranes)

For most women, once labour has been established, it advances without medical intervention. Artificial rupture of membranes is a surgical intervention and thus

Box 38.2 ARM terminology

- ARM—amniotomy or artificial rupture of membranes
- SROM—spontaneous rupture of membranes
- PROM—prelabour or premature rupture of membranes
- PPROM—pre-term, prelabour rupture of membranes

requires the woman's consent, but for years has been the first medical treatment option for a pathological prolonged labour (Walsh, 2012) (Box 38.2). As Cohain (2013) suggests, this seemingly 'routine' procedure may not always be beneficial and has associated risks. According to the latest available evidence, ARM is no longer recommended as a routine practice for shortening spontaneous labour (Smyth et al., 2013); in this review, amniotomy was associated with an increased risk of birth by caesarean section compared with women in the control group, although the difference was not statistically significant. Neither was there any statistical difference in length of the first stage of labour, maternal satisfaction with childbirth experience, or Apgar scores less than 7 at 5 minutes. Consequently, the New Zealand College of Midwives consensus statement (2016) does not support the use of routine ARM if labour is progressing physiologically. Until recently, early amniotomy was advocated as a component of the active management of labour, to accelerate the progress of labour by increasing the frequency and quality of contractions (Fraser et al., 1999).

ARM (often used in combination with an oxytocic infusion) is used to augment labour if labour progress is considered to be slower than expected, because 'prolonged labour' is associated with birth by caesarean section and a low cord pH in the fetus. There is, however, a lack of evidence to support or refute these assertions. ARM may also be performed to obtain access to the fetus for a scalp pH assessment, to attach a fetal scalp electrode or to assess the status of the liquor.

Complications of ARM

As soon as the membranes are ruptured there is an increased risk of umbilical cord prolapse, fetal compromise and chorioamnionitis (Smyth et al., 2013). Once an ARM has been performed, birth should occur within 12–24 hours. Prelabour rupture of the membranes at or near term (term PROM) increases the risk of infection for the woman (chorioamnionitis); however, the effect on the fetus is less certain (Middleton et al., 2017). The routine use of antibiotics for women at the time of term PROM is thought to reduce this risk. However, a systematic review (Wojcieszek et al., 2014) found no convincing evidence of benefit for the routine use of antibiotics for term PROM and concluded that they should not be used in the absence of confirmed infection. Nevertheless, many clinicians still prescribe intravenous antibiotics if the membranes were ruptured for more than 12 hours, though this is not common practice in New Zealand hospitals.

The amniotic sac and its liquor protect the fetal head; once the membranes rupture, this effect is removed. Compression of the fetal head leads to increased moulding and changes in the fetal heart rate—early decelerations. Variable decelerations, the result of increased cord compression from the loss of liquor following an ARM, are often apparent on the electronic fetal heart rate trace (Peru et al., 2020). Following are listed some of the potential but rare consequences of an amniotomy that may require emergency intervention.

Maternal risk factors include:

- prolapse of the umbilical cord leading to operative birth
- chorioamnionitis
- sepsis
- significant umbilical cord compression leading to operative birth
- rupture of a vasa praevia.

Fetal risk factors include:

- pre-term birth
- infection
- cord prolapse
- malpresentation (Smyth et al., 2013).

Indications for amniotomy

- Prior to the commencement of oxytocin augmentation.
- Placement of a fetal spiral electrode (Vincent, 2005).

Contraindications for amniotomy

- Woman refuses the procedure.
- Presentation unknown or unstable.
- Cervix dilated <4 cm.
- Unengaged fetal head.
- Non-vertex position of the fetal head.
- Woman is HIV positive.
- Presence of active genital herpes simplex virus.

CLINICAL POINT

Before performing an ARM, the midwife:

- ensures the woman has consented to the procedure
- ensures that the position of the placenta is known (see Ch. 22)
- ensures that there is indication for the intervention and there are no contraindications
- performs an abdominal palpation and vaginal examination to determine the stage of labour, presentation, position, cervical dilation and position of the fetal head relative to the ischial spines
- during a vaginal examination, assesses the progress of labour by cervical dilation; unless the fetal head is well engaged in the pelvis, ARM is not advocated
- introduces the amniohook through the cervix and makes a small tear in the membranes lying in front of the fetal head.

After the procedure, the midwife:

- checks and records the colour, odour and quantity of the liquor and the fetal heart rate
- ensures that the woman is dry and comfortable, and informs her of the findings
- documents findings.

CRITICAL THINKING EXERCISE

You are the midwife for Maria, a primigravida who has been in labour for 15 hours. Maria's mother Henrietta asks you to 'break the waters—my midwife broke mine'. What will you say and do?

Augmentation of labour with synthetic oxytocin

Labour augmentation usually involves the stimulation of uterine contractions to hasten birth after the onset of labour following an ARM. How effective augmentation of labour with oxytocin actually is to assist women to achieve a vaginal birth is questionable (Bugg et al., 2013). As discussed earlier in this chapter, the long-term effects of maternal exposure to synthetic oxytocin may impact upon both the mother and baby.

Before intravenous oxytocics are administered, cephalopelvic disproportion needs to be excluded by careful abdominal palpation and vaginal examination. The most frequent complications of oxytocin-augmented labours are uterine hyperstimulation leading to excessive maternal pain, fetal compromise, umbilical cord compression and, rarely, uterine rupture. Consequently, most hospitals have a policy of continuous electronic fetal monitoring once augmentation or induction of labour with oxytocin begins. After birth, postpartum haemorrhage from uterine atony is a significant risk (Loscul et al., 2016).

INDUCTION OF LABOUR

Induction of labour (IOL) is artificial initiation of labour before its spontaneous onset for the purpose of birthing the baby. The rate of IOL varies between countries and between centres, and ranges from 10% to 30%. Enkin et al. (2000, p. 375) make the point that 'the decision to bring pregnancy to an end before the spontaneous onset of labour is one of the most drastic ways of intervening in the natural history of pregnancy and childbirth'. Induction of labour is not 'risk free' and may negatively affect a woman's experience of birth through increased pain, restriction of movement and concern for her infant (Hildingsson et al., 2011).

There are two forms of labour stimulation. The first, augmentation, has been discussed earlier in this chapter. It involves the stimulation of uterine contraction in a labour that has already begun. If the rhythms of labour are ineffective, contractions may be stimulated by augmenting labour with a combination of ARM and an infusion of an oxytocic drug such as Syntocinon. It should only be used once non-invasive strategies, such as positioning and ambulation, emptying the bladder, relief of unbearable pain and anxiety (perhaps with hydrotherapy) and correcting dehydration and ketosis with fluid and nutrition, have been tried. There is some evidence to suggest that acupressure (Mollart et al., 2015) or nipple stimulation (Suresh & Soni, 2019) may also be of benefit. The rates of augmentation of labour are rising; up to 45% of women with an uncomplicated pregnancy, who labour spontaneously at full term, will have their labours artificially accelerated (Zhang et al., 2010). In contrast, induction of labour refers to the artificial induction of labour with or without rupturing the amniotic sac before the spontaneous onset of labour for the purpose of accomplishing birth. In Australia over a third of women (34%) had their labours induced in 2018 (Australian Institute of Health and Welfare (AIHW), 2020).

The UK National Institute for Health and Care Excellence (NICE) guidelines (currently under review) on induction of labour state that:

> *Although a variety of specific clinical circumstances may indicate the need for induction of labour with a greater or lesser degree of urgency, the essential judgment that the clinician and the pregnant woman must make is whether the interests of the mother or the baby, or both, will be better served by ending or continuing the pregnancy.*
>
> (National Collaborating Centre for Women's and Children's Health, 2008, p. 2)

Indications for induction

Induction of labour is indicated if the health of both mother and baby would be compromised if pregnancy continues; that is, the benefits of imminent birth outweigh the risks associated with the induction of labour. Table 38.2 summarises the current clinical indications for the induction of labour. The list is not exhaustive and there may be other issues such as social conditions or mental health status that may be legitimate indications for induction, however these should be considered on an individual basis. Women are an integral part of the decision-making process and should be informed of the risks and benefits of an induction of labour as well as the difficulties associated with accurate determination of gestational age.

Two indications for induction of labour have resulted in significant debate and controversy, and are discussed in more detail here.

Induction and postdates pregnancies

The most frequent indication for an induction of labour and the most difficult to assess is the postdates or post-term pregnancy. There is considerable debate about the definitions of a term and a post-term pregnancy. Commonly accepted midwifery and obstetric language used

Table 38.2 Indications for induction of labour

Reasons to consider IOL	Recommendation
Post dates	Offer induction of labour between 41 + 0 and 42 + 0 weeks gestation to women with an uncomplicated pregnancy, to reduce the risks of perinatal death, caesarean section, 5-minute Apgar <7 and meconium aspiration syndrome.
Prelabour rupture of membranes	In women with prelabour rupture of membranes at $\geq$ 37 weeks gestation, offer planned early birth* (within 24 hours), to reduce the risks of maternal infectious morbidity, definite or probable early-onset neonatal sepsis, and NICU admission. In these circumstances share information to support informed decision making and avoid digital vaginal examination. If there are risk factors for early onset group B *Streptococcus* or meconium-stained liquor then offer immediate induction.
Suspected small for gestational age or growth restriction	If EFW is 3rd centile or more and other investigations such as uterine artery Doppler studies are normal offer induction at 40 weeks. Offer induction between 37 and 38 weeks depending on availability and outcomes of uterine artery Doppler studies, or earlier if there are other concerns.
Diabetes in pregnancy	If there is good glycaemic control, normal fetal growth and no obstetric complications then continue expectant management to at least 40 weeks gestation. Type 2 diabetes—continue expectant management to 39 weeks unless there are obstetric or fetal indications for earlier births or diabetes complications. Type 1 diabetes—management to be individualised.
Maternal obesity	Do not offer induction for women with maternal obesity, in the absence of other risk factors or pregnancy complications.
Advanced maternal age	Consider offering induction at around 40 weeks gestation.
Reduced fetal movements	In the presence of normal maternal and fetal assessment, continue expectant management.
Hypertension in pregnancy	Chronic hypertension and low risk of adverse outcomes, consider expectant management beyond 37 weeks gestation with increased monitoring. Gestational hypertension diagnosed after 37 + 0 weeks gestation, consider induction of labour, to reduce the risks of severe hypertension, severe preeclampsia, HELLP syndrome, abruptio placenta, pulmonary oedema, severe renal impairment, and fetal growth restriction. Preeclampsia diagnosed after 37 + 0 weeks gestation, offer induction of labour.
Antepartum haemorrhage of unknown origin	For antepartum haemorrhage of unknown origin, in the presence of normal maternal and fetal assessment, consider expectant management.
Suspected fetal macrosomia	In the absence of pregnancy complications, consider expectant management.
Artificial reproductive technology	In the absence of pregnancy complications, consider expectant management.
Multiple pregnancy	For women with an uncomplicated monochorionic diamniotic twin pregnancy, consider offering induction of labour between 36 and 37 weeks gestation. For women with an uncomplicated dichorionic twin pregnancy, consider offering induction of labour between 37 and 38 weeks gestation.
Reduced liquor $<$ 41 weeks gestation	In women with reduced liquor as an isolated finding at $<$ 41 weeks gestation, in the presence of normal maternal and fetal assessment, consider expectant management.
Obstetric cholestasis	For women with obstetric cholestasis, if symptomatic or if serum bile acid concentration $\geq$ 100, consider induction of labour; otherwise consider expectant management.
Previous stillbirth	For women with previous stillbirth, consider expectant management or induction of labour, based on a review of risk factors for recurrence and any other antenatal risk factors, and guided by maternal choice.
No medical indication	Do not offer induction of labour in the absence of a medical indication. The management of induction of labour for maternal request is to be individualised.

(Source: NZCOM et al., 2019)

to describe the indication for induction of labour from 37 completed weeks to 42 weeks gestation include 'term pregnancy', 'prolonged', 'post-mature', 'postdates' and 'post-term', which many assume are synonymous albeit vague terms that differentiate between the 'normal' and 'abnormal' range of pregnancy. This terminology contributes to the confusion about options for optimum best care at this time. The New Zealand guidelines for induction of labour (draft) (RANZCOG, 2019) recommend that induction of labour in low-risk women occurs between 41 and 42 weeks (with known certainty) of pregnancy to avoid a prolonged pregnancy. It recommends that an informed discussion occurs with the woman in regard to why, where and how the induction will occur, risks and benefits, analgesia options, alternative options if induction is declined and that induction might not work (see Ch. 39 for further information). The Safer Baby Bundle initiative, designed to reduce rates of term stillbirth, also includes recommendations for induction of labour at 41 weeks amongst the five elements within the bundle (Andrews et al., 2020). The timing for induction may occur at earlier gestations based on assessment of risk factors such as reduction or changes in fetal movements. However, some have cautioned that since high-quality trials have highlighted some limitations on the use of fetal movements as a measure of risk (Norman et al., 2018), such approaches may also increase the incidence of otherwise early and unnecessary induction if strict audits of the introduction of the bundle are not undertaken (Swannell, 2020).

Three recent large RCTs have explored routine induction versus waiting for spontaneous labour in low-risk women and the effect on stillbirth rates (Grobman et al., 2018; Keulen et al., 2019; Wennerholm et al., 2019). The largest of these trials, in which 6106 nulliparous women participated, found no difference in stillbirth rates between induction at 39 weeks and expectant management up to 41 completed weeks (Grobman et al., 2018). Two other trials compared elective induction at 41 weeks versus expectant management until 42 completed weeks and both reported a significant reduction in stillbirth rates when women were induced at 41 weeks (Keulen et al., 2019; Wennerholm et al., 2019). However, it is interesting to note that in both of these trials stillbirth only occurred in nulliparous women. None of the multiparous women whose pregnancies extended beyond 41 weeks suffered a stillbirth or perinatal loss (Keulen et al., 2019; Wennerholm et al., 2019). These studies may suggest that whilst induction of labour at 41 weeks is a means of reducing postdates stillbirth this intervention could be more selectively applied to nulliparous women.

A limitation in all of the three studies mentioned above was that of the thousands of women who were eligible to participate over 70% declined to do so. In one study, 60% of the women who declined did so because they preferred expectant management, whereas only 14% expressed a preference for early induction of labour (Keulen et al., 2019). This does raise the question of how representative of 'low-risk' women the trials are if the majority of pregnant women meeting this criteria declined to participate. The generalisability, or external validity, of a trial's results is dependent on how representative the trial participants are of the broader population. If the majority of a group of potential participants to a trial decline to participate, this may mean that those that do consent could be a particular subset of the population that have something in common. That particular trait may not be measured within the research but still independently affect the trial outcomes, particularly if the outcome researched is uncommon. For example, if women with a higher level of anxiety about pregnancy and birth were more likely to participate in the induction of labour trials this may potentially alter the results, as psychological stress during pregnancy has been associated with higher rates of stillbirth (Wisborg et al., 2008). This then means that the trial results would be more applicable to the subset of women expressing anxiety in pregnancy and not the general population.

A Cochrane review also examined the benefits and harms of induction of labour policy at term or post-term in comparison with waiting for spontaneous labour or a later induction. The findings were that the absolute risk of perinatal death is small but that an induction of labour policy is associated with fewer perinatal deaths in comparison to expectant management (Middleton et al., 2018).

The RCT by Grobman et al. (2018) also reported a significant reduction in caesarean sections in the early induction group compared to expectant management. However, reviews of the study have pointed out that of the 'low-risk' women who took part, 53% had a BMI greater than 30, which calls into question the classification of 'low-risk' (Ghi et al., 2019). This may also have contributed to the higher incidence of hypertension in the post-term women and resulting higher caesarean section rate (Ghi et al., 2019). The Cochrane review by Middleton et al. (2018) and an earlier meta-analysis of induction of labour trials (Wood et al., 2014) also suggested that induction at term may result in fewer caesarean sections. However, other studies have questioned this result, finding that induction of labour is associated with an increased risk of caesarean section (Mahomed et al., 2016; Zhao et al., 2017; Dahlen et al., 2021). The article by Mahomed et al. (2016) provides a good explanation for the differences in results and is recommended reading. It is important to remember that much of the 'evidence' surrounding the indications for induction of labour is 'weak'. In other words, there are few if any high-quality randomised controlled trials to support the recommendations (see also Ch. 39).

Austin & Benn's (2006) investigation of decision making around induction of labour for primigravid women suggests that the reason/s for induction of labour were perceived differently for women and their lead maternity carer (LMC). They also identified that it was the hospital system of bookings that most often influenced the timing of an induction, possibly resulting in unnecessary induction for 'postdates', and suggested that midwives should develop a greater trust in the timing of the onset of labour for a well woman and baby. Further research about women's choice with regards to induction of labour presented in a directive or non-directive way found that women were more likely to opt for induction if given information in a directive way and from a medical viewpoint (Stevens & Millar, 2012),whereas women who felt more involved in their decision making had lower rates of induction (Attanasio, 2016). However, Keirse (2010) remarks that the boundaries between what is elective induction, what is medically indicated or not, and what is persuasive coercion or maternal request with regards to induction, are as 'vague' as ever!

CLINICAL POINT

All women should be offered information about the risks associated with pregnancies that last longer than 42 weeks at the 38-week antenatal assessment and asked for their opinions, thus enabling them to be partners in the decision-making process.

Induction for maternal request

Labour is sometimes induced for 'social' or 'geographical' reasons without a medical or obstetric indication. In Australia, as many rural and remote maternity settings close, once their pregnancies reach 36 weeks women have no choice but to travel to cities to await the birth. It is not surprising that they opt for an induction rather than be away from home for an extended but indeterminate period of time. In some Australian states this affects up to a quarter of birthing women (Sweet et al., 2015). An unintended consequence of this is a significant rise in the number of babies being born before arrival at a maternity unit, contributing to increased risks for mother and baby (Kildea et al., 2015).

An induction of labour is not an isolated intervention and it frequently results in a cascade of interventions (Box 38.3) that have the potential to affect the childbirth process and its outcomes negatively (Tracy et al., 2006).

Box 38.3 Cascade of intervention

The cascade of intervention that usually follows induction of labour includes:

- intravenous lines
- enforced bed rest
- continuous electronic fetal heart rate monitoring
- amniotomy
- increased pain and discomfort
- epidural analgesia
- operative birth
- prolonged hospital stay.

Whilst the risks and benefits of synthetic oxytocic induction remain inconclusive, as discussed earlier in this chapter, maternal exposure to synthetic oxytocin may have long-term health consequences for mother and baby.

Contraindications for induction

Many clinical contraindications to spontaneous onset of labour and vaginal birth are also contraindications for the induction of labour. Contraindications include (NICE, 2008):

- any maternal or fetal condition that precludes vaginal birth
- malpresentation—transverse or oblique lie, compound or shoulder presentation
- previous major uterine surgery—'classical' caesarean section
- absolute cephalopelvic disproportion
- cord prolapse
- active genital herpes
- placenta praevia
- invasive carcinoma of the cervix
- a severely compromised fetus.

Relative contraindications include:

- non-reassuring fetal heart rate trace
- breech presentation
- unknown fetal presentation
- polyhydramnios
- presenting part above the pelvic brim
- severe maternal hypertension
- maternal heart disease.

Risks of induction

Induction of labour is perceived by many midwives as the first step in an often-irreversible cascade of interventions (see Box 38.3) that culminates in an increased need for epidural analgesia, operative birth and caesarean section, particularly among primigravid women (Akinsipe et al., 2012). IOL is steadily becoming more common; in New Zealand in 2017, 25.5% were induced, and the induction rate increases with age to 42.3% of women aged 40 years or over (Ministry of Health (MOH), 2017). In Australia, rates of induction exceed 34% (AIHW, 2020).

IOL may increase the risk of:

- cord prolapse
- uterine rupture
- postpartum haemorrhage
- requiring an epidural
- requiring an operative vaginal birth
- requiring a caesarean section.

Benefits of induction of labour

Depending on the indication for the induction there are considerable benefits to be gained from inducing labour. For example, IOL at 41 weeks or beyond compared with awaiting spontaneous labour for at least 1 week is associated with fewer perinatal deaths and lower risk of meconium aspiration syndrome (Middleton et al., 2018). Other studies have found that women prefer IOL at 41 weeks over serial antenatal monitoring (Heimstad et al., 2006).

Prerequisites for induction

The mother must be given full disclosure of the procedure, its risks and benefits, as well as information about any limitations of the birthing unit—for example, perhaps there is no 24-hour epidural service, or if she requires a caesarean section 'out of hours' she will have to be transferred to another hospital with these facilities. In addition, the following criteria should be met:

- There is documented evidence that the procedure has been discussed with the woman, that the risks and benefits of induction of her labour have been discussed and that she has given her consent for the procedure.
- There is a documented indication for the induction of labour as well as the presence of any contraindications.
- Parity is confirmed.
- The gestational age is confirmed.
- There is documented assessment of cervical favourability, fetal position and presentation and relationship of the fetal head to the pelvic brim.
- Membrane status has been assessed—intact or ruptured.
- The adequacy of the pelvis has been considered.
- The presence of uterine activity is known.
- The fetal heart rate has been recorded with cardiotocography (CTG).

Midwifery support prior to induction

Induction of labour may result in maternal feelings of loss of control, and loss of continuity of midwifery care if the maternity unit is some distance from the woman's place of residence, as well as other physical complications. Discussion about the indications for an induction of labour during pregnancy aids informed decision making at a time when a woman who is already compromised in her ability to cope with the physical discomforts of late pregnancy is more vulnerable than usual to others' coercion in her decision making. However, obtaining the woman's informed consent for the procedure lies with the medical practitioner who is going to perform the procedure, not the midwife.

A MIDWIFE'S STORY

As a core midwife working in a tertiary maternity unit on the delivery suite, I was allocated a woman who was coming in from an outlying area at 08:00 for an induction of labour. This was the first time I or the doctor on duty in the labour ward had met her. It was the woman's first baby and she was exactly 39 weeks gestation by sure dates. I welcomed her into the birthing room and completed her baseline observations, an abdominal palpation and assessment. Her uterine fundus was equal to dates; the baby was felt to be about 3500 g and on palpation I found a cephalic presentation with a right occipitolateral position, and a well-engaged flexed head deep in the pelvis. The baby's heart rate ranged from 120 to 140 b.p.m. Her baby had been moving well and there did not appear to be any medical indication for an induction of labour. I asked her what she understood was the reason for the induction and what she had been told about the procedure. She told me that her midwife, who was not in attendance due to distance, had made her a hospital appointment after seeing her at 38 weeks 1 week ago and she had been booked for induction today after seeing a doctor in another antenatal clinic 3 days before. She said that 'it was necessary to bring the labour on because she was overdue'. The woman gave no indication that she was aware she had alternative choices and options, or that she wanted to know about them. Nor did the woman seem to have much understanding about what was going to happen today or the risks and benefits of an induction of labour.

REFLECTIVE THINKING EXERCISE

Consider the above story, and reflect on your responsibilities and subsequent actions, taking into consideration your philosophy of practice, research findings, hospital guidelines, standards for practice and codes of ethics. You might like to consider the ethical principle of 'best interests' (see also Ch. 14).

The process of induction

'Natural methods'

There are various 'natural' methods for non-invasive induction of labour. These include: cod liver oil, herbal remedies such as blue and black cohosh, acupuncture, nipple stimulation, sexual intercourse (because semen has natural prostaglandins), and the use of raspberry leaf tea during the latter stages of pregnancy. The risks and benefits of these methods are unknown because the quality of evidence is based on a long tradition of use and on anecdotal case reports rather than on good-quality research. The NICE (2008) guidelines on induction of labour therefore do not recommend their use by health professionals. In any case, the New Zealand and Australian Colleges of Midwives both recommend that, before using these therapies, the woman should seek advice from a registered therapist unless her midwife has undertaken a recognised education program that entitles her to use or recommend these treatments.

Bishop's score

Before induction takes place, assessment of the cervix to determine readiness for labour is essential, and is done using the Bishop's score (Bishop, 1964). A Bishop's score (Table 38.3) is ascertained by assigning points to the parameters of cervical readiness (ripeness) for labour. The higher the Bishop's score the greater is the likelihood of a successful induction of labour. Although this is an attempt at objectivity, the care provider still makes a subjective assessment of the cervix. Induction should not be attempted unless a mother has a favourable Bishop's score. If the cervix is unfavourable (Bishop's score <6), cervical ripening prior to the induction with vaginal endogenous prostaglandin (PGE_2) or a balloon catheter is warranted, because if the cervix does not readily dilate then a long labour ending in a caesarean section with resulting potential complications is more likely (Beckmann et al., 2017). A score of 8 or 9 would indicate that the cervix was very ripe and induction has a high probability of success.

Women with a Bishop's score ≥5 generally labour more easily than do those with a score <5. Women with a low Bishop's score (primiparous and multiparous) experience higher rates of unsuccessful induction and caesarean section.

Pharmacological cervical ripening

Prostaglandins have been used for cervical ripening and induction of labour since the 1970s. The goal of the administration of prostaglandins in the process of induction of labour is to achieve cervical ripening before the onset of contractions. Prostaglandins have been administered via various routes, including local (extra-amniotic, intracervical, intravaginal) and general administration (oral, intramuscular and intravenous). A 2008 systematic review (Boulvain et al., 2008) found of a total of 56 trials (7738 women) that, although the intracervical route of administration is effective, it offers no advantages compared with other methods of administration, namely the vaginal route. The NICE guidelines on induction of labour (2008) do not recommend the use of the following pharmacological methods of induction: oral PGE_2, intravenous PGE_2, extra-amniotic PGE_2, intracervical PGE_2, intravenous oxytocin alone, hyaluronidase, corticosteroids, oestrogen and vaginal nitric oxide donors. A review by Bakker et al. (2013) looked at the difference in outcomes between a morning or evening induction and found no strong evidence that either was superior in regards to timing in use of oxytocin, but suggested that women preferred to have prostaglandins in the morning.

Synthetic forms of prostaglandins—PGE_2 as either a gel or pessaries (dinoprostone: Prepidil, Cervidil, Prostin)—are marketed for cervical ripening. Prostaglandins facilitate cervical ripening (softening and effacing the cervix) via a number of different mechanisms.

Types of PGE_2

Midwives should be aware of the clinical implications of each of the pharmacological agents used for cervical ripening. The types of exogenous PGE_2 are:

- intravaginal insert containing dinoprostone
- intracervical dinoprostone gels
- hospital-compounded intravaginal gels.

A normal CTG should be evident prior to the insertion of PGE_2 and the CTG trace continued for at least half an hour after its insertion. Prostaglandin (PGE_2)—Prostin comes as a 1-mg or 2-mg gel and is administered vaginally into the posterior fornix. The prescribed dose is determined by parity and the obstetrician's preferences, but the gel may be reapplied every 6–12 hours if necessary. The manufacturers recommend an initial dose of 1 mg followed by a second 1-mg or 2-mg dose 6 hours later if necessary, up to a maximum of three doses.

Dinoprostone (Cervidil) comes as a 10-mg controlled-release (over 24 hours) vaginal pessary, which has a removable cord for easy removal if necessary. A single dose of 10 mg of dinoprostone pessary (Cervidil) (releases approximately 0.3 mg dinoprostone per hour over 24 hours) is inserted into the posterior vaginal fornix. After administration, the woman remains semirecumbant for 30 minutes before ambulating (Medsafe, 2018).

Dinoprostone pessary (Cervidil) precautions for use

- Remove pessary if:
  - uterine hyperstimulation occurs
  - labour becomes established

Table 38.3 Modified Bishop cervical score system

Cervical feature	Modified Bishop score			
	0	1	2	3
Dilation (cm)	<1	1–2	2–4	>4
Length of cervix (cm)	>4	2–4	1–2	<1
Station (relative to ischial spines)	−3	−2	−1/0	+1/+2
Consistency	Firm	Average	Soft	—
Position	Posterior	Mid/anterior	—	—

(Source: Royal College of Obstetricians and Gynaecologists (RCOG), Clinical Effectiveness Support Unit. *Induction of Labour.* Evidence-based Clinical Guideline Number 9. London: RCOG Press; 2001. ©Royal College of Obstetricians and Gynaecologists; reproduced with permission.)

- after spontaneous rupture of membranes or before performing ARM.
- Oxytocin augmentation should not be commenced within 30 minutes of removal of dinoprostone pessary (Cervidil).

Misoprostol (Cytotec) is a synthetic PGE_1 analogue. Although it has been suggested as a useful agent for pre-induction cervical ripening and labour induction, it has not been approved or licensed for use in Australia and New Zealand and should be used only in the context of clinical trials until it is approved by the appropriate authorities.

Possible adverse effects include:

- gastrointestinal (e.g. nausea, vomiting), back pain, fever
- increased intraocular pressure in women with a history of glaucoma
- uterine tachysystole (more than five contractions in 10 minutes, or contractions lasting more than 2 minutes) (El-Din & El-Morghatz, 2000)
- placental abruption or uterine rupture.

Management of uterine tachysystole (hyperstimulation)

A study reporting cases of tachysystole associated with dinoprostone pessary (Cervidil) observed reversal of tachysystole 2–13 minutes after removal of product. Tocolytics were administered in one in five cases. Uterine tachysystole occurs more frequently with dinoprostone gel (Prostin) gel than with intravenous oxytocin (Enkin et al., 2000).

The following interventions may be instituted:

- If dinoprostone pessary (Cervidil) is in situ: remove pessary by pulling the withdrawal tape.
- If dinoprostone gel (Prostin) is used, consider manually removing the gel.
- Change maternal position.
- Continuous CTG monitoring.
- Prepare and administer emergency tocolysis of salbutamol or terbutaline.
- Consider fetal scalp blood sampling (where possible and available).
- Consider caesarean section if tachysystole and fetal compromise persist.

Mechanical ways to ripen the cervix

Mechanical induction of labour dates back to Hippocrates' description of breast stimulation and digital dilation of the cervix (Chodankar et al., 2017). Other procedures included the insertion of Bougies (a cylinder of celluloid or gum elastic) or inflatable bags into the vagina and cervix (Nabi et al., 2014). Most of these methods relied on forcibly stretching and dilating the cervix in an attempt to stimulate contractions. In modern maternity care the use of membrane sweeping and balloon catheters are common methods to prepare the cervix for induction.

Membrane stripping/sweeping

This practice has long been advocated as a relatively non-invasive, albeit uncomfortable, means to stimulate a 'spontaneous labour', but is an intervention in a physiological process. The amniotic fetal membrane is separated from the decidua of the lower uterine segment. It is believed that this process increases the release of prostaglandin $F_{2\alpha}$ production from the decidua and adjacent fetal membrane, thereby stimulating the onset of 'spontaneous' labour. According to the Cochrane database (Finucane et al., 2020), a review of 44 randomised controlled trials (6940 women) demonstrates that this procedure increases the rate of spontaneous labour and potentially reduces the incidence of formal induction of labour, but does not increase the rate of unassisted births. The procedure does not seem to increase the risks associated with known group B *Streptococcus* (GBS) colonisation (Kabiri et al., 2015).

Cervical ripening—balloon catheter

The use of a transcervical balloon catheter for pre-induction cervical ripening has been shown to be an efficient, safe, cost-effective, reversible method with similar caesarean section rates to prostaglandins, and a lower risk of hyperstimulation and infection (Du et al., 2017). Transcervical catheters are either single (Foley's) or double balloon. In some instances tension may be applied to single-balloon catheters; however, this appears only to shorten the time the balloon is in place in multiparous women (Fruhman et al., 2017). Double-balloon catheters apply force to the internal and external cervical os between the two inflated balloons. There is little evidence to support the use of one type over another other than maternal comfort (Katukuri et al., 2017). In nulliparous women, transcervical balloon catheters are more effective than prostaglandins in achieving vaginal birth within 24 hours (Suffecool et al., 2014). However, in multiparous women there appears to be little advantage (Løkkegaard et al., 2015). A randomised controlled trial found that ripening an unfavourable cervix in nulliparous women with a double balloon catheter inflated with 80 mL rather than 30 mL provided a more effective dilation (Hoppe et al., 2016).

Induction of labour with oxytocin

Oxytocin is the most commonly used agent to induce labour (Table 38.4). It has been used alone, in combination with amniotomy, or following cervical ripening with other pharmacological or non-pharmacological methods (Mozurkewich et al., 2011; Thomas et al., 2014). Prior to the introduction of prostaglandin agents, oxytocin was used as a cervical ripening agent as well. In developed countries, oxytocin alone is more commonly used in the presence of ruptured membranes whether spontaneous or artificial. In developing countries where the incidence of HIV is high, delaying amniotomy in labour reduces vertical transmission rates and hence the use of oxytocin with intact membranes warrants further investigation.

Amniotomy was considered earlier in this chapter in the section on augmentation of labour. Intravenous oxytocin has been widely used to induce and augment labour for more than 50 years (Chodankar et al., 2017).

Table 38.4 Oxytocin administration

Consideration	Administration
Administration	Use a volumetric pump to ensure an accurate rate of infusion Consider the need for sideline/secondary IV access as per local protocols A standard dilution of oxytocin should always be used Individual protocols should specify maximum doses The dose should be titrated against uterine contractions Titration should occur at 30-minute or greater intervals Aim for 3–4 contractions in a 10-minute period with duration of 40–60 seconds and resting period not less than 60 seconds Use the minimum dose required to establish and maintain active labour Record the dose in milliunits per minute Mark changes to dose clearly and contemporaneously on the CTG and/or intrapartum record
Maximum dose	Review by an obstetrician should occur before exceeding a dose of 20 milliunits per minute
Side effects	Cardiovascular disturbances (e.g. bradycardia, tachycardia) Headache Gastrointestinal disorders (e.g. nausea, vomiting)
Cease infusion if: • uterine activity becomes hypertonic • resting uterine tone increases • fetal compromise occurs (any concerning FHR abnormality)	Consult with an obstetrician before recommencing infusion

CTG = cardiotocograph; FHR = fetal heart rate; IV = intravenous.
(Sources: MIMS Online. Syntocinon solution for injection http://www.mims.com.au/ and Society of Obstetricians and Gynaecologists of Canada (SOCG), 2013)

Once the cervix is ripe, oxytocin is still the favoured pharmacological agent for inducing labour. Endogenous oxytocin, an octapeptide hormone, is secreted in the hypothalamus and transported to the posterior pituitary gland, where it is stored. It is chemically related to vasopressin (antidiuretic hormone, ADH). Its effects are enhanced by high levels of oestrogen—the highest levels occur just prior to term. Released in a pulsatile fashion, oxytocin stimulates both the frequency and the strength of uterine contractions and has antidiuretic properties. Synthetic oxytocin—e.g. Syntocinon—maintains these properties.

CLINICAL POINT

Monitoring during induction of labour with oxytocin

- Administer the drug in the birth suite (or room) where the fetal heart rate (FHR) and uterine activity can be monitored simultaneously through one-to-one midwifery care.
- There is no clear evidence for continuous FHR monitoring (Alfirevic et al., 2013), but because of the increased risks to mother and fetus many units recommend continuous electronic FHR monitoring and evaluation of the trace at least hourly during the first stage of labour and every 5 minutes during the second stage.
- Before each increase in the rate of oxytocin infusion, assess FHR baseline, variability, presence of accelerations, and periodic or non-periodic decelerations.
- Unless an intrauterine pressure transducer is in situ, the uterine contraction pattern should be manually palpated every 15–30 minutes.
- If intermittent auscultation is used, determine and record the FHR at least every 15 minutes during the first stage and at least every 5 minutes during the second stage.
- Maternal vital signs, response to contractions and urinary output are recorded either at each incremental dose of oxytocin or at least every 4 hours.
- Ascertain the mother's response to contractions.

Complications

Oxytocin has a short half-life and is generally well tolerated by mother and baby, although induction of labour is never without some risk (Mozurkewich et al., 2011). Uterine tachysystole is common when synthetic oxytocin is used (Kunz et al., 2013). Though definitions vary, uterine tachysystole can be described as more than five contractions in 10 minutes, whereas uterine hypertonus refers to contractions lasting more than 2 minutes, or insufficient resting tone (RANZCOG, 2014). Both uterine tachysystole and hypertonus can reduce placental perfusion and contribute to abnormal fetal heart patterns (Kunz et al., 2013). This complication underscores the importance of close FHR monitoring. The need for close assessment of uterine activity and maternal and fetal wellbeing necessitates one-to-one midwifery care.

If fetal compromise is suspected (perhaps the trace shows variable decelerations but other features indicating fetal compromise are not apparent), the oxytocin dosage can usually be lowered rather than stopped completely. This allows the fetus to recover without unnecessarily slowing the entire labour. Other steps include changing the mother's position, assessing maternal blood pressure, and increasing intravenous fluid administration. In emergency situations, the infusion is discontinued. A vaginal examination is performed to assess the progress of labour and rule out umbilical cord prolapse.

The intensity of uterine activity and the rapid onset of contractions, often from the start of labour, mean that the pain relief method of choice is frequently an epidural (Jacobsen et al., 2018). An actively managed third stage of labour is recommended owing to the increased risk of PPH.

Midwifery assessments for induction of labour

Preinduction assessments:

- ensure that the woman has given informed consent for the labour to be induced
- identify indications for, contraindications to, or risk factors for the procedure
- determine lie, presentation of the fetus and the relationship of the fetal head to the pelvis
- ensure that the Bishop's score has been calculated
- assess amniotic membrane status
- obtain a baseline CTG if hospital policy requires this, and analyse it for non-reassuring features.

CLINICAL POINT

Uterine tachysystole or hypertonus

Uterine tachysystole or hypertonus results in decelerations in the FHR and/or other signs of fetal compromise.

If tachysystole or hypertonus occurs with signs of fetal compromise:

- slow or discontinue oxytocin infusion
- position the woman on her left side
- consider increasing infusion rate in the main line
- notify the lead carer
- prepare for possible caesarean section if the fetal heart rate does not return to normal
- consider tocolysis: IV nitroglycerin 50–200 mg, or 1–2 metered doses of a sublingual spray (400–800 mg), terbutaline 250 µg subcutaneously or intravenous salbutamol
- palpate the uterus to determine uterine response to management
- if intrauterine resuscitation is successful, restart oxytocin infusion at half the last dose.

CRITICAL THINKING EXERCISE

You are a midwife in a busy maternity unit caring for Eunice (gravida 3, para 2) during an induction of her labour. The induction began 4 hours ago. You examine Eunice and find that the fetal head is deeply engaged in the pelvis and ROA. The uterine contractions are occurring every 3 minutes; they are strong and last 70 seconds. The FHR shows average variability and there are no abnormal features; the rate ranges from 130 b.p.m. to 150 b.p.m. Eunice's cervix is 7 cm dilated and effaced and +1 below the ischial spines. The oxytocin infusion is now running at 6 mU/min. Will you continue the same infusion rate? If yes, why and if no, why not?

PRE-TERM LABOUR

Pre-term labour or, as it is often referred to, premature labour (PTL), is defined as one that begins after 20 weeks but before 37 completed weeks of pregnancy (259 days). Most mortality and morbidity occur in babies born before 34 weeks. Despite new diagnostic and therapeutic modalities, efforts to prevent the onset of PTL have largely been ineffective and it remains the leading cause of neonatal mortality and morbidity (Norman & Shennan, 2013). The following sections focus on pre-term labour rather than the collaborative and ongoing care of women at risk of pre-term labour and the management of the pre-term baby. Chapters 18, 36, 39 and 42 deal with these topics in more depth.

Epidemiology of pre-term labour

Approximately 5%–10% of all births are pre-term. For example, the 2010 New Zealand Ministry of Health (MOH) maternity report showed a 7.4% rate of premature births (MOH, 2012), the same rate as in 2004. Pre-term birth rates in Australia have increased in the last 20 years, primarily owing to the rise in late pre-term births (Verburg et al., 2018). Late pre-term births (34–36 weeks) comprise 70% of all pre-term births. The causes for this trend are unclear; however, possible aetiologies include increasing maternal age, increased use of artificial reproductive technologies and increased multiple births (Box 38.4). Compared with term-born children, late pre-term children have not only increased mortality and in-hospital morbidity including respiratory difficulties, but also long-term cognitive, school performance, behaviour and psychiatric problems (Cheong et al., 2017). The New Zealand Perinatal and Maternal Mortality Review Committee report (PMMRC, 2013) recommended that all women having assisted reproduction are offered single-embryo transfer in order to reduce perinatal-related mortality.

Whilst a history of pre-term birth or second trimester miscarriages is recognised as the strongest predictor of pre-term birth, risks of spontaneous pre-term birth are invariably linked to the mother's age, lifestyle, level of

Box 38.4 Risk factors for premature birth

Risk factors for premature delivery are:

- anaemia (haemoglobin <11 and S-ferritin 12–15 μg/L)
- abnormal uterine anatomy
- abruptio placentae (placental abruption)
- cervix insufficiency
- drug use (heroin and cocaine)
- fetal anomalies
- iatrogenic
- infections (UTIs, infections caused by GBS, intra-uterine infections, bacterial vaginosis)
- low maternal weight
- low social status
- multiple gestations
- placenta praevia
- polyhydramnios
- premature rupture of membranes
- previous pre-term birth
- smoking
- stressful lifestyle
- young mother (<15–19 years)
- domestic violence.

GBS = group B *Streptococcus*; UTI = urinary tract infection.
(Source: Haram et al., 2003, p. 689)

education, nutritional status and access to healthcare (Di Renzo et al., 2017). Low socioeconomic status is strongly associated with increased incidence of pre-term birth (Braveman et al., 2015). Pre-term birth has also been associated with psychological stress, with one study reporting a fourfold increase in risk for women with major depressive disorders or post-traumatic stress disorder (Yonkers et al., 2014).

Prevention, identification and management

The interventions that have been demonstrated to effectively diminish the risk of pre-term birth or improve outcomes for pre-term babies born to asymptomatic women are: smoking cessation counselling for smokers (Lumley et al., 2009), intramuscular progesterone for women with prior pre-term birth now carrying a singleton fetus (Dodd et al., 2013), ultrasound-indicated cervical cerclage in women with both a prior pre-term birth and shortening of cervical length less than 25 mm prior to 24 weeks of pregnancy in a singleton pregnancy (Berghella et al., 2005), and history-indicated cervical cerclage (Conde-Agudelo et al., 2013). Other studies have suggested that continuity of midwifery care may reduce the incidence of pre-term birth in at-risk populations such as adolescents and young adults (Allen et al., 2015).

The identification of women at risk of PTL, and its prevention and management, have been widely studied and are important challenges in reducing the number of pre-term births and improving outcomes for mothers and babies. Two recent research projects have reported reductions in pre-term birth rates employing quite different approaches. A multi-faceted pre-term birth prevention program was introduced into Western Australia in 2014 consisting of routine cervical length measurement, vaginal progesterone supplementation (cervical length <25 mm), cervical cerclage (cervical length <10 mm), smoking cessation program and pre-term birth prevention clinics at tertiary centres for high-risk women (Newnham et al., 2020). The study reported a 7.6% reduction in pre-term birth statewide and a 20% reduction in tertiary centres. One of the most significant reductions occurred amongst Australian Indigenous women in the Kimberley region (Newnham et al., 2020). An urban Birthing on Country service comprising Indigenous governance, partnership and leadership, midwifery continuity of care, increased Indigenous workforce, and a focus on family wellbeing and parenting was established in Brisbane, Queensland in 2013 (Kildea et al., 2019). Compared to similar women receiving standard maternity care there was a significant difference in pre-term birth rates for those women attending the Birthing on Country model (11.6% standard care vs 6.9% Birthing on Country) (Kildea et al., 2019). These studies suggest that addressing both biophysical and sociocultural risk factors can successfully reduce the rates of pre-term birth, particularly in vulnerable groups.

Maternal physical health is not usually adversely influenced by pre-term labour, although psychosocial morbidities are high and include increased levels of anxiety and the potential for feelings of failure often if there were medical and/or obstetric indications such as preeclampsia or cardiac disease.

Assessing risk of PTL in pregnancy

Assessing a woman's risk of PTL and birth is part of the midwife's scope of practice. Beginning with a comprehensive booking history early in pregnancy, the midwife assesses for and documents risk factors for pre-term labour and birth, making an appropriate early referral after consultation and with consent from the woman to a specialist if necessary. Because in 60% of cases PTL will occur in women with no risk factors, the midwife should inform the woman that if, at any time, signs of labour are apparent before 37 weeks she should contact her LMC immediately. This is of particular importance for women residing in rural and remote areas with limited access to secondary or tertiary maternity and paediatric services, as PTL may mean a transfer of considerable distance to an appropriate facility.

Later, as the midwife's relationship with the woman grows, the midwife gathers information about the woman's past and present births, her physical and social histories including stressors (such as housing and food availability), social support, cultural safety, financial stressors, history of family violence, the presence of infections or the earlier diagnosis of antiphospholipid syndrome, anticardiolipin antibodies and lupus anticoagulant antibodies as well as the presence of structural abnormalities.

CLINICAL POINT

Many pregnant women experience symptoms that suggest pre-term labour. These may include uterine contractions, changes in vaginal discharge, backaches, pelvic pressure, cramping and cervical dilation. Not all symptomatic women will actually have a pre-term birth.

Tests for pre-term labour

No risk-assessment tool has proved effective in lowering the incidence of PTL. The most common clinical tests used to determine the risk of PTL are transvaginal ultrasonography (TVS) to measure the length of the endocervix (the shorter the cervix the greater the risk of PTL and birth), cervicovaginal fetal fibronectin (fFn) and Actim Partus tests. Fetal fibronectin is an extracellular matrix glycoprotein localised at the maternal–fetal membrane (Berghella et al., 2008). In healthy pregnancies fFn is found at very low levels in cervicovaginal secretions. Levels greater than or equal to 50 mg/mL at or after 22 weeks of pregnancy are associated with an increased risk of spontaneous pre-term birth (Berghella et al., 2008). The Actim Partus test examines levels of phosphorylated insulin-like growth factor binding protein-1 (phIGFBP-1), synthesised by maternal decidual cells (Khambay et al., 2012). Women with a negative fFn or Actim Partus are unlikely to give birth in the next 14 days, hence it is the negative predictability of these tests that is often most accurate and useful (Singhal et al., 2017). This finding may provide a woman with the confidence to stay in her community and support for a decision not to commence immediate tocolytic therapy or administer corticosteroids to mature fetal lungs. There does not seem to be a role for either test to be used as a routine screening test for PTL.

CLINICAL POINT

Biochemical tests such as fetal fibronectin are used to screen pregnant women who are within 26 weeks and 34 weeks of gestation and are having symptoms of premature labour. The test may be beneficial in predicting the risk of premature birth.

The tests should be used only on those who:

- have intact amniotic membranes
- have a cervix that has not dilated more than 3 cm
- do not have more than slight vaginal bleeding
- do not have cervical cerclage
- have not had sexual intercourse or a pelvic examination in the past 24 hours.

The tests are not recommended for screening asymptomatic women even if they are considered to be at high risk for premature labour and birth.

Signs of pre-term labour

Many of the early signs of PTL are common in normal pregnancy. They include:

- abdominal pain or increased uterine contractions
- dull, low back pain
- painful menstrual-like cramps
- vaginal bleeding
- change in character of or increased vaginal discharge
- suprapubic and pelvic pressure with a sensation of 'heaviness'
- urinary frequency
- diarrhoea.

Tests to determine whether the membranes have broken

PROM (pre-term rupture of the membranes) is normally diagnosed by speculum vaginal examination of the cervix and vaginal cavity; however, the presence of cervical mucous discharge or infection may make such a finding difficult or equivocal. Biochemical tests for placental alpha microglobulin-1 (PAMG-1) have been demonstrated to have a high degree of accuracy and reliability when testing for liquor (Abdelazim & Makhlouf, 2013). Previously the presence of liquor could also be established through ferning of the dried fluid under microscopic examination, and alkalinity of the fluid as determined by nitrazine paper or by Amnicator confirm the diagnosis. Blood contamination of the nitrazine paper may produce false-positive results. For prolonged PROM, an ultrasonographic examination may then show absence of or very low amounts of amniotic fluid in the uterine cavity. Nearly all women with PROM and PPROM (pre-term, premature rupture of the membranes) proceed to active labour and birth soon after PPROM (Pasquier & Bujold, 2007). With appropriate therapy and conservative management, approximately 50% of all remaining pregnancies birth each subsequent week after PPROM (Pasquier & Bujold, 2007). Thus, very few women remain pregnant more than 3–4 weeks after PPROM. This is important information to give the woman considering expectant management remote from viability and/or need referral to a tertiary centre with a neonatal intensive care unit (NICU) (see Ch. 42).

CLINICAL POINT

Women are valuable resources in making diagnoses in relation to pre-term labour but they must know what to expect. For example, some women can have 'spotting' in pregnancy and think this is not serious. Others may pass cramping or painful uterine contractions off as normal. Midwives need to help women acquire the knowledge they require in order to know when to contact their lead carer. All pregnant women should be able to recognise symptoms of pre-term labour, which can be stimulated by:

- vomiting and diarrhoea
- dehydration
- trauma (including family violence, see Chs 37 and 40)
- infection.

Collaborative support

When a woman who has not completed 37 weeks of pregnancy reports any of the above signs, she needs to be referred to a hospital-based specialist medical team who will decide whether she is in 'true' labour. The diagnosis of PTL is usually made in the presence of four uterine contractions in 20 minutes plus the presence of cervical changes—dilation and effacement. A sterile speculum examination is performed to estimate cervical length and dilation, look for signs of bleeding or amniotic liquor and obtain endocervical and rectovaginal swabs for microbiological examination. If possible, digital vaginal examination is avoided. A CTG trace is useful to assess fetal wellbeing; however, uterine contractions may be difficult to demonstrate particularly if the woman is overweight or obese. Fetal tachycardia and reduced baseline variability are often the first signs of maternal and fetal infection, such as chorioamnionitis. Nevertheless, interpretation of a CTG trace at early gestation is difficult.

Diagnostic data that can be used to guide management decisions are:

- complete blood cell count with differential and platelet counts, C-reactive protein
- midstream specimen to rule out urinary tract infection
- cervical, high vaginal and anorectal swabs for bacterial vaginosis, GBS, gonorrhoea, chlamydia and *Trichomonas vaginalis*, to rule out infection
- fetal surveillance studies to determine signs of fetal compromise
- ultrasonography to determine biometry, fetal size, presentation, amniotic fluid volume, fetal anomalies, and placentography
- Doppler studies of the umbilical artery
- biochemical evaluation to determine risk of PTL
- transvaginal ultrasound to determine cervical length.

Sterile speculum examination if rupture of membranes is suspected

First, perform an abdominal palpation to determine fetal size and presentation. Speculum examination is undertaken to:

- exclude cord prolapse
- visualise pooling of liquor (note presence of vernix)
- collect cervical and vaginal microbiological swabs (including GBS)
- estimate cervical dilation
- look for biochemical markers for pre-term labour or rupture of membranes.

Ongoing care and support of the woman with threatened or actual pre-term labour takes place in collaboration with midwifery, obstetric and paediatric secondary/tertiary services. Management depends on gestation, the availability of a NICU, stage of labour, and evidence of complicating factors such as cause of the pre-term labour, viability of the fetus, presence of infection, state of the membranes, or maternal illness. Thus, if there is evidence of maternal or fetal infection, management centres on treating the infection. Tocolytic drugs are considered to inhibit labour to allow for administration of corticosteroids and transfer to a hospital with suitable neonatal facilities.

McNamara (2003, p. 82) describes some of the critical issues concerned with PTL and maternal transport. She contends that the critical issue is the clarification of which team is 'sending' or 'receiving', and is responsible for the woman while she is in transit. McNamara (2003) makes the crucial point that the best location for a pre-term birth is in a tertiary referral centre and the worst is in a transport vehicle en route to the hospital. The following factors influence decisions about when to transfer, how it will take place and where the woman will be transferred to:

- availability of NICU beds/neonatal care
- length of time before birth
- transfer time
- availability of space for the mother at a tertiary centre/perinatal care facility
- fetal weight
- gestational age
- availability of two qualified transporting staff—one for the mother and one for the baby—should complicated birth take place en route
- cervical dilation—reassess immediately prior to transport; if the cervix is >6 cm dilated, transport is generally not advised (McNamara 2003, p. 82).

REFLECTIVE CASE STUDY

- It is afternoon, you are recently qualified and the only midwife on duty in a rural health centre about 40 minutes from the nearest maternity unit. A woman arrives at the front door exhibiting signs of advanced labour. It is her third baby and she says she is 32 weeks pregnant. You take baseline observations, and assess the strength, length and regularity of her contractions, which appear to be 2–3 minutes apart, becoming expulsive and strong. Abdominal palpation reveals a breech presentation, deeply engaged, with a fetal heart rate of 140–160 b.p.m. There are no signs of bleeding and the membranes are intact.
- You inform the woman and her support persons of your findings and what you plan to do, also taking into account her birth plan, which is rather sketchy at this stage. You resist the urge to panic, and ask

an enrolled nurse to quickly telephone the maternity unit and a medical practitioner for consultation. He suggests that you perform a vaginal examination to determine the degree of cervical dilation and, depending on these findings, transfer the woman to the referral centre. The hospital contacts the referral team for you. Vaginal examination reveals that the woman's cervix is 8–9 cm dilated with a breech presentation at the ischial spines. Shortly afterwards she begins to push, shouting loudly, 'I can't stop!' even though you advise her not to push. Quickly you prepare for birth, heating the room and checking resuscitation equipment.

- She stands up, the membranes rupture and the baby births, with you gently supporting the buttocks once they come out, to prevent sudden birth of the head and the added risk of a tentorial tear. The baby is born with Apgar scores of 8 at 1 minute and 9 at 5 minutes; the baby is carefully wrapped, and nestled close to mum's skin to keep warm. A physiological third stage occurs after 5 minutes, with minimal blood loss, and then you carefully examine the baby, noting indicators for gestational age and signs of respiratory distress.
- The paediatric retrieval team phones to tell you it is 10 minutes away. Documentation is completed and you accompany the family to the hospital.

REFLECTIVE THINKING EXERCISE

Read the Reflective Case Study above. Then answer the following questions.

- On reflection, what would you have done differently? In this situation, what are your legal and professional responsibilities? Are there particular learning points for you in this story?

Inhibition of pre-term labour

In up to 50% of women, uterine contractions will stop spontaneously and the pregnancy will continue to term without any medical treatment. Clinicians need to discern those in whom drug therapy (**tocolysis**) is warranted and whether it is the drug of choice. Tocolytic therapy can successfully, albeit temporarily, inhibit labour. Its main function is to delay labour for 24–48 hours to enable the woman and her fetus to be transferred to a suitable facility and to allow maximal effect of corticosteroids used to induce pulmonary surfactant in the fetal lungs. Generally, if the pregnancy is between 24 and 34 weeks gestation, and the baby has an estimated weight of >2500 g, it is recommended that uterine action be suppressed with drug therapies. After 34 weeks it is reasonable to let labour continue although tocolysis may still be considered to enable transport to a suitable hospital.

CLINICAL POINT

In symptomatic women, corticosteroids (betamethasone 11.4 mg intramuscularly in two doses 24 hours apart between 23 and 33 weeks is preferred if available) given to the mother prior to pre-term birth are effective in preventing respiratory distress syndrome, intraventricular haemorrhage and neonatal mortality. Tocolysis is often used to inhibit labour until the corticosteroids have been administered.

(Source: Roberts & Dalziel, 2006)

A Cochrane review by Flenady et al. (2014) found that, when indicated, calcium-channel blockers are preferable to other comparable tocolytic agents, mainly beta-mimetics, which have significant side effects. These drugs should not be used if the fetus is not viable, if fetal wellbeing is in jeopardy, or if maternal health is severely compromised, such as with an abruption. Following diagnosis, maintenance treatment with beta-mimetics has not yet been proved to be effective. Magnesium sulfate is now widely used in obstetric practice, in particular to reduce eclamptic seizures, but has not been proved to be comparably more effective than other tocolytics for treating pre-term labour (Flenady et al., 2014). Atosiban (Tractocile) has recently been developed to avoid the side effects of some of the other tocolytic drugs, but it is more expensive than the XYZ-adrenergic receptor agents; it acts as an oxytocin antagonist but has not been found to be more effective in practice than either beta-mimetics or placebo in terms of tocolytic efficacy or infant outcomes (Papatsonis et al., 2010).

Calcium-channel blockers

Calcium-channel blockers prevent the entry of calcium through cell membranes, which inhibits contractions of the smooth muscle of the uterus (Doyle et al., 2009). Nifedipine (Adalat) in slow-release form is an effective oral tocolytic agent and increasingly popular. Side effects are less distressing than those occurring with the beta-adrenergic receptor agents; maternal tachycardia, headache and dizziness are the most common. One regimen involves an initial dose of 10 mg sublingually every 20 minutes for three doses and then 10–30 mg every 6 hours orally. Nifedipine is commonly the drug of choice in the treatment of pre-term labour as it can be easily administered prior to transfer, if necessary, and has fewer side effects than previous therapies (Flenady et al., 2014).

Magnesium sulfate for neuroprotection of the fetus

(See also Ch. 40.)

Controlled trials show that fetal exposure to magnesium sulfate given before pre-term birth has a neuroprotective role (Doyle et al., 2009). The number of women needed to be treated to benefit one baby by avoiding cerebral palsy is 63 (Doyle et al., 2009). This systematic review also showed a significant reduction in the rate of gross motor dysfunction in early childhood (Doyle et al., 2009). These benefits have been supported in more recent trials (Wolf et al., 2020).

Indications include neuroprotection of the fetus in women at risk of pre-term birth who are at least 24 + 0 weeks of gestation and <30 + 0 weeks of gestation, when birth is anticipated within 24 hours or in cases of expected planned delivery as close to 4 hours before expected time of birth and regardless of:

- plurality
- why the woman is at risk of pre-term birth
- parity
- anticipated mode of birth
- whether antenatal corticosteroids have been given.

Antimicrobial therapy

The relationship between infection (chorioamnionitis, bacterial vaginosis and GBS infections as well as urinary tract infection) and PTL is well documented (see also Chs 37 and 41). Consequently, the use of therapeutic and prophylactic broad-spectrum antibiotics has become popular in some centres. Randomised studies and two meta-analyses have demonstrated that in the presence of ruptured membranes, especially in mothers who have GBS infections, antibiotic therapy prolongs pregnancy and reduces the incidence of chorioamnionitis, and postpartum and neonatal sepsis. In a Cochrane review, Kenyon et al. (2013) concluded that the administration of antibiotics after PROM is associated with a delay in birth and a reduction in maternal and neonatal morbidity. The findings are not so clear in the presence of intact membranes; a Cochrane review by Flenady et al. (2013) failed to demonstrate a clear overall benefit from prophylactic antibiotic treatment for pre-term labour with intact membranes on neonatal outcomes. The review did report the finding of short- and long-term harm in children of mothers exposed to certain types of antibiotic prophylactically.

Antimicrobial therapy if there is no evidence of chorioamnionitis

Commence antibiotic prophylaxis (below is an example regimen; always follow your local guideline):

1. Benzylpenicillin 3 g IV loading dose, then 1.2 g IV every 4 hours for 48 hours or until delivery if this occurs earlier. If the woman is allergic to penicillin, other antibiotics such as lincomycin 600 mg IV in 100 mL over 1 hour every 8 hours or azithromycin 500 mg IV once daily for 48 hours or until birth if this occurs earlier.
2. Oral erythromycin 250 mg 4 times a day for 10 days or until birth if this occurs earlier.

   If there are signs of chorioamnionitis:

- diagnosis of chorioamnionitis relies on the clinical presentation
- maternal fever >38°C with any two of the following:
  - increased white cell count ($>15 \times 10^9$/L)
  - maternal tachycardia (>100 b.p.m.)
  - fetal tachycardia (>160 b.p.m.)
  - uterine tenderness
  - offensive smelling vaginal discharge
  - C-reactive protein >40
- histological examination of placenta and membranes with evidence of acute inflammation may confirm the diagnosis after birth.

Antibiotics

- Ampicillin (or amoxycillin) 2 g IV initial dose, then 1 g IV every 4 hours.
- Gentamicin 5 mg/kg IV daily.
- Metronidazole 500 mg IV every 12 hours.
- If allergic to penicillin, give lincomycin 600 mg IV in 100 mL over 1 hour every 8 hours or clindamycin 450 mg IV in 50–100 mL over at least 20 minutes until birth.
- Do not inhibit labour, but consider hastening birth under intravenous antibiotic cover.
- Consider optimal mode of birth (lower-segment caesarean section versus vaginal birth) on the basis of the findings and the anticipated duration until birth. After birth antibiotic therapy is continued.

Midwifery support

The midwife's role in supporting women at risk of or in PTL is to administer the prescribed treatments according to local protocols, make ongoing regular assessments of maternal and fetal wellbeing, provide psychological and emotional support, and take appropriate action if labour continues, ensuring that the documentation is up to date. If labour does proceed, tocolysis will be discontinued and the labouring woman will be offered labour support and pain relief if required, although narcotic analgesia, in particular pethidine, is not recommended because of the respiratory suppressant effect upon the pre-term baby. Midwives need to take the time to provide psychological as well as physical support and education on the processes of labour, especially if, as is often the case, no childbirth preparation sessions have been accessed.

Continuous CTG is recommended to monitor fetal wellbeing during labour to detect fetal compromise, as the premature baby has less tolerance to stress and has an increased risk of hypoxia at birth. The midwife should carefully observe and assess the woman in PTL, as the progress of labour may vary from that expected for a term baby, and specialist help including a paediatrician should be present at the birth. Timely preparations for transfer to and receiving at the newborn unit after immediate resuscitation is required. Pre-term uterine contractions are not as easily palpated as those at term and the CTG monitor will not accurately indicate the presence of contractions, which depend upon maternal position. There are too few data to support the use of hydration as a specific treatment for women presenting with pre-term labour unless the woman is already dehydrated. Nor is there any evidence to support bed rest either in hospital or at home if labour 'stops' (Sosa et al., 2015).

There is still controversy over the mode of birth recommended for pre-term babies. Caesarean section is often advocated, to decrease fetal trauma associated with vaginal birth, but these assumptions have never been substantiated (Alfirevic et al., 2013). Moreover, an elective caesarean does not reduce fetal mortality or morbidity if the presentation is cephalic and the birth may lead to additional complications. Due to the associated psychological disruption of PTL for both mother and baby, the LMC should remain in contact if possible as this person may be the only known 'face' and trusted healthcare practitioner at this challenging time.

RESEARCH ACTIVITY

1. Use a search engine such as Google, PubMed or Ovid to research a specific complication discussed in this chapter.
2. Use the information you gain from these sites to help you create teaching–learning activities for the women you work in partnership with during pregnancy and birthing.

Conclusion

Despite the very best of care and support, not all labours proceed as planned and an exploration of the causes, associations and management of these deviations from the usual birthing journey is the overall aim of this chapter. For the vast majority of women, pregnancy follows a routine course. Nevertheless some women will develop one or more difficulties related to their health or the health of their baby. This does not mean that *all* women should be treated as if they have or may develop complications.

For a number of reasons, interventions during pregnancy and birth have increased in recent years and these are discussed elsewhere in this text. Our concern about this has led to a renewed focus on promoting normality in labour and birth. Invasive interventions prior to the onset of labour, during labour and birth such as induction of labour, epidural anaesthesia, instrumental birth including caesarean section involve exposure to additional risks so should be used only in circumstances where there is good evidence that the benefit of the intervention outweighs its potential harm. A caesarean can be a life-saving operation, and some babies will not be born vaginally under any circumstances; however, it is still major surgery. The evidence is unequivocal—*unnecessary* caesareans expose more mothers and babies to risks, without any clear gains for maternal and infant health overall. Women have a legal right to know the risks associated with their treatment and the right to accept or decline it. It is important for midwives to work with the woman as she weighs up the risks and benefits of planned procedures. Sometimes the benefits will outweigh the risks, and sometimes the procedure's risks will outweigh its benefits.

The chapter begins with a review of what a 'normal' birth journey is and what it is not. The chapter explores the ways that an appropriate balance can be struck between maximising safety for the mother and for the baby, in the current and in subsequent pregnancies, achieving a range of additional optimal health outcomes and whenever possible ensuring a positive experience for the woman and a positive start in life for the baby. The chapter describes the factors that disturb the rhythms of labour, leading to what is commonly called dystocia (difficult labour)—such as prolonged labour, and pre-term labour, as well as the interventions used to manage these, such as augmentation and induction of labour. In summary, the keys to safe and effective maternity care are first to provide care that reflects the belief that birth is a normal physiological process for the majority of women and secondly to minimise intervention for women with normal pregnancies and labours. Thirdly, irrespective of their place of practice, midwives must have the skills to support women whose labours do not follow the expected rhythms. Finally, it is important to remember that women require:

- care that is consistent with the best available research on quality, safety and effectiveness
- an environment and treatments that support and enhance, rather than interfere with, the natural rhythms of pregnancy and birth
- individualised, woman-focused care that takes into account the woman and her family's needs as well as those of her baby, and meets her personal preferences and values
- accurate, appropriate evidence-informed and abundant support, comfort and information
- care that enables women to seamlessly access, either directly or through efficient referral mechanisms, treatments for complications, should the need arise.

Review questions

1. Discuss the advantages and disadvantages of amniotomy during a 'normal' labour.
2. Describe the impact of selected interventions in labour on the childbearing woman and her support team.
3. How might a midwife support a woman dealing with a slower than expected labour?
4. Should women be offered fluids during labour? Provide arguments for and against. If a woman asks your advice on this issue, what will you tell her?
5. How do you describe the progress of labour? As an exercise, ask 10 of your colleagues how they recognise progress during labour.
6. You are asked to give a talk to a group of pregnant women about what to expect in terms of the progress or natural rhythm of labour. Outline the main points you would cover and provide references to back up the points you make.

Acknowledgements

The author would like to acknowledge the work of Carol Thorogood and Catherine Donaldson, who contributed to the previous editions of the text.

Online resources

American Academy of Family Physicians: https://www.aafp.org/home.html.

Association of Radical Midwives: http://www.midwifery.org.uk/.

Australian College of Midwives: https://www.midwives.org.au/.

Healthcare Quality Improvement Partnership (HQIP)—CEMACH and CEMACE reports: https://www.hqip.org.uk/national-programmes/a-z-of-clinical-outcome-review-programmes/cmace-reports/.

Improvements in the Maternity Services: http://www.aims.org.uk/.

Midwifery Journal—women's experiences of labour: http://www.midwiferyjournal.com/article/S0266-6138(13)00100-9/references.

New Zealand College of Midwives: http://www.midwife.org.nz/.

References

Abdelazim IA, Makhlouf HH. Placental alpha microglobulin-1 (AmniSure test) versus insulin-like growth factor binding protein-1 (Actim PROM test) for detection of premature rupture of fetal membranes. *J Obstet Gynaecol Res*. 2013;39(6):1129–1136.

Akinsipe C, Villalobos L, Ridley R. A Systematic review of implementing an elective labor induction policy. *J Obstet Gynecol Neonatal Nurs*. 2012;41:5–16. doi:10.1111/j.1552-6909.2011.01320.

Albers L. The duration of labour in healthy women. *J Perinatol*. 1999;19(2):114–119.

Alfirevic Z, Devane D, Gyte GM. Continuous cardiotocography (CTG) as a form of electronic fetal monitoring (EFM) for fetal assessment during labour. *Cochrane Database Syst Rev*. 2013;(5):CD006066, doi:10.1002/14651858.CD006066.pub2.

Algovik M, Kivinen K, Peterson H, et al. Genetic evidence of multiple loci in dystocia—difficult labour. *BMC Medical Genetics*. 2010;11(1):105. doi:10.1186/1471-2350-11-105.

Allen J, Gibbons K, Beckmann M, et al. Does model of maternity care make a difference to birth outcomes for young women? A retrospective cohort study. *Int J Nurs Stud*. 2015;52(8):1332–1342.

Allman AC, Genevier ES, Johnson MR, et al. Head-to-cervix force: an important physiological variable in labour. 2. Peak active force, peak active pressure and mode of delivery. *BJOG*. 1996;103:769–775.

American College of Obstetricians and Gynecologists (ACOG). Obstetric care consensus no. 1: safe prevention of the primary cesarean delivery. *Obstet Gynecol*. 2014;123(3):693–711.

Ames AC, Cobbold S, Maddock J. Lactic acidosis complicating treatment of ketosis of labour. *BMJ*. 1975;4:611–613.

Andrews CJ, Ellwood DA, Gordon A, et al. Stillbirth in Australia 2: Working together to reduce stillbirth in Australia: The Safer Baby Bundle initiative. *Women and Birth*. 2020;33(6):514–519. doi:10.1016/j.wombi.2020.09.006

Ängeby K. *Prolonged latent phase of labour: Prevalence, labour outcomes, quality of care, women's experiences and preferences, and psychometric properties of a questionnaire*. Sweden: Karlstads universitet; 2018.

Anim-Somuah M, Smyth RM, Jones L. Epidural versus non-epidural or no analgesia in labour. *Cochrane Database Syst Rev*. 2011;(12):CD000331.

Arrowsmith S, Wray S, Quenby S. Maternal obesity and labour complications following induction of labour in prolonged pregnancy. *BJOG*. 2011;118(5):578–588.

Attanasio L. *Characteristics of the Patient-Provider Relationship and Use of Labor Induction and Cesarean Delivery*; 2016. Online: https://conservancy.umn.edu/handle/11299/200233.

Austin D, Benn C. Induction of labour: the influences on decision making. *NZCOM J*. 2006;34:6–10.

Australian College of Midwives (ACM). *National Midwifery Guidelines for Consultation and Referral*. Issue 2. 3rd ed. 2013. Online: https://www.midwives.org.au/shop/national-midwifery-guidelines-consultation-and-referral-3rd-edition-issue-2-book.

Australian Institute of Health and Welfare (AIHW). *Australia's Mothers and Babies 2018—in Brief*. Canberra: AIHW; 2020.

Bakker J, van der Goes B, Pel M, et al. Morning versus evening induction of labour for improving outcomes. *Cochrane Database Syst Rev*. 2013;(2):CD007707, doi:10.1002/14651858.CD007707.pub2.

Bates C, ed. *Midwifery Practice: Ways of Working in Pregnancy, Birth and Maternity Care. Feminist Perspectives*. London: Books for Midwives; 2004.

Beckmann M, Gibbons K, Flenady V, et al. Predictors of mode of birth and duration of labour following induction using prostaglandin vaginal gel. *Aust N Z J Obstet Gynaecol*. 2017;57(2):168–175. doi:10.1111/ajo.12588.

Berghella V, Odibo AO, To MS, et al. Cerclage for a short cervix on ultrasonography: meta-analysis of trials using individual patient-level data. *Obstet Gynecol*. 2005;106:181–189.

Berghella V, Hayes E, Visintine J, et al. Fetal fibronectin testing for reducing the risk of preterm birth. *Cochrane Database Syst Rev*. 2008;(4):CD006843, doi:10.1002/14651858.CD006843.pub2.

Bernitz S, Dalbye R, Zhang J, et al. The frequency of intrapartum caesarean section use with the WHO partograph versus Zhang's guideline in the Labour Progression Study (LaPS): a multicentre, cluster-randomised controlled trial. *The Lancet*. 2019;393(10169):340–348.

Bishop E. Pelvic scoring for elective induction. *Obstet Gynecol*. 1964;24(2):267.

Blackburn ST. *Maternal, Fetal and Neonatal Physiology: A Clinical Perspective*. 5th ed. Washington, DC: Elsevier; 2017.

Bohren MA, Hofmeyr GJ, Sakala C, et al. Continuous support for women during childbirth. *Cochrane Database Syst Rev*. 2017;(7):CD003766, doi:10.1002/14651858.

Boulvain M, Kelly AJ, Irion O. Intracervical prostaglandins for induction of labour. *Cochrane Database Syst Rev*. 2008;(1):CD006971, doi:10.1002/14651858.CD006971.

Braveman PA, Heck K, Egerter S, et al. The role of socioeconomic factors in black-white disparities in preterm birth. *Am J Public Health*. 2015;105(4):694–702.

Brown HC, Paranjothy S, Dowswell T, et al. Package of care for active management in labour for reducing caesarean section rates in low-risk women. *Cochrane Database Syst Rev*. 2013;(9):CD004907, doi:10.1002/14651858.CD004907.pub3.

Buckley S. Undisturbed birth—nature's hormonal blueprint for safety, ease and ecstasy. *Midwifery Today Int Midwife*. 2004;14(2):203–209.

Bugg GJ, Siddiqui F, Thornton JG. Oxytocin versus no treatment or delayed treatment for slow progress in the first stage of spontaneous labour. *Cochrane Database Syst Rev*. 2011;(7):CD007123, doi:10.1002/14651858.CD007123.pub2.

Bugg GJ, Siddiqui F, Thornton JG. Oxytocin versus no treatment or delayed treatment for slow progress in the first stage of spontaneous labour. *Cochrane Database Syst Rev*. 2013;(6):CD007123, doi:10.1002/14651858.CD007123.pub3.

Burvill S. Midwifery diagnosis of labour onset. *Br J Midwifery*. 2002;10(10):600–605.

Carlsson I-M, Ziegert K, Sahlberg-Blom E, et al. Maintaining power: women's experiences from labour onset before admittance to maternity ward. *Midwifery*. 2012;28(1):86–92. doi:10.1016/j.midw.2010.11.011.
Cheong JL, Doyle LW, Burnett AC, et al. Association Between Moderate and Late Preterm Birth and Neurodevelopment and Social-Emotional Development at Age 2 Years. *JAMA Pediatrics*. 2017;171(4):e164805-e164805. doi:10.1001/jamapediatrics.2016.4805.
Cheyne H, Terry R, Niven C, et al. 'Should I come in now?': a study of women's early labour experiences. *Br J Midwifery*. 2007; 15(10):604–609.
Chodankar R, Sood A, Gupta J. An overview of the past, current and future trends for cervical ripening in induction of labour. *TOG*. 2017;19(3):219–226.
Ciardulli A, Saccone G, Anastasio H, et al. Less-restrictive food intake during labor in low-risk singleton pregnancies: a systematic review and meta-analysis. *Obstet Gynecol*. 2017;129(3): 473–480. doi:10.1097/AOG.0000000000001898.
Clark SL, Simpson KR, Knox GE, et al. Oxytocin: new perspectives on an old drug. *Am J Obstet Gynecol*. 2009;200(1):35:e1–e6.
Cluett ER, Pickering RM, Getliffe K, et al. Randomised controlled trial of labouring in water compared with standard of augmentation for management of dystocia in first stage of labour. *BMJ*. 2004;328(7435):314.
Cohain JS. The less studied effects of Amniotomy. *The Journal of Maternal-Fetal & Neonatal Medicine*. 2013;26(17):1687–1690.
Conde-Agudelo A, Romero R, Nicolaides K, et al. Vaginal progesterone vs cervical cerclage for the prevention of preterm birth in women with a sonographic short cervix, previous preterm birth, and singleton gestation: a systematic review and indirect comparison metaanalysis. *Am J Obstet Gynecol*. 2013;208(1): 42, e1–e18.
Dahlen H, Thornton C, Downe S, et al. Intrapartum interventions and outcomes for women and children following induction of labour at term in uncomplicated pregnancies: a 16-year population-based linked data study. *BMJ Open*. 2021;*0:e047040*. doi:10.1136/bmjopen-2020-047040.
Dalbye R, Bernitz S, Olsen IC, et al. The Labor Progression Study: The use of oxytocin augmentation during labor following Zhang's guideline and the WHO partograph in a cluster randomized trial. *Acta Obstetricia et Gynecologica Scandinavica*. 2019;98(9):1187–1194. doi:https://doi.org/10.1111/aogs.13629.
Dawood F, Dowswell T, Quenby S. Intravenous fluids for reducing the duration of labour in low risk nulliparous women. *Cochrane Database Syst Rev*. 2013;(6):CD007715, doi:10.1002/14651858.CD007715.pub2.
Deakin B-A. Alternative positions in labour and childbirth. *Br J Midwifery*. 2001;9(10):620–625.
Desgranges FP, Simonin M, Barnoud S, et al. Prevalence and prediction of higher estimated gastric content in parturients at full cervical dilatation: A prospective cohort study. *Acta Anaesthesiologica Scandinavica*. 2019;63(1):27–33. doi:10.1111/aas.13220.
Di Renzo GC, Pacella E, Di Fabrizio L, et al. Preterm birth: risk factors, identification and management. In: Malvasi A, Tinelli A, Di Renzo GC, eds. *Management and Therapy of Late Pregnancy Complications: Third Trimester and Puerperium*. Champaign, IL: Springer International; 2017:81–94.
Dick-Read G. *Childbirth Without Fear: The Principles and Practice of Natural Childbirth*. 2nd ed. London: Heinemann; 1946.
Dixon L, Foureur M. The vaginal examination during labour: is it of benefit or harm? *NZCOM J*. 2010;42:21–26.
Dixon L, Skinner J, Foureur M. Women's perspectives of the stages and phases of labour. *Midwifery*. 2013;29:10–17.
Dodd JM, Jones L, Flenady V, et al. Prenatal administration of progesterone for preventing preterm birth in women considered to be at risk of preterm birth. *Cochrane Database Syst Rev*. 2013;(7):CD004947, doi:10.1002/14651858.CD004947.pub3.
Doyle LW, Crowther CA, Middleton P, et al. Magnesium sulphate for women at risk of preterm birth for neuroprotection of the fetus. *Cochrane Database Syst Rev*. 2009;(1):CD004661, doi:10.1002/14651858.CD004661.pub3.
Du Y, Zhu LY, Cui LN, et al. Double-balloon catheter versus prostaglandin E2 for cervical ripening and labour induction: a systematic review and meta-analysis of randomised controlled trials. *BJOG*. 2017;124(6):891–899.
El-Din NMN, El-Morghatz DAM. Cervical ripening and induction of labor with misoprostol, prostaglandin E2 or prostaglandin E2 gel: a randomized comparative clinical trial. In: *XVI FIGO World Congress of Obstetrics and Gynecology (Book 4)*; 2000 September 3–8. Washington, DC: FIGO; 2000.29.
Enkin M, Keirse M, Neilson J, et al. *A Guide to Effective Care in Pregnancy and Childbirth*. New York: Oxford University Press; 2000.
Finucane EM, Murphy DJ, Biesty LM, et al. Membrane sweeping for induction of labour. *Cochrane Syst Rev*. Online: https://www.cochrane.org/CD000451/PREG_membrane-sweeping-induction-labour.
Flenady V, Hawley G, Stock OM, et al. Prophylactic antibiotics for inhibiting preterm labour with intact membranes. *Cochrane Database Syst Rev*. 2013;(12):CD000246.
Flenady V, Wojcieszek AM, Papatsonis DNM, et al. Calcium channel blockers for inhibiting preterm labour and birth. *Cochrane Database Syst Rev*. 2014;(6):CD002255, doi:10.1002/14651858.CD002255.pub2.
Fong A, Serra AE, Caballero D, et al. A randomized, double-blinded, controlled trial of the effects of fluid rate and/or presence of dextrose in intravenous fluids on the labor course of nulliparas. *Am J Obstet Gynecol*. 2017;217(2):208.e201–208.e207. doi:10.1016/j.ajog.2017.03.010.
Fraser W, Turcot L, Kraus I, et al. Amniotomy for shortening spontaneous labour. *Cochrane Database Syst Rev*. 1999;(4): CD000015, doi:10.1002/14651858.CD000015.
Freedman D, Brown AS, Shen L, et al. Perinatal oxytocin increases the risk of offspring bipolar disorder and childhood cognitive impairment. *J Affect Disord*. 2015;173:65–72.
Friedman EA. Primigravid labor: a graphicostatistical analysis. *Obstet Gynecol*. 1955;6:567–589.
Fruhman G, Gavard JA, Amon E, et al. Tension compared to no tension on a Foley transcervical catheter for cervical ripening: a randomized controlled trial. *Am J Obstet Gynecol*. 2017;216(1): 67.e1–67.e9. doi:10.1016/j.ajog.2016.09.082.
Ghi T, Dall'Asta A, Fieni S. Elective induction of labour in low risk nulliparous women at term: Caution is needed. *Eur J Obstet Gynecol Reprod Biol*. 2019;239:64–66. doi:10.1016/j.ejogrb.2019.05.037.
Gould D. Normal labour: a concept analysis. *J Adv Nurs*. 2000; 31(2):418–427.
Greulich B, Tarrant B. The latent phase of labour: diagnosis and management. *J Midwifery Womens Health*. 2007;52(3):190–198.
Grobman W, Rice M, Reddy U, et al. Labor Induction versus Expectant Management in Low-Risk Nulliparous Women. *New Engl J Med*. 2018;379(6):513–523. doi:10.1056/NEJMoa1800566.
Gross M, Haunschild T, Stoxen T, et al. Women's recognition of the spontaneous onset of labor. *Birth*. 2003;30(4):267–271.
Gross M, Drobnic S, Keirse M, et al. Influence of fixed and time-dependent factors on duration of normal first stage labor. *Birth*. 2005;32(1):27–33.
Gross M, Hecker H, Matterne A, et al. Does the way women experience the onset of labour influence the duration of labour? *BJOG*. 2006;113:289–294.
Hall M, Moran V, Dykes F. *Maternal and Infant Nutrition and Nurture. Controversies and Challenges*. Malta: MA Healthcare; 2006.

Handelzalts JE, Fisher S, Sadan O, et al. Object relations, unconscious defences and fear of childbirth, as reflected in maternal-request caesarean section. *J Reproduct Infant Psychol.* 2017;35(1):91–102. doi:10.1080/02646838.2016.1253832.

Haram K, Helge-Mortensen J, Wollen A. Preterm delivery: an overview. *Acta Obstet Gynecol Scand.* 2003;82:687–704.

Heimstad R, Romundstad P, Eik-Nes S, et al. Outcomes of pregnancy beyond 37 weeks of gestation. *Obstet Gynecol.* 2006; 108(3 Pt1):500–508.

Hildingsson I, Karlström A, Nystedt A. Women's experiences of induction of labour–findings from a Swedish regional study. *Aust N Z J Obstet Gynaecol.* 2011;51(2):151–157. doi:10.1111/j.1479-828X.2010.01262.x.

Hoppe KK, Schiff MA, Peterson SE, et al. 30 mL Single- versus 80 mL double-balloon catheter for pre-induction cervical ripening: a randomized controlled trial. *J Matern Fetal Neonatal Med.* 2016;29(12):1919–1925.

Institute for Safe Medical Practices. *High alert medications.* 2015. Online: http://www.ismp.org/Tools/highAlertMedicationLists.asp.

Jacobsen LK, Haslund H, Brock C, et al. Medically induced labor: Epidural analgesia and women's perceptions of pain in early labor. *Eur J Midwifery.* 2018;2(November). doi:10.18332/ejm/99545.

Janga D, Bickerton N. Labour precipitate. In: Hollingworth T, ed. *Differential Diagnosis in Obstetrics and Gynaecology: An A–Z.* London: CRC Press; 2015:200.

Kabiri D, Hants Y, Yarkoni TR, et al. Antepartum membrane stripping in GBS carriers, Is it safe? (The STRIP-G Study). *PLoS ONE.* 2015;10(12):e0145905.

Katukuri V, Blue NR, Holbrook BD, et al. 747: double balloon is not superior to single balloon trans-cervical catheter for induction of labor: a meta-analysis. *Am J Obstet Gynecol.* 2017;216(1):S434.

Keirse M. Elective induction, selective deduction and caesarean section. *Birth.* 2010;37(3):252–256.

Kenkel WM, Yee JR, Carter CS. Is oxytocin a maternal–foetal signalling molecule at birth? Implications for development. *J Neuroendocrinol.* 2014;26(10):739–749.

Kenyon S, Boulvain M, Neilson JP. Antibiotics for preterm rupture of membranes. *Cochrane Database Syst Rev.* 2013;(12):CD001058, doi:10.1002/14651858.CD001058.pub3.

Keulen JK, Bruinsma A, Kortekaas JC, et al. Induction of labour at 41 weeks versus expectant management until 42 weeks (INDEX): multicentre, randomised non-inferiority trial. *BMJ.* 2019 Feb 20;364:l344. doi:10.1136/bmj.l344. PMID: 30786997; PMCID: PMC6598648.

Khambay H, Bolt L, Chandiramani M, et al. The Actim Partus test to predict pre-term birth in asymptomatic high-risk women. *J Obstet Gynaecol.* 2012;32(2):132–134.

Kildea S, Gao Y, Hickey S, et al. Reducing preterm birth amongst Aboriginal and Torres Strait Islander babies: a prospective cohort study, Brisbane, Australia. *EClinicalMedicine.* 12;43–51.

Kildea S, McGhie AC, Gao Y, et al. Babies born before arrival to hospital and maternity unit closures in Queensland and Australia. *Women Birth.* 2015;28(3):236–245.

Kubli M, Scrutton M, O'Sullivan G, et al. An evaluation of isotonic 'sport drinks' during labor. *Anesth Analg.* 2002; 94:404–408.

Kunz MK, Loftus RJ, Nichols AA. Incidence of uterine tachysystole in women induced with oxytocin. *J Obstet Gynecol Neonatal Nurs.* 2013;42(1):12–18. doi:10.1111/j.1552-6909.2012.01428.x.

Lavender T, Alfirevic Z, Walkinshaw S. Effect of different partogram action lines on birth outcomes: a randomized controlled trial. *Obstet Gynecol.* 2006;108(2):295–302.

Lavender T, Alfirevic Z, Walkinshaw S. Partogram action line study: a randomised trial. *BJOG.* 1998;105(9):976–980.

Lavender T, Hart A, Smyth R. Effect of partogram use on outcomes for women in spontaneous labour at term. *Cochrane Database Syst Rev.* 2013;7:CD005461, doi: 10.1002/14651858.CD005461.pub4.

Lavender T, Cuthbert A, Smyth RM. Effect of partograph use on outcomes for women in spontaneous labour at term and their babies. *Cochrane Database Syst Rev.* 2018;(8).

Lee NJ, Neal J, Lowe NK, et al. Comparing different partograph designs for use in standard labor care: a pilot randomized trial. *Matern Child Health* J. 2018;22(3):355–363. doi:10.1007/s10995-017-2366-0.

Leeners B, Görres G, Block E, et al. Birth experiences in adult women with a history of childhood sexual abuse. *J Psychosom Res.* 2016;83:27–32. doi:10.1016/j.jpsychores.2016.02.006.

Løkkegaard E, Lundstrøm M, Kjær MM, et al. Prospective multicentre randomised trial comparing induction of labour with a double-balloon catheter versus dinoprostone. *J Obstet Gynaecol.* 2015;35(8):797–802.

Loscul C, Chantry AA, Caubit L, et al. Association between oxytocin augmentation intervals and the risk of postpartum haemorrhage. *J gynecol, obstet biologie de la reprod.* 2016;45(7): 708–715. doi:10.1016/j.jgyn.2015.12.005.

Lowe NK. The nature of labour pain. *Am J Obstet Gynecol.* 2002; 186:s16–s24.

Lowe NK. A review of factors associated with dystocia and cesarean section in nulliparous women. *J Midwifery Womens Health.* 2007;52(3):216–228.

Lumley J, Chamberlain C, Dowswell T, et al. Interventions for promoting smoking cessation during pregnancy. *Cochrane Database Syst Rev.* 2009;(3):CD001055, doi:10.1002/14651858.CD001055.pub3.

McDonald S, Magill-Cuerden J. *Mayes' Midwifery: A Textbook for Midwives.* 14th ed. London: Ballière Tindall; 2013.

McNamara H. Problems and challenges in the management of preterm labour. *BJOG.* 2003;110(suppl 20):79–85.

McNiven PS, Williams JI, Hodnett E, et al. An early labor assessment program: a randomized, controlled trial. *Birth.* 1998; 25(1):5–10.

Mahomed K, Pungsornruk K, Gibbons K. Induction of labour for postdates in nulliparous women with uncomplicated pregnancy—is the caesarean section rate really lower? *J Obstet Gynaecol.* 2016;36(7):916–920.

Mauad-Filho F, Morais END, Parente JV, et al. Effect of glucose infusion on the maternal and fetal acid-base equilibrium during labor. *J Perinatal Med.* 1982;10(2):99–104. doi:10.1515/jpme.1982.10.2.99.

Medsafe. *Cervidil® 10mg pessary. New Zealand data sheet.* 2018. Online: http://www.medsafe.govt.nz/profs/Datasheet/c/Cervidilpessary.pdf.

Middleton P, Shepherd E, Flenady V, et al. Planned early birth versus expectant management (waiting) for prelabour rupture of membranes at term (37 weeks or more). *Cochrane Database Syst Rev.* 2017;(1):CD005302, doi:10.1002/14651858.CD005302.pub3.

Middleton P, Shepherd E, Crowther CA. Induction of labour for improving birth outcomes for women at or beyond term. *Cochrane Database Syst Rev.* 2018;(5):CD004945, doi:10.1002/14651858.CD004945.pub4.

Midwifery Council of New Zealand (MCNZ). *Competencies for Entry to the Register of Midwives.* Wellington: MCNZ; 2007.

Midwifery Council of New Zealand (MCNZ). *Scope of Practice.* Wellington: MCNZ; 2010. Online: https://www.midwiferycouncil.health.nz/sites/default/files/for-midwives/Gazette%20Notice%202010%20-scope%20%26%20quals%20new%20form.pdf.

Ministry of Health (MOH). *Report on Maternity, 2010.* Wellington: Ministry of Health; 2012. Online: https://www.health.govt.nz/publication/report-maternity-2010.

Ministry of Health (MOH). *Report on Maternity, 2015.* Wellington: Ministry of Health; 2017. Online: https://www.health.govt.nz/publication/report-maternity-2015.

MirzaeeRabor F, Mirzaee F, MirzaiiNajmabadi K, et al. Respect for woman's decision-making in spontaneous birth: a thematic synthesis study. *Iranian J Nurs Midwifery Res.* 2016;21(5): 449–457. doi:10.4103/1735-9066.193389.

Mollart LJ, Adam J, Foureur M. Impact of acupressure on onset of labour and labour duration: a systematic review. *Women Birth.* 2015;28(3):199–206. doi:10.1016/j.wombi.2015.03.007.

Mozurkewich EL, Chilimigras JL, Berman DR, et al. Methods of induction of labour: a systematic review. *BMC Pregnancy Childbirth.* 2011;11:84.

Murray ML. Uterine activity impacts fetal/neonatal outcomes. *Int J Childbirth.* doi:10.1891/IJCBIRTH-D-19-00037.

Nabi HA, Aflaifel NB, Weeks AD. A hundred years of induction of labour methods. *Eur J Obstet Gynecol Reprod Biol.* 2014;179: 236–239.

Nahaee J, Abbas-Alizadeh F, Mirghafourvand M, et al. Pre- and during- labour predictors of dystocia in active phase of labour: a case-control study. *BMC Pregnancy Childbirth.* 2020;20(1), 425. doi:10.1186/s12884-020-03113-5.

National Collaborating Centre for Women's and Children's Health. *Induction of Labour.* London UK: RCOG Press; 2008. Online: https://www.nice.org.uk/guidance/cg70/evidence/full-guideline-241871149.

National Institute for Health and Clinical Excellence (NICE). *Inducing labour. Clinical guideline CG70.* London: NICE; 2008. Online: https://www.nice.org.uk/guidance/cg70/.

National Institute for Health and Care Excellence (NICE). *Intrapartum Care: Care of Healthy Women and Their Babies During Childbirth (CG190).* London: National Institute for Health and Care Excellence; 2014. Online: http://www.nice.org.uk/guidance/cg190/resources. updated 2017.

Neal J, Lowe NK. Physiologic partograph to improve birth safety and outcomes among low-risk, nulliparous women with spontaneous labor onset. *Med Hypotheses.* 2012;78(2):319–326. doi:10.1016/j.mehy.2011.11.012.

Neal JL, Lowe NK, Ahijevych KL, et al. "Active labor" duration and dilation rates among low-risk, nulliparous women with spontaneous labor onset: a systematic review. *J Midwifery Womens Health.* 2010a;55(4):308–318. doi:10.1016/j.jmwh.2009.08.004.

Neal J, Lowe N, Patrick T, et al. What is the slowest-yet-normal cervical dilation rate among nulliparous women with spontaneous labour onset? *J Obstet Gynecol Neonatal Nurs.* 2010b;39(4):361–369. doi:10.1111/j.1552-6909.2010.01154.x.

Neal JL, Lamp JM, Buck JS, et al. Outcomes of nulliparous women with spontaneous labor onset admitted to hospitals in preactive versus active labor. *J Midwifery Womens Health.* 2014;59(1): 28–34. doi:10.1111/jmwh.12160.

Neal JL, Ryan SL, Lowe NK, et al. Labor dystocia: uses of related nomenclature. *J Midwifery Womens Health.* 2015;60(5): 485–498. doi:10.1111/jmwh.12355.

Neerland CE. Maternal confidence for physiologic childbirth: a concept analysis. *J Midwifery Womens Health.* 2018;63(4):425–435. doi:10.1111/jmwh.12719.

New Zealand College of Midwives (NZCOM). *Consensus Statement on Normal Birth.* Christchurch: NZCOM; 2006, updated 2009.

New Zealand College of Midwives (NZCOM). *Consensus Statement on Assessment of Fetal Wellbeing During Pregnancy.* Christchurch: NZCOM; 2012.

New Zealand College of Midwives (NZCOM), Royal Australian and New Zealand College of Obstetrics and Gynaecology (RANZCOG), and Royal Australasian College of Physicians. *Induction of Labour in Aotearoa New Zealand: A clinical practice guideline.* RANZCOG; 2019.

Newnham JP, White SW, Lee H.-S, et al. The elements of success in a comprehensive state-wide program to safely reduce the rate of preterm birth. *PloS ONE.* 2020;15(6): e0234033.

Norman JE, Shennan AH. Prevention of preterm birth—why can't we do any better? *Lancet.* 2013;381(9862):184–185.

Norman JE, Heazell AE, Rodriguez A, et al. Awareness of fetal movements and care package to reduce fetal mortality (AFFIRM): a stepped wedge, cluster-randomised trial. *Lancet.* 2018;392(10158):1629–1638.

Oladapo OT, Diaz V, Bonet M, et al. Cervical dilatation patterns of 'low-risk' women with spontaneous labour and normal perinatal outcomes: a systematic review. *BJOG.* 2017; doi:10.1111/1471-0528.14930. [Epub ahead of print].

O'Driscoll K, Stronge JM, Minogue M. Active management of labour. *BMJ.* 1973;3(5872):135–137.

Olza Fernández I, Marín Gabriel M, Malalana Martínez A, et al. Newborn feeding behaviour depressed by intrapartum oxytocin: a pilot study. *Acta Paediatr.* 2012;101(7):749–754.

Papatsonis D, Flenady V, Cole S, et al. Oxytocin receptor antagonists for inhibiting preterm labour. *Cochrane Database Syst Rev.* 2010;(3):CD004452, doi:10.1002/14651858.C004452.pub2.

Pasquier JC, Bujold E. A systematic review of intentional delivery in women with preterm prelabor rupture of membranes. *J Matern Fetal Neonatal Med.* 2007;20(7):567–568.

Perinatal and Maternity Mortality Review Committee (PMMRC). *Reporting Mortality 2013.* 2013. Online: https://www.hqsc.govt.nz/assets/PMMRC/Publications/Ninth-PMMRC-report-FINAL-Jun-2015.pdf.

Peru J, Garabedian C, Drumez E, et al. Does rupture of membranes have an impact on the fetal heart rate during spontaneous labor? *Gynecologie, obstetrique, fertilite & senologie.* 2020;48(10): 715–721. doi:10.1016/j.gofs.2020.02.008.

Philpott R, Castle W. Cervicographs in the management of labour in primigravidae. The alert line for detecting abnormal labour. *BJOG.* 1972;79:592–598.

Powell-Kennedy H, Shannon M. Keeping birth normal: research findings on midwifery care during childbirth. *J Obstet Gynecol Neonatal Nurs.* 2004;33:554–560.

Prevost M, Zelkowitz P, Tulandi T, et al. Oxytocin in pregnancy and the postpartum: relations to labor and its management. *Front Public Health.* 2014;2:1. doi:10.3389/fpubh.2014.00001.

Rankin J. Physiology in *Childbearing: With Anatomy and Related Biosciences.* 4th ed. Edinburgh: Elsevier; 2017.

RANZCOG. *Induction of Labour in New Zealand: A clinical practice guideline (draft).* Online: https://mhsfaculty.auckland.ac.nz/inductionNZ/.

Roberts D, Dalziel S. Antenatal corticosteroids for accelerating fetal lung maturation for women at risk for preterm birth. *Cochrane Database Syst Rev.* 2006;(3):CD004454.

Rohwer AC, Khondowe O, Young T. Antispasmodics for labour. *Cochrane Database Syst Rev.* 2013;(6):CD009243, doi:10.1002/14651858.CD009243.pub3.

Roshanfekr D, Blakemore KJ, Lee J, et al. Station at onset of active labor in nulliparous patients and risk of cesarean delivery. *Obstet Gynecol.* 1999;93:329–331.

Royal Australian and New Zealand College of Obstetricians and Gynaecologists (RANZCOG). *Intrapartum Fetal Surveillance. Clinical Guideline.* 3rd ed. 2014. Online: https://www.ranzcog.edu.au/RANZCOG_SITE/media/RANZCOG-MEDIA/Women%27s%20Health/Statement%20and%20guidelines/Clinical-Obstetrics/Intrapartum-Fetal-Surveillance-Guideline-Third-edition-Aug-2014.pdf?ext=.pdf.

Royal College of Obstetricians and Gynaecologists (RCOG). *Clinical Effectiveness Support Unit. Induction of Labour. Evidence-based Clinical Guideline Number 9*. London: RCOG Press; 2001.

Scott-Pillai R, Spence D, Cardwell CR, et al. The impact of body mass index on maternal and neonatal outcomes: a retrospective study in a UK obstetric population, 2004–2011. *BJOG*. 2013;120(8):932–939. doi:10.1111/1471-0528.12193.

Singata M, Tranmer J, Gyte GML. Restricting oral fluid and food intake during labour. *Cochrane Database Syst Rev*. 2013;(8):CD003930, doi:10.1002/14651858.CD003930.pub3.

Singhal S, Sarda N, Dhiman N, et al. Double blinded study on comparison of phosphorylated insulin like growth factor binding protein 1 test and fetal fibronectin test for prediction of preterm delivery. *Int J Reprod Contracept Obstet Gynecol*. 2017;6(4):5.

Smyth RMD, Alldred SK, Markham C. Amniotomy for shortening spontaneous labour. *Cochrane Database Syst Rev*. 2013;(6):CD006167, doi:10.1002/14651858.CD006167.pub4.

Society of Obstetricians and Gynaecologists of Canada (SOGC). Induction of labour. SOGC clinical practice guideline no. 296. *J Obstet Gynaecol Can*. 2013;(September):840–842. (replaces no. 107, August 2001). Online: https://sogc.org/wp-content/uploads/2013/08/September2013-CPG296-ENG-Online.

Sosa CG, Althabe F, Belizán JM, et al. Bed rest in singleton pregnancies for preventing preterm birth. *Cochrane Database Syst Rev*. 2015;(3):CD003581, doi:10.1002/14651858.CD003581.pub3.

Stevens G, Miller Y. Overdue choices: how information and role in decision-making influence women's preferences for induction for prolonged pregnancy. *Birth*. 2012;39(3):248–257.

Striebich S, Mattern E, Ayerle GM. Support for pregnant women identified with fear of childbirth (FOC)/tokophobia: a systematic review of approaches and interventions. *Midwifery*. 2018;61:97–115. doi:10.1016/j.midw.2018.02.013.

Suffecool K, Rosenn BM, Kam S, et al. Labor induction in nulliparous women with an unfavorable cervix: double balloon catheter versus dinoprostone. *J Perinat Med*. 2014;42(2):213–218. doi:10.1515/jpm-2013-0152.

Suresh V, Soni R. A quasi experimental study to assess the effectiveness of nipple stimulation in the progress of labour among primipara women during first stage of labour in selected hospital of Jabalpur (MP). *Indian Holist Nurs*. 2019;10(1):1–7.

Swannell C. Caution needed implementing Safer Baby Bundle. *Med J Aust*. 2019;1.

Sweet LP, Boon VA, Brinkworth V, et al. Birthing in rural South Australia: the changing landscape over 20 years. *Aust J Rural Health*. 2015;23(6):332–338. doi:10.1111/ajr.12214.

Thomas J, Fairclough A, Kavanagh J, et al. Vaginal prostaglandin (PGE_2 and PGF_2) for induction of labour at term. *Cochrane Database Syst Rev*. 2014;(6):CD003101, CD003101, doi:10.1002/14651858.pub3.

Thornton J. Active management of labour. BMJ. 1996;313:378.

Toohill J, Soong B, Flenady V. Interventions for ketosis during labour. *Cochrane Database Syst Rev*. 2008;(3). doi:10.1002/14651858.CD004230.pub2.

Tracy SK, Sullivan E, Wang Y, et al. Birth outcomes associated with interventions in labour amongst low risk women: a population-based study. *Women Birth*. 2006;20(2):41–48.

Verburg PE, Dekker GA, Venugopal K, et al. Long-term trends in singleton preterm birth in South Australia from 1986 to 2014. *Obstet Gynecol*. 2018;131(1):79–89. doi:10.1097/aog.0000000000002419.

Vincent V. Amniotomy: to do or not to do? *Midwives*. 2005;8(5):228–229.

Walsh D. We should go with the rhythm of labour. *Br J Midwifery*. 2003;11(11):656.

Walsh D. How long is too long? Prohibitions on the length of labour. *Br J Midwifery*. 2005;13(12):756.

Walsh D. *Evidence and Skills for Normal Labour and Birth—A Guide for Midwives*. London: Routledge; 2012.

Wennerholm UB, Saltvedt S, Wessberg A, et al. Induction of labour at 41 weeks versus expectant management and induction of labour at 42 weeks (SWEdish Post-term Induction Study, SWEPIS): multicentre, open label, randomised, superiority trial. *BMJ: Bri Med J (Online)*. 2019;367. doi:http://dx.doi.org/10.1136/bmj.l6131.

Wisborg K, Barklin A, Hedegaard M, et al. Psychological stress during pregnancy and stillbirth: prospective study. *BJOG*. 2008;115(7):882–885.

White L, Lee N, Beckmann M. First stage of labour management practices: a survey of Australian obstetric providers. *Aust N Z J Obstet Gynaecol*. 2017;57(3):266–271. doi:10.1111/ajo.12510.

Wojcieszek AM, Stock OM, Flenady V. Antibiotics for prelabour rupture of membranes at or near term. *Cochrane Database Syst Rev*. 2014;(10):CD001807, doi:10.1002/14651858.CD001807.pub2.

Wolf H, Brok J, Henriksen T, et al. Antenatal magnesium sulphate for the prevention of cerebral palsy in infants born preterm: a double-blind, randomised, placebo-controlled, multi-centre trial. *BJOG*. 2020;127(10):1217–1225. doi:10.1111/1471-0528.16239.

Wood S, Cooper S, Ross S. Does induction of labour increase the risk of caesarean section? A systematic review and meta-analysis of trials in women with intact membranes. *BJOG*. 2014;121(6):674–685.

World Health Organization (WHO). *The application of the WHO partograph in the management of labour. Report of a WHO multicentre study*. Geneva, Switzerland: WHO; 1994:1990–1991.

World Health Organization (WHO). *WHO recommendations on intrapartum care for a positive childbirth experience*. World Health Organization; 2018.

Wuntakai R, Kaler M, Hollingworth T. Women with a high BMI: should they be managed differently due to antagonizing action of leptin in labour? *Med Hypotheses*. 2013;80(6):767–768.

Yonkers KA, Smith MV, Forray A, et al. Pregnant women with posttraumatic stress disorder and risk of preterm birth. *JAMA Psychiatry*. 2014;71(8):897–904.

Zhang J, Troendle J, Yancey M. Reassessing the labor curve. *Am J Obstet Gynecol*. 2001;185(suppl 6):71–72.

Zhang J, Troendle JF, Yancey MK. Reassessing the labor curve in nulliparous women. *Am J Obstet Gynecol*. 2002;187(4):824–828.

Zhang J, Landy HJ, Branch DW, et al. Consortium on Safe Labor. Contemporary patterns of spontaneous labor with normal neonatal outcomes. *Obstet Gynecol*. 2010;116(6):1281–1287. doi:10.1097/AOG.0b013e3181fdef6e.

Zhao Y, Flatley C, Kumar S. Intrapartum intervention rates and perinatal outcomes following induction of labour compared to expectant management at term from an Australian perinatal centre. *Aust N Z J Obstet Gynaecol*. 2017;57(1):40–48. doi:10.1111/ajo.12576.

Further reading

Mahomed K, Pungsornruk K, Gibbons K. Induction of labour for postdates in nulliparous women with uncomplicated pregnancy—is the caesarean section rate really lower? *J Obstet Gynaecol*. 2016;36(7):916-920.

Nobis P. *Clinical Methods in Obstetrics and Gynaecology*. 2nd ed. New York: Churchill Livingstone; 2014.

Breech birth article. https://www.midwifery.org.uk/articles/breech-birth/.

CHAPTER 39

Interventions in pregnancy, labour and birth

Sally K Tracy

LEARNING OUTCOMES

Learning outcomes for this chapter are:

1. To describe interventions in birth in relation to the normal physiology of birth
2. To explore the cascade of interventions that may result in operative birth
3. To outline the aetiology of cerebral palsy
4. To discuss the use of electronic fetal monitoring and the cardiotocograph during labour and birth including indications and contraindications in relation to current evidence and best practice
5. To describe the implications of epidurals and combined spinal epidurals for birth
6. To explore indications for and outcomes of birth by caesarean section
7. To explore indications for and outcomes of birth by forceps or vacuum extraction.

CHAPTER OVERVIEW

In Australia, less than half of all childbearing women have spontaneous vaginal births. In Aotearoa New Zealand the rate for spontaneous vaginal birth is considerably higher and it is accompanied by a predominance of maternity care offered by midwives in the community (MOH, 2021). Even though we live in an age of evidence-informed practice, it has become routine to offer women many interventions for which the evidence is either non-existent or very weak. There are mounting global concerns regarding the wasteful spending on the overuse of interventions and rising rates of interventions during birth in high-income countries like ours (Betran et al., 2018; Hanson et al., 2020; Miller et al., 2016). The difficulty for midwives is in separating practices based on sound evidence from those driven by opinion, authority, dogma, market or business principles or other needs. This chapter will discuss common interventions that occur during labour and birth in the light of findings from recently published research.

KEY TERMS

biophysical profile
caesarean section
cascade of interventions
electronic fetal monitoring
epidural analgesia and anaesthesia
forceps
intermittent auscultation
operative birth
placenta accreta spectrum
vacuum extraction
vaginal birth after caesarean (VBAC)

INTRODUCTION

Routine use of interventions during pregnancy, labour and childbirth is common in both Australia and New Zealand. These interventions include induction of labour, electronic fetal monitoring (EFM), epidurals, oxytocin, episiotomies, instrumental birth with either forceps or vacuum, and caesarean section (CS). Some say the first major intervention is moving women to hospital to give birth rather than their giving birth at home.

Evidence is available to guide practice on a number of interventions during pregnancy, labour and childbirth, such as restricting the use of episiotomy, promotion or discontinuation of active management of the third stage of labour, routine amniotomy, electronic fetal heart rate (FHR) monitoring, epidural analgesia and use of oxytocin/ergometrine to prevent postpartum haemorrhage. However, there is no good evidence for the routine use of many interventions and technologies such as EFM, epidurals, oxytocin or episiotomies in women who have normal, uncomplicated pregnancies (WHO, 2018). Evidence does exist for alternatives such as intermittent auscultation of the fetal heart, non-pharmacological measures for pain relief, and low-technology strategies such as walking and baths for comfort and stimulation in labour. Further evidence is required on how women cope emotionally with the consequences of labour interventions.

As confusing as this may seem, there are several other factors worth considering. Physiologists claim that a woman should not be removed from her safe environment for labour because this will invariably result in inhibition of uterine contractions. Over thirty years ago, in the first edition of the famous work by Chalmers et al. *Effective Care in Pregnancy and Childbirth* published in Oxford in 1989, the wise observation was made concerning the safest way to help labouring women, to 'respect nature and not to interfere with spontaneous events unless there is clear evidence that to do so would be beneficial' (Naaktgeboren, 1989, p. 796). Since then, however, some modern obstetric commentators have moved an opposing view—that labour might be best avoided altogether and babies delivered routinely by abdominal operation (Dietz, 2017; Hannah, 2004).

THE GOLDEN RULES FOR AVOIDING UNNECESSARY INTERVENTION

There are two golden rules for midwives faced with the plethora of routine interventions found in most hospitals in New Zealand and Australia today:

- There must be a good reason for intervening in a woman's labour and birth. This means that you must be able to describe and support with good evidence the 'clinical indications' that require you to do anything that would interfere with the normal physiological process of labour and birth. Then you must weigh up the evidence to show that the intervention you are about to undertake will *not* cause more harm than good.
- By supporting a woman fully with appropriate and adequate information, you will find that many unnecessary interventions can be avoided.

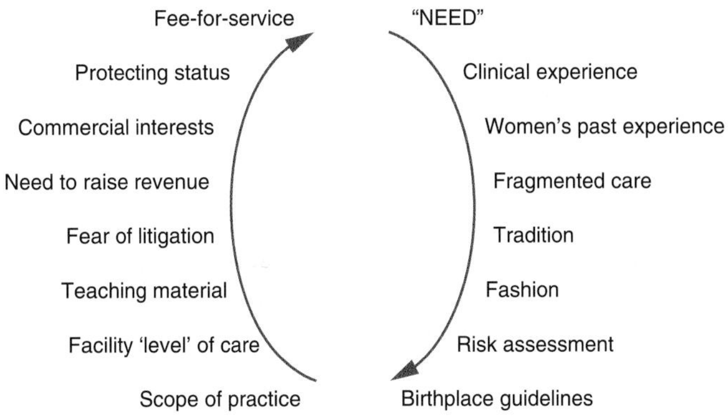

FIGURE 39.1 The Intervention Circle
(Based on Chalmers I,1991)

Much of the intervention that is routinely used in hospitals today evolved from the use of technology to 'save' mothers or babies when they were in distress during birth. 'Distress' itself is a subjective term and now there are parameters—or measurements—that enable us to see whether or not a woman may need medical intervention. Fig. 39.1 shows an intervention circle based on an 'intervention clock', which was presented in the journal *Birth* in 1991. Even though it is over 30 years old, it still resonates for many of us. Professor Iain Chalmers described the need to intervene in pregnancy and childbirth in terms of a 'decision to intervene' clock:

> *As you go around the clock ... from unambiguous 'need' at 1 o'clock to 'commercial interests' at 11 o'clock, the factors that influence the decision to intervene become less and less defensible.*
>
> (Chalmers, 1991, p. 137)

Several important studies demonstrate that there is still a need to question the effect of non-clinical factors on the rates of operative intervention during childbirth (Cary, 1990; Dahlen et al., 2012, 2014, 2021; Roberts et al., 2000; Shorten & Shorten, 1999; Tracy et al., 2007a).

There are two other influences that must be considered when addressing the rates and role of intervention in childbirth: the 'seductive' nature of technology and the belief that all forms of intervention will avert or prevent an adverse outcome such as brain damage or cerebral palsy. Our technocratic society places great value on intervention and the use of machines and monitors and, as a result, midwives and obstetricians are confronted with an ever-expanding array of technologies, both reproductive and information based, that have a significant impact on the level and nature of care provided.

CEREBRAL PALSY

A major influence on the use of intervention was the belief that intervention in birth would be effective in preventing cerebral palsy (Blair & Stanley, 1997). In some cases this might be so, but the birth prevalence of cerebral palsy in high-income countries has barely declined since the mid 1950s, in contrast to perinatal mortality. Most aetiological paths leading to cerebral palsy are likely to commence before labour and birth. Approximately 8–10% of cases are believed to be causally linked with adverse intrapartum events. The current trend is to assume a prenatal cause in the absence of clear evidence for a perinatal or postnatal cause. See Fig. 39.2 for the risk factors and population rates of cerebral palsy (Blair & Stanley, 1997; Reddihough & Collins, 2003; Sadowska et al., 2020). Cerebral palsy (CP) is a term of convenience applied to a group of motor disorders or motor impairment stemming from a malfunction of the brain (rather than spinal cord or muscles). CP is not a diagnosis, because it infers nothing about pathology, aetiology or prognosis. Rather, it is an umbrella term covering a wide range of cerebral disorders (Badawi et al., 1998) that are chronic, non-progressive (interference, lesion or abnormality), appear early in life, and in which the defining symptoms are abnormal control of movement, posture, motor function, or a combination, and where the interference, lesion or abnormality arose in the developing or immature brain (Shepherd et al., 2017).

Research suggests that spastic quadriplegia and, less often, dyskinetic CP are the only types of CP associated with hypoxic intrapartum events but that neither of these

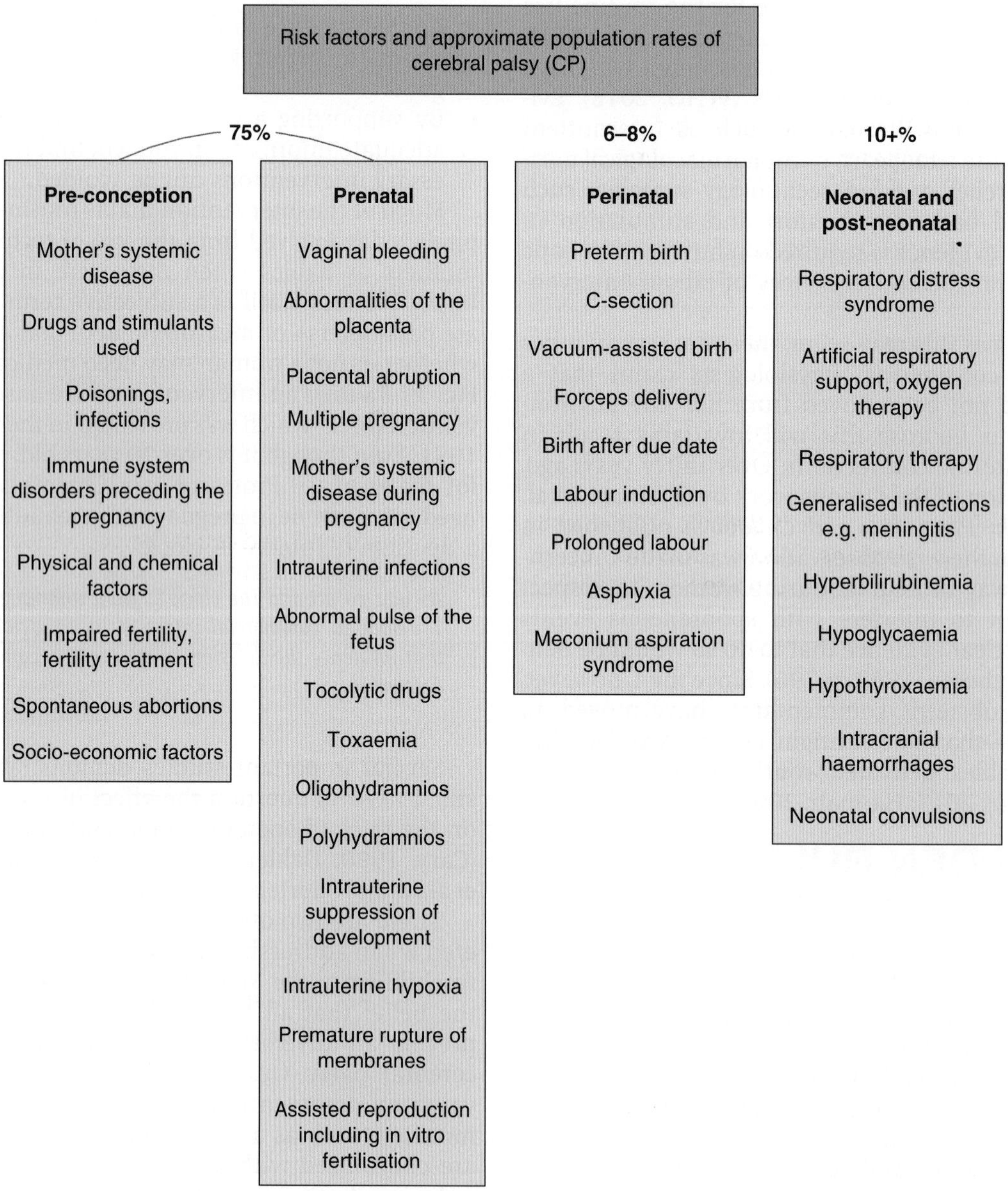

FIGURE 39.2 Risk factors and approximate population rates of cerebral palsy (CP)

Box 39.1 Classification of cerebral palsy

Cerebral palsy types are classified by the number of limbs involved:

- hemiplegia
- quadriplegia
- hemiparesis

and the type of movement disorder:

- spastic
- athetoid/dyskinetic
- akinetic
- ataxic
- mixed.

(Source: Hankins & Speer, 2003)

types of CP is specific to intrapartum asphyxia (Box 39.1). However, hemiplegic CP, spastic diplegia and ataxia are not associated with intrapartum asphyxia in term infants (Fahey & King, 2005). CP affects 2 in 1000 live-born children—in Australia, 1 in 700 Australian children—with pre-term birth being the leading risk factor for CP and with the risk increasing substantially with decreasing gestational age at birth (Keir et al., 2021). It is the most common physical disability in childhood (Jacobsson et al., 2008). There are a number of antenatal factors that have been associated with CP in both the pre-term and the term infant, with birth asphyxia playing a minor role (Fig. 39.2).

Due to the increasing survival of the very pre-term and very low-birth-weight infant secondary to improvements in neonatal and obstetric care, the incidence of CP may be increasing (Longo & Hankins, 2009; Crowther et al., 2017). Global estimates suggest that up to 8% of pre-term babies have neurological impairments, of which 5% are mild and 3% moderate or severe (Blencowe et al., 2013).

Since publication of the results of an Australian study by Crowther et al. (2003), the BEAM Trial (Rouse et al., 2008) and the Cochrane meta-analysis (Shepherd et al., 2017), the clinical use of magnesium sulfate for the prevention of cerebral palsy has become increasingly widespread in Australia and New Zealand. Magnesium sulfate ($MgSO_4$) has been shown to prevent cerebral palsy among children born to women at high risk of early pre-term birth (Box 39.2).

Maternal receipt of this fetal neuroprotective medication before pre-term birth reduces the risk of death or CP (relative risk (RR) 0.85, 95% CI 0.74 to 0.98), and of CP alone (RR 0.68, 95%CI 0.54 to 0.87) for exposed pre-term born children (Keir et al., 2021). Guidelines have now been developed for the use of magnesium sulfate to prevent cerebral palsy, as three large, randomised placebo-controlled trials and a subsequent Cochrane review suggest that this intervention can decrease rates of cerebral palsy by 32% with a number needed to treat of 63 to prevent one case (Rouse & Hirtz, 2016).

Box 39.2 Magnesium sulfate ($MgSO_4$) for the prevention of cerebral palsy

The following two treatment protocols have been published.

1. Treatment protocols based around the BEAM trial (Rouse et al., 2008):
   - Women in the magnesium sulfate group received a 6 g intravenous loading dose, followed by 2 g/h intravenously for up to 12 h. If, at 12 h, the baby had not been born the magnesium sulfate was discontinued, to be resumed if pre-term birth threatened prior to 33 weeks, 6 days.
2. Treatment protocol based on Crowther et al. (2003) in their Australian study:
   - Women in the magnesium sulfate group received $MgSO_4$ as a 4-g intravenous bolus, and then a constant infusion of 1 g/h for up to 24 h.

(Sources: Crowther et al., 2003, 2016; Rouse & Hirtz, 2016; Rouse et al., 2008; Shepherd et al., 2017)

RESEARCH ACTIVITY

What is the treatment protocol for magnesium sulfate in your health district?

A study that reviewed data from the West Australian Cerebral Palsy Register found:

- CP proportions are not falling in spite of significant increases in obstetric and neonatal interventions aimed at reducing asphyxia
- CP proportions in low-birth-weight infants are rising in most developed countries, coincident with increases in the neonatal survival of low-birth-weight babies
- few cases of CP seem to be caused by birth asphyxia, and those that are may not have been preventable by obstetric care.

The study concluded that parents will continue to sue if obstetricians keep promising perfection from obstetric care in the face of 2.0–2.5 cases of CP per 1000 children born (Stanley & Blair, 1991).

In pregnancy, the risk of CP is inversely associated with birth-weight ratio (Blair & Stanley, 1997; Palmer et al., 1995). Researchers agree, however, that it is not low birth weight alone that increases the risk of CP, but rather birth weight in association with intrauterine growth restriction (IUGR) (Blair & Stanley, 1997; Dahlseng et al., 2014).

The latest Cochrane systematic review summarised CP in the following way:

> *Cerebral palsy is usually due to events before, during, or after childbirth that lead to injury in babies' developing brains. There is no single cause of cerebral palsy. For many children, the cause of cerebral palsy is unclear, however, there are many known risk factors. The biggest risk factor is birth before 37 weeks of pregnancy (preterm birth). Other risk factors for mothers include some medical conditions (including thyroid*

problems), abnormalities of the placenta, pre-eclampsia (high blood pressure and protein in the urine), and some bacterial and viral infections. For babies, risk factors include congenital and genetic abnormalities, having a low birthweight or growth restricted as a fetus, being a twin or triplet, some infections, and prolonged loss of oxygen during birth.

(Shepherd et al., 2017, online summary: http://cochranelibrary-wiley.com/doi/10.1002/14651858.CD012077.pub2/full).

CLINICAL POINT

Risk factors

Risk factors cannot be assumed to be causes, even when they do have a causal potential. Risk factors are markers that we interpret as needing further intervention or assistance.

Intrapartum factors

Intrapartum factors producing hypoxia and/or trauma have traditionally been assumed to be the principal cause of CP. This has, no doubt, contributed to the increasing use of obstetric intervention and is responsible for malpractice suits being brought against perinatal caregivers (Tito, 1995). (The most frequently observed FHR patterns associated with CP are those with multiple late decelerations and decreased beat-to-beat variability. However, these patterns should not be used to predict CP as they have a false-positive rate of 99% (Nelson et al., 1996)).

Four essential criteria are considered prerequisites to moderate to severe neonatal encephalopathy that subsequently results in CP. If intrapartum hypoxic–ischaemic insult is held to be the cause then all four criteria must be met:

1. evidence of metabolic acidosis in fetal umbilical cord arterial blood obtained at birth (pH less than 7 and base deficit of 12 mmol/L or more)
2. early onset of severe or moderate neonatal encephalopathy in infants born at ≥34 weeks gestation
3. CP of the spastic quadriplegic or dyskinetic type
4. exclusion of other identifiable aetiologies, such as trauma, coagulation disorders, infectious conditions or genetic disorders (Hankins & Speer, 2003).

Birth asphyxia occurs in a newborn baby who may have had significant reduction in oxygenation or perfusion in utero and prior to birth. The clinical features are described in the clinical syndrome of hypoxic–ischaemic encephalopathy (HIE) (Box 39.3). Currently in the UK, hypoxic–ischaemic encephalopathy was the largest contributor to term brain injury, and intraventricular/periventricular haemorrhage was the largest contributor to pre-term brain injury (Gale et al., 2017).

Box 39.3 What are the features of hypoxic–ischaemic encephalopathy (HIE)?

The measurement of hypoxic stress (or peripartum asphyxia) includes:

- Newborn infant of 35 weeks gestation or greater
- Apgar score of 5 or less at 10 minutes
- Mechanical ventilation or resuscitation at 10 minutes
- Cord pH <7.1, or an arterial pH <7.1, or
- Base deficit of 12 or more within 60 minutes of birth
- The baby may have seizures or be in a coma, together with multisystem organ failure
- Need for prolonged resuscitation and moderate to severe encephalopathy
- No major congenital abnormalities recognisable at birth

(These babies are treated with therapeutic hypothermia.)

(Adapted from Jacobs SE, Berg M, Hunt R, et al. Cooling for newborns with hypoxic ischaemic encephalopathy. *Cochrane Database Syst Rev.* 2013;1:CD003311. doi: 10.1002/14651858.CD003311.pub3)

Anti-D—a success story in the prevention of cerebral palsy

Anti-D immunoglobulin is now administered to Rh-negative women at risk of an Rh-positive fetomaternal haemorrhage. This prevents the possibility of maternal Rh isoimmunisation producing maternal Rh antibodies, which can cause kernicterus and choreoathetosis with deafness in a subsequent Rh-positive fetus. This anti-D injection has almost eliminated choreoathetosis with deafness in developed countries (Blair & Stanley, 1993). (See also Chs 37 and 40.)

Postneonatal cerebral palsy

After birth, the causes of CP are known to be infective, anoxic or traumatic, with septicaemia and meningitis accounting for the majority of cases, particularly in developing countries. In developed countries, there is a greater variety of postneonatal aetiology, with trauma accounting for up to 24% of cases (including motor vehicle accidents and non-accidental injury) and cerebrovascular accident and postoperative causes accounting for up to another 25%. Because these are the most aetiologically obvious, they may also be the most preventable (Blair & Stanley, 1997).

INTERVENTIONS BEFORE BIRTH

Assessing the wellbeing of the fetus

Interventions to assess the wellbeing of the baby while it is in utero are intended to provide midwives, obstetricians and mothers with the best information about the optimal time for birth. Fetal hypoxemia and acidosis which constitute the most common pathway to fetal death in many high-risk pregnancies may be detected through changes in amniotic fluid, fetal movements, and fetal heart rate characteristics. Antenatal fetal surveillance is offered to individuals whose pregnancies are complicated by conditions associated with increased risk for stillbirth; however, there is a paucity of evidence-based recommendations on the timing and frequency of antenatal fetal surveillance (ACOG, 2021).

IUGR affects approximately 10% of pregnancies and is associated with significant adverse perinatal outcomes. Severe IUGR results from multiple causes, such as genetic syndromes, aneuploidy and congenital infections, and is thought to be the result of a 'compromised' placenta. When a placenta is not functioning optimally, there is a risk that the fetus will suffer from a lack of oxygen (known as 'placental respiratory failure' or 'fetal hypoxaemia'). Obstetricians believe that the inherent risks of delaying delivery of the severely growth-restricted fetus include those of worsening hypoxia, long-term neurodevelopmental complications and even perinatal death. Antenatal tests of fetal wellbeing are performed with the intention of identifying severely growth-restricted fetuses with early signs of compensatory failure and fetuses most at risk of adverse outcomes. However, the optimal antenatal test to guide obstetricians about the timing of delivery for the pre-term fetus with severe IUGR remains uncertain (see also Chs 37 and 40).

Fetal movements

Fetal movements (FMs) are one of the first signs of fetal life and are an indirect measure of central nervous system integrity and function. Pregnant women usually sense FM from 18 to 20 weeks of gestation in a first pregnancy and at about 16 weeks of gestation in the second or subsequent pregnancy. As pregnancy proceeds, the weekly number of FMs increases (Olesen & Svare, 2004). The movements are related to neuromuscular development and a normal metabolic state of the central nervous system of the fetus (Olesen & Svare, 2004). On average, the fetus is active between 9% and 18% of the time in late pregnancy (Olesen & Svare, 2004), having about 4 to 100 movements an hour (Mangesi et al., 2015).

The Cochrane database suggests that 'Fetal movement counting may allow the clinician to make appropriate interventions in good time to improve outcomes. On the other hand, fetal movement counting may cause unnecessary anxiety to pregnant women, or elicit unnecessary interventions' (Mangesi et al., 2015, p. 1).

For further guidance on what to do when a pregnant woman reports reduced fetal movements, see the care pathway endorsed by all the professional associations of midwives and obstetricians in Australia and New Zealand (Fig. 39.3) (Flenady et al., 2019).

The most recent published systematic review which contained a large sample from the AFFIRM trial found: 'Instructing pregnant women on fetal movement counting compared with no instruction is not associated with a clear improvement in pregnancy outcomes. There are weak associations with some secondary outcomes such as pre-term delivery, induction of labor, and cesarean delivery' (Bellussi et al., 2020).

On ultrasound it can be observed that babies display chest wall movements that appear to be 'breathing'

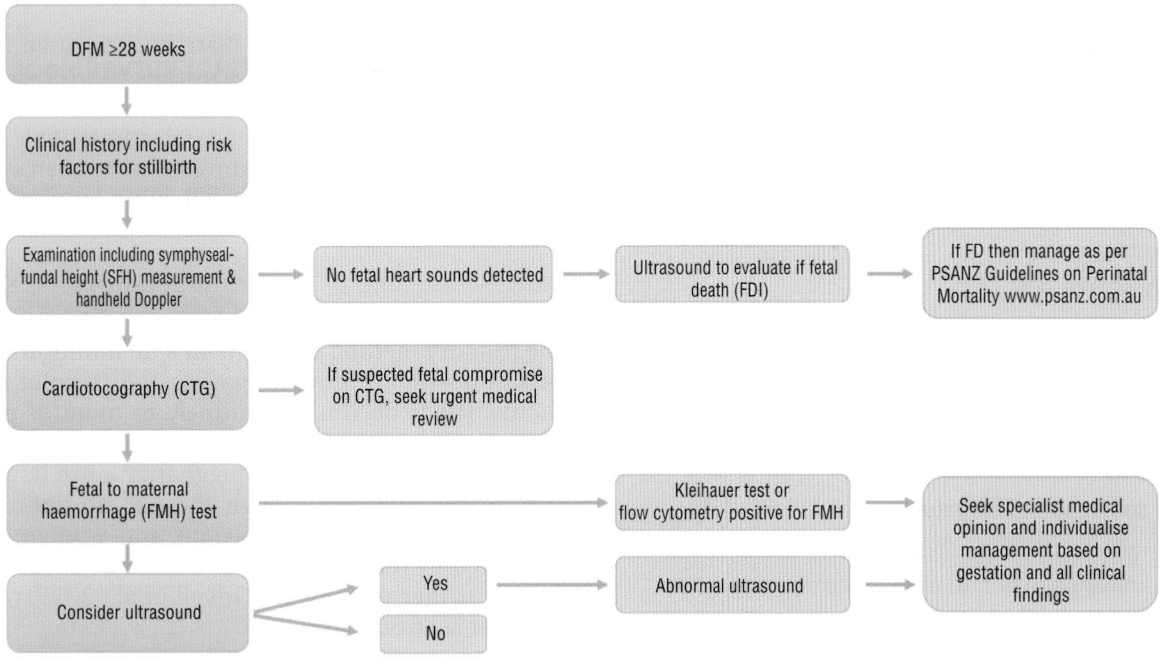

FIGURE 39.3 Care pathway for women presenting with decreased fetal movements from 28 weeks gestation
(Source: Gardener et al., 2017)

movements. During the last couple of months in a normal pregnancy, these 'breathing' movements may become irregular and have a frequency between 10 and 200 breaths/minute (Adelson et al., 1999). The complete absence of breathing is observed in some normal fetuses for up to 122 minutes (fetal apnoea), which indicates that monitoring of respiratory movements may require a long observation time (Adelson et al., 1999; Rayburn, 1990). Women often report fetal hiccup movements that can be very intense, but there is no known pathology associated with this.

CLINICAL POINT

Clinical practice points for women presenting with decreased fetal movements from 28 weeks gestation

Advice to pregnant women

- Be aware of baby's movements daily.
- Provide PSANZ patient information brochure (https://sanda.psanz.com.au/parent-centre/pregnancy/).
- Women with concerns about decreased or absent fetal movements should be advised to contact their midwife or health care provider immediately.
- Women with concerns about decreased or absent fetal movements should be assessed by their midwife or healthcare provider immediately.
- For Australian midwives and women: see the Centre of Research Excellence in Stillbirth, *Raising awareness and improving care for women with decreased fetal movements,* 2019, available from https://stillbirthcre.org.au/about-us/our-work/the-safer-baby-bundle/decreased-fetal-movements/.

Risk factors for stillbirth

- Previous stillbirth
- Fetal growth restriction and small for gestational age (SGA)
- Antepartum haemorrhage
- Diabetes
- Hypertension
- Parity of 0 or >3
- Advanced maternal age (>35 years)
- In vitro fertilisation (IVF)
- Indigenous ethnicity
- Maternal obesity (BMI >25)
- Smoking or illicit drug use
- Low socioeconomic status

Examination

- Abdominal palpation to assess uterine tone and tenderness, fetal lie/presentation.
- Symphyseal fundal height (SFH) to be measured in centimetres and plotted on growth chart.
- Handheld ultrasound Doppler is recommended, not auscultation with a stethoscope or Pinards.
- Record maternal pulse rate and confirm as different to fetal heart rate.
- Blood pressure and temperature.

Cardiotocography

- Perform within 2 hours of presentation.
- Perform for at least 20 min or until satisfactory.
- Use maternal fetal movement recorder during CTG.

Ultrasound

- Consider ultrasound within 24 hours.
- Include fetal biometry, amniotic fluid volume and morphology (if not already performed).
- Placental and fetal Doppler assessment, as indicated.
- The time frame to perform this investigation will depend on the clinical circumstances and availability of appropriate expertise.

Fetal to maternal haemorrhage

- Perform Kleihauer test or flow cytometry test, where feasible.
- Middle cerebral artery Doppler assessment may be performed where expertise in ultrasonography is available.

(*Source:* Gardener et al., 2017, p. 7)

The most commonly used methods for the assessment of fetal wellbeing in high-risk pregnancies include the non-stress test (NST) or antenatal cardiotocography (CTG) (Grivell et al., 2015), the fetal biophysical profile (BPP) (Lalor et al., 2008) and Doppler velocimetry (DV) studies of the fetal circulation. Earlier methods of detecting fetal wellbeing depended largely on the mother recognising FMs.

Methods of antenatal fetal surveillance

For each admission to hospital for birth in Australia, there are about 15–20 antenatal admissions (Adelson et al., 1999). During these admissions, women very often undergo one or other of the following tests to ascertain fetal wellbeing.

Non-stress test and antenatal cardiotocography

Antenatal CTG (or NST) has become widely accepted as the primary method of antenatal fetal monitoring in conjunction with ultrasound imaging and Doppler measurements. It has been used routinely to monitor post-term pregnancies, reduced FM, hypertensive disease, growth restriction and bleeding in pregnancy since its introduction in the 1980s. Although there is no definitive evidence of their efficacy, clinicians and women are often reassured by the findings of antenatal CTGs (Box 39.4.)

For further reading see Grivell et al., 2015, p. 13, and Thacker & Stroup (2003).

Fetal biophysical profile

There are some conditions that may alert the midwife to consider the wellbeing of the fetus through measurement

Box 39.4 Antenatal cardiotocography/non-stress test

Cardiotocography (CTG) is a continuous recording of the fetal heart rate obtained via an ultrasound transducer placed on the mother's abdomen. It is widely used in pregnancy as a method of assessing fetal wellbeing, predominantly in pregnancies with increased risk of complications.

The non-stress test (NST) is widely used for antenatal surveillance in an effort to detect intrauterine fetal compromise. During an NST a baby's heart rate is monitored to see how it responds to the baby's movements. The term 'non-stress' refers to the fact that nothing is done to place stress on the fetus during the test. The results of the NST are:

- *Reactive*: before week 32 of pregnancy, results are considered normal (reactive) if the baby's heartbeat accelerates to a certain level above the baseline twice or more for at least 10 seconds each within a 20-minute window. At week 32 of pregnancy or later, if the baby's heartbeat accelerates to a certain level above the baseline twice or more for at least 15 seconds each within a 20-minute window, the results are considered reactive.
- *Non-reactive*: if the baby's heartbeat doesn't meet the criteria described above, the results are considered non-reactive. Non-reactive results might occur because the baby was inactive or asleep during the test.

There is no clear evidence from studies that computerised or other antenatal CTG improves perinatal outcome.

(Source: Grivell et al., 2015)

of the **biophysical profile (BPP)**. Tables 39.1 and 39.2 describe the maternal conditions that may cause chronic hypoxia, leading to a depressed central nervous system in the fetus. This will manifest as reduced heart rate variability, decreased movement, decreased tone, and fewer than usual breathing movements. If the degree of cardiovascular compensation to protect vital organs (such as the brain and heart) is severe, depressed renal blood flow also results in oligohydramnios (Sarris, Bewley et al., 2012).

The BPP combines the use of CTG with the ultrasound assessment of FM, fetal tone, fetal breathing movements and amniotic fluid volume. Each parameter is scored 0–2 points, with a maximum total score of 10. A normal score (8) is reassuring, has a high negative predictive value and is associated with a low stillbirth rate (0.8%) (Thompson et al., 2012) (Table 39.2).

The impact of the BPP on other interventions such as length of hospitalisation, serious short-term and long-term neonatal morbidity and parental satisfaction requires further evaluation. At present, there is insufficient evidence from randomised trials to support the use of BPP as a test of fetal wellbeing in high-risk pregnancies (Everett & Peebles, 2015; Lalor et al., 2008).

Umbilical artery Doppler velocimetry (DV)

Doppler ultrasonography is used to assess the flow velocity waveforms in the fetal umbilical artery. Some clinicians also observe the maternal vessels supplying the placental intervillous space and (especially since the development of colour flow imaging) other fetal vessels, including aorta and cerebral arteries (Alfirevic et al., 2015). The study of the umbilical artery has remained the most widely used approach, however, because less-experienced operators can achieve highly reproducible results with simple, inexpensive continuous-wave equipment.

Umbilical artery DV has been adapted as a fetal surveillance technique because it is believed that flow velocity waveforms in the umbilical artery of fetuses with normal growth differ from those in fetuses with growth restriction. The waveform in a normally growing fetus has high-velocity diastolic flow, whereas in cases of Intrauterine Growth Restriction (IUGR) this flow is diminished. With extreme IUGR, the flow may be absent or even reversed.

The assessment of umbilical artery waveforms by Doppler ultrasonography in *high-risk pregnancies* (e.g. in

Table 39.1 Conditions that may predispose the fetus to chronic hypoxia and alert the clinician to undertake a biophysical profile

Maternal conditions	Pregnancy-related conditions
Antiphospholipid syndrome	Pregnancy-induced hypertension
Poorly controlled hyperthyroidism	Decreased FM
Haemoglobinopathies such as thalassaemia	Oligohydramnios
Cyanotic heart disease	Polyhydramnios
Systemic lupus erythematosus	IUGR
Chronic renal disease	Post-term pregnancy
Type 1 diabetes mellitus	Moderate to severe isoimmunisation
Hypertensive disorders	Previous fetal demise (unexplained or recurrent risk)
	Multiple gestation with significant growth discrepancy

Table 39.2 Components of the biophysical profile		
Biophysical variable	Normal score = 2	Abnormal score = 0
Non-stress test (reactive fetal heart rate pattern on CTG)	Reactive is >2 accelerations in a 20-minute period (15 beats per minute × 15 seconds above baseline heart rate)	Non-reactive (abnormal) is ≤2 accelerations
Fetal breathing	At least one episode of breathing >30 seconds in 30 minutes	Absent breathing
Fetal movement	Three or more discrete body or limb movements within 30 minutes	Absent fetal movement
Fetal tone	One or more episodes of extension of a fetal extremity with return to flexion, or opening or closing of a hand within 30 minutes	Absent
Amniotic fluid	A single vertical pocket of amniotic fluid exceeding 2 cm is considered evidence of adequate amniotic fluid	Absent or insufficient
Each of the components is given a score of 2 (normal or present as defined previously) or 0 (abnormal, absent or insufficient). A composite score of 8 or 10 is normal, a score of 6 is equivocal and a score of 4 or less is abnormal. In the presence of oligohydramnios, further evaluation is warranted regardless of the composite score.		

fetuses with IUGR or those at risk, such as hypertensive pregnancies) may reduce the odds of perinatal death by 38% (Alfirevic et al., 2017a) and has also been shown to lead to fewer caesarean sections and inductions of labour. It has not, however, altered the rate of births using forceps or ventouse and there is no clear difference in the number of stillbirths or of babies with a low Apgar score 5 minutes after birth (Alfirevic et al., 2017a; Everett & Peebles, 2015).

Assessment of low-risk pregnancies to determine babies at risk of birth asphyxia is currently an area requiring more study, given that possibly over 60% of babies who suffer fetal asphyxia occur in this apparently 'low-risk' population. Five Cochrane systematic reviews have shown a lack of effective strategies for identifying the 'at-risk' baby prior to birth in 'low-risk' women at term (Alfirevic et al., 2015, 2017a; Bricker et al., 2015; Devane et al., 2017; Grivell et al., 2015). See Fig. 39.4 for steps to take when suspecting a small for gestational age (SGA) fetus antenatally. See also the New Zealand guideline showing the integration of most of the tests mentioned here for assessing babies at risk (New Zealand Maternal Fetal Medicine Network (NZMFMN), 2014). And also https://www.nationalwomenshealth.adhb.govt.nz/assets/Womens-health/Documents/Policies-and-guidelines/Small-for-Gestational-Age-SGA-and-Fetal-Growth-Restriction-from-34-weeks-Detection-and-Management.pdf.

INTERVENTIONS IN LABOUR

Electronic fetal monitoring/cardiotocography

It is beyond the scope of this chapter to do other than introduce the subject of **electronic fetal monitoring** and the midwife is advised to refer to Gibb & Arulkumaran's very comprehensive book *Fetal Monitoring in Practice* (2008) and a review by Pinas & Chandraharan (2016).

Electronic fetal monitoring is defined as 'the use of electronic fetal heart-rate monitoring for the evaluation of fetal wellbeing in labour' (National Institute for Health and Care Excellence (NICE), 2017). The word cardiotocography translated means 'a technical means of recording (-graphy) the fetal heartbeat (cardio-) and the uterine contractions (-toco-) during labour'. Thus, CTG records changes in the fetal heart rate and their temporal relationship to uterine contractions.

There are two methods for FHR monitoring:

External FHR monitoring uses a device to listen to or record the fetal heartbeat through the mother's abdomen. Continuous and/or intermittent electronic fetal monitoring may be used during labour. An ultrasound transducer placed on the mother's abdomen conducts the sounds of the fetal heart to a computer. The rate and pattern of the fetal heart are displayed on the computer screen and printed onto special graph paper.

Internal FHR monitoring uses an electronic transducer connected directly to the fetal scalp. A wire electrode is attached to the fetal scalp through the cervical opening and is connected to the monitor. This type of electrode is sometimes called a spiral or scalp electrode. The ST waveform of the fetal electrocardiogram (ECG) provides continuous information on the ability of the fetal heart muscle to respond to stress of labour. Internal monitoring may be used when external monitoring of the FHR is inadequate, or closer surveillance is needed.

Direct risks associated with (internal) fetal scalp electrodes

In about 10% of cases, the use of an internally inserted electrode is attached to the fetal scalp to measure the electric currents from the baby's heart. It necessitates rupture of membranes and may contribute to the following:

- bruising or scratching of the baby's scalp
- the risk of infection to the mother or baby from an outside source

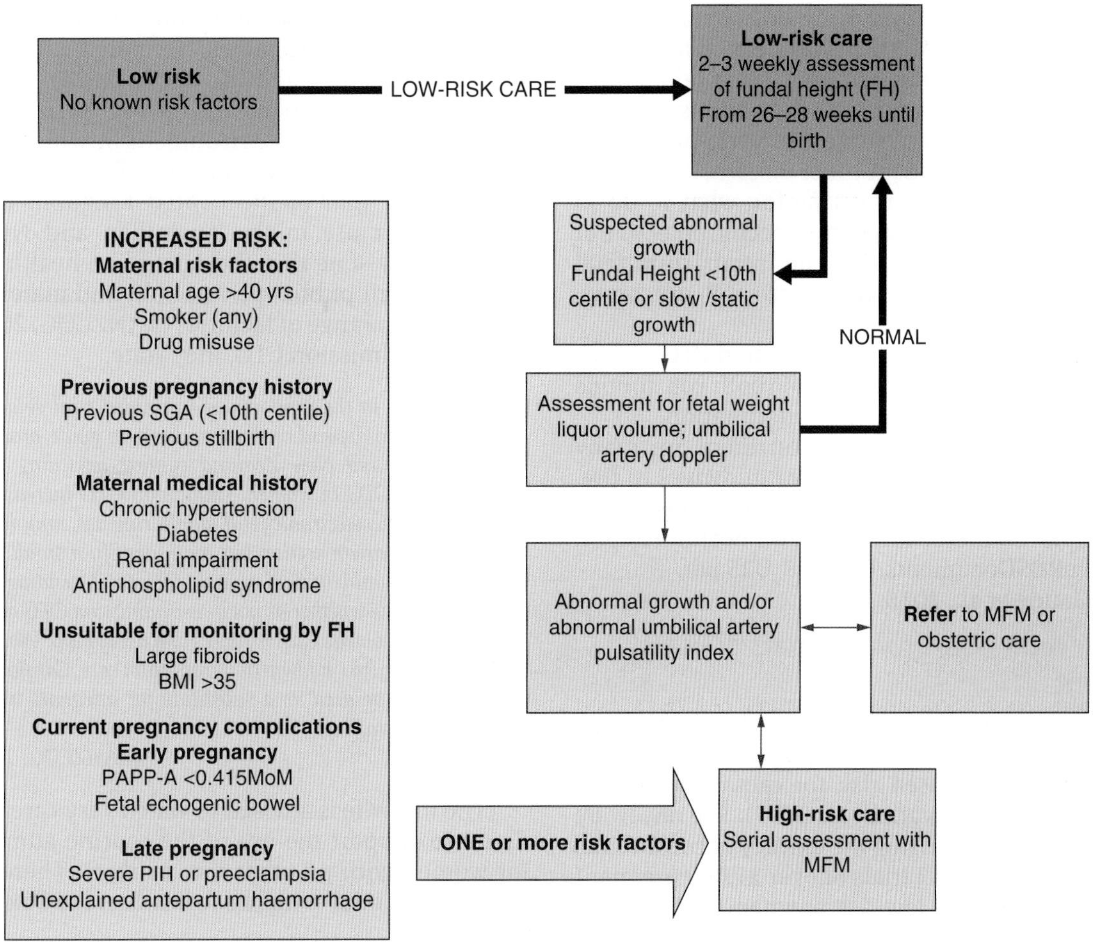

FIGURE 39.4 Fetal surveillance algorithm and management of suspected SGA

- the restriction of movement for the mother, which can make labour more painful and difficult
- the risk of infection from mother to child (internal monitoring is contraindicated in women with HIV, herpes or hepatitis).

The procedure has attracted controversy among some practitioners who believe it is unnecessarily invasive. Some studies have suggested that its use is associated with higher, rather than lower, rates of caesarean births and forceps delivery.

The aim of fetal monitoring is to identify babies who may be short of oxygen (hypoxic) to guide additional assessments of fetal wellbeing, or to determine whether intervention is called for and the baby needs to be delivered by CS or instrumental vaginal birth (Alfirevic et al., 2017b). Fetal monitoring allows detection and analysis of the FHR (via Doppler ultrasound with external transducers, or direct measurement with a fetal scalp electrode) and a semiquantitative analysis of uterine muscle activity and contractions. FHR pattern recognition, including the relationship between the uterine contractions and FHR decelerations, is fundamental to the use of continuous CTG monitoring. Algorithms have been developed in a bid to assess and record what may be considered abnormal, necessitating urgent delivery of the baby. However, CTG traces are often interpreted differently by different caregivers. The visual interpretation of CTG based on 'pattern recognition' is fraught with inter- and intra-observer variability (Devane & Lalor, 2005; Pinas & Chandraharan, 2016).

Although CTG was initially developed as a screening tool to predict fetal hypoxia, its positive predictive value for intrapartum fetal hypoxia is approximately only 30% with a corresponding false positive rate of (60%) (Pinas & Chandraharan, 2016):

> *CTG during labour is associated with reduced rates of neonatal seizures, but no clear differences in cerebral palsy, infant mortality or other standard measures of neonatal wellbeing. However, continuous CTG was associated with an increase in caesarean sections and instrumental vaginal births. The challenge is how best to convey these results to women to enable them to make an informed decision without compromising the normality of labour.*
> (Alfirevic et al., 2017b, p. 2)

EFM was introduced with the aim of reducing perinatal mortality and cerebral palsy; however, systematic reviews of randomised controlled trials (RCTs) have not demonstrated its effectiveness in the 50 years since it was introduced (NICE, 2017; Pinas & Chandraharan, 2016). Along with the use of EFM, there has been a significant increase in caesarean section and operative vaginal birth rates (Pinas & Chandraharan, 2016). Both admission CTG and continuous EFM are the subject of widespread concern in midwifery. The student must discern, in collaboration with the woman she is caring for, what to do in practice. This section will address the specific objective of reducing inappropriate or inadequate intrapartum fetal surveillance and reducing adverse perinatal outcomes, with specific reference to:

- decisions relating to the use of admission CTG
- decisions relating to the use of EFM (both continuous and intermittent) or intermittent auscultation.

For further advice and information there are many national and state-based guidelines for midwives to use. The 'NSW Maternity—Fetal heart rate monitoring guide' is one example of these: https://www1.health.nsw.gov.au/pds/ActivePDSDocuments/GL2018_025.pdf.

See also Maude et al., 2016.

Measuring fetal heart rate as part of initial assessment

Current evidence from the Cochrane Library finds *no benefit* for the use of admission CTG in *low-risk pregnancy* and an associated increased risk for caesarean of 20% (Alfirevic et al., 2017b; Devane et al., 2017). The review by Alfirevic et al. (2017), assessing the efficacy of continuous EFM in labour, included 13 trials of over 37,000 pregnant women in both high- and low-risk pregnancies.

- Overall, a statistically significant decrease in neonatal seizures was associated with routine continuous EFM compared with intermittent auscultation (RR 0.50; 95% CI 0.31–0.80).
- No significant differences were observed in perinatal deaths or cerebral palsy.
- An increase associated with the use of continuous EFM was observed in the rate of:
  - caesarean birth (RR 1.63, 95% CI 1.29–2.07)
  - operative vaginal birth (RR 1.15, 95% CI 1.01–1.33).

The authors concluded that the only clinically significant benefit from the use of routine continuous EFM was in the reduction of neonatal seizures. In view of the increase in caesarean and operative vaginal deliveries, the long-term benefit of this reduction must be evaluated in the decision reached jointly by the pregnant woman and her clinician to use continuous EFM or intermittent auscultation during labour.

NICE (2017) recommends offering auscultation of the FHR at first contact with a woman in labour, and at each further assessment using either a Pinard stethoscope or Doppler ultrasound, carrying out the auscultation immediately after a contraction for at least 1 minute and recording it as a single rate. In addition to this, record accelerations and decelerations if heard and palpate the maternal pulse to differentiate between the maternal and fetal heartbeats (NICE, 2017, p. 23).

For women at low risk of complications there is insufficient evidence about whether CTG as part of the initial assessment either improves outcomes or results in harm for women and their babies, compared with intermittent auscultation alone (NICE, 2017, p. 24). However, the Guideline Development Group for Australia and New Zealand feel that the environment in which obstetrics is practised in Australia and New Zealand differs sufficiently from that of the United Kingdom to require a guideline for use in the Australian and New Zealand setting. They state that the Australian healthcare system has a different public/private split and maternity care is provided in a range of facilities (RANZCOG, 2019). On the subject of admission CTG, they state:

> *Limitations in the randomised controlled trial evidence make it difficult to depend on that evidence to guide practice in the Australian and New Zealand context regarding the use of admission CTG in women. Admission CTG increases the rate of continuous electronic fetal monitoring use, may increase the rate of caesarean section but may identify a small number of previously unidentified at risk fetuses. Attending clinicians should decide whether or not to use admission CTG according to individual women's circumstances and decisions ... Women should receive 1,Äâ;Äâ1 midwifery intrapartum care. Cardiotocography should not be used as a substitute for adequate intrapartum midwifery staffing.*
>
> (RANZCOG, 2019, p.12)

(The midwife is advised to watch very carefully for evidence to support the use of the routine admission trace for women with no other risk markers. There appears to be no substantial evidence for its use; see Box 39.5.)

Continuous EFM

The use of continuous EFM for intrapartum fetal surveillance has now become entrenched in obstetric practice without robust RCT evidence to support it. The RCTs that have been undertaken confirm that the use of continuous EFM significantly increases the rate of **operative birth**.

Continuous electronic FHR monitoring in labour may be interpreted through computerised systems designed to objectively detect abnormalities in FHR patterns during labour that are associated with asphyxia and bring them to the attention of birth attendants. These systems, known as ST-Analyser or STAN, analyse the fetal ECG using a computerised system. Decision support software designed to improve the identification of abnormal FHR patterns and reduce the rates of unnecessary intervention was tested in a large randomised trial of more than 46,000 women in the

Box 39.5 CTG settings

It is recommended that settings on cardiotocographs in institutions in Australia and New Zealand show:

- paper speed of 1 cm/min
- sensitivity displays of 20 b.p.m./cm
- FHR range displays of 50–210 b.p.m.

(Source: RANZCOG, 2014)

UK (INFANT Collaborative Group, 2017). The trial found no evidence that the use of decision-support software in conjunction with CTG reduced the likelihood of poor neonatal outcomes compared with CTG alone; the researchers concluded that 'use of computerised interpretation of CTG in women who have continuous electronic fetal monitoring in labour does not improve clinical outcomes for mothers or babies' (INFANT Collaborative Group, 2017, p. 1719). The authors noted that the quality of care in labour is a major concern for women, their families and the health professionals providing care for them. Technologies to improve intrapartum monitoring that identify early signs of fetal hypoxia during labour are needed so that clinicians can intervene and attempt to prevent poor neonatal outcomes. The results of the INFANT trial showed that the method of decision support tested did not achieve this aim (INFANT Collaborative, 2017).

When should continuous fetal monitoring in labour be recommended?

Notwithstanding the results of the INFANT trial (2017), the intrapartum guidelines from the NICE group in the UK (NICE, 2017) advise changing from intermittent to continuous CTG if any of the following risk factors are present:

- maternal pulse over 120 beats/minute on two occasions 30 minutes apart
- temperature of 38°C or above on a single reading, or 37.5°C or above on two consecutive occasions 1 hour apart
- suspected chorioamnionitis or sepsis pain reported by the woman that differs from the pain normally associated with contractions
- the presence of significant meconium
- fresh vaginal bleeding that develops in labour
- severe hypertension: a single reading of either systolic blood pressure of 160 mmHg or more or diastolic blood pressure of 110 mmHg or more, measured between contractions
- hypertension: either systolic blood pressure of 140 mmHg or more or diastolic blood pressure of 90 mmHg or more on two consecutive readings taken 30 minutes apart, measured between contractions
- a reading of 2+ of protein on urinalysis and a single reading of either raised systolic blood pressure (140 mmHg or more) or raised diastolic blood pressure (90 mmHg or more)
- confirmed delay in the first or second stage of labour
- contractions that last longer than 60 seconds (hypertonus)
- more than five contractions in 10 minutes (tachysystole) when oxytocin is used.

The guidelines further note:

- Do not offer continuous CTG to women who have non-significant meconium if there are no other risk factors (NICE, 2017).
- Do not regard amniotomy alone for suspected delay in the established first stage of labour as an indication to start continuous CTG (NICE, 2017).

FHR monitoring is a highly complex task, often undertaken in a stressful working environment. It requires:

- a sound understanding of fetal physiological responses to hypoxia
- good pattern-recognition skills
- the ability to integrate this knowledge with each clinical situation.

The baseline FHR is analysed over 5–10 min and expressed in beats per minute (b.p.m.):

> *The normal range is considered to be 110–160 b.p.m. It is regulated by the combined action of the sympathetic and parasympathetic nervous systems. Consequently, preterm fetuses with a less developed parasympathetic system will commonly show a higher baseline rate compared with term or post-term fetuses when the parasympathetic system is well developed, and they will usually have baseline rates between 110 and 130 b.p.m. It is not uncommon for a post-term fetus to have a baseline heart rate between 90 and 110 b.p.m. as a consequence of maturity of the parasympathetic nervous system. This should be considered as normal if other parameters on the CTG trace are reassuring.*
>
> (Pinas & Chandraharan, 2016, p. 35)

An increase in the baseline rate of greater than 160 b.p.m. persisting for more than 10 min is called baseline tachycardia (Pinas & Chandraharan, 2016). A baseline FHR of less than 100 b.p.m. lasting for more than 10 min is called baseline bradycardia (Pinas & Chandraharan, 2016).

EFM was introduced in the 1960s as an alternative to the traditional auscultation by stethoscope or fetoscope; it involves monitoring the FHR by either internal or external methods. Sampling of the fetal scalp blood during labour and delivery and testing it for pH (a measure of acid–base balance) complements the external and internal methods. EFM diffused rapidly into practice in the 1970s; it was used in the majority of deliveries in the United States by 1975. The INFANT study (2017) is the most comprehensive systematic assessment of EFM to date.

REFLECTIVE THINKING EXERCISE

You are encouraged to read an account of the attempts to assess the technology, and reactions to the assessment, as well as some factors that might have prevented the assessment from influencing practice substantially, recounted in a paper by Banta & Thacker (2002), entitled 'Electronic fetal monitoring: lessons from a formative case of health technology assessment'.

Intermittent auscultation in labour

In a pregnancy where women are at low risk of complications in established labour, the preferred method for assessing the wellbeing of babies is through **intermittent auscultation** (NICE, 2017) using a Pinard stethoscope or Doppler ultrasound.

- Based upon the Dublin trial (MacDonald et al., 1985) the NICE and FIGO guidelines recommend 15-minute intervals of intermittent auscultation. However, given the lack of robust evidence to support this recommendation, the widespread established standard practice in Australia and New Zealand is as follows. Intermittent Auscultation should be undertaken and documented:

- every 15–30 minutes in the active phase of the first stage of labour
- with each contraction or at least every five minutes in the active second stage of labour (RANZCOG, 2019). Use either a Pinard stethoscope or Doppler ultrasound.

- Carry out intermittent auscultation immediately after a contraction for at least 1 minute, and record it as a single rate.
- Record accelerations and decelerations if heard.
- Palpate the maternal pulse hourly or more often if there are any concerns, to differentiate between the maternal and fetal heartbeats (NICE CG 190, 2017, p. 33).
- The FHR should be auscultated at specified intervals (usually every 15 minutes in the first stage and every 5 minutes in the second stage; this of course depends on whether the woman is comfortable with this arrangement).
- Any intrapartum events that may affect the FHR should be noted, at the time that they happen, in the mother's notes and signed, and the time noted as usual.

The latest evidence for recommendations on fetal heart assessment and reasons for transfer to continuous EFM in the UK (NICE CG 190, 2017) concludes that:

- current evidence does not support the use of the admission CTG in low-risk women and it is not recommended
- intermittent auscultation of the FHR is recommended for low-risk women in established labour in any birth setting; for a woman who is healthy and has had an otherwise uncomplicated pregnancy, intermittent auscultation should be offered and recommended in labour to monitor fetal wellbeing
- initial auscultation of the fetal heart is recommended at first contact in early labour and at each further assessment undertaken to determine whether labour has become established
- once a woman is in established labour, intermittent auscultation of the fetal heart after a contraction should be continued, for at least 1 minute and recorded as a single rate:
  - every 15–30 minutes in the first stage
  - every 5 minutes in the second stage.

Changing to continuous EFM in low-risk women should be advised for the following reasons:

- significant meconium-stained liquor; for light meconium-stained liquor, consider the whole clinical picture to decide whether to change to continuous EFM
- abnormal FHR detected by intermittent auscultation (less than 110 b.p.m.; greater than 160 b.p.m.; any decelerations after a contraction)
- if there is evidence on auscultation of any decelerations
- if any intrapartum risk factors develop.
- maternal pyrexia (defined as 38.0°C once or 37.5°C on two occasions 2 hours apart)
- fresh bleeding developing in labour
- oxytocin use for augmentation
- at the woman's request.

Appropriate monitoring in an uncomplicated 'normal' pregnancy according to the Royal Australian and New Zealand College of Obstetricians and Gynaecologists (RANZCOG) EFM policy is summarised in Box 39.6.

If a woman is advised to have continuous fetal monitoring (when she had previously been intermittently auscultated), be aware of any concerns that the woman has about continuous CTG, and give her and her birth companion(s) the following information:

- Explain that continuous CTG is used to monitor the baby's heartbeat and the labour contractions.
- Explain that it may restrict her mobility.
- Give details of the types of findings that may occur. Explain that a normal trace indicates that the baby is coping well.
- Explain that changes to the baby's heart rate pattern during labour are common and do not necessarily cause concern.
- Explain that if the trace is not normal (Tables 39.3, 39.4) there will be less certainty about the condition of the baby and so continuous monitoring will be advised.
- Explain that decisions about her care during labour and birth will be based on an assessment of several factors, including her preferences, her condition and

Box 39.6 EFM policy—things to do when monitoring using EFM

Before any form of fetal monitoring is undertaken:

- Palpate the maternal pulse simultaneously with FHR auscultation in order to differentiate between the maternal and fetal heart rates.
- Check the date and time settings on CTG machine.
- Label the CTG trace with the mother's name, hospital number, date and time of commencement and include the maternal observations.
- Note contemporaneously any intrapartum events that may affect the fetal heart rate (e.g. vaginal examination, obtaining an FBS, insertion/top-up of an epidural). Include the date, time and signature.
- For continuous CTG, the trace should be reviewed at least every 15–30 minutes and should be acted upon. It should be regularly recorded by either written or electronic entry in the medical record that the CTG has been reviewed.
- Be aware that machines from different manufacturers use different vertical axis scales, and this can change the perception of FHR variability.

CTG = cardiotocography; EFM = electronic fetal monitoring; FBS = fetal blood sample; FHR = fetal heart rate.
(Adapted from Royal Australian and New Zealand College of Obstetricians and Gynaecologists (RANZCOG). *Intrapartum Fetal Surveillance Clinical Guideline*. 3rd ed., 2014)

Table 39.3 Describing the classifications on the CTG

Cardiotocograph (CTG) classification	
NORMAL	A CTG where all four features fall into the reassuring category
SUSPICIOUS	A CTG whose features fall into one of the non-reassuring categories and the remainder of the features are reassuring
PATHOLOGICAL	A CTG whose features fall into two or more non-reassuring categories or one or more abnormal categories

Fetal heart-rate feature classification

	Baseline b.p.m.	Variability b.p.m.	Decelerations	Accelerations
Reassuring	110–160	≥5	None	Present
Non-reassuring	100–109 161–180	<5 for ≥40 but <90 minutes	Early deceleration Variable decelerations Single prolonged deceleration up to 3 minutes	The absence of accelerations with an otherwise normal CTG is of uncertain significance
Abnormal	<100 b.p.m. >180 b.p.m. Sinusoidal pattern for ≥10 minutes	<5 for ≥90 minutes	Atypical variable decelerations Late decelerations Single prolonged deceleration for greater than 3 minutes	

(Based on Oats & Abraham, 2004, E-Book p. 165)

Table 39.4 Definitions and descriptions of individual features of fetal heart rate (FHR) traces

Term	Definition
RATE	
Baseline fetal heart rate (FHR)	The average (mean) level of the FHR when this is stable, excluding accelerations and decelerations. It is determined over a time period of 5 or 10 minutes and expressed in b.p.m. Pre-term infants tend to have values towards the upper end of this range. A trend to a progressive rise in the baseline is important as well as the absolute values
Normal baseline FHR	110–160 b.p.m.
Moderate bradycardia	100–109 b.p.m.
Moderate tachycardia	161–180 b.p.m.
Abnormal bradycardia	<100 b.p.m.
Abnormal tachycardia	>180 b.p.m.
VARIABILITY	
Baseline variability	The minor fluctuations in baseline FHR occurring at three to five cycles per minute. It is measured by estimating the difference in beats per minute (b.p.m.) between the highest peak and lowest trough of fluctuation in a one-minute segment of the trace
Normal baseline variability	Greater than or equal to 5 b.p.m. between contractions
Non-reassuring baseline variability	Less than 5 b.p.m. for 40 minutes or more but less than 90 minutes
Abnormal baseline variability	Less than 5 b.p.m. for 90 minutes or more
ACCELERATIONS	
Normal accelerations	Transient increases in FHR of 15 b.p.m. or more and lasting 15 seconds or more. (The significance of no accelerations on an otherwise normal CTG is unclear)
Decelerations	Transient episodes of slowing of FHR below the baseline level of more than 15 b.p.m. and lasting 15 seconds or more
Early decelerations	Uniform, repetitive, periodic slowing of FHR with onset early in the contraction and return to baseline at the end of the contraction
Late decelerations	Uniform, repetitive, periodic slowing of FHR with onset mid to end of the contraction and the lowest point more than 20 seconds after the peak of the contraction and ending after the contraction. (May also include any pattern of decelerations above)

Continued

Table 39.4 Definitions and descriptions of individual features of fetal heart rate (FHR) traces—cont'd

Term	Definition
Variable decelerations	Variable, intermittent periodic slowing of FHR with rapid onset and recovery. Time relationships with contraction cycle are variable and they may occur in isolation. Sometimes they resemble other types of deceleration patterns in timing and shape
Atypical variable decelerations	Variable decelerations with any of the following additional components: • loss of primary or secondary rise in baseline rate • slow return to baseline FHR after the end of the contraction • prolonged secondary rise in baseline rate • biphasic deceleration • loss of variability during deceleration • continuation of baseline rate at lower level
Prolonged deceleration	An abrupt decrease in FHR to levels below the baseline that lasts at least 60–90 seconds. These decelerations become pathological if they cross two contractions, i.e. greater than 3 minutes
Sinusoidal pattern	A regular oscillation of the baseline long-term variability resembling a sine wave. This smooth, undulating pattern, lasting at least 10 minutes, has a relatively fixed period of 3–5 cycles per minute and an amplitude of 5–15 b.p.m. above and below the baseline. Baseline variability is absent

(Compiled from Guidelines published by Canadian, UK, Australian and New Zealand. National Institute for Health and Clinical Excellence (NICE) 2017. *Intrapartum Care for Healthy Women and Babies* (CG190))

that of her baby, as well as the findings from CTG (NICE, 2017).

- If continuous CTG has been started because of concerns arising from intermittent auscultation, but the trace is normal after 20 minutes, return to intermittent auscultation unless the woman asks to stay on continuous CTG (NICE, 2017).

Measuring lactate through fetal blood sample (FBS)

The scalp blood pH analysis is the standard technique of determining metabolic acidosis in the fetus during labour. However, it may be time consuming and there are difficulties in getting adequate samples of blood, as a minimum sample of 35–50 mL is needed for most machines for automated analysis. The analysis of pH does not discriminate between respiratory and metabolic acidaemia, the latter being associated with neonatal morbidity.

Lactate analysis as an alternative for detecting acidosis is preferred in some centres because less blood is required and can usually be obtained with a single scalp incision and sampling attempt (Okosun & Arulkumaran, 2005; Pennell & Tracy, 1999). Lactate is a metabolite in anaerobic metabolism and reflects tissue hypoxia. Fetal blood analysis using lactate levels is comparable to pH in fetal scalp blood in predicting fetal compromise (Allanson et al., 2017; Wiberg-Itzel et al., 2008). The procedure for measuring lactate has been shown to be more successful than that for pH, because the sample volume needed for this bedside analysis is 5 mL or less. All scalp pH estimations should be interpreted by taking into account the previous pH or lactate measurement, the rate of progress in labour and the clinical features of the mother and baby. FBS should not be taken during or immediately after a prolonged deceleration, and the woman should be in the left-lateral position. (See Box 39.7 and Table 39.5 for summaries of fetal blood analysis.)

Contraindications to FBS include:

- cord prolapse or suspected placental abruption
- risk of maternal-to-fetal transmission of infection (e.g. HIV, hepatitis viruses and HSV virus)
- fetal bleeding disorders (e.g. haemophilia)
- pre-term less than 34 weeks.

Epidural analgesia and anaesthesia

The popularity of epidural anaesthesia for childbirth is a relatively recent phenomenon. It blocks pain without rendering the mother unconscious. No other current drug or technique has that degree of selectivity. Epidural anaesthesia is also adaptable to the wide variety of pain patterns encountered during the course of a normal labour (Caton et al., 2002) (Box 39.8). The character and neurological basis of childbirth pain change during the course of labour. During the first stage, the primary nerves mediating pain are small fibres of the sympathetic division of the autonomic nervous system. This pain is also known as visceral pain, mediated by the nerve fibres from T10 to L1 of the spine (Eltzschig et al., 2003). Women typically perceive this pain as diffuse abdominal cramps, in phase with each uterine contraction. In contrast, pain of the second stage of labour is more continuous than rhythmic, sharper in character, and sensed in the perineum rather than in the abdomen or back. It is mediated by larger, somatic

Box 39.7 Things to consider when taking fetal blood samples

- When seeking a woman's consent to fetal blood sampling it is important to take into consideration the whole context of her labour so far—whether she is progressing well, how tired she is, what the CTG is showing and whether she would prefer to have this intervention or not. Explain the relevance to her of measuring the acid level in the baby's blood.
- Explain the risks and benefits of taking a fetal blood sample.
- Explain that the procedure is invasive and involves using a speculum to visualise the baby's head. It will require making a small scratch on the baby's head and the results may help to inform the next steps to take.
- Fetal blood sampling should be undertaken when the woman is lying comfortably in the left-lateral position.
- Deciding whether to take a pH or a lactate reading will depend on the availability of equipment such as a blood gas machine or a lactate hand-held meter.
- Table 39.4 provides an outline of the interpretation of the fetal blood sample and suggested clinical management.
- If a fetal blood sample cannot be obtained, and the CTG reading has not improved, the lead clinician will assess the situation and may advise a caesarean section or instrumental birth (forceps or ventouse).

CTG = cardiotocograph.
(Based on NSW Health. *Maternity—Fetal Heart Rate Monitoring GL2016_001 Policy*. 2018 (review date 06-Jan-2021); and NSW Health 'Between the Flags—keeping patients safe' policy: http://www1.health.nsw.gov.au/pds/ActivePDSDocuments/GL2016_001.pdf; see also NICE, 2017)

sensory fibres from sacral portions of the spinal cord (Caton et al., 2002) mediated by fibres from S1 to S4 of the spinal cord (Eltzschig et al., 2003).

Other types of pain may superimpose on the basic patterns described above. For example, when the head of the fetus is pushed hard against a large nerve against the posterior wall of the pelvis, the woman may experience intense pain in the lower back or in a discrete area of a hip or leg. If this pressure is prolonged or severe, it may result in temporary or even permanent nerve damage. A full, distended bladder may cause continuous suprapubic pain that may be confused with the pain of labour. Other patterns of pain may be caused by placental abruption or a ruptured uterus. An experienced midwife may easily evaluate the distribution and character of labour pain, but judging its severity may be far more difficult. Individuals respond to pain differently according to personal, familial and cultural factors (Caton et al., 2002).

In Australia, each year approximately 32% of all women who give birth experience either an epidural or a spinal block as analgesia during labour (Australian Institute of Health and Welfare, (AIHW), 2021). In New Zealand, each year nearly 26% of all women giving birth have an epidural (Ministry of Health (MOH), 2017; NZCOM MMPO, 2017).

Mechanism of epidural and spinal anaesthesia

Labour pain is transmitted through lower thoracic, lumbar and sacral nerve roots, which are amenable to epidural blockade (Eltzschig et al., 2003). Epidural analgesia is achieved by placement of a catheter into the lumbar epidural space or the space between the dura mater and the ligamentum flavum at spinal cord levels C7 to C10. The space is filled with loose adipose tissue lymphatics and blood vessels, and the solution tends to remain localised at the level where injected. The solution does not contact the spinal cord or the cerebrospinal fluid, so there is less risk of central nervous system infection than with a spinal injection. Postoperative urinary retention is common, as parasympathetic nerves are blocked (Bryant, 2003, p. 229). Solutions of a local anaesthetic, opioid or both can then be administered as intermittent rapid doses or as a continuous infusion (Box 39.9). In the alternative technique of combined spinal–epidural analgesia a single bolus of an opioid, sometimes in combination with local anaesthetic, is injected into the subarachnoid space, in addition to the placement of an epidural catheter (Eltzschig et al., 2003, p. 319).

In spinal anaesthesia, the local anaesthetic is injected into the cerebrospinal fluid in the subarachnoid space below the level of termination of the spinal cord—at

Table 39.5 Interpreting fetal blood samples during labour[a]

Fetal blood sample	Lactate (mmol/L)	pH	Action
Normal	≤4.1	≥7.25	Repeat in an hour if FHR abnormality persists
Pre-acidotic range (Suspicious / Borderline)	4.2–4.8	7.21–7.24	Repeat within 30 minutes if FHR abnormality persists
Acidotic range (Abnormal)	>4.8	≤7.20	The baby should be delivered as soon as possible.

[a]Interpretation of fetal blood samples should always take into account the changes from a previous sample of pH or lactate and the rate of progress of labour.
(Sources: NSW Health, 2018; The Women's Hospital, 2017)

Box 39.8 Common terms

Commonly used terms in analgesia/anaesthesia:

- *Analgesia*—the use of medication to decrease or alter the normal sensation of pain
- *Anaesthesia*—the use of medication to provide partial or complete loss of sensation with or without the loss of consciousness
- *Combined spinal/epidural*—the simultaneous combination of both spinal and epidural anaesthesia
- *Local anaesthetic agent*—a pharmacological agent capable of producing a loss of sensation in an area of the body
- *Epidural (lumbar or peridural) block*—injection of an anaesthetic again with or without added opioid and/or adrenaline (epinephrine) into the epidural space (lumbar spinous interspace between L4 and L5) as intermittent boluses or a continuous infusion
- *Neuraxial analgesia*—administration of analgesic agents (local anaesthetic or opioids) either continuously or intermittently into the epidural or intrathecal space to relieve visceral pain
- *Patient-controlled epidural analgesia*—a technique that allows the woman to self-administer a dose of epidural medication
- *Regional (as opposed to general) anaesthetic*—the use of local anaesthetic agents to induce anaesthesia through the effect onto the spinal cord and nerve roots. Techniques include epidural, spinal and combined epidural and spinal. Obstetric regional generally refers to a partial or complete loss of sensation below the T8 to T10 level
- *Spinal anaesthesia (saddle block)*—an injection of an anaesthetic agent with or without added opioid and/or adrenaline into the subarachnoid space (lumbar spinous interspace between L4 and L5) as single-dose intermittent boluses or as a continuous infusion

(Sources: Poole, 2003a, 2003b)

Box 39.9 Commonly used drugs in childbirth

Opioids

- *Morphine*—crosses placenta rapidly; fetal effects are dose and gestational age dependent; decreased FHR variability; maternal and neonatal CNS depression; inhibits oxytocin release and decreases uterine contractions
- *Fentanyl*—potent respiratory depressant; cumulative effect with large dose over time; crosses placenta rapidly; excreted in breast milk; has a fast onset and a short duration of action (2 min and 30 min, respectively)
- *Meperidine (pethidine)*—a synthetic opioid, related to fentanyl; more lipid soluble than morphine and crosses the placenta readily; metabolised to normeperidine (norpethidine) by the liver
- *Remifentanil patient-controlled intravenous analgesia*—can provide adequate analgesia and is useful when epidural analgesia is contraindicated; remifentanil patient-controlled analgesia requires close monitoring to avoid maternal hypoxia due to respiratory depression
- *Practice note:* All parenteral opioids will cause a degree of maternal sedation, respiratory depression, dysphoria, nausea and vomiting. All opioids cross the placenta and have effects on the FHR variability, neonatal sedation and respiratory depression.

Analgesia/anaesthesia

- *Procaine/novocaine*—slow onset with short duration; poor spreading and penetrating properties; has been used for spinals but because of short duration is generally combined with another agent for labour
- *Lignocaine (lidocaine)/Xylocaine*—relatively fast onset with intermediate duration; produces profound motor blockade; generally used for surgical block; crosses the placenta rapidly; fetus and newborn can metabolise; elimination half-life in newborns is approx. 3 hours; may produce CNS depression in newborn; small amounts excreted into breast milk but considered compatible with breastfeeding
- *Ropivacaine*—moderate onset with long duration; less potent than bupivacaine but with similar blocking properties; intensity and duration of motor blockade shorter than that of bupivacaine when used for caesarean
- *Bupivacaine/Marcaine or Sensorcaine*—moderate onset and long duration; used for subarachnoid blockade for caesarean birth; duration and extent of blockade is dose related; approx. four times as potent as lignocaine; duration is enhanced if adrenaline is added; accidental IV administration can cause acute cardiovascular collapse

CNS = central nervous system; FHR = fetal heart rate; IV = intravenous.
(Sources: Phillips et al., 2017; Poole, 2003a, 2003b)

about the level of L3–L4 or L4–L5. The needle and solution come into contact with the cerebrospinal fluid, necessitating strict aseptic techniques in order to prevent infections such as meningitis occurring (Bryant, 2003, p. 229). The use of a subarachnoid bolus of opioids results in the rapid onset of regional anaesthesia with virtually no motor blockade. In contrast to epidural local anaesthetics, spinal opioids do not cause impairment of balance, giving the labouring woman the option to continue moving around (Eltzschig et al., 2003).

Combined spinal–epidural (CSE) analgesia blocks both low thoracic and sacral nerve roots with minimal maternal and umbilical cord blood concentrations of analgesics because of the low doses of local anaesthesia and opioid required to initiate spinal analgesia (Sng et al., 2017). Some studies have suggested that there may be an increase in the frequency of non-reassuring patterns in the FHR, particularly bradycardia, with combined spinal–epidural analgesia, and such patterns may lead to emergency caesarean delivery (Clarke et al., 1994; Eltzschig et al., 2003; Gambling et al., 1998). The Cochrane systematic review also reports these studies and found an increased risk of assisted vaginal birth in the epidural group (RR 1.44, 95% CI 1.29 to 1.60; 30 studies and 9948 women; studies = 30 . However, in studies undertaken since 2005 and included in this Cochrane review there was not a higher incidence of forceps or vacuum assisted birth possibly associated with the use of lower concentrations of local anaesthetic and more modern epidural techniques such as patient-controlled epidural analgesia (PCEA) Anim-Somuah et al., 2018. In the latest Cochrane review (Anim-Somuah et al., 2018) the CS rate did not reach a statistically significant difference (RR 1.07, 95% CI 0.96 to 1.18; including 33 studies and 10,350 women).

Although there are insufficient data to establish whether there is a causal association, there are no studies suggesting that combined spinal–epidural analgesia is associated with an increase in adverse outcomes for the fetus (Eltzschig et al., 2003, p. 321).

For many years there has been debate about the efficacy of an epidural offered early in labour. There is a widely held opinion that having an epidural early in labour—before about 4–5 cm dilation—increases the risk of operative intervention. The results of a French study published in 2005 demonstrated that the placement of an epidural when cephalic presentation was still 'high' was associated with a higher percentage of occiput posterior and transverse positions during labour independently of other risk factors studied (Le Ray et al., 2005). Lieberman et al. (2005), in studying the position changes of the fetus during labour, concluded that the consistently higher rate of instrumental vaginal birth associated with epidural analgesia in randomised trials (Lieberman & O'Donoghue, 2002) could result from an increase in abnormal fetal position complicating delivery. Use of epidural analgesia for pain relief has been consistently associated with a lower rate of spontaneous vaginal birth (Anim-Somuah et al., 2018; Howell et al., 2001; Lieberman & O'Donoghue, 2002; Roberts et al., 2000, 2002).

However, the latest pragmatic randomised controlled trial of over 3000 women having a first baby in the UK found that lying down compared with being upright in the second stage of labour with a low-dose epidural increased the chance of spontaneous vaginal birth (41.1% versus 35.2%). This represents a 5.9% absolute increase in the chance of spontaneous vaginal birth in the lying-down group. There didn't appear to be any differences in the rate of instrumental vaginal birth, obstetric anal sphincter injury, infant Apgar score less than 4 at 5 minutes or maternal faecal incontinence at 1 year (Epidural and Position Trial Collaborative Group, BUMPES trial, 2017). This report of the optimal position for women to achieve a non-instrumental vaginal birth indicates that a policy of adopting a lying-down position in the second stage of labour in women having their first baby with epidural analgesia increases the chances of a spontaneous vaginal birth (number needed to treat: 17 women (95% CI 11–40) to achieve one additional spontaneous vaginal birth (Epidural and Position Trial Collaborative Group, 2017).

NB. The Cochrane review including the BUMPES study and published in 2018 found that amongst high-quality studies there appeared to be clear harm from upright positions (3 trials, 3609 women). There was evidence of an increased risk of operative birth (instrumental or caesarean birth combined) and an increase in caesarean births (Walker et al., 2018).

Managing an epidural

Midwives will be guided in their management of the epidural by the policies and procedures of each institution. Box 39.10 is an example of the most commonly used techniques in NSW using population data. There are no hard-and-fast rules about epidurals—it is another area of practice that has evolved through expert opinion and received wisdom. As far as research-based evidence goes, there is very little to guide midwives in the best way to look after a woman who has requested an epidural. Most facilities have their own policies to guide practice.

CLINICAL POINT

Find the epidural management guidelines that assist midwifery practice in your institution or facility.

This section outlines for the midwife the most commonly used techniques for managing epidurals and some of the most commonly observed side effects. Figs 39.5 and 39.6 show the mechanism and the pathways affected by the epidural and spinal analgesia / anaesthesia.

Eltzschig et al. (2003) describe the pathways of labour pain and its blockage as follows:

> *Labour pain has both a somatic and visceral component. Bradykinin, potassium, serotonin and histamine are released when uterine contractions cause myometrial ischemia. In addition, distension and stretching of the lower sections of the*

Box 39.10 Epidural management for first-time mothers in New South Wales[a]

Before progressing to an epidural, the woman may be offered a choice of a non-pharmacological option, an opioid (pethidine) or nitrous oxide.

When an epidural is decided upon, the following interventions are undertaken:

- An IV line is inserted to administer IV fluids.
- A urinary catheter is inserted.
- A continuous CTG monitor is applied.
- The woman is confined to bed.
- Regular BP recordings are made (to watch for low BP).
- Most women (62% of primiparous women) are augmented with synthetic oxytocin in the drip.
- The delay before 'pushing' in the second stage varies from 0 to 3 hours (median 2 hours) to no time limit (depending on hospital policy).
- The duration of the second stage varies from 1.54 hours to no time limit (depending on hospital policy).

[a]This work is based on a study of the 'standard' primiparous woman having an epidural in labour in New South Wales, in 2000 (findings from population-based research).
BP = blood pressure; CTG = cardiotocograph; IV = intravenous.
(Source: Roberts et al., 2003)

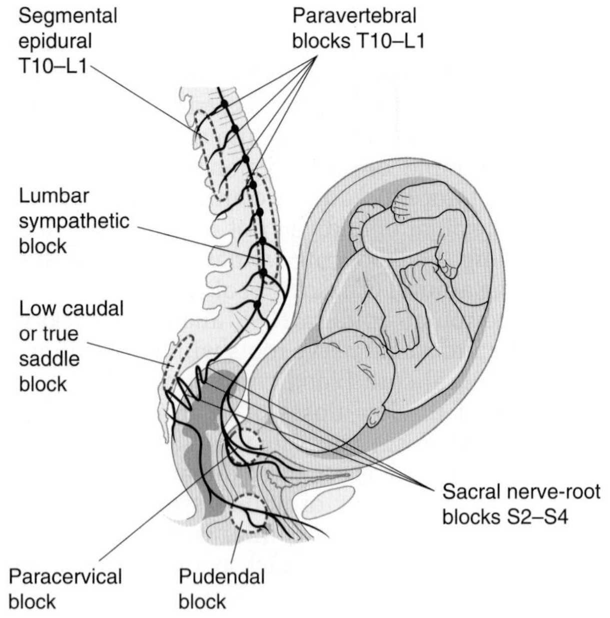

FIGURE 39.5 Pathways of analgesics and anaesthetics used in labour
(Based on Eltzschig et al., 2003)

uterus and the cervix stimulate mechanoreceptors. Pain impulses follow sensory nerve fibres that accompany nerve endings, then travel through the paracervical region and the hypogastric and pelvic plexus to enter the lumbar sympathetic chain. The T10, T11, T12 and L1 spinal nerves allow the impulses to enter the dorsal horn of the spinal cord [see Fig. 39.5]. These pathways could be mapped by a demonstration that blockade at different points along this path (sacral nerve-root blocks S2–S4, paracervical block, lumbar sympathetic block, pudendal block, true saddle or low caudal block, paravertebral blocks T10–L1 and segmental epidural blocks T10–L1) can improve the visceral component of labour pain.

(Adapted from Eltzschig et al., 2003, p. 320)

Epidural analgesia [see Fig. 39.6a] involves placing a catheter into the lumbar epidural space. After the intervertebral space between L3 and L4 has been identified, local anaesthetic is infiltrated into the space followed by a hollow epidural needle which is placed into the intervertebral ligaments. The connected syringe allows the anaesthetist to confirm the resistance to penetration of these ligaments. Entry into the epidural space will be characterized by a sudden loss of resistance. An epidural catheter is then advanced into the space. Solutions of opioids, local anaesthetic or a combination of the two can now be administered. When combining spinal–epidural analgesia the lumbar epidural space is also identified with an epidural needle. A thin spinal needle can now be introduced through the epidural needle into the subarachnoid space. A free flow of cerebrospinal fluid will confirm that the catheter is in the correct place. A single bolus of local anaesthetic, opioid or a combination of both can be injected through this needle. The needle is then removed, and a catheter is advanced into the epidural space through the epidural needle. When the spinal analgesic wears off, the epidural catheter can be used for continual pain management.

(Adapted from Eltzschig et al., 2003, p. 322)

Siting an epidural or a spinal block

The method for siting an epidural or spinal block differs according to the practice of each anaesthetist. Women will be given instructions by the anaesthetist, and the midwife is primarily called on to help position and attend to the comfort of the woman as she tries to position herself as directed by the anaesthetist. Depending on the stage of labour and the level of distress the woman is feeling, this could be a gruelling procedure for all concerned.

Additional interventions before placement of the epidural catheter

Intravenous fluids are commenced prior to the introduction of spinal or epidural anaesthetics. This is to prevent the onset and effects of maternal hypotension. The most commonly used solutions include warmed (37.8°C) Ringer lactate solution IV before the induction of anaesthesia. The Cochrane recommendation for IV fluids (preload) is that 500–1000 mL of a non-glucose balanced sodium chloride solution may be administered 15–30 minutes before the procedure, to minimise the effect of hypotension. Glucose solutions are contraindicated because of the

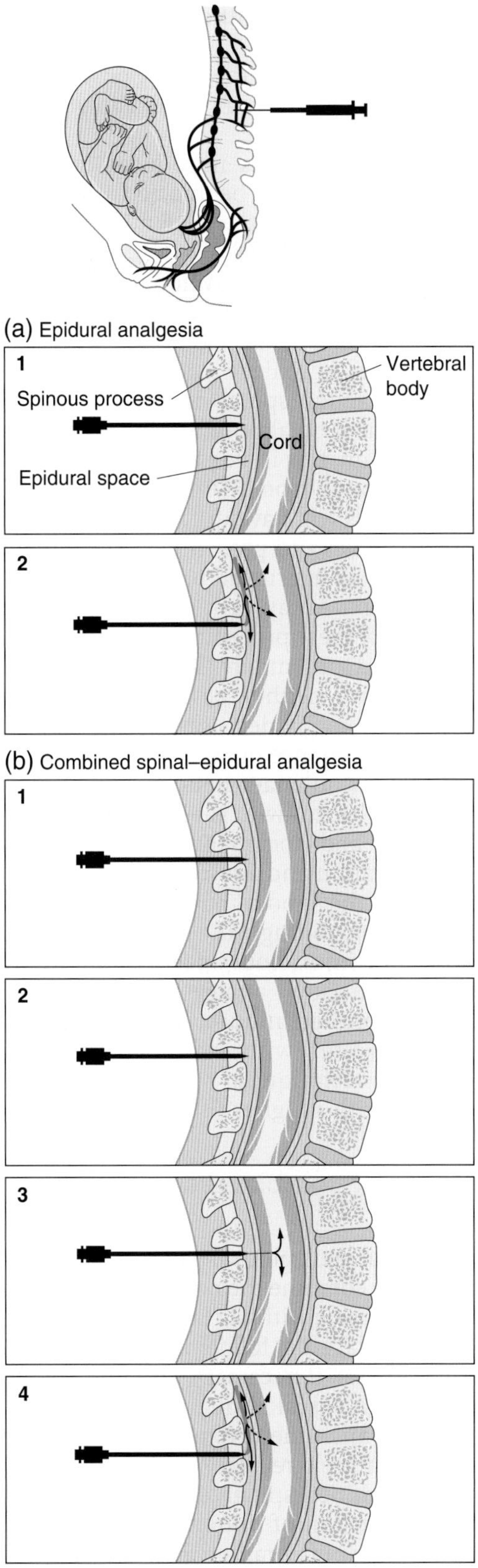

FIGURE 39.6 Epidural and combined spinal–epidural anaesthesia
(Based on Eltzschig et al., 2003)

risk of fetal hyperglycaemia and rebound hypoglycaemia in the infant. A Cochrane review of studies designed to assess the effect of prophylactic IV fluid preloading before epidural analgesia concluded that there may be beneficial fetal and maternal effects of this approach to minimising maternal hypotension (Hofmeyr et al., 2004). Low-dose epidural and combined spinal–epidural analgesia techniques may reduce the need for preloading. Studies so far have been too small to determine whether preloading is beneficial for women having regional analgesia during labour using the lower-dose local anaesthetics or opioids. Further investigation is required of low-dose epidural or combined spinal–epidural (including opioid only) blocks, and the risks and benefits of intravenous preloading for women with pregnancy complications (Hofmeyr, 2004).

Most maternity hospitals will expect midwives to follow the policies and protocols that have been developed for that specific context. The following instructions are very general—and may or may not be followed depending on the context and particular policies in use at the time. It is always important to be familiar with the policies and guidelines of the place where you attend women in childbirth.

If the woman is having an elective CS, she may be prescribed an antibiotic prophylactic; this is not routine, although most hospitals have local policy and guidelines for these matters.

A urinary catheter is inserted. Before initiating an epidural, women should be encouraged to void because the sensation of a full bladder will not be felt after the introduction of intrathecal anaesthetic. Catheterisation ensures an empty bladder, preventing concerns about a full bladder impeding uterine contractility and the risk of bladder trauma during surgery. There may be a lack of postpartum bladder tone, and therefore it is most important to keep an eye on this following birth or CS where a woman has had an epidural or combined epidural–spinal block. Urinary catheterisation poses an additional risk for the development of subsequent postpartum infection (Mayberry et al., 2002).

The fetal heart is usually monitored continuously. Again, this will be explicit in some hospital policies and not in others.

A blood-pressure cuff is placed (in a permanent position) so that the maternal blood pressure can be measured at 2-minute intervals (using an automatic cycling device, if the hospital has one) and following insertion of the block; the maternal blood pressure is measured every 5 minutes in some hospitals for the first 30 minutes following insertion. With a 'walking epidural' (where the block is lighter or the drugs do not have such a powerful anaesthetising effect on the nerve endings), it is not necessary to monitor so regularly. Again, each maternity hospital will outline the policies and procedures expected.

An oxygen saturation monitor may be attached to the woman (if the hospital has one) to measure the heart rate and peripheral oxygen saturation continuously.

Combined spinal and epidural block

Most maternity hospitals will expect midwives to follow the policies and protocols that have been developed for that specific context. Again, the following instructions are very general—and may or may not be followed depending on the context and particular policies in use at the time. It is always important to be familiar with the policies and guidelines of the place where you attend women in childbirth. See Fig. 39.6b for siting combined epidural and spinal analgesia.

The anaesthetist will perform a lumbar puncture at the L2–L3 or L3–L4 interspace with the woman in a sitting (or lying) position. The dural puncture is usually made with a 27 G (you may use a 29 G) pencil-point needle after the introduction of a Tuohy needle and identification of the epidural space. Once correct placement of the spinal needle has been confirmed by the aspiration of cerebrospinal fluid, 1.5–1.8 mL of 0.5% hyperbaric bupivacaine are given (varying with each woman's height: 1.5 mL for women under 1.65 m tall; 1.8 mL for those 1.65 m tall or taller) over 30 seconds. A 20 G epidural catheter is inserted 3–4 cm into the epidural space and secured in place with adhesive tape after withdrawal of the spinal needle, and the woman is positioned supine with a 15° left-lateral tilt achieved by placing a wedge under her right hip. Uterine displacement by either lateral tilt positioning or wedging the right hip minimises the maternal–fetal effects of compression of the aorta or inferior vena cava. Compression of these vessels decreases the blood return to the right side of the heart, which in turn contributes to maternal hypotension, which then contributes to a decrease in uteroplacental perfusion (Conklin & Backus, 1999; Poole, 2003a). If the block does not reach the T4 level after about 10 minutes, 10 mL of 0.25% plain bupivacaine plus 50 mg fentanyl (top-up) may be given epidurally in addition. The aim of this technique is to raise the level of spinal block to T8–T9 by using low doses of local anaesthetic, and to cause it to reach the T4 level by means of a low epidural top-up dose given in the next 10 minutes. There is not as yet any consensus about the nature of the mechanism by which the epidural top-up dose works (Karaman et al., 2005).

It takes about 10 minutes to achieve a block using the combined method. If the woman is having an elective CS, it may be about 15 minutes before surgery begins.

NB. This description is one way of inserting a spinal epidural block. There are many variations—different anaesthetists will use different-sized needles and catheters, and different cocktails of anaesthetic. There is very little robust evidence in this area concerning drugs and dosage!

Epidural block

Again, most maternity hospitals will expect midwives to follow the policies and protocols that have been developed for that specific context. The following instructions are very general—and may or may not be followed depending on the context and particular policies in use at the time. It is always important to be familiar with the policies and guidelines of the place where you attend women in childbirth.

The woman is placed in the sitting position and a lumbar puncture is made with an 18 G Tuohy needle at the L2–L3 or L3–L4 interspace.

An epidural catheter is introduced, and 3 mL 2% lignocaine (lidocaine) may be injected as a test dose. The epidural solution may consist of 16 mL 0.5% bupivacaine mixed with 100 mg fentanyl.

After an initial dose, an additional 2 mL 0.5% bupivacaine per unblocked segment may be given until a sensory block extending to the T4 level is achieved. It takes about 20 minutes to achieve a good block using the epidural (without added spinal) method, and for women having a CS it may be about 25 minutes before surgery begins. Once again, this is a description of one way of inserting an epidural block. Different anaesthetists and different hospitals will have different policies and protocols for anaesthetics and procedures. The midwifery student will always be instructed on what to do in assisting in this procedure. Always ask if you are in any doubt about any part of these procedures. Anaesthetics is a very complicated and potentially life-threatening business, and midwives are neither permitted nor expected to make any autonomous decisions concerning the insertion or safe maintenance of an anaesthetic. The midwife will always follow an anaesthetic policy or guideline on these matters. The midwife is always expected to safely monitor, report and document anything that she feels calls for consultation and advice.

Maintaining the labour analgesia by a continuous epidural infusion through the infusion pump reduces the number of clinical hours needed in topping up. Although more consistent analgesia is ensured with continuous infusion techniques, local anaesthetic consumption is greater with infusion than with bolus administration techniques; thus infusion techniques are associated with a higher risk of motor blockade (Sng et al., 2017).

Advantages of combined spinal and epidural blocks

Combined spinal and epidural blocks have become popular because they combine the rapid onset and intensity of a subarachnoid block with the facility of having an epidural catheter in place for follow-up intraoperative extension of anaesthesia, if necessary, and post-caesarean epidural analgesia. A spinal lumbar block requires a smaller amount of local anaesthetic to produce an effective block with complete muscle relaxation (Karaman et al., 2005). The use of combined spinal–epidural analgesia (which involves the injection of minimal doses of medications directly into the spinal, rather than the epidural, space) has facilitated profound analgesia without concomitant motor block; moreover, the ability of women to ambulate while receiving this method of pain relief has added even greater flexibility to analgesic options (Camann, 2005).

The disadvantages of spinal lumbar anaesthesia, such as the risk of an extensive block, the fixed duration of anaesthesia, hypotension and the risk of postdural puncture headache (PDPH), gave rise to the use of epidural anaesthesia as an alternative method (Thoren et al., 1994). In placing an epidural, the anaesthetist is able to target the exact level to which the block will extend and to maintain the block with supplementary doses. The catheter can remain in place for surgical anaesthesia and subsequently for postoperative pain relief. However, epidural anaesthesia is more time consuming and involves a higher incidence of insufficient or superficial block, especially of the motor roots, despite the use of larger doses of local anaesthetic agent (Karaman et al., 2005). The use of epidural anaesthesia for caesarean sections has been criticised because of the 25%–38% rate of ineffective anaesthesia. It is difficult to obtain complete anaesthesia during this operation in pregnant women because of the anatomical changes in the epidural space (Choi et al., 2000). This is why fentanyl, adrenaline (epinephrine) and sodium bicarbonate ($NaHCO_3$) with proven effects of potentiating the effects of local anaesthetics, are used to increase the efficacy of epidural analgesia (Choi et al., 2000; Davies et al., 1997; Karaman et al., 2005).

The Cochrane review of CSE versus epidural analgesia in labour (Simmons et al., 2012) found that, of the CSE versus traditional epidural analyses, CSE was more favourable in relation to: the speed of onset of analgesia from time of injection, the need for rescue analgesia, the rate of urinary retention and rate of instrumental delivery, and for umbilical venous pH. For CSE versus low-dose epidurals, CSE had a faster onset of effective analgesia from time of injection but was associated with more pruritus. Although no differences between CSE and epidural were seen for maternal satisfaction, there is a lack of data on this aspect for CSE versus traditional epidural analgesia (Simmons et al., 2012, p. 2).

Patient-controlled epidural analgesia and low-dose epidural solutions

Patient-controlled epidural analgesia (PCEA) has become a more popular method for the administration of epidural anaesthetic because it allows the woman to control the rate of anaesthetic drug according to her needs rather than having to call someone to 'top up' the epidural. The current technique consists of a continuous background infusion supplemented by patient-controlled bolus doses. It differs from continuous epidural infusions in reducing the dose of local anaesthetic used. PCEA is thought to provide equivalent analgesia with lower anaesthetic usage, lower rates of supplementation and higher patient satisfaction. Currently, there is no consensus on the most appropriate PCEA solutions, basal infusion rates, lockout intervals and demand dosing (Halpern & Carvalho, 2009; Sng et al., 2017). Threats to maternal safety, including hypotension, catheter misplacement, high blocks and respiratory depression, appear to be lessened with PCEA. Hypotension is more common following the initial placement of the epidural with the initial sympathetic blockade. PCEA maintains a more stable maternal haemodynamic status and hypotension is rare, even after self-administered boluses (Poole, 2003a). The Comparative Obstetric Mobile Epidural Trial (COMET) showed a lower assisted vaginal birth rate with a low-dose epidural infusion (0.1% bupivacaine) compared with a higher dose (0.25% bupivacaine). Amongst first-time mothers, low-dose epidural analgesia resulted in significantly more normal vaginal births than traditional techniques. Although methods of initiating analgesia (CSE versus epidural technique), initial doses, maintenance techniques (continuous infusion or intermittent bolus), drug concentrations and group size differed in that trial, almost one in four operative vaginal births appeared to be prevented by the introduction of low-dose epidural analgesia (Comparative Obstetric Mobile Epidural Trial (COMET) Study Group UK, 2001).

NB. The midwife is advised to be familiar with the individual policies and guidelines of the facility in which she is supporting the labouring woman.

The future of PCEA epidurals

Computerised modelling will undoubtedly feature in the future of epidural technology. As Sng et al. (2017) hypothesise in their paper 'Maintenance of epidural labour analgesia: the old, the new and the future' (p. 20):

> *The role of computerised advances in pump technology have allowed clinicians to better individualise and optimise analgesia. It is imperative to evaluate how these innovations will improve childbirth outcomes and experience, including long-term outcomes. The role of data analytics and probabilistic modelling in providing labour analgesia remains to be explored.*

Remifentanil

Remifentanil has been used for anaesthesia for many years, providing effective and controllable analgesia for different kinds of surgical procedures. Due to its characteristics (fast onset, short half-life), it can be administered in a patient-controlled mode, giving the woman the opportunity of pain relief when required. (Small doses of opioids lead to a steady state of plasma concentration of drug.) Remifentanil patient-controlled analgesia (PCA) for labour analgesia is becoming increasingly popular in some countries and is considered a safe alternative to other opioids and to epidural analgesia.

Weibel et al. (2017) studied pharmacological pain management for all women in labour, including high-risk groups with planned vaginal birth, comparing remifentanil given via a PCA device with other opioids given via the same method or via an intramuscular (IM) or intravenous (IV) injection, with epidural analgesia, with different regimens of remifentanil (PCA) or with remifentanil as a continuous IV infusion; they also compared PCA methods with inhalational analgesia or with no analgesia during birth. The review reported that women who received PCA with remifentanil were more satisfied with their pain relief than women receiving other opioids by either IV or IM injection. Remifentanil (PCA) provided stronger pain relief at 1 hour than the other opioids by IV or IM injection, and using remifentanil (PCA) was associated with a reduced need for additional analgesia compared with other IV or IM opioids (Weibel et al., 2017).

More recently trials have been undertaken to assess the comparative effectiveness between using manual intermittent boluses or continuous infusion alongside PCEA or a combination of these techniques (Morau et al., 2019; Roofthooft et al., 2020). Given the lack of robust data on drugs and mode of administration of epidurals in labour it is important to familiarise yourself with the guidelines and protocols for the administration of epidurals during labour at your institution.

Positions during labour with an epidural

After the insertion of an epidural, depending on the type, some women may be advised to move cautiously during labour (walking epidural). Other women may find the trailing leads of IV fluids, catheter bags and CTG leads too cumbersome to contemplate moving from a stationary position for the duration of the labour. A controversial area of management of epidurals in labour has to do with how long a woman remains in 'second stage' without pushing the baby out. Downe et al. (2004) used an RCT to study the different positions women might best use for the second stage of labour with an epidural. Women are normally encouraged to sit up, to maximise the use of gravity in encouraging descent of the fetus (Downe et al., 2004). However, the women randomised to the lateral position had a greater chance of a spontaneous birth, and of avoiding an episiotomy, than those randomised to the sitting position. The number-needed-to-treat calculation indicates that, for every five women using the lateral position (as opposed to the sitting position), one more experienced a normal birth, and one less an episiotomy (Downe et al., 2004). Evidence from the BUMPES study now strongly supports a lying-down position to achieve a spontaneous vaginal birth (Epidural and Position Trial Collaborative Group, 2017).

Side effects of epidural and spinal anaesthesia

Side effects of epidural and spinal anaesthetic in childbirth range from moderately mild to catastrophic. Lumbar epidural block provides safe obstetric analgesia and anaesthesia, but inadvertent intravascular, intrathecal or subdural injection is potentially life threatening.

The signs of catastrophic side effects described by Jenkins (2005) are as follows:

- *Intravascular injection* is diagnosed when the woman complains of perioral paraesthesia, visual disturbance or tinnitus, usually following the test dose or an incremental dose of low-concentration local anaesthetic. Intravascular injection of local anaesthetic may lead to convulsions, loss of consciousness and cardiac arrest. However, these symptoms are frequently preceded by premonitory signs, such as minor auditory or visual symptoms and complaints of a metallic taste. The incidence is 1 in 5000 epidurals.
- *Intrathecal injection* is diagnosed when injection of local anaesthetic, usually the test dose or an incremental dose of low concentration local anaesthetic, leads to a rapid onset of dense sensory and motor block with sacral involvement. The incidence is 1 in 2900 epidurals.
- *Subdural injection* is diagnosed when injection of local anaesthetic leads to an unexpectedly high block, often asymmetric and involving the arms and face nerve roots. Subdural block is slower in onset than subarachnoid block, taking 15–30 minutes, and motor block and hypotension may be minimal or absent. However, it can also lead to life-threatening collapse with hypotension and apnoea. The incidence is 1 in 4200 epidurals.
- *High or total spinal block due to subarachnoid or subdural injection* of local anaesthetic is diagnosed in the presence of a rapidly progressing motor and sensory block followed by respiratory paralysis requiring intubation, hypotension and loss of consciousness occurring within seconds to 20 minutes. High spinal block may occur after an apparently normal test dose. The incidence is 1 in 16,200 epidurals.

Headache caused by 'dural tap'

A common and very unpleasant side effect of an epidural is known as a 'dural tap'. Insertion of an epidural needle for obstetric epidural analgesia or anaesthesia is complicated by dural puncture in 1 in 50,250 cases (Paech et al., 2001), or a 1.5% risk of accidental dural puncture (Agerson et al., 2012), with the rate among maternity units in the United Kingdom ranging from 0.19% to 3.6% (Baraz & Collis, 2005). Accidental dural puncture is the most common major complication of epidural pain relief, and the headache following this complication can be very distressing and extremely disabling to the mother who is trying to nurse her newborn in the postnatal period.

Postdural puncture headache following a dural tap may involve at least 80% of women. Although serious morbidity is rare, severe and prolonged headache is common, and the healthcare costs are enormous, often requiring an additional postnatal hospital stay of 2–3 days. As the use of epidurals is burgeoning, and the incidence of dural tap has not improved much, this poses a real cost to women and the healthcare system. PDPH has implications for the mental and physical health of the mother. It often lasts several days, prolongs hospitalisation, and may be associated with auditory and visual disturbances, nausea and vomiting, and cranial nerve palsy.

PDPH usually presents within 72 h after meningeal puncture in 90% of women and is evident by a headache typically worsening within 15 min of standing and resolving within 30 min of recumbency (International Headache Society (IHS)).

Despite a variety of definitions, most women report that the PDPH is severe.

The headache is usually dull in nature and frontal in location (75% of the time), but occipital pain also occurs which may, or may not, radiate into the neck and shoulder area (Sachs & Smiley, 2014).

Many symptomatic therapies have been tried during expectant management, including systemic opioids, nonsteroidal anti-inflammatory drugs and cerebral vasoconstrictors such as caffeine. Pain may be accompanied by neck stiffness, photophobia, nausea or tinnitus. It typically resolves spontaneously within 1 week or within 48 hours after treatment of the dural leak; however, symptoms can persist for months to years (Agerson et al., 2012). Headaches can be severe and debilitating, limiting interaction between mother and baby during the postpartum period, in addition to prolonging hospitalisation and increasing healthcare costs. Almost 40% of affected women with PDPH experience greater than 1 week of impairment in activities of daily living. Chronic headache following meningeal puncture is a serious problem that is probably underreported and has been implicated in permanent disability, including cranial nerve palsy and chronic headache (sometimes necessitating surgical closure). It has been cited as the third most common cause of lawsuits against anaesthetists in the US by obstetric patients (approximately 12%) (Sachs & Smiley, 2014).

There is no evidence that the advice to 'lie flat for a day', or that bed rest, patient positioning (prone, supine, head-up, head-down, etc.), immobilisation, or supplemental IV fluid administration following meningeal puncture helps prevent a PDPH (Arevalo-Rodriguez et al., 2013).

Evidence from randomised trials of either prophylactic or therapeutic epidural blood patching is lacking and does not allow reliable assessments of the effectiveness of this intervention in the prevention or treatment of PDPH (Agerson et al., 2012). The therapeutic blood patch is thought to exert its effect by sealing the dural leak, which in turn acts to propel cerebrospinal fluid into the cranium, thus increasing the intracranial pressure and mitigating vasodilation. Reports of therapeutic effectiveness range from 73% to 93% (Agerson et al., 2012). Despite the paucity of randomised evidence, epidural blood patches are used widely for the treatment of PDPH (Agerson et al., 2012). Contraindications to blood patch are fever and risk of bleeding.

Inserting a blood patch:

- The woman is usually placed in the left lateral position and the procedure carried out under strict aseptic conditions, including skin preparation and the wearing of mask, gloves and gown when identifying the epidural space, and mask and gloves when performing venipuncture.
- Autologous blood is collected by the second anaesthetist and handed to the first, who injects slowly into the epidural space until 15–20 mL are delivered, or a feeling of intense pressure or pain is reported by the woman. Women are advised to remain recumbent for 2 hours (Banks et al., 2001).
- All patients are reviewed after the blood patch and discharged within a few hours. Patients are routinely informed that they should report back to the hospital with any concerns after discharge (Banks et al., 2001).
- Serious complications associated with epidural blood patch include lumbovertebral syndrome, arachnoiditis (thought to be due to injection of blood into the subarachnoid space via an intrathecally placed catheter), acute meningeal irritation, deterioration of mental status, seizures, subdural haematoma, acute exacerbation of PDPH and transient bradycardia (Banks et al., 2001). The incidence of these events is unknown, but case reports are sporadic and infrequent. Nevertheless, because they may have serious consequences for the patient, such complications should be discussed when obtaining informed consent for a blood patch (Banks et al., 2001).

Hypotension associated with epidural or spinal blocks

A drop in blood pressure usually happens soon after the introduction of an epidural, owing to sympathetic block secondary to the local anaesthetic administration into the epidural space. The resulting vasodilation of the lower limbs reduces venous return (Peyronnet et al., 2017).

The incidence of hypotension among women having an epidural is between 0% and 50%, and hypotension is described as maternal systolic arterial blood pressure either below 90–100 mmHg or a 20%–30% decrease below baseline (Mayberry & Clemmens, 2002). Blood pressure is carefully monitored in all patients receiving epidurals regardless of the technique or drug combination / dosage regimen. It should be assessed frequently (as often as every 5 minutes during the first 30 minutes and every 15 minutes thereafter with stabilisation, and then continued frequently throughout the remainder of labour). Each hospital will have a local policy for the management of fluids for women having epidurals; it is important for the student to be aware of local guidelines and standard procedures.

The development of orthostatic hypotension when women move to an upright position or get out of the labour bed is also a potential risk for women receiving epidurals. Appropriate positioning to relieve potential aortal and inferior vena caval compression is necessary to minimise the risk of hypotension and the reduction of blood return to the heart, lowering of cardiac output and reduction of placental perfusion associated with recumbent positions in labour (Mayberry & Clemmens, 2002). The lateral position is preferable to a supine position if there are problems with hypotension. If the hypotension persists and is not alleviated with positional changes after administration of an epidural, sometimes vasopressors may be required.

A recent study in France of 300 women who either wore compression stockings or did not found that lower limb compression with medical stockings (20–36 mmHg) significantly reduced the incidence of maternal hypotension within 15 min and within 1 hour following epidural induction in women in spontaneous labour at term (Peyronnet et al., 2017). Until now the efficiency of leg compression in preventing the occurrence of hypotension after neuraxial anaesthesia has been demonstrated only in the context of scheduled CS with spinal anaesthesia or epidural anaesthesia (Peyronnet et al., 2017).

Overuse of electronic FHR monitoring has been an issue in obstetric care for at least the past 5 years, but the increased epidural rate is likely to be a primary reason for its continued use. Standard hospital protocols require that women be monitored using electronic FHR monitors throughout the duration of labour. One reason is that a potential FHR change in response to a decrease in uterine blood flow is a risk associated with maternal hypotension (Mayberry & Clemmens, 2002).

Most facilities will have guidelines and policies based on standard management of epidurals requiring women to have IV fluids and regular CTG monitoring.

Shivering

Shivering occurs in at least 20% of women during labour without neuraxial analgesia, and about 35% with epidural analgesia. Shivering can be distressing for women and can interfere with monitoring. Its impact can be minimised by warming IV fluids, and administering epidural fentanyl can reduce its incidence and severity (Karaman et al., 2005).

It is curious that shivering is observed so often, because increased energy expenditure during labour presumably requires heat dissipation rather than heat production (Mayberry & Clemmens, 2002). Physiologists believe that the shivering in labour is largely non-thermoregulatory, and the causes of these responses remain unknown (Panzer et al., 1999).

Pruritus associated with epidural and spinal blocks

Epidural morphine is used widely for pain relief because it has a prolonged analgesic effect, but it produces many side effects such as pruritus, nausea, vomiting, respiratory depression and difficulty in micturition. Epidural morphine produces better analgesia than does IV morphine, but also more severe pruritus. The exact mechanism of pruritus is not clear; medullary dorsal horn activation may be related (Jeon et al., 2004).

The treatment of opioid-induced side effects remains a challenge. From a systematic review of the side effects of epidurals, Mayberry & Clemmens (2002) found that the incidence of pruritus among women who were given drug combinations containing one or the other opioids (with or without anaesthetics) ranged between 8% and 100%, with an average of 62%. The highest incidences were noted in study groups in which the highest doses of narcotics were administered. The incidence of pruritus within studies in which women were not given a drug combination including either fentanyl or sufentanil was 0%–4%. The average length of discomfort was not specified in the studies, but most investigators reported symptoms of pruritus that were not considered severe enough to require treatment. Women who have 'fentanyl-only' epidurals experienced more widespread body distribution of pruritus than the other groups, in which only facial symptoms predominated.

Treatments for pruritus may consist of IV opioid antagonist or diphenhydramine. Effectiveness in terms of the extent of relief (i.e. complete or not) and how long the medications took to work are not known.

Nausea and vomiting

The risk of nausea and vomiting in CSs performed under local anaesthesia depends on the technique used, the severity of hypotension, the surgical stimulus, the woman's position and any medications given. The incidence varies from about 30% to 35% of women who have an epidural (Davies et al., 1997; Karaman et al., 2005) and between 20% and 25% of women who have a combined spinal and epidural block (Davies et al., 1997; Karaman et al., 2005). Severe nausea accompanied by vomiting may be an added risk for hypoglycaemia associated with prolonged fasting, particularly for women who have spent a lengthy period in the labour and delivery ward without food (Mayberry & Clemmens, 2002).

Maternal and neonatal outcomes

Randomised studies show that compared with other forms of analgesia, epidurals are associated with increased length of labour, oxytocin augmentation, instrumental deliveries, perineal trauma and maternal fever / neonatal sepsis evaluation (Leighton & Halpern, 2002). The BUMPES study recommends that women with low-dose epidurals give birth lying down (Epidural and Position Trial Collaborative Group, 2017).

In 2000, 2005 and 2012 research was undertaken in Australia using population data to determine the association between epidurals and other interventions in labour and birth (Dahlen et al., 2012; Dahlen et al., 2021; Roberts et al., 2000; Tracy et al., 2007a). These population data studies showed that the **cascade of interventions** that follows the introduction of an epidural indicates that interventions such as epidurals during labour and birth should have been evaluated more thoroughly before their 'wholesale' introduction into maternity practices. Women are very often given no indication of the rate of risk associated with having an epidural for pain relief in labour (Table 39.6).

Several population-based studies from Australia have been undertaken over the past twenty years showing the association between interventions such as having induction or augmentation of labour with or without an epidural for labour, and the resulting use of forceps or vacuum instrumental birth or CS, for primiparous and multiparous women respectively. Interestingly, the studies show that over the past twenty years there has been a steady increase in the unintended effects on the outcome of labour and birth as interventions are introduced during labour. This phenomenon, where one intervention leads to another in an attempt to solve problems, is called a *cascade of intervention* (see Dahlen et al., 2012; Dahlen et al., 2021; Roberts et al., 2000; Tracy et al., 2007a).

Figs 39.7 and 39.8 were derived from a population-based study in NSW (Roberts et al., 2000). They show the change in the rate of spontaneous vaginal birth amongst low-risk women who had no identified risk factors at the time of birth and were offered various interventions during labour. As you can see in Fig. 39.7, amongst 100 low-risk first-time mothers who had public hospital care, only one

Table 39.6 Explaining epidural anaesthetic risks to women

Risk level	Risk expressed in everyday terms	Epidural complication
1 in 1	Something happens every time	
1 in 10	Something happening to one person in a family	Progress to instrumental birth Difficulty moving legs Itching Difficulty passing urine
1 in 100	Something happening to someone in your street	Headache 'Failure' of epidural
1 in 1000	Death from smoking >10 a day Death in car accident in your lifetime	Severe fall in blood pressure Neurological injury from spinal Neurological injury from epidural
1 in 5000		Intrathecal injection Intravascular injection of local anaesthetic
1 in 10,000		Total spinal block Meningitis Nerve damage
1 in 100,000	Being murdered	Spinal haematoma after spinal or epidural Paralysis
1 in 1,000,000	Death due to the Pill	
1 in 10,000,000	Struck by lightning	Maternal death from anaesthesia
1 in 100,000,000	Something happening to someone in Europe	
1 in 1,000,000,000	Something happening to one person in the world	

(Source: adapted from Adams & Smith, 2001 and Bethune et al., 2004)

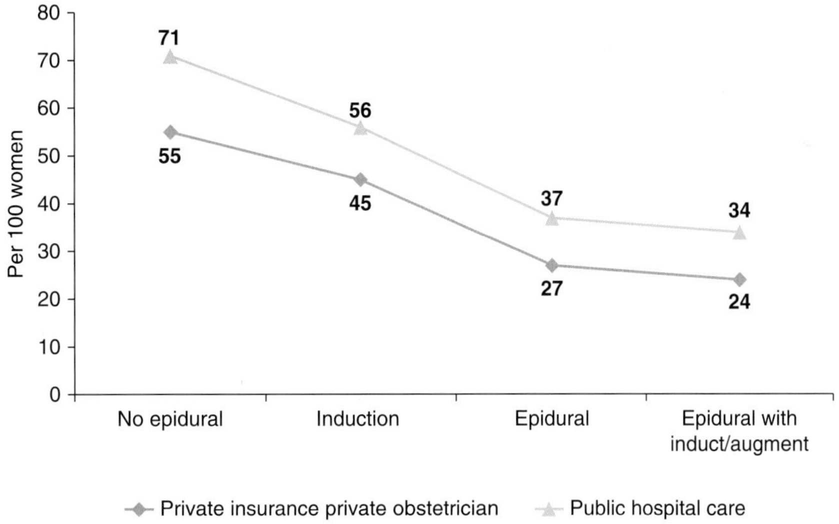

FIGURE 39.7 Cascade of interventions in primipara

in three women (34 per 100 women) had an unassisted vaginal birth without an episiotomy. Even fewer low-risk first-time mothers, one in four women, had a similar outcome if they had private obstetric care and private health insurance (24 per 100 women). (See the studies by Dahlen et al., 2012; Dahlen et al., 2021, Roberts et al., 2000; Tracy et al., 2007a and note how there have been no improvements in the cascade of labour interventions over the years and the rate of intervention in the private sector remains considerably higher than that in the public hospital system). Box 39.11 summarises the barriers to birthing without an epidural, from the perspectives of staff and of women.

Side effects for the baby

Many factors may influence neonatal acid–base balance at CS, such as a direct effect resulting from placental drug

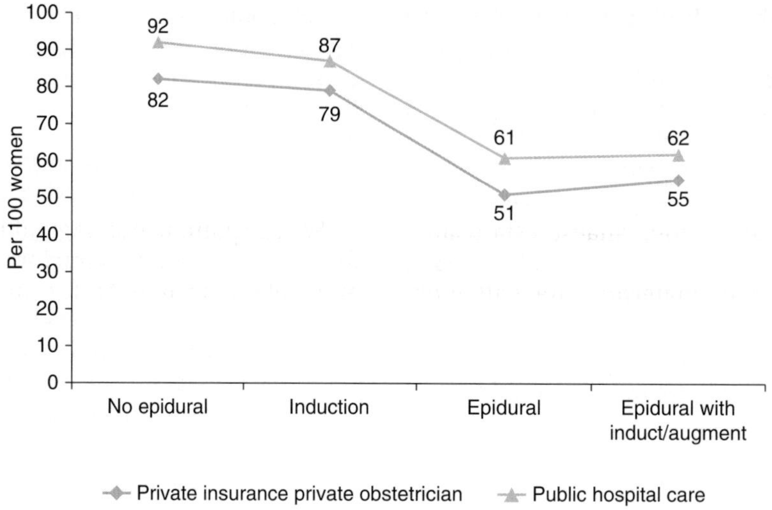

FIGURE 39.8 Cascade of intervention in multipara

Box 39.11 Barriers to birth without an epidural

A qualitative exploratory study from Canada aimed to explore barriers to and facilitators to birth without epidural in a tertiary centre, from the perspectives of staff and patients. They found that the tendency toward intervention in the tertiary environment makes birth without epidural a rare event.

Resources may be prioritised towards the acute care needs of high-risk patients causing financial constraints and limiting the resources for one-to-one continuity.

A 24-hour dedicated anaesthetic service contributes to a lack of exposure to birth without epidural.

This in turn results in a lack of skills for supporting birth without epidural, and a heightened sensitivity to expressions of pain and discomfort when witnessing labour without epidural.

Discrepancies exist between professional and patient attitudes about childbirth pain. This also influences epidural use.

The following four main themes emerged from the study:

- differing perceptions of pain
- being ready for things to go wrong
- labour support is more labour intensive
- having insufficient resources for birth without epidural.

The researchers recommended allocating dedicated resources to better support birth without an epidural. Specifically, support could be improved through the implementation of guidelines for assessment and management of labour pain, provision of a variety of pain management options and labour support training for healthcare professionals.

(Source: Knox et al., 2017)

transfer or an indirect effect resulting from maternal physiological or biochemical changes. There are numerous aspects of management that may affect the baby indirectly, including IV fluid loading, the use of vasopressors, maternal position or uterine displacement, the presence and extent of sympathetic blockade, inspired oxygen concentration, skin incision and uterine incision, delivery intervals and previous use of sedative drugs (Reynolds & Seed, 2005).

(It is remarkable that spinal anaesthesia can induce a significant increase in fetal metabolic acidosis over the normally short time interval between administration of anaesthesia and delivery of the baby by CS. Maternal blood pressure cannot be used as a surrogate for fetal outcome, as the changes may be too short lived. Moreover, placental intervillous blood flow is dependent not solely on maternal blood pressure but also on maternal cardiac output and its distribution. It has been shown that spinal but not epidural anaesthesia is associated with a reduction in cardiac output even in the presence of a normal blood pressure (Reynolds & Seed, 2005).)

Breastfeeding

A dose–response relationship between fentanyl and artificial feeding has been reported. When well-established determinants of infant feeding are accounted for, intrapartum fentanyl may impede establishment of breastfeeding, particularly at higher doses (Jordan et al., 2005).

General anaesthesia

General anaesthesia is most likely to be used for a caesarean birth when there are no obstetric anaesthetists available to administer a spinal or epidural anaesthetic, or during an emergency, or if the woman has a contraindication to the use of regional anaesthesia. Pregnant women respond differently from non-pregnant women to the pharmacological agents used for general anaesthesia. Cricoid pressure may be called for to reduce the risk of aspiration of gastric contents.

Many units have their own individual policy regarding what to give before women have a general anaesthetic. To reduce gastric acidity, an H_2-receptor antagonist, proton pump inhibitor, and/or metoclopramide and/or a clear antacid administered orally may be given (Poole, 2003b). Although maternal mortality from anaesthesia-related causes has declined since the mid 1980s (Poole, 2003b), anaesthetic-related deaths in maternity are still more likely to be related to general anaesthetic than to epidural or spinal anaesthetic.[a]

OPERATIVE BIRTH

When spontaneous vaginal birth is not possible, instrumental vaginal birth may be attempted. An operative or instrumental delivery is performed if it is necessary to expedite the birth of the baby. Chamberlain & Steer (1999) subdivide operative deliveries into abdominal methods (CS) and vaginal assisted births (forceps deliveries and vacuum extractions). This section focuses on vaginal assisted births, both vacuum and forceps. The incidence of forceps deliveries declines as the rate of CS continues to rise (Patel & Murphy, 2004).

Before any operative procedure is performed, it is crucial to obtain the woman's consent, which involves an active participation in the discussion about the risks and benefits of the procedure and alternative treatments (expectant observation and expedited delivery by CS).

Controversy continues concerning whether and when to conduct operative vaginal deliveries and which instruments are best. In many centres, over 50% of women have a vaginal assisted birth. Tracy et al. (2007a) published an important study that showed the magnitude of the increase in operative births among Australian women. Irrespective of 'risk' status, fewer than 56.8% of primiparous Australian women gave birth spontaneously (10% had a forceps delivery, 13% were delivered by vacuum extraction and just over 19% were by CS). Almost 80% of multiparous women gave birth spontaneously. As the authors point out, assisted deliveries are preceded by and follow a cascade of interventions (epidurals, oxytocin therapy, episiotomies, uterine scar, etc.). In a repeat study, the authors found that 10 years later the cascade of interventions had in fact increased by 5% for women in public hospitals and by over 10% for women in private hospitals (Dahlen et al., 2012).

When spontaneous vaginal birth is not possible, both forceps and vacuum extractors (ventouse) are acceptable and safe instruments for operative vaginal delivery. Although the procedures fall outside the scope of midwifery practice, it is important that all clinicians understand the indications for an assisted vaginal delivery, the risks and benefits associated with both, and the principles of management.

Choice between vacuum extraction and forceps deliveries

The decision to use a vacuum extractor instead of forceps in assisted vaginal delivery is based on the clinical situation and the experience and expertise of the accoucheur (Table 39.7). For many clinicians these two instruments are interchangeable and the choice will depend on the clinical situation, while others feel more comfortable with one or the other.

Lack of skill, failure to obtain the woman's consent, an inability to accurately assess fetal position or station, degree of cephalopelvic disproportion (CPD), progress of labour and uterine contractions, engagement of the fetal head and malpresentation are contraindications to an operative vaginal delivery.

Forceps

The history of obstetric **forceps** is long and colourful. Sanskrit writings from approximately 1500 bc contain evidence of single and paired instruments. However, these were designed to deliver the baby only after it had died. The credit for the invention of the precursor of the

Table 39.7 Comparison between the advantages of vacuum extractions and forceps deliveries

Vacuum extractions	Forceps deliveries
Easier skill to learn and is easier to place than the forceps	Fewer neonatal injuries, including cephalohaematoma, retinal haemorrhage and transient lateral rectus palsy
Less maternal genital trauma—perineal lacerations and episiotomies Less risk of rectal sphincter and bladder dysfunction	Higher rate of successful vaginal delivery
Can be performed comfortably without analgesia or anaesthesia	May be a quicker delivery
Vacuum extraction exposes the baby to less traction in comparison to forceps delivery	Success rates higher
May occasionally be performed before the cervix is completely dilated	The cervix must be completely dilated

modern forceps used on live infants goes to Peter Chamberlen (1575–1628), an English man-midwife. The family kept his invention a secret for more than 100 years and only his sons were privy to their design and use. Even when the design became public knowledge, their use was restricted to man-midwives (the forerunner of today's obstetrician) and used primarily as a measure to save the life of the mother once the fetus was dead. In 1845, Sir James Simpson developed a forceps that was designed to appropriately fit both cephalic and pelvic curves.

According to Patel & Murphy (2004, p. 1302), there are more than 700 types of obstetric forceps. Each of the three main types (outlet, midcavity or rotational) is designed for specific clinical situations and requires different levels of expertise (Fig. 39.9a). Three of the most common are Wrigley's, Simpson's and Kielland's, used for rotational deliveries (Fig. 39.9b–d). The criteria for an outlet forceps delivery are that the vertex (the bony skull) is visible at the introitus and the sagittal suture is in the anteroposterior position of the pelvis. For a low (outlet) forceps application, the vertex must be at station +2 or more below the ischial spines but on the pelvic floor. The fetus must be lying in an occipitoanterior position. In a midcavity delivery, which often requires rotation of the fetal head, the head must be engaged in the pelvis and the vertex positioned at station +1 or +2. There is no place for a 'high forceps'—where the biparietal diameter of the fetal head is above the pelvic inlet—in modern obstetrics.

Structure of forceps

Forceps have four major components (Fig. 39.9b):

- blades—this is the portion of the instrument that fits around the fetal head (each blade is curved so that it fits around the head)
- shanks—these connect the blades to the handles and are either parallel or crossing
- lock—this is the articulation between the shanks
- handles—these are for the accoucheur to hold when applying traction to the fetal head.

Indications for forceps delivery

Indications for the use of forceps include the presence of any condition that threatens the wellbeing of the mother or fetus if she proceeds to a spontaneous vaginal birth. Absolute and relative conditions that put the woman at risk include the following.

Maternal factors include:

- need for prophylactic shortening of the second stage of labour (cardiovascular disease and hypertension, including severe preeclampsia)
- pulmonary oedema
- infection
- neurological disease (spinal cord injury, myasthenia gravis).

Obstetric factors include:

- maternal distress and exhaustion
- malposition of the fetus
- forceps to the aftercoming head in a breech birth
- controlled delivery of the head in a CS

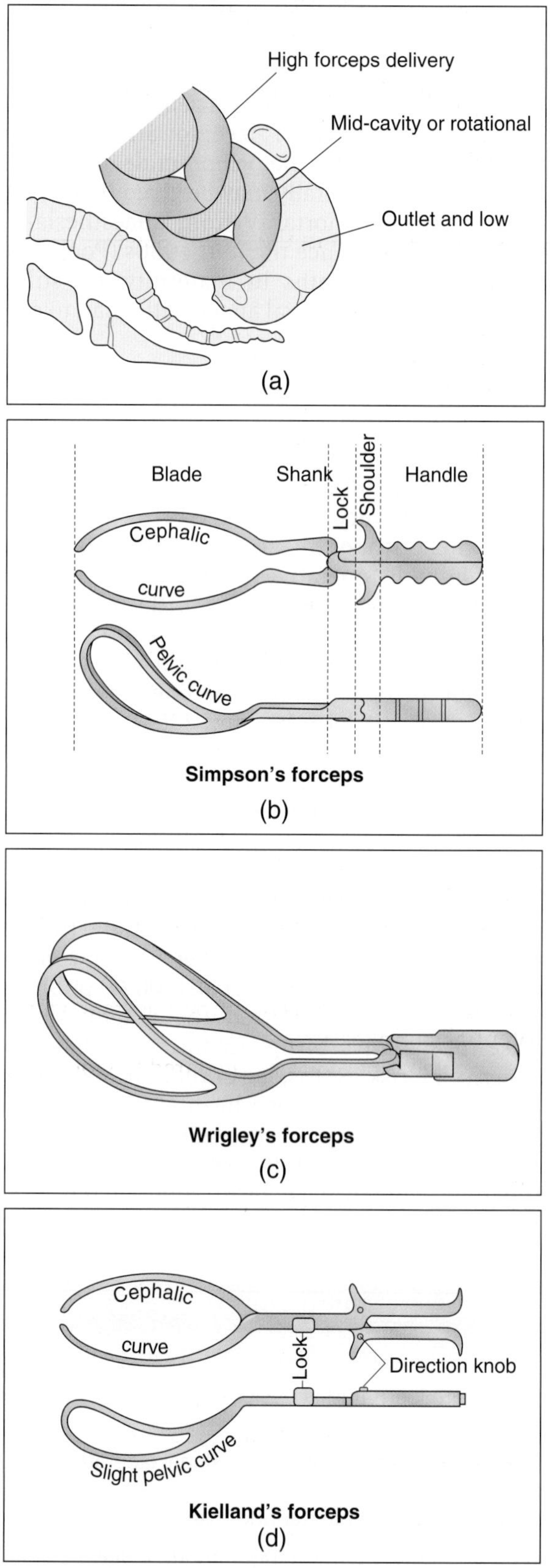

FIGURE 39.9 Obstetric forceps. The top panel shows the station of the head when the forceps is applied.
(Source: Oats & Abraham, 2004)

- cord prolapse in the second stage of labour
- lack of advance of the fetal head in the second stage of labour
- dense epidural block (ineffective pushing efforts in second stage).

Fetal factors include:

- signs of fetal compromise (non-reassuring fetal heart rate)
- placental abruption in the second stage.

Contraindications

Contraindications for forceps delivery include:

- incompletely dilated cervix
- unknown fetal position
- station higher than +1 or >1 / 5 palpable abdominally
- inexperienced accoucheur
- evidence of absolute CPD.

Prerequisites

Prerequisites for forceps delivery include the following:

- As with any invasive procedure, the woman must consent to the procedure.
- Adequate anaesthesia must be administered.
- The head must be engaged in the pelvis.
- The station, presentation and position of the head must be known.
- The cervix must be fully dilated.
- The amniotic membranes must be ruptured.
- The bladder should be empty.
- There should be no evidence of absolute CPD.
- Episiotomy should be performed.
- Adequate facilities and supportive elements should be available.
- The accoucheur should be competent in the use of the instruments and the recognition and management of potential complications.
- The accoucheur should be prepared to stop (i.e. to not 'force the issue').

CRITICAL THINKING EXERCISE

How will you respond to a woman who asks the following questions?

1. Why are forceps deliveries and vacuum extractions necessary?
2. What can I do to avoid them?
3. If I do need one, which is safer and less traumatic?

Complications

The medical literature contains considerable information about the risks and complications of forceps delivery. Reports of maternal and fetal complications vary depending on the skill and judgement of the accoucheur. The most common are associated with increased perineal and vaginal trauma (Patel & Murphy, 2004). Other maternal complications associated with forceps-assisted vaginal deliveries are:

- postpartum haemorrhage (third stage should be actively managed)
- intrapartum rupture of the unscarred uterus
- late complications, which are mainly related to injury to the pelvic support tissues and organs, often leading to faecal and urinary incontinence (Box 39.12).

Evidence evaluating neonatal morbidity is inconsistent (Patel & Murphy, 2004).

Neonatal complications include:

- transient facial forceps marks, bruising, lacerations and cephalhaematoma
- facial nerve palsy (cranial nerve VII)
- skull fractures, intracranial haemorrhage with falx, or tentorial lacerations
- an increased incidence of shoulder dystocia.

Box 39.12 Can we prevent obstetric anal sphincter injuries?

Obstetric anal sphincter injuries (OASIS) are associated with a two- to threefold increase in the risk of faecal incontinence after vaginal birth. Women suffer the lifelong impact of faecal incontinence when these injuries are sustained. Given the often disappointing results of its treatment, primary prevention of OASIS is of the utmost importance (van Bavel et al., 2018).

A study of all births in the Netherlands recorded in the Dutch Perinatal Registry (Perined) of almost all births between 2000 and 2010 in the Netherlands found that amongst a cohort of 170,969 primiparous and multiparous women the use of a mediolateral episiotomy during both vacuum delivery and forceps delivery is associated with a five- to 10-fold reduction in the rate of OASIS in primiparous and multiparous women (van Bavel et al., 2018).

The Royal College of Obstetricians and Gynaecologists (RCOG) guidelines state that 'there is evidence that a mediolateral episiotomy should be performed with instrumental deliveries as it appears to have a protective effect on OASIS' (RCOG, 2015a, p. 7).

(Sources: van Bavel et al., 2018; RCOG, 2015a)

Vacuum extraction (ventouse)

A **vacuum extraction** is an obstetric procedure used to facilitate the birth of the fetus by applying suction to the fetal head (Fig. 39.10). The indications for its use are mostly the same as for a forceps delivery. In general a vacuum extraction aims to correct a malpositioned fetal head. Assistance from normal 'forces' of labour is used to deliver the baby. A 5 cm cup with vacuum of 600 mmHg provides more than enough traction force (16 kg) to properly orient the head and deliver the fetus. Thus any traction must be of minimal force and duration.

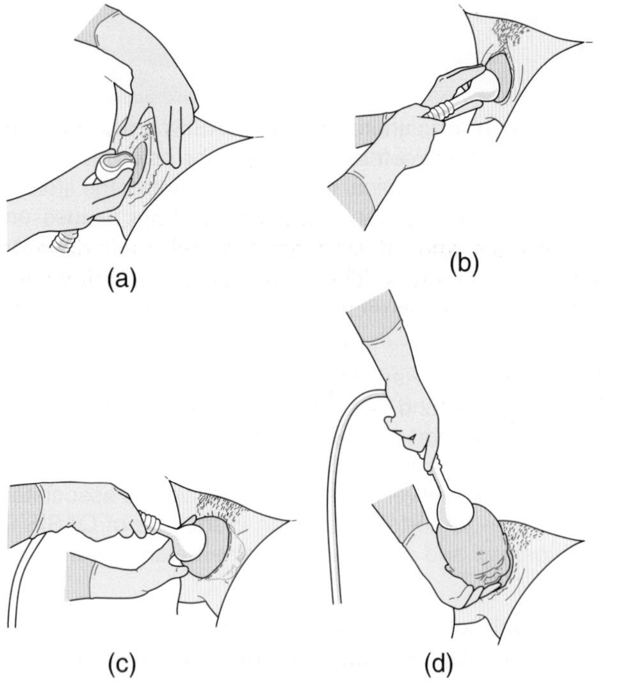

FIGURE 39.10 Ventouse extraction. (a) Application of the vacuum cup so that the centre of the cup is placed over the flexion point of the fetal skull (1 cm anterior to the posterior fontanelle). (b–d) With each contraction, traction is applied in a line perpendicular to the plane of the cup's ring. The fetal head is slowly lifted out of the vagina. Only two or three pulls should be required for the fetal head to birth
(Based on Henderson & Macdonald, 2004)

Vacuum extractions are contraindicated in pre-term births (less than 34 weeks gestation) and malpresentations, including a face presentation. Cups are available in various sizes. Some (Bird cup) are metal and the newer ones consist of a plastic or silastic cup connected to silastic tubing, which in turn is attached to a hand- or foot-controlled pump or wall-connected device that produces the negative pressure necessary to create a vacuum (approximately 60–80 kPa or 600–800 cmH_2O). The suction creates an artificial caput or 'chignon' as the scalp is pulled into the cup (Fig. 39.11) (see also Ch. 31). It is important that the accoucheur ensures that no vaginal tissue (if the cervix is not completely dilated) is caught by the cup. With maternal expulsive aid during contraction, the accoucheur applies traction to the fetal head. If there is no evidence of bony descent after three pulls, or if the baby is not born after 20 minutes, the procedure is stopped.

CLINICAL POINT

'Pop-offs'

The vacuum cup will 'pop off' if it is applied incorrectly, if traction is excessive or applied in the wrong direction, or if CPD is present.

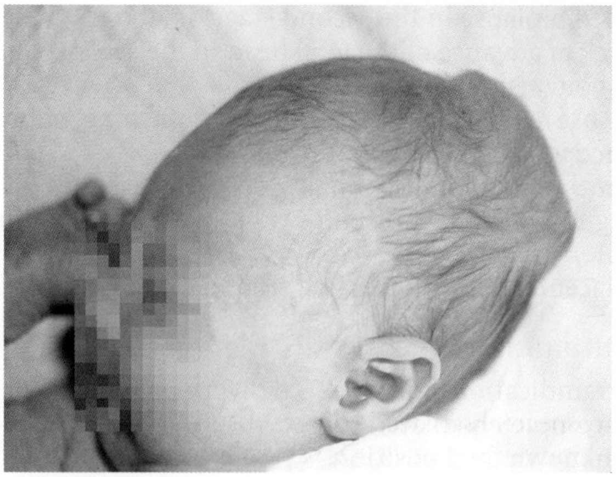

FIGURE 39.11 Baby with a chignon
(Source: Henderson & Macdonald, 2004)

Maternal and neonatal complications of vacuum extraction

Data addressing reproductive morbidity after instrumental vaginal delivery or CS are scarce. Maternal complications associated with vacuum extraction are comparable to those associated with spontaneous vaginal births. Complications do not vary with the type of vacuum extractor used. In the immediate postpartum period, forceps have been associated with increased rates of primary and secondary haemorrhage, perineal and vaginal trauma and a greater requirement for analgesia compared with vacuum extractors. Cervical laceration, postpartum infection and prolonged hospital stay are also more common in women who had forceps delivery compared with those who had vacuum-assisted delivery or a spontaneous vaginal birth.

Maternal complications

- Complications of anaesthesia
- Lacerations:
  - extension of the episiotomy
  - perineal tear
  - vaginal tears
  - cervical lacerations
- Bladder injury
- Ureteric injury
- Ruptured uterus
- Bone injuries: to pelvic joints, coccyx or symphysis pubis
- Pelvic nerve injuries
- Postpartum haemorrhage due to lacerations or atony
- Puerperal infections
- Rare effects: genital prolapse, stress incontinence, cervical incompetence and genitourinary fistulas

Neonatal complications

Vacuum extraction can injure the fetus.

Direct injury:

- cephalhaematoma
- intracranial haemorrhage (parenchymal, subdural, intraventricular, subarachnoid)

- nerve injury
- scalp laceration, abrasion, ecchymoses, necrosis
- skull fracture
- subgaleal haemorrhage.

Indirect injury:
- anaemia, hyperbilirubinaemia
- brachial plexus injury
- scalp infection or abscess.

Subgaleal haemorrhage

Subgaleal haemorrhage is a serious neonatal complication. It is reported to occur in 0.3%–0.76% of vacuum extractions in retrospective studies, though prospective studies report a higher incidence (4.14%–21%) (Colditz et al., 2014). Blood can accumulate in a large potential space between the galea aponeurotica and the periosteum of the cranial bones (Fig. 39.12) after vacuum extraction. An infant with subgaleal haemorrhage will exhibit a boggy scalp, with swelling that crosses the suture lines and expands head circumference, and may also have signs of hypovolaemia, pallor, tachycardia and a falling haematocrit. (See also Ch. 42.)

Documentation

Documentation is the most important witness to any intervention in labour. Following a vacuum extraction or a forceps delivery, the following must be documented:
- indication for the procedure
- course of labour
- anaesthesia
- personnel present
- instruments used
- position and station of the fetal head
- force and duration of traction
- complications, including how they were recognised and managed
- immediate condition of the baby and mother
- all steps taken in resuscitation.

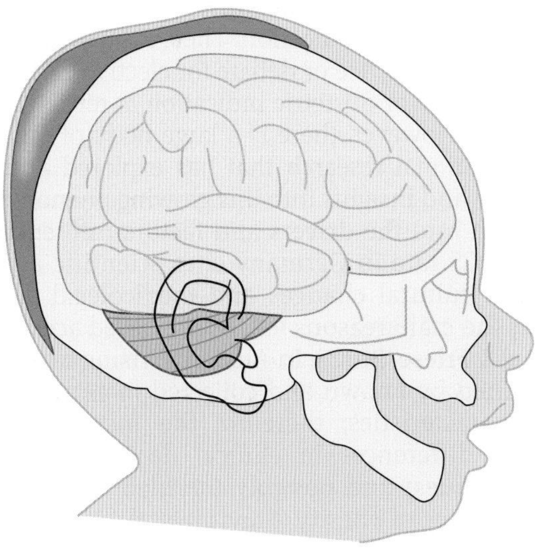

FIGURE 39.12 Subgaleal haemorrhage

Mothers' perspectives on operative delivery

Most women anticipate a spontaneous vaginal birth in a joyous atmosphere, and so unexpected outcomes can often lead to disappointment and regret. Women's experience of birth determines their attitudes and feelings towards subsequent ones, and affects what they tell their daughters, friends and relatives. The challenge is for midwives to ensure that, in pregnancy, women are empowered to make informed choices about their care and that they have an opportunity to create realistic birth plans. Moreover, all women should be given the chance to discuss the events leading up to, during and after the birth.

Care of the mother and baby following an instrumental birth

Midwives should always remember that when the natural process and movements of birthing are disrupted, as with an instrumental birth, there is always a higher risk of shoulder dystocia and postpartum haemorrhage caused by uterine atony, retained placenta fragments and trauma. Prolonged labour, immobility and assisted delivery (especially midcavity forceps) are risk factors for thromboembolism. It may be necessary to commence thromboprophylaxis. Paracetamol and ibuprofen are effective pharmaceutical analgesics following instrumental births (see also Chs 40 and 41).

Care is required to ensure appropriate bladder function. Bladder dysfunction is more common following an instrumental birth, especially if regional analgesia has been used (Chaliha, 2006). Early diagnosis and intervention are required to prevent irreversible bladder damage. The timing and volume of the first void urine should be monitored. All women who have had a midcavity forceps delivery should have a fluid balance chart, for at least 24 hours, to detect postpartum urinary retention. Post-void residual urinary catheterisation may be necessary if retention is suspected. Physiotherapy-directed strategies will help to prevent urinary incontinence.

Operative vaginal birth can be associated with fear of subsequent childbirth, and in a severe form may manifest as a post-traumatic stress type syndrome that has been referred to as 'tokophobia' (Bakshi et al., 2008). Post-traumatic stress disorder after childbirth is a poorly recognised phenomenon. Women who experienced both a high level of obstetric intervention and dissatisfaction with their birthing are more likely to develop trauma symptoms than women who receive a high level of obstetric intervention or women who perceive their care to be inadequate.

Compared with forceps delivery, the vacuum extractor is associated with an increased incidence of neonatal cephalhaematoma, retinal haemorrhage and jaundice. Immediately after the delivery the newly born infant's head should be carefully examined and then assessed at regular intervals for the next 24 hours to exclude bleeding into the scalp. If a hat has been placed on the baby's head to reduce the risk of hypothermia, it should be removed to inspect the scalp. On the day after the delivery, the clinician who performed the procedure should examine the baby in the mother's presence, answer her questions and allay any concerns.

CAESAREAN BIRTH

The rates of caesarean birth continue to rise globally. In 2019 in Australia 36% (107,543 women) had a **caesarean section** birth (AIHW, 2021). In New Zealand caesarean section rates have also increased over the last ten years to 28.4% of all births in 2018, the highest ever recorded. In 2018, a corresponding decrease in spontaneous vaginal birth (62.2%) and no change to rates of assisted vaginal birth (9.5%) was recorded (MOH, 2021). However, in New Zealand most women giving birth (92.9%) received care from a community-based Lead Maternity Carer (MOH, 2021). This notable fact may explain some of the differences between Australia and New Zealand's rate of operative birth. In Australia, Dahlen et al. (2012) showed that less than 12% of Australian childbearing women have risk markers that suggest an intervention may be required. Why, then, has the rate of caesarean surgery climbed so dramatically in the past 30 years?

The rise cannot be fully explained by changing demographics or an increase in maternal age; it is therefore of public health importance that the short- and long-term consequences of caesarean birth are well understood. The only intervention to date that has reduced the rate of caesareans in low-risk women is caseload midwifery care (Sandall et al., 2016).

According to a study of responses to open-ended questions collected through a 6-week postnatal survey in the M@NGO trial in Australia, the caseload model provided midwives with the motivation and capacity to go 'above and beyond' and to be 'empowering and endorphic' (Allen et al., 2017) (Fig. 39.13). These concepts highlight some of the active ingredients that moderate or mediate the effects of the midwifery care within the M@NGO trial (Tracy et al., 2013) and may in the future be found to be associated with reducing surgical intervention in birth. The concept of an 'endorphic midwife' (Allen et al., 2017) makes a useful contribution to midwifery theory as it enhances our understanding of how the complex intervention of caseload midwifery may influence normal birth rates and experiences.

Systematic reviews and research based mainly in high-income countries has shown us that midwife-led continuity of care offers a middle path by reducing the likelihood of potentially harmful interventions (Betran et al., 2018; Edmonds et al., 2020; Sandall et al., 2016; WHO, 2018). Without a significant change in the current trajectory of health spending maternity systems will become harder to sustain due to increasing costs and inefficiencies including wasteful spending on the overuse of interventions and rising rates of caesarean section. The problem is how to implement or adopt evidence-based interventions factoring in the dynamic complexity of both the intervention and the system in which the intervention takes place (Shiell et al., 2008). Experience shows us that introducing new ways of doing things is not simply a function of reallocating resources or directing change from the top down.

Why caesarean birth?

Beyond clinical complications that necessitate a CS the drivers are diverse, complex and often interrelated via complex social factors and processes. Caesareans are undoubtedly lifesaving and necessary at times. For example:

- cord prolapse
- placenta praevia
- placental abruption
- persistent transverse lie of the fetus.

These life-threatening conditions occur in approximately less than 1% of all births (Wolf, 2017), which suggests that surgical delivery is happening at a rate more often than is medically necessary.

CS rates are affected by:

- sociodemographic factors including health insurance status, institutional culture including clinicians' attitudes and preferences, social norms including family and social pressures, the legal system and fear of litigation (Box 39.13)
- access to services and the availability of technology
- women's requests, and women's role models, in particular portrayal of celebrity birth (O'Leary et al., 2007).

The main drivers of CS have been reported as:

- private health insurance (AIHW, 2021; Dahlen et al., 2012, 2014; Roberts et al., 2000)
- previous CS (AIHW, 2021)
- increasing maternal age associated with the presence of medical conditions or previous pregnancy complications rather than age alone (Morris et al., 2018)
- non-Caucasian, non-indigenous ethnicity (O'Leary et al., 2007; Thomas & Paranjothy, 2001)
- nulliparity (McCarthy et al., 2007; O'Leary et al., 2007)
- socioeconomic advantage (O'Leary et al., 2007).

There are increasing rates of CS before the onset of labour for no clinical indication. There is no evidence from RCTs to inform practice or debate for elective CS in the absence of medical or obstetric indication at term (Lavender et al., 2012). However, there is a large body of qualitative and observational research that has explored and offers explanation and insights into this growing phenomenon.

Research into the drivers and factors influencing the increasing CS rate in Germany cites scientific advances, social and cultural changes and medicolegal considerations as the main reasons for the increased acceptability (Mylonas & Friese, 2015). In Australia, rising rates cannot be explained by known and collected maternal or pregnancy characteristics; therefore the increase may be related to differences in clinical decision making or maternal request and possibly the high and increasing Australian rates of obesity (Stavrou et al., 2011). There is growing concern, however, from all corners of the globe regarding the overmedicalisation of birth and the increasing level of intervention and consequent morbidity

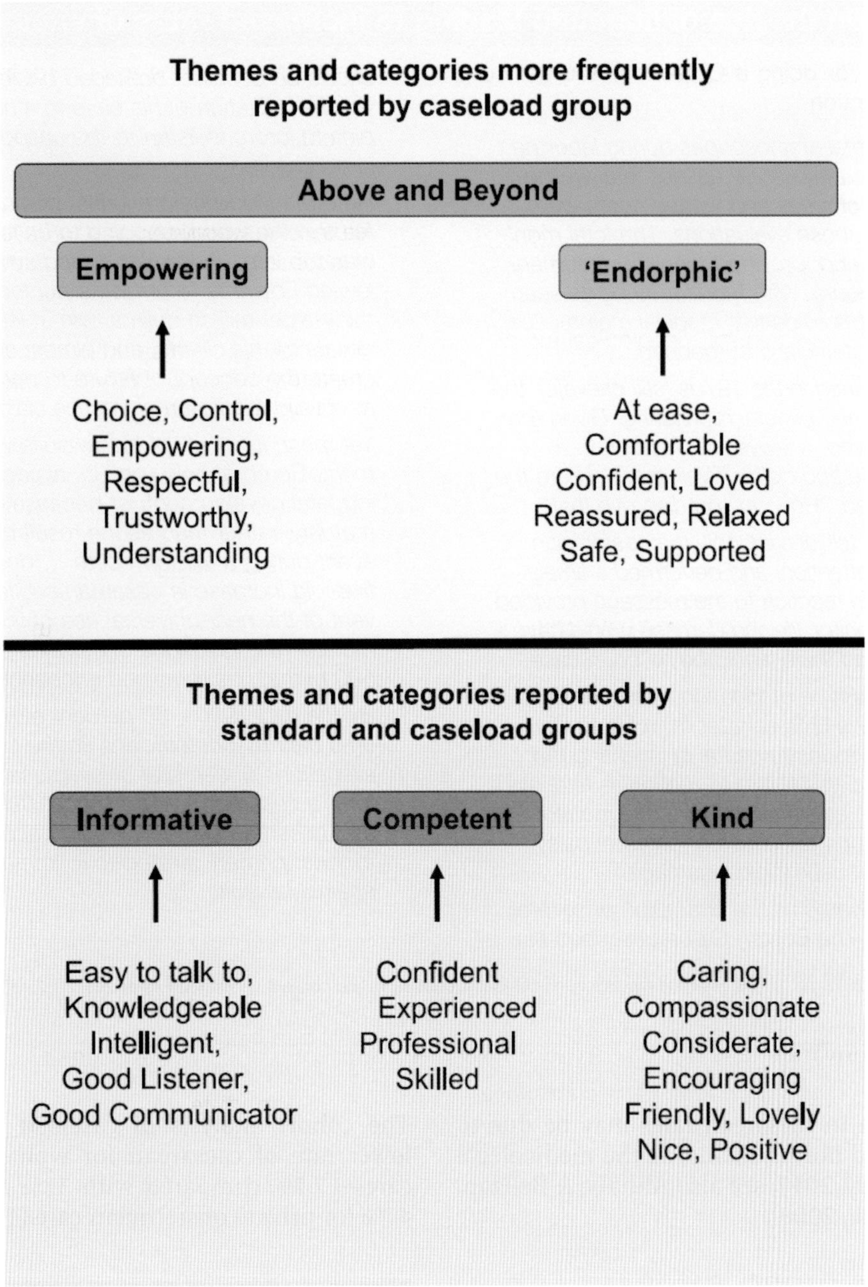

FIGURE 39.13 Athematic map of the overarching theme 'above and beyond' explaining the association between the five categories of midwife attributes
(Source: Allen et al., 2017)

amongst childbearing women (Betran et al., 2021; Miller et al., 2016; see also Kotaska, n.d.).

The evidence to support the relative safety of different surgical modes of delivery is complex, often controversial and remains conflicting. Other than one trial of vaginal compared with caesarean birth for term breech presentation, little evidence from RCTs exists to compare the safety of caesarean with vaginal birth (Bell et al., 2001). With the growing trend towards 'patient choice' or 'purely elective' caesarean deliveries, there is a need for better understanding of the risks of all forms of delivery to enable informed consent (Black et al., 2005) (Fig. 39.14).

Although CS rates have increased over the past 20 years, the major clinical determinants of the CS rate have not changed (Farquhar et al., 2017). Maternal demographics have changed in that women giving birth are likely to be heavier and possibly older than 20 years ago. Infant birth weight has also changed over the past 20 years. Maternal preferences may account for a small proportion of caesarean births; however, it seems that

Box 39.13 On the rise of litigation leading to increased rates of caesarean section

'You don't get sued for doing a C-section. You get sued for not doing a C-section.'

While the use of fetal stethoscopes during labor had allowed doctors to periodically assess fetal wellbeing, physicians' memories and written notes were the only record of those evaluations. The fetal monitor, on the other hand, provided tangible documentation of entire labours. With monitor strips as seemingly incontrovertible evidence, medical malpractice claims against obstetricians burgeoned …

An obstetrician trained in the 1970s 'still grieve[s]' the litigiousness spawned by fetal monitoring. Given the device, she observed, a lawyer could point to a squiggle on a page and claim, 'Well, that's where the baby was damaged.' How do you disprove that?

Lawyers began to tell juries: if only the obstetrician had been paying attention, and performed a timely cesarean section in reaction to the message provided by the stalwart monitor, lifelong damage would have been prevented and there would be no court case.

The pioneer of this type of litigation was John Edwards—eventually a U.S. senator from North Carolina … Edwards was instrumental in inventing the claim that a physician's failure to recognize fetal hypoxia during labor, as signalled by a fetal monitor printout, was the primary cause of cerebral palsy and other forms of neurological damage.

Admirers cast Edwards as the champion of severely disabled children. The Boston Globe described his efforts on behalf of damaged babies as going 'beyond a recitation of his case to a heart-wrenching plea to jurors to listen to the unspoken voices of injured children'.

He often stood before juries, playing the role of the fetus in the womb begging to be let out before it was too late. Juries responded sympathetically, allowing Edwards to amass a personal fortune of thirty-eight million dollars, win at least 205 million dollars for his clients, and almost single-handedly create the concept of failure to perform a cesarean as a valid medical malpractice claim …

Yet most, if not all, of his lawsuits were without merit. Cerebral palsy occurs almost exclusively during fetal development, or because of extreme prematurity, rather than as the result of an untoward event during a full-term birth … despite a more than five-fold increase in cesarean sections since the advent of the near-universal use of the electronic fetal monitor, the incidence of cerebral palsy, at one in 500 births, has remained unchanged …

By the mid-1990s, 60 percent of malpractice premiums paid by obstetricians (in the US) went to cover allegations of cerebral palsy caused by failure to perform a cesarean … The successful claims ensured that cesarean sections would become one of obstetricians' primary strategies to immunize themselves against lawsuits …

(Source: Jacqueline H Wolf (2017, pp. 22–23) Risk and reputation: obstetricians, cesareans, and consent. *J Hist Med Allied Sci*. 2017;73(1):7–28, by permission of Oxford University Press)

much of the increase in caesarean rates may be due to cultural pressures and norms, including the medicolegal environment (Caughey, 2017; see also Althabe & Belizan, 2006; Bourgeault et al., 2008).

Lowering caesarean rates

New Zealand has a significantly lower national CS rate than Australia, and in particular the primary units (where women are attended mainly by midwives) in both countries are showing real gains in lowering the CS rate. Place of birth has a significant effect on the rate of caesarean birth (see Ch. 7). Reduction in interventions are associated with home birth, one-to-one support in labour and induction of labour for uncomplicated pregnancies beyond 41 weeks. Women deemed low risk and receiving caseload midwifery also have demonstrated a decrease in caesarean rate (McLachlan et al., 2012). An RCT of caseload care versus standard care at two tertiary level Australian hospitals demonstrated a substantial fall in the rate of CS compared with pretrial levels among all women regardless of risk status within the trial (Tracy et al., 2013). The cohort analysis of caseload care demonstrated a lower rate of caesarean for women receiving caseload care—17.2% compared with 33% for standard care and 47% for private obstetrician care (Tracy et al., 2014).

CRITICAL THINKING EXERCISE

Make a note of the neonatal and maternal outcomes from midwife-led units and primary-level units that are documented in the literature so far. Draw a comparison table of the rates of intervention (CS/instrumental birth) in relation to the perinatal mortality of those countries. Report data from your own practice concerning caesarean birth rates and prevention, vaginal birth after caesarean and elective caesarean.

Indications for caesarean section

Caesarean birth is the delivery of the infant through an abdominal and uterine incision. The method originated

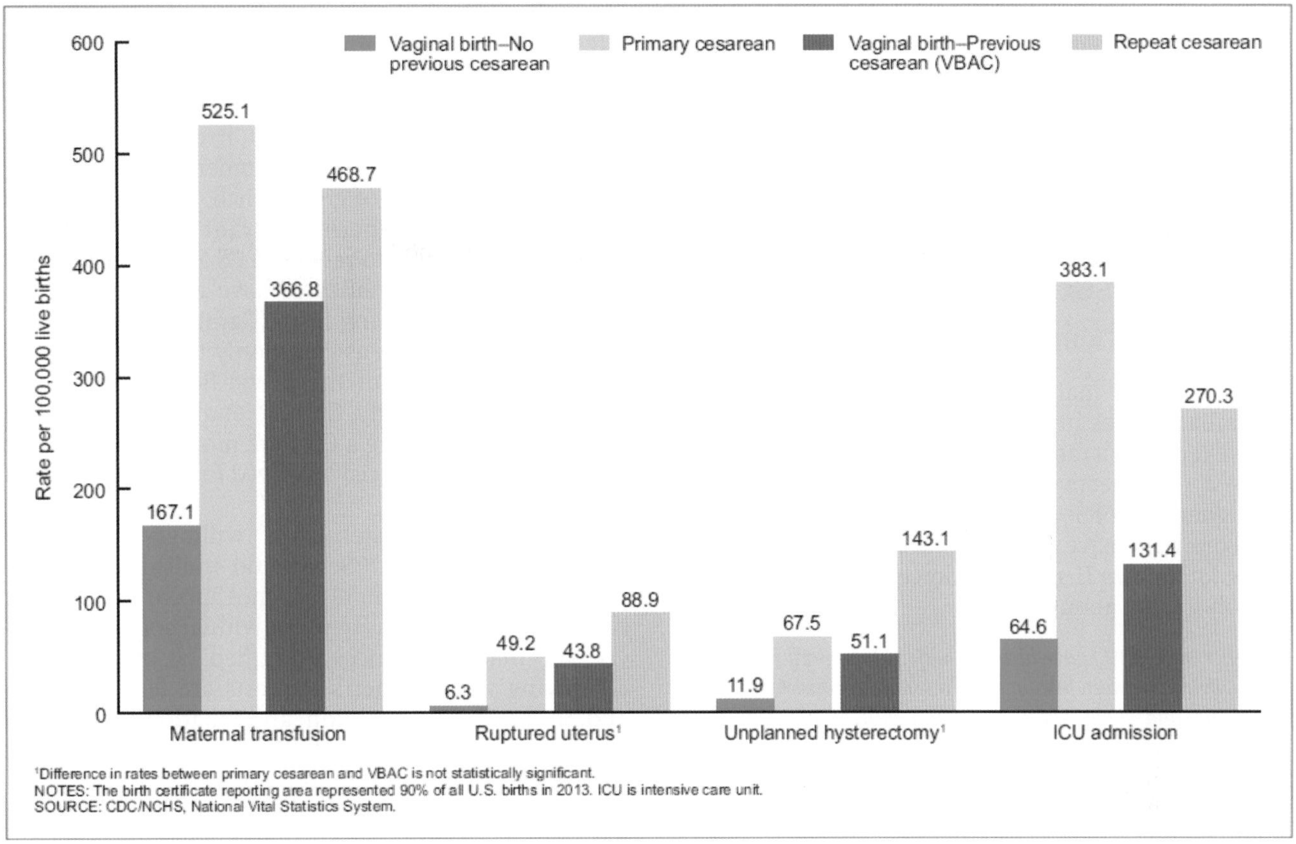

FIGURE 39.14 Maternal morbidity, by method of birth and previous caesarean history, US 2013
(Source: CDC Vital Statistics https://www.cdc.gov/nchs/data/nvsr/nvsr64/nvsr64_04.pdf)

as a salvage procedure to rescue a child from a dying or dead mother. Technological and medical advances have altered society's attitude towards caesarean birth, from considering it a 'procedure of last resort' to an 'alternative birth method'. Nevertheless, it is often a traumatic and difficult decision for all concerned, and the risks and benefits of surgical birth should always be thoroughly discussed with each woman and her midwife and obstetric colleagues. (Shoe size, maternal height and estimations of fetal size (ultrasound or clinical examination) do not accurately predict CPD and should not be used to predict 'failure to progress' during labour.) The decision to perform a CS is based primarily on the question of what is best for or may save the lives of the mother and child. The indications for CS can therefore be divided into absolute and relative indications. Elective CS, performed solely at the wish of the mother and without any medical indication, is considered a separate indication.

The main indications for a caesarean surgery (overlapping in some cases) can be divided into absolute and relative indications (adapted from Mylonas & Friese, 2015, pp. 490–91):

Absolute indications for CS include:

- *absolute disproportion*: small maternal pelvis, making vaginal birth impossible
- *chorioamnionitis* (amniotic infection syndrome): infection of the placenta and possibly of the fetus, requiring immediate delivery
- *maternal pelvic deformity*: anatomical malformation, making vaginal birth impossible
- *eclampsia and HELLP syndrome*: life-threatening complications of pregnancy, usually leading to caesarean delivery
- *fetal asphyxia or fetal acidosis*: life-threatening situations for the fetus that can lead to fetal hypoxia
- *umbilical cord prolapse*: prolapse of the umbilical cord between the head of the fetus and the vaginal opening, which can lead to fetal asphyxia
- *placenta praevia*: anomalous placental position, impeding vaginal birth
- *abnormal lie and presentation*: anomaly of fetal position that makes vaginal birth impossible
- *uterine rupture*: acute situation threatening the life of both mother and fetus, requiring immediate delivery by CS.

Relative indications for CS include:

- *pathological CTG*: may provide indication of acute hypoxia or fetal asphyxia; if fetal acidosis occurs, the birth should be completed either as an instrumental delivery (suction and / or forceps) or by CS

- *failure to progress in labour* (prolonged labour, secondary arrest): delayed delivery or cessation of labour can result in an adverse outcome for the fetus or newborn
- *previous CS*: it is widely assumed that having had one CS makes it impossible to have a vaginal birth in subsequent pregnancies; however, this indication is changing as more evidence accumulates on the safety of vaginal birth following a previous CS.

Caesarean section 'on demand' (maternal choice?)

The rates of CS for maternal request are poorly reported. In Australia, studies utilising prospective consumer surveys have reported a rate of 0.3% (Gamble & Creedy, 2001) whereas a retrospective obstetrician survey reported a much higher rate, of 3% of births (Robson et al., 2009).

The comprehensive and landmark study from the US, *Listening to Mothers II study* (Declercq et al., 2007) found in the cohort that about:

> *1 mother in 3 (32%) gave birth by major abdominal surgery, evenly divided between first time and repeat cesareans. Although the media and some health professionals have given much attention to the phenomenon of 'maternal request' cesareans, just 1 mother among the 252 survey participants with an initial (primary) cesarean reported having had a planned cesarean at her own request with no medical reason. Similarly, just 1 mother (in a repeat cesarean) reported having a cesarean in the belief that it would help avoid incontinence later in life, despite extensive media and professional focus on cesarean as a purported preventive measure for long-term pelvic floor problems. A small proportion of mothers with a previous cesarean (11%) had a VBAC (vaginal birth after cesarean), though quite a few would have liked to have had the choice but had providers or hospitals unwilling to support their vaginal births.*
>
> (Extract from the *Listening to Mothers II Report*, Declercq et al., 2007, p. 11)

In the subsequent study Listening to Mothers III (Declercq et al., 2013) almost six in ten respondents strongly agreed (34%) or agreed (25%) with the statement, 'Giving birth is a process that should not be interfered with unless medically necessary' (p. 34).

The reasons women give for requesting a CS are diverse. Some women cite a family history of difficult labour or history of previous CS (Kornelsen et al., 2010; Schimpf et al., 2011); others cite the presence of a medical condition, a sense of vulnerability due to age, especially when conception was challenging, and influences of family and friends (Kornelsen et al., 2010). Fear of pain or fear of an adverse outcome associated with a vaginal birth have also been identified as reasons (Fenwick et al., 2010; Kornelsen et al., 2010) with some women perceiving greater risk to their baby's wellbeing with a vaginal birth than if they have a CS (Kornelsen et al., 2010).

Women if given the option, and irrespective of whether they have had a previous caesarean birth or not, are more likely to prefer to have a normal birth than an elective CS (Gamble & Creedy, 2001; Schimpf et al., 2011). Women also believe that elective CS on maternal request is not advisable and that normal birth is safer for mother (Schimpf et al., 2011) and baby (Pevzner et al., 2008). In contrast, an Australian study exploring cultural norms of the acceptance of CSs found that, irrespective of individual sociodemographic factors, women perceived CS as an easy, convenient way of giving birth (Walker et al., 2004) or a sign of 'good mothering' (Bryant et al., 2007).

Those more likely to request a CS are those who have a complication of pregnancy or have experienced a previous complication during birth (Gamble & Creedy, 2001). Women are not likely, as commonly thought, to choose a CS for maintenance of the pelvic floor (Schimpf et al., 2011). Not surprisingly, Gamble et al. (2001) also found that women preferring a CS were more anxious, and had less knowledge of the risk involved in a CS while overstating the safety.

Differences in obstetricians' willingness to support women requesting a CS with no indication varies between countries and there does not appear to be a correlation of this willingness with individual countries' rates of CS. The main influences identified by obstetricians in complying with women's requests are fear of litigation and, in the European region, an affiliation with a university hospital (Habiba et al., 2006). One study reported that obstetricians interpreted women's concerns about childbirth anxieties and the health of the baby as maternal request (Hopkins, 2000); in particular the exchange of evidence and information on the procedure was suggested to be constrained, sanitised or absent, with women reporting that the decision for caesarean was because of medical recommendation.

Women have been reported to be resolute about their decision for CS at maternal request (patient initiated). Primiparous women having an elective CS expressed that there was a lack of rigor in discussion for informed consent; however, they were likely to view clinicians who declined or resisted their request as obstructive and unsupportive (Kornelsen et al., 2010). So it seems possible and plausible that maternal pressure for caesarean on request may be influencing obstetric practice particularly in the private sector (O'Leary et al., 2007; Stavrou et al., 2011).

Michel Odent makes the observation, in his booklet on caesarean sections (Odent, 2004, p. 7), that at the end of the 20th century we were wondering whether it was ethical for women to 'demand' to have a CS on request (without known medical indicators), and at the beginning of the 21st century we are wondering whether all women should give birth by CS!

The phenomenon of elective CS on demand began in Italy and in the largest Latin American cities (Behague et al., 2002; Belizan et al., 1999; Potter et al., 2001). There has been vigorous debate about the ethical and biological 'need' for women to have an elective CS on demand. In Australia, several factors have influenced the prevalence of elective caesarean birth. These include the belief that CS is protective of urinary and faecal incontinence, that elective CS is safe, and that women's autonomy around birth translates into their right to choose an elective CS regardless of clinical indication. (For further discussion of the concept of a woman's right to choose CS, see Bewley & Cockburn (2002), Clement (1995), O'Neill (2002), Odent (2004) and Wolf (2017) in Further reading.)

CRITICAL THINKING EXERCISE

How would you suggest lowering the rate of CS in your health facility—given the most common indications for surgical birth are a prior caesarean, inadequate progress of labour and abnormal FHR tracing?

The following summaries will give you an idea of how contentious the subject is (see also Box 39.14, for the statement by the American College of Obstetricians and Gynecologists (ACOG)).

- The National Institute of Health and Clinical Excellence (NICE) guidelines that appeared in November 2011 contain the following recommendations concerning CS by maternal request (NICE, 2011, pp. 58–9):
    - *For women requesting a CS, if after discussion and offer of support (including perinatal mental health support for women with anxiety about childbirth), a vaginal delivery is still not an acceptable option, offer a planned CS.*
    - *An obstetrician unwilling to perform a CS should refer the woman to an obstetrician who will carry out the CS.*

Box 39.14 Elective caesarean section[a]

We conclude that beneficence-based, justice-based and autonomy-based considerations do not support routinely recommending or even offering elective caesarean delivery.

The physician should respond to questions with a thorough informed consent process and a suggestion that the woman reconsider her request in order to ensure that her autonomy is being meaningfully exercised.

In these cases, implementing her request is ethically permissible. The physician should beware of the potentially insidious influence of economic and other forms of conflict of interest. Acting on self-interest in increased income or convenience distorts clinical judgement and undermines the physician's fiduciary obligations to patients. However, by neither dismissing a patient's informed desire regarding caesarean delivery, nor automatically acquiescing to it, the physician maintains both a responsibility to professional integrity and a respect for the patient's autonomy.

[a]Statement made by a group of physicians, obstetricians and medical ethicists in the United States and published by the American College of Obstetricians and Gynecologists.
(Source: Minkoff et al., 2004)

- The International Federation of Gynecology and Obstetrics (FIGO) stated that it is unethical to perform a CS without a medical reason because of inadequate evidence to support a net benefit (Schenker & Cain, 1999).
- To maintain objective decision making in the face of a barrage of medicolegal, media and emotional concerns is difficult, and it would be easy for women and doctors to slip into a short-term approach of doing CS as the easy way out: 'the belief that a caesarean delivery is the easy way does not appear to come from facts about caesarean birth itself but rather from deeply rooted fears about vaginal childbirth' (Clement, 1995, Introduction). Is it fear, or simply that obstetricians are rightly more relaxed about the dangers of CS and focusing more on the recently and incompletely researched complications of vaginal delivery (Bump & Norton, 1998, cited in Bewley & Cockburn, 2002).
- The Canadian Association of Midwives argued that presenting interventions such as CS as 'options' puts maternity care providers and women in a consumerist relationship, and treats childbirth as a problem to be solved rather than a process to be respected (Canadian Association of Midwives (CAM), 2004).
- From an anonymous survey sent to all gynaecologists and registrars in the Netherlands in 1999, the researchers concluded that 'in The Netherlands, a woman can always find a gynaecologist willing to perform a CS for non-medical reasons. This willingness increases with the age of the doctor. There is a need for guidelines when handling these cases' (Kwee et al., 2004, online abstract: https://www.ncbi.nlm.nih.gov/pubmed/15063958).
- Research undertaken by the author with a team from the University of New South Wales found that women identified themselves as good or bad mothers and felt obliged to choose what is set up as the most obvious and sensible option: safe, ordered caesareans. In this way, caesareans can be positioned as a preferential means of birth (Bryant et al., 2007).

REFLECTIVE THINKING EXERCISE

Ethical issues in elective caesarean birth force us to examine our obligations of justice (treating women fairly, and allocating healthcare resources fairly), respect for autonomy (self-governance, privacy and individual choice), non-malfeasance (offering only treatments that have a benefit, doing no harm) and beneficence (promoting good and preventing harm).

Can you make a 'case' for and against the right to have a CS 'on demand'?

Preventing urinary incontinence

Many caesarean sections are performed in the belief that avoiding vaginal birth is a means of avoiding future urinary incontinence. However, the finding that the prevalence of urinary incontinence in postmenopausal nuns who had never been pregnant is similar to that reported in parous, postmenopausal women appears to be contrary to the conventional wisdom that nulliparity protects against stress urinary incontinence (Buchsbaum et al., 2002). It is clear that our understanding of factors leading to pelvic floor disruption over a woman's lifetime is limited, and that the topic is extremely complex. Pregnancy itself may predispose to mechanical changes, hormonal changes or both that can lead to urinary incontinence (Rortveit et al., 2003).

In an editorial in the *British Journal of Obstetrics and Gynaecology* the editor remarked on the fact that it is pregnancy itself, and not childbirth, that has the greater effect on the frequency of pelvic floor dysfunction in the population (Grant, 2000). One in eight women who had never been pregnant had some form of pelvic floor dysfunction, compared with one-half of the women who had had a CS or a spontaneous vaginal delivery and two-thirds of the women who underwent an instrumental vaginal delivery (Grant, 2000). Meanwhile, in the United States, Diony Young, a past editor of *Birth*, lamented:

> *What is a woman's chance of having a caesarean delivery? Certainly these days she's at high risk if she's too big or too small; too early or too late; too old or too fearful; too tired of being pregnant or too tired of being in labour; if she's having twins, if she's breech, if she's previously had a caesarean; or if she's due and so is the weekend, Christmas ....*
>
> (Young, 2003)

Breech presentation at term

Breech presentation is one of the contributing factors to the rate of CS in Australia. Consequently, midwifery and obstetric exposure in the management of vaginal breech birth has significantly diminished (NSW Health, 2017). This means that, among singleton pregnancies (and the first of twins), 1 in every 23 babies (12,984 babies) is breech and 90% of these result in a CS. Breech presentation is considered a primary indication for CS; however, there is increasing evidence to show that vaginal breech must be reconsidered as a safe option for uncomplicated vaginal birth (Kotaska et al., 2009). (See also Ch. 36.)

External cephalic version

Interventions to promote cephalic version of babies in the breech position include external cephalic version (ECV), moxibustion and postural management. ECV involves applying pressure to the mother's abdomen to turn the fetus in either a forward or backward 'somersault' to achieve a vertex presentation. (See also Ch. 36.)

The risk of maternal morbidity following caesarean section

Not only does a surgical birth increase the rate of longer hospital stays postpartum for the mother and the baby, but also serious morbidity following caesarean birth now includes the rising rate of placental disorders in the next pregnancy. (See also Ch. 40.)

An increased risk of uterine rupture can occur for women with a previous CS irrespective of whether they have planned repeat CS or not. For women attempting labour the risk is increased when induction of labour is performed, in particular among women with prostaglandin-induced labour (Lydon-Rochelle et al., 2001a). There is significant maternal risk in the immediate post-surgery period. Women have been reported to have nearly twice the risk of hospital re-admission following a CS than if they have had a vaginal birth (Liu et al., 2005; Lydon-Rochelle et al., 2000). Research has shown that the increase in re-admission is attributable to an increased presentation of venous disorders and thromboembolism, obstetric surgical complication, pelvic injury or wound infection as a result of the surgery (Lydon-Rochelle et al., 2000) and puerperal infection for women post CS operation (Liu et al., 2005). In addition women are more likely to be re-admitted for mental health, cardiopulmonary, gastrointestinal and urogenital problems (Liu et al., 2005). Women who had a CS and were re-admitted to hospital generally had a longer length of stay compared with women who gave birth vaginally (Liu et al., 2005; Lydon-Rochelle et al., 2000). Studies have shown that, in terms of general wellbeing, primiparous women at 7 weeks post CS had less vitality in performing simple life tasks, and were more likely to score lower in mental health status, have pain that interfered with day-to-day functioning and state that their health interfered with their social activities than women who had an unassisted vaginal birth (Lydon-Rochelle et al., 2001b).

Little is known about the impact of CS on normal physiology for the mother; however, it has been demonstrated that maternal neuroendocrine function in breastfeeding mothers is altered post CS. The postbirth secretion of the hormones oxytocin and prolactin is decreased and this influences breastfeeding efficiency and success and also the promotion of maternal–infant attachment (Nissen et al., 1996). The association of CS and delayed initiation of breastfeeding postbirth and lowered exclusive breastfeeding rates has also been demonstrated (Zanardo et al., 2010).

Abnormalities of placentation

One of the major maternal morbidities associated with the growing global rate of CS is the rising incidence of abnormal placentation, which falls under the broad term of **placenta accreta spectrum** (Jauniaux et al., 2018). Women who have undergone a previous caesarean are at risk in subsequent pregnancies of placenta accreta spectrum (PAS) (Jauniaux et al., 2018), which carries significant morbidity for women and their babies (see Box 39.15 and Figs 39.15 and 39.16). PAS is a histopathological term that defines abnormally adherent and invasive placentation and is the consequence of damage to the endometrium–myometrial interface of the uterine wall. When first described 80 years ago, it mainly occurred after manual removal of the placenta, uterine curettage or endometritis.

Box 39.15 Abnormal placentation

Abnormal placental implantation with myometrial penetration can be a potentially life-threatening condition. Placenta accreta, increta and percreta represent a continuum under the broader category of placental implantation disorders.

The grading classification of abnormal placentation is according to the depth of villous invasiveness inside the myometrium and falls into the following three categories:

- placenta creta when the villi simply adhere to the myometrium
- placenta increta when the villi invade the myometrium
- placenta percreta when the villi invade the full thickness of the myometrium through the serosal layer of the uterus with potential invasion of adjacent organs.

Abnormal implantation of the placenta in or through the uterine wall can precipitate profuse haemorrhage, often at the time of birth. The most common treatment for this is a hysterectomy performed immediately following birth. The incidence of emergency hysterectomy after childbirth is reported to range from 1.55 per 1000 deliveries in the United States to 0.2 per 1000 deliveries in Norway.

(Source: Engelsen et al., 2001; Jauniaux et al., 2018)

Superficial damage leads primarily to an abnormally adherent placenta, and is diagnosed as the complete or partial absence of the decidua on histology. Today, the main cause of placenta accreta spectrum is uterine surgery and, in particular, 'uterine scar secondary to cesarean delivery' (Jauniaux et al., 2018, p. 1). Amongst women giving birth for the first time the independent risk factors for placenta accreta are advanced maternal age and a current multiple pregnancy. Amongst multiparous women the risk factors are a previous CS and a current placenta praevia (Farquhar et al., 2017). Following a first CS, women having their second or subsequent birth are at an increased risk of placental abruption and placenta praevia compared with first-time mothers who give birth vaginally (Lydon-Rochelle et al., 2001c). The rising CS rate over the past 20 years has been accompanied by a 10-fold rise in the incidence of placenta accreta (Jauniaux et al., 2018).

The incidence of placenta accreta in a study of the combined rate in Australia and New Zealand was 44.2 / 100,000 women giving birth (Farquhar et al., 2017). This is similar to the rates reported previously from single-centre studies in individual hospitals in New Zealand (60.2 / 100,000) (Wong et al., 2008) and Australia (38.8 / 100,000) (Grace et al., 2013).

Although the condition remains relatively rare, it is associated with a high risk of severe morbidity, and the rare risk of maternal death. These facts underlie the significance of an incidence rate of 1 in 2000 women giving birth in Australia and New Zealand (Farquhar et al., 2017). With the increased incidence of CS worldwide, we can expect to see peripartum hysterectomy becoming a major morbidity among women who have previously had CS (Jauniaux et al., 2018).

Neonatal outcomes

Neonatal outcomes following CS vary in seriousness and long-term morbidity. Although birth asphyxia is the most worrying outcome, both initially and because of the long-term sequelae (see Cerebral palsy, earlier in the chapter), serious morbidity is experienced in other forms of birth trauma. Serious trauma has been defined as subdural or cerebral haemorrhage, fractured clavicle, other injuries to the skeleton, injury to the spine or spinal cord, facial nerve palsy, brachial plexus injury, subarachnoid haemorrhage,

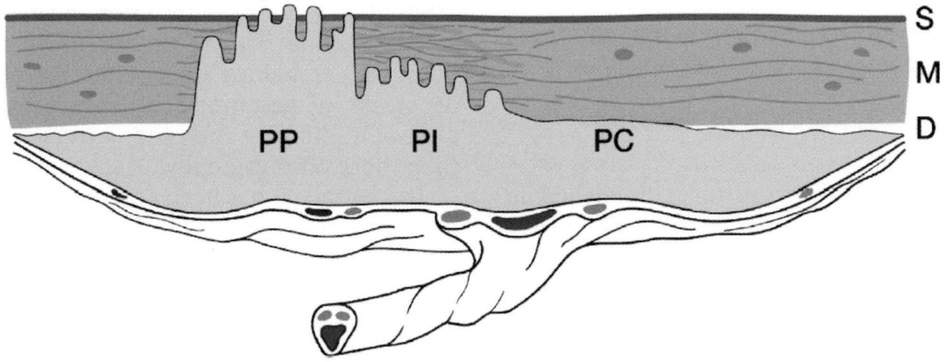

Anterior placenta previa accreta combining areas of abnormal adherence and invasion to the uterine wall: creta, increta, and percreta.

D, decidua; *M*, myometrium; *PC*, placenta creta; *PI*, placenta increta; *PP*, placenta percreta; *S*, serosa.

FIGURE 39.15 Placenta accreta spectrum
(Reproduced from Jauniaux et al. *Am J Obstet Gynecol.*, 2018)

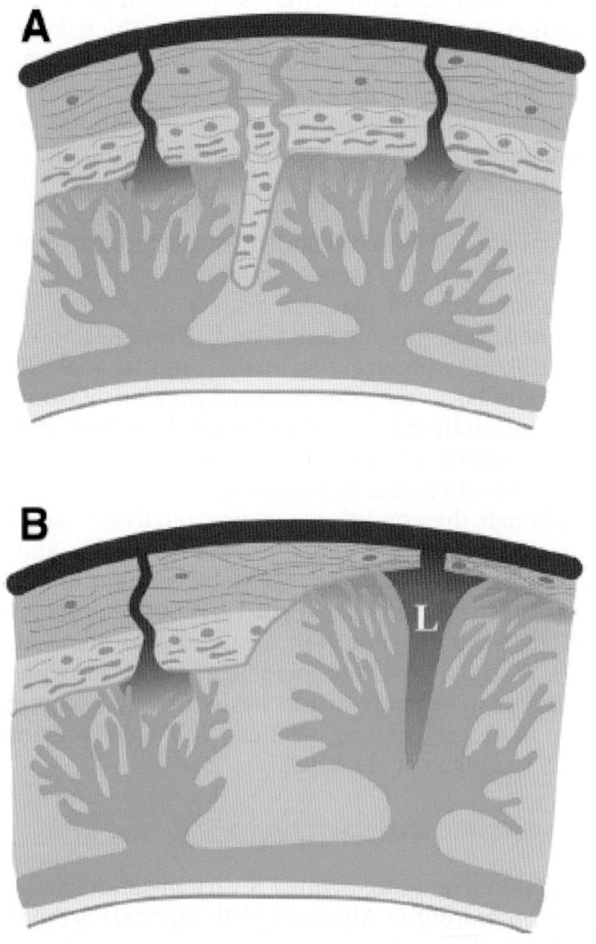

FIGURE 39.16 Normal and accreta cotyledons. Placental cotyledon in A, normal and B, increta placentation reaching deep myometrial circulation. Note distortion of normal cotyledon anatomy in increta placentation with loss of intercotyledon septa and formation of lacuna (L)
(Reproduced from Jauniaux et al. *Am J Obstet Gynecol*. 2018)

convulsions, other and unspecified cerebral irritation, or cerebral depression/coma.

Short-term neonatal morbidity following caesarean section

A large linked data study from Australia published in 2014 (Dahlen et al., 2014) found that the continual rise in obstetric intervention for low-risk women in Australia, especially in private hospitals, may be contributing to increased morbidity for babies at a higher cost for healthcare. Rates of CS among low-risk women having their first baby were higher in private versus public hospitals (24.7% versus 15.6%) with the rate of elective CS (before the onset of labour) (8.8% versus 3.0%). In addition to this these women had an epidural rate of 70.8% versus 35.4%. In association with such high rates of obstetric intervention within the first 28 days, there were higher rates of admission for babies born in private hospitals for reasons such as birth trauma (mainly scalpel related), jaundice, feeding difficulties and respiratory conditions (Dahlen et al., 2014). The study found that regardless of this unexplained variation in intervention and admission rates the perinatal mortality did not differ between the groups (Dahlen et al., 2014). Further research by Dahlen et al. (2021) using large, linked data sets showed that the rate of intervention in birth rises in both first-time mothers and those women having a second or subsequent baby following the introduction of induction of labour, which is clearly associated with a consequent rise in rates of intervention. The paper also found that following induction, incidences of neonatal birth trauma, resuscitation and respiratory disorders were higher, as were admissions to hospital for infections (ear, nose, throat, respiratory and sepsis) up to 16 years (Dahlen et al., 2021).

In an Australian population-based study of over a million low-risk babies born between 37 and 41 weeks gestation, Tracy et al. (2007b) found that after an elective CS the odds of admission to a neonatal intensive care unit (NICU) or special-care nursery were significantly increased for all gestations less than 40 weeks regardless of parity. Among babies born to first-time mothers at 37 weeks, the adjusted odds of admission to a NICU or special-care nursery were 12 times greater than those for babies born at 40 weeks gestation (Tracy et al., 2007b) (Fig. 39.17). To understand the benefit of gestational maturity, see also Every Week Counts: http://www.everyweekcounts.com.au.

Several studies have shown that, in addition to the risk of being born via CS, infants born by CS at term without experiencing labour experience further risk factors. One of the major problems for infants born before the onset of labour is an increased risk of respiratory distress syndrome. Studies in the United Kingdom undertaken by Morrison et al. (1995) found that among term babies born via CS the risk of neonatal respiratory distress was higher (35.5 with prelabour caesarean, versus 12.2 with caesarean during labour, versus 5.3 with vaginal birth, per 1000 live births). This relationship was maintained week by week up to 40 weeks gestation (Morrison et al., 1995). Being born before term as well as by elective CS confers further risks to the infant. In the US a study of over 13,000 babies born after an elective CS before 39 weeks of gestation, the babies experienced higher rates of respiratory and other adverse neonatal outcomes than those born vaginally (Tita et al., 2009a) (Table 39.8).

In Australia it has been demonstrated that if babies are born by any means other than an unassisted vaginal birth, particularly if the CS is performed before the onset of labour, there is a stronger association with specialist neonatal intensive care (Tracy et al., 2007b). In addition to respiratory comprise, other neonatal physiological changes that occur as a result of CS and need specialist neonatal intensive care support include an impaired thermoregulation response causing lowered neonatal body temperature immediately postpartum (Christensson et al., 1993). There are other identified short-term physiological differences for the newborn associated with CS compared with vaginal birth. These include altered

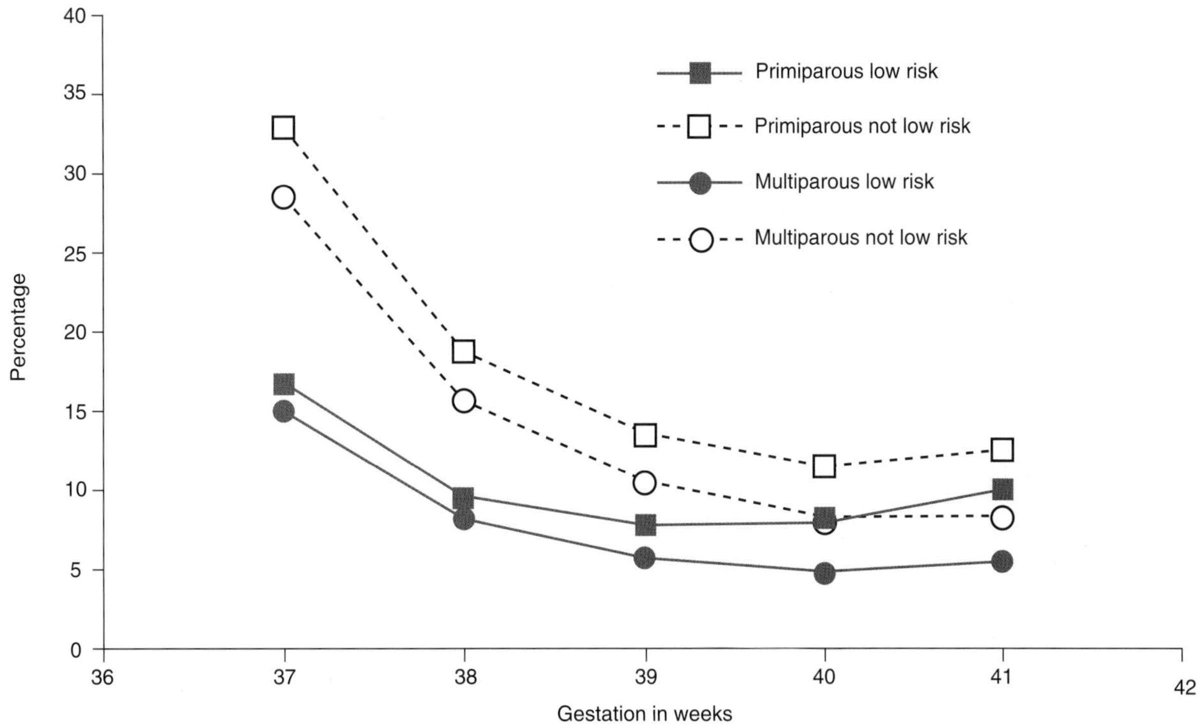

FIGURE 39.17 Rate of admission to neonatal intensive care in Australia (1999–2002), for term singleton infants, among 'low-risk' and 'not-low-risk' women
(Source: Tracy et al., 2007a)

glucose metabolism, altered immune cell populations and reduced systolic and diastolic blood pressures (Hyde et al., 2012, pp. 3–4).

Long-term neonatal morbidity following caesarean section

A growing body of evidence is emerging around the altered physiology of newborns due to CS that may influence health in later life, in particular where surgery has occurred prior to the onset of labour (Hyde et al., 2012). It has been postulated that normal vaginal birth and the physiological adaptation that occurs during this is a catalyst to long-term health 'programming' and hence the by-pass of these through CS could have health consequences (Hyde et al., 2012).

Is there an association between caesarean section and asthma?

An association between birth by CS and the later development of asthma was explored in a large population-based cohort study of over one and a half million singleton babies recorded in the birth registry of Norway between 1967 and 1998, and followed up to the age of 18 years. The researchers found that children born via CS had a 52% increased risk of asthma compared with spontaneously vaginally born children, with a possibly stronger association with emergency than with planned CS (Tollånes et al., 2008). Similar findings have been published from large epidemiological studies using linked data sets (Thilaganathan et al., 1994).

Is there an association between caesarean section and type 1 (insulin-dependent) diabetes?

A European study investigating the evidence of an increased risk of childhood-onset type 1 (insulin-dependent) diabetes in children born by caesarean section found a significant (23%) increased risk of type 1 diabetes in children born by CS that could not be explained by known confounders (Cardwell et al., 2008). The increased risk of type 1 diabetes after CS was only slightly altered after adjustment for gestational age, birth weight, maternal age, birth order, breastfeeding and maternal diabetes. The researchers hypothesised in their discussion that the explanation for the observed increase in the risk of type 1 diabetes in children born by CS could be explained by a few plausible theories:

- The difference in gut microbiotic composition could increase the risk of type 1 diabetes. The gut microbiota are known to play an important role in stimulating the development of the immune system, and recent studies have shown that the gut microbiotic composition differs in children born by CS compared with vaginally born children, perhaps because children born by CS are first exposed postpartum to bacteria originating from the hospital environment rather than to maternal bacteria. Colonisation of the gastrointestinal tract of newborn

Table 39.8 Incidence of adverse neonatal outcomes according to completed week of gestation at birth after an elective caesarean section (US)[a]

	Number/total number (%)						
Outcome	Wk 37 (*n* = 834)	Wk 38 (*n* = 3909)	Wk 39 (*n* = 6512)	Wk 40 (*n* = 1385)	Wk 41 (*n* = 505)	Wk ≥42 (*n* = 113)	*p* for trend[b]
Admission to the NICU	107/833 (12.8)	316/3905 (8.1)	382/6510 (5.9)	66/1381 (4.8)	40/504 (7.9)	16/113 (14.2)	<0.001
Hospitalisation ≥5 days	76/831 (9.1)	221/3904 (5.7)	237/6503 (3.6)	56/1381 (4.1)	38/504 (7.5)	13/113 (11.5)	<0.001
Newborn sepsis[c]	58/833 (7.0)	156/3904 (4.0)	163/6508 (2.5)	37/1381 (2.7)	19/504 (3.8)	12/113 (10.6)	<0.001
Proved case	3/833 (0.4)	3/3904 (0.1)	7/6508 (0.1)	2/1381 (0.1)	2/504 (0.4)	0/113	0.260
Adverse respiratory outcome							
Respiratory distress syndrome	31/833 (3.7)	75/3904 (0.9)	58/6510 (0.9)	13/1381 (0.9)	4/504 (0.8)	2/113 (1.8)	<0.001
Respiratory distress syndrome or transient tachypnoea of the newborn	68/833 (8.2)	213/3904 (5.5)	221/6510 (3.4)	42/1381 (3.0)	26/504 (5.2)	9/113 (8.0)	<0.001
Transient tachypnoea of the newborn	40/833 (4.8)	153/3904 (3.9)	178/6508 (2.7)	34/1381 (2.5)	24/504 (4.8)	7/113 (6.2)	<0.001
Ventilation in 1st 24 h	16/833 (1.9)	34/3904 (0.9)	27/6509 (0.4)	5/1381 (0.4)	2/504 (0.4)	0/113	<0.001
CPR or ventilation in 1st 24 h	16/833 (1.9)	35/3904 (0.9)	27/6509 (0.4)	5/1381 (0.4)	2/504 (0.4)	0/113	<0.001
Other							
Treated hypoglycaemia	20/833 (2.4)	35/3904 (0.9)	44/6508 (0.7)	11/1381 (0.8)	8/504 (1.6)	2/113 (1.8)	<0.001
Any adverse outcome or death	128/834 (15.3)	430/3909 (11.0)	524/6512 (8.0)	101/1385 (7.3)	57/505 (11.3)	22/113 (19.5)	<0.001

[a]Amongst a group of women who underwent an elective caesarean delivery (i.e. a delivery performed in the absence of labour or other recognised medical or obstetrical indications for delivery) of a viable infant at 37 weeks of gestation or later.
[b]The *p* value was calculated by the Cochran–Armitage test for trend for the period from 37 to 39 weeks only.
[c]Newborn sepsis includes both suspected infections (with clinical findings suggesting infection) and proved infections (as confirmed in a subgroup of neonates with positive cultures of blood, cerebrospinal fluid, or urine obtained by catheterisation or suprapubic aspiration; cardiovascular collapse; or an unequivocal radiograph confirming infection in a neonate with clinical sepsis).
CPR = cardiopulmonary resuscitation; NICU = neonatal intensive care unit.
(Adapted from Tita et al. Timing of elective repeat cesarean delivery at term and neonatal outcomes. *N Engl J Med.* 2009a;360:111–120)

infants starts immediately after birth and occurs within a few days. Initially, the type of delivery (passage through the birth canal versus CS) and the type of diet (breast-feeding versus formula feeding) might affect the colonisation pattern. The initial colonisation is therefore very relevant to the final composition of the permanent flora (Guarner & Malagelada, 2003).

- The incidence of childhood type 1 diabetes mellitus has risen in parallel with that of childhood asthma, and the hygiene hypothesis proposes that this is due to reduced stimulation of the immune system by early intercurrent infection. According to this hypothesis, as children born by CS may have a reduced exposure to infections compared with children born vaginally, this could increase their diabetes risk (Gale, 2002).

Is there an association between caesarean section and the development of the immune system?

In a recently published Swedish cohort study, researchers found a strong association between mode of birth and the formation of neonatal lymphocytes; compared with vaginal birth, CS was associated with 32% higher risk of having an infant with a lower number of newly formed T-lymphocytes (Schlinzig et al., 2017). Given that labour and birth stress may act as primers and regulators of the neonatal immune system, and given that stress of being born is strongly related to mode of birth, with a much lower sympathoadrenal activation after elective CS than after vaginal birth, it appears that mode of birth may be an important determinant of the postnatal adaption of the offspring immune system (Schlinzig et al., 2017).

A 14-year follow-up population-based study from Denmark concluded that the newborn delivered by elective CS does not acquire microbial colonisation from the birth canal where the membranes are usually intact, which is in contrast to the situation in acute CS where the child might already be colonised with the maternal vaginal microflora in utero. They found that children delivered by CS are at increased risk of disease associated with immune function and, in particular those diseases involving the mucosal immune system (Kristensen & Henriksen, 2016).

The gastrointestinal tract of the newborn infant is considered to be sterile. Bacteria from the environment, mainly from the mother, colonise the infant gut immediately following birth. Dominant members of anaerobic *Firmicutes* and *Bacteroidetes* do not appear to grow outside the gut and hence need to be transmitted between human hosts. Bacterial colonisation is necessary for the development of the immune system and immune regulation. The microbiota composition differs between infants born by CS and those born vaginally, with a delayed colonisation of the genus *Bacteroides* (Jakobsson et al., 2014).

What is the effect of operative birth on the human genome?

In 2013 Dahlen et al. published the Epigenetic Impact of Childbirth (EPIIC) hypothesis and proposed that when physiological labour and birth occurs (primarily without intervention) a healthy, positive form of stress (eustress) is exerted on the mother and baby (Dahlen et al., 2013). They argued that this could have a physiological epigenomic effect on specific genes, such as those that program immune responses, weight regulation, etc. Excessively high levels of stress during labour and birth (dys-tress) and excessively low levels (astress) were hypothesised to be associated with pathological priming. The authors suggest a middle range of stress is physiologically optimal and may enable optimal epigenetic priming (Dahlen et al., 2013).

Prophylaxis for caesarean section

Women undergoing CS have a five- to 20-fold greater chance of getting an infection compared with women who give birth vaginally (Smaill & Grivell, 2014). These infections can be in the urine, surgical incision or the lining of the womb (endometritis). The infections can become serious causing, for example, an abscess in the pelvis or infection in the blood, and very occasionally can lead to the mother's death (Gyte et al., 2014). Both ampicillin and first-generation cephalosporins have similar efficacy in reducing postoperative endometritis. There does not appear to be any added benefit from using a broad-spectrum agent or a multiple-dose regimen. There is need for an appropriately designed randomised trial to test the optimal timing of administration (immediately after the cord is clamped versus preoperative). There is general consensus that prophylactic antibiotics should be routinely administered to all women undergoing CS to prevent infection. Compared with placebo or no treatment, the use of prophylactic antibiotics in women undergoing CS reduced the incidence of wound infection, endometritis and serious infectious complications by 60%–70% (Smaill & Grivell, 2014). However, there is uncertainty about the consequences for the baby. There is a dearth of data estimating the effect of maternal administration of antibiotics on infant outcomes. No studies in the current Cochrane review systematically report on adverse infant outcomes nor on the effect of antibiotics on the developing infant immune system. There appear to be few data on the incidence of oral candidiasis (thrush) in babies or maternal adverse effects following antibiotic prophylaxis (Smaill & Grivell, 2014). If the rising rate of CS continues, the health and economic burden of post-CS infection will probably continue to rise. Infections remain among the top five causes of pregnancy-related mortality and account for a disproportionate contribution to maternal morbidity around the world. The most common post-CS infections are surgical site infection (SSI) (endomyometritis and wound infection); infection of the urinary tract; pelvic abscess, septic pelvic phlebitis, pneumonia and sepsis, although rare, are also increased and are associated with considerable health and economic burdens (Tita et al., 2009b).

Based on the best currently available evidence, 'antistaphylococcal cephalosporins' and 'broad spectrum penicillins plus betalactamase inhibitors' may have similar efficacy at caesarean section when considering immediate postoperative infection, although we did not have clear evidence for several important outcomes. Most trials administered antibiotics at or after cord clamping, or postoperatively, so results may have limited applicability to current practice, which generally favours administration prior to skin incision. We have no data on any infant outcomes, nor on late infections (up to 30 days) in the mother; these are important gaps in the evidence that warrant further research. Antimicrobial resistance is very important but more appropriately investigated by other trial designs (Williams et al., 2021). See also NICE Guideline on CS, 2021.

Caesarean section and maternal obesity

A recent study in the US found that the increasing rate of obesity is associated with increased risk of SSI following caesarean delivery. The study, published in *JAMA*, found that the optimal perioperative antibiotic prophylactic regimen in this high-risk population undergoing caesarean birth is unknown (Valent et al., 2017). Among obese women undergoing caesarean birth who received the standard preoperative cephalosporin prophylaxis, a postoperative 48-hour course of oral cephalexin and metronidazole reduced the rate of SSI within 30 days after delivery, compared with placebo treatment. The study recommended that prophylactic oral cephalexin and metronidazole may be warranted for the prevention of SSI among obese women after caesarean delivery.

Preparing the woman for a caesarean section

These issues were discussed fully in the earlier section on fluids and surveillance for epidural and spinal blocks. When the decision to move to CS is made, there may not be much time to lose; however, it is of paramount importance that you are aware not only that the birth has become a major surgical procedure, but also that it is the beginning of a special relationship between a woman and her baby. As the midwife you will facilitate a discussion of the options surrounding CS between the obstetrician and the woman, and the anaesthetist and the woman (a paediatrician may also be involved depending on the circumstances). It is important that the partner or husband is also included in the discussion and information-sharing session. Often you will be called upon to recount the events leading up to and including the caesarean birth of a baby. This is often crucial to the reconciliation of the fact that a CS has had to be performed where the mother and her significant others were not planning for an emergency. Many women feel a sense of loss and grief when they have had a CS. Some women feel guilty that they were unable to experience a normal, natural vaginal birth. For whatever reason women have a CS, it is important to remember that this is a special event in a woman's life. There are ways of making it memorable for her without succumbing to the depersonalising effect of technology.

REFLECTIVE THINKING EXERCISE

What is the average number of caesarean sections in your country or state? What does the World Health Organization recommend? Can you think of 10 ways to lower the CS rate in your maternity unit or in your own practice?

Classification of caesarean sections

In an attempt to globally audit the rates of caesarean section, a classification system has been adopted so that data is comparable. The global classification recommended by the WHO is known as the Robson classification, or the Ten Group Classification System (TGCS) (Robson, 2001) (Box 39.16). The system classifies all women into one of 10 categories that are mutually exclusive. The categories are based on five basic obstetric characteristics that are routinely collected in all maternities:

- parity (nulliparous, multiparous with and without previous caesarean section)
- onset of labour (spontaneous, induced or prelabour caesarean section)
- gestational age (pre-term or term)
- fetal presentation (cephalic, breech or transverse)
- number of fetuses (single or multiple).

The classification is simple, robust, reproducible, clinically relevant, and prospective—which means that every woman admitted for delivery can be immediately classified

Box 39.16 Robson's 10-group classification

1. Nulliparous, single cephalic, ≥37 weeks, in spontaneous labour
2. Nulliparous, single cephalic, ≥37 weeks, induced or caesarean section (CS) before labour
3. Multiparous (excluding previous CS), single cephalic, ≥37 weeks, in spontaneous labour
4. Multiparous (excluding previous CS), single cephalic, >37 weeks, induced or CS before labour
5. Previous CS, single cephalic, ≥37 weeks
6. All nulliparous breeches
7. All multiparous breeches (including previous CS)
8. All multiple pregnancies (including previous CS)
9. All abnormal lies (including previous CS)
10. All single cephalic, <37 weeks (including previous CS)

into one of the 10 groups based on these few basic characteristics. This allows a comparison and analysis of caesarean section rates within and across these groups (WHO, 2015).

Birth following previous caesarean section

In Australia the total cost of birth for women according to the national hospital funding authority was approximately $1.51 billion in 2014–15 (Independent Hospital Pricing Authority (IHPA), 2017). Caesarean birth represents approximately one-third of all these births and accounts for almost half the birth funding annually (IHPA, 2017). Caesarean sections cost, on average, 26% more to the health system over the first 1000 days of the perinatal journey compared with non-instrumental vaginal delivery (Callander et al., 2019; Fox et al., 2021). Similar figures have been reported in the US, making it therefore most appropriate to consider the safe use of caesarean and **vaginal birth after caesarean (VBAC)** not only at an individual level but increasingly as a national health policy concern (Guise et al., 2010).

Having a prior caesarean birth is the most common indication for CS, accounting for at least two-thirds of CSs in Australia in 2018 (AIHW, 2021). There is now increasing evidence that having a VBAC is a reasonable option for women given the growing evidence of serious morbidity that is associated with multiple caesareans—a result of the increased use of elective caesarean birth over VBAC (Dodd et al., 2013; Guise et al., 2010).

When caring for women who are attempting a VBAC, the strongest indicator that all is not well is an abnormality in the FHR. Other signs may be vaginal bleeding, pain and disturbances of uterine contractions. Most of the information concerning the success or failure rate of VBAC has been forthcoming from tertiary institutions in the developed world.

Of major concern is the possible maternal morbidity and mortality (mainly the risk of uterine rupture) resulting from a trial of labour after caesarean birth. Guise et al. (2010) provide the most comprehensive analysis of uterine rupture to date. Overall, evidence regarding the rate of uterine rupture for women with a prior caesarean delivery is moderate in strength and indicates that the risk of uterine rupture for women with prior caesarean is 0.3%. Compared with women undergoing an elective repeat caesarean, women undergoing a trial of labour (TOL) have a significantly higher risk of uterine rupture. This translates to 5.1 additional ruptures per 1000 women undergoing TOL. To date, there have been no maternal deaths reported because of uterine rupture, and the risk of perinatal death due to uterine rupture in term birth studies is 2.8% of all uterine ruptures (Guise et al., 2010).

Similar findings were published in a study of births recorded in the population-based data from the Scottish birth registry, where the risk of uterine rupture was a rare event occurring in just 3.5 per 1000 trials of labour (Smith et al., 2004). In the Scottish study (Smith et al., 2004), women who gave birth in a hospital with fewer than 3000 births per annum did not experience a significantly increased rate of uterine rupture; however, the 'risk of perinatal death due to uterine rupture was also higher in women who had not previously given birth vaginally and in women who had been induced with prostaglandins but not with other methods of induction' (p. 376), and among 'women who had not previously given birth vaginally, the risk of uterine rupture without induction of labour with prostaglandin was one in 210 and with induction of labour with prostaglandin was one in 71' (p. 377).

Guise et al. (2010) set out to address the practice policy question: what additional risks does a woman who has had a caesarean birth assume if she chooses to attempt VBAC rather than have a repeat CS? Most of the literature focuses on the risk of uterine rupture in those attempting a VBAC, with an implicit assumption that this risk would be eliminated by elective repeat caesarean birth. However, elective repeat caesarean birth is not guaranteed to prevent uterine rupture (Fig. 39.18).

Overall, the strength of evidence regarding the rate of mortality for women with a prior caesarean birth and a trial of labour compared with elective caesarean birth is high (Guise et al., 2010). Although maternal mortality is rare, with an overall rate of 10.1 per 100,000 for all women with prior caesarean, the risk of maternal mortality is significantly increased with elective repeat caesarean birth. Amongst births where the analysis is limited to term studies, the combined risk of maternal deaths for a trial of labour is 1.9 per 100,000, and for repeat elective caesarean birth is 9.6 per 100,000 (Guise et al., 2010). Among four studies that focused exclusively on women giving birth at term, the maternal mortality risk was similarly lower for those undergoing a trial of labour: 7.0 less deaths per 100,000 compared with the elective repeat CS group (Guise et al., 2010).

Ideally, women should be informed of all the morbidity associated with CSs and repeat CSs, and this of course includes not only the rare event of a uterine rupture, but also the risk of the baby dying if such an event should happen, and that of hysterectomy in a subsequent pregnancy following a first CS (see Abnormalities of placentation section).

The existing evidence is sufficient to conclude that there is an increased risk of symptomatic uterine rupture for TOL over elective repeat caesarean and that caesarean birth is not completely protective. However, uterine ruptures do not always have serious consequences, and women may wish to base decisions on the likelihood of significant morbidity or mortality for the mother and baby rather than on the occurrence of uterine rupture itself.

Remaining issues of concern are the increased risks of placenta praevia and placenta accreta for pregnancies subsequent to elective repeat caesarean births.

Amongst women who have a high BMI above or equal to 30, the risks related to perinatal morbidity and

Likelihood of	**Overall**
Successful VBAC (one previous caesarean delivery, no previous vaginal birth)	3 out of 4 or 72–75%
Successful VBAC (one previous caesarean delivery, at least one previous vaginal birth)	Almost 9 out of 10 or up to 85–90%
Unsuccessful VBAC more likely in: Induced labour, no previous vaginal delivery, body mass index (BMI) greater than 30 and previous caesarean for labour dystocia. If all of these factors are present, successful VBAC is achieved in 40% of cases.	

Likelihood of	**VBAC**	**ERCS**
	Maternal	
Uterine rupture	5 per 1000/0.5%	< 2 per 10 000/< 0.02%
Blood transfusion	2 per 100/2%	1 per 100/1%
Endometritis	No significant difference in risk	
Serious complications in future pregnancies	Not applicable if successful VBAC	Increased likelihood of placenta praevia/ morbidly adherent placenta
Maternal mortality	4 per 100 000/0.004%	13 per 100 000/0.013%
	Fetal/newborn	
Transient respiratory morbidity	2–3 per 100/2–3%	4–6 per 100/4–6% (risk reduced with corticosteroids, but there are concerns about potential long-term adverse effects)
Antepartum stillbirth beyond 39^{+0} weeks while awaiting spontaneous labour	10 per 10 000/0.1%	Not applicable
Hypoxic ischaemic encephalopathy (HIE)	8 per 10 000/0.08%	< 1 per 10 000/< 0.01%

Information leaflet(s) provided: VBAC ☐ ERCS ☐ Other ☐

Discussed:

Continuous electronic fetal monitoring at the onset of regular uterine contractions

Birth on the labour suite

Need for intravenous (IV) access in labour

FIGURE 39.18 Discussing the risks of vaginal birth after caesarean (VBAC) versus elective repeat caesarean section (ERCS)
(Source: Royal College of Obstetricians and Gynaecologists (RCOG). *Birth After Previous Caesarean Birth*. Green-top Guideline No. 45. London: RCOG Press; 2015b, updated 2017)

maternal morbidity are notably higher (Yao et al., 2017). The risk of blood transfusion, hysterectomy, ICU admission and uterine rupture were higher amongst those women who tried but didn't achieve a VBAC. The main benefit of trying for a VBAC is to succeed in following pregnancies with a vaginal birth and reduce surgery-related complications. Obese women should be counselled that the rate of successful vaginal birth appears to be lower than that quoted for normal weight women; however, it is not clear what the significance of maternal and neonatal complications associated with multiple repeat caesarean birth is in future pregnancies (Yao et al., 2017) (see Fig. 39.14).

A CS is major abdominal surgery and so the woman faces the same risks of complications as those following any abdominal surgery. These are increased if she requires general anaesthesia, has had a prolonged, difficult labour or has complications such as diabetes, severe hypertension or is obese. In these instances, recovery may be prolonged. Unlike patients recovering from major surgery, women recovering from a CS are expected to take on the exhausting role of new mother at the same time.

In the immediate postoperative phase, the woman should be observed on a one-to-one basis by a qualified member of theatre staff until she has regained airway control, cardiorespiratory stability and is able to communicate.

She should not be transferred from a high-dependency unit to a postnatal ward until the vital signs (respiratory rate, oxygen saturation, heart rate and blood pressure) are stable, and her blood loss (vaginal and wound), her pain level and sedation are assessed. In the first hours after surgery, assessments are made after 15 minutes, then every half hour for 2 hours, and then hourly thereafter provided the observations are stable. If not, more frequent observations and medical review may be warranted. (Refer to the local policies and guidelines appropriate to your area of practice.)

Postoperative complications and associated preventative measures

- *Haemorrhage and shock*—hypoperfusional postoperative shock is usually related to postpartum haemorrhage (Fullerton et al., 2013) (see Ch. 37). On admission to the ward after CS, the wound dressing is observed for signs of oozing and the vaginal loss assessed at least half-hourly. Regular assessment of the respiratory rate, heart rate, blood pressure, pulse and oxygen saturation together with urinary output and pain levels continues for at least 24 hours. Many hospitals record these observations according to Modified Early Obstetric Warning Score (MEOWS) guidelines. If intrathecal opioids are used hourly, assessments of the respiratory rate, sedation and pain scores for at least 12 hours are necessary. For women who have been given epidural opioids or have ongoing PCA with opioids, hourly monitoring of respiratory rate, sedation, pain scores and blood loss is warranted.
- *Wound infection*—local infection of the operative field is prevented by asepsis, but wound infection is still a risk. A UK study estimated that 1 in 10 women develop a postsurgical infection following a CS, with 1.2%–5% of women developing the infection during their inpatient stay (Wloch et al., 2012). Even minor infections can still result in pain and discomfort for the woman and may spread to affect deeper tissues. Postoperative infection can seriously affect a woman's quality of life at a critical time when she is recovering from an operation and has a newborn baby to look after. The more serious infections will require extended hospital stays or re-admission to hospital. Preoperative prophylactic antibiotics that are effective against endometritis and wound infection remain a controversial issue. Usually the wound dressing is removed 24 hours after surgery. The wound is observed for signs of infection (e.g. redness, discharge and increased pain). Removal of drains should be according to the surgeon's instructions. As soon as practicable, women can be encouraged to take over the care of their wound and advised how to clean and dry the area when they go home. Wound infection is a much higher risk amongst obese women following caesarean surgery (Valent et al., 2017).
- *Paralytic ileus (short-term paralysis of the bowel)*—rarely temporary paralysis of a portion of the intestines occurs after surgery. As the intestinal content of this portion is unable to move forward, food or drink should be avoided until peristaltic sound is heard from auscultation of the bowel. Most women having a CS are young and healthy and so, if there are no complicating factors and providing they are not experiencing nausea and vomiting, they may eat and drink when they wish as soon as bowel sounds are heard. IV fluids are discontinued once the woman is tolerating oral fluids and has begun a postpartum diuresis.
- *Venous thromboembolism and pulmonary thromboembolism*—women having a CS are frequently offered thromboprophylaxis because of the increased risk of venous thromboembolism. The choice of method of prophylaxis (e.g. graduated and correctly fitted stockings, hydration, early mobilisation, low-molecular-weight heparin) depends on the risk of thromboembolic disease (see Ch. 37) and institutional guidelines. Early mobilisation, adequate hydration and devices such as Flowtron boots may be useful preventative measures. Nevertheless, there is a paucity of quality studies investigating the efficacy of thromboprophylaxis during CS. No clinical trials using compression stockings and/or pneumatic-compression stockings have been conducted. (See study by Peyronnet et al. (2017) on reducing the incidence of maternal hypotension following epidural analgesia with compression stockings.) Particular attention needs to be paid to women who have chest symptoms (e.g. shortness of breath) or leg symptoms (e.g. painful swollen calves), as well as those who have a history of thromboembolic disease, because these are early-warning signs of thromboembolic disease. Most women will continue to wear stockings at home.
- *Bladder injury and urinary infection*—urinary infections occur in about 8% of women who have had a CS (see Ch. 41; Lusardi et al., 2013). The significance of urinary catheter-associated urinary tract infections following CS is that, whereas the infections are usually asymptomatic, they can result in a myriad of short- and long-term complications (i.e. pyrexia, acute and chronic pyelonephritis, and bacteraemia) (Lusardi et al., 2013). The urinary bladder catheter is removed when the woman is mobile and when full sensation returns following regional anaesthesia. A fluid balance chart is maintained until removal of the urinary catheter and the woman has voided twice with volumes of at least 300 mL.
- *Postoperative pain*—postoperatively women should be offered opioid analgesia, which may be required for up to 48 hours. Oral analgesics such as paracetamol and anti-inflammatory medication should also be offered and the woman should be prescribed a supply of analgesics to take home on discharge.
- *Chest infection*—early mobilisation improves respiratory function. Routine respiratory physiotherapy does not need to be routinely offered to women even after a CS under general anaesthesia. Coughing, phlegm, pyrexia and respiratory auscultatory changes may indicate respiratory infection.

Baby care and infant feeding

Early skin contact between mother and baby should be encouraged and facilitated because it improves maternal perceptions of the infant, mothering skills, maternal behaviour and breastfeeding outcomes, and reduces infant crying. Women who have had a CS are less likely to start breastfeeding in the first few hours after birth, but when breastfeeding is established they are as likely to continue as women who have had a vaginal birth. Therefore it is important that they are offered additional breastfeeding support as soon as possible after giving birth. Women should also be given assistance with baby care and personal hygiene until able to mobilise and care for their babies and themselves independently. All care planned and implemented should be documented in the maternal records.

Babies born by CS are more likely to have a lower temperature and develop TTN, and thermal care should be in accordance with good practice for thermal care of the newborn baby. (See also Chs 31 and 42.)

Preparation for discharge

Women who have had a CS require the same support and education as all new mothers (see Chs 25, 30 and 41). In addition, it is important for the midwife to ensure that the woman has a clear understanding of the reason for the caesarean, its impact on the transition to motherhood and the possible effects of CS surgery for future pregnancies. Women require information about the resumption of normal activities (e.g. driving, lifting, sexual activity), the signs of infections or complications after discharge from hospital, exercises for the prevention of venous thromboembolism, and follow-up with their LMC. Midwives should inform women that after a CS they are not at increased risk of difficulties with breastfeeding and should provide contact details for ongoing support.

Summary: caesarean section

Caesarean section has become one of the most common surgical procedures in both Australia and New Zealand. (For current rates see the mothers and babies yearly report for your country—the AIHW, the New Zealand MOH and the NZCOM MMPO publish yearly rates.) Decisions to give birth via CS can be made before the onset of labour (elective caesarean) or after the onset of labour (emergency caesarean). Delivery by caesarean may be appropriate in a range of circumstances related to the clinical characteristics of women where a vaginal birth is not possible. Some of the reasons for this may include breech or transverse presentation, cephalopelvic disproportion, placenta praevia, placental insufficiency, a prolapsed cord, multiple pregnancy and dangerously high blood pressure in the mother. However, studies across the world have shown that non-clinical factors also contribute to the rising rates of CS. These include women's requests for delivery by elective CS when they perceive that the benefits of a planned elective caesarean outweigh the risks, the different practice patterns of individual doctors, unexplained clinical variation in health districts and the private health insurance status of women.

The escalation in the total caesarean rate is fuelled by both the rise in the primary caesarean rate and the low uptake of VBAC. In Australia, the rates have increased in both public and private hospitals, although they remain consistently higher in the private sector. Higher rates of electronic fetal monitoring, induction and epidural analgesia have been implicated in the rise in caesareans, but other factors are also contributing. Randomised controlled trials and some multicentre trials (Hannah et al., 1992, 2000) concluded that professional management guidelines should promote CS for breech birth. Greater access to private hospitals and changes in practice responding to the medical indemnity crisis have also contributed to rising rates.

A review of comparable statistics provided by the OECD indicates that Australia, New Zealand and Canada have similar perinatal outcomes overall. The lower rate of growth in interventions in New Zealand (CS, instrumental births, induction and epidurals) and higher levels of patient satisfaction have been linked to the introduction of the midwife-led contracting model (IHPA, 2017).

Implications

What are the risks of caesarean birth? One of the most significant risks is the need for a subsequent caesarean birth (Colmorn et al., 2017; Guise et al., 2010). There is steady growth in the research evidence that illustrates the seriousness of the rising CS phenomenon in terms of maternal and infant complications, and the importance of the debate about the appropriateness of caesarean birth in maternity care.

REFLECTIVE THINKING EXERCISE

What are the known risk factors that predispose women to the risk of uterine rupture? Where should these women give birth? Can we establish definitive risk criteria for women wanting to give birth vaginally following a previous CS?

Framing risk

How should we frame risk in conditions of uncertainty?

In their Nobel Prize-winning work, Tversky & Kahneman discovered that framing of outcomes, choices and contingencies influences decision making (Kahneman & Tversky, 1979; Tversky & Kahneman, 1981). The reference points and language chosen by providers and policy-making organisations influence public perceptions, policy formulation and the climate for practice and research. Whether discussions highlight benefits or risks and whether the portrayal is relative or absolute can affect perceptions. Society often behaves as if the risk threshold were set at perfection and no risk is acceptable. Modern technology and superior medical care cannot remove all risk completely. Therefore, to decide on thresholds for risk for vaginal birth and repeat CS we need to look at rates for harms such as uterine rupture and benefits, and also to ensure consistency with other issues when we interpret the thresholds (Guise et al., 2010).

CS also requires a longer recovery time, and operative complications such as lacerations, bleeding and infection have been discussed. Babies are also implicated in risks associated with CS. Australia, New Zealand and the United States rank highly in terms of rates of CS for resource-rich countries, especially compared with the Nordic countries and Europe (Central Intelligence Agency (CIA) US, 2017).

Box 39.17 Global changes in maternity care provision during the COVID-19 pandemic

During the COVID-19 pandemic there have been rapid and substantive changes to maternity care provision globally. This includes a substantial decrease in the number of scheduled and unscheduled antenatal care visits, hospitalisations for urgent care, a reduction in antenatal care screening uptake (including but not limited to ultrasound and prenatal genetic testing), and delayed attendance at the planned place of care when labour starts. There has been a global increase in virtual or remote consultations and a decrease in face-to-face appointments. Inequalities and inequities have been highlighted amongst people with fewer resources who may have had less access to telehealth. In addition to these changes there has been a reduction in companionship allowed during birth, and a reduction in postpartum hospital length of stay, regardless of mode of birth.

(Townsend et al., 2021)

Conclusion

Routine use of multiple childbirth procedures—that is, the overtreatment of normal childbirth—is neither fiscally nor medically defensible. Each procedure adds more costs to intrapartum care (IHPA, 2017; Tracy & Tracy, 2003), has potential adverse health effects for mother and baby and necessitates use of still more technical care measures (Dahlen et al., 2012, 2014, 2021; Tracy et al., 2007a, 2007b). Reducing unnecessary intervention requires midwives to challenge the prevailing norm of overtreatment in hospital settings. Ideally, a safe birth and optimal health of the new mother are both necessary goals, for which spontaneous vaginal birth and an intact genital tract are key elements. Such a mother will have the best postnatal health, including fewer hospital re-admissions for post-delivery morbidity, less perineal pain and a stronger pelvic floor, and better sexual function and overall physical functioning (Lydon-Rochelle et al., 2001b; Thompson et al., 2002). The mother's optimal health should be a high priority of caregivers, because newborn wellbeing depends so greatly on her health and functional status, which help equip her to undertake the complex and demanding task of mothering an infant with confidence (Albers, 2005, p. 68).

Common obstetric interventions are often for 'convenience' rather than for clinical indications. Before proceeding, it should be made clear in whose interests the intervention is made. The midwife must make every effort to make sure that women and their partners have a full understanding of what is known about the associated risks, benefits and alternative approaches of the proposed intervention. Thorough and accurate information allows a woman to choose what is best for her and her infant on the basis of the individual clinical situation. Ideally, this discussion takes place during the antenatal time when there is ample opportunity to ask questions, reflect on the potential implications and confer with partners and family members. Although the interventions outlined above often are medically indicated for the wellbeing of mothers and infants, the evidence supporting their benefits when used electively may not be based on rigorous research and in many cases remains controversial.

See Box 39.17 for the rapid and substantive changes to maternity care provision globally that have occurred as a result of the COVD-19 pandemic.

Review questions

1. What are two points that midwives must consider with regards to the use of interventions as routine practice?
2. What factors are associated with cerebral palsy in the antenatal period, during labour and in the postpartum period?
3. What is the evidence for the use of CTG assessment of fetal wellbeing in pregnancy?
4. What is the evidence for the use of routine CTG assessment on admission in labour?
5. What is the most appropriate form of fetal monitoring in an uncomplicated labour?
6. What are the 'protective' aspects of vaginal birth?
7. List four characteristics of a non-reassuring CTG tracing.
8. What is the evidence in relation to the timing of induction of labour?
9. What are the risks of CS to mother and infant?
10. List six possible reasons for the increasing CS rate in Western healthcare systems.

NOTE

a. Although the majority of caesarean births are now carried out under regional anaesthesia, thus reducing a significant cause of maternal mortality, the spectre of pain during caesarean delivery is the most common negligence claim against obstetric anaesthetists in the UK. The figures are unavailable in Australia or New Zealand at present. However, in the UK between 2000 and 2010, the damages awarded for claims relating to obstetric anaesthesia and the association with 'pain complaints' exceeded £19 million, representing 3.8% of all successful obstetric claims to the NHS Litigation Authority (McCombe et al., 2018).

Online resources

Babycentre (UK): https://www.babycentre.co.uk/.
CDC births and natality statistics: https://www.cdc.gov/nchs/fastats/births.htm.
Health Direct: https://www.healthdirect.gov.au/.
March of Dimes: https://www.marchofdimes.org/.
Midwife Thinking: https://midwifethinking.com/about/.
Ministry of Health NZ. Report on Maternity 2015: https://www.health.govt.nz/publication/report-maternity-2015.
National Institute of Health and Care Excellence (NICE): https://www.nice.org.uk/.
Royal College of Midwives (RCM), UK: https://www.rcm.org.uk/news-views-and-analysis/analysis/auscultation-the-art-of-listening.
Up to Date: https://www.uptodate.com/home.

References

Adelson PL, Child AG, Giles WB, et al. Antenatal hospitalisations in New South Wales, 1995–96. *Med J Aust.* 1999;170:211–215.
Agerson AN, Scavone BM. Prophylactic epidural blood patch after unintentional dural puncture for the prevention of postdural puncture headache in parturients. *Anesth Analg.* 2012; 115(1):133–136.
Albers L. Overtreatment of normal childbirth in US hospitals. *Birth.* 2005;32(1):67–68.
Alfirevic Z, Stampalija T, Medley N. Fetal and umbilical Doppler ultrasound in normal pregnancy. *Cochrane Database Syst Rev.* 2015;(4):CD001450, doi:10.1002/14651858.CD001450.pub4.
Alfirevic Z, Stampalija T, Dowswell T. Fetal and umbilical Doppler ultrasound in high-risk pregnancies. *Cochrane Database Syst Rev.* 2017a;(6):CD007529, doi:10.1002/14651858.CD007529.pub4.
Alfirevic Z, Devane D, Gyte GML, et al. Continuous cardiotocography (CTG) as a form of electronic fetal monitoring (EFM) for fetal assessment during labour. *Cochrane Database Syst Rev.* 2017b;(2):CD006066, doi:10.1002/14651858.CD006066.pub3.
Allanson ER, Waqar T, White CRH, et al. Umbilical lactate as a measure of acidosis and predictor of neonatal risk: a systematic review. *BJOG.* 2017;124(4):584–594. doi:10.1111/1471-0528.14306.
Allen J, Kildea S, Hartz DL, et al. The motivation and capacity to go 'above and beyond': qualitative analysis of free-text survey responses in the M@NGO randomised controlled trial of caseload midwifery. *Midwifery.* 2017;50:148–156.
Althabe F, Belizan JM. Caesarean section: the paradox. *Lancet.* 2006;368:1472–1473.
Amin-Zaki L, Majeed MA, Elhassani SB, et al. Prenatal methylmercury poisoning. Clinical observations over five years. *Am J Dis Child.* 1979;133(2):172–177.
Anim-Somuah M, Smyth RMD, Cyna AM, Cuthbert A. Epidural versus non-epidural or no analgesia for pain management in labour. *Cochrane Database Syst Rev.* 2018;5:CD000331. doi:10.1002/14651858.CD000331.pub4.
Arevalo-Rodriguez I, Ciapponi A, Munoz L, Roque i Figuls M, Bonfill Cosp X. Posture and fluids for preventing post-dural puncture headache. *Cochrane Database Syst Rev.* 2013;7: CD009199. 7.
Australian Institute of Health and Welfare (AIHW). *Australia's Mothers and Babies.* Cat no. PER 101. Canberra: AIHW; 2021. https://www.aihw.gov.au/reports/mothers-babies/australias-mothers-babies/contents/about
Badawi N, Watson L, Petterson B, et al. What constitutes cerebral palsy? *Dev Med Child Neurol.* 1998;40(8):520–527.
Bakshi R, Mehta A, Mehta Sharma B. Tokophobia: fear of pregnancy and childbirth. *Int J Gynecol Obstet.* 2008;10:1.
Banks S, Paech M, Gurrin L. An audit of epidural blood patch after accidental dural puncture with a Tuohy needle in obstetric patients. *Int J Obstet Anesth.* 2001;10:172–176.
Banta HD, Thacker SB. Electronic fetal monitoring: lessons from a formative case of health technology assessment. *Int J Technol Assess Health Care.* 2002;18:762–770.

Baraz R, Collis RE. The management of accidental dural puncture during labour epidural analgesia: a survey of UK practice. *Anaesthesia*. 2005;60(7):673–679.

Behague DP, Victora CG, Barros FC. Consumer demand for caesarean sections in Brazil: informed decision making, patient choice, or social inequality? A population based birth cohort study linking ethnographic and epidemiological methods. *BMJ*. 2002;324:942–945.

Belizan JM, Althabe R, Barros FC, et al. Rates and implications of caesarean sections in Latin America: ecological study. *BMJ*. 1999;319:1397–1400.

Bell JS, Campbell DM, Graham WJ, et al. Do obstetric complications explain high caesarean section rates among women over 30? A retrospective analysis. *BMJ*. 2001;322:894–895.

Betran AP, Temmerman M, Kingdon C, et al. Interventions to reduce unnecessary caesarean sections in healthy women and babies. *Lancet*. 2018;392(10155):1358–1368.

Betran AP, Ye J, Moller A-B, et al. Trends and projections of caesarean section rates: global and regional estimates. *BMJ Glob Health*. 2021;6(6).

Bewley S, Cockburn JI. The unethics of 'request' Caesarean section. *BJOG*. 2002;109:593–596.

Black C, Kaye JA, Jick H. Caesarean delivery in the United Kingdom. Time trends in the general practice research database. *Obstet Gynecol*. 2005;106:151–155.

Blair E, Stanley F. Aetiological pathways to spastic cerebral palsy. *Paediatr Perinat Epidemiol*. 1993;7:302–317.

Blair E, Stanley F. Issues in the classification and epidemiology of cerebral palsy. *Ment Retard Dev Disabil Res Rev*. 1997;3: 184–193.

Blencowe H, Lee AC, Cousens S, et al. Preterm birth-associated neurodevelopmental impairment estimates at regional and global levels for 2010. *Pediatr Res*. 2013;74(suppl 1): 17–34.

Bourgeault IL, Declercq E, Sandall J, et al. Too posh to push? Comparative perspectives on maternal request caesarean sections in Canada, the US, the UK and Finland. *Adv Med Sociol*. 2008; 10:99.

Bricker L, Medley N, Pratt JJ. Routine ultrasound in late pregnancy (after 24 weeks' gestation). *Cochrane Database Syst Rev*. 2015;(6):CD001451.

Bryant J, Porter M, Tracy SK, et al. Caesarean birth: consumption, safety, order, and good mothering. *Soc Sci Med*. 2007;65: 1192–1201.

Bryant SA. Making culture visible: an examination of birthplace and health status. *Health Care Women Int*. 2003;24(2):103–114.

Buchsbaum GM, Chin M, Glantz C, et al. Prevalence of urinary incontinence and associated risk factors in a cohort of nuns. *Obstet Gynecol*. 2002;100:226–229.

Bump H, Norton P. Epidemiology and natural history of pelvic floor dysfunction. *Obstet Gynecol Clin North Am*. 1998;2:723–746.

Callander EJ, Fenwick J, Donnellan-Fernandez R, et al. Cost of maternity care to public hospitals: a first 1000-days perspective from Queensland. *Aust Health Rev*. 2019;43:556–64.

Camann W. Pain relief during labour. *N Engl J Med*. 2005;352(7): 718–720.

Canadian Association of Midwives (CAM). Statement on caesarean section by Board of Directors. *Birth Matters*. 2004;8(3):14.

Cardwell CR, Stene LC, Joner G, et al. Caesarean section is associated with an increased risk of childhood-onset type 1 diabetes mellitus: a meta-analysis of observational studies. *Diabetologia*. 2008;51:726–735.

Cary AJ. Intervention rates in spontaneous term labour in low-risk nulliparous women. *Aust N Z J Obstet Gynaecol*. 1990;30(1): 46–51.

Caton D, Frölich MA, Euliano TY. Anesthesia for childbirth: controversy and change. *Am J Obstet Gynecol*. 2002;186:S25–S30.

Caughey A. Evidence-based labor and delivery management can we safely reduce the cesarean rate? *Obstet Gynecol Clin North Am*. 2017;44:523–533.

Central Intelligence Agency (CIA). *The World Factbook*. 2017. Online: https://www.cia.gov/library/publications/resources/the-world-factbook/index.html.

Chaliha C. Postpartum bladder dysfunction. *Rev Gynaecol Perinat Pract*. 2006;6(3–4):133–139.

Chalmers I. The perinatal research agenda: whose priorities? *Birth*. 1991;18(3):137–141.

Chamberlain G, Steer P. ABC of labour care: operative delivery. *BMJ*. 1999;318:1260–1264.

Choi DH, Kim JA, Chung S. Comparison of combined spinal epidural anesthesia and epidural anesthesia for caesarean section. *Acta Anaesthesiol Scand*. 2000;44:214–219.

Christensson K, Siles C, Cabrera T, et al. Lower body temperatures in infants delivered by caesarean section than in vaginally delivered infants. *Acta Paediatr*. 1993;82(2):128–131. [Comparative Study Research Support, Non-U.S. Gov't].

Clarke VT, Smiley RM, Finster M. Uterine hyperactivity after intrathecal injection of fentanyl for analgesia during labor: a cause of fetal bradycardia? *Anesthesiology*. 1994;81:1083.

Clement S. *The Caesarean Experience*. London: Pandora; 1995.

Colditz MJ, Lai M, Cartwright D, et al. Subgaleal haemorrhage in the newborn: a call for early diagnosis and aggressive management. *J Paediatr Child Health*. 2014;51(2):140–146. doi:10.1111/jpc.12698.

Colmorn LB, Krebs L, Klungsøyr K, et al. Mode of first delivery and severe maternal complications in the subsequent pregnancy. *Acta Obstet Gynecol Scand*. 2017;96:1053–1062.

Comparative Obstetric Mobile Epidural Trial (COMET) Study Group UK. Effect of low-dose mobile versus traditional epidural techniques on mode of delivery: a randomised controlled trial. *Lancet*. 2001;358:19–23.

Conklin K, Backus A. Physiologic changes in pregnancy. In: Chestnut D, ed. *Obstetric Anesthesia: Principles and Practice*. 2nd ed. St Louis, MO: Mosby; 1999:17–42.

Crowther CA, Hiller JE, Doyle LW, et al. Effect of magnesium sulfate given for neuroprotection before preterm birth. A randomized controlled trial. *JAMA*. 2003;290:2669–2676.

Crowther CA, Middleton PF, Voysey M, et al. Assessing the neuroprotective benefits for babies of antenatal magnesium sulphate: an individual participant data meta-analysis. *PLoS Med*. 2017;14(10):e1002398. doi:10.1371/journal.pmed.1002398.

Dahlen HG, Tracy SK, Tracy MB, et al. Rates of obstetric intervention among low-risk women giving birth in private and public hospitals in NSW: a population-based descriptive study. *BMJ Open*. 2012;2(5):doi:10.1136/bmjopen-2012-001723. pii:e001723.

Dahlen HG, Kennedy HP, Anderson CM, et al. The EPIIC hypothesis: intrapartum effects on the neonatal epigenome and consequent health outcomes. *Med Hypotheses*. 2013;80(5):656–662. doi:10.1016/j.mehy.2013.01.017.

Dahlen HG, Tracy SK, Tracy MB, et al. Rates of obstetric intervention and associated perinatal mortality and morbidity among low-risk women giving birth in private and public hospitals in NSW (2000–2008): a linked data population-based cohort study. *BMJ Open*. 2014;4:e004551. doi:10.1136/bmjopen-2013-004551.

Dahlen HG, Thornton C,Downe S, et al. Intrapartum interventions and outcomes for women and children following induction of labour at term in uncomplicated pregnancies: a 16-year population-based linked data study. *BMJ Open*. 2021;11:e047040. doi:10.1136/bmjopen-2020-047040.

Dahlseng MO, Andersen GL, Irgens LM, et al. Risk of cerebral palsy in term-born singletons according to growth status at birth. *Dev Med Child Neurol*. 2014;56(1):53–58. doi:10.1111/dmcn.12293.

Davies SJ, Paech MJ, Welch H, et al. Maternal experience during epidural or combined spinal-epidural anesthesia for Cesarean section: a prospective, randomized trial. *Anesth Analg.* 1997;85: 607–613.

Declercq E, Sakala C, Corry M, et al. *Listening to Mothers II: 2007 Report of the Second National US Survey of Women's Childbearing Experiences. Pregnancy and Birth.* New York: Childbirth Connection; 2007.

Declercq ER, Sakala C, Corry MP, et al. *Listening to Mothers LSM III: Pregnancy and Birth.* New York: Childbirth Connection; 2013.

Devane D, Lalor J. Midwives' visual interpretation of intrapartum cardiotocographs: intra- and inter-observer agreement. *J Adv Nurs.* 2005;52(2):133–141.

Devane D, Lalor JG, Daly S, et al. Cardiotocography versus intermittent auscultation of fetal heart on admission to labour ward for assessment of fetal wellbeing. *Cochrane Database Syst Rev.* 2017;(1):CD005122, doi:10.1002/14651858.CD005122.pub5.

Dietz HP. Women and babies need protection from the dangers of normal birth ideology: FOR: the recent maternity review risks making the situation even worse. *BJOG.* 2017;124(9):1384. doi:10.1111/1471-0528.14666.

Dodd JM, Crowther CA, Huertas E, et al. Planned elective repeat caesarean section versus planned vaginal birth for women with a previous caesarean birth. *Cochrane Database Syst Rev.* 2013; (12):CD004224, doi:10.1002/14651858.CD004224.pub3.

Downe S, Gerrett D, Renfrew MJ. A prospective randomised trial on the effect of position in the passive second stage of labour on birth outcome in nulliparous women using epidural analgesia. *Midwifery.* 2004;2:157–168.

Edmonds, JK, Ivanof J, Kafulafula U. Midwife led units: transforming maternity care globally. *Ann Glob Health.* 2020;86(1):44.

Eltzschig HK, Lieberman ES, Camann WR. Regional anesthesia and analgesia for labour and delivery. *N Engl J Med.* 2003; 348(4):319–332.

Engelsen IB, Albrechtsen S, Iversen OE. Peripartum hysterectomy—incidence and maternal morbidity. *Acta Obstet Gynecol Scand.* 2001;80(5):409–412.

Epidural and Position Trial Collaborative Group. Upright versus lying down position in second stage of labour in nulliparous women with low dose epidural: BUMPES randomised controlled trial. *BMJ.* 2017;359:j4471. doi:10.1136/bmj.j4471.

Everett TR, Peebles DM. Antenatal tests of fetal wellbeing. *Semin Fetal Neonatal Med.* 2015;20:138–143.

Fahey J, King TL. Intrauterine asphyxia: clinical implications for providers of intrapartum care. *J Midwifery Womens Health.* 2005;50(6):498–506.

Farquhar CM, Li Z, Lensen S, et al. Incidence, risk factors and perinatal outcomes for placenta accreta in Australia and New Zealand: a case–control study. *BMJ Open.* 2017;7:e017713. doi:10.1136/bmjopen-2017-017713.

Fenwick J, Staff L, Gamble J, et al. Why do women request caesarean section in a normal, healthy first pregnancy? *Midwifery.* 2010;26(4):394–400. doi:10.1016/j.midw.2008.10.011.

Flenady et al. My Baby's Movements: a stepped wedge cluster randomised controlled trial to raise maternal awareness of fetal movements during pregnancy study protocol. *BMC Pregnancy Childbirth.* 2019;19:430. doi:org/10.1186/s12884-019-2575-1.

Fox H, Callander E et al., Is there unwarranted variation in obstetric practice in Australia? Obstetric intervention trends in Queensland hospitals. *Aust Health Rev.* 2021;45:157–166. doi:10.1071/AH20014.

Fullerton G, Danielian PJ, Bhattacharya S. Outcomes of pregnancy following post partum haemorrhage. *BJOG.* 2013;20(5): 621–627.

Gale C, Statnikov Y, Jawad S, et al. Neonatal brain injuries in England: population-based incidence derived from routinely recorded clinical data held in the National Neonatal Research Database. *Arch Dis Child Fetal Neonatal Ed.* 2017;doi:10.1136/archdischild-2017-313707. pii:fetalneonatal-2017-313707.

Gale EA. A missing link in the hygiene hypothesis? *Diabetologia.* 2002;45:588–594.

Gamble JA, Creedy DK. Women's preference for a cesarean section: incidence and associated factors. *Birth.* 2001;28(2):101–110.

Gambling DR, Sharma SK, Ramin SM, et al. A randomized study of combined spinal–epidural analgesia versus intravenous meperidine during labour: impact on caesarean delivery rate. *Anesthesiology.* 1998;89:1336–1344.

Gardener G, Daly L, Bowring V, et al. *Clinical Practice Guideline for the Care of Women With Decreased Fetal Movements.* Brisbane: Centre of Research Excellence in Stillbirth; 2017. Online: https://stillbirth.centre.uq.edu.au/files/1162/DFM-Clinical-Practice-Guideline-10-August-2017.pdf.

Gibb D, Arulkumaran S. *Fetal Monitoring in Practice.* London: Churchill Livingstone; 2008.

Grace Tan SE, Jobling TW, Wallace EM, et al. Surgical management of placenta accreta: a 10-year experience. *Acta Obstet Gynecol Scand.* 2013;92:445–450.

Grant JM. Pregnancy, not childbirth, causes pelvic floor dysfunction (Editorial). *BJOG.* 2000;107:viii.

Grivell RM, Alfirevic Z, Gyte GM, et al. Antenatal cardiotocography for fetal assessment. *Cochrane Database Syst Rev.* 2015;(9): CD007863.

Guarner F, Malagelada JR. Gut flora in health and disease. *Lancet.* 2003;361:512–519.

Guise J-M, Eden K, Emeis C, et al. Vaginal Birth After Cesarean: New Insights. Evidence Report / Technology Assessment No.191. (Prepared by the Oregon Health and Science University Evidence-based Practice Center under Contract No. 290-2007-10057-I.) AHRQ Publication No. 10-E003. Rockville, MD: Agency for Healthcare Research and Quality; 2010.

Gyte GML, Dou L, Vazquez JC. Different classes of antibiotics given to women routinely for preventing infection at caesarean section. *Cochrane Database Syst Rev.* 2014;(11):CD008726, doi:10.1002/14651858.CD008726.pub2.

Habiba M, Kaminski M, Da Frè M, et al. Caesarean section on request: a comparison of obstetricians' attitudes in eight European countries. *BJOG.* 2006;113(6):647–656. doi:10.1111/j.1471-0528.2006.00933.x.

Halpern SH, Carvalho B. Patient-controlled epidural analgesia for labor. *Anesth Analg.* 2009;108(3):921–928.

Hankins GDV, Speer M. Defining the pathogenesis and pathophysiology of neonatal encephalopathy and cerebral palsy. *Obstet Gynecol.* 2003;102:628–636.

Hannah ME. Planned elective Caesarean section: a reasonable choice for some women? *CMAJ.* 2004;170:813.

Hannah ME, Hannah WJ, Hellmann J, et al.; The Canadian Multicenter Post-Term Pregnancy Trial Group. Induction of labor as compared with serial antenatal monitoring in postterm pregnancy: a randomized controlled trial. *N Engl J Med.* 1992;326: 1587–1592. Published correction appears in 327:368.

Hannah ME, Hannah WJ, Hewson SA, et al. Term Breech Trial Collaborative Group. Planned caesarean section versus planned vaginal birth for breech presentation at term: a randomised multicentre trial. *Lancet.* 2000;356:1375–1383.

Harrison J. *Auscultation: The Art of Listening.* London: Royal College of Midwives; 2008. Online: https://www.rcm.org.uk/news-views-and-analysis/analysis/auscultation-the-art-of-listening.

Henderson C, Macdonald S. *Mayes' Midwifery: A Textbook for Midwives.* London: Baillière Tindall; 2004.

Hofmeyr GJ. Evidence-based intrapartum care. *Best Pract Res Clin Obstet Gynaecol.* 2004;19(1):103–115.

Hofmeyr GJ, Cyna AM, Middleton P. Prophylactic intravenous preloading for regional analgesia in labour. *Cochrane Database Syst Rev.* 2004;(4):CD000175, doi:10.1002/14651858.CD000175.pub2.
Hopkins K. Are Brazilian women really choosing to deliver by cesarean? *Soc Sci Med.* 2000;51(5):725–740.
Howell CJ, Kidd C, Roberts W, et al. A randomised controlled trial of epidural compared with non-epidural analgesia in labour. *BJOG.* 2001;108:27–33.
Hyde MJ, Mostyn A, Modi N, et al. The health implications of birth by Caesarean section. *Biol Rev Camb Philos Soc.* 2012;87(1): 229–243. doi:10.1111/j.1469-185X.2011.00195.x.
Independent Hospital Pricing Authority (IHPA). Bundled Pricing for Maternity Care. Final Report of IHPA and the Bundled Pricing Advisory Group. November 2017. Online: https://www.ihpa.gov.au/sites/g/files/net636/f/bundled_pricing_for_maternity_care_-_final_report.pdf.
INFANT Collaborative Group. Computerised interpretation of fetal heart rate during labour (INFANT): a randomised controlled trial. *Lancet.* 2017;389:1719–1729. doi:10.1016/S0140-6736(17)30568-8.
Jacobs SE, Berg M, Hunt R, et al. Cooling for newborns with hypoxic ischaemic encephalopathy. *Cochrane Database Syst Rev.* 2013;(1):CD003311, doi:10.1002/14651858.CD003311.pub3.
Jakobsson HE, Abrahamsson TR, Jenmalm MC, et al. Decreased gut microbiota diversity, delayed *Bacteroidetes* colonisation and reduced Th1 responses in infants delivered by caesarean section. *Gut.* 2014;63:559–566.
Jauniaux E, Collins S, Burton GJ. Placenta accreta spectrum: pathophysiology and evidence-based anatomy for prenatal ultrasound imaging. *Am J Obstet Gynecol.* 2018;218(1):75–87. doi:10.1016/j.ajog.2017.05.067.
Jenkins JG. Some immediate serious complications of obstetric epidural analgesia and anaesthesia: a prospective study of 145,Ää550 epidurals. *Int J Obstet Anesth.* 2005;14:37–42.
Jeon Y, Hwang J, Kang J. Effects of epidural naloxone on pruritus induced by epidural morphine: a randomized controlled trial. *Int J Obstet Anesth.* 2004;14:22–25.
Jordan S, Emery S, Bradshaw C. The impact of intrapartum analgesia on infant feeding. *BJOG.* 2005;112(7):927–928.
Kahneman D, Tversky A. Prospect theory: an analysis of decision under risk. *Econometrica.* 1979;47:263–291.
Karaman S, Akercan F, Akarsu T, et al. Comparison of the maternal and neonatal effects of epidural block and of combined spinal-epidural block for Caesarean section. *Eur J Obstet Gynecol Reprod Biol.* 2005;121(1):18–23.
Keir AK, Shepherd E, McIntyre S, et al. Antenatal magnesium sulfate to prevent cerebral palsy Arch Dis Child Fetal Neonatal Ed Epub ahead of print 2021: doi:10.1136/ archdischild-2021-321817
Knox A, Rouleau G, Semenic S, et al. Barriers and facilitators to birth without epidural in a tertiary obstetric referral center: perspectives of health care professionals and patients. *Birth.* 2017;1–8. doi:10.1111/birt.12327. Epub ahead of print.
Kornelsen J, Hutton E, Munro S. Influences on decision making among primiparous women choosing elective caesarean section in the absence of medical indications: findings from a qualitative investigation. *J Obstet Gynaecol Can.* 2010;32(10): 962–969. [Research Support, Non-U.S. Gov't].
Kotaska A. *Caesarean section or vaginal delivery in the 21st century.* nd. https://www.euro.who.int/__data/assets/pdf_file/0006/277737/Cesarean-Section-or-Vaginal-Delivery-in-the-21st-Century.pdf.
Kotaska A, Menticoglou S, Gagnon R, et al. Vaginal delivery of breech presentation. *J Obstet Gynaecol Can.* 2009;31(6): 557–566, 567–578.
Kristensen K, Henriksen L. Cesarean section and disease associated with immune function. *J Allergy Clin Immunol.* 2016; 137:587–590.
Kwee A, Cohlen BJ, Kanhai HH, et al. Caesarean section on request: a survey in The Netherlands. *Eur J Obstet Gynecol Reprod Biol.* 2004;113:186–190.
Lalor JG, Fawole B, Alfirevic Z, et al. Biophysical profile for fetal assessment in high risk pregnancies. *Cochrane Database Syst Rev.* 2008;(1):CD000038. doi:10.1002/14651858.CD000038.pub2.
Lavender T, Hofmeyr GJ, Neilson JP, et al. Caesarean section for non-medical reasons at term. *Cochrane Database Syst Rev.* 2012;(3):CD004660, doi:10.1002/14651858.CD004660.pub3.
Le Ray C, Carayol M, Jaquemin S, et al. Is epidural analgesia a risk factor for occiput posterior or transverse positions during labour? *Eur J Obstet Gynecol Reprod Biol.* 2005;123(1):22–26.
Leighton BL, Halpern SH. The effects of epidural analgesia on labor, maternal, and neonatal outcomes: a systematic review. *Am J Obstet Gynecol.* 2002;186(suppl):S69–S77.
Lieberman E, Davidson K, Lee-Parritz A. Changes in fetal position during labor and their association with epidural analgesia. *Obstet Gynecol.* 2005;105:974–982.
Lieberman E, O'Donoghue C. Unintended effects of epidural analgesia during labor: a systematic review. *Am J Obstet Gynecol.* 2002;186(suppl):S31–S68.
Liu S, Heaman M, Joseph KS, et al. Risk of maternal postpartum readmission associated with mode of delivery. *Obstet Gynecol.* 2005;105(4):836–842.
Longo M, Hankins GD. Defining cerebral palsy: pathogenesis, pathophysiology and new intervention. *Minerva Ginecol.* 2009; 61(5):421–429.
Lusardi G, Lipp A, Shaw C. Antibiotic prophylaxis for short-term catheter bladder drainage in adults. *Cochrane Database Syst Rev.* 2013;(7):CD005428, doi:10.1002/14651858.CD005428.pub2.
Lydon-Rochelle M, Holt VL, Martin DP. Association between method of delivery and maternal rehospitalization. *JAMA.* 2000;283:2411–2416.
Lydon-Rochelle M, Holt VL, Easterling TR, et al. Risk of uterine rupture during labor among women with a prior Cesarean delivery. *N Engl J Med.* 2001a;345(1):3–8.
Lydon-Rochelle MT, Holt VL, Martin DP. Delivery method and self-reported postpartum general health status among primiparous women. *Paediatr Perinat Epidemiol.* 2001b;15:232–240.
Lydon-Rochelle M, Holt VL, Easterling TR, et al. First birth Cesarean and placental abruption or previa at second birth. *Obstet Gynecol.* 2001c;97(5 Pt 1):765–769.
MacDonald D, Grant A, Sheridan-Pereira M, Boylan P, Chalmers I. The Dublin randomized controlled trial of intrapartum fetal heart rate monitoring. *Am J Obstet Gynecol.* 1985;152(5):524–39.
Maude R, et al. Putting intelligent structured intermittent auscultation (ISIA) into practice. *Women Birth.* 2016;29: 285–292.
McCarthy F, Rigg L, Cady L, et al. A new way of looking at caesarean section births. *Aust N Z J Obstet Gynaecol.* 2007;47:316–320.
McCombe K, Bogod DG. Learning from the law. A review of 21 years of litigation for pain during caesarean section. *Anaesthesia.* 2018; 73(2):223–230. doi:10.1111/anae.14119.
McLachlan H, Forster D, Davey M, et al. Effects of continuity of care by a primary midwife (caseload midwifery) on caesarean section rates in women of low obstetric risk: the COSMOS randomised controlled trial. *BJOG.* 2012;19(12):1483–1492.
Mangesi L, Hofmeyr GJ, Smith V, et al. Fetal movement counting for assessment of fetal wellbeing. *Cochrane Database Syst Rev.* 2015;(10):CD004909, doi:10.1002/14651858.CD004909.pub3.
Mayberry LJ, Clemmens D, De A. Epidural analgesia side effects, co-interventions, and care of women during childbirth: a systematic review. *Am J Obstet Gynecol.* 2002;186(5 supplNature):S81–S93.
Miller S, Abalos E, Chamillard M Ref: https://www.thelancet.com/journals/lancet/article/PIIS0140-6736(16)31472-6/fulltext et al. Beyond too little, too late and too much, too soon: a pathway towards evidence-based, respectful maternity care worldwide. *Lancet.* 2016;388(10056):2176–2192.

Ministry of Health (MOH). *Report on Maternity 2015*. Wellington, NZ: MOH; 2017. Online: https://www.health.govt.nz/system/files/documents/publications/report-on-maternity-2015-updated_12122017.pdf.

Ministry of Health (MOH). *Report on Maternity 2018*. Wellington, NZ: MOH; 2021. Online: https://www.health.govt.nz/publication/report-maternity-web-tool.

Minkoff H, Powderly KR, Chervenak F, et al. Ethical dimensions of elective primary cesarean delivery. *Obstet Gynecol*. 2004;103(2): 387–392.

Morau E, Jaillet M, Storme B, et al. Does programmed intermittent epidural bolus improve childbirth conditions of nulliparous women compared with patient-controlled epidural analgesia?: A multicentre, randomised, controlled, triple-blind study. *Eur J Anaesthesiol*. 2019 Oct;36(10):755–762. doi: 10.1097/EJA.0000000000001053. PMID: 31335447.

Morris JM, Totterdell J, Bin YS, et al. Contribution of maternal age, medical and obstetric history to maternal and perinatal morbidity/mortality for women aged 35 or older. *Aust N Z J Obstet Gynaecol*. 2018;58(1):91–97. doi:10.1111/ajo.12674.

Morrison JJ, Rennie JM, Milton PJ. Neonatal respiratory morbidity and mode of delivery at term: influence of timing of elective caesarean section. *BJOG*. 1995;102(2):101–106.

Mylonas I, Friese K. The indications for and risks of elective cesarean section. *Dtsch Arztebl Int*. 2015;112:489–495. doi:10.3238/arztebl.2015.0489.

Naaktgeboren C. The biology of childbirth. In: Chalmers I, Enkin M, Keirse MJ, eds. *Effective Care in Pregnancy and Childbirth*. Oxford: Oxford University Press; 1989:795–804.

National Institute for Health and Care Excellence (NICE). *Caesarean Section*. Clinical guideline. London: NICE; 2021. Online: https://www.nice.org.uk/guidance/ng192/resources/caesarean-birth-pdf-66142078788805

National Institute for Health and Care Excellence (NICE). *Intrapartum Care for Healthy Women and Babies (CG190)*. London: NICE; 2017. Online: https://www.nice.org.uk/guidance/cg190/resources/intrapartum-care-for-healthy-women-and-babies-pdf-35109866447557.

Nelson KB, Dambrosia JM, Ting TY, et al. Uncertain value of electronic fetal monitoring in predicting cerebral palsy. *N Engl J Med*. 1996;334:613–618.

New South Wales (NSW) Health. *Maternity—Supporting Women Planning a Vaginal Breech Birth*. Guideline GL2017_008. Sydney. NSW Health; 2017.

New South Wales (NSW) Health. *Maternity—Fetal Heart Rate Monitoring GL2016_001 Policy*. Sydney: NSW Health; 2018 (review date 06-Jan-2021). Online: http://www1.health.nsw.gov.au/pds/ActivePDSDocuments/GL2016_001.pdf.

New Zealand College of Midwives and the Midwifery and Maternity Providers Organisation (NZCOM MMPO). *Report on New Zealand's MMPO Midwives Care Activities and Outcomes*. Christchurch, NZ: NZCOM / MMPO; 2017. Online: https://www.midwife.org.nz/midwives/publications/midwifery-outcomes/ .

New Zealand Maternal Fetal Medicine Network (NZMFMN). *Guideline for the Management of Suspected Small for Gestational Age Singleton Pregnancies After 34 Weeks Gestation*. Auckland: NZMFMN; 2014. Online: https://www.cdhb.health.nz/Hospitals-Services/Health-Professionals/maternity-care-guidelines/Documents/NZMFM-SGA-Guideline.pdf.

Nissen E, Uvnas-Moberg K, Svensson K, et al. Different patterns of oxytocin, prolactin but not cortisol release during breastfeeding in women delivered by caesarean section or by the vaginal route. *Early Hum Dev*. 1996;45(1–2):103–118. (Research Support, Non-U.S. Gov't).

Oats S, Abraham J. *Llewellyn-Jones Fundamentals of Obstetrics and Gynaecology*. 8th ed. London: Mosby; 2004.

Odent M. Are caesareans the future? *RCM Midwives J*. 2004;7(7): 276.

Okosun H, Arulkumaran S. Intrapartum fetal surveillance. *Curr Obstet Gynaecol*. 2005;15(1):18–24.

O'Leary C, de Klerk N, Keogh J, et al. Trends in mode of delivery during 1984–2003: can they be explained by pregnancy and delivery complications? *BJOG*. 2007;114:855–864.

Olesen AG, Svare JA. Decreased fetal movements: background, assessment, and clinical management. *Acta Obstet Gynecol Scand*. 2004;83:818–826.

Paech M, Banks S, Gurrin L. An audit of accidental dural puncture during epidural insertion of a Tuohy needle in obstetric patients. *Int J Obstet Anesth*. 2001;10(3):162–167.

Palmer L, Blair E, Petterson B, et al. Antenatal antecedents of moderate and severe cerebral palsy. *Paediatr Perinat Epidemiol*. 1995; 9:171–184.

Panzer O, Ghazanfari N, Sessier D, et al. Shivering and shivering-like tremor during labor with and without epidural analgesia. *Anesthesiology*. 1999;90:1609–1616.

Patel R, Murphy D. Forceps delivery in modern obstetric practice. *BMJ*. 2004;328:1302–1305.

Pennell CE, Tracy MB. A new method for rapid measurement of lactate in fetal and neonatal blood. *Aust N Z J Obstet Gynaecol*. 1999;39(2):227–233.

Peyronnet V, Roses A, Girault A, et al. Lower limbs venous compression reduces the incidence of maternal hypotension following epidural analgesia during term labor. *Eur J Obstet Gynecol Reprod Biol*. 2017;219:94–99.

Pevzner L, Goffman D, Freda MC, et al. Patients' attitudes associated with cesarean delivery on maternal request in an urban population. *Am J Obstet Gynecol*. 2008;198(5):e35–e37.

Phillips SN, Fernando R, Girard T. Parenteral opioid analgesia: does it still have a role? Small doses of opioids leads to a steady state of plasma concentration of drug. *Best Pract Res Clin Anaesthesiol*. 2017;31:3–14.

Pinas A, Chandraharan E. Continuous cardiotocography during labour: analysis, classification and management. *Best Pract Res Clin Obstet Gynaecol*. 2016;30:33–47.

Poole J. Neuraxial analgesia for labor and birth: implications for mother and fetus. *J Perinat Neonatal Nurs*. 2003a;17(4): 252–267.

Poole J. Analgesia and anesthesia during labor and birth: implications for mother and fetus. *J Obstet Gynecol Neonatal Nurs*. 2003b;32(6):780–794.

Potter JE, Berquo E, Perpetuo IH, et al. Unwanted caesarean sections among public and private patients in Brazil: prospective study. *BMJ*. 2001;323:1155–1158.

Rayburn WF. Fetal body movement monitoring. *Obstet Gynecol Clin North Am*. 1990;17:95–110.

Reynolds F, Seed PT. Anaesthesia for caesarean section and neonatal acid-base status: a meta-analysis. *Anaesthesia*. 2005;60: 636–653.

Roberts CL, Algert C, Peat B, et al. Trends in labour and birth interventions among low-risk women in an Australian population. *Aust N Z J Obstet Gynaecol*. 2002;42(2):176–181.

Roberts CL, Raynes-Greenow CH, Upton A, et al. The management of labour among women with epidural analgesia. *Aust N Z J Obstet Gynaecol*. 2003;43:78–81.

Roberts CL, Tracy S, Peat B. Rates for obstetric intervention among private and public patients in Australia: population based descriptive study. *BMJ*. 2000;321(7254):137–141.

Robson MS . Can we reduce the caesarean section rate? *Best Pract Res Clin Obstet Gynaecol* 2001;15:179–94. doi:10.1053/beog.2000.0156

Robson S, Tan W, Adeyemi A, et al. Estimating the rate of cesarean section by maternal request: anonymous survey of obstetricians in Australia. *Birth*. 2009;36(3):208–212.

Roofthooft et al. Programmed intermittent epidural bolus for labour analgesia. *Anaesthesia.* 2020;75:1635–1642.
Rortveit G, Daltveit AK, Hannestad YS, et al. Norwegian EPINCONT Study. Urinary incontinence after vaginal delivery or cesarean section. *N Engl J Med.* 2003;348:900–907.
Rouse DJ, Hirtz DG, Thom E, et al. A randomized, controlled trial of magnesium sulfate for the prevention of cerebral palsy. *N Engl J Med.* 2008;359(9):895–905.
Rouse DJ, Hirtz DG. What we learned about the role of antenatal magnesium sulfate for the prevention of cerebral palsy. *Semin Perinatol.* 2016;40:303–306.
Royal Australian and New Zealand College of Obstetricians and Gynaecologists (RANZCOG). *Intrapartum Fetal Surveillance Clinical Guideline.* 3rd ed. Melbourne: RANZCOG; 2014.
Royal Australian and New Zealand College of Obstetricians and Gynaecologists (RANZCOG). *Intrapartum Fetal Surveillance Clinical Guideline.* 4th ed. Melbourne: RANZCOG; 2019. Online: https://ranzcog.edu.au/RANZCOG_SITE/media/RANZCOG-MEDIA/Women%27s%20Health/Statement%20and%20guidelines/Clinical-Obstetrics/IFS-Guideline-4thEdition-2019.pdf?ext=.pdf.
Royal College of Obstetricians and Gynaecologists (RCOG). *The Management of Third- and Fourth-Degree Perineal Tears.* Green-top Guideline no. 29. London: RCOG Press; 2015a. Online: https://www.rcog.org.uk/globalassets/documents/guidelines/gtg-29.pdf.
Royal College of Obstetricians and Gynaecologists (RCOG). *Birth After Previous Caesarean Birth.* Green-top Guideline no. 45. London: RCOG Press; 2015b, updated 2017. Online: https://www.rcog.org.uk/globalassets/documents/guidelines/gtg_45.pdf.
Schenker JG, Cain JM. FIGO Committee report. FIGO Committee for the Ethical Aspects of Human Reproduction and Women's Health. International Federation of Gynecology and Obstetrics. *Int J Gynaecol Obstet.* 1999;64:317–322.
Schimpf MO, Tulikangas PK, O'Sullivan DM, et al. Characteristics of nulliparous women who would consider cesarean delivery on maternal request. *Conn Med.* 2011;75(4):207–218.
Schlinzig T, Johansson S, Stephansson O, et al. Surge of immune cell formation at birth differs by mode of delivery and infant characteristics—a population-based cohort study. *PLoS ONE.* 2017;12(9):e0184748. doi:10.1371/journal.pone.0184748.
Shepherd E, Salam RA, Middleton P, et al. Antenatal and intrapartum interventions for preventing cerebral palsy: an overview of Cochrane systematic reviews. *Cochrane Database Syst Rev.* 2017;(8):CD012077, doi:10.1002/14651858.CD012077.pub2.
Shiell A, Hawe P, Gold L. Complex interventions or complex systems? Implications for health economic evaluation. *BMJ.* 2008. 336(7656):1281–1283.
Shorten A, Shorten B. Episiotomy in NSW hospitals 1993–1996: towards understanding variations between public and private hospitals. *Aust Health Rev.* 1999;22(1):18–32.
Simmons SW, Taghizadeh N, Dennis AT, et al. Combined spinal–epidural versus epidural analgesia in labour. *Cochrane Database Syst Rev.* 2012;(10):CD003401. doi:10.1002/14651858.CD003401.pub3.
Smaill FM, Grivell RM. Antibiotic prophylaxis versus no prophylaxis for preventing infection after cesarean section. *Cochrane Database Syst Rev.* 2014;(10):CD007482. doi:10.1002/14651858.CD007482.pub3.
Smith GC, Pell JP, Pasupathy D, et al. Factors predisposing to perinatal death related to uterine rupture during attempted vaginal birth after caesarean section: retrospective cohort study. *BMJ.* 2004;329:375–380.
Sng BL, Sia ATH. Maintenance of epidural labour analgesia: the old, the new and the future. *Best Pract Res Clin Anaesthesiol.* 2017;31:15–22. doi:10.1016/j.bpa.2017.01.002.
Stanley FJ, Blair E. Why have we failed to reduce the frequency of cerebral palsy? *Med J Aust.* 1991;154(9):623–626.
Stavrou E, Ford J, Shand A, et al. Epidemiology and trends for caesarean section births in New South Wales, Australia: a population-based study. *BMC Pregnancy Childbirth.* 2011;11(1):8.
Thilaganathan B, Meher-Homji N, Nicolaides KH. Labor: an immunologically beneficial process for the neonate. *Am J Obstet Gynecol.* 1994;171(5):1271–1272.
Thomas J, Paranjothy S. *National Sentinel Caesarean Section Audit Report. Royal College of Obstetricians and Gynaecologists Clinical Effectiveness Support Unit.* London: RCOG Press; 2001.
Thompson JF, Roberts CL, Currie M, et al. Prevalence and persistence of health problems after childbirth: associations with parity and method of birth. *Birth.* 2002;29:83–94.
Thompson JL, Kuller JA, Rhee EH. Antenatal surveillance of fetal growth restriction. *Obstet Gynecol Surv.* 2012;67:554–565.
Thoren T, Holmstrom B, Rawal N, et al. Sequential combined spinal epidural block versus spinal block for cesarean section: effects on maternal hypotension and neurobehavioral function of the newborn. *Anesth Analg.* 1994;78:1087–1092.
Tita A, Landon M, Spong C, et al. Timing of elective repeat cesarean delivery at term and neonatal outcomes. *N Engl J Med.* 2009a;360:111–120.
Tita ATN, Rouse DJ, Blackwell S, et al. Emerging concepts in antibiotic prophylaxis for cesarean delivery. A systematic review. *Obstet Gynecol.* 2009b;113:675–682.
Tito F. *Review of Professional Indemnity Arrangements for Health Care Professionals: Compensation and Professional Indemnity in Health Care: Report.* Canberra: AGPS; 1995.
Tollånes M, Moster D, Daltveit A, et al. Cesarean section and risk of severe childhood asthma: a population-based cohort study. *J Pediatr.* 2008;153:112–116.
Townsend R, Chmielewska B, et al. Global changes in maternity care provision during the COVID-19 pandemic: A systematic review and meta-analysis. E Clinical Medicine. 2021;37: 100947.
Tracy SK, Tracy M. Costing the cascade: estimating the cost of increased obstetric intervention in childbirth using population data. *BJOG.* 2003;110:717–724.
Tracy SK, Sullivan ES, Wang YA, et al. Birth outcomes associated with interventions in labour amongst low risk women: a population-based study. *Women Birth.* 2007a;20:41–48.
Tracy SK, Tracy MB, Sullivan EA. Admission of term infants to neonatal intensive care: a population-based study. *Birth.* 2007b;34(4):301–307.
Tracy SK, Hartz DL, Tracy MB, et al. Caseload midwifery care versus standard maternity care for women of any risk: M@NGO, a randomised controlled trial. *Lancet.* 2013;382(9906):1723–1732.
Tracy SK, Welsh A, Hall B, et al. Caseload midwifery compared to standard or private obstetric care for first time mothers in a public teaching hospital in Australia. *BMC Pregnancy Childbirth.* 2014;14:46. doi:10.1186/1471-2393-14-46.
Tversky A, Kahneman D. The framing of decisions and the psychology of choice. *Science.* 1981;211:453–458.
Valent AM, DeArmond C, Houston JM, et al. Effect of post–cesarean delivery oral cephalexin and metronidazole on surgical site infection among obese women a randomized clinical trial. *JAMA.* 2017;318(11):1026–1034.
van Bavel J, Hukkelhoven CWPM, de Vries C, et al. The effectiveness of mediolateral episiotomy in preventing obstetric anal sphincter injuries during operative vaginal delivery: a ten-year analysis of a national registry. *Int Urogynecol J.* 2018;29(3): 407–413. doi:10.1007/s00192-017-3422-4.
Walker KF, Kibuka M, Thornton JG, Jones NW. Maternal position in the second stage of labour for women with epidural anaesthesia. *Cochrane Database Syst Rev.* 2018;11:CD008070, doi:10.1002/14651858.CD008070.pub4.

Walker R, Turnbull D, Wilkinson C. Increasing cesarean section rates: exploring the role of culture in an Australian community. *Birth.* 2004;31(2):117–124.

Weibel S, Jelting Y, Afshari A, et al. Patient-controlled analgesia with remifentanil versus alternative parenteral methods for pain management in labour. *Cochrane Database Syst Rev.* 2017;(4):CD011989, doi:10.1002/14651858.CD011989.pub2.

Wiberg-Itzel E, Lipponer C, Norman M, et al. Determination of pH or lactate in fetal scalp blood in management of intrapartum fetal distress: randomised controlled multicentre trial. *BMJ.* 2008;336:1284–1287.

Wloch C, Wilson J, Lamagni T, et al. Risk factors for surgical site infection following caesarean section in England: results from a multicentre cohort study. *BJOG.* 2012;19(11):1324–1333. doi:10.1111/j.1471-0528.2012.03452.x.

Wolf J. Risk and reputation: obstetricians, cesareans, and consent. *J Hist Med Allied Sci.* 2017;73(1):7–28.

Wong HS, Hutton J, Zuccollo J, et al. The maternal outcome in placenta accreta: the significance of antenatal diagnosis and non-separation of placenta at delivery. *N Z Med J.* 2008;121:30–38.

World Health Organization. *WHO recommendations: intrapartum care for a positive childbirth experience.* Geneva: World Health Organization; 2018. Licence: CC BY-NC-SA 3.0 IGO.

Yao R, Crimmins SD, Contag SA, et al. Adverse perinatal outcomes associated with trial of labor after cesarean section at term in pregnancies complicated by maternal obesity. *J Matern Fetal Neonatal Med.* 2017;1–6. doi:10.1080/14767058.2017.1404023.

Young D. The push against vaginal birth (Editorial). *Birth.* 2003; 30(3):149–152.

Zanardo V, Svegliado G, Cavallin F, et al. Elective cesarean delivery: does it have a negative effect on breastfeeding? *Birth.* 2010;37(4):275–279.

Further reading

Bewley S, Cockburn JI. The unethics of 'request' Caesarean section. *BJOG.* 2002;109:593–596.

Clement S. *The Caesarean Experience.* London: Pandora; 1995.

Everett TR, Peebles DM. Antenatal tests of fetal wellbeing. *Semin Fetal Neonatal Med.* 2015;20:138–143.

See particularly the *middle cerebral artery (MCA) Doppler* as an important indicator of fetal anemia; the 'cerebro:placental' or 'cerebro:umbilical' ratio to determine fetuses with a low *cerebro:placenta ratio (C:P)* who may have failed to reach their growth potential; the utility of the *ductus venosus (DV) waveform* to determine cardiac function in the very premature fetus with IUGR, or in the pre-term fetus.

Finer NN, Robertson CM, Richards RT, et al. Hypoxic ischemic encephalopathy in term neonates: perinatal factors and outcome. *J Pediatr.* 1981;98(1):112–117.

Gibb D, Arulkumaran S. *Fetal Monitoring in Practice.* London: Churchill Livingstone; 2008.

Odent M. Are caesareans the future? *RCM Midwives J.* 2004;7(7):276.

O'Neill O. *Autonomy and Trust in Bioethics.* Cambridge: Cambridge University Press; 2002.

Pinas A, Chandraharan E. Continuous cardiotocography during labour: analysis, classification and management. *Best Pract Res Clin Obstet Gynaecol.* 2016;30:33–47.

Sarnat HB, Sarnat MS. Neonatal encephalopathy following fetal distress. A clinical and electroencephalographic study. *Arch Neurol.* 1976;33(10):696–705.

Thacker SB, Stroup DF. Revisiting the use of the electronic fetal monitor. *Lancet.* 2003;361(9356):445–446.

Wolf J. Risk and reputation: obstetricians, cesareans, and consent. *J Hist Med Allied Sci.* 2017;73(1):7–28.

CHAPTER 40

Life-threatening emergencies

Lesley Dixon and Elaine Gray

LEARNING OUTCOMES

Learning outcomes for this chapter are:

1. To discuss those factors that indicate a potential for emergency life-threatening situations for woman and baby in pregnancy, birth and the puerperium
2. To describe the aetiology and management of a range of emergency situations in pregnancy, labour, birth and the puerperium, whilst recognising that some actions and initial management may depend on the place of onset and context of care
3. To identify the current evidence in relation to the identification, assessment and collaborative management of maternal and fetal/newborn emergencies.

CHAPTER OVERVIEW

For most women, childbirth is a healthy event. However, some women may develop complications requiring complex levels of medical and technological intervention, and it is these women who are the focus of this chapter. This chapter discusses the most frequent life-threatening complications, which can often transpire with little or no warning. It is not designed to be a definitive guide to the management of midwifery/obstetric emergencies. Readers are advised to supplement the information they gain from this chapter with other more specialised texts and review other chapters in this textbook (specifically Chs 20, 24, 29, 37, 38 and 41). A thorough understanding of the biosciences and pathophysiology underpinning emergency conditions in midwifery is important. Life-threatening emergencies discussed in this chapter include umbilical cord presentation and prolapsed cord, shoulder dystocia, postpartum haemorrhage, eclampsia, amniotic fluid embolism, uterine rupture and inversion, maternal collapse and cardiopulmonary resuscitation. The chapter provides an overview on how midwives can identify, assess and seek support when faced with these emergencies that threaten the life of either the woman or her baby.

KEY TERMS

amniotic fluid embolism
cardiopulmonary resuscitation
disseminated intravascular coagulopathy
eclampsia
placenta accrete
placenta praevia
postpartum haemorrhage
shoulder dystocia
trauma
umbilical cord prolapse
uterine inversion
uterine rupture

INTRODUCTION

Life-threatening emergencies can occur with little or no warning, so it is crucial that all midwives can recognise and manage a range of midwifery / obstetric emergencies until they can access medical support and / or the woman is transferred to an appropriate facility. This chapter commences with a discussion on the essential elements of any emergency and the potential for that emergency to cause emotional trauma for all involved. It then moves on to specific life-threatening conditions that affect fetal health followed by emergencies that affect the woman's health and have the potential to affect fetal health if the woman remains pregnant.

ESSENTIAL ELEMENTS OF EMERGENCY CARE

When complications arise, a multidisciplinary approach is usually required and so there must be a system of escalation in place for access to consultation and referral to medical facilities, personnel and emergency transport. Effective communication is pivotal to best practice in maternity care, but never more so than when emergencies arise. In Aotearoa New Zealand, midwives are required by the Midwifery Council to attend annual education to maintain skills and knowledge of the most common obstetric emergencies as part of their recertification requirements. There are several multiprofessional training packages available in Australia and New Zealand and many obstetric hospitals regularly hold courses designed to support multidisciplinary groups to practise and update their skills in preparation for life-threatening emergency situations.

There are essential elements of any emergency (Box 40.1), although these will vary dependent on the place and context of the emergency. If the emergency develops during a home birth, for instance, then calling for help would involve ambulance and paramedic support until transfer into a suitable facility. However, being prepared, identifying, assessing and treating the emergency quickly and collaborating with the multidisciplinary team are essential skills necessary for any emergency situation.

Keeping the woman and her partner informed and updated is also necessary regardless of the situation. Life-threatening emergencies are often traumatic for all involved, which includes the woman, her partner, her family / whanau and each of the clinicians providing the various aspects of clinical care.

Box 40.1 Essential elements of any emergency situation for midwives

- Be prepared—have emergency equipment available and tested
- Call for help—to initiate additional support
- Assess condition
- Provide initial emergency management
- Communicate and collaborate with multidisciplinary team
- Keep the woman and her partner / family / whanau aware and updated

Women's experiences of obstetric emergencies

A traumatic birth can have a profound impact on a woman's sense of self and identity. Post-traumatic stress disorder (PTSD) is an emotional response that can be triggered by a traumatic event such as threatened death and serious injury. Following a traumatic experience, the individual may have difficulty relaxing and have nightmares, flashbacks, numbness, mood changes, loss of appetite, lack of concentration and difficulty socialising. PTSD is diagnosed if these symptoms last longer than a month following the incident, or they are causing difficulties in functioning. PTSD can occur for the woman and others who have witnessed the traumatic event (see https://www.healthnavigator.org.nz/health-a-z/p/post-traumatic-stress-disorder-ptsd/).

De la Cruz et al. (2013) interviewed 15 women who had an emergency peripartum hysterectomy, finding seven themes that encompassed the women's experiences. The women described their fear during the event, with some having high levels of pain; some described thinking they were dying, whilst others realised their closeness to death after the event; many described numbness and / or a delay in their emotional reaction and there were concerns about bonding with their baby. The women identified the need for clear communication and information and that compassion, respect and sensitivity from their care providers during their follow-up care was important. They described how during the emergency they had faced their own mortality and had lost their expected birth experience. Their psychological upset was often delayed with women needing to have more follow-up so that they could fill in the gaps in their understanding and memory of the events. The authors identified three phases of care to consider based on their findings; these have been adapted and may be useful to consider during any life-threatening emergency (Fig. 40.1).

Debriefing and counselling for the woman and her family

There are two main types of debriefing, one is the informal debriefing that occurs postnatally with midwives discussing and filling in the gaps for women following their birth. The second is a formal structured psychological debriefing aimed at preventing longer term issues. At present there is insufficient high-quality evidence to support debriefing as

During the emergency	• Calm atmosphere, team work. • Communicate what is happening with the woman as well as others. • Manage the woman's pain. • Reassurance for the woman and her family. • Compassionate, respectful care.
During hospital recovery	• Communication—what has happened and recovery pathway. • Early and regular contact with baby. • Flexible vists from partner and family—support partner rooming in. • Manage pain. • Debrief with clinicians. • Referal for follow up psychological support.
Discharge home and follow up	• Follow-up appointments—as many as needed. • Referral for community psychological support. • A detailed debriefing of events for the woman and her family. • Compassionate and respectful care.

FIGURE 40.1 What do women need during an emergency?
(Adapted from de la Cruz et al., 2013)

having a positive or negative effect (Bastos, 2015). This may be due to the poor quality of the evidence and the lack of clarity around definitions of debriefing. For women who have experienced a life-threatening emergency, talking through the events with clinicians at follow-up meetings can be helpful as a way of understanding what happened to them. Follow-up counselling can also be helpful and may support the woman to make sense of her ongoing feelings about the traumatic event. Partners and other family members can also be affected and may need emotional support and debriefing (Box 40.2).

Box 40.2 Effect of life-threatening event on partners and family members

Other members of the family can also be deeply affected by the woman's life-threatening experience and will need immediate information and support during the emergency. Ways to help are:

- Provide personal touches of support (these can make a real difference to how partners and family members cope).
- Partners and family members will often remember more about events than the woman who is ill, but they will still appreciate repeated explanations.
- Partners/fathers and family members can find seeing their partner in a high-dependency or intensive care unit very traumatic and may need support from midwives to help them:
  - visit their partner and understand her condition
  - understand that the situation is not hopeless—their partner may recover
  - come to terms with what has happened.
- Partners/fathers may experiences long-term emotional health problems too and families may need additional support in this event.
- Partners/fathers who experience emotional health symptoms do not necessarily seek help, although they do feel that counselling, if offered, could be beneficial.

(Adapted from Knight et al., 2016)

Debriefing and counselling for midwives

Midwives are frequently exposed to stress and trauma in their day-to-day work, which can have a toll on the midwives' own emotional health. In their survey of 233 Australian midwives, Toohill et al. (2019) found that 93.6% had experienced a traumatic birth mostly during their professional role, with 97 (41.6%) also experiencing trauma during their own labour. Organisational stressors that contributed to these midwives' professional trauma included: witnessing the disrespect of women, being disrespected as a midwife and being complicit in poor care practices. Improving women-centred care and improving professional relationships may enhance midwives' resilience.

Elmir et al. (2017) used a meta-ethnographic approach to explore midwives' experiences of adverse events. Eleven qualitative studies were reviewed with four major themes identified, these were:

- feeling the chaos
- powerless, responsible and a failure
- it adds another scar to my soul
- finding a way to deal with it.

Clearly, life-threatening events have an impact on all clinicians involved; being able to discuss and review the case and the responses in a non-judgmental, collaborative and supportive meeting is often helpful. Many employers also provide an employee assistance program (EAP) for their employees; this service can provide counselling and support for midwives and other clinicians following a traumatic experience.

EMERGENCY SITUATIONS THAT MAY IMPACT ON NEWBORN HEALTH

In any emergency situation there is the potential for the situation to result in fetal compromise and require newborn resuscitation. Hence, it is important to have equipment and additional personnel available to provide assessment and resuscitative support.

Cord presentation and prolapse

Umbilical cord presentation

An umbilical cord presentation (Fig. 40.2) is the presence of the umbilical cord between the presenting part of the fetus and the uterine cervix with intact amniotic membranes. Cord presentation is difficult to identify clinically but may be identified during vaginal examination. Once the membranes break, the risk that the cord will prolapse through the cervix into the vagina increases significantly. In an occult cord presentation, a loop of cord lies alongside the presenting part and is not felt on vaginal examination.

Umbilical cord prolapse

Umbilical cord prolapse is defined as descent of the umbilical cord through the cervix alongside (occult) or past (overt) the presenting part in the presence of ruptured membranes (see Fig. 40.2). It occurs when the cord drops down through the cervix into the vagina and can sometimes be seen at the introitus. An occult prolapse occurs when the membranes rupture and the cord is trapped between the presenting part and the maternal pelvis.

Much more is known about cord prolapse than cord presentation, because the former is dramatically apparent and the latter is usually diagnosed by sonography or during a 'routine' vaginal examination of a clinically asymptomatic woman. If the umbilical cord prolapses through the cervix, or even between the presenting part and the pelvis, during uterine contractions it will be exposed to intermittent compression during contractions, which compromises the fetal circulation. Depending on the duration and the degree of compression, fetal hypoxia, neurological damage and even fetal death may occur. Dramatic changes in the fetal heart rate are often the first signs of a cord prolapse.

As Table 40.1 shows, risk factors for cord prolapse are mostly due to an ill-fitting presenting part (Royal College of Obstetricians and Gynaecologists (RCOG), 2014).

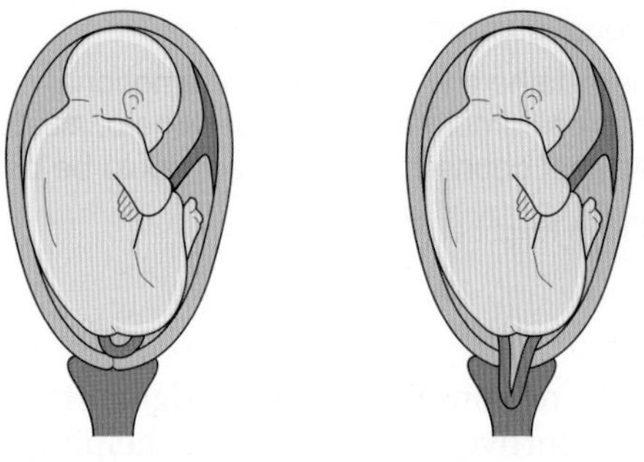

FIGURE 40.2 Cord presentation and cord prolapse
(Based on Henderson & Macdonald, 2004)

Incidence

The incidence of cord prolapse ranges from 0.1% to 0.6%, with an increased frequency (1%) for breech presentation (RCOG, 2014). Iatrogenic obstetric intervention such as induction of labour and artificial rupture of membranes have been identified as being responsible for 50% of cases (Kawakita et al., 2018). In their retrospective cohort study involving 57,204 women who had an artificial rupture of the membranes (ARM), Kawakita et al. (2018) identified a cord prolapse incidence of 0.2% (113 women). For these women, a dilatation of between 6–10 cm and a high head (station -3) or dilatation of less than 6 cm (any station) was associated with a higher risk of cord prolapse (Kawakita et al., 2018), suggesting that clinicians need to balance the increased risk of cord prolapse against the benefits of ARM before 6 cm or when the head is not engaged after 6 cm.

Table 40.1 Risk factors for cord prolapse

General	Procedure related
Multiparity	Artificial rupture of the membranes
Low birth weight, less than 2.5 kg	Vaginal manipulation of the fetus with ruptured membranes
Prematurity less than 37 weeks	External cephalic version (during procedure)
Fetal congenital anomalies	External cephalic version (during procedure)
Breech presentation	Stabilising induction of labour
Transverse, oblique and unstable lie especially when the longitudinal axis of the fetus changes repeatedly	Insertion of uterine pressure transducer
Second twin	External cephalic version
Polyhydramnios	Large balloon catheter during labour
Unengaged presenting part	
Low-lying placenta, other abnormal placentation	

(Source: RCOG 2014 Green-top Guideline No. 50 Umbilical Cord Prolapse. ©Royal College of Obstetricians and Gynaecologists; reproduced with permission)

The risks of umbilical cord presentation and prolapse increase in frequency with malpresentation and with poorly fitting presenting parts, such as in a transverse lie, or shoulder or breech presentation (RCOG, 2014) (see Table 40.1). A flexed or footling breech poses the most risk for cord prolapse owing to the increased space through which the umbilical cord can fall into the vagina. Prematurity is also a risk factor for cord prolapse because pre-term babies are more likely to present as a malpresentation, and their small size in relation to the maternal pelvis means there is more room for loops of cord to escape through the cervix. Additionally, there is usually more liquor volume in relation to fetal size than for the term fetus.

Any structural abnormalities of the placenta, uterus or pelvis may also stop the presenting part from descending into the pelvis and increase the risk of cord prolapse (e.g. **placenta praevia**, succenturiate placental lobe or contracted pelvis). Repeated pregnancies interfere with the integrity of the abdominal musculature, which means that some multiparous women have lax abdominal muscles, increasing the likelihood of an ill-fitting presenting part at term. Finally, cord prolapse is a rare complication of ECV to turn a breech presentation, so the procedure should ideally be conducted in an environment where fetal wellbeing can be assessed and resources are available to proceed to an emergency caesarean section.

Whenever the presenting part is not fully engaged, an amniotomy (artificial breaking of the membranes)—especially in the presence of polyhydramnios—poses a real risk of an iatrogenic cord prolapse. Spontaneous rupture of the membranes can also trigger cord prolapse and so it is important for the midwife to auscultate the fetal heart prior to and immediately after amniotomy and as soon as is practical following a spontaneous rupture of membranes. Women with a known risk of cord prolapse (e.g. malpresentation prematurity) should be advised to go to the nearest maternity unit for assessment for cord prolapse as quickly as possible if the membranes rupture.

CLINICAL POINT

Artificial rupture of the membranes (ARM) has been associated with cord prolapse in the presence of an unengaged presenting fetal part. It should never be a routine procedure. In the presence of an unengaged fetal part a controlled ARM in theatres may be performed prior to induction of labour (IOL). The operating theatres provide a safe place for an immediate caesarean section should the cord prolapse. If the ARM is successful, the woman can be transferred back to the birthing unit to continue the IOL.

Diagnosis of cord presentation and prolapse

Unresolved ongoing cord compression may result in some level of fetal hypoxia, an increase in the severity of the fetal heart decelerations and, depending on the ability of the fetus to withstand episodic hypoxia, eventually to prolonged fetal bradycardia. A fetal heart rate pattern with a prolonged deceleration may be the first obvious sign that the cord has prolapsed.

The presence of repetitive, early FHR decelerations on an electronic fetal heart tracing may be indicative of umbilical cord compression or occult cord presentation, especially in the presence of oligohydramnios. Listening to the FHR through contractions via a Doppler or a Pinard stethoscope may also pick up these ominous changes in the FHR and guidelines recommend immediate vaginal examination to exclude cord prolapse. In about 50% of cases, however, the decelerations occur because the umbilical vein is thinner than the arterial walls and therefore more susceptible to compression. Seemingly dramatic heart rate accelerations often resolve rapidly after the contraction is finished and may cease altogether if the woman changes her position. Expectant management is often the best choice. See Box 40.3.

CLINICAL POINT

Prolapse of the umbilical cord is a maternity emergency demanding immediate attention. Delay in management is associated with significant perinatal morbidity and mortality, due mainly to complications associated with birth asphyxia.

If the umbilical cord is presenting and the amniotic membranes are still intact, the midwife may palpate a pulsating membrane at the same rhythm and rate as the fetal heart. It is important to differentiate this rate from the maternal pulse, which may also be felt through the vaginal fornices. Once the umbilical cord prolapses through the cervix, the cord may be felt during a vaginal examination (rope-like and pulsing). At times the cord is visible at the introitus.

Box 40.3 Clinical diagnosis of cord presentation and prolapse

- Cord presentation—loops of cord are palpated through the membranes. The presence of umbilical cord lying in front of the presenting part can also be visualised using colour Doppler studies.
- Cord prolapse—diagnosis is made by visual inspection or palpation of a pulsing umbilical cord during a vaginal examination. The umbilical cord is felt below or beside the presenting part.
- Occult prolapsed cord—is rarely felt on vaginal examination and the only indication may be fetal heart rate changes.
- Overt prolapse—the umbilical cord can be seen protruding from the introitus or loops of cord palpated within the vaginal canal.
- Cord prolapse is often associated with changes in the fetal heart rate such as tachycardia, a prolonged deceleration or an ongoing fetal bradycardia, and is an obstetric emergency.

Management of cord prolapse in labour

The aim of management is to elevate the presenting part to prevent/alleviate compression on the cord and then to expedite the birth. Elevating the presenting part can be undertaken by placing the woman in either an exaggerated Sims position (Fig. 40.3) or a knee-chest position (Fig. 40.4) and applying digital pressure to lift the fetus away from the cord. This can also be achieved through filling the woman's urinary bladder.

Emergency management depends on the fetus being a viable gestation and on discussion with the woman. If no cord pulsation or fetal heart beat is heard, it is important to confirm the presence or absence of the fetal heart with a portable ultrasound to help guide further management.

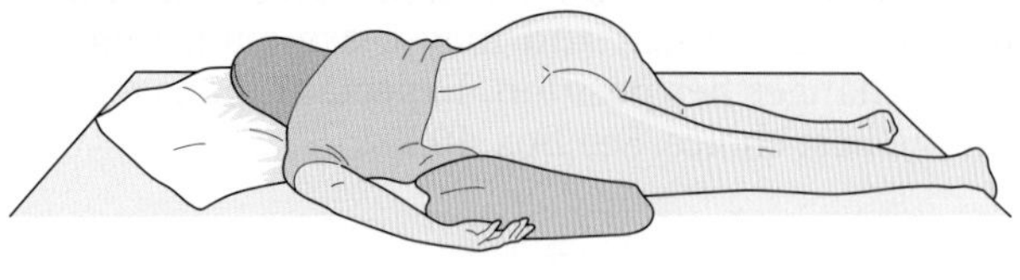

FIGURE 40.3 Exaggerated Sims' position
(Based on Henderson & Macdonald, 2004)

During labour contractions, if the umbilical cord prolapses through the cervix or even lies between the presenting part and the pelvis it will be exposed to intermittent compression, compromising the fetal circulation. Exposure of the umbilical cord to cool air and/or too much handling in an overt prolapse can lead to vasospasm of the cord vessels, causing a significant reduction in placental fetal blood flow and leading to ongoing fetal hypoxia and acidosis.

Perinatal asphyxia may also result in hypoxic–ischaemic encephalopathy and cerebral palsy for the newborn. The principal causes of asphyxia in this context are thought to be:

- cord compression that reduces the blood flow capacity to and from both the placenta and fetus
- umbilical arterial vasospasm secondary to exposure to vaginal fluids and/or air causing the same disruption to placental–fetal blood flow.

If the fetus is viable and the cervix is not completely dilated, prompt birth via caesarean section is recommended

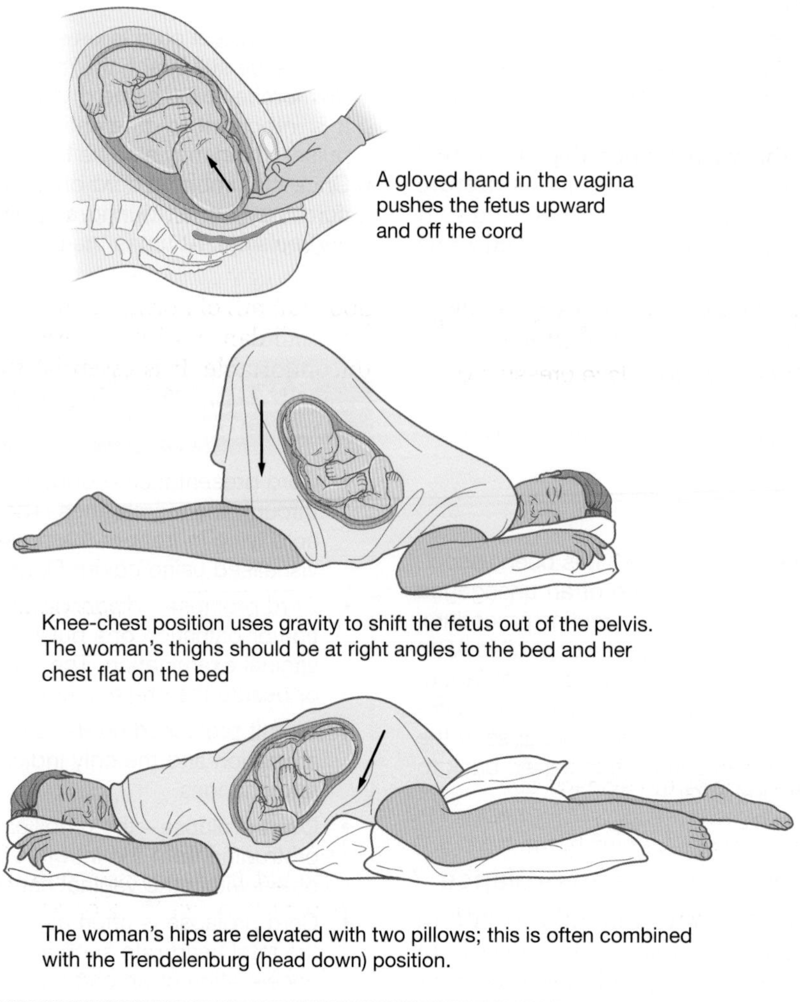

FIGURE 40.4 Knee-chest position

(RCOG, 2014). If the cord prolapse is associated with a pathological heart rate pattern then a caesarean section should be undertaken as soon as possible and within 30 minutes of diagnosis. If the fetal heart rate pattern is normal, a continuous FHR should be commenced (cardiotocograph), tocolysis may be considered and a caesarean section may be undertaken.

A vaginal birth may still be possible if the birth is imminent—that is, the cervix is completely dilated, the presenting part is engaged and there are no contraindications that will slow the birth. This has to be a considered assessment and evaluation by the clinician providing care. It is an option only if the birth can be expedited very quickly—as such it may be suitable only for those women who have had a previous vaginal birth. If the fetus is very pre-term and non-viable or has died (confirmed by ultrasound) then the woman should be supported to have a vaginal birth.

Immediate management until help is accessed

The strategies outlined in Box 40.4 are designed to improve placental–fetal blood flow through the umbilical cord. If the fetus is viable and birth is not imminent, the midwife supports the woman to assume an exaggerated Sims' position (her hips can be elevated on pillows; see Fig. 40.3) or knee-chest position (Fig. 40.4) and inserts (or keeps) two fingers into the vagina to push the presenting part up and away from the cord and applies continuous pressure to keep the presenting part clear of the cord. A variation and less commonly used manoeuvre is to remove the hand from the vagina once the presenting part has been pushed above the pelvic brim and apply continuous suprapubic pressure upwards. Excessive displacement may encourage more of the cord to prolapse. This manoeuvre is maintained until help arrives or the baby is born. If the cord is visible at the introitus, it is important to reduce potential umbilical cord spasm by minimal handling of the cord, and preventing the cord becoming cold or drying. Some clinicians recommend that it should be replaced gently in the vagina, to minimise chilling and vasospasm. An alternative recommendation is to gently wrap the cord in warm saline-soaked swabs to prevent reactive vasoconstriction and the onset of fetal hypoxia–acidosis.

Once pressure on the umbilical cord is relieved, the midwife makes a rapid assessment to determine the degree of cervical dilation, fetal position and descent of the presenting part as well as signs of fetal compromise—management now depends on the viability of the fetus, the stage of labour and whether or not birth is imminent. Auscultation of the FHR is a valuable adjunct to decision making regarding the positioning of the woman and the elevation of the presenting part. Whichever manoeuvre maintains a normal FHR is the best position for the woman while decisions and planning are made regarding birth.

Box 40.4 Cord prolapse management summary

- Change the woman's position to relieve pressure on the cord.
- Call for help—a full obstetric/midwifery team is required.
- Note time of diagnosis of cord presentation/prolapse, confirm viability and presence of fetal heart sounds and maintain a contemporaneous record of events until birth occurs.
- Minimise compression of the cord between the fetal head and the pelvis (via finger displacement or bladder filling).
- Administer 100% oxygen via a Hudson mask at 6–8 L/min. Note that there is no recent, good-quality evidence that supports the efficacy of giving supplemental oxygen, but neither is there any evidence to suggest that it causes harm.
- Obtain intravenous access.
- Give a brief explanation to the woman and her family.
- Prepare the woman for transfer to theatre and an operative birth unless birth is imminent, the fetus is not viable or there is fetal demise.

Bladder filling

If the decision to birth interval is likely to be prolonged, particularly if it involves ambulance transfer from home or a midwifery-led unit, umbilical cord compression may also be relieved by first pushing the fetal head out of the pelvis and then inserting a Foley catheter into the maternal bladder, which is filled with normal saline. This can be achieved quickly by inserting the end of a blood-giving set into the catheter. The catheter should be clamped once 500–750 mL of normal saline has been instilled. Transfer via ambulance with a very full bladder can be very uncomfortable. It is essential to empty the bladder just before birthing the baby, whether by vaginal birth or caesarean section (RCOG, 2014).

If oxytocin is being given intravenously during the labour, (e.g. induction of labour) then this should be stopped immediately.

Another useful therapy is to decrease the force and frequency of contractions using subcutaneous terbutaline if there will be a prolonged interval of time from diagnosis to birth; this should be undertaken in consultation with an obstetrician. Whenever possible, expediting the birth is the treatment of choice, provided the fetus still is viable and alive.

CLINICAL POINT

Following a diagnosis of cord prolapse, where the fetus is alive but it is not possible to birth vaginally, it is a high priority to move the woman to the operating room. The aim should be to expedite the birth of the baby in a manner that provides for safe anaesthesia for the woman.

- Depending on local circumstances, some procedures (e.g. intravenous cannulation, blood tests for ABO and

Rh testing, and urinary catheterisation) can be delayed until the woman is in the operating theatre.

- The usual prophylaxis to prevent the adverse effects of the aspiration of gastric contents should still be given to the woman (e.g. sodium citrate plus ranitidine).
- Informed consent should be obtained from the woman.
- If delay in C/S then use of tocolytics and cease oxytocin if in use.
- Paired umbilical cord blood samples should be collected following the birth.
- Documentation of the timing of events and treatments can occur immediately following the birth.

Cord prolapse in the community

Women should be informed if they have risk factors for cord prolapse. If a woman's membranes rupture when at home (in the absence of the midwife) and if she suspects cord prolapse she should assume a knee-to-chest face-down position (or exaggerated Sims' position), call an ambulance and state that it is a life-threatening emergency so that she can be transferred to the nearest maternity unit with facilities for emergency caesarean section and neonatal resuscitation.

If cord prolapse occurs during a planned home birth or midwifery-led unit birth and a vaginal examination by the lead midwife reveals that a spontaneous vaginal birth is imminent, preparations for transfer should still be made because it is likely that the baby will require active resuscitation. If birth is not imminent, the presenting part should be elevated during transfer by either the manual or the bladder-filling method (see previous section) and the exaggerated Sims' position. It is a good idea for community-based midwives to consider carrying a Foley catheter and equipment for fluid infusion for this purpose.

During emergency ambulance transfer, the knee-to-chest position will be unsafe so the left-lateral or exaggerated Sims' position is preferable.

CLINICAL POINT

- Cord prolapse is a frightening event for women. They and their family will require ongoing explanations and reassurance.
- Document the time of cord prolapse, immediate management, ongoing care and treatment at the time or as soon as possible after the event (retrospectively).

CRITICAL THINKING EXERCISE

Ella is a 30-year-old woman who is in labour with her fourth baby. You are providing labour care in a midwifery-led unit which is 30 minutes from the nearest obstetric unit.

Ella's membranes rupture and you hear a fetal bradycardia when you auscultate the fetal heart. A vaginal examination reveals a cord prolapse; the cervix is 5 cm dilated.

1. What are your next steps?
2. How will you alleviate pressure on the cord?
3. How will you access more help and support?
4. What do you tell the woman and her partner?
5. What will you document?

Summary: cord prolapse

Umbilical cord prolapse is an infrequent obstetric emergency which can lead to increased perinatal morbidity and/or mortality. The aim of management is to relieve pressure on the cord until the birth can be expedited. Referral and transfer to a multidisciplinary team are essential to minimise maternal and fetal risks.

Shoulder dystocia

Shoulder dystocia, although rare, is a dramatic, anxiety-provoking emergency both for clinicians and for women and their families. It is associated with a high risk of physical and psychological complications for the woman and neonate, is unpredictable and has potentially catastrophic consequences. It is important that clinicians practise manoeuvres to release the shoulders and have an action plan in place to guide them as they manage this complication.

Shoulder dystocia occurs as a result of disproportion between the bisacromial diameter of the fetus and the anteroposterior diameter of the pelvic inlet. After the head births, the posterior shoulder descends past the sacral promontory and enters the true pelvis. The fetal anterior shoulder begins its descent but becomes impacted behind the symphysis pubis. Rarely, the posterior shoulder also impacts above the sacral promontory and very rarely both shoulders are obstructed. It is important to remember that the point of obstruction occurs at the inlet of the pelvis; therefore no amount of pulling on the baby's head will release this bony obstruction. Instead manoeuvres which widen the diameters of the pelvis and/or alter the position of the shoulders in relation to the pelvis need to be undertaken.

Shoulder dystocia occurs unexpectedly during birth; it can occur during a spontaneous or instrumental birth (ventouse or forceps) or occasionally at caesarean section.

The best way to determine the degree of **shoulder dystocia** is to describe clearly the manoeuvres needed to release the shoulders and birth the baby. There are a number of clinical signs that lead clinicians to suspect a possible shoulder dystocia including prolonged second stage, slow descent of the fetal head, appearance of the 'turtle' sign of the fetal head following birth (slow extension of the head with the chin remaining tight against the maternal perineum) and the absence of signs of restitution of the baby's head.

CLINICAL POINT

There are differing perspectives on how shoulder dystocia should be defined, resulting in difficulty defining the incidence. RCOG (2012) define shoulder dystocia as a vaginal cephalic birth that requires additional manoeuvres to deliver the shoulders after gentle traction has failed. Menticoglou (2018) argues that it should be defined as the failure to deliver the shoulders with maternal effort during the contraction after the birth of the head. Ansell et al. (2019) identified shoulder dystocia as when either one or both shoulders do not enter the pelvic cavity.

What do you consider is the optimal way of defining shoulder dystocia?

Incidence and risk factors

The diagnosis of shoulder dystocia is poorly defined and dependent on recognition by clinicians and the reported use of manoeuvres to dislodge the shoulders. Michelotti et al. (2018) in their review of 38,088 Australian births found an incidence of 5.3% between the years 2007 and 2015 (in one tertiary centre). Ansell et al. (2019) reviewed 52,055 births between 2006 and 2013, in a tertiary centre in New Zealand, finding an incidence of 0.81%. The incidence of shoulder dystocia increased from 0.54% in 2006 to 1.26% in 2013. Whether this increase is due to better recognition of the condition or other factors is as yet unknown.

Risk factors for shoulder dystocia include increasing maternal age, maternal obesity, maternal diabetes, induction of labour, use of epidural analgesia during labour/birth, prolonged labour and assisted birth (Michelotti et al, 2017; Overland et al., 2014 ; Zhang et al., 2017) (Box 40.5). Despite the association between fetal size and shoulder dystocia, fetal size is not a good predictor of shoulder dystocia (RCOG, 2012). This is because most cases occur in fetuses of normal birth weight and are unanticipated, which limits the clinical usefulness of risk factor identification. While there are predisposing risk factors for shoulder dystocia, approximately half occur in the absence of any known risk factors.

Anticipation of shoulder dystocia

Although a number of antenatal and intrapartum risk factors (perhaps better called associations) have been reported to be associated with shoulder dystocia, these have a low positive predictive value both singly and in combination (Ouzounian et al., 2014) because many women with multiple risk factors do not experience it, and conversely many women without risk factors experience it. Moreover, severe shoulder dystocia can occur during birth with a small-for-gestational-age infant (Ruis et al., 2011). This poor predictability is because shoulder dystocia is caused by dynamic or evolving mechanical events, with variations in diagnosing shoulder dystocia resulting in many false positives. Identifying fetal weight is difficult with current methods—both uterine height measurement and ultrasound scanning having poor predictive value (Boulvain et al., 2016).

Box 40.5 Risk factors associated with shoulder dystocia

Maternal

- Increasing maternal age
- Maternal obesity BMI >35
- Maternal birth weight
- Abnormal pelvic anatomy
- Gestational diabetes
- Prolonged pregnancy
- Previous shoulder dystocia
- Short stature

Fetal

- Suspected macrosomia >4500 g
- Asymmetric accelerated fetal growth

Labour

- Assisted vaginal delivery (forceps or ventouse)
- Precipitous second stage (<20 min)
- Epidural block
- Protracted active phase of first-stage labour
- Protracted second-stage labour
- Epidural analgesia—relaxes pelvic floor

Therefore, it is not possible to anticipate which babies will develop shoulder dystocia with certainty. Early induction of labour for women with suspected fetal macrosomia who do not have gestational diabetes does not improve either maternal or fetal outcome (Boulvain et al., 2016). Women who have had a previous shoulder dystocia are advised to discuss birth options with an obstetrician. Factors such as the severity of any previous neonatal or maternal injury, including psychological trauma, predicted fetal size and maternal choice should all be discussed with the woman when she and her family are making plans for their next birth. There is no evidence that the use of the McRoberts' manoeuvre before birth of the fetal head prevents shoulder dystocia (Mollberg et al., 2007).

Avoiding shoulder dystocia

An Australian midwife, Rachel Reed, argues that supporting the woman's physiology, avoiding intervention (augmentation) and epidurals and working with women to birth 'actively' may help them to avoid shoulder dystocia (https://midwifethinking.com/2015/05/13/shoulder-dystocia-the-real-story/). Reed argues that the baby needs time to move into the best position for birth. When the second stage is hurried the baby may not be able to make these adjustments and shoulder dystocia may occur. Induction and augmentation of labour and instrumental birth as well as 'directed pushing' may also interrupt the baby's positioning. She also considers that epidural analgesia 'completely alters the physiology of birth' and because of it the woman is unable to actively birth her baby. Similarly, birthing in the semirecumbent position increases the risk of shoulder dystocia because the pelvic diameters do not 'open the pelvis'. Anecdotal evidence from experienced midwives over many years supports the latter recommendation. Midwives can encourage women to assume a range of positions during labour and birth—standing, squatting, side-lying and all-fours positioning—rather than the semirecumbent position.

Maternal diabetes, macrosomia and shoulder dystocia

Current guidelines in New Zealand advise that for women with good glycaemic control and no other complexity, planned birth (IOL) before 40 weeks is *not* recommended (MOH, 2014). For women with poor control and a large-for-gestational-age baby, timing of the birth should be individualised.

Management of shoulder dystocia

Timely management of shoulder dystocia requires prompt recognition and action. The midwife should routinely observe for warning signs of impending shoulder dystocia (Box 40.6). Gentle traction in an axial direction (in line with the fetal spine) can be used to support shoulder delivery but any other traction should be avoided. Midwives are the only maternity clinicians who attend all births and are therefore more likely to experience and gain expertise in shoulder dystocia. Robson (2019) argues that because obstetricians are not constantly present in birthing suites, they are unlikely to develop expertise in shoulder dystocia. Midwives are the primary clinicians dealing with shoulder dystocia, and this should be formally recognised in their role.

Many countries teach a set of systematic manoeuvres (and a mnemonic) known as HELPERR to assist birth of a baby with shoulder dystocia (see Box 40.7 and next section). Although nomenclature of these manoeuvres (and mnemonics) may change, the principles of management remain the same.

Box 40.6 Warning signs of impending shoulder dystocia

- Prolonged second stage—bobbing of the fetal head
- Difficulty birthing the face and chin
- The head remains tightly applied to the vulva or even retracts—'turtle' sign
- Failure of restitution of the fetal head
- Failure of the shoulders to descend into the pelvis
- Normal birth manoeuvres fail to birth the shoulders

Box 40.7 The HELPERR mnemonic (ALSO)

H Call for help
E Evaluate for episiotomy
L Legs (McRoberts manoeuvre)
P Suprapubic pressure (Rubin I)
E Enter manoeuvres (internal rotation)
R Remove the posterior arm
R Roll the woman on to all fours (Gaskin manoeuvre)

(Adapted from Gobbo, 2000)

In New Zealand, educators are now describing the set of shoulder dystocia manoeuvres as the three Ps (CDHB, 2021). The first P refers to the change of *position* for the woman to open the pelvis; the second P refers to *pressure* above the symphysis pubis to release the shoulders; and the third P is for *per vaginum*, which signals the need to commence internal manoeuvres.

Ansell et al. (2019) found that 46% of the shoulder dystocias in her study were resolved with a position change (McRoberts) and / or suprapubic pressure, whereas Michelotti et al. (2018) found that 77% of cases were resolved with McRoberts and suprapubic pressure alone.

Wherever the place of birth and whatever resources are available, it is vital that the midwife summons help and prepares to resuscitate the baby. In a hospital, additional midwives, an obstetrician, neonatologist or other clinicians available to resuscitate the baby should be called. Allocating someone to document times and the manoeuvres used is also important.

CLINICAL POINT

Whenever the normal events and progress of labour are disturbed by obstetric intervention—epidural block, induction of labour or interfering with the normal progress of the second stage of labour with forceps and vacuum extraction—think about the increased risk of shoulder dystocia. Following a shoulder dystocia the woman is at risk of a postpartum haemorrhage and the baby is at risk of asphyxia.

Emergency manoeuvres

Emergency manoeuvres for the management of shoulder dystocia are designed to increase the diameter of the pelvis and dislodge the shoulders. This is done by position, pressure or 'per vaginum' (internal manoeuvres).

Position. The midwife asks the woman to change her position to increase the functional size of the bony pelvis by flattening of the lumbar lordosis and cephalad rotation of the symphysis. This can be done by undertaking the McRoberts manoeuvre if the woman is semi-cumbent

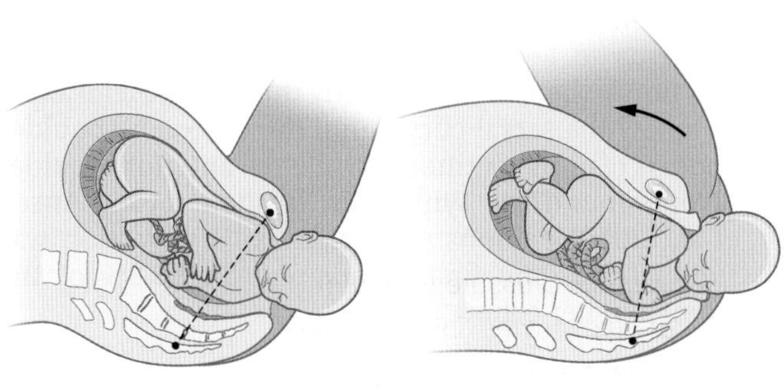

FIGURE 40.5 Shoulder dystocia: increasing the diameter of the pelvis
(Source: © Christy Krames 2020)

(Fig. 40.5), or asking the woman to adopt a deep hands and knees position, or a running start position—all of which will be dependent on the existing position of the woman and her level of mobility.

1. *McRoberts*—support the woman into a supine position, ensure she is completely flat and all the pillows have been removed from under her head or back. Removing or lowering the bottom of the bed and / or manipulating the woman's buttocks to the extreme edge of the bed provides more room for the internal manoeuvres. Two assistants hyperflex the woman's thighs against her abdomen (knees to nipples). This raises the symphysis pubis by about 9 mm and flattens out the lumbosacral spine, which may provide sufficient clearance to release the anterior shoulder from behind the symphysis. By flattening the lumbosacral spine, McRoberts positioning may also advance the posterior fetal shoulder into the hollow of the sacrum.
2. *Hands and knees (all fours) position*—an exaggerated knee-to-chest position can also be achieved by rolling the woman into an all-fours (reverse McRoberts) position. Both femora are abducted, rotated outwards and flexed, so that the thighs touch the woman's abdomen, with the aid of the two assistants. This allows the sacrum to rotate backwards. The midwife then applies gentle traction to the baby's head. Unfortunately for some women rolling over on to all fours may not be possible particularly if the woman has a deep epidural block. Rolling the woman to the all-fours position can often dislodge the posterior shoulder and this may be sufficient to dislodge the impaction. Rotation of the woman also facilitates birth by increasing the pelvic diameters and provides improved access to the posterior shoulder through the sacral hollow.
3. *The 'running start' position*—this is very useful if the woman is standing or on all fours during her birth. She lifts one leg and places her foot flat on the mattress (floor) where she is birthing. Her knee should be up near her ribs (almost to her arm pit). In the positioning of the leg, the knee isn't away from her body; it is important that the 'running start' leg does not swing out to one side but rather remains in alignment with the woman's torso. In other words, this is similar to a 'half-McRoberts manoeuvre'. For women in a birthing pool, standing and lifting a leg onto the side of the pool is similar to a half McRoberts.

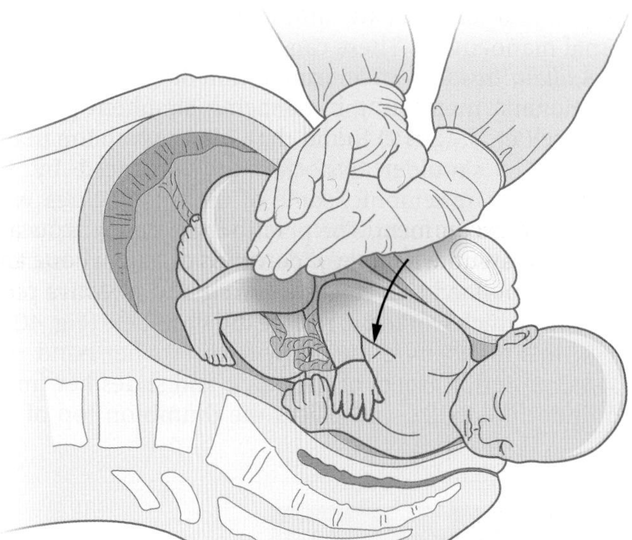

FIGURE 40.6 Suprapubic pressure on the posterior aspect of the impacted shoulder
(Source: © Christy Krames 2020)

Pressure. The midwife attempts to decrease the bisacromial diameter of the fetus (i.e. the breadth of the shoulders) of the fetus through application of suprapubic pressure on the posterior aspect of the impacted shoulder. This can only be done if the woman is in the McRoberts position.

Suprapubic pressure combined with the McRoberts manoeuvre improves success rates. This manoeuvre reduces the fetal bisacromial diameter and promotes rotation of the anterior fetal shoulder into the wider oblique pelvic diameter (Fig. 40.6). The shoulder is then freed to slip underneath the symphysis pubis with the aid of routine axial traction. An assistant applies continuous suprapubic pressure over the fetal anterior shoulder, in a cardiopulmonary resuscitation style with a downward and lateral motion on the posterior aspect of the anterior fetal shoulder to disimpact the shoulder. Suprapubic pressure helps to adduct the fetal shoulders—that is, decrease the bisacromial diameter. This manoeuvre should be attempted while continuing downward traction to birth the shoulders. If birth is unsuccessful, a rocking motion may be applied. Initially the procedure should be continuous for 30 seconds, followed by a rocking motion for another 30 seconds. If birth is still not possible, the internal manoeuvres should be attempted.

Per vaginum—commence internal manoeuvres. The midwife attempts to change the relationship of the bisacromial diameter within the bony pelvis through internal manoeuvres. These can be:

1. *Axillary traction*—in an exploration of five expert practitioners' methods for managing shoulder dystocia, Ansell et al. (2012) found that, although the management of shoulder dystocia was influenced by the HELPERR mnemonic, some of the manoeuvres were difficult to perform. The practitioners described using a manoeuvre which they identified as axillary traction and explained that it was a simple and effective technique which worked to release the shoulders (Fig. 40.7). In this manoeuvre the midwife inserts her hand into the posterior aspect of the pelvis and slides her finger under the axilla, and places the thumb on top of the shoulder. A second finger is placed alongside the fetal humerus to keep the arm against the baby's body. Traction is then applied directly through the fetal axilla to follow the sacral curve until the posterior shoulder appears over the perineum while the anterior shoulder pivots around the symphysis. In their review Ansell et al. (2012) demonstrated that axillary traction was successful as the first manoeuvre for 95.8% of the women in her cohort.

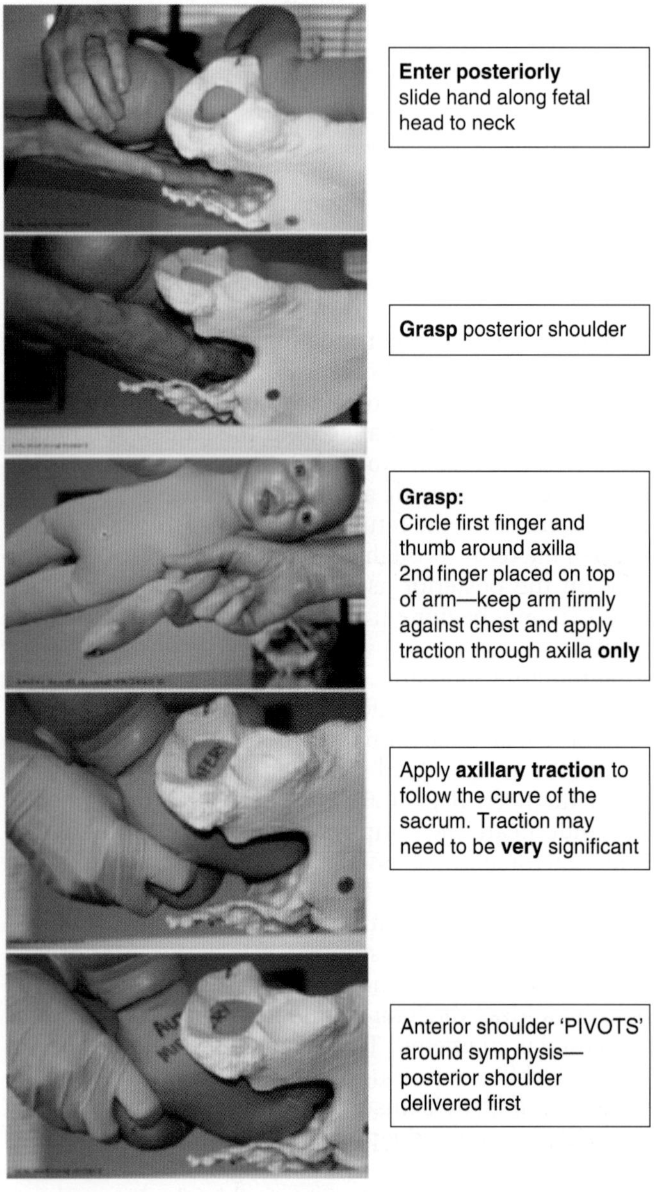

FIGURE 40.7 Axillary traction: an effective method of resolving shoulder dystocia
(Source: Ansell et al., 2019)

2. *Removal of the posterior arm*—freeing the posterior arm reduces the diameter of the fetal shoulders by the width of the arm. Removing the posterior arm from the birth canal (Fig. 40.8, Fig. 40.9) aims to shorten the bisacromial diameter, allowing the fetus to drop into the sacral hollow and freeing the impaction. If the woman is not in the all-fours position, it may be helpful to ask her to move into a McRoberts position before attempting to remove the posterior arm. Insert your hand into the sacral hollow to identify the posterior shoulder, and follow the arm down to the cubital fossa to grasp the fetal arm, and flex at the baby's elbow, encouraging the arm to sweep over the baby's chest and out ('cat lick' manoeuvre). Grasping and pulling directly on the fetal arm may fracture the humerus. Ansell et al. (2012) found that removing the posterior arm was successful as a first manoeuvre for 85.7% of the woman in her cohort, while Michelotti et al. (2018) found it was used successfully in 13% of their cohort.
3. *Other manoeuvres:*
   a. *Rubin II* (Fig. 40.8)—this manoeuvre attempts to provide internal adduction to the anterior fetal shoulder to encourage the fetus to rotate its anterior shoulder into an oblique plane and under the maternal symphysis. Two fingers are inserted posteriorly into the vagina behind the baby's back stretching the fingers up to reach the posterior aspect of the anterior shoulder and then rotating it in an anterior direction, attempting to push the shoulder towards the fetal chest, for another 30 seconds. Once the midwife sees the fetal shoulder move, traction can be applied to the fetal head to support birth of the shoulders.
   b. *'Wood screw' manoeuvre* (the only manoeuvre using two hands) (Fig. 40.8)—this involves another attempt to disimpact the anterior shoulder from under the symphysis pubis by still rotating the fetal shoulders into the oblique, so that the upper, impacted, shoulder will drop beneath the pubic arch. So, if the fetus is left occipitolateral (LOA; 'looking' towards the maternal right), the right, upper shoulder of the fetus is anterior, and is the impacted one. While maintaining pressure on the posterior aspect of the anterior shoulder, two fingers of the second hand are placed into the vagina and placed on the anterior aspect of the posterior shoulder. Both hands now apply pressure in an effort to rotate the posterior shoulder in the same direction as before. The midwife again attempts birth once the shoulders move into the oblique diameter. If this does not work, the midwife moves to the next manoeuvre.

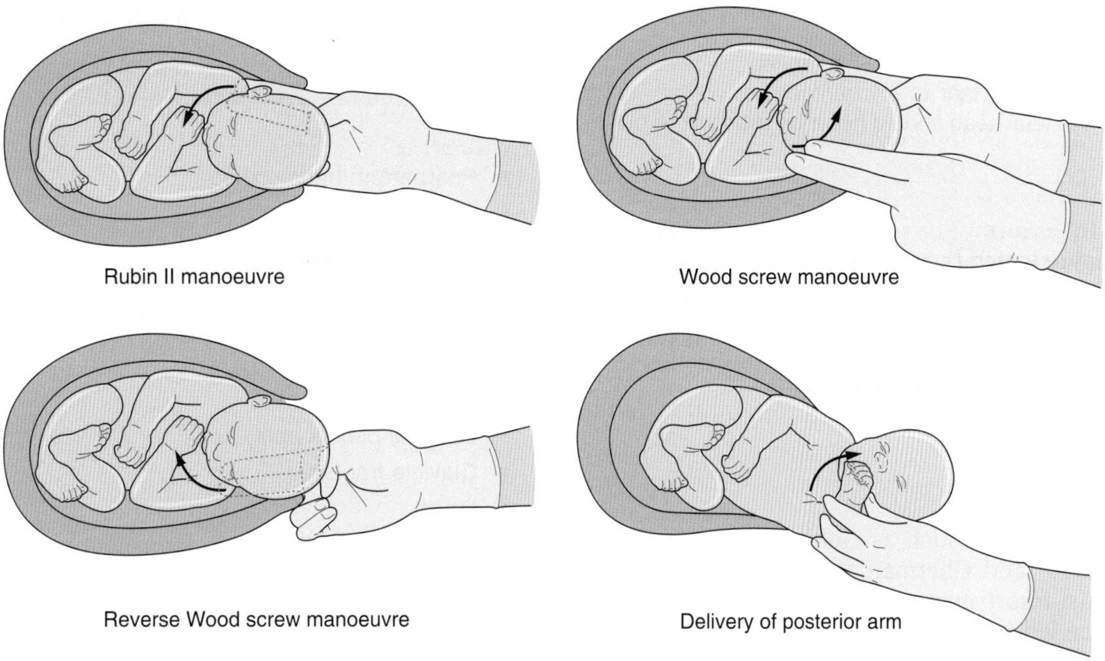

FIGURE 40.8 HELPERR manoeuvres for shoulder dystocia
(Based on Oats & Abraham, 2004)

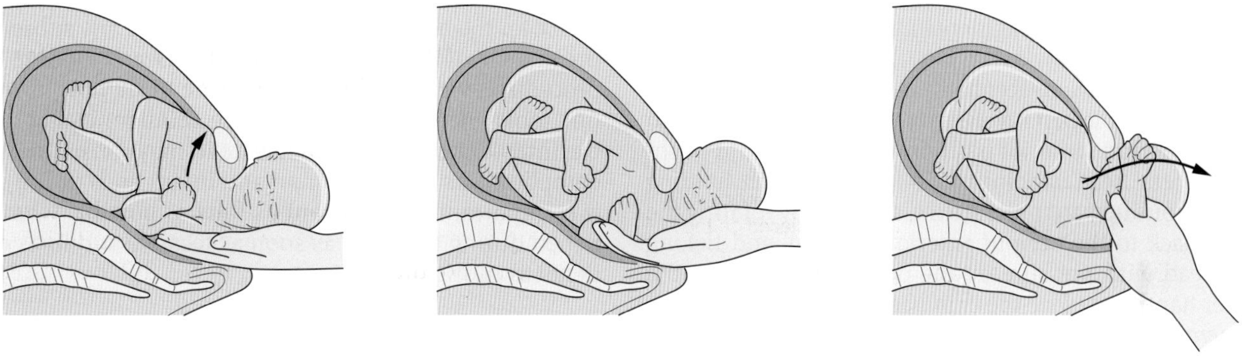

FIGURE 40.9 Shoulder dystocia: delivery of the posterior arm
(Based on Henderson & Macdonald, 2004)

c. *'Reverse Wood screw' manoeuvre*—the fingers on the posterior shoulder (Fig. 40.8) are removed from the vagina, and the two fingers on the anterior shoulder moved down and along the fetal back to the posterior aspect of the posterior shoulder. The midwife attempts to rotate the shoulder in the opposite direction to the wood screw manoeuvre for 30–60 seconds.

The HELPERR mnemonic

The HELPERR mnemonic was developed by Advanced Life Support in Obstetrics (ALSO, 2017). Each of the manoeuvres that comprise the HELPERR mnemonic focus on increasing the diameters of the maternal pelvis, decreasing the bisacromial diameter or rotating the fetal shoulders into a larger available pelvic diameter. There is no reason why the steps should be followed in order with the order of manoeuvres dependent on the woman's position—whether she is semirecumbent, on her side, on her hands and knees or in a birthing pool will often dictate the first manoeuvre that can be undertaken (Souter, 2002). Episiotomy should be considered, but only because it makes more room for the clinician to perform internal rotational manoeuvres. An episiotomy may also provide more room for birth of the posterior shoulder. Episiotomy can be more difficult to do once the baby's head has been born.

CLINICAL POINT

During all manoeuvres used when trying to release the shoulders it is important to encourage the woman not to push; also the fetal head should never be grasped or pulled.

Midwifery Practice Scenario

With colleagues and a torso and doll, practise using the various manoeuvres discussed during a 'mock' shoulder dystocia.

Manoeuvres of last resort

A number of authors, such as Gobbo & Baxley (2000), Sandberg (1999) and Gherman et al. (1997), describe a number of 'last-resort' manoeuvres. These are manoeuvres that would be led by a multidisciplinary team, although there is little or no evidence to support their use; they are briefly summarised below.

- *Deliberate clavicle fracture (surgical division of the clavicle or bending with a finger)*—the anterior clavicle is pressed against the ramus of the pubis. Theoretically, a fracture of the clavicle is less serious than a brachial nerve injury and often heals rapidly. The danger of this procedure is that bone fragments may pierce the underlying lung or the subclavian blood vessels.
- *Zavanelli manoeuvre*—cephalic replacement is followed by caesarean birth; it involves rotating the fetal head into a direct occiput anterior position, then flexing and pushing the fetal head back into the birth canal, while holding continuous upward pressure. This is done by rotating the head back to the occiput anterior position, and flexing the head with pressure on the occiput while using the other hand to replace the chin back into the vagina.
- *General anaesthesia*—musculoskeletal or uterine relaxation with a general anaesthetic may bring about enough uterine relaxation to effect the birth. Oral or intravenous nitroglycerine may be used as an alternative to general anaesthesia.
- *Symphysiotomy*—intentional division of the fibrous cartilage of the symphysis pubis under local anaesthesia is used more widely in developing than in developed countries. It should be used only when all other manoeuvres have failed and caesarean birth is unavailable. There is a high incidence of serious maternal morbidity and poor neonatal outcome.

Complications

The complications associated with shoulder dystocia are listed in Box 40.8.

Box 40.8 Complications of shoulder dystocia

Maternal

- Postpartum haemorrhage
- Rectovaginal fistula
- Symphyseal separation or diastasis, with or without transient femoral neuropathy
- Third- or fourth-degree episiotomy or tear
- Uterine rupture

Fetal

- Brachial plexus palsy
- Clavicle fracture
- Death
- Hypoxia, with or without permanent neurological damage
- Fracture of the humerus

Documentation

If there have been any manoeuvres necessary to support the birth of the shoulders, then it is important to document what was done to resolve the problem. Having accurate data supports midwives to continue to identify the incidence and success rates of the various manoeuvres used and to improve outcomes for women and their babies. Box 40.9 provides a guide to what should be documented during the emergency. These details can provide clear evidence for the planning and management of any subsequent pregnancies. Documentation should clearly outline what procedures were used to expedite the birth, how long each one took, and their effect. Because shoulder dystocia (and the interventions used to alleviate it) may cause significant complications for the woman and infant and/or litigation, it is important to document as fully as possible what happened during the birth as soon as feasible and in as much detail as possible.

Summary—shoulder dystocia

Sooner or later every midwife will be confronted with shoulder dystocia. The key to management is that the clinicians in the room work as a team, and proceed through a logical series of steps designed to disimpact the anterior shoulder from behind the symphysis pubis. It is important to explain the occurrence of dystocia to the parents of the infant, offer debriefing and ongoing counselling.

CRITICAL THINKING EXERCISE

Shoulder dystocia

1. Is shoulder dystocia predictable?
2. Can shoulder dystocia be prevented?
3. What manoeuvres can be performed?
4. What are the sequelae of shoulder dystocia for woman and baby?

Box 40.9 Documentation of shoulder dystocia

Note and document the following:

- The time of birth of the head
- The direction the head is facing after restitution
- The manoeuvres performed, their timing and sequence—the HELPERR mnemonic is very useful
- Approximate length of time each manoeuvre was tried
- Duration of attempts to resolve the dystocia
- The time of delivery of the body
- The staff in attendance and the time they arrived
- The condition of the baby and resuscitative measures
- The baby's weight
- Debriefing and counselling for the woman and her caregivers

Outcomes

Fetal

- The condition of the baby (Apgar score)—especially if the Apgar score is less than 7 at 5 minutes
- Response to neonatal resuscitation
- Evidence of:
  - asphyxia
  - meconium aspiration—hypoxic–ischaemic encephalopathy
- Umbilical cord blood acid–base measurements
- Newborn birth injuries, including brachial plexus injuries, clavicular and humeral fractures

Maternal

After the shoulder dystocia has been resolved, assess and document:

- Postpartum blood loss/haemorrhage
- Any soft tissue damage—cervix and vagina
- Any trauma resulting from application of manoeuvres, including:
  - symphyseal separation and sacroiliac dislocation—episiotomy and/or laceration (degree)
  - pain/discomfort
  - any uterine rupture
  - any bladder trauma/haematuria
- Psychological outcomes (including postnatal depression)

If both woman and baby are well they may need additional support to ensure optimal woman–baby connection and interaction.

MATERNAL LIFE-THREATENING CONDITIONS

This section identifies life-threatening conditions that primarily effect maternal health; but if the emergency occurs during pregnancy, it is also likely to impact fetal health.

Major postpartum haemorrhage

Across the world, **postpartum haemorrhage** (PPH) is one of the leading causes of maternal mortality. It remains a major cause of maternal mortality and morbidity within Australia and New Zealand, with early recognition and action essential to ensure effective treatment (Ministry of Health (MOH), 2022). Postpartum haemorrhage is defined as a blood loss of 500 mL or more following birth or any amount where the woman shows signs of compromise. In New Zealand it is further defined as blood loss of more than a 1000 mL following a caesarean section (MOH, 2022). The timing of the haemorrhage will determine whether it is a primary or secondary PPH (Box 40.10). Secondary PPH is discussed more fully in Chapter 41. Haemorrhage is further defined as moderate and severe.

REFLECTIVE THINKING EXERCISE

Visual estimation of blood loss at childbirth is difficult because the blood mixes with amniotic fluid and urine. Trends of overestimating blood loss at the lower levels and underestimating blood loss at higher loss levels have been identified (Cheerranichanunth & Poolnoi, 2012). Methods to improve blood loss identification have included weighing pads and sheets and improving clinicians' skills in estimation through workshops; however, skill decay is experienced within 9 months of training completion (Toledo et al., 2012). Blood loss estimation is an unreliable tool because of this inaccuracy.

- What other tools could be used when seeking to identify unusual blood loss that requires further action?
- Consider how you would identify ongoing insidious blood loss.

Box 40.10 Definitions of PPH

- A primary PPH—within the first 24 hours following the birth
- A secondary (late) PPH—from 24 hours to the first 6 weeks after birth

Blood loss volumes:

- PPH is a blood loss of >500 mL
- moderate >1001–2000 mL
- severe > 2000 mL

CLINICAL POINT

Although most PPH occurs immediately at the time of birth, some women can have ongoing insidious bleeding for several hours following the birth. For some women a slow, steady blood loss occurs over some hours after the birth until their blood loss becomes problematic (Centre for Maternal and Child Enquiries (CMACE), 2011). Given the relative hypervolaemia of pregnancy, the clinical signs of haemorrhage and shock such as hypotension, tachycardia and oliguria may not appear until the woman has lost over 1500 mL—that is, just before she becomes haemodynamically unstable.

Incidence

The incidence of PPH is reported as between 5% and 15% of all births, but severe or life-threatening PPH is estimated to occur in 3.7 per 1000 pregnancies (Dahlke et al., 2015). Life-threatening PPH is defined by RCOG (Ford et al., 2015) as:

- estimated blood loss of more than 2.5 litres
- treatment with 5 or more units of blood products
- treatment for coagulopathy.

It is now recognised that saturation of the oxytocin receptors and subsequent desensitisation may occur for women who have their labour induced or augmented and this may be dose dependent. In a review of 31,837 vaginal births in a Danish hospital, Graugaard & Maimburg (2021) found that 5.7% experienced a severe PPH (>1000 mL). Induction of labour, augmentation of labour, irregular fetal position, maternal age >40, instrumental birth and infant birthweight >4000g were risk factors for severe PPH. For women with vaginal tears a vaginal tear of >3 cm also increased the risk of severe PPH. Other risk factors for PPH are outlined in Box 40.11.

Box 40.11 Risk factors for postpartum haemorrhage

Risk factors for primary postpartum haemorrhage are:

- antepartum haemorrhage (especially placental abruption and placenta praevia)
- postpartum haemorrhage during a previous birth
- known placenta accreta (associated with catastrophic haemorrhage)
- multiple pregnancy
- coagulopathies
- anaemia
- preeclampsia
- fetal macrosomia
- obesity (BMI >35)
- elective or previous lower segment caesarean section
- induction/augmentation of labour (Balki et al., 2016; Grotegut et al., 2011)
- prolonged labour (second stage in particular)
- episiotomy
- retained placenta (RCOG, 2016).

Treatment of PPH

In New Zealand a National Consensus Guideline and treatment flow chart provide guidance on the principles for early identification and treatment of PPH (MOH, 2022). These principles include:

- Call for additional help.
- Measure, assess and arrest the bleeding.
- Resuscitation—minimise the impact of blood loss.
- Maternal observations and clinical assessments to ensure response to treatment.

Documentation of the blood loss and treatment provided and early and ongoing communication with the woman and her family and other health professionals is essential.

Action should be undertaken as soon as an abnormal blood loss is suspected—which may be before the woman has lost more than 500 mL of blood. Although the presentation of PPH is most often dramatic, bleeding may be slower but can still ultimately result in critical loss and shock (Table 40.2). This is more likely to be true of bleeding secondary to retained tissue or trauma. Hancock et al. (2021) found that reaction to blood loss was often intuitive when the bleeding was fast and with visible blood flow but slower bleeding was less clearly recognised. In their simulations they found that clinicians would often initiate treatment with blood volumes of less than 200 mL when the loss was fast and heavy, but fewer treated slower blood loss despite a similar blood loss volume.

Table 40.2 Blood loss and clinical signs and symptoms

Blood volume loss	Blood pressure (systolic)	Symptoms and signs	Degree of shock
500–1000 mL (10%–15%)	Normal	Palpitations, tachycardia, dizziness	Compensated
1000–1500 mL (15%–25%)	Slight fall (80–100 mmHg)	Weakness, tachycardia, sweating	Mild
1500–2000 mL (25%–35%)	Moderate fall (70–80 mmHg)	Restlessness, pallor, oliguria	Moderate
2000–3000 mL (35%–50%)	Marked fall (50–70 mmHg)	Collapse, air hunger, anuria	Severe

(Adapted from American Congress of Obstetricians and Gynecologists (ACOG). ACOG Practice Bulletin Number 76. Postpartum Hemorrhage. *Obstet Gynecol.* 2006a;108(4):1039–1048)

Table 40.3 The four Ts of postpartum haemorrhage

	Frequency (%)	Causes	Risk factors
Tone	80	Uterine atony—uterus does not contract fully or maintain contraction	Fetal macrosomia, polyhydramnios, multiple pregnancy, fetal abnormality, uterine abnormality, prolonged labour, rapid forceful labour, use of drugs that inhibit contractions, placenta implantation site in lower uterine segment , bacterial toxins, hypoxia, hypothermia
Trauma	10	Vaginal or cervical lacerations, haematoma or uterine rupture	Uterine inversion, caesarean section (prolonged labour)
Tissue	9	Retained products of conception (placenta, membranes)	Succenturiate or additional lobe, pre-term birth, placenta praevia, placenta accreta
Thrombin/ thrombus	1	Coagulation disorders	Pre-existing (familial) or acquired (DIC) HELLP syndrome, sepsis, amniotic fluid embolism

DIC = disseminated intravascular coagulopathy; HELLP = Haemolysis, Elevated Liver enzymes, Low Platelet count.
(Adapted from Anderson J, Etches DJ. Postpartum haemorrhage: third stage emergency. In: Damos JD, Eisinger SH, Baxley EG, eds. *Advanced Life Support in Obstetrics Course Syllabus*. 4th ed. Leawood, Kan: American Academy of Family Physicians; 2008)

The four Ts

In order to treat PPH effectively it is important to identify and treat the underlying cause of bleeding. As a way of remembering the causes of PPH, several sources have suggested using the 'four Ts' as a mnemonic: tone, trauma, tissue and thrombin (Society of Obstetrics and Gynecology of Canada (SOGC), 2008) (Table 40.3).

Uterine atony (first T—tone). The vast majority of PPHs are caused by uterine atony, so the midwife's first action is to check the tone and position of the uterus and, if necessary, massage it or 'rub up the fundus' to promote uterine contractions and control of bleeding. An empty and contracted uterus will not bleed (except where coagulopathy occurs). The finding of a 'boggy' uterus indicates that it is not well contracted and the blood vessels or 'living ligatures' are not compressed, resulting in excessive postpartum bleeding. The midwife's first action is to massage or 'rub up the fundus' until it is firm and contracted and pooled blood or clots are expelled. A uterus that is not centrally located suggests that a full bladder has pushed it to one side. If the woman continues to bleed vaginally even though the uterus is contracted and centrally located, the cause of the haemorrhage is due to one of the other factors—trauma, retained placental fragments or coagulopathy.

Genital trauma (second T—trauma). Genital tract trauma is the most likely cause of PPH when the fundus is well contracted. Table 40.4 outlines treatment for genital trauma.

Tissue—retained placenta and membranes (third T—tissue). Retained placental fragments are a common cause of primary PPH and the most frequent cause of late haemorrhage (Dossou et al., 2015). Retention of fragments is usually caused by partial separation of the placenta during massage of the uterine fundus prior to

Table 40.4 Genital trauma

Clinical aspects	Practice points
Condition stable	• Attempt clamping of obvious arterial bleeding prior to repair • Position woman to maximise visualisation and maternal comfort • Repair—ensuring bleeding at the apex of the laceration is secured

Condition compromised	• Treat shock:
	  • Apply pressure on the wound or bimanual compression
	  • Assess analgesia requirements
	  • Urgently transfer to OT for repair under anaesthetic

Suboptimal wound visualisation	• Transfer to OT
	• Maximise lighting and position in lithotomy
	• Under anaesthetic:
	  • Apply retractors to optimise visualisation, utilise assistants
	  • Check uterine cavity is empty and uterus is intact

Anaesthetic ineffective	• Assess rate of bleeding and weigh options of:
	  • Top up local or regional anaesthetic
	  • Transfer to OT for general anaesthetic

Puerperal haematoma	• Large non-haemostatic haematoma:
	  • Treat shock
	  • Transfer to OT for evacuation and repair

OT = operating theatre.

spontaneous placental separation. Following birth, the placenta and membranes should always be checked for completeness. The midwife should always look on the maternal side of the placenta for missing placental fragments or cotyledons. On the fetal side, blood vessels that traverse the edge of the placenta and then outwards into the membranes are suggestive of a succenturiate lobe.

Coagulopathies (fourth T—thrombin). Coagulopathy is the condition in which the ability of blood to clot is impaired. It can occur due to pre-eclampsia and thrombocytopenia (low levels of platelets) and following placental abruption and amniotic fluid embolism. Dilutional coagulopathy can also happen following blood loss replacement with crystalloid and colloid infusion.

Clinical signs include (Burtelow et al., 2007):

- blood that no longer clots
- oozing from puncture / cannulation / injection sites or surgical field
- haematuria
- petechial, subconjunctival and mucosal haemorrhage
- uterine atony secondary to increased fibrin degradation products.

If clinical signs are present, clinicians should not wait for blood results to begin treatment (Burtelow et al., 2007).

Initial early recognition and action for PPH

Abnormal bleeding can occur within any setting (home, birthing unit or obstetric hospital). The midwife is the first responder and will need to do the following (Box 40.12):

1. Call for help (more hands are needed to treat the blood loss and stabilise the woman).
2. Consider the cause of the bleeding (tone, trauma, tissue, thrombin).
3. Assess and arrest the bleeding (massage the uterus, administer uterotonics, empty bladder).
4. Minimise the impact of the blood loss (gain IV access and start rapid IV fluid replacement, take blood for group and hold, coagulation and blood count, give oxygen). Undertake observations and continue full clinical assessment (BP, pulse, respiratory rate, temperature, cumulative blood loss, fluid input).
5. If the blood loss exceeds 500 mL, Tranexamic acid treatment should be considered.

If the bleeding continues and is significant, it is important to escalate care and involve the senior obstetric team response (MOH, 2022).

If the PPH occurs at home or in a primary (midwife-led) unit, follow above actions but in addition organise transfer to secondary / tertiary obstetric service and:

- commence IV oxytocin infusion of 40 units in sodium chloride 0.9% 500 mL over four hours

Box 40.12 Initial early recognition and action of PPH

Call for help

- Allocate roles.

Assess and arrest bleeding

- Lie the woman flat.
- Deliver the placenta.
- Massage the uterus and expel clots.
- Place baby skin to skin (to support maternal oxytocin release).
- Administer uterotonics:
    - Syntocinon 10 IU IM or 5 IU IV or Syntometrine 1 mL IM (total dose should not exceed 3mL in 24 hours)
- Empty bladder (catheter).
- Measure cumulative blood loss and assess woman's condition.

Identify cause

- Consider the four Ts and treat depending on cause.

Minimise impact of blood loss

- Insert large-bore IV cannula (16 G or 18 G).
- Take blood for full blood count, group and hold, coagulation.
- Consult with obstetrician (regarding emergency transfer if at home or in midwifery-led unit).
- Start rapid IV fluid replacement with crystalloids (sodium chloride 0.9% or Hartmann's solution).
- Consider tranexamic acid (1 g/10 mL IV at 1 mL per minute).

Maternal observations and clinical assessment

- Use Maternal Early Warning System (MEWS) to assess and document: blood pressure, pulse, respiratory rate, temperature, cumulative blood loss and fluid balance.

If the blood loss stops and the woman's condition is stable:

- Continue observations and clinical assessments using MEWS.
- Document plan for ongoing care (including care location).
- Ensure adequate level of observation by health practitioner or partner or whānau with access to health practitioner or emergency services.
- Watch for further blood loss.
- Check haemoglobin via FBC.
- After the event, consider a culturally safe opportunity to discuss, reflect and debrief.

(Source: MOH, 2021)

- reconsider the four Ts to identify and ensure treatment is effective
- apply bimanual compression to arrest blood loss (see Fig. 40.10)
- consult with obstetric team and ensure senior obstetric and midwifery team are present on arrival at hospital.

If the blood loss stops at this time and the woman's condition is stabilised, she will need to have continued observation and clinical assessment along with consideration of best place for ongoing care, observation of further blood loss and a haemoglobin check.

Ongoing significant bleeding

If significant ongoing bleeding continues the midwife will work as part of the team and continue with the principles outlined above along with additional treatment as outlined in Box 40.13.

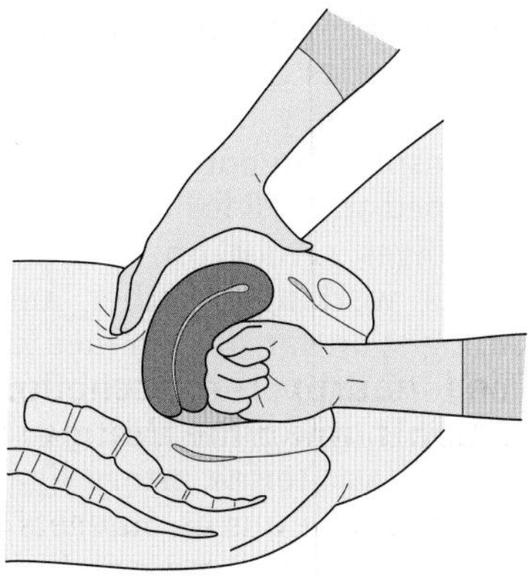

FIGURE 40.10 Bimanual compression
(Adapted from Anderson J, Etches D, Smith D. Postpartum hemorrhage. In: Baxley E. *Advanced Life Support in Obstetrics* course syllabus. 4th ed. Leawood, Kan.: American Academy of Family Physicians; 2001)

Box 40.13 Ongoing significant bleeding

- If birth at home or birthing unit—don't delay—transfer to secondary/tertiary obstetric service.
- Allocate care of baby to suitable person and ensure that partner and whānau are supported.
- Commence oxytocin infusion (40 units in sodium chloride 0.9% 500 mL over 4 hours).
- Reconsider the four Ts and apply bimanual compression to arrest blood loss.
- Request senior obstetric and midwifery team to attend immediately or be immediately available on arrival if transfer to a secondary/tertiary obstetric service.

Call for additional support

- Consult with obstetric team and anaesthetist.
- Prepare theatre team.
- Inform laboratory of major PPH.
- Send blood to lab on arrival: FBC, cross-match, APTT and fibrinogen.
- Point of care testing of haemoglobin and coagulation, where available.
- Request blood for transfusion.

Assess and arrest bleeding

- Reconsider the four Ts.
- Measure cumulative blood loss and assess woman's condition.
- Insert second large IV cannula (16 G or 18 G).
- Massage fundus, expel clots, consider bimanual compression.
- Insert indwelling catheter.
- Administer syntometrine 1ml IM if not already given
- Consider tranexamic acid (1g/10mL IV at 1mL per minute) if ongoing bleeding after 30 minutes and if has not already been administered.
- Administer carboprost 250 µg IM or intrauterine every 15 minutes (maximum of 8 doses)
- Consider examination under anaesthesia for:
  - removal of retained placenta
  - repair of tears
  - intrauterine balloon packing.

Resuscitation

- Give crystalloids (maximum 2–3 L).
- Give red cell transfusion as soon as possible (may require O-negative until type specific blood is available).

Maternal observations and clinical assessment

- Use MEWS to assess and document blood pressure, pulse, respiratory rate, temperature, cumulative blood loss, fluid balance.

If the blood loss stops and the woman's condition is stable then:

- Continue observations and clinical assessment.
- Document plan for ongoing care.
- Ensure one-to-one midwifery care is provided.
- Observe for further blood loss.
- Check haemoglobin via full blood count.
- Consider IV iron replacement promptly applying a low threshold for prescribing.
- After the event arrange a culturally safe opportunity to discuss, reflect and debrief.

(Source: MOH, 2022)

Ongoing uncontrolled bleeding

If the bleeding continues and is uncontrolled then the massive transfusion policy (MTP) should be triggered. The majority of hospitals in both New Zealand and Australia have developed an MTP for maternity units.

The MTP involves senior obstetricians, midwives and anaesthetists working together and consulting with a haematologist or transfusion medicine specialist to correct blood loss, support resuscitation and correct coagulopathy. At this time other treatment options will be considered such as uterine artery ligation, uterine balloon or packing of the uterus, internal iliac embolisation, aortic compression or hysterectomy. Box 40.14 provides an overview of medical management of ongoing uncontrolled bleeding. The woman will need to be transferred to theatre for ongoing management of bleeding, resuscitation and treatment until the woman's condition is stable. It is important to keep the woman and her family fully informed of the situation at all times.

Tranexamic acid

There is now high-quality evidence on the effectiveness of tranexamic acid for reducing mortality from PPH with no major adverse effect. A large randomised controlled trial involving 20,060 women who had a PPH in 193 hospitals from 21 countries explored whether early administration of tranexamic acid (TXA) had an effect on maternal death and/or hysterectomy in women with PPH (Shakur et al., 2017). Subsequent trials and meta-analysis have confirmed that TXA increases overall survival from bleeding, with earlier administration (within 15 minutes of the bleeding) associated with improved outcomes for mortality and hysterectomy (Della Corte et al., 2020; Gayet-Ageron, 2018). Administration of tranexamic acid reduces bleeding by inhibiting the enzymatic breakdown of fibrinogen and fibrin by plasmin. Morbidity is significantly reduced in women given tranexamic acid, if given within 3 hours of the blood loss. The World Health Organization recommends the early use (within 3 hours of birth) of intravenous tranexamic acid in addition to standard care for women with clinically diagnosed postpartum haemorrhage following a vaginal or caesarean birth (WHO, 2017).

Many of the interventions described for ongoing life-threatening PPH may not be within the scope of midwifery practice but it is important that midwives know about them so that when they are confronted with intractable haemorrhage they can support other members of the medical team. When administering any medications,

Box 40.14 Ongoing uncontrolled bleeding

Call for additional support

- Transfer clinical responsibility for care to senior obstetrician and senior anaesthetist.
- Consult with haematologist/transfusion medicine specialist.
- Transfer to operating theatre.
- Ensure that partner and whānau are supported.

Assess and arrest bleeding

- Reconsider the four Ts and AFE.
- Consider other options if appropriate:
  - uterine compression suture (+/- tamponade balloon/packing)
  - uterine artery ligation
  - internal iliac embolisation
  - aortic compression
- Consider laparotomy.
- Consider early recourse to hysterectomy.

Resuscitation

- Initiate massive transfusion protocol where available.
- Assess coagulation status including fibrinogen.
- Administer blood and blood products guided by laboratory and point of care tests of haemoglobin and coagulation (aim for APTT <40s, PR <1.5, platelets >75x109/L, fibrinogen >2 g/L).
- Avoid hypothermia, hypocalcaemia and acidosis by keeping patient warm and warming all fluids and blood products (if warming facilities are available).
- Consider cell salvage.

Maternal observations and clinical assessments

- Consider arterial line or central venous line.
- Use MEWS to assess and document blood pressure, pulse, respiratory rate, temperature, oxygen saturation:
  - document cumulative blood loss and accurate fluid balance (hourly urine output)
  - FBC and coagulation studies at least hourly until blood loss stops.

Blood loss stops and the woman's condition is stable

- Make plan for ongoing care.
- Consider transfer to Intensive Care Unit, High Dependency Unit or Acute Observation Unit.
- Consider IV iron replacement promptly, applying a low threshold for prescribing.
- After the event, ensure that a culturally safe opportunity to discuss, reflect and debrief occurs.

(Source: MOH, 2022)

midwives need to understand the mechanism of action, the correct dose and route of administration, the length of time until effectiveness, the side effects and reactions with other drugs before they administer them.

Haemorrhagic shock

Haemorrhagic shock can result in a combination of anaemic and ischaemic tissue hypoxia (Rajan & Wing, 2010). Tissue hypoxia causes a progressive failure of cellular metabolism. Compensatory mechanisms and different oxygen requirements in various tissue beds cause a range of complications. These include organ damage, which may result in early or late multiorgan dysfunction and death. Haemorrhagic shock may coexist with other types of shock, such as following trauma or septic shock (most often from wound contamination or genital infection). Clinically hypovolaemic shock is classified as mild, moderate or severe depending on the blood volume loss (Rajan & Wing, 2010). In mild or uncompensated shock less than 20% of blood volume is lost. Vasoconstriction begins and redistribution of blood flow is shunted to vital organs. In moderate shock 20%–40% of the blood volume is lost and there is decreased perfusion of organs such as kidneys, spleen and pancreas. In severe shock the woman loses more than 40% of her blood volume; there is decreased perfusion of the brain and heart. Hypovolaemic shock produces compensatory physiological responses in almost all organ systems.

Secondary postpartum haemorrhage

Secondary postpartum haemorrhage is defined as excessive blood loss from the genital tract occurring more than 24 hours and up to 6 weeks after birth (see also Ch. 41). Secondary PPH is a clinical diagnosis of exclusion, which may present as slight to heavy bleeding (rarely catastrophic haemorrhage and hypovolaemic shock) usually 7–14 days after birth (Ambrose & Repke, 2011). Women who have had a primary PPH are seven times more likely to have a secondary PPH (Humphrey, 2005) (Box 40.15). In addition, women who have had a manual removal of their placenta are four times more likely to have a secondary PPH (Humphrey, 2005).

Box 40.15 Risk factors for secondary postpartum haemorrhage

- Primary postpartum haemorrhage
- Active management of the third stage
- Prolonged third stage
- Actual or suspected incomplete third stage
- Subinvolution of the placental site
- Retained products of conception
- Placenta accreta
- Pre-term birth and low-birth-weight fetus
- Not breastfeeding
- Maternal smoking
- Genital infection, endometritis, myometritis, parametritis, dehiscence of caesarean scar
- Trauma

(Based on MOH, 2013)

Placenta accreta spectrum

During pregnancy the placenta attaches to the uterine wall. Placenta accreta spectrum is a pathological condition involving abnormal attachment of the placenta. It is characterised by adherence of or invasion of the trophoblast into the myometrium (Jauniaux et al., 2019). **Placenta accreta** spectrum is rare with rates ranging between 0.01 to 1.1%, although accurate estimation of the incidence and prevalence is limited by the differing clinical criteria used to define the condition and a lack of detailed pathological examination (Jauniaux et al., 2019).

- Placenta accreta occurs when the trophoblastic villi are superficially attached to the myometrium (You & Zahn, 2006). This is the most common form, accounting for approximately 75% of all cases.
- Placenta increta occurs when the villi invade the myometrium. Thus the chorionic villi penetrate into the uterine muscle. This accounts for approximately 15% of all cases.
- Placenta percreta occurs when there is full penetration through the myometrial wall with possible invasion into the adjacent structures such as the bladder. This is the least common of the three conditions, accounting for approximately 5% of all cases (Eller et al., 2011).

Both adherent and invasive types of the condition result in parts of, or the whole placenta being unable to separate spontaneously from the uterine wall following birth. There is a strong association between caesarean section and the incidence of accreta placentation (Keag et al., 2018). Other risk factors for the various forms of placenta accreta include (Aiken et al., 2011):

- placenta praevia with or without previous uterine surgery
- prior myomectomy
- prior caesarean delivery—two or more
- Asherman syndrome
- submucous leiomyomata
- maternal age older than 35 years
- multiparity—gravida four or more births.

Profuse and life-threatening haemorrhage can occur when attempting to separate the placenta. Caesarean section and access to specialist centres with access to blood products and an intensive care unit are essential. The safest treatment in this circumstance is prompt hysterectomy.

Women who decline blood products

Most women faced with an objective, informed and clear explanation of the need to use blood products in the advent of massive obstetric haemorrhage will consent to their use as a life-saving measure. Others do not consent to blood transfusions because of religious, personal or cultural beliefs. The right to refuse medical treatment is a requirement of the Code of Health and Disability Consumers Rights in New Zealand.

Each hospital/health service provider should have policies and protocols to guide care providers when developing appropriate plans of care if women refuse all or some blood products. Consideration will need to be given to discussing ways of remedying anaemia or other risk factors for PPH. In addition the clinician will need to consider and discuss the woman's wishes in relation to all aspects of labour and birth. During labour, other clinicians involved (obstetrician and anaesthetist) will need to be informed of the woman's wishes in relation to blood products. In the event of haemorrhage, the focus should be on pharmacological interventions such as the administration of vitamin K, tranexamic acid and early surgical intervention, as well as further discussion with the woman and her family if there is a medical indication for blood transfusion. The woman's right to decline treatment should always be respected and the midwife should provide care within professional standards.

Postnatal considerations following PPH

After any PPH the woman should be monitored carefully for 24–48 hours. Table 40.5 provides an overview of essential postpartum care. Regular assessment of the woman's hemodynamic status is necessary. A urinary indwelling catheter is usually left in situ to promote adequate drainage of the bladder and to further aid uterine contractions, as well as to provide a means to accurately measure and document urinary output. Women who have experienced an obstetric haemorrhage are predisposed to renal tubular necrosis and may become anuric. Following a PPH the woman is at increased risk of infection and lactation may be delayed.

It is important to discuss the events with the woman and her support people so that they can understand what has occurred and ask questions. Postpartum haemorrhage has been associated with a high incidence of post-traumatic stress disorder (PTSD) related symptoms for the woman and her partner (Ricborg et al., 2015).

Following life-threatening PPH, any subsequent pregnancies will require specialist care and counselling to prevent/manage recurrence. Women who survive PPH are more likely to suffer from long-term anaemia and other complications. Because their health is already compromised, such women often need blood transfusions but are susceptible to the associated risks of transfusion reactions or infection with HIV or hepatitis.

Uterine inversion

Uterine inversion is a rare but potentially life-threatening complication of childbirth (Fig. 40.11). It is defined as the folding of the fundus into the uterine cavity in varying degrees, turning the uterus partially or completely inside out. Uterine inversion may occur with the third stage of labour or, less frequently, postpartum. Women's survival rate is about 85% (Belfort & Dildy, 2011). The most frequent cause of death is intractable haemorrhage and associated shock. These complications are minimised by prevention, prompt recognition and management.

Incidence

The incidence of uterine inversion varies owing to its rarity. In their review of 2427 cases in the USA between 2004 and 2013, Coad et al. (2017) found an incidence of 2.9 per 10,000 births.

Pathophysiology

For uterine inversion to occur, relaxation of the lower uterine segment must combine with the simultaneous downward movement of the uterine fundus. A portion of the uterine wall either indents towards or prolapses through the dilated cervix. Thus a patulous cervix, uterine relaxation (uterine atony) combined with simultaneous downward fundal pressure (Credé's manoeuvre), and/or with additional traction applied to the umbilical cord before the placenta has separated from the uterine wall, causes the fundus of the uterus to prolapse. Encouraging the woman to push to help expel the unseparated placenta increases the risk of uterine inversion. There are case reports of uterine inversions occurring without cord traction even during caesarean birth, via the myometrial incision after the neonate is born but before the placenta is delivered.

Associated factors

According to Varney (2004), there are a number of other reported associations (not causations) with uterine inversion. Inversion is so infrequent that a number of otherwise common factors must act in concert to result in an inversion.

These factors include:

- a short umbilical cord
- multiparity
- sudden increase in abdominal pressure, as in coughing
- placenta accreta/increta/percreta
- fundal implantation of the placenta
- chronic endometritis
- fetal macrosomia
- use of magnesium sulfate
- 'trials' of vaginal birth following caesarean section
- myometrial weakness/uterine sacculation
- congenital abnormalities of the uterus
- precipitate labour
- tocolysis with nitroglycerine or other potent agents.

Most frequent precipitating causes during the third stage

Premature or excessive cord traction during active management of the third stage (Mirza & Gaddipati, 2009) and/or a combination of fundal pressure and cord traction to deliver the placenta, or the use of fundal pressure when the uterus is atonic during placental delivery, often precipitates the inversion.

Table 40.5 Postnatal care following postpartum haemorrhage

Clinical aspects	Good practice points
Interhospital transfer	• Transfer to high-dependency/intensive care unit for observation

Monitoring: haemodynamic state	• If condition not critical:
	  • Observe in birth suite for 2 hours—once stable transfer to postnatal area
	  • First 24 hours post birth—monitor vital signs, uterine tone and blood loss at least 4-hourly
	  • After 24 hours post birth—monitor as per clinical condition

Haemoglobin (Hb)	• Take 6 hours after stabilisation—repeat within 24 hours of birth • If Hb <70 g/L and/or the woman is symptomatic: offer evidence-based information about RBC transfusion • If refusal on basis of beliefs: consider IV iron therapy • If Hb <70 g/L and asymptomatic: commence iron therapy with vitamin C supplement • Provide information on ways to increase dietary iron and consultation with dietitian • Inform woman when discharging home that iron tablets need to be kept out of the reach of infants and young children • If Hb <70–80 g/L in the postnatal period and where there is no continuing or threat of bleeding, the decision to transfuse should be made on an informed individual basis
Venous thromboembolism (VTE)	• Increased risk after PPH—consider offering pharmacological VTE prophylaxis to postnatal women who have had excess blood loss or blood transfusion (refer to Ch. 37) • If spinal/epidural catheter is still in situ: apply sequential compression device • After removal—proceed to graduated elastic compression stockings and/or pharmaceutical prophylaxis • Encourage early mobilisation, rest and avoid dehydration • Observe for signs of deep vein thrombosis and pulmonary embolism
Parenting	• Support maternal and infant bonding • Facilitate regular skin-to-skin contact under direct supervision • Support breastfeeding—offer midwifery/lactation consultant assistance • If unable to lactate or persistent hypotension consider Sheehan's syndrome • Discuss risks and advise against co-sleeping and bed sharing given possible fatigue associated with anaemia

Preparation for discharge	• Offer social worker/psychologist review and ongoing support services
	• Offer woman and family clinical disclosure/debriefing with senior clinician, preferably present at time of the event
	• Educate woman about signs, symptoms and self-referral to midwife and general practitioner (GP) for:
	  • infection—risk of secondary PPH
	  • warning signs of secondary PPH, infection, etc.
	  • PND—risk associated with anaemia
	  • risks of post-traumatic stress syndrome
	  • VTE—risk associated with PPH
	• Encourage follow-up with midwife and GP (e.g. monitor Hb, lactation, mental health, parenting skills, maternal/infant attachment)
	• Complete discharge summary
	• Referral to appropriate, local child health services for lactation support and close follow-up in view of anaemia and PND risk
	• Offer advice regarding maintaining bowel functions if using iron supplements and if woman has had perineal repair or evacuation of haematoma
	• Inform woman of increased risk of PPH in subsequent pregnancies and the need to inform future maternity care providers of PPH complication

PND = postnatal depression; PPH = postpartum haemorrhage; RBC = red blood cells; VTE = venous thromboembolism.
(Adapted from Aiken et al., 2011; Anderson & Etchens, 2008; RCOG, 2011)

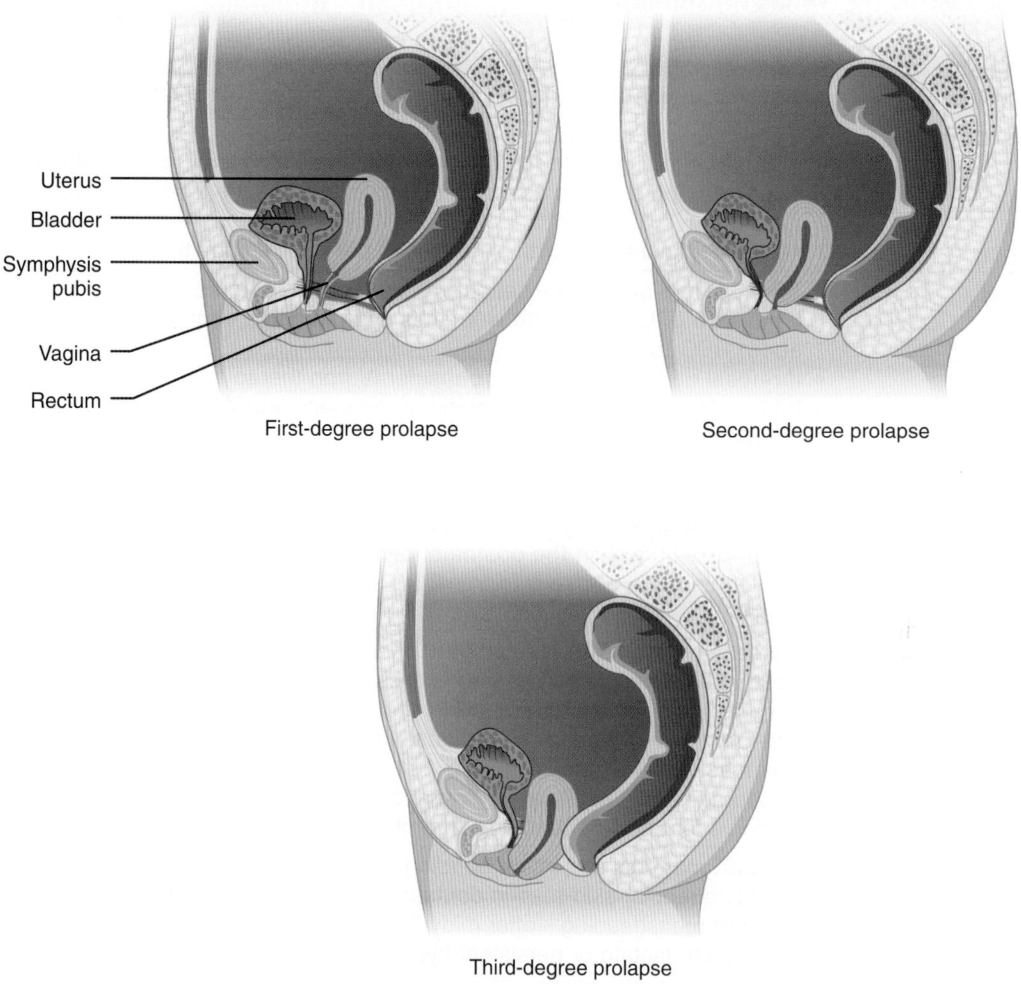

FIGURE 40.11 Classification of uterine inversion can be identified by the severity of the inversion and by the timing of the inversion
(Source: From Goodman CC, Fuller KS: Pathology: implications for the physical therapist, ed 4, St Louis, 2013, Elsevier.)

Classification

Classification of uterine inversion can be identified by the severity of the inversion and by the timing of the inversion (Belfort & Dildy, 2011; Mirza & Gaddipati, 2009).

Severity

The uterus is partially (first degree) or completely (second and third degrees) turned inside out. Second-degree inversion refers to cases in which the fundus has passed through the cervix but not outside the vagina (Belfort & Dildy, 2011). The inside of the fundus protrudes through the cervical os (incomplete), descends to the vaginal introitus (complete) or extrudes beyond the vulva (prolapsed).

- *First degree*—the fundus reaches the internal os.
- *Second degree*—the body or corpus of the uterus is inverted to the internal os.
- *Third and fourth degree*—the uterus, cervix and vagina are inverted and are visible.

Timing

- *Acute*—occurs within 24 hours of birth.
- *Subacute*—occurs after 24 hours, within 4 weeks.
- *Chronic*—occurs after 4 weeks, rare.

Clinical presentation and recognition

Early recognition is key to initiating prompt treatment and reducing associated morbidity and improve outcomes. Acute uterine inversion is often associated with severe, acute lower abdominal pain in the third stage of labour, or severe shock of neurogenic and haemorrhagic origin (Belfort & Dildy, 2011; Mirza & Gaddipati, 2009).

About 93% of women will have a postpartum haemorrhage and profound neurogenic shock. The degree of clinical shock is usually out of proportion to the blood loss. The shock is thought to be due primarily to the parasympathetic effect of traction on the ligaments supporting the uterus, and may be associated with maternal bradycardia (rather than the tachycardia usually associated with hypovolaemic shock). However, this description of the characteristics of shock is not well supported by the literature, and may mislead emergency management (Belfort & Dildy, 2011). The placenta may or may not be attached. The diagnosis is usually established clinically when it is noted the uterus is lying outside the vulva immediately after birth, perhaps when the fundus of the uterus cannot be palpated after the delivery of the placenta (second degree). Bimanual pelvic examination reveals a mass in the vagina (first or second degree) or outside the introitus (third degree) (Belfort & Dildy, 2011).

Management

Due to the relatively low incidence, experience in managing this maternity emergency is sparse. Early recognition and management provides the best prognosis (Leal et al., 2014). Because the principal features of this complication are haemorrhage and shock, immediate management depends on minimising the effects of these. The initial step regardless of context/place of birth is to call for help—for midwifery, senior obstetric and anaesthetic assistance. The first priority is always to implement the DRSABCDs (see section on Cardiac arrest in pregnancy). The amount of blood loss depends on the inversion–reversion interval and can exacerbate haemodynamic instability. Thus, simultaneous resuscitation of the woman should occur while a skilled practitioner attempts uterine re-inversion as quickly as possible before the cervix constricts. Skilled assistance and immediate access to the operating room are important components of success.

In general, treatment for inversion employs parenteral tocolytics to permit immediate uterine replacement (Leal, 2014; Mirza & Gaddipati, 2009), treatment of shock, fluid replacement and oxytocic drugs to maintain normal uterine positioning. Use of glyceryl trinitrate can help facilitate uterine relaxation for prompt replacement. Beta-agonist tocolytics and magnesium sulfate have also been used successfully. If intravenous measures fail, rapid-sequence induction of general anaesthesia and use of a volatile anaesthetic agent may help to achieve adequate relaxation. Rarely, a laparotomy may be necessary to replace the inverted uterus. Following replacement, an oxytocic infusion will increase uterine tone and minimise further blood loss.

The optimal technique for rapid uterine replacement is contentious. Theoretically, in the presence of neurological shock, further stretching of the pelvic viscera as the uterus is replaced has the potential to worsen shock (Mirza & Gaddipati, 2009). In practice, however, once the diagnosis is recognised, the best management is still immediate replacement, because the longer the delay the more firmly contracted the lower uterine segment/cervix becomes, making replacement increasingly difficult (Leal et al., 2014). Consequently, the administration of oxytocin is withheld until after successful correction of inversion. Wherever possible, an obstetrician is usually the best-placed practitioner to attempt to replace the uterus by re-inverting it. The clinician inserts a hand into the vagina and holds the inverted uterus so that the fundus is positioned in the palm of the hand (Fig. 40.12). Pressure is then applied to lift the uterus upwards and anteriorly through the pelvis into the abdominal cavity to the level of the umbilicus (Belfort & Dildy, 2011). The clinician's hand remains in the uterus to stop repeated inversion until an intravenous oxytocic infusion can be commenced (Mirza & Gaddipati, 2009). If possible, an indwelling urinary catheter is inserted to keep the bladder empty.

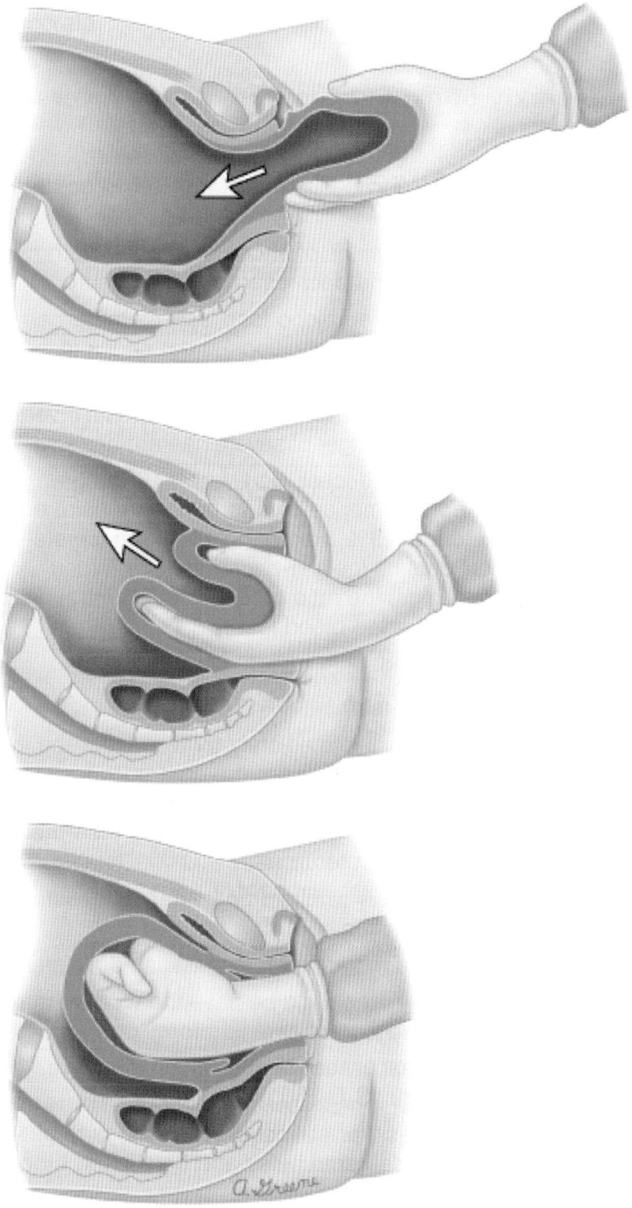

FIGURE 40.12 Correcting uterine inversion
(Based on World Health Organization (WHO) n.d. Correcting uterine inversion. Department of Reproductive Health and Research, WHO, Geneva. http://apps.who.int/iris/bitstream/handle/10665/43972/9241545879_eng.pdf?sequence1)

In most cases, the placenta will not have separated before manual or surgical replacement is attempted. Furthermore, in the increasingly common event of a placenta accreta/increta/percreta, separation is very difficult or impossible. If the placenta remains adherent to the inverted uterus, no attempt should be made to remove it because it significantly increases the risk of haemorrhage (American Congress of Obstetricians and Gynecologists (ACOG), 2006b). If immediate replacement is not possible, or if two or more attempts at this very painful procedure fail, surgery is indicated. The woman is stabilised and then transferred to theatre immediately.

CLINICAL POINT

Summary of management of uterine inversion

If at home or in a primary unit then:

- Call emergency services to assist transfer to obstetric hospital.
- Assess for clinical signs of shock, e.g. cool, clammy, pale, rapid pulse and decreased blood pressure.
- Observe for increased blood loss, assess maternal condition (maternal observations), treat shock (if required).
- Do not attempt to remove the placenta from an inverted uterus—there is a danger of severe haemorrhage.
- Obtain intravenous access via two 14–16-gauge cannulae and commence an appropriate IV fluid, e.g. sodium chloride 0.9%, Hartmann's solution (crystalloids) or Gelofusine (gelatin-based colloid). When using crystalloids, the ratio of resuscitative intravenous fluid required to blood lost is 3:1.

In the hospital setting:

- Call the obstetric team.
- The obstetrician will immediately try to correct the inversion: with sterile gloves on, the obstetrician grasps the uterus and inserts it through the cervix towards the umbilicus to its normal position, using the other hand to support the uterus.
- Synthetic oxytocin is withheld until after successful correction of inversion.
- 100% oxygen via rebreather facemask is administered.
- The head of the bed should be flat—the woman may remain with her legs bent or in lithotomy position.
- Continue maternal assessment of blood pressure, pulse, respirations, S_pO_2.
- Continue to assess for clinical signs of shock, e.g. cool, clammy, pale, rapid pulse and decreased blood pressure.
- Intravenous access via two 14–16-gauge cannulae is obtained (if not already in situ) and commence appropriate intravenous fluid, e.g. sodium chloride 0.9%, Hartmann's solution (crystalloids) or Gelofusine (gelatin-based colloid). When using crystalloids, the ratio of resuscitative intravenous fluid required to blood lost is 3:1.
- To resuscitate more quickly, intravenous fluids may be administered using a pressure infusion device.
- Blood is taken for group- and cross-match for at least 4 units of blood and a complete blood picture.
- If the uterus is successfully returned to its normal position, then the placenta can be manually removed in an operating theatre under anaesthesia.
- Insert an indwelling urinary catheter.
- Following removal of the placenta, 10 IU of oxytocin intravenously followed by an oxytocic infusion (40 IU in 1000 mL of Hartmann's solution or sodium chloride 0.9%) are administered.
- If the above measures fail, O'Sullivan's hydrostatic manoeuvre is employed.

(Adapted from Belfort & Dildy, 2011; Mirza & Gaddipati, 2009.)

Alternative non-surgical techniques

In 1945, O'Sullivan described a method for the correction of partial uterine inversion using hydrostatic pressure by infusing saline into the vagina. If the uterus cannot be replaced manually then O'Sullivan's hydrostatic method may be used to replace the inverted uterus. The hydrostatic method does not always require anaesthesia and may be performed while waiting for theatre or on the way to theatre (Ogueh & Ayida, 1997). The clinician prepares two 1-litre bags of warmed irrigation fluid (e.g. sodium chloride 0.9%) attached to a wide-bore giving set (or cystoscopy irrigation set). The clinician (obstetrician) places one hand in the vagina and obtains a seal at the vaginal entrance with the wrist/hand and the use of vaginal packs. The warmed saline is run in, in copious amounts by gravity. (Up to 4 L may be required in total.) The fluid pushes the uterine fundus upwards until it resumes its correct position. An oxytocic infusion maintains uterine contraction. In most cases this reduces the inversion, with rapid resolution of the shock. The placenta can then be removed under anaesthesia.

Surgical approaches

Laparotomy with open reduction of the uterine inversion may be necessary if the previous methods have not worked. It may be necessary to relax the uterus, perhaps with:

- glyceryl trinitrate spray 400 μm sublingual (works within 2 minutes and has a short half-life) *or*
- intravenous salbutamol up to 250 μm *or*
- subcutaneous terbutaline 250 μm
- general anaesthesia followed by laparotomy or incision of the contracted cervix if necessary to replace the uterus.

Regardless of the procedure employed to replace the uterus, uterine atony and PPH are common after replacement. The prompt administration of 15-methyl prostaglandin $F_2\alpha$ (Haemabate), high-dose oxytocin infusions and perhaps ergometrine (provided there are no contraindications), or misoprostol (Cytotec) per rectum is recommended to control PPH.

Many clinicians administer a single prophylactic dose of a broad-spectrum first-generation cephalosporin or a similar drug at the time of repositioning, for example cefazolin 2 g intravenously, one dose only, plus metronidazole 500 µg intravenously, one dose only.

Postpartum

It is important to remember that re-inversion may also occur. Indeed, uterine inversion can occur in the acute (less than 24 hours after birth) or chronic (greater than 1 month) phases. The clinician's only clues to chronic uterine inversion may be persistent vaginal bleeding or sight of the uterus at the introitus. Occasionally the midwife may detect a partial inversion when palpating the uterine fundus in the postpartum period.

Summary—uterine inversion

Uterine inversion is often accompanied by massive haemorrhage and shock. Timely diagnosis, replacement of the inverted uterus and prompt, expert management are mandatory. Judicious replacement of the inverted uterus by vaginal manipulation is recommended. Careful clinical observation following replacement and the administration of oxytocic drugs prevents most re-inversions. In the rare case when the inversion is longstanding or if manual replacement fails, surgical replacement is required. The risk of recurrence of inversion in subsequent births is unknown.

Rupture of the uterus

Uterine rupture in pregnancy is a rare and life-threatening event with a high incidence of fetal and maternal mortality. The term 'uterine rupture' is used to describe trauma to the uterus in a continuum of events, from a 'weak' spot in the uterine wall seen by the obstetrician at the time of a caesarean section to a full rupture of the uterus so that the fetus and placenta are expelled into the peritoneal cavity.

Incidence

Uterine rupture is a rare occurrence, but is more common when there is a scar on the uterus due to a caesarean section or other uterine surgery. The majority of cases occur in women who have had a previous caesarean section. Fitzpatrick et al. (2012) found an incidence of 0.2 per 1,000 maternities in a case control study undertaken between 2009 and 2010. Women who had a previous caesarean section had an incidence of 2.1 per 1000 maternities, the odds of rupture increased for women who had two or more previous caesarean sections (aOR 3.02, CI 95% 1.16 –7.85) or where there had been less then twelve months since the last caesarean section (aOR 3.12, 95% CI 1.62–6.02). The risks also increased with labour induction and oxytocin use (aOR 3.92 95% CI 1.00–15.33). The risk of uterine rupture is higher in women having a trial of labour (<1%) than in women having an elective repeat caesarean delivery (0.03%) (Yang et al., 2017).

Classification

There are two types of uterine rupture: complete and incomplete. Rupture of the uterus during labour is more dangerous than one occurring in pregnancy, because the shock is greater and infection is almost inevitable.

Complete uterine rupture refers to a full-thickness tear through the myometrium and serosa and may occur in a previously intact uterus or in one with a previous caesarean or myomectomy scar. The entire thickness of the uterine wall and usually the overlying broad ligament rupture so the uterine contents, including the fetus and occasionally the placenta, extrude into the peritoneal cavity. Uterine rupture most often occurs in the lower uterine segment, with the most common site of rupture being the anterior uterine wall. Longitudinal rupture of the lateral wall is also relatively common and may extend upwards into the fundus of the uterus or downwards into the vagina. Posterior ruptures are the least common and are usually transverse.

Different terms used to describe an *incomplete rupture of the uterus* include partial separation (dehiscence) and healing defects (windows) of uterine scars. It seldom results in major maternal or fetal complications (Rogers & Chang, 2006). Uterine scar dehiscence is a separation of a pre-existing scar that does not disrupt the overlying visceral peritoneum (uterine serosa) and that does not significantly bleed from its edges. In addition, the fetus, placenta and umbilical cord are contained within the uterine cavity.

> **CLINICAL POINT**
>
> Following uterine rupture, in more than 75% of cases, signs of compromise will appear before pain or bleeding. Prolonged, late or variable decelerations and bradycardia seen on FHR monitoring are the most common—and often the only—manifestation of uterine rupture.

Risk factors

Uterine rupture may develop as a result of pre-existing injury, such as a scar from uterine surgery, perforation or anomaly. In resource-poor countries, uterine rupture is most often caused by obstructed labour related to cephalopelvic disproportion (CPD), grand multiparity and malpresentation. In contrast, in resource-rich countries the most common cause of uterine rupture is dehiscence of a previous caesarean section scar. Injudicious use of oxytocin and traumatic rupture from obstetric manipulative procedures such as internal podalic version are also contributing factors. Box 40.16 provides a list of associated risk factors.

Diagnosis

Rupture at the site of a previous uterine scar may occur with few warning signs because the scar is relatively avascular. A number of studies on VBAC report that prolonged fetal bradycardia is the first sign in over 70% of cases of uterine rupture (Martel & MacKinnon, 2004). Variable or

Box 40.16 Associated risk factors for uterine rupture

Associations—*not* causes—for uterine rupture include (Kaczmarczyk et al., 2007):

- BMI (high or low)
- short interval between births <24 months (Yang, 2017)
- gestational age >40 weeks (Yang, 2017)
- estimated fetal weight >4000 g (Yang, 2017)
- extremes of age
- short maternal stature <159 cm
- previous vaginal birth
- uterine scars
- prior caesarean section
- prior uterine rupture
- trauma
- injury from instrumentation during a termination of pregnancy
- significant myomectomy
- any cause of uterine perforation or cervical laceration
- uterine anomalies (e.g. undeveloped uterine horn)
- prior invasive molar pregnancy
- history of placenta percreta or increta
- difficult forceps delivery
- malpresentation
- podalic version
- fetal anomaly
- obstructed labour
- induction of labour (suspected association) (Dekker et al., 2010)
- excessive uterine stimulation:
    - prostaglandin E_1 (misoprostol)
    - prostaglandin E_2 (dinoprostone)
    - synthetic oxytocin, especially high infusion rates
    - alkaloidal / crack-cocaine abuse
- manual removal of the placenta (placenta percreta and increta)
- conditions causing overdistension of uterus:
    - hydramnios
    - macrosomia
    - multiple pregnancy
    - choriocarcinoma.

late fetal heart decelerations may be a sign of impending rupture. Box 40.17 provides a list of potential warning signs of complete rupture. If there is an atypical pattern of pain, or pain previously controlled by analgesia (epidural or otherwise) that becomes more severe, complete clinical reassessment by an experienced obstetrician is required (Lieberman et al., 2004; Martel & MacKinnon, 2004).

Box 40.17 Warning signs of complete rupture

- Severe constant abdominal pain
- Sudden cessation of uterine contractions
- Vaginal bleeding
- Maternal tachycardia
- Maternal hypotension / shock
- Haematuria (bladder injury can occur)
- Severe fetal distress / intrauterine death
- Chest pain or shoulder tip pain
- Sudden onset shortness of breath

(Adapted from Mid Essex Hospital Services NHS: *Management of Ruptured Uterus, Clinical Guideline* 2017, http://www.meht.nhs.uk/about-us-/policies-and-guidelines/)

Management

The consequences of uterine rupture during pregnancy or in labour depend on the time that elapses from the rupture until the institution of definitive therapy. Principles of management are:

1. Resuscitate the woman while arranging urgent laparotomy / caesarean section.
    a. Monitor vital signs as maternal condition dictates: blood pressure, pulse (attach pulse oximeter, ECG), neurological status, respirations and temperature. Urinary output is measured and the vaginal loss recorded.
    b. Insert two large-bore catheters (16 G or above), take blood for cross match (4–6 units), full blood count (FBC), urea and electrolytes, liver function tests and clotting screen.
    c. Administer rapid IV fluids such as Hartmann's and, when available, blood and blood products and / or inotropes as required.
2. Repair of the uterus is preferable, but in some cases hysterectomy may be required.
3. Provide standard postoperative and postnatal care.
4. Provide adequate counselling as soon as possible and arrange further follow-up. It is important that the woman be counselled about future pregnancies and given evidence-based information.

In the event that a laparotomy and hysterectomy is required, the most experienced medical clinician should explain the procedures fully, outline any risks involved and obtain the woman's consent. Sensitive postsurgery counselling is crucial.

If the rupture was confined to the lower segment and repaired, the risk of rupture in a subsequent pregnancy is similar to that of someone with a previous caesarean. If there are extensive tears involving the upper segment, future pregnancy may be contraindicated. Women with a history of uterine rupture are usually advised to have a planned elective caesarean section (37–8 weeks gestation) in their next pregnancy.

Amniotic fluid embolism

Amniotic fluid embolism (AFE) is a poorly understood phenomenon usually occurring without warning and is a major cause of direct maternal mortality in New Zealand and Australia (McDonnell et al., 2015). AFE is unpredictable, unpreventable and rapidly progressive. It carries a high probability of life-threatening sequelae including cardiac arrest, adult respiratory distress syndrome (ARDS), coagulopathy with massive haemorrhage, encephalopathy, seizures and both maternal and infant mortality. AFE is rare and can be difficult to diagnose but in recent years there have been significant improvements in both the morbidity and the mortality of AFE in many countries due to increased awareness and responsiveness to the condition and to developments in resuscitation and treatment.

Amniotic fluid embolism is defined differently depending on the country. It is generally understood to be as a result of the amniotic fluid and/or fetal cells entering the maternal circulation, causing an allergic-type reaction usually around the time of birth (Perinatal and Maternal Mortality Review Committee (PMMRC), 2017). The term AFE and in particular 'embolism' creates confusion. Although some of the typical features of an AFE may resemble the mechanical obstruction of the pulmonary blood flow observed in a typical pulmonary embolism, a number of other features do not fit with this model (Benson, 2012). For this reason, possible immune-mediated mechanisms have also been suggested. The term AFE does not reflect the underlying condition, with suggested alternatives being 'anaphylactoid syndrome of pregnancy' or 'sudden obstetric collapse syndrome' (Benson, 2012).

CLINICAL POINT

AFE should always be considered if /when a woman collapses during labour or birth (within 30 minutes), or presents with acute behavioural changes such as sudden anxiety, agitation and dyspnoea (PMMRC, 2017).

If any of the following occur during labour or caesarean birth or within 30 minutes postpartum and there is no other obvious explanation, the midwife should consider the possibility of AFE.

Signs of AFE are:

- acute hypotension
- cardiac arrest
- acute hypoxaemia or respiratory distress
- severe haemorrhage or coagulopathy.

Other common signs are:

- premonitory symptoms such as restlessness, numbness, agitation and tingling
- chest pain, vomiting
- shortness of breath, respiratory dyspnoea, bronchospasm, pulmonary oedema, acute respiratory distress
- cardiovascular cyanosis, hypotension, transient hypertension, chest pain, cardiopulmonary arrest
- neurological seizures, headache, loss of consciousness
- haematological coagulopathy, disseminated intravascular coagulation
- fetal bradycardia.

Management

Early recognition and aggressive resuscitation are important and are thought to improve outcomes for women and babies. If the woman is at home or in a birthing unit it is essential to transfer urgently if there are any of the above signs or symptoms. Within a secondary/tertiary setting it is vital to involve senior obstetric, anaesthetic, intensive, midwifery and neonatal staff as soon as possible.

If maternal collapse occurs:

- Commence/continue cardiopulmonary resuscitation (CPR) if there has been a cardiac arrest, profound hypotension or loss of consciousness.
- Ensure there is left uterine displacement in women with a palpable uterus.
- Perimortem caesarean section needs to be considered if there has been cardiac arrest at the start of resuscitation, with the aim of birth of the baby within 5 minutes.
- Initiate the massive transfusion protocol, including the use of cryoprecipitate.
- Life-saving interventions such as defibrillation and medication should not be withheld in the setting of pregnancy.

AFE requires vigilance, a high level of clinical suspicion, and rapid all-out resuscitative efforts by a multidisciplinary expert team that is practised in emergency management (PMMRC, 2017).

Incidence

A review of prospectively collected data from Australia, France, the Netherlands, Slovakia and the UK were pooled and examined to identify an incidence of 0.8 to 1.8 per 100,000 maternities (Fitzpatrick et al., 2019). The proportion of women who died from AFE or had permanent neurological injury ranged from 30% to 41% dependent on the case definition. Mortality was more likely for women who presented with cardiac arrest (89% versus 40%, aOR 10.58, 95% CI 3.93–28.48 $p<0.001$). Having an obstetrician and/or anaesthetist present at the time of the AFE reduced the odds of mortality (61% versus 75%, aOR 0.38, 95% CI 0.16–0.90, $p=0.027$) and interventions to correct coagulopathy (including an adequate dose of

Table 40.6 Amniotic fluid embolism—associated risk factors	
Sociodemographic and maternal characteristics	Adjusted odds ratio (95% CI, p value)
Maternal age 35 or more	2.40 (1.71–3.37, <0.001)
Multiple pregnancy	6.28 (3.23–12.22, <0.001)
Polyhydramnios	5.04 (1.90–13.36, <0.001)
Placenta praevia	13.26 (6.35–27.69, <0.001)
Placental abruption	14.14 (3.52–56.86, <0.001)
Induction of labour (any method)	2.37 (1.68–3.34 <,0.001)
Instrumental birth	9.82 (3.93–24.49, <0.001)
Cesarean section	14.02 (6.25–31.42, <0.001)
Source: Fitzpatrick et al. (2019)	

tranexamic acid) were also found to improve maternal outcomes.

Despite a relatively unchanged incidence, it has been noted that the mortality associated with AFE has decreased significantly in the recent past, which is thought to be due to improvements in the provision of critical care. AFE should no longer be considered to be a universally fatal condition (Society for Maternal–Fetal Medicine, 2016). Risk factors are identified in Table 40.6.

CLINICAL POINT

The syndrome develops without warning, usually during the birth, as amniotic fluid enters the systemic maternal circulation during an apparently normal labour and birth not associated with prebirth complications. If the AFE occurs during labour and prior to birth, there is a risk that the baby will become anoxic.

Pathophysiology

The pathophysiology of AFE is still poorly understood, but what is known is that amniotic fluid must first enter the maternal circulation for an anaphylactoid reaction to occur (Fig. 40.13). The amniotic fluid is normally separated from the maternal circulation by the intact fetal membranes but in AFE there is a breach in this barrier, perhaps through endocervical veins or the site of placentation when labour was induced. It has also been suggested that perhaps the uterine hypertonus sometimes observed prior to the onset of clinical signs of AFE occurs because of the AFE. To confuse understanding of AFE further, it is known that in some women amniotic fluid may enter the maternal circulation as a relatively normal aspect of childbirth and not trigger any adverse reaction. Findings such as this indicate that amniotic fluid triggers AFE in only a few women (Benson, 2012). Amniotic fluid contains a number of potentially vasoactive substances as well as substances that may interfere with coagulation and probably leads to the profuse haemorrhage and disseminated intravascular coagulopathy (DIC) that often occur in AFE (Kaur, 2016).

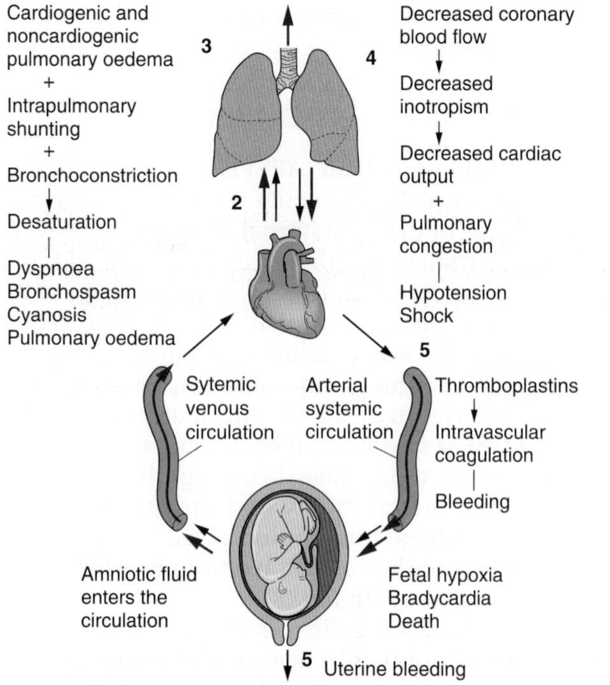

Sequence of events:

(1) For reasons not completely understood, amniotic fluid reaches the maternal intravascular compartment (systemic venous system).

(2) The amniotic fluid enters pulmonary circulation via the pulmonary artery. This contaminated blood crosses to the left atrium through a patent foramen and probably through intrapulmonary shunts once the embolism is significant, as shown in cases of massive amniotic fluid embolism at autopsy.

(3) The exposure of the pulmonary vasculature to both soluble (leucotrienes, surfactant, thromboxane A_2, endothelin, etc.) and insoluble components (squames, vernix, hair, mucin, etc.) of the amniotic fluid and possibly other mediators released locally induces capillary leak, negative inotropism, and bronchospasm. This results in sudden onset of respiratory distress and cyanosis.

(4) Within minutes, the negative inotropic effect becomes prevalent (probably due to myocardial ischaemia). Pulmonary venous pressure (congestion) increases and a drop in cardiac output are manifested by pulmonary oedema and hypotension to the point of shock.

(5) The exposure of the intravascular compartment to amniotic fluid thromboplastin and to other mediators freed in the circulation by the presence of amniotic fluid induces a consumptive coagulopathy in a large proportion of the first-phase survivors. This disseminated intravascular coagulation often results in severe uterine bleeding.

(6) The resultant systemic hypotension decreases the uterine perfusion. Abnormalities of the fetal heart tracing will rapidly follow and may result in fetal death.

FIGURE 40.13 Pathophysiology of amniotic fluid embolism (Adapted from Hic et nunc, Amniotic fluid embolism, https://commons.wikimedia.org/wiki/File:Amniotic_fluid_embolism.png. CC BY SA 3.0)

REFLECTIVE CASE STUDY

Direct maternal death caused by amniotic fluid embolism

A multiparous woman was induced because of polyhydramnios. Induction was followed by vaginal bleeding and blood-stained liquor. During labour she collapsed with no recordable blood pressure, a feeble pulse and a low Glasgow Coma Score. Collapse was accompanied by fetal bradycardia, and she was resuscitated in the hope this would assist the fetal condition. She appeared to improve a little but then collapsed again and developed DIC after an emergency caesarean section.

(Source: CEMACE, 2011)

In most cases, AFE occurs in the intrapartum and immediate postpartum periods; occasional cases have been described during amniocentesis, termination of pregnancies and abdominal trauma and after caesarean delivery (Knight et al., 2012). The classic description is one of a sudden and severe deterioration that is rapidly fatal. Hypotension is a common and first sign in severe episodes of AFE, followed by acute respiratory distress and perhaps respiratory arrest. Coagulation disturbances (DIC) often occur very rapidly in AFE and, in some cases, may be the initial presenting sign (see section on DIC). The pathophysiology of AFE occurs in a two-phase process but the precise pathway is still unknown.

Phase one

This usually occurs within 30 minutes. Under certain conditions, when amniotic fluid and its fetal components enter the maternal circulation, endogenous mediators (e.g. prostaglandins, leucotrienes, histamine, bradykinin, cytokines, thromboxane, complement-activating factors and platelet-activating factors) are released. This causes severe pulmonary hypertension secondary to pulmonary vasoconstriction with resulting right heart failure, hypotension and hypoxaemia. The hypoxaemia can lead to ischaemic myocardial injury followed by non-cardiogenic pulmonary oedema and bronchospasm.

Phase two

Phase two is characterised by haemodynamic instability and/or DIC. Many women will die in phase one from left heart failure and ARDS caused by mechanical circulatory obstruction or inflammatory/immunological mechanisms (Gist et al., 2009). Death often occurs within the first hour. If they survive most women develop coagulopathy resulting in massive bleeding, which may be one of the most prominent signs of AFE and which usually appears within 4 hours of the initial presentation.

Fetal signs and symptoms

Profound fetal respiratory acidosis and associated FHR changes occur in response to maternal hypoxia and hypertonic uterine contractions. Prolonged late decelerations followed by baseline fetal bradycardia can result in neurological injury. A fetal heart rate of 60 b.p.m. or less for more than 3 minutes may indicate a terminal bradycardia. A short interval between cardiac arrest and birth correlates positively with neonatal survival.

CLINICAL POINT

Classic presenting signs and symptoms may include sudden anxiety, agitation, dyspnoea, cough, hypotension, cyanosis, cardiopulmonary arrest, coagulopathy and seizures. A sudden change in the woman's behaviour may be an early feature of the onset of hypoxia heralding AFE. Sometimes this is followed by a toxic confusional state.

Clinical diagnosis

Currently no definitive test exists to diagnose or confirm AFE. The diagnosis of AFE is a clinical one, based on the presence of cardiovascular and respiratory compromise and coagulopathy after the exclusion of other causes (Society for Maternal–Fetal Medicine, 2016). The diagnosis can be made at autopsy by examining for the presence of fetal material in the maternal pulmonary circulation. However, given that fetal material may be present in otherwise well women, the sensitivity of this finding may not confirm the diagnosis. In Australia and New Zealand AFE is defined as:

> *. . . a clinical diagnosis following acute hypotension or cardiac arrest, acute hypoxia and coagulopathy in the absence of any other potential explanation for the symptoms and signs observed or as a post mortem diagnosis with the presence of fetal squames/debris in the pulmonary circulation.*
>
> (Fitzpatrick et al., 2019)

CLINICAL POINT

The 2003 report of maternal deaths within the UK found that women who died from AFE frequently had premonitory symptoms before complete collapse including feeling cold, restlessness and respiratory distress (Weindling, 2003). This may give a clue to diagnosis, before cardiac arrest and DIC occur. In a New Zealand review, premonitory symptoms such as restlessness, numbness, agitation and tingling occurred in 11 of the 18 cases reviewed and were the presenting signs in two of the cases (PMMRC, 2016).

Management

Recognition of the condition followed by prompt and aggressive treatment of AFE is necessary to achieve better outcomes (Leighton et al., 2011). The three main goals of treatment are: (1) oxygenation, (2) maintaining cardiac output and blood pressure, and (3) correcting coagulopathy.

As soon as the woman's condition is stabilised, the birth of the baby should be expedited. An emergency bedside caesarean delivery may be necessary to improve the woman's chances for a good outcome because the weight of the gravid uterus on the inferior vena cava impedes blood return to the heart and decreases systemic blood pressure; it may also save the life of the baby (Society of Maternal–Fetal Medicine, 2016).

In the event of cardiac arrest, the resuscitation team should follow standard Advanced Cardiac Life Support protocols. Administration of blood transfusions and blood components is considered the first line of treatment for correcting coagulopathy associated with AFE. Ideally, overall management should take place in an obstetric unit or failing that a medical or surgical intensive care unit. Blood products including packed red blood cells, fresh frozen plasma, platelets and cryoprecipitate are used to maintain organ perfusion and urinary output until bleeding from DIC resolves.

Postpartum

Apart from ongoing care of women and their babies who survive, those with AFE will need to be monitored for any future neurological impairment by the appropriate neurology teams and have annual reviews with their GP. Counselling and debriefing should be offered before they go home and then as required. If the woman and baby do have ongoing neurological sequelae, for instance paresis or problems with speech or mobilisation, they will require ongoing care.

CRITICAL THINKING EXERCISE

You are a midwifery student undertaking a routine postpartum assessment of Mary's health 1 hour after Mary's beautiful spontaneous vaginal birth following an ARM induction of labour. You find Mary's pulse rate is 120 b.p.m., and her BP is 70/50 mmHg.

- What other observations would you undertake?
- Would you escalate care?

Summary—amniotic fluid embolism

Amniotic fluid embolism is a catastrophic condition with high fatality for both woman and baby. It can occur during labour, birth or immediately following birth and is characterised by the sudden development of hypotension, respiratory distress, shock, cardiac arrest and uncontrolled bleeding. AFE can be neither predicted nor prevented but premonitory signs appear to be a common feature. Many women succumb to cardiorespiratory failure, but if they survive the initial insult some will still die after developing DIC. Early diagnosis, optimal resuscitation and immediate treatment are important components that support survival. Some survivors develop neurological impairments.

Disseminated intravascular coagulopathy

Disseminated intravascular coagulopathy (DIC) is characterised by systemic activation of blood coagulation (clotting cascade), which results in generation and deposition of fibrin, leading to microvascular thrombi in various organs and contributing to multiple organ dysfunction syndrome (MODS) (Vincent & De Backer, 2005). Consumption and ensuing exhaustion of coagulation proteins and platelets (from ongoing activation of coagulation mechanisms) may induce severe bleeding, although microclot formation may follow in the absence of relentless clotting factor depletion and haemorrhage (Levi & ten Cate, 1999). DIC is not a specific diagnosis, and its presence always indicates another underlying issue such as trauma or sepsis. It is defined as an acquired syndrome of disseminated intravascular coagulopathy with widespread development of thromboses, mainly within the capillaries of the microcirculation, usually seen in association with well-defined clinical disorders (Box 40.18). In obstetrics, DIC is always a secondary complication of a condition that initiates coagulation-promoting factors into the maternal circulation.

Incidence and management

It is difficult to determine the exact incidence of DIC in obstetrics although Hizkiyahu et al. (2018) identify an incidence of 0.03–0.35% of pregnancies and 15–20% of cases of HELLP syndrome. DIC is thought to be a contributory cause of up to 25% of all maternal deaths (Cunningham & Nelson, 2015). If there is any suspicion of DIC arising from either clinical or laboratory findings, the woman should be carefully monitored with ongoing clinical assessment and frequent haematological tests to identify the progression of the coagulopathy. In most cases the disease can be ameliorated in the initial stages, for example in cases of DIC induced by abruptio placentae (placental abruption). Management is focused on stabilising maternal health whilst identifying and treating the underlying disorder.

Box 40.18 Disseminated intravascular coagulopathy—associated risk factors

- Placental abruption
- Placenta praevia
- Preeclampsia
- Eclampsia
- HELLP syndrome
- Retained fetus syndrome
- Infection

HELLP = Haemolysis, Elevated Liver enzymes, Low Platelet count.

Pathophysiology

Several concurrent mechanisms play a role in the pathogenesis of DIC and review of the 'clotting pathway' is recommended to understand the pathophysiology (see Ch. 20 or textbooks such as Rankin, 2017 or Blackburn, 2013).

In the healthy body a balance between coagulation and fibrinolysis is maintained. Pregnant women are said to be in a hypercoagulable state owing to increases in procoagulant factors associated with a decrease in anticoagulant proteins and fibrinolysis. Normal haemostatic mechanisms include the vasculature, cellular components, circulating procoagulants, anticoagulants and fibrinolytic factors. During pregnancy the platelet count declines slightly, although it remains in the normal range. However, in less than 10% of pregnancies, incidental mild thrombocytopenia occurs. The precise mechanism is not clearly understood. Nevertheless, normal platelet function including aggregation is slightly enhanced during pregnancy. Circulating levels of factor VII, X and fibrinogen increase substantially during the first trimester. In contrast, factor XI levels slightly fall while those of factor V remain unchanged. Fibrinolytic activity is reduced, perhaps owing to an increase in plasminogen activator inhibitors PAI-1 and PAI-2. Circulating AT-III activity is unchanged during pregnancy, as are levels of protein C and total protein S, although free protein S levels decrease by about 50% (proteins C and S work together to inhibit excessive blood clotting).

After birth, there are striking changes in maternal haemostasis. Platelet aggregation increases, thrombin generation increases, contact factors drop and fibrin/fibrinogen degradation products (FDPs) go up. FDPs are potent circulating anticoagulants that contribute further to the bleeding manifestations of DIC. However, within a few hours, fibrinolytic activity normalises, probably because of the decrease in PAI-1 and PAI-2. DIC occurs following a triggering event, and is due to the processes that support coagulation and fibrinolysis being dysregulated, resulting in widespread clotting and bleeding.

DIC is:

- primarily a thrombotic process
- a systemic process producing both thrombosis and haemorrhage
- also called consumption coagulopathy and defibrination syndrome.

Its clinical manifestation may be widespread haemorrhage in acute, fulminant cases. DIC usually arises in one of four clinical circumstances:

- *obstetric catastrophes*—where uterine material with tissue factor activity (TFA) gains access to the maternal circulation (e.g. in abruptio placentae, retained dead fetus syndrome and following AFE)
- *shock*—from any cause including PPH, probably because of the generation of TFA on monocytes and endothelial cells
- *bacterial infection*—particularly with Gram-negative organisms; Gram-negative endotoxins cause generation of TFA on the plasma membrane of monocytes and endothelial cells
- *malignancy*—particularly mucin-secreting adenocarcinomas in which hypergranular, leukaemic cells are thought to release material from their granules with TFA.

The mechanisms by which DIC is triggered are not entirely understood and are too complex to be considered in detail in this chapter. In brief, several simultaneously occurring mechanisms play a role in the pathogenesis of DIC (Fig. 40.14). For some reason, maternal blood is exposed to large amounts of the tissue factor VIIa system. Two proteolytic enzymes, thrombin and plasmin, are activated and released into the systemic circulation. In normal circumstances the balance between these two substances determines a bleeding or thrombotic tendency. Thrombin cleaves fibrinogen to form fibrin monomers. The fibrin deposition is a result of tissue factor-mediated thrombin generation that is insufficiently balanced by physiological anticoagulant mechanisms such as the antithrombin system and the protein C system. In addition to enhanced fibrin formation, fibrin removal is impaired as a result of depression of the fibrinolytic system. This leads to small- and large-vessel thrombosis, with the end result of multiorgan failure. As a result, large amounts of thrombin are generated, leading to a hypercoagulable state. In the normal physiological state, plasmin is responsible for breaking fibrin into fibrin split products, thereby limiting the formation of fibrin clots. In DIC, the quantity of plasmin is significantly increased, leading to the generation of significant quantities of fibrin degradation products. This results in the catastrophic bleeding seen in DIC.

Acute DIC

In acute DIC:

- blood is exposed to large amounts of tissue factor in a short period of time, creating large amounts of thrombin
- coagulation factors are consumed at a rate in excess of the capacity of the liver to synthesise them
- platelets are consumed in excess of the capacity of bone marrow megakaryocytes to release them.

CLINICAL POINT

Warning signs of DIC

- Profound haemorrhage.
- Blood fails to clot.
- Petechiae appear.
- Bleeding from the woman's eyes, nose, gums or vagina and from venipuncture, surgical and episiotomy sites occurs.
- Haematomas, flank pain, abdominal distension, swollen extremities, neurological abnormalities, hypotension, tachycardia, cool skin temperature, pallor and diaphoresis may indicate profuse internal bleeding.

Chronic or subacute DIC

Features of chronic or subacute DIC include:

- retained dead fetus
- exposure to small amounts of tissue factor.

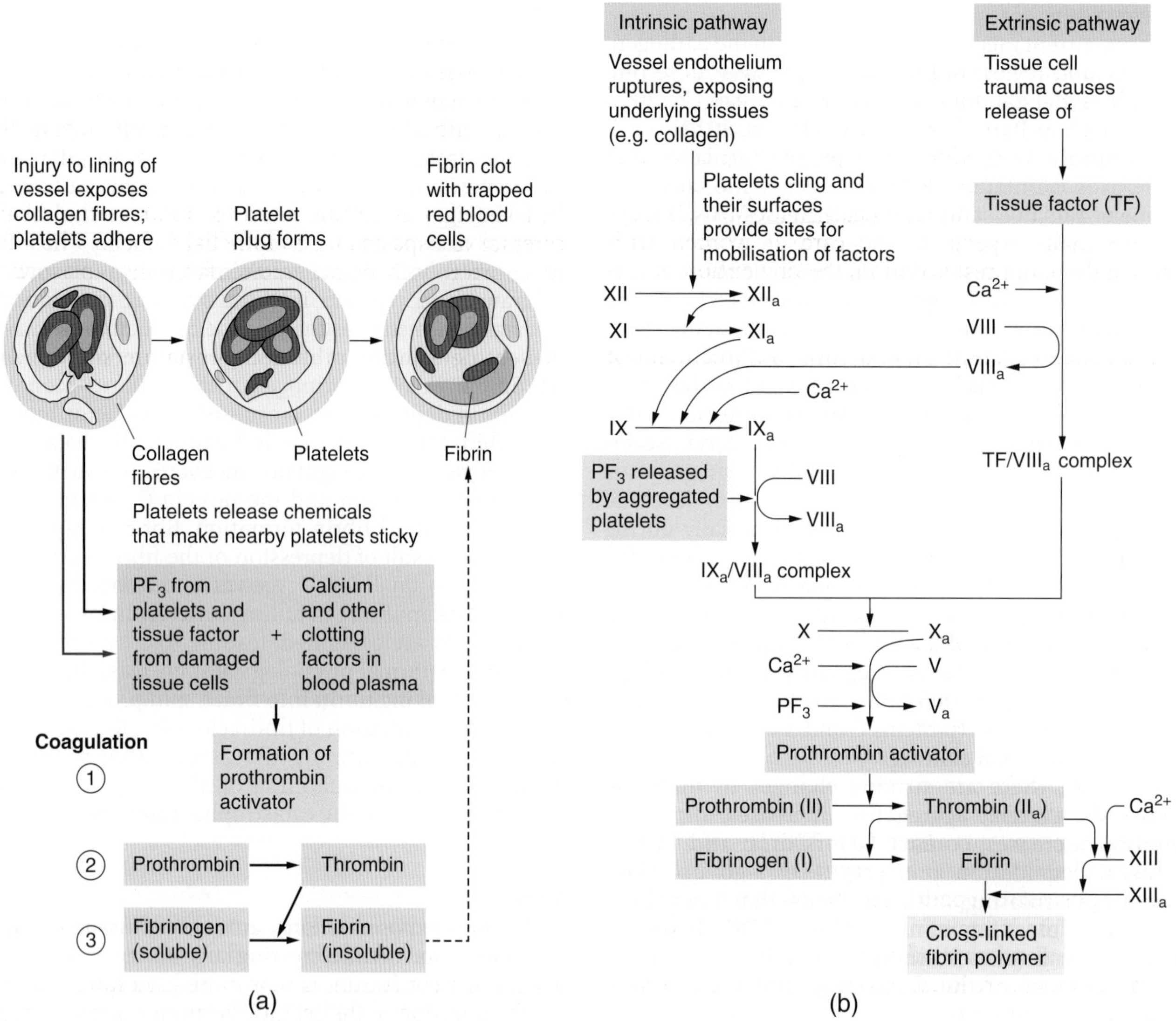

FIGURE 40.14 Platelet formation and blood clotting: (a) Simplified overview of events. Steps 1 to 3 are the major events. (b) Detailed flow chart indicating intermediates and events involved in platelet plug formation and the intrinsic and extrinsic mechanisms of clotting (Note: subscript a denotes activated procoagulant.)
(Based on Marieb, 2004)

CLINICAL POINT

- DIC always has an underlying aetiology.
- The condition must be identified and eliminated to treat the coagulopathy successfully.
- The development of DIC in many disorders is associated with an adverse outcome.
- DIC mortality rate approaches 40%–80%.

Treatment

Treatment includes:
- identifying the underlying cause and treating; all other therapies are temporising
- for women who are actively bleeding or who are at high risk of bleeding:
  - blood component treatments
  - transfusions of platelets
  - treatment for thrombocytopenia—fresh frozen plasma
  - replacement of consumed coagulation factors and correction of the prolonged PT and aPTT
- anticoagulants:
  - may be used to block thrombin and secondary fibrinolysis
  - might exacerbate the bleeding tendency
  - but they are usually reserved for forms of DIC manifested by thrombosis, acrocyanosis, cancer, vascular malformations, retained dead fetus, acute promyelocytic leukaemia
- restoration of anticoagulant pathways.

Eclampsia

Eclampsia is a serious consequence of pre-eclampsia (see Ch. 37). It is a pregnancy-specific, multiorgan disorder usually associated with hypertension, thrombocytopenia and proteinuria, and which may progress to eclamptic seizures (Hutcheon et al., 2011). The Society of Obstetric Medicine of Australia and New Zealand (SOMANZ) identifies four main aspects to the care of women with eclampsia; these are resuscitation, the prevention of further seizures, control of hypertension and expediting the birth of the baby (Lowe et al., 2015). In New Zealand a clinical practice guideline on diagnosis and treatment of hypertension and preeclampsia also covers the development of HELLP and eclampsia (MOH, 2022). Eclampsia is included here because it is a life-threatening emergency for woman and baby.

Definition

Eclampsia has been defined as: a generalised seizure in the setting of preeclampsia, in the absence of another more likely cause (Pollock et al., 2020). It typically occurs during or after the 20th week of gestation or in the postpartum period and can be the presenting feature of preeclampsia for some women Hutcheon et al., 2011.

The convulsions of eclampsia are directly associated with the effects of severe preeclampsia such as decreased vascular resistance and increased intracellular fluid load. The most common cause of seizures during pregnancy is pre-existing epilepsy (see Ch. 37). De-novo-onset seizures in the latter half of pregnancy or during the immediate postpartum period are most frequently caused by eclampsia. Other causes of new-onset seizures can be classified as either secondary to neurological pathology or complications of critical illness (e.g. stroke, tumours or infection).

Incidence

The estimated incidence of eclampsia has been identified as 2.2% (95% CI 1.9–2.7) per 10,000 women giving birth (Pollock et al., 2020) with up to 44% of seizures occurring after birth (MOH, 2022).

> **REFLECTIVE CASE STUDY**
>
> Samantha, a primigravid woman at 38 weeks, attends a rural maternity centre with a severe headache. On assessment her blood pressure is found to be 170/120. She has diminished urine output, a urine analysis of 3+ protein, epigastric pain and hyperreflexia. The FHR is within normal limits.
>
> - What further assessment would you undertake?
> - Would you escalate care and organise transfer?
> - What initial management would you provide?

Pathophysiology

Preeclampsia / eclampsia is part of a multisystem disorder of unknown aetiology characterised by vasoconstriction and hypercoagulability. Most women with eclampsia present with a history of hypertension, although in about 20% of cases eclampsia may occur without warning in women who have no history of hypertension. It is believed that eclamptic seizures occur as the result of cerebral vasospasm and endothelial damage, which leads to cerebral ischaemia, microinfarctions and oedema. Eclampsia is a severe manifestation of preeclampsia and can occur before, during or after birth. It can be the presenting feature of preeclampsia in some women (MOH, 2022).

Imminent eclampsia: signs and symptoms

Most women report premonitory symptoms of eclampsia (Cooray et al., 2011):

- *severe frontal headache*—cerebral oedema (83%)
- *hyperreflexia*—cardinal signal of impending eclampsia (80%)
- *diminished urinary output*—renal failure: most important clinical feature (52%)
- *visual disturbances*—retinal oedema (44%)
- *epigastric pain*—haemorrhage of the subcapsular parts of the liver (19%)
- *vomiting and nausea*—related to cerebral oedema and liver damage
- *oedema*—not considered an important clinical sign of impending eclampsia (49%).

Course of an eclamptic seizure

Eclampsia initially manifests as a grand-mal seizure or more, with each seizure generally lasting 60–75 seconds; in general the convulsion is self-limiting. Respiration ceases for the duration of the seizure. Eclamptic seizures may be divided into two phases. *Phase 1* lasts 15–20 seconds and begins with facial twitching. The body becomes rigid, leading to generalised muscular (tonic–clonic) contractions. *Phase 2* lasts about 1 minute. The seizure moves to the jaw, then to the muscles of the face and eyelids, and then spreads throughout the body. The muscles begin alternating between contracting and relaxing in rapid tonic–clonic sequence. A coma or short period of unconsciousness follows phase 2. The woman gradually regains some consciousness, and she may become extremely agitated and amnesiac. A period of hyperventilation follows the tonic–clonic seizure. This compensates for the respiratory and lactic acidosis that develops during the apnoeic phase. Seizure-induced complications can include tongue biting, head trauma, broken bones and aspiration.

Management of severe preeclampsia and prevention of eclampsia

Early detection and prevention of severe preeclampsia is the key to prevention of eclampsia. The main aims of treatment are focused on prevention or treatment of seizures, resuscitation, control of hypertension, treatment of complications, prompt consultation and expediting the birth of the baby and placenta.

The suppression of eclamptic seizures does not solve the underlying multisystem disease. Nevertheless, it helps to protect the woman and baby from complications such as cerebral haemorrhage, antepartum haemorrhage, fetal asphyxia and death while the maternal condition is stabilised, and enables a multidisciplinary team to plan future care including referral to a tertiary (level III) hospital and the mode of birth. Box 40.19 provides a summary of care provision if an eclamptic seizure occurs.

Box 40.19 Management of eclamptic seizure

- Immediate consultation with obstetric team

During the seizure:

- Airway, breathing, circulation, disability, exposure management (ABCDE).
- Do not leave the woman alone.
- Summon assistance.
- Ensure a patent airway by:
  - turning the woman onto her left side (left-lateral positioning)—decreases the risk of aspiration and will help to improve uterine blood flow by relieving obstruction of the vena cava by the gravid uterus
  - gently suctioning the mouth to clear any saliva, mucus, blood and/or vomitus if needed.
- Protect the woman from injury:
  - do not restrain the woman
  - do not place tongue or airway guards into the mouth during the seizure.
- Administer 100% oxygen at 6–8 L/min via a Hudson facemask.
- Apply oxygen saturation monitoring and attach an ECG as soon as possible.
- Note the features and duration of seizure:
  - time of onset
  - progress of the seizure
  - body involvement
  - signs of cyanosis
  - presence of incontinence
  - time of cessation.
- Commence fluid balance chart and record input and output.
- Assess and monitor fetal wellbeing (cardiotocography).
- Perform a secondary survey including a neurological examination.
- As soon as possible, measure blood glucose levels, electrolytes and if needed antiepileptic drug titres.

Prevention and control of seizures

Magnesium sulfate ($MgSO_4$) should be the first-line drug treatment to prevent further eclamptic seizures and for recurrent seizures (MOH, 2022). Although the exact mechanism is unknown, $MgSO_4$ is thought to act as a physiological calcium antagonist and may act by blocking calcium channels in smooth muscle, resulting in the reversal of cerebral vasospasm. Continuous infusion improves the maintenance of serum levels compared with intermittent bolus doses. Magnesium has been shown to be superior to phenytoin and diazepam for the management of eclamptic seizures (Cahill et al., 2007).

Magnesium sulfate administration. Following consultation with the obstetric team, magnesium sulfate may be prescribed. Goals are to reduce morbidity, prevent complications and correct eclampsia. The drug of choice to treat and prevent eclampsia is magnesium sulfate (Lowe et al., 2015). Regimes may vary regionally and within organisations. In New Zealand the MOH national guideline (MOH, 2022) has established a standard Magnesium Sulphate Protocol for Eclampsia.

Ongoing management

A transfer to the nearest high-dependency unit (HDU) once the woman's condition stabilises is necessary, with the woman requiring one-to-one care.

- Ongoing assessment should include:
  - frequent blood pressure monitoring, pulse and respirations
  - arterial oxygen saturation levels with pulse oximetry and ECG
  - urine output and fluid balance
  - fetal heart rate—continuous cardiotocograph (CTG)
  - level of consciousness
  - presence of restlessness and twitching
  - assessment and treatment of any injuries sustained during the seizure
  - observation for uterine contractions—for signs of labour; this may start spontaneously and go unnoticed
  - vaginal loss (blood and/or amniotic liquor).
- The woman should be nil by mouth until medical assessment.
- Minimise external stimuli (e.g. bright lights, noise and handling, visitors).
- An indwelling urinary catheter (IDC) should be inserted with output measured hourly.
- Arrange blood tests as required. These may include:
  - full blood count
  - electrolytes
  - creatinine
  - liver function tests
  - coagulation studies
  - blood group and hold
  - blood gas analysis.
- Provide counselling, information and support to the woman and her family about the seizure and ongoing management plans.

CLINICAL POINT

$MgSO_4$ has no sedative effect, so once the woman has recovered from the postictal phase she should be alert and oriented. Box 40.20 identifies the ongoing observations required once a woman has commenced $MgSO_4$.

$MgSO_4$ depresses neuromuscular transmission at the myoneural junction, causing muscular paralysis as serum levels are increased. The rationale for clinical monitoring is that loss of the patellar reflex (knee jerk) precedes respiratory depression and respiratory arrest. Frequent monitoring of the patellar reflex and respiratory rate are therefore essential if complications of therapy are to be minimised (Box 40.21). If patella reflexes are absent but the respiratory rate is not depressed, further doses of $MgSO_4$ are withheld until the reflexes return. The absence of patellar reflexes should be documented and senior personnel notified. If, however, respiration is depressed then call for urgent help, cease the infusion of $MgSO_4$ and administer calcium gluconate IV as per protocol, give facial oxygen and maintain the airway by placing the woman in the 'recovery' position. In consultation with senior staff the $MgSO_4$ can be restarted if considered necessary once reflexes have returned, but at a reduced dose unless there have been further convulsions.

$MgSO_4$ signs of toxicity are summarised in Table 40.7.

REFLECTIVE CASE STUDY

A woman presented to an emergency department during her second trimester with abdominal pain and vomiting. Previously normotensive at the antenatal clinic, her blood pressure rose from 191/110 to 210/130 mmHg while in the emergency department. She had proteinuria +++. She developed a severe headache and pain on breathing and was transferred to the labour ward where she was given a calcium-channel blocker and opiate analgesia. Following an eclamptic seizure, treatment with $MgSO_4$ and hydralazine infusion was started. First hands-on consultant involvement occurred around 8–10 hours after admission, at which time her blood pressure was still extremely high (systolic pressure still >200 mmHg) and she was unrousable. She died shortly after from a large intracranial bleed.

(Source: CEMACE, 2011, p. 69)

CLINICAL POINT

To treat toxicity, stop the infusion and consult with obstetric team. Treatment is usually calcium gluconate. Blood should be taken to assess magnesium levels and to confirm that the altered state is due to $MgSO_4$ toxicity and not another cause.

Box 40.20 Assessment and monitoring during magnesium sulfate infusion

The woman should be assessed for:

- respiratory depression
- drowsiness
- loss of consciousness
- half-hourly blood pressure, pulse, respiratory rate in the acute phase
- 1-hourly patellar reflexes
- 1-hourly urine output measurement plus 4-hourly testing of urinary protein
- 2-hourly temperature
- continuous electronic fetal monitoring.

ECG and oxygen saturation monitoring should also be considered

Box 40.21 Deep tendon reflex grading scale

4+ Hyperactive; very brisk, jerky—includes clonus if present; abnormal

3+ Brisker than average; may not be abnormal

2+ Average response, normal

1+ Diminished response; low normal

0 No response; abnormal

Table 40.7 Potential complications of increased magnesium sulfate levels

Observed condition	Target levels (i.e. normal levels) (mmol/L)
Normal plasma level	0.75–1
Therapeutic range	2.0–3.0
ECG changes	2.5–5
Loss of deep tendon reflex	5
Sinoatrial and atrioventricular block	7.5
Respiratory paralysis	7.5
Cardiac arrest	12.5

Control of hypertension

Severe hypertension is diagnosed when the diastolic pressure is ≥100 mmHg and the systolic pressure is ≥170 mmHg, with immediate management required to lower the blood pressure (Lowe et al., 2015). In New Zealand, once the systolic pressure reaches ≥160 mmHg and the diastolic pressure is ≥110 mmHg, urgent antihypertensive treatment should be commenced (MOH, 2022). In Australia these values may differ dependent on regional and organisational guidelines (Safer Care Victoria, 2020). The aim of antihypertensive therapy is to reduce and stabilise the blood pressure. It is important not to decrease the blood pressure too quickly or by too much, as this may further reduce placental perfusion. The aim is to decrease the systolic pressure by about 20–30 mmHg and the diastolic pressure by 10–15 mmHg.

Calcium channel blockers such as nifedepine, betablockers such as labetalol and vasodilators such as hydralazine are recommended as options for treating severe hypertension during pregnancy and the postpartum (MOH, 2022). Box 40.22 identifies the different drugs, dosage and frequency of use for women with severe hypertension.

Fluid balance

Acute pulmonary oedema is a significant cause of morbidity and mortality in severe preeclampsia. Fluid balance should be monitored very closely. If the urinary output is <100 mL in 4 hours the $MgSO_4$ infusion should be ceased immediately.

Severe preeclampsia / eclampsia is associated with high peripheral resistance, haemoconcentration, reduction and central distribution of plasma volume and oliguria. Pulmonary oedema from excessive fluid administration is a major cause of maternal morbidity and mortality in cases of severe preeclampsia / eclampsia. A strict limit to fluid intake should be adhered to and input / output carefully monitored and documented. Tightly controlled maintenance fluids should still be given to prevent maternal hypotension and fetal compromise especially prior to epidural analgesia or giving hydralazine (Brown & Garovic, 2011).

Box 40.22 Antihypertensive agents for acute lowering of severe hypertension

Nifedipine
- 10 mg immediate release tablet (oral)
- Onset of action: 30–45 minutes
- Onset of maximum effect: 30 minutes
- Repeat: after 30–45 minutes (if needed)
- Maximum: 80 mg daily

Labetalol
- Initially 20 mg IV bolus over 2 minutes
- Onset of action: 5 minutes
- Onset of maximum effect: 10–15 minutes
- Repeat with 40–80 mg
- Repeat: every 10 minutes (if needed)
- Maximum: 300 mg

Hydralazine
- 5–10 mg IV bolus over 3–10 minutes (5 mg if fetal compromise)
- Onset of action: 20 minutes
- Onset of maximum effect: 10–80 minutes
- Repeat: every 20 minutes
- Maximum: 30 mg
- Consider IV bolus of crystalloid fluid before or when administering first IV hydralazine dose (usually 200–300 mL)

Source: MOH, 2018)

Birth

Birth is the definitive treatment for eclampsia after the woman's condition has been stabilised. No attempt should be made to expedite the birth either vaginally or by caesarean until the acute phase of the seizure or coma has passed. The timing and place of birth depend on the maternal and fetal condition. Referral to a tertiary / regional centre for advice and / or assistance is crucial in all cases of severe preeclampsia or eclampsia. Expediting the birth by caesarean section or induction of labour may be appropriate. If pre-term, corticosteroids for fetal lung maturation should be administered.

The mode of birth should be based on obstetric indications but should be chosen with awareness that vaginal birth is preferable from a maternal standpoint. Adequate maternal analgesia is vital and may be provided with either systemic opioids or epidural anaesthesia (in the absence of coagulopathy). In the absence of fetal malpresentation or signs of fetal compromise, oxytocin or prostaglandins may be administered to induce labour.

Postpartum management

$MgSO_4$ should be continued for at least 24 hours after the last seizure. In part because of the large amount of IV fluids the woman will have received plus the potential for renal insufficiency, the woman is at risk of fluid overload. It is vital to monitor and assess fluid input and output and document these on a fluid balance chart (Lowe et al., 2015). Pulse oximetry and frequent pulmonary auscultation are important, especially in women with pre-existing chronic hypertension, abnormal renal function or placental abruption. Antihypertensive medications are continued and titrated as required.

Al-Safi et al. (2011) suggest that the first week after birth is the most critical period for the development of postpartum eclampsia. Hence timing of discharge should take into account the risk of late seizures. Before discharge a full medical review is required.

Follow-up care

According to SOMANZ (Lowe et al., 2015), studies of the risk of recurrent preeclampsia in women with a history of a pregnancy-related disorder in a prior pregnancy show variable results. Women with a history of preeclampsia have about a 14% risk of developing preeclampsia in subsequent pregnancies. However, it is clear (Lowe et al., 2015) that women with a history of hypertensive disease in pregnancy are at considerable risk of subsequent cardiovascular morbidity. Discussing the risks and educating the woman and her family about the possibility of delayed postpartum preeclampsia is important, regardless of whether she already has hypertensive disease or develops it prior to discharge (Al-Safi et al., 2011).

Aftercare includes the following:

- A recommendation that women stay in a secondary/tertiary hospital for at least 72 hours following the birth. Discharge decisions should be individually based and contingent on the ability to ensure ongoing monitoring and follow-up arrangements (MOH, 2022).
- Appropriate and timely communication with the lead maternity carer/community health provider.
- Blood pressure should be assessed, at home 24 hours post discharge, then at one week and approximately weekly dependent on BP stability and condition severity (MOH, 2022).
- Postnatal review at 6 weeks postpartum to discuss the events of the pregnancy should be offered to women whose pregnancies have been complicated by severe preeclampsia.
- Referral to appropriate specialists if there is persistent hypertension or proteinuria.
- Pre-conceptual counselling should be offered, where risk factors and preventative therapies (e.g. calcium supplementation, low-dose aspirin) can be discussed.
- Screening for pre-existing hypertension, underlying renal disease and thrombophilia should be offered to women with a history of severe preeclampsia.
- Ongoing assessment of traditional cardiovascular risk markers is of benefit to women who are normotensive but who had a hypertensive disorder of pregnancy.
- Overweight women should be encouraged to attain a healthy BMI <25 for long-term health and to decrease the risk of complication in future pregnancies.
- The woman's general practitioner should be sent a comprehensive discharge summary.

Outcomes and complications

In recent years the incidence of eclampsia has declined in industrialised countries (Liu et al., 2011). However, many women will experience short- and long-term deficits. About 56% of women who have experienced eclampsia have transient deficits including cortical blindness (Liu et al., 2011). Studies suggest that there is an increased risk for cerebrovascular accidents (CVAs) and coronary artery disease (CAD) in eclamptic women later in life.

Other potential complications of eclampsia include the following:

- permanent neurological damage from recurrent seizures or intracranial bleeding
- renal insufficiency and acute renal failure
- fetal changes—intrauterine growth restriction, abruptio placentae, oligohydramnios
- hepatic damage and rarely hepatic rupture
- haematological compromise and DIC
- increased risk of recurrent preeclampsia/eclampsia with subsequent pregnancy
- maternal or fetal/neonatal death (Liu et al., 2011).

Summary—eclampsia

Eclampsia remains a major, albeit rare and declining, cause of maternal and perinatal morbidity and mortality in Australia and New Zealand. It is often associated with other morbidity, such as pre-term birth. The relationship between the onset of preeclampsia and eclampsia is not fully understood. Optimal emergency management of seizures, hypertension and fluid balance and subsequent safe transfer are essential to minimise morbidity and mortality. It is important that midwives are able to manage an eclamptic seizure until they are able to access support.

CRITICAL THINKING EXERCISE

In a simulated learning environment, role-play the management of a term pregnant woman having an eclamptic seizure. Make you sure that you note when:

- seizure starts
- seizure ends
- help is called, etc.
- arrival of:
  - midwives
  - obstetric specialist registrar or consultant
  - anaesthetic specialist registrar or consultant
- correct positioning (left lateral)
- airway assessment and management
- delivery of oxygen
- intravenous access
- pharmacological intervention
- monitoring: oxygen saturation in arterial blood, blood pressure (non-invasively), heart rate and rhythm (electrocardiography), blood glucose concentration, fetal wellbeing (cardiotocography), renal function (urinary catheter), fluid balance, signs of magnesium toxicity
- birth plan
- documentation
- debriefing.

HELLP syndrome

HELLP syndrome is a rare but life-threatening liver disorder that is thought to be a severe manifestation of severe preeclampsia. Not all women who develop preeclampsia will develop HELLP, which has an incidence of 0.5–0.9% of all pregnancies and in 10–20% of those with severe preeclampsia.

It is characterised by **H**aemolysis (destruction of red blood cells), **E**levated **L**iver enzymes (which indicate liver damage) and **L**ow **P**latelet count.

Many hypotheses attempt to define the pathogenesis of HELLP syndrome, but the true pathology remains unclear. HELLP syndrome has been shown to share histopathologic placental morphologic and changes in gene expression with early onset preeclampsia (Oliveira et al., 2016). Both HELLP and preeclampsia occur during the later stages of pregnancy, and sometimes after childbirth. Women may experience non-specific symptoms including malaise, fatigue, right upper quadrant or epigastric pain, nausea and/or vomiting, jaundice, flu-like symptoms or visual disturbances

On examination, oedema, hypertension and proteinuria are often found and sometimes tenderness over the liver. Early diagnosis is critical to prevent liver distension, rupture and haemorrhage and the onset of DIC. Indicators of HELLP are identified in Box 40.23.

Diagnosis of HELLP syndrome relies on recognising haemolysis with fragmented red cells on the blood film and a raised lactate dehydrogenase (LDH) >600 IU/L with a raised bilirubin. Liver enzymes are raised, with an aspartate aminotransferase (AST) or alanine aminotransferase (ALT) level of >70 IU/L; levels of >150 IU/L are associated with increased maternal morbidity and mortality. Alkaline phosphatase (ALP) is another liver enzyme that may be raised in HELLP syndrome and is often still raised after other liver enzymes have returned to normal.

Treatment

The optimal treatment is to expedite the birth of the baby, commence anti-hypertensive drugs and magnesium sulfate (as per protocol) (MOH, 2018). Monitoring, intrapartum care and postpartum care are all similar to that for eclampsia.

Box 40.23 Indicators of HELLP

In a woman with preeclampsia, the presence of any of the following is an indicator of HELLP:

- Maternal platelet count of less than 100×10^9/L
- Elevated transaminases (elevated blood concentrations of liver enzymes to twice normal concentration)
- Microangiopathic haemolytic anaemia with red cell fragments on blood film

HELLP = Haemolysis, Elevated Liver enzymes, Low Platelet count.

(Source: Diagnosis and Treatment of Hypertension and Preeclampsia in Pregnancy in New Zealand: A Clinical Practice Guideline (MOH, 2022))

Outcomes and complications

The risk of maternal mortality and morbidity are increased. The most common cause of maternal death is liver rupture.

Maternal complications of HELLP syndrome may include the following:

- haematological—thrombocytopenia (maternal platelet count of less than 100×10^9/L), haemolysis, DIC, bleeding, hepatic haematoma
- cardiac—cardiac arrest, myocardial ischaemia
- pulmonary—pulmonary oedema, respiratory failure, pulmonary embolism, ARDS
- CNS—haemorrhage / stroke, cerebral oedema, central venous thrombosis, seizures, retinal detachment
- renal—acute renal failure, chronic renal failure requiring dialysis
- hepatic—elevated liver enzymes (elevated transaminases), hepatic (usually subcapsular) haematoma with possible rupture, ascites, nephrogenic diabetes insipidus, infection (Lichtman et al., 2010).

Cardiac arrest in pregnancy

Pregnant women can experience cardiac arrest as a result of life-threatening conditions that occur in pregnancy, during labour and birth and in the immediate postpartum period. The physiological changes of pregnancy affect the process of resuscitation as well as outcomes for the woman and baby. The most common causes of cardiac arrest in pregnancy are related to haemorrhage, infection and complications of hypertension.

Cardiac arrest in pregnancy is most commonly caused by:

- cardiac disease
- pulmonary embolism
- poisoning and self-harm
- hypertensive disorders of pregnancy
- sepsis
- haemorrhage
- amniotic fluid embolism
- haemorrhage and shock from a ruptured ectopic pregnancy.

Pregnant women can also have the same causes of cardiac arrest as females of the same age group (e.g. anaphylaxis, drug overdose, trauma perhaps from self-harm or motor vehicle accidents, family violence).

Resuscitation in pregnancy

Cardiac arrest occurs about once in every 30,000 pregnancies, and maternal and fetal survival from this catastrophic event is rare. All maternity care providers, irrespective of their place of work, have a duty of care to the woman in need of resuscitation and should therefore be competent in both basic life support (BLS) (Fig. 40.15) and advanced cardiac life support (ACLS) (Fig. 40.16) (Bennett et al., 2016). Certain circumstances require different interventions or slight alterations to these protocols (see below), but the principles remain the same. The following is a brief summary of the most important issues to highlight during adult BLS training.

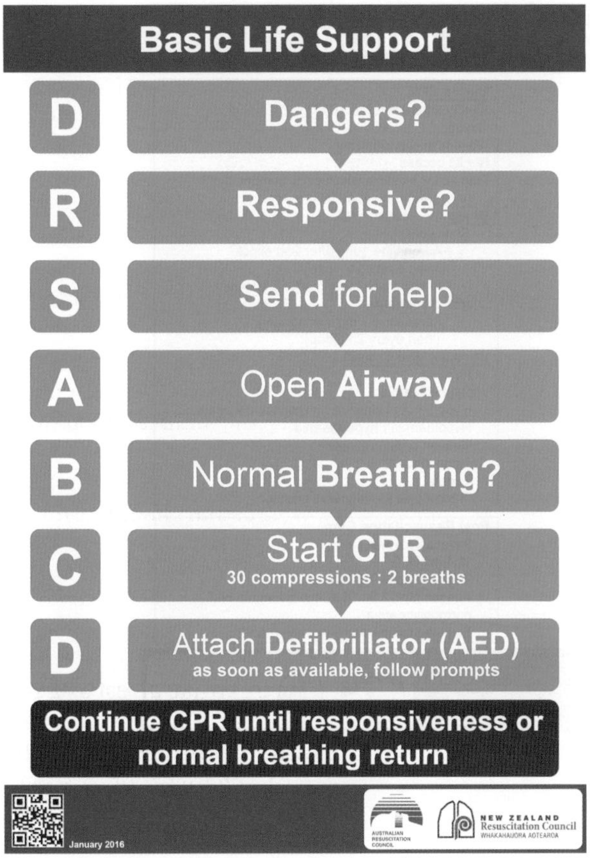

FIGURE 40.15 Basic life support for adults
(Reproduced with permission of the Australian Resuscitation Council, www.resus.org.au)

The International Liaison Committee on Resuscitation (ILCOR) publishes international recommendations and guidelines on maternal resuscitation on their website http://www.ilcor.org/home/. These are contextualised and guidelines are provided for Australia and New Zealand through each country's national resuscitation councils. Fig. 40.17 demonstrates the steps to follow during resuscitation of a pregnant woman.

The optimal management of a cardiac arrest during pregnancy must take into account the physiological changes of pregnancy as they relate to resuscitation. In summary there are significant changes in the airway (A), breathing (B) and circulation (C) during pregnancy, and therefore important resuscitation modifications must be made to maximise the chance of a successful resuscitation. Some texts/policies refer to the mnemonic acronym 'DRSABCD Action Plan'. The letters DRSABCD stand for:

- **D** Check for **D**anger
- **R** Check for **R**esponse
- **S** **S**end for help
- **A** Open the **A**irway
- **B** Check **B**reathing; if not, need to give two rescue breaths at this point
- **C** **C**ompressions; rescuers to perform 30 compressions to victims who are unresponsive and not breathing normally, followed by 2 breaths. If unwilling/unable to perform rescue breathing, then perform compression-only CPR.
- **D** **D**efibrillator; directs rescuers to attach an automated external defibrillator (AED) as soon as it is available.

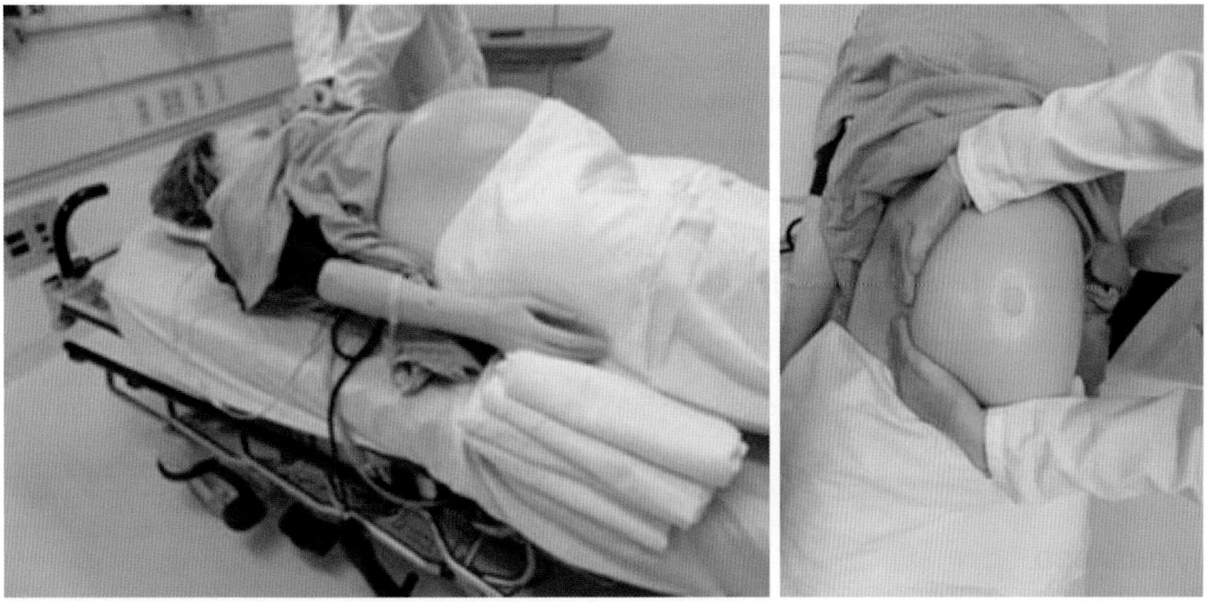

FIGURE 40.16 Starting chest compressions and pulling the gravid uterus laterally
(Source: Saksena & Camm, 2012. Figure 73-8B. *Electrophysiological Disorders of the Heart*. 2nd ed. ©2005, 2012 by Saunders, an imprint of Elsevier Inc.)

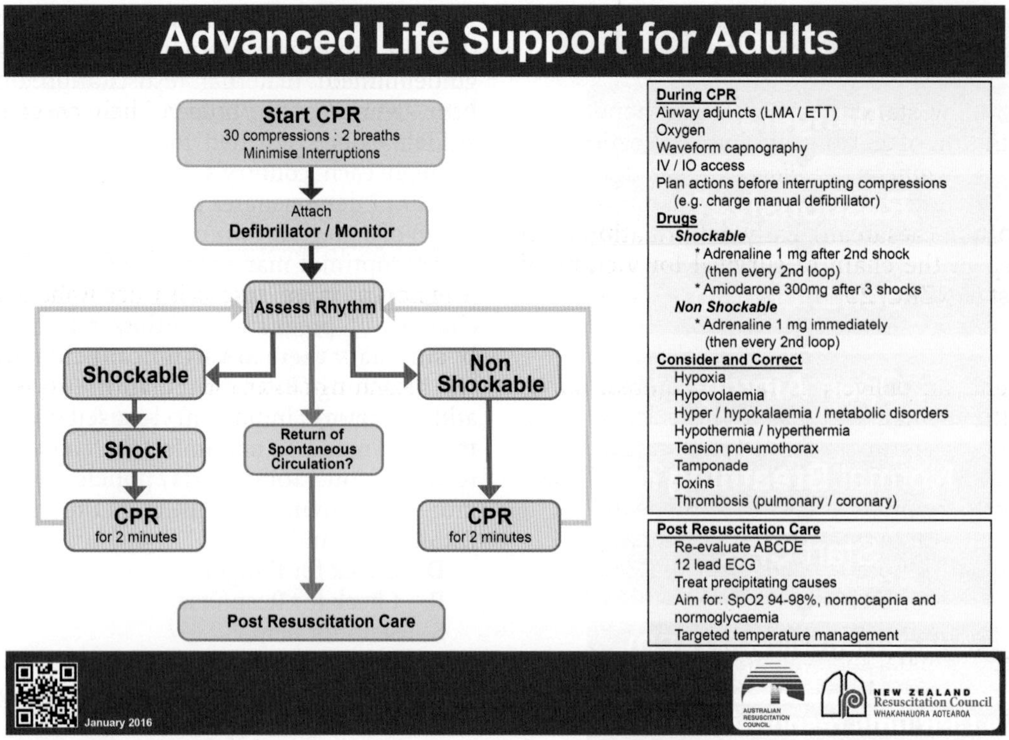

FIGURE 40.17 Advanced life support for adults
(Reproduced with permission of the Australian Resuscitation Council, www.resus.org.au)

There are a number of physiological reasons why CPR is more difficult and less successful in pregnancy. These include the increased cardiac output, blood volume, minute ventilation, oxygen consumption and reduced lung volumes which make management of the ABCs more difficult. Women become hypoxic mores quickly, intubation is more difficult and gastric reflux is more likely. The size of the uterus can compress the abdominal organs and major blood vessels when the woman is in the supine position, which can result in reduced cardiac output and hypotension.

During a cardiac arrest, all the principles of basic and advanced life support apply, but with adaptations. These involve the following.

- Manually displace the uterus to the left to remove caval compression. Add left lateral tilt if this is feasible (the optimal angle of tilt is unknown).
- The angle of tilt used needs to allow high-quality chest compressions.
- Caesarean delivery of the fetus may be considered by the obstetric team.

Modifications to standard basic life support and advanced cardiac life support guidelines

Primary DRSABCD.

- *Primary survey*—assess for *danger* and *safety* to rescuers prior to resuscitation—ensure it is safe to commence resuscitation and not put rescuers at risk of ill health or death.
- *Responsiveness*—determine whether the woman is conscious or unconscious. This can be done by tactile and verbal stimulation.
- *Shout* (call for help)—if the woman is unresponsive, she is considered to be unconscious and assistance should be sought using an appropriate 'code'.
- *Airway*—no modifications.
- *Breathing*—no modifications; assess whether the woman is breathing normally and if not then commence CPR immediately.
- *Circulation*—chest compressions are ineffective when a woman in her last trimester lies on her back because the gravid uterus blocks the return of blood from the inferior vena cava. Start chest compressions after placing the woman on her left side with her back at an angle from the floor using a ratio of 30 compressions to 2 breaths.

  Start chest compressions after placing a wedge under the woman's right side (so that she lies on her left side), or have one rescuer kneel next to the woman on her left side and gently pull the gravid uterus laterally to relieve pressure on the inferior vena cava (Fig. 40.17).
- *Defibrillation*—no modifications; defibrillatory shocks transfer no significant current to the fetus in utero.

Secondary ABCD.

- *Airway*—no modifications to intubation techniques, although intubation is often more difficult.
- *Breathing*—no modifications secondary to confirmation of successful intubation; a gravid uterus is known

to push up the diaphragm and therefore decrease ventilator volumes and make positive-pressure ventilation difficult.
- *Circulation*—follow standard ACLS recommendations for administration of all resuscitation medications.
- *Defibrillation* and *differential diagnosis and decisions*—decide whether to perform emergency caesarean section (perimortem caesarean). Early defibrillation is an essential step in the chain of survival for victims of cardiac arrest (ANZRC, 2016).

Perimortem caesarean delivery

Perimortem caesarean delivery is rarely required, but is performed on the woman who has a viable fetus where maternal resuscitation is unsuccessful. Expediting the birth improves thoracic compliance, which improves the efficacy of chest compressions and the ability to ventilate the lungs. According to the '4-minute rule', if maternal resuscitation is unsuccessful after 4 minutes of CPR the fetus should be delivered by the fifth minute. CPR is continued throughout the procedure and afterwards, in a final effort to improve the maternal and perinatal survival rate.

A few cases of maternal survival after the birth of the baby during unsuccessful cardiopulmonary resuscitation (CPR) have been reported. It is also possible to commence transabdominal cardiac massage or, if the chest wall is opened, open-chest cardiac massage (OCM).

Trauma in pregnancy

Trauma during pregnancy can cause maternal and fetal morbidity and mortality. Where it results in mortality, it is identified as coincidental death by the perinatal and maternal mortality review groups and includes accidental injury and motor vehicle accidents. The number of deaths from these causes is small and difficult to identify due to other causes of death being included in the category. Types of injury may include:
- head injury—major cause of death
- pelvic fractures—can result in severe haemorrhage and fetal death
- other injuries:
  - diaphragmatic tear
  - urinary bladder injury
  - uterine injury
  - fetal injury.

Trauma and maternal and neonatal mortality

Motor vehicle accidents (MVA) and domestic violence/intimate partner violence are the most common mechanisms of traumatic injury during pregnancy (Mendez-Figueroa et al., 2013). Vivian-Taylor et al. (2012) in their population cohort study of 600,000 Australian women explored the incidence of MVA during pregnancy and outcomes. They found an incidence of 3.5 women per 1000 maternities were admitted to hospital following an MVA. For women who were less than 20 weeks gestation immediate birth was uncommon (0.4%) but for women who were more than 20 weeks 96% continued with their pregnancy and had similar pregnancy outcomes as other women not involved in an MVA. For the 3.5% who gave birth immediately, there was increased risk of antepartum haemorrhage, preterm birth, caesarean section and perinatal death.

Relationships between the physiological changes in pregnancy and trauma

The non-pregnant uterus is thick walled and protected by the pelvic girdle but loses this protection as it expands out of the pelvis from about 12 weeks gestation (Box 40.24). By the second trimester the growing fetus is protected somewhat by amniotic fluid (Oxford & Ludmir, 2009). By the third trimester the uterus is thin walled, and by the 36th week of pregnancy the head may engage in the pelvis.

Box 40.24 Trauma in pregnancy

Unique problems of the pregnant woman with trauma:
- The placenta is devoid of elastic tissue but the myometrium is very elastic, predisposing to shearing from the uterine wall.
- After 12 weeks gestation, the bladder is displaced upwards and forwards by the enlarging uterus, leading to an increased risk of bladder injury from blunt or penetrating trauma.
- The trachea is displaced to the right. Upward displacement of the diaphragm and viscera decreases chest compliance and ventilation and makes chest compression in CPR more difficult.
- Because of the enlarging uterus, the diaphragm rises by about 4 cm and the diameter of the chest enlarges by about 2%.
- As pregnancy progresses, there is a decrease in the functional residual capacity of the lungs, coupled with a 20% increase in oxygen consumption, making women more prone to hypoxia. Further, 30% of pregnant women have airway closure during normal tidal ventilation if they are placed in a supine position. All these alterations predispose pregnant women to a rapid decrease in maternal P_aO_2 during periods of apnoea or airway obstruction.
- Changes in the gastrointestinal tract and increased levels of progesterone make pregnant women more prone to regurgitation of gastric contents and Mendelson's syndrome.
- Enlarged breast tissue also makes chest compression more difficult.
- From 16 weeks gestation following trauma, the most common cause of pre-term labour is abruptio placentae (the most common complication following blunt injury).
- Fetal skull injury is the most common fetal injury, with a mortality rate of 42%.

When full, the bladder also becomes an abdominal organ and therefore prone to trauma. An increase in heart rate and stroke volume leads to an increase in cardiac output by about 50% in pregnancy. Blood volume has increased by as much as 50% by the 28th week of gestation. The protective effects of hypervolaemia allow the woman to lose up to 30% (1500 mL) of her circulating blood volume before signs associated with hypotension appear (Cusick & Tibbles, 2007). However, it is not uncommon for a pregnant woman to have what is often called 'low blood pressure'—perhaps 80/40 mmHg in early pregnancy, although late in the second trimester the blood pressure returns to 'normal' levels.

Maternal posture, haemodynamics and their relationships to trauma and resuscitation

In the third trimester, the heavy gravid uterus compresses the descending aorta and the inferior vena cava. This results in a greater tendency for pooling of venous blood in the lower limbs, decreasing venous return from the heart, a fall in cardiac output and hypotension (Oxford & Ludmir, 2009). One of the first signs of supine hypotension is a non-reassuring FHR caused by decreased uteroplacental perfusion. If the woman is supine, cardiac return may be reduced by as much as 30%. This affects the woman's cardiac output. It is therefore important to tilt the pregnant woman to the left by about 30°; alternatively manually displace the uterine fundus to the woman's left (Fig. 40.18). However, it should be remembered that airway control and efforts to reduce the risk of supine hypotension must be balanced against the need to stabilise the cervical spine (Sugrue et al., 2004).

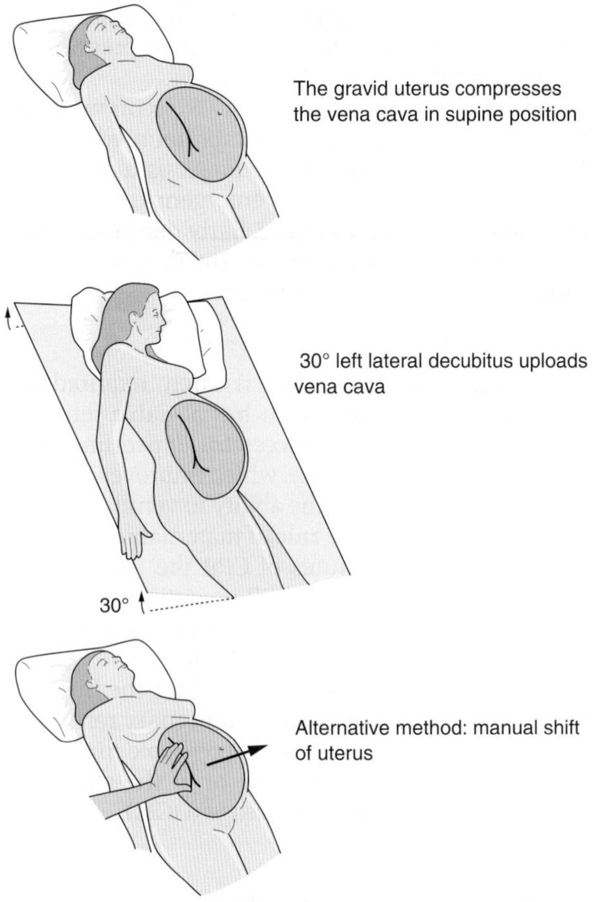

FIGURE 40.18 Management of supine hypotension

Management

Principles of first-line management in the emergency department

Women with minor trauma and who are at less than 20 weeks gestation do not require pregnancy-specific intervention or monitoring. After 20 weeks gestation the pregnant woman with serious traumatic injury requires a multidisciplinary team, which includes an obstetrician, a trauma surgeon, a neonatologist and skilled nurses and midwives. All pregnant women who are more than 20 weeks pregnant who have direct or indirect abdominal trauma should undergo at least 4 hours of cardiotocographic monitoring before discharge, ensuring a normal fetal heart rate pattern is recorded prior to discharge. Resuscitation must always focus on the woman because the most common causes of fetal death are associated with maternal shock or maternal death. The woman will sustain her vital signs at the cost of the fetus because the woman shunts blood away from the uterus. Plasma volume is increased 50%, and maternal shock may not be noticeable until maternal blood loss exceeds 30%.

If the woman is more than 24 weeks pregnant, she should be tilted 15–30° to the left. If she does not require spinal immobilisation, she can be asked to assume the left-lateral position.

Resuscitation. If the woman is haemodynamically compromised, so too is the blood supply to the fetus, which rapidly becomes hypoxic and acidotic. Consequently, the key to resuscitation of the fetus is resuscitation of the woman. The woman cannot be resuscitated until blood flow to her right ventricle is restored, and therefore prevention of supine hypotension caused by the gravid uterus pressing on the woman's major blood vessels must be prevented. Blood pressure can, however, be a distraction; if low it confirms the woman is significantly hypovolaemic but conversely a normal BP does not necessarily imply a normovolaemic, fully resuscitated woman.

Once the woman is haemodynamically stable the following radiological tests can be performed. The following plain films are taken:

- chest
- pelvis
- lateral C spine.

Complications of trauma

The most common complication of trauma in pregnancy is uterine contractions and the onset of labour. Myometrial and decidual cells damaged by contusion or placental separation release prostaglandins, which stimulate uterine contractions (Oxford & Ludmir, 2009). These may or may not be painful. Occasional uterine contractions are very common after trauma and in the vast majority of cases will resolve in a few hours, and are therefore not associated with adverse perinatal outcomes. Progression to true labour depends on the extent of uterine trauma, the amount of prostaglandins released and the gestational age of the fetus (Muench & Canterino, 2007).

- Rupture of amniotic membranes can lead to chorioamnionitis, pre-term labour and cord prolapse.
- Retroperitoneal haemorrhage, uterine rupture (diagnosed with maternal hypotension, palpation of fetal part, radiographic findings) and amniotic fluid embolism may lead to acute respiratory distress syndrome.

Definitive care

Ongoing management of any further injuries should be undertaken at the closest trauma centre as soon as possible. A history of abdominal trauma (particularly with ultrasound evidence of intraperitoneal fluid), persistent hypotension and tachycardia despite appropriate fluid resuscitation is an indication for immediate midline laparotomy to definitively control intra-abdominal bleeding (abruption, uterine rupture, splenic rupture, vascular injury, etc.). If a caesarean section is necessary, trauma surgeons should be present to assess and treat any maternal injuries. The trauma team may consider venous thromboembolism prophylaxis. If required, Rh (D) immunoglobulin (625 IU CSL for gestation >12 weeks) is administered (if the woman is Rhesus negative and has no pre-existent Rh (D) antibodies). In most cases, all women suffering trauma in pregnancy (irrespective of degree) should be admitted to a maternity unit for fetal assessment if the gestational age is thought to be ≥20 weeks. It is safe to administer tetanus toxoid in pregnancy (Oxford & Ludmir, 2009).

Placental abruption

Maternal trauma may be associated with placental abruption. Placental abruption occurs when shearing forces lead to a separation of the rigid placenta from the elastic uterus. Up to 30%–50% of pregnant women with major traumatic injuries and about 5% with minor injuries have placental abruption after trauma (Muench & Canterino, 2007). It is the most common cause of fetal death when the woman survives the trauma. Placental abruption may be delayed for as long as 24–48 hours after the traumatic incident, although most cases of abruption become evident within several hours after trauma.

Box 40.25 Discharge following fetomaternal haemorrhage

- Before discharge: ensure all Rh (D)-negative women with abdominal trauma have received a dose of 625 IU CSL Rh D immunoglobulin even if the Kleihauer test is negative
- The woman is counselled to return if:
  - any signs of pre-term labour
  - abdominal pain and/or vaginal bleeding
  - any change in fetal movements.

KB = Kleihauer–Betke; Rh = Rhesus.

Fetomaternal haemorrhage

Blunt trauma to the abdomen increases the risk of fetomaternal haemorrhage (FMH)—the transplacental haemorrhage of fetal blood into the normally separate maternal circulation. It is a rare but severe complication that can result in fetal anaemia, fetal hypoxia, intrauterine death or neonatal neurological damage (Taronen et al., 2011). The reported incidence of FMH after trauma is 8%–30%. Complications of FMH include Rhesus sensitisation in the woman, fetal anaemia, fetal atrial tachycardia and fetal death from exsanguination (Taronen et al., 2011). FMH is most likely to occur after 12 weeks gestation, when the uterus rises above the pelvis and becomes more susceptible to direct trauma. FMH is primarily detected by the Kleihauer test.

Box 40.25 provides discharge criteria following fetomaternal haemorrhage.

Summary

Grossman (2004, p. 1309) comments that, despite advances in trauma management, fetal and maternal mortality rates from traumatic injury have not declined. Prevention is therefore the key to increasing maternal and fetal survival. Both motor vehicle accidents and domestic assault are preventable causes of trauma in pregnancy. Even in countries where seatbelt use is compulsory, pregnant women have lower rates of seatbelt use than non-pregnant women.

Conclusion

Although childbirth is, for most women, a healthy event, some may develop life-threatening complications requiring complex levels of medical and technological intervention. The most important of these emergencies are: umbilical cord presentation and prolapse, shoulder dystocia, uterine inversion, amniotic fluid embolism, disseminated intravascular coagulation, eclampsia, rupture of the uterus, maternal trauma, cardiac arrest and postpartum haemorrhage.

As these emergencies frequently arise with little or no warning, midwives and all healthcare practitioners must ensure that their clinical practice and life-support skills are kept up to date and are based on the best available evidence.

Review questions

1. Identify the major causes of postpartum haemorrhage, and for each one describe the appropriate strategies to prevent or manage it should it occur.
2. Describe the identification and assessment of a woman who has developed an amniotic fluid embolism.
3. Discuss the manoeuvres that may be used during a shoulder dystocia.
4. Discuss five interventions you would initiate for a woman who appears to have a cord prolapse.
5. Make a directory of the support networks available near you for women who have had a traumatic pregnancy and birth.

Acknowledgements

The authors would like to acknowledge the work of Carol Thorogood and Helen Cooke, who contributed to the previous edition of this text.

Online resources

Australian Action on Pre-eclampsia: https://www.aapec.org.au/.
Australian College of Midwives: http://www.midwives.org.au.
Australian Institute of Health and Welfare (AIHW). National Perinatal Data Collection: https://www.aihw.gov.au/about-our-data/our-data-collections/national-perinatal-data-collection.
Australian Nursing and Midwifery Council (ANMC). 2006. National Competency Standards for the Midwife: http://www.anmc.org.au/. [L'D: AQ? Or replace with: 'https://anmac.org.au/standards-and-review/midwife']
Australian Resuscitation Council https://resus.org.au/.
Cochrane Library—contains high-quality, independent evidence to inform healthcare decision-making: http://www.cochrane.org.
Health Navigator New Zealand. Post-traumatic Stress Disorder: https://www.healthnavigator.org.nz/health-a-z/p/post-traumatic-stress-disorder-ptsd/.
Midwifery Council of New Zealand (MCNZ): http://www.midwiferycouncil.health.nz/.
New Zealand Resuscitation Council https://www.nzrc.org.nz.
Perinatal and Maternal Mortality Review Committee (PMMRC): http://www.hqsc.govt.nz/our-programmes/mrc/pmmrc/.

References

Advanced Life Support in Obstetrics (ALSO). *Provider Manual.* 8th ed. Kansas: ALSO; 2017.
Aiken CEM, Mehasseb MK, Prentice A, et al. *A Comprehensive Textbook of Postpartum Hemorrhage: An Essential Clinical Reference for Effective Management.* 2nd ed. London: Sapiens; 2011.
Al-Safi Z, Imudia AN, Filetti LC, et al. Delayed postpartum preeclampsia and eclampsia: demographics, clinical course, and complications. *Obstet Gynecol.* 2011;118(5):1102–1107.
Ambrose A, Repke JT. Puerperal problems. In: James DK, Steer PJ, Weiner CP, et al., eds. *High Risk Pregnancy.* 3rd ed. Philadelphia: Elsevier; 2011:1313–1329.
American Congress of Obstetricians and Gynecologists (ACOG). Clinical findings in obstetric haemorrhage. *Obstet Gynecol.* 2006a;108:1039–1047.
American Congress of Obstetricians and Gynecologists (ACOG). ACOG practice bulletin: clinical management guidelines for obstetrician-gynecologists number 76, October 2006: postpartum hemorrhage. *Obstet Gynecol.* 2006b;108(4):1039–1047.
Anderson J, Etches DJ. Postpartum haemorrhage: third stage emergency. In: Damos JD, Eisinger SH, Baxley EG, eds. *Advanced Life Support in Obstetrics Course Syllabus.* 4th ed. Leawood, Kansas: American Academy of Family Physicians; 2001.
Ansell Irving L, McAra-Couper J, Smythe E. Shoulder dystocia: a qualitative exploration of what works. *Midwifery.* 2012; 28(4):E461–E468. doi:10.1016/j.midw.2011.05.007.
Ansell L, Ansell D, McAra-Couper J, et al. Axillary traction: An effective method of resolving shoulder dystocia. *Aust Maternity Outcomes Surveill Sys.* 2019;59:627–633.
Balki M, Ramachandran N, Lee S, et al. The recovery time of myometrial responsiveness after oxytocin-induced desensitization in human myometrium in vitro. *Anesth Analg.* 2016;122(5): 1508–1515. doi:10.1213/ane.0000000000001268.
Bastos M, Furuta M, Small R, et al. Debriefing interventions for the prevention of psychological trauma in women following childbirth. *Cochrane Database Syst Rev.* 2015;4: CD007194. doi: 10.1002/14651858.CD007194.pub2.
Belfort MA, Dildy GA III. Postpartum haemorrhage and other problems of the third stage. In: James DK, Weiner CP, Steer PJ, et al., eds. *High Risk Pregnancy Management Options.* 4th ed. St Louis: Elsevier Saunders; 2011:1307–1308.
Bennett TA, Katz VL, Zelop CM. Cardiac arrest and resuscitation unique to pregnancy. *Obstet Gynecol Clin North Am.* 2016; 43(4):809–819.
Benson MD. Current concepts of immunology and diagnosis in amniotic fluid embolism. *Clin Dev Immunol.* 2012;2012: 946576.
Blackburn S. *Maternal, Fetal and Neonatal Physiology: A Clinical Perspective.* 4th ed. London: WB Saunders; 2013.
Boulvain M, Irion O, Dowswell T, et al. Induction of labour at or near term for suspected fetal macrosomia. *Cochrane Database Syst Rev.* 2016;5:CD000938, doi:10.1002/14651858.CD000938.pub2.
Brown CM, Garovic VD. Mechanisms and management of hypertension in pregnant women. *Curr Hypertens Rep.* 2011;13: 338–346. doi:10.1007/s11906-011-0214-y.
Burtelow M, Riley E, Druzin M, et al. How we treat: management of life-threatening primary postpartum hemorrhage with a standardized massive transfusion protocol. *Transfusion.* 2007; 47:1564–1572.
Cahill AG, Macones GA, Odibo AO, et al. Magnesium for seizure prophylaxis in patients with mild pre-eclampsia. *Obstet Gynecol.* 2007;110:601–607.
Canterbury DHB Te Poari Hauora o Waitaha (CDHB). Christchurch Women's Hospital Maternity Guidelines, Shoulder Dystocia, GLM0011; 2021.
Centre for Maternal and Child Enquiries (CMACE). Confidential Enquiries into Maternal Deaths in the United Kingdom (CMACE) 8th report. Reviewing maternal deaths to make womanhood safer: 2006–2008. *BJOG.* 2011;118(suppl 1): 1–203.
Cheerranichanunth P, Poolnoi P. Using blood loss pictogram for visual blood loss estimation in cesarean section. *J Med Assoc Thail.* 2012;95(4):550–556.

Coad SL, Dahlgren LS, Hutcheon JA. Risks and consequences of puerperal uterine inversion in the United States, 2004 through 2013. *Am J Obstet Gynecol.* 2017;217(3):377.e1–377.e6. doi:10.1016/j.ajog.2017.05.018.

Cooray SD, Edmonds SM, Tong S, et al. Characterization of symptoms immediately preceding eclampsia. *Obstet Gynecol.* 2011; 118(5):995–999.

Cunningham FG, Nelson DB. Disseminated intravascular coagulation syndromes in obstetrics. *Obstet Gynecol.* 2015;126(5): 999–1011. doi:10.1097/AOG.0000000000001110.

Cusick SS, Tibbles CD. Trauma in pregnancy. *Emerg Med Clin North Am.* 2007;25(3):861–872, xi.

Dahlke JD, Mendez-Figueroa H, Maggio L, et al. Prevention and management of postpartum hemorrhage: a comparison of 4 national guidelines. *Am J Obstet Gynecol.* 2015;213(1): 76.e1–76.e10. doi:10.1016/j.ajog.2015.02.023.

Dekker GA, Chan A, Luke CG, et al. Risk of uterine rupture in Australian women attempting vaginal birth after one prior caesarean section: a retrospective population-based cohort study. *BJOG.* 2010;117:1358–1365.

Della Corte L, Saccone G, Locci M, et al. Tranexamic acid for treatment of primary postpartum hemorrhage after vaginal delivery: A systematic review and meta-analysis of randomized controlled trials. *J Matern Fetal Neonatal Med.* 2020;33(5):869–874.

De la Cruz C, Coulter M, O'Rourke K, et al. Women's experiences, emotional responses and perceptions of care after emergency peripartum hysterectomy: A qualitative survey of women from 6 months to 3 years postpartum. *Birth.* 2013;40(4):256–263.

Dossou M, Debost-Legrand A, Déchelotte P, et al. Severe secondary postpartum hemorrhage: a historical cohort. *Birth.* 2015;42(2): 149–155. doi:10.1111/birt.12164.

Eller AG, Bennett MA, Sharshiner M, et al. Maternal morbidity in cases of placenta accreta managed by a multidisciplinary care team compared with standard obstetric care. *Obstet Gynecol.* 2011;117:331–337.

Elmir R, Pangas J, Dahlen H, et al. A meta-ethnographic synthesis of midwives' and nurses' experiences of adverse labour and birth events. *J Clin Nurs.* 2017;26(23–24):4184–4200. doi:10.1111/ jocn.13965.

Fitzpatrick K, Kurinczuk J, Alfirevic Z et al. Uterine rupture by intended mode of delivery in the UK: A national case control study. *PloS Med.* 2012;9(3):e1001184. doi:10.1371/journal.pmed.1001184.

Fitzpatrick K, van den Akker T, Bloemenkamp K, et al. Risk factors, management, and outcomes of amniotic fluid embolism: A multicountry, population-based cohort and nested case-control study. *PLoS Med.* 2019:16(11):e1002962. doi:10.1371/journal. pmed.1002962.

Ford J, Patterson JA, Seeho S, et al. Trends and outcomes of postpartum haemorrhage, 2003–2011. *BMC Pregnancy Childbirth.* 2015;15(334):1–10. doi:10.1186/s12884-015-0788-5.

Gherman RB, Goodwin TM, Souter I, et al. The McRoberts' maneuver for the alleviation of shoulder dystocia: how successful is it? *Am J Obstet Gynecol.* 1997;176(3):656–661.

Gayet-Ageron A, Prieto-Merino D, Ker K, et al. Effect of treatment delay on the effectiveness and safety of antifibrinolytics in acute severe haemorrhage: A meta-analysis of individual patient-level data from 40 138 bleeding patients. *Lancet.* 2018;391(10116): 125–132. doi:10.1016/S0140-6736(17)32455-8.

Gist RS, Stafford IP, Leibowitz AB, et al. Amniotic fluid embolism. *Anesth Analg.* 2009;108:1599–1602.

Gobbo R, Baxley E, eds. Shoulder dystocia. In: *ALSO: Advanced Life Support in Obstetrics Provider Course Syllabus.* Leawood, KS: American Academy of Family Physicians; 2000.

Grossman NB. Blunt trauma in pregnancy. *Am Fam Physician.* 2004;70(7):1303–1310.

Graugaard H. Maimburg R. Is the increase in postpartum haemorrhage after vaginal birth because of altered clinical practice?: A register-based cohort study. *Birth.* 2021:48 338–346.

Grotegut C, Paglia M, Johnson L, et al. Ocytocin exposure during labour among women with post partum haemorrhage secondary to uterine atony. *Am J Obstet Gynecol.* 2011;204:56.e1–56.e6.

Hancock A, Weeks A, Fuber C, et al. The recognition of excessive blood loss at childbirth (REACT) study: a two-phase exploratory, sequential mixed methods inquiry using focus groups, interviews and a pilot randomised crossover study. *BJOG.* 2021;128(11):1843–1854.

Henderson C, Macdonald S. *Mayes' Midwifery.* 13th ed. London: Baillière Tindall; 2004.

Humphrey M. *Management of Secondary Postpartum Haemorrhage.* Melbourne: Victorian Perinatal Emergency Referral Services; 2005.

Hutcheon J, Lisonkova S, Joseph KS. Epidemiology of pre-eclampsia and the other hypertensive disorders of pregnancy. *Best Pract Res Clin Obstet Gynaecol.* 2011;25(4):391–403.

Jauniaux E, Bunce C, Gronbeck L, et al. Prevalence and main outcomes of placenta accreta spectrum a systematic review and meta analysis. *Am J Obstet Gynecol.* 2019;221(3):208–218.

Kaczmarczyk M, Sparén P, Terry P, et al. Risk factors for uterine rupture and neonatal consequences of uterine rupture: a population-based study of successive pregnancies in Sweden. *BJOG.* 2007;114:1208–1214.

Kaur K, Bhardwaj M, Kumar P, et al. Amniotic fluid embolism. *J Anaesthesiol Clin Pharmacol.* 2016;32(2):153–159.

Keag O. Norman J. Stock S. Long-term risks and benefits associated with caesarean delivery for mother, baby, and subsequent pregnancies: Systematic review and meta-analysis. *PLoS Med.* 2018; 15(1):e1002494. doi:10.1371/journal.pmed.1002494.

Knight M, Berg C, Brocklehurst P, et al. Amniotic fluid embolism incidence, risk factors and outcomes: a review and recommendations. *BMC Pregnancy Childbirth.* 2012;12:7.

Knight M, Acosta C, Brocklehurst P, UKNeS coapplicant group, et al. *Unheard Voices. Beyond Maternal Death: Improving the Quality of Maternal Care Through National Studies of 'Near-miss' Maternal Morbidity.* Southampton: NIHR Journals; 2016.

Leal R, Mano R, Pinto de Almeida J, et al. Total and acute uterine inversion after delivery: a case report. *J Med Case Rep.* 2014;8:347.

Leighton BL, Wall MH, Lockhart EM, et al. Use of recombinant factor VIIa in patients with amniotic fluid embolism: a systematic review of case reports. *Anesthesiology.* 2011;115(6):1201–1208.

Levi M, ten Cate H. Disseminated intravascular coagulation. *N Engl J Med.* 1999;341(8):586–592.

Lichtman M, Kipps T, Seligsohn U, et al. Hemolytic anemia resulting from physical injury to red cells. In: Kaushansky K, Lichtman MA, Beutler E, et al., eds. *Williams Hematology.* 8th ed. New York: McGraw-Hill; 2010:8.

Lieberman E, Ernst EK, Rooks JP, et al. Results of the national study of vaginal birth after caesarean in birth centres. *Obstet Gynecol.* 2004;104(5 Pt 1):933–942.

Lipitz S, Frenkel Y Puerperal inversion of the uterus. *Eur J Obstet Gynecol Reprod Biol.* 1988;27(3):271. Online: https://www.uptodate.com/contents/puerperal-uterine-inversion#:~:text=INTRODUCTION%20Uterine%20inversion%20occurs%20when,a%20life%2Dthreatening%20obstetric%20emergency.

Liu L, Joseph J, Liston R, et al. Incidence, risk factors, and associated complications of eclampsia. *Obstet Gynecol.* 2011;118(5): 987–994.

Lowe SA, Bowyer L, Lust K, et al. SOMANZ guidelines for the management of hypertensive disorders of pregnancy 2014. *Aust N Z J Obstet Gynaecol.* 2015;55:e1–e29. doi:10.1111/ ajo.12399.

McDonnell N, Knight M, Peek MJ, et al. Amniotic fluid embolism: an Australian–New Zealand population-based study. *BMC Pregnancy Childbirth.* 2015;15(1):352. doi:10.1186/s12884-015-0792-9.

Marieb E. *Human Anatomy and Physiology.* 6th ed. New York: Pearson; 2004.

Martel MJ, MacKinnon CJ. Guidelines for vaginal birth after caesarean birth. *J Obstet Gynaecol Can.* 2004;27(7):660–683.

Mendez-Figueroa H, Dahlke JD, Vrees RA, et al. Trauma in pregnancy: an updated systematic review. *Am J Obstet Gynecol.* 2013;209(1):1–10. doi:10.1016/j.ajog.2013.01.021.

Menticoglou S. Shoulder dystocia: incidence, mechanisms, and management strategies. *Int J Womens Health.* 2018;10:723–732.

Michelotti F. Flatley C. Kumar S. Impact of shoulder dystocia, stratified by type of manoeuvre, on severe neonatal outcome and maternal morbidity. *Aust NZ Obstet Gynecol.* 2018;58:298–305.

Ministry of Health (MOH). *National Consensus Guideline for Treatment of Postpartum Haemorrhage.* Wellington, NZ: MOH; 2013. Online: https://www.health.govt.nz/system/files/documents/publications/national-consensus-guideline-for -treatment-of-postpartum-haemorrhage-nov13-v2_0.pdf.

Ministry of Health. (MOH). *Diabetes in Pregnancy: Quick reference guide for health professionals on the screening, diagnosis and treatment of gestational diabetes in New Zealand.* Wellington, NZ: MOH; 2014.

Ministry of Health (MOH). *Diagnosis and Treatment of Hypertension and Pre-eclampsia in Pregnancy in New Zealand: A Clinical Practice Guideline.* Wellington, NZ: MOH; 2018. Online: https://www.health.govt.nz/publication/diagnosis-and-treatment-hypertension-and-pre-eclampsia-pregnancy-new-zealand-clinical-practice.

Ministry of Health (MOH). *National Consensus Guideline for Treatment of Postpartum Haemorrhage.* Wellington, NZ: MOH; 2022. Online: https://www.health.govt.nz/system/files/documents/publications/national-consensus-guideline-for-treatment-of-postpartum-haemorrhage-nov13-v2_0.pdf.

Mirza FG, Gaddipati S. Obstetric emergencies. *Semin Perinatol.* 2009;33:97–103.

Mollberg M, Wennergren M, Bager B, et al. Obstetric brachial plexus palsy: a prospective study on risk factors related to manual assistance during the second stage of labor. *Acta Obstet Gynecol Scand.* 2007;86:198–204.

Muench MV, Canterino JC. Trauma in pregnancy. *Obstet Gynecol Clin North Am.* 2007;34(3):555–583.

Oats I, Abraham S. Lllewellyn-Jones' *Fundamentals of Obstetrics.* Sydney: Elsevier; 2004.

Ogueh O, Ayida G. Acute uterine inversion: a new technique of hydrostatic replacement. *BJOG.* 1997;104:951–952.

Oliveira N, Poon L, Nicolaides K, et al. First trimester prediction of HELLP syndrome. *Prenat Diagn.* 2016;36(1):29–33.

Ouzounian J, Sanchez M, Opper N, et al. 554: Clinical risk factors do not predict shoulder dystocia. *Am J Obstet Gynecol.* 2014;210(1):S273. doi:10.1016/j.ajog.2013.10.587.

Overland EA, Vatten LJ, Eskild A. Pregnancy week at delivery and the risk of shoulder dystocia: a population study of 2,014,956 deliveries. *BJOG.* 2014;121(1):34–41. doi:10.1111/1471-0528.12427.

Oxford CM, Ludmir J. Trauma in pregnancy. *Clin Obstet Gynaecol.* 2009;52(4):611–629. doi:10.1097/GRF.0b013e3181c11edf.

Perinatal and Maternal Mortality Review Committee (PMMRC). *Tenth Annual Report of the Perinatal and Maternal Mortality Review Committee: Reporting Mortality and Morbidity 2014.* Wellington, NZ: Health Quality & Safety Commission; 2016. Online: https://www.hqsc.govt.nz/assets/PMMRC/Publications/tenth-annual-report-SUMMARY-Jun-2016.pdf.

Perinatal and Maternal Mortality Review Committee (PMMRC). *Eleventh Annual Report of the Perinatal and Maternal Mortality Review Committee: Reporting Mortality and Morbidity 2015.* Wellington, NZ: Health Quality & Safety Commission; 2017. Online: https://www.hqsc.govt.nz/assets/PMMRC/Publications/2017_PMMRC_Eleventh_Annual_Report.pdf.

Pollock W, Peek M. Wang A, et al Eclampsia in Australia and New Zealand: A prospective population-based study. *ANZJOG.* 2020;60:533–540.

Rankin J. *Physiology in Childbearing with Anatomy and Related Biosciences.* 4th ed. London: Elsevier; 2017.

Ricborg A, Gosme C, Gayat E, et al. Emotional impact of severe post partum haemorrhage on women and their partners: an observational, case-matched, prospective, single-centre pilot study. *Eur J Obstet Gynecol Reprod Biol X.* 2015;193:140–143.

Robson M. Shoulder dystocia: Is it time to think differently? *Aus NZ J Obstet Gynaecol.* 2019; 59:605–607.

Rogers MS, Chang AMZ. Post partum hemorrhage and other problems of the third stage. In: James DK, Weiner CP, Steer PJ, et al., eds. *High Risk Pregnancy.* 3rd ed. Philadelphia: Elsevier; 2006:1559–1579.

Royal College of Obstetricians and Gynaecologists (RCOG). *Shoulder Dystocia. Green-top Guideline no. 42.* 2nd ed. London: RCOG; 2012. Online: https://www.rcog.org.uk/media/ewgpnmio/gtg_42.pdf.

Royal College of Obstetricians and Gynaecologists (RCOG). *Umbilical Cord Prolapse. Green-top Guideline no. 50.* London: RCOG; 2014. Online: https://www.rcog.org.uk/globalassets/documents/guidelines/gtg-50-umbilicalcordprolapse-2014.pdf.

Royal College of Obstetricians and Gynaeocologists (RCOG). *Prevention and Management of Postpartum Haemorrhage. Green-top Guideline no. 52.* London: RCOG; 2016. Online: https://obgyn.onlinelibrary.wiley.com/doi/epdf/10.1111/1471-0528.14178.

Ruis KA, Allen RH, Gurewitsch ED. Severe shoulder dystocia with a small-for-gestational-age infant: a case report. *J Reprod Med.* 2011;56(3–4):178–180.

Safer Care Victoria. *Hypertension in pregnancy.* 2020. Online: https://www.bettersafercare.vic.gov.au/clinical-guidance/maternity/hypertension-in-pregnancy.

Saksena S, Camm AJ, eds. *Electrophysiological Disorders of the Heart.* 2nd ed. Philadelphia: Saunders; 2012.

Sandberg E. The Zavanelli manoeuvre: 12 years of recorded experience. *Obstet Gynecol.* 1999;93:312–317.

Shakur H, Roberts I, Fawole B, et al. Effect of early tranexamic acid administration on mortality, hysterectomy, and other morbidities in women with post-partum haemorrhage (WOMAN): an international, randomised, double-blind, placebo-controlled trial. *Lancet.* 2017;389(10084):2105–2116. doi:10.1016/S0140-6736(17)30638-4.

Society for Maternal–Fetal Medicine (SMFM), Pacheco LD, Saade G, et al. Amniotic fluid embolism: diagnosis and management. *Am J Obstet Gynecol.* 2016;215:B16–B24. Online: https://www.ajog.org/article/S0002-9378(16)00474-9/pdf.

Society of Obstetrics and Gynecology of Canada (SOGC). Postpartum hemorrhage. In: *ALARM Manual.* 15th ed. Ottawa, ON: SOGC; 2008.

Souter C. Shoulder dystocia. *NZCOM J.* 2002;27:16–20.

Taronen M, Ulander VM, Suvai L, et al. (summary translated) Minor trauma during pregnancy can cause severe fetomaternal haemorrhage. *Duodecim.* 2011;127(16):1727–1731.

Toledo P, Eosakul S, Goetz K, et al. Decay in blood loss estimation skills after web-based didactic training. *Simul Healthc.* 2012; 7(1):18–21. doi:10.1097/SIH.0b013e318230604f.

Varney H. *Varney's Midwifery.* 3rd ed. New York: Jones & Bartlett; 2004.

Vincent JL, De Backer D. Does disseminated intravascular coagulation lead to multiple organ failure? *Crit Care Clin.* 2005;21(3):469–477.

Vivian-Taylor J, Roberts C, Chen J, et al. Motor vehicle accidents during pregnancy: a population-based study. *BJOG.* 2012;119(4):499–501. doi:10.1111/j.1471-0528.2011.03226.x.

World Health Organization (WHO). n.d. *Correcting uterine inversion. Department of Reproductive Health and Research.* WHO, Geneva. Online: http://apps.who.int/iris/bitstream/handle/10665/43972/9241545879_eng.pdf?sequence=1.

World Health Organization (WHO). *WHO recommendation on tranexamic acid for the treatment of postpartum haemorrhage.* WHO: Geneva; 2017.

Yang YZ, Ye X-P, Sun X-X. Maternal and neonatal morbidity: repeat cesarean versus a trial of labour after previous Cesarean delivery. *Clin Invest Med.* 2017;40(3): e135–e145.

You WB, Zahn CM. Postpartum haemorrhage: abnormally adherent placenta, uterine inversion, and puerperal hematomas. *Clin Obstet Gynecol.* 2006;49(1):184–197.

Further reading

Boyle M. *Emergencies Around Childbirth: A Handbook for Midwives.* 3rd ed. London: Routledge; 2016.

James DK, Steer PJ, Weiner CP, et al., eds. *High Risk Pregnancy With Online Resource.* Vol. 1. 5th ed. Management Options. St Louis, MO: Elsevier Saunders; 2018.

Marshall J, Raynor M. *Myles Textbook for Midwives.* 16th ed. London: Elsevier; 2016.

Paterson-Brown S. Obstetric emergencies. In: Edmonds DK, eds. *Dewhurst's Textbook of Obstetrics and Gynaecology.* 8th ed. Oxford, UK: Wiley-Blackwell; 2012:296–310, [Ch. 25].

World Health Organization (WHO). *Correcting Uterine Inversion.* Geneva: Department of Reproductive Health and Research, WHO, n.d.

Wylie L, Bryce H. *The Midwives' Guide to Key Medical Conditions: Pregnancy and Childbirth.* London: Elsevier; 2016.

CHAPTER 41

Complications in the postnatal period for the mother

Jane Morrow

LEARNING OUTCOMES

Learning outcomes for this chapter are:

1. To describe the range and prevalence of physical health problems women may experience following childbirth in the days, weeks and months following birth
2. To discuss factors associated with postpartum physical morbidity
3. To discuss the various emotional responses to childbirth, and psychosocial factors that place women at risk for emotional distress.

CHAPTER OVERVIEW

This chapter discusses physical and psychological morbidity for the mother after childbirth. Commonly the postpartum period is considered to be the 6–8 weeks following birth, although it is known that some women will experience ongoing health problems that persist beyond this time frame. Poor maternal physical health can have a profound and ongoing impact on the woman's emotional health and the health of the whole family, with the health of the mother being intrinsically linked to the health of her children. The health challenges faced by women following birth can occur in the early postpartum period or may develop and become identifiable in the later weeks and months, either of which can have long-term consequences. This chapter will use these time periods (early and later) to address the most common postnatal health challenges, including known risk factors and evidence-based recommendations for care (where available).

KEY TERMS

dyspareunia
faecal incontinence
fatigue
haemorrhoids
morbidity
pelvic floor dysfunction
postnatal depression
secondary postpartum haemorrhage
thromboembolism

INTRODUCTION

The postpartum period is generally considered to be the 6–8 weeks following the birth, during which time postnatal care is provided by a health professional—most commonly a midwife (National Institute for Health and Care Excellence (NICE), 2015; New Zealand College of Midwives (NZCOM), 2021). It is a time of physical recovery and emotional adaptation to parenthood for women and their families (see Ch. 30). There are a range of health problems that can occur during this time that have an ongoing effect on the woman's health, with recovery from childbirth often taking longer than the defined postnatal period. There is growing recognition that the complexity of health issues in developed countries such as chronic disease, increased caesarean section and severe perineal trauma are contributing to long-term health issues for women following birth (Schmied & Bick, 2014).

It is important that midwives understand the impact that birth can have on the woman's health, that they identify **morbidity** and refer to other health professionals when appropriate. The impact on women's health will also impact on their family so midwives can make a difference to family outcomes by caring for women. This chapter explores postnatal health issues and evidence-based recommendations for provision of maternity care.

POSTPARTUM MORTALITY AND MORBIDITY

Maternal mortality has reduced significantly over the past century in the majority of countries, but the measurement of maternal health problems following birth continues to be sporadic (Vanderkruik et al., 2013). The importance of maternal health was identified by the United Nations (UN) in 2000 by the Millennium Development Goals (MDGs) and continues with global strategies identified to support maternal health and prevent maternal mortality (UN, 2015; World Health Organization (WHO), 2015). Complications of pregnancy, birth and the postnatal period may cause morbidities that can affect women's health in the short and long term, and potentially her whole life (Vanderkruik et al., 2013).

The major morbidities of postnatal health that can lead to maternal death include:

- haemorrhage
- deep vein thrombosis
- pulmonary embolism
- eclampsia
- postpartum infection (Australian Institute of Health and Welfare (AIHW), 2020; Heath Quality & Safety Commission (NZ), 2019; WHO, 2013).

Studies of postnatal morbidity conducted in Victoria, Australia regularly since 1993 initially reported that 94% of women had one or more health problems in the six months following birth and this has remained constant (Brown & Lumley, 1998; Brown, 2013). The most common problems identified by the women were extreme tiredness and exhaustion, backache, sexual problems, haemorrhoids, urinary incontinence, faecal incontinence, perineal pain and scores using the Edinburgh Postnatal Depression Scale (EPDS) indicating possible postnatal depression (Brown & Lumley, 1998; Brown et al., 2005; Brown, 2013; Thompson et al., 2002). The limitations of these findings are that they rely on self-reporting and recall at six months postpartum using a list of complications which may be incomplete.

Chronic physical symptoms following childbirth are likely to affect the mother's psychological wellbeing, as well as have a direct influence on her ability to parent (Winter et al., 2001) and on her quality of life (Van der Woude et al., 2015). As the severity of the problem increases the ability of the woman to look after their child, work or complete tasks decreases (Webb et al., 2008). The health status of infants is linked to the health of the mother (McLeish & Redshaw, 2017) and often maternal health problems are undetected because the focus of care moves from the mother to the infant during the postnatal period. The mood and behaviour of the baby can have an enormous influence on the mother's psychological wellbeing in the early postnatal period, with a baby that sleeps and feeds well increasing the woman's self-confidence (Wilkins, 2006) as she becomes more skilled at parenting (Kristensen et al., 2018).

Seeking help for postpartum issues

A number of studies have investigated postpartum women's health-seeking behaviours (Brown & Lumley, 1998; NICE, 2015). These studies highlight the prevalence of health problems after childbirth and the importance of providing accurate information to women to support them to access health professionals when needed. Without exception, studies recommend that clinicians talk to women during pregnancy and after birth about common problems and health concerns that women may develop postnatally (Brown & Lumley, 1998; NICE, 2015).

A number of studies have demonstrated that long-term maternal health problems that persist beyond the postnatal period may go undetected and unreported, possibly because health professionals did not ask about them (Albers, 2000; Brown & Lumley, 1998). Albers (2000) suggests that problems such as bowel, urinary and sexual problems may be embarrassing to discuss with clinicians and are accepted by mothers as part of giving birth, so many women may think that nothing can be done about them. In a 1993 survey of new mothers in Victoria, almost 50% said they would have liked more help or advice, with one-quarter saying they had not discussed their issues with a health professional (Brown & Lumley, 1998); despite the frequent contact the women had with their GPs, the majority did not recall discussing their own health issues. Despite these studies in the early 1990s identifying that women do not discuss these issues with their health practitioner (MacArthur et al., 1991;

Brown & Lumley, 1998), there appears to be little follow-up to explore whether access to services has improved.

A possible explanation for the lack of detection of health problems could be that the timing of postnatal care provided by midwives does not coincide with the period when women are ready to report these complications of childbirth, or that the relationship (communication) between the care provider and the woman is insufficient for her to feel comfortable discussing these issues.

A development since the last publication of this chapter is the proliferation of online / mobile applications for support in the postpartum period. Sardi et al. (2020) analysed 48 postnatal mobile applications covering topics such as health and fitness, baby tracking and parenting. They scored the applications and concluded that the quality of support and advice was variable. The study did not attempt to compare advice or guidance with evidence-based guidelines for postnatal care so currently there are no recommendations for use.

Documentation, referral and ongoing communication

When women do disclose postnatal issues, the midwife needs to refer to the appropriate services and ensure that these issues are communicated with ongoing health services on the woman's discharge from maternity services. In Victoria, communication between the hospital and the Maternal and Child Health service is addressed through the use of the child health record, which is given to all mothers in Victoria shortly after the time of birth, whilst in hospital.

In Aotearoa New Zealand information about the woman's maternity care and referral to Well Child services and general practitioner should occur when the midwife completes her care (see Ch. 30). The New Zealand College of Midwives (NZCOM), Well Child and the Royal New Zealand College of General Practitioners have developed a referral form for midwives to use to support referral between these services.

EARLY COMPLICATIONS (FIRST FEW DAYS) OF THE POSTNATAL PERIOD

In the early postpartum period, the midwife is responsible for the provision of care most often in a maternity facility setting. In Australia this is followed by a short period of support in the home environment (Forster et al., 2016), whereas in New Zealand postnatal care is provided in the woman's home for up to 6 weeks (NZCOM, 2021). In New Zealand, the *Midwives Handbook for Practice* identifies the need for midwives to undertake physical assessment and observations of the woman in the postnatal period (NZCOM, 2015). The NICE guideline for routine postnatal care for healthy women and babies recommends the care detailed in Box 41.1 in the first 24 hours to detect the most common complications (NICE, 2015).

Box 41.1 Recommended care for the first 24 hours

- Take blood pressure within 6 hours of birth
- Document the first urine void within the first 6 hours
- Encourage gentle mobilisation
- Provide an opportunity to talk about birth
- Be alert to life-threatening conditions, i.e. postpartum haemorrhage, sepsis, preeclampsia/eclampsia, pulmonary embolism and deep vein thrombosis
- Women who are obese should receive individualised care because of increased risk of thromboembolism

(Source: NICE, 2015)

Preeclampsia and eclampsia

Pre-eclampsia and eclampsia can present for the first time in the postnatal period. (See Chs 37 and 40 for discussion of these conditions.) It is therefore recommended that women's blood pressure is checked within the first six hours of the birth (NICE, 2015). If a woman complains of a headache then she should be evaluated for preeclampsia. If the diastolic blood pressure is above 90 mmHg then it should be repeated in 4 hours unless there are other symptoms of preeclampsia, in which case a full assessment should take place (NICE, 2015).

Management

For women with hypertension or preeclampsia (PE) diagnosed during pregnancy New Zealand guidelines advise that blood pressure should be monitored regularly during the postnatal period (MOH, 2022). Women should be advised to remain within a maternity facility for regular blood pressure monitoring for 72 hours following the birth. For women with preeclampsia the blood pressure will frequently increase between days 3 and 5, with a return to normal within 16 days of the birth. Once stable the blood pressure should be assessed within 24 hours of discharge home, then weekly for 6 weeks.

Women who have been treated with antihypertensive medication may need to continue for several weeks following birth and will require regular review of the medication. Hypertension and other signs of PE should resolve by 6–12 weeks postpartum. Women should also be advised that there are increased longer term health risks as well as an increased risk of gestational hypertension in future pregnancies.

Urinary retention / difficult voiding

Urinary retention or difficulty with voiding is a relatively common phenomenon in the early postpartum period, although the incidence is uncertain owing to varied definitions and a lack of studies carried out on this topic. The importance of early recognition and appropriate

Box 41.2 Risk factors for urinary retention and difficulties with voiding following birth

- Epidural and regional anaesthesia
- Prolonged first and second stage of labour
- Instrumental births
- Primiparity
- Birth weight >3800 grams

(Source: Lim, 2010)

management is essential to avoid long-term difficulties such as denervation, detrusor atony and long-term difficulties with voiding (Lim, 2010; Zaki et al., 2004). NICE (2015) recommend that women should pass urine within the first 6 hours after birth and if not successful there should be a fuller assessment to determine the need for catheterisation and referral. The causes are likely to be multifactorial, involving psychological, mechanical and neurological factors. Box 41.2 summarises the risk factors.

Diagnosis

Women may complain of a complete inability to void, voiding small volumes frequently, slow or intermittent stream, urgency, bladder pain or discomfort, incontinence or no sensation to void.

Management

Management of these conditions varies from measurement of voids, strict fluid balance recording, postvoid residual volumes and use of ultrasound to measure residual bladder volumes (Lim, 2010). Failure to manage this complication promptly may lead to persistent bladder dysfunction requiring catheterisation for many weeks. Rarely, the damage can be permanent (Zaki et al., 2004). Women should be encouraged to do pelvic floor exercise to support improved bladder function and control.

CRITICAL THINKING EXERCISE

What measures have you observed being used to aid voiding in clinical practice?

What do you understand by the term 'Trial of Void'?

Venous thromboembolism

Pulmonary thromboembolism (PTE) and deep vein thrombosis (DVT) are the two components of a single condition called venous thromboembolism (VTE) (see also Ch. 37). Women are at higher risk of VTE during pregnancy, and in particular during the postpartum period, than when not pregnant, with failure to recognise this being reported to contribute to maternal mortality (Queensland Clinical Guidelines, 2020). The report of maternal deaths in Australia from the period 2009–18 reported 20 maternal deaths from **thromboembolism** (AIHW, 2020). In a similar timeframe (2006–16) New Zealand reported six maternal deaths due to thromboembolism (Health Quality & Safety Commission, 2019).

Diagnosis

Acute VTE should be suspected in women with signs and symptoms of possible VTE, in particular if they have other known risk factors (Box 41.3). Regardless of risk for VTE, immobilisation and dehydration should be minimised (Queensland Clinical Guidelines, 2020). Gentle early mobilisation is recommended as a preventive measure to avoid thrombotic conditions in the early postpartum period (NICE, 2015). Signs and symptoms include leg pain and swelling (usually unilateral—90% in the left calf), pitting oedema, increased calf / thigh circumference particularly of 2 cm or more, increased temperature and prominent superficial veins (Queensland Clinical Guidelines, 2020). A pulmonary embolism may also present with dyspnoea, palpitations / tachycardia, chest pain, haemoptysis, hypoxia / cyanosis, tachypnoea, hypotension and collapse (Queensland Clinical Guidelines, 2020).

Clinical diagnosis is unreliable; therefore diagnosis of VTE should be made using doppler ultrasound, compression ultrasonography or contrast venography (King Edward Memorial Hospital (KEMH), 2016). For the diagnosis of PTE, ventilation perfusion (*V/Q*) scanning or computerised tomography pulmonary angiography (CTPA) is recommended according to local practice (see Ch. 37). Reliance on D-dimer without pretest probability assessment is not recommended as D-dimer can also be elevated owing to physiological changes in healthy pregnant women and to other conditions such as preeclampsia (RCOG, 2010).

Management

Any women with signs and symptoms suggestive of VTE should be referred for medical assessment. They will normally be commenced on low-molecular-weight heparin (LMWH) until the diagnosis of VTE is excluded (KEMH, 2016; RCOG, 2010). There is insufficient data on optimal timing and dosage of LMWH; however, they are commonly used in pregnancy for women with a history of idiopathic proximal VTE, thrombophilia or other high-risk factors. Anticoagulant therapy should be continued for 6 weeks after calf vein thrombosis and for 3 months in proximal DVT or PTE. Both heparin and warfarin are satisfactory for use postpartum and are not contraindicated in breastfeeding (Queensland Clinical Guidelines, 2020). The optimum therapeutic dose will depend on body weight and warfarin should not be commenced until 2–3 days after birth owing to the risk of postpartum haemorrhage. Graduated elastic stockings should be worn on the

Box 41.3 Risk factors for venous thrombosis

VTE may occur at any time during pregnancy; however, the puerperium is the time of highest risk.

Risk factors include:

- Age over 35 years
- Caesarean birth
- Excessive blood loss (>1000 mL)
- Forceps (mid-cavity or rotational)
- Inflammatory disorders and infection
- Malignancy
- Maternal heart disease
- Multiparity >3
- Multiple pregnancy
- Nephrotic syndrome
- Obesity
- Ovarian hyperstimulation syndrome/hyperemesis/dehydration
- Personal/family history of thrombosis
- Preeclampsia
- Pregnancy/puerperium
- Prolonged immobilisation—including paraplegia, pelvic trauma, long-distance travel
- Prolonged labour (>24 h)
- Sickle cell disease
- Smoker
- Surgical procedure
- Thrombophilia
- Antithrombin deficiency
- Protein S or C deficiency
- Activated protein C resistance/factor V Leiden
- Prothrombin gene mutation
- Antiphospholipid antibodies/lupus anticoagulant
- Varicose veins

(Source: Virkus R.A., 2014)

affected leg, however there is limited evidence of the necessary duration of this intervention (Queensland Clinical Guidelines, 2020).

Hormonal contraception should be discussed with women following an episode of VTE. Currently there is debate about the safety of using the combined oral contraceptive pill (COCP) (Royal Australian and New Zealand College of Obstetricians and Gynaecologists (RANZCOG), 2016). Consensus opinion is that the risk of VTE can be minimised by avoiding prescribing COCPs for women at high risk (i.e. women who are obese, who smoke, have a family history of VTE or who are at increased cardiovascular risk).

REFLECTIVE THINKING EXERCISE

'Lisa', a 35-year-old primigravid, arrived in the birth suite from home following induction with Prostin 5 hours earlier in the day assessment unit. Her pregnancy had been uneventful, although she had been told by an obstetrician at 36 weeks gestation, at a routine antenatal visit, that the baby appeared to be quite large and the obstetrician had questioned Lisa's ability to achieve a vaginal birth. Lisa had commenced pregnancy with a body mass index (BMI) of 30 and had gained 20 kilograms in the pregnancy but had been well with no other risk factors identified. She was then 40 weeks plus 10 days, this being the indication for induction of labour.

Lisa had been reluctant to be induced and had tried various methods she had heard about from friends and relatives (i.e. walking, intercourse, hot curry and finally castor oil). She had had no response from these attempts and had decided that she would take medical advice as she also had in the back of her mind the comment about the size of the baby.

On admission to the birth suite, Lisa was contracting 5-minutely with contractions lasting 40–50 seconds. All baseline observations (temperature, pulse and blood pressure) were within normal limits. An admission cardiotocograph was reassuring. The admission vaginal examination revealed a breech presentation, 5 cm dilated and fully effaced. Lisa was confused and frightened with the information with which she was presented. The medical staff did not support vaginal breech birth so Lisa felt pressured to choose a caesarean section. She underwent a caesarean section and gave birth to a live boy weighing 3200 g and returned to the postnatal ward in the late evening.

Overnight Lisa reported frequently that she was in pain and this prevented her from sleeping and made attempting to breastfeed difficult. She was unable to move freely and required assistance to lift the baby and to move around the bed. The next day, due to the busyness of the postnatal ward, Lisa remained in her bed until late in the afternoon. At this time she was visited by a member of the pain management team and finally received effective assistance with her pain. This allowed her to move from her bed, shower and feed her baby whilst sitting up. Her intravenous infusion and indwelling urinary catheter were removed.

The following day Lisa was more comfortable and moving freely; however, she reported that her lower left leg was swollen and painful. On examination Lisa's calf was red and swollen. A diagnosis of DVT was made using ultrasound and treatment commenced with LMWH (enoxaparin (Clexane); 1 mg/kg twice a day) and thromboembolism-deterrent (TED) stockings.

- What were the risk factors for development of DVT?
- Was there anything that could have been done differently to prevent this occurrence?
- What advice does Lisa need for the future?

Postnatal vaginal bleeding

Blood loss following birth has been found to be variable for each woman and often continues for several weeks following the birth. A systematic review of what matters to women in the postnatal period reported that women experience anxiety about vaginal bleeding and would like more information from health professionals (Finlayson et al., 2020). The BLiPP (Blood Loss in the Postnatal Period) study, involving two districts in the UK in 1995, explored the patterns of involution of the uterus and experience of blood loss following birth in an apparently normal puerperium (Marchant et al., 1999). The aim of the study was to have women describe their vaginal loss from 24 hours after birth until 3 months postnatally. The study involved 524 women completing two questionnaires and two separate diaries, the first one from day 2 until day 10, and the second on days 14, 21 and 28 postpartum. The findings were reported as more variable than the researchers had anticipated, and they noted that the experiences of the women did not reflect the descriptions of vaginal loss within the midwifery texts. Vaginal loss continued for longer than expected, with almost 25% of women reporting vaginal loss for up to 6 weeks after birth. A further study of postnatal vaginal loss was undertaken in the Philippines including 477 breastfeeding women. In this study, vaginal loss was experienced for a median of 27 days after birth, with a range of 5–90 days—once again much longer than the time described in most textbooks of the era (Visness et al., 1997). Similarly, in an Australian study, 20% of women reported excessive or prolonged bleeding at 8 weeks postpartum and, although this problem had resolved to a large extent by 24 weeks postpartum, 2% of women continued to experience prolonged or excessive bleeding (Thompson et al., 2002). Chapter 40 explores primary postpartum haemorrhage in more detail.

Secondary postpartum haemorrhage

Secondary postpartum haemorrhage (PPH) is traditionally defined as excessive bleeding at any time from the first 24 hours following birth until 6 weeks postpartum (Safer Care Victoria, 2019). The majority of secondary PPHs are a result of sub-involution of the uterus caused by infection and / or retained products (Safer Care Victoria, 2019). Other causes include uterine polyps or fibroids, coagulopathies or trauma. Although this can be a life-threatening emergency as described for primary PPH (Ch. 40), it is more often a problem of morbidity. Morbidity includes anaemia and iron deficiency, which have been shown to impact on a woman's postpartum adaptation including fatigue, delayed healing, low breast-milk supply (Bergmann et al., 2010), postnatal depression (Bergmann et al., 2010; Khalafallah et al., 2012) and reduction in breastfeeding duration (Khalafallah et al., 2012). Postnatal anaemia and iron deficiency are therefore contributors to significant health problems for childbearing women, which may cause difficulties for the early mothering role and predispose women to adjustment disorders, depression and early cessation of breastfeeding.

Box 41.4 Other risk factors for secondary postpartum haemorrhage

- Endometritis
- Retained products of conception
- Lower genital tract trauma
- Placental abnormalities (placenta accreta, increta and percreta)
- Uterine abnormities (fibroids)
- Choriocarcinoma
- Caesarean section wound dehiscence/surgical injury
- Bleeding disorders (von Willebrand disease, carriers of haemophilia and factor XI deficiency)

(Source: Aiken et al., 2012)

Diagnosis

The incidence of secondary PPH determined by hospital admission is low although, as there is no specific amount of blood loss that determines the definition, there is variation in the incidence reported (Aiken et al., 2012). Additionally, because postpartum vaginal loss is managed primarily in the community, calculating the incidence of secondary PPH from hospital admissions data may underreport the problem. Most women present in the second week after birth and significant risk factors include a history of primary postpartum haemorrhage and manual removal of placenta (Hoveyda & MacKenzie, 2001; Marchant et al., 2006) (Box 41.4).

CRITICAL THINKING EXERCISE

Define subinvolution of the uterus. 'Retained products' in the uterus is associated with bleeding early in the postpartum period. What does this mean and why do retained products occur?

Assessment

Initial assessment of the woman should include a thorough history and a complete set of observations (heart rate, blood pressure, respiratory rate, oxygen saturation and temperature)—a deterioration of vital signs will signify a significant acute haemorrhage (Aiken et al., 2012). Clinical signs may include offensive-smelling lochia, abdominal cramping, uterine tenderness, pyrexia (temperature >37.5°C) and enlarged uterus. There is a lack of evidence to support assessing the symphysis–fundal distance;

however, in an acute setting a high or deviated uterine fundus associated with uterine tenderness can be a valuable clinical sign.

CRITICAL THINKING EXERCISE

What clinical investigations may be performed for a woman admitted to hospital with a secondary PPH? Make sure that you can identify 'normal' and 'abnormal' findings. Identify the most common causative bacteria.

Management

Evidence regarding the management of secondary PPH is limited, but depending on the clinical assessment the management may be conservative, medical or surgical. Safer Care Victoria (2019) have produced recent guidance and recommend if the woman's condition is unstable the management should be as per primary postpartum haemorrhage (see Chapter 40). If the woman's condition is stable then investigations should be undertaken to identify extent of the blood loss on maternal health. These include blood tests for full blood count (FBC), C-reactive protein (CRP) and blood group (to hold and / or cross match). To identify if infection is the cause of the blood loss, vaginal swabs and a mid-stream specimen of urine should be taken and blood cultures may also be required. If retained tissue is suspected then a pelvic ultrasound and Doppler may be undertaken (Safer Care Victoria, 2019). More research is required to assess the extent and impact of secondary PPH on women during the postpartum period.

CLINICAL POINT

Possible antibiotic regimen for secondary postpartum haemorrhage

The antibiotics are administered intravenously for 48 hours then switched to oral if no longer febrile or septic:

- Ampicillin 2 g IV initial dose then 1 g IV every 6 hours, and
- Gentamicin 5 mg/kg IV daily, and
- Metronidazole 500 mg IV every 12 hours.

Penicillin allergy:

- Clindamycin or Lincomycin 900 mg 8 hourly
- =/− Gentamicin 5 mg/kg daily.

Postpartum infection

Postpartum infections often complicate the recovery from birth and, as discussed previously, can lead to further complications such as secondary PPH. The most common sites of infection in the postpartum period are uterine (endometritis), urinary (urinary tract infection), trauma sites (caesarean section scar, episiotomy or perineal tear); breast (mastitis or breast abscess) and post-abortion. Recently the World Health Organization (WHO) Global Maternal Sepsis Study (GLOSS) Research Group reported that the contribution of infection to direct and indirect maternal death was much higher than previously reported (Bonet et al., 2020). They called for earlier recognition and treatment for women across the world. One leading cause of severe, life-threatening maternal sepsis is group A *Streptococcus* (GAS) (see also Chs 37 and 40).

Group A *Streptococcus* maternal sepsis (puerperal fever)

The incidence of puerperal sepsis declined following the introduction of antibiotics in developed countries (Busowski et al., 2013), but has recently re-emerged as the main contributor to maternal morbidity and mortality in Australia, with 23 maternal deaths reported in the period 2009–18, and in New Zealand, with six maternal deaths due to it in the period 2006–16 (AIHW, 2020; Bowyer et al., 2017; PMMRC, 2018). Up to 30% of people in the community are asymptomatic carriers of GAS, usually in the throat or the surface of the skin (AIHW et al., 2020).

Diagnosis

The onset is most commonly within a few days of birth (Busowski et al., 2013) and clinical features are listed in Box 41.5. Most women complain of a preceding upper respiratory tract infection, have had contact with young children and the majority of cases occur in winter/early spring (Tennant, 2013). Presentation usually includes peritonitis, toxic shock and necrotising fasciitis—this may appear as skin infection with pain out of proportion to the clinical appearance, mild gastrointestinal symptoms and a feeling of general malaise (Tennant, 2013). Persistent tachycardia, tachypnoea and raised C-reactive protein should alert the clinician to possible sepsis.

Box 41.5 Clinical features of GAS maternal sepsis

- Fever of more than 38°C
- Tender, subinvoluted (slow to return to normal size following birth) uterus
- Chills and general malaise
- Lower abdominal pain
- Diarrhoea
- Purulent and foul-smelling lochia (vaginal discharge after birth)
- Vaginal bleeding
- Hypothermia, tachypnoea and neutropenia
- Signs of shock such as hypotension and sustained tachycardia (>100 b.p.m.)

(Source: New South Wales (NSW) Government Health Department. *Maternal Sepsis (Puerperal Fever) due to Group A Streptococcus—Information for Clinicians* fact sheet. 2016 ©State of New South Wales NSW Ministry of Health. For current information go to www.health.nsw.gov.au.)

Management

Treatment must be aggressive and should include broad-spectrum antibiotics commenced immediately after obtaining appropriate samples for culture (bloods, high and low vaginal swabs, wound swabs, and a midstream urine sample).

Prevention is problematic because infection is rare and generally occurs in a healthy woman, and may progress rapidly (Busowski et al., 2013). There is a point where antimicrobial treatment cannot prevent death (Tennant, 2013, p. 58). Populations at higher risk include women who have had: caesarean section, long labour or prolonged ruptured membranes, frequent vaginal examinations in labour, traumatic birth, retained products, a sore throat, and poor personal or perineal hygiene in the early postpartum period. Australian Aboriginal women have a higher rate of GAS sepsis, as do women with other chronic diseases, immunosuppression or injecting drug use (NSW Government Health Department, 2016).

Other infections

Endometritis (inflammation of the lining of the uterus) may occur owing to other organisms and is frequently linked to uterine infection (Alexander et al., 2002). Women with endometritis may be febrile, with possibly only a low-grade temperature, and report abdominal / pelvic pain. On palpation, the uterus may be tender and subinvoluted (delayed or absent involution in the postpartum period). The vaginal loss might be an unusual colour and frequently has an offensive smell. Bowel and bladder function may be disturbed and other possible infection or inflammation sites such as the breast (mastitis), urinary tract and surgical incisions (wound infections) need to be excluded.

Other common health problems in the early postpartum period

NICE (2015) recommend that, in the first 3 days following birth, information and reassurance should be offered in regard to common conditions experienced by women that cause pain and concern. Sources for postpartum pain include perineal pain, caesarean section, afterbirth pains, headache, diastasis of the rectus abdominis muscle (DRAM), dyspareunia, backache, haemorrhoids, constipation and persistent fatigue.

Headaches

Headaches are common (incidence ranging from 11% to 80%) and may be associated with life changes such as sleep deprivation, irregular food intake and dehydration (Stella et al., 2007).

Women who have had an epidural or spinal anaesthesia are at risk of a dural puncture headache, which should be differentiated from a general headache. A dural puncture headache is severe and has a rapid onset following the birth, generally when the woman sits or stands. If this occurs the woman will need immediate assessment by an anaesthetist (NICE, 2015) and may require treatment. A range of treatments include hydration, caffeine-containing drinks or medications, simple analgesia and epidural blood patch (Russell et al, 2019).

Turner and colleagues explored the predictors of headache during pregnancy and after the birth in 2434 women who gave birth in one of four university hospitals in the United States and Europe (Turner et al., 2012). They found that 10% of their cohort experienced headache during pregnancy, 3.7% experienced a headache within 72 hours of the birth and 3.6% had experienced headaches when asked at 8 weeks following the birth. When compared with women who did not have a history of headaches, the history of headache prior to pregnancy was the strongest predictor that the woman would experience a headache during pregnancy and following the birth. Headaches may be due to tension, lack of sleep and increased stress. Women who previously suffered from migraine headaches may find these recurring in the postnatal period (Bick et al., 2009). Women who experience headaches should explore ways of alleviating tension and ensuring sufficient sleep. If headaches are problematic following the birth, analgesia such as paracetamol may be helpful.

CRITICAL THINKING EXERCISE

Describe the procedure of epidural blood patch.

Diastasis of the rectus abdominis muscle

Diastasis of the rectus abdominis muscle (DRAM) is common during and after pregnancy owing to stretching and thinning of the linea alba (Benjamin et al., 2019). The degree of separation may be measured with a tape measure, caliper devices or ultrasound, or estimated using palpation—and is considered to be clinically meaningful if greater than 2.2–2.3 cm (Benjamin et al., 2019). Predisposing factors include obesity, multiparity, fetal macrosomia, flaccid abdominal muscles, polyhydramnios and multiple pregnancies. In their systematic review analysing eight studies of varying designs, Benjamin et al. (2013) concluded that there is insufficient evidence to recommend antenatal exercise to prevent or reduce DRAM. All included studies examined the effect of postnatal exercise of the transverse abdominis muscle and two additionally recommended the use of external support garments (Tubigrip or corset) (Benjamin et al., 2013). Consistent classification is needed along with more research to evaluate a single intervention either in the antenatal period to prevent or reduce occurrence or in the postnatal period as an effective treatment.

Perineal pain

Perineal pain is common in the initial postpartum period regardless of perineal trauma, with increased perineal trauma associated with greater pain scores and higher use of analgesia (Macarthur & Macarthur, 2004). The midwife should offer to visually assess the perineum if the woman has pain or discomfort (NICE, 2015). For a detailed analysis of optimum care of the perineum see Chapter 26.

LONGER-TERM POSTPARTUM COMPLICATIONS

As discussed at the beginning of the chapter, many women experience long-term consequences of childbirth, which until relatively recently have been ignored or accepted as a normal change associated with giving birth. Women usually receive limited information about these long-lasting problems and therefore may be unprepared for such health issues (Schytt et al., 2005). Such complications include: pelvic floor dysfunction, dyspareunia (painful sexual intercourse), urinary incontinence, faecal incontinence, pain from the caesarean section scar, and haemorrhoids (Brown & Lumley, 1998; Glazener et al., 1995; MacArthur et al., 1991; Schytt et al., 2005). The most commonly reported longer term health problems following birth are tiredness, fatigue and back pain (Woolhouse et al., 2014).

Tiredness and fatigue

Following the birth of a baby many parents report tiredness and fatigue due to frequently disrupted sleep due to infant night-time waking, feeding and care (Loutzenhiser et al., 2015). Postpartum **fatigue** can be defined as an overwhelming sustained sense of exhaustion, a decreased capacity for physical and mental activity, lack of energy and / or impairment in concentration (Henderson et al., 2019; Loutzenhiser et al., 2015). In a large observational study of 10,000 women 3 months following birth, Henderson et al. (2019) found that 38% identified fatigue at 10 days postpartum, 27% at 1 month and 11.4% at 3 months postpartum (Henderson et al., 2019). The proportions varied dependent on the woman's age, level of deprivation, education and parity with women reporting depression, anxiety, sleep problems and breastfeeding at higher risk of fatigue at 3 months. A systematic review (Kurth et al., 2011) explored the relationship between infant crying and maternal tiredness and fatigue. Women who reported more infant crying described an increase in tiredness / fatigue. The emotional effects of fatigue were described by women as difficulty in concentrating, reduced patience, frustration, guilt, resentment, feelings of incompetence and concerns about becoming aggressive towards the baby. Kurth and colleagues (2011) suggest that the consequences of infant crying can be seen as cyclical, in that prolonged infant crying impairs the parent's ability to rest and increases tiredness / fatigue; this fatigue can then interfere with the parent's empathetic care for the crying infant, leading to more crying.

In a qualitative, exploratory study, Taylor & Johnson (2010) explored how women managed fatigue following birth. The women described self-care practices such as going to bed early, getting more sleep and rest, and looking after themselves. They also talked about balancing the work to be done with the aim of managing the fatigue and having realistic expectations along with juggling tasks; this also included getting help from other members of the family. Taylor & Johnson (2010) discuss the finding that the women's expectations of themselves were high and involved feeling that they should be able to cope with looking after the baby, the family and the housework. The authors suggest that this reflects contemporary representations of mothers as 'superwomen', and in later work they found that high levels of maternal anxiety were associated with fatigue (Taylor & Johnson, 2010, 2013).

Tiredness and fatigue can be caused by physical factors such as anaemia (which can be remedied with iron therapy once diagnosed) or infection, thyroid disorder or depression (Bick et al., 2009). Women who have experienced a caesarean section are more likely to report exhaustion / extreme tiredness than women who have had a spontaneous vaginal birth at 6 weeks postpartum (Jansen et al., 2007), possibly because of postpartum pain or greater blood loss at the time of birth. Discussing the woman's feelings about her fatigue and what she thinks may be the cause can be helpful in identifying ways to reduce it. In their review of tiredness and fatigue, McQueen & Mander (2003) suggest that postnatal adjustment could be enhanced if childbirth education focused more on realistic expectations of motherhood. They suggest that women should seek help from support people for routine household tasks and activities in the postpartum period (McQueen & Mander, 2003). Fatigue may also contribute to emotional distress.

REFLECTIVE THINKING EXERCISE

Sophie gave birth to her second son in a metropolitan hospital where discharge after six hours was encouraged. The pregnancy, labour and birth were uneventful so Sophie felt well prepared to go home. She had successfully breastfed her first son who was now 3 years old and was keen to fully breastfeed her new baby. Due to the global pandemic in 2020 (COVID-19), her partner was working at home and she no longer had access to any childcare for her first son. The first few days at home were difficult as she could have no visitors to her home and she was experiencing difficulties with breastfeeding. The new baby was unsettled and her other son was experiencing difficulty with accepting his new place in the family. Overnight Sophie became very distressed due to the exhaustion she was feeling and realised she needed help but was unsure of where to find it.

1. What resources would be available to Sophie in your community?
2. What support could you offer Sophie?
3. What advice would you give Sophie regarding her other child?

Back pain

Many women experience back pain during pregnancy and this may persist into the postpartum period. Studies have commonly explored the association between backache and receiving an epidural and there is no consensus in the findings, with some reporting epidural as a risk factor (Brown & Lumley, 1998; Russell et al., 1993) and others refuting this (Howell et al., 2001; Koughnan et al., 2002). The NICE guidelines (2015) recommend that back pain should be managed as in the general population—a combination of analgesia and other therapies.

Backache is a common disorder among the general population. It is difficult to assess whether there is an increase in complaints about backache following childbirth (Bick et al., 2009). An acute onset of backache should be referred to an appropriate practitioner for investigation immediately. For ongoing postpartum backache, women can be advised to remain active and try localised applications of heat and mild oral analgesia; if the backache does not improve or continues for up to 6 weeks, referral to an appropriate practitioner such as a GP, physiotherapist, osteopath or chiropractor is advised (Bick et al., 2009).

Haemorrhoids

Haemorrhoids (piles) are swollen veins near the anus, to which women are predisposed during pregnancy and the puerperium. The incidence has been reported to be up to 40% in pregnancy, usually the third trimester or the first month following birth (Hollingshead & Phillips, 2016). Women may have symptoms without prolapse (first degree) to consistently prolapsed (fourth degree) (Poskus, et al., 2014).

Women with haemorrhoids may experience bleeding, itching and pain; however, this is usually mild and transient. Self-help strategies include eating a high-fibre diet, increasing fluid intake and water immersion. Pharmacological management involves localised treatments such as anesthetic ointments, phlebotonics or glucocorticosteroids which can be used alone or in a combination depending on the severity of the heamorrhoids. Phlebotonics have a beneficial effect in treating haemorrhoid symptoms (Parera, et al., 2012). Conservative management includes prevention of constipation through dietary modifications (increased fibre and water in the diet) (NICE, 2015). Further measures may include mild laxatives and local treatment such as salt baths, witch hazel compresses and ointments/creams which may contain steroids to assist with the reduction in the size of the haemorrhoid or anaesthetic to alleviate the discomfort (Hollingshead & Phillips, 2016). It is rare in pregnancy or the early postnatal period for surgical intervention or rubber-band ligation to be recommended.

Pelvic floor dysfunction

Pelvic floor dysfunction is the inability of the pelvic floor to fulfil its supportive role to the pelvic organs and includes urinary and faecal incontinence, perineal pain and dyspareunia.

Urinary incontinence

The incidence of urinary incontinence is high for women as they age, but more so for women who have experienced pregnancy and birth (MacLennan et al., 2000); Box 41.6 lists the particular risk factors. The most common type suffered by postpartum women is stress incontinence (between 0.3% and 44%) (Lemos et al., 2008), which is defined as involuntary leakage of urine on effort or exertion, or on sneezing or coughing (Abrams et al., 2002). Urge incontinence is the involuntary leakage accompanied by or immediately proceeded by urgency (Abrams et al., 2002) and is also common; and many women experience a combination of different types of incontinence (Press et al., 2007).

Other factors identified as increasing the risk include smoking, incontinence during pregnancy, high BMI (Burgio et al., 2003; Wesnes & Lose, 2013); chronic constipation and episiotomy in at least one birth (Ewings et al., 2005); and maternal body weight over 75 kg (Diez-Itza et al., 2009). A review of studies reporting reduced risk of urinary incontinence for women having caesarean section compared with women having a vaginal birth suggests that caesarean birth may be protective (Nygaard, 2006); however, other research suggests that this effect may be only short term, with the difference not evident in surveys of women beyond 6 months postpartum (MacLennan et al., 2000; Thompson et al., 2002). Examination of the research is complex owing to some studies examining either any urinary incontinence or only stress incontinence, making comparisons between studies challenging. However, the message is clear that a

Box 41.6 Risk factors for urinary incontinence

- Vaginal birth (OR 2.08, 95% CI 1.72–2.52)
- Advanced age at gestation (OR 1.06, 95% CI 1.04–1.08)
- Advanced maternal BMI (OR 1.04, 95% CI 1.03–1.06)
- Excess weight gain during pregnancy (OR 1.13, 95% CI 1.00–1.26)
- Diabetes (OR 1.91, 95% CI 1.53–2.38)
- Episiotomy (OR 1.76, 95% CI 1.06–2.94)
- Forceps birth (OR 2.69, 95% CI 1.25–5.76)
- Gestational urinary incontinence (OR 5.04, 95% CI 2.07–12.28)
- Gestational stress urinary incontinence (OR 4.28, 95% CI 2.61–7.01)
- Prenatal urinary incontinence (OR 8.54, 95% CI 3.52–20.70)

(Source: Wang et al., 2020)

large proportion of women experience urinary incontinence following childbirth and a study including women from the UK and New Zealand confirms that this is persistent and long term (MacArthur et al., 2016).

Pelvic floor muscle training (PFMT) (pelvic floor exercise) is commonly recommended for women, particularly during pregnancy and after birth for prevention and treatment of urinary incontinence (Boyle et al., 2012; NICE, 2015; Woodley et al., 2020) (Fig. 41.1). PFMT increases the resting tone and the ability to contract the muscles of the pelvic floor when coughing (Wesnes & Lose, 2013). A Cochrane review of PFMT for prevention and treatment of urinary and faecal incontinence concluded that, for women having their first baby, PFMT can prevent urinary incontinence for up to 6 months after birth and that it is appropriate treatment for women with persistent postnatal urinary incontinence (Woodley et al., 2020).

PFMT is described as a program of repeated voluntary pelvic floor muscle contractions taught and supervised by a health professional (Woodley et al., 2020). Systematic reviews have recommended close follow-up and intensive training. Bø & Haakstad (2011) reported that more than 30% of women are not able to perform the correct contraction at their first consultation; therefore it is important that there is a checking process for correct pelvic floor muscle contraction, which consists of two components: squeeze around the pelvic openings and inward lift as described by Kegel in 1952 (Bø & Mørkved, 2015).

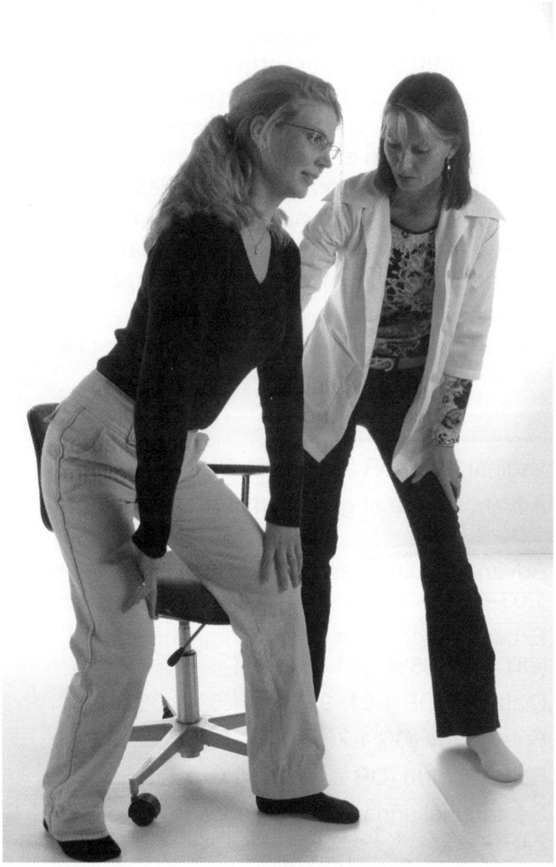

FIGURE 41.1 The woman sits on an armrest with legs apart, feet on the floor, flexed hips and straight back with the perineum resting on the armrest. The instruction is to squeeze around the pelvic openings and lift the skin away from the armrest without rising up or putting any pressure on the feet
(Source: Bø K & Mørkved S, 2015)

Other options for treatment may include surgery, in particular if the incontinence is complicated by prolapse (displacement of the uterus or vagina downward) where conservative treatments have not helped (NICE, 2019).

Faecal incontinence

Faecal incontinence is the involuntary loss of faecal material; however, as suggested by Birch et al. (2006), it may be more pertinent to examine the involuntary loss of faeces and / or gas when researching the incidence following birth. The true prevalence is probably not known as often women do not seek or receive professional help (MacArthur et al., 1997). Only 14% (5 / 36) of women interviewed about their faecal incontinence (on average 45 weeks following birth) by MacArthur et al. (1997) reported that they had consulted a doctor, with the most common reason for not consulting being they thought the symptoms would eventually improve and that it hadn't been happening long enough to go to the doctor. Comparing studies is difficult owing to the differences in what has been measured (i.e. gas and / or faeces or faeces only). There are no measures for the severity and studies have been conducted at different times postnatally, ranging from immediately after birth to 6 years later. NICE (2015) recommends assessing for severity, duration and frequency of symptoms when reported. The risk factors and treatment are the same as for urinary incontinence, with the addition of anal sphincter trauma during birth as a risk factor (see Box 41.6). Women with third- and fourth-degree tears are at risk of faecal urgency and incontinence (Birch et al., 2006).

CRITICAL THINKING EXERCISE

1. How have certain birthing practices affected pelvic floor function? (You may wish to consider the effects of Valsalva 'coached' pushing, birthing positions, and use of traction for controlled cord traction delivery of the placenta.)
2. How might teaching pelvic floor control in pregnancy, not just strengthening exercises (i.e. ability to relax pelvic floor for birth, not just lifting pelvic floor for strengthening), affect postpartum pelvic floor function and other birth outcomes?

Dyspareunia

Dyspareunia (pain during sexual intercourse) may occur with or without perineal trauma, with 16% of women reporting dyspareunia at 12 months postpartum (Manresa, et al., 2019).

Dyspareunia is a subjective experience of painful or difficult sexual intercourse that may result from perineal damage and is possibly complicated by other factors such as tiredness and lack of desire (Thompson et al., 2002). Other terms exploring sexual difficulties including 'sexual dysfunction' and 'sexual morbidity' have been used in the literature to include difficulties such as: vagina feeling too tight or lax; lack of lubrication; unwanted leakage of flatus, urine or faeces during intercourse; and lack of sensation (numbness) during sexual intercourse (Williams et al., 2007). Glazener et al. (1995) reported that 53% of women reported problems with intercourse in the first 8 weeks after birth and 49% after the first 2 months. Brown & Lumley (1998) in a study of postnatal health in Victoria, Australia reported that 21% of women continued to experience problems with perineal pain during intercourse 6–7 months postpartum. Similar rates have been reported in other studies (Lumley et al., 2006; Thompson et al., 2002). Women who have had instrumental births (forceps or vacuum) have an increased incidence of vaginal and perineal trauma and subsequent sexual problems (Brown & Lumley, 1998; Thompson et al., 2002). The NICE clinical guidelines for routine postnatal care recommend that women are asked at each postnatal contact whether they have any concerns about dyspareunia and that an offer should be made to examine the woman's perineum if there is pain or discomfort; however, they report that there have been no studies evaluating the management of dyspareunia (NICE, 2015). Women are advised to use lubricant gels or oils, relaxation techniques and at times ultrasound.

SHORT AND LONGER TERM EMOTIONAL AND PSYCHOLOGICAL COMPLICATIONS

This section will address the short and longer term emotional and psychological complications that occur following birth. There is increased recognition that these conditions are major health issues that have long-term consequences for the family as well as the woman.

Childbirth is a complex life event characterised by rapid biological, social and emotional transition that can be associated with a range of short- and long-term emotional consequences. Many women experience significant somatic (physical) and cognitive–affective (thinking–feeling) changes following childbirth, but may not be clinically depressed. Changes in mood may be part of normal postpartum adjustment.

Early postpartum emotional health

Postpartum affective disorders may be divided into three categories: postpartum blues, postpartum depression and postpartum psychosis. Both postpartum blues and postpartum psychosis occur close to the time of birth, whereas postpartum depression generally becomes apparent later in the postpartum period.

Postpartum blues, commonly called the 'baby blues', occurs in up to 84% of women with symptoms including mood lability, irritability, dysmorphic mood, crying, generalised anxiety, insomnia and loss of appetite (O'Hara & Wisner, 2014). These symptoms generally peak by days 4 to 5 and will have largely diminished by days 10 to 12 following birth. NICE (2015) recommends that if symptoms do not resolve after 10–14 days the woman should be assessed for postnatal depression, and if symptoms persist then further evaluation is required.

Debriefing

NICE (2015) guidelines for postnatal care recommend that caregivers provide an opportunity to talk about the birth and give information on normal patterns of emotional change. Various terms have been used to describe how midwives discuss birth experiences with women postnatally, including debriefing, counselling, supporting and reviewing experiences. Although these terms have been used interchangeably in the midwifery literature, debriefing refers to a psychological approach to help people cope with a traumatic event (Bastos & McCourt, 2010). Some interventions, structured or unstructured, have been offered universally to women following birth, whereas others have targeted groups of women considered to be at risk of psychological distress (Sheen & Slade, 2015). The question has been raised as to who is the right person to undertake the review of the birth experience, and at this point there is insufficient evidence to support any one profession or intervention (Bastos et al., 2015). More research is needed about postnatal interventions for women who experience birth trauma. It is important that midwives are aware of and able to refer women who may suffer post-traumatic stress disorder (PTSD), and may need information about problems such as depression (Bastos et al., 2015).

Puerperal psychosis

Postpartum (or puerperal) psychosis is the most severe and uncommon form of postnatal affective illness, occurring in one to two of every 1000 childbearing women (O'Hara & Wisner, 2014). Risk factors include a past history of a psychotic condition. The clinical onset is rapid and is most commonly observed within the first 2 weeks following birth.

Symptoms include:

- Mood disturbances
  - Persistently high or elevated mood, alternatively an irritable mood
  - Decreased need for sleep
  - Increasingly talkative (in volume and amount of talk)
  - Racing thoughts and rapid changes of topic
  - Not being aware of the baby's needs
  - Rapid changes of intense feelings—from laughter to tears, to anger and back

- Psychosis
  - Delusions—unusual beliefs
  - Thought disturbances—feeling that thoughts are being taken or put into the head
  - Hallucinations—hearing, feeling, seeing, smelling something that is not there
  - Changed perceptions (colours and sounds may seem very intense)

(Mental Health Foundation of New Zealand, 2019)

Assessment

A full clinical assessment is required by the maternal mental health team (if available) or the local mental health team.

Management

Women with psychoses will require close physical monitoring, and support from a skilled health professional. Generally, they are hospitalised within a mother and baby unit. Treatment includes medication options and psychotherapy. A full recovery is usual, however, these women are at risk of further episodes of bipolar affective disorder (Austin et al., 2017).

Anxiety and depression

The postnatal period and transition to parenthood is recognised as a stressful life event. Global studies concerning perinatal mental health have demonstrated that one in ten women experience depression during pregnancy and up to one in seven in the year following birth (Austin et al., 2017). Other mental health illnesses such as schizophrenia, bipolar disorders and borderline personality disorders exist less frequently, but all can have a negative impact on maternal and infant outcomes. Additionally, women with mental health issues have been reported to experience a higher rate of life-threatening obstetric complications (Easter et al., 2021), which highlights how important it is to provide holistic care to women during pregnancy and the postpartum period. Anxiety disorders are also prevalent with around one in five women experiencing this, often in conjunction with depression.

Anxiety

Anxiety is a broad term used to refer to a wide range of conditions (COPE, 2021). See Box 41.7 for common symptoms. A systematic review by Dennis et al. (2017) reported that the prevalence was high throughout pregnancy (18–24%) and into the postpartum period (15%) with rates being higher in low- to middle-income countries.

Box 41.7 Common symptoms of anxiety

- Feelings of fear and worry which begin to 'take over' your thinking
- Feeling irritable, restless, tense or constantly 'on edge'
- Racing heart / strong palpitations—sometimes panic attacks
- Reoccurring worrying thoughts such as that you are not doing things right and / or that something terrible will happen
- Unable to sleep—even when you have the opportunity
- Avoiding situations for fear something bad will happen

(Source: COPE, 2021)

Predisposing factors

A study including 918 women 6 months after birth from South Australia and Victoria reported that 21% (189/918) of women were scoring positive for anxiety alone, with a further 38% (344/918) experiencing both anxiety and depression (Yelland et al., 2010). This study explored the association with social health issues such as moving house, new employment, serious illness of a family member or death and called for health professionals to recognise the impact of these factors on women's social health. Further to this there is a reported association with childbirth fear; a preference for caesarean section; decreased effective coping strategies; higher rates of eating disorders; an increased risk of suicide and adverse outcomes for children in terms of development (Dennis et al., 2017).

The studies of anxiety depend on self-reporting which have inherent limitations. There is a perception of anxiety being more prevalent, however this was not supported by the findings of the systematic review by Dennis et al. (2017).

Management

Anxiety may be treated with behavioural therapies aiming to change patterns of thinking and behaviour, which may be just as effective if delivered online (beyondblue, 2021). The importance of recognising and treating maternal anxiety is paramount to providing good mental healthcare as it is common to experience postnatal depression alongside postnatal anxiety (Austin et al., 2017).

Postnatal depression

The term '**postnatal depression**' (PND) is used in clinical practice to describe depression presenting any time during the first year after giving birth (Austin et al, 2017). PND is the most prevalent mood disorder associated with childbirth and presents in a similar pattern to depression at other stages of life, although during postpartum it is characterised by irritability, anger, having low energy levels and loss of interest, and feelings of guilt (Buist et al., 2008).

Prevalence

The prevalence rates are reported to be between 10% and 16% depending on when the assessment is undertaken and the diagnostic criteria (Austin et al., 2017; Schmied et al., 2013). The Growing Up in New Zealand cohort study identified an antenatal depression rate of 12.1%, which reduced to 7.9% at 9 months postnatally (Underwood et al., 2016).

Predisposing factors

Factors associated with PND include financial hardship, being single, and migration to a country where the mother's primary language is not spoken, association with three or more stressful life events (Dennis et al., 2004; Yelland et al., 2010), social isolation, poor partner relationship and previous history of depression (Dennis et al., 2004; NICE, 2015). NICE (2015) recommends that all women are assessed 10–14 days after birth about resolution of baby blues (discussed previously) and if symptoms are not resolved the woman should be assessed for PND.

Diagnosis

The most common tool used for self-reporting of postnatal depression is the EPDS (Cox et al., 1987) (Box 41.8). This

Box 41.8 Edinburgh Postnatal Depression Scale

As you have recently had a baby, we would like to know how you are feeling. Please UNDERLINE the answer that comes closest to how you have felt IN THE PAST 7 DAYS, not just how you feel today.

Here is an example, already completed.

I have felt happy:

Yes, all the time

<u>Yes, most of the time</u>

No, not very often

No, not at all

This would mean: 'I have felt happy most of the time' during the past week. Please complete the other questions in the same way.

In the past 7 days:

1. I have been able to laugh and see the funny side of things
   As much as I always could
   Not quite so much now
   Definitely not so much now
   Not at all
2. I have looked forward with enjoyment to things
   As much as I ever did
   Rather less than I used to
   Definitely less than I used to
   Hardly at all
3. *I have blamed myself unnecessarily when things went wrong
   Yes, most of the time
   Yes, some of the time
   Not very often
   No, never
4. I have been anxious or worried for no good reason
   No, not at all
   Hardly ever
   Yes, sometimes
   Yes, very often
5. * I have felt scared or panicky for no very good reason
   Yes, quite a lot
   Yes, sometimes
   No, not much
   No, not at all
6. * Things have been getting on top of me
   Yes, most of the time I haven't been able to cope at all
   Yes, sometimes I haven't been coping as well as usual
   No, most of the time I have coped quite well
   No, I have been coping as well as ever
7. * I have been so unhappy that I have had difficulty sleeping
   Yes, most of the time
   Yes, sometimes
   Not very often
   No, not at all
8. * I have felt sad or miserable
   Yes, most of the time
   Yes, quite often
   Not very often
   No, not at all
9. * I have been so unhappy that I have been crying
   Yes, most of the time
   Yes, quite often
   Only occasionally
   No, never
10. * The thought of harming myself has occurred to me
    Yes, quite often
    Sometimes
    Hardly ever
    Never

Administered/Reviewed by ______________________
Date ______________

Response categories are scored 0, 1, 2, 3 according to increased severity of the symptoms. Items marked with an asterisk are reverse scored (i.e. 3, 2, 1, 0). The total score is calculated by adding together the scores for each of the ten items.

(Source: Cox et al., 1987; reproduced with permission)

scale has been translated into many languages and validated for use with different populations at various time points in both the antenatal and the postnatal period. The EPDS has been trialled with Aboriginal and Torres Strait Islander women and at this stage is the recommended tool with the proviso that the tool be implemented in a culturally appropriate way preferably by an Aboriginal health worker known to the woman (Austin et al., 2017).

It is important to remember that the EPDS has not been translated into the vast majority of Aboriginal languages and for many of these women English may be their second, third or even fourth language, which is also true for other culturally and linguistically diverse groups. A study in 2014 developed the Kimberley Mum's Mood Scale (KMMS) to be used with Aboriginal women in the Kimberley region of Western Australia (Carlin et al., 2019). Exploration of the use of this tool reported that the outcome was significantly linked to the relationship formed by the healthcare professional using the tool (Carlin et al., 2019). The professional needed to form a trusting relationship using 'yarning' and be non-judgmental as they actively listened to women.

The EPDS has been validated for use with Samoan and Tongan women in one study (Ekeroma et al., 2012) and has been used without specific cultural validation in other studies (Deverick & Guiney, 2016; Waldie et al., 2015).

The use of the EPDS has been called into question by some researchers. Other tools that have been validated include the HADS (Hospital Anxiety and Depression Scale); PHQ-9 (Patient Health Questionnaire-9) (Austin et al., 2017; NICE, 2015); shorter versions of the PHQ-9 (PHQ-2), the Whooley Questions and the K-10 (Austin et al., 2017). It is always difficult making comparisons between studies when different tools or different cut-off criteria along with different timing of assessments are used. A high proportion of women identified as 'at risk' may never develop PND and, equally, women identified as 'low risk' may develop PND, with potential harm resulting from late diagnosis or lack of diagnosis (Yelland et al., 2010).

As the EPDS is most frequently used and is recommended by the most recent Australian guideline (Austin et al., 2017), the use of the tool will be explained. Each item in the EPDS is scored on a scale of zero to three resulting in a possible score range of 0 to 30. (Note: some items are reverse scored.) Austin et al. (2017) suggest the following for considering the total score:

0–9	The likelihood of depression is considered low.
10–12	The woman should be monitored and the EPDS repeated 2-4 days later.
≥13	The likelihood of depression can be considered to be high

Collaborative care in Australia

In Australia an evidence-based guideline for mental healthcare in the perinatal period has been developed (Austin et al., 2017). Not all recommendations are supported by empirical evidence (EBR), so where this has not been available the group have consensus-based recommendations (CBR) and practice points (PP). The main points are the following:

- The guideline recognises the variety and number of individuals providing care to women across the maternity continuum with a recommendation for continuity of care wherever possible (Austin et al., 2017).
- It is recommended (CBR) that all individuals providing care should have training in 'woman-centred communication skills, psychological assessment and culturally safe care' (p. 7).
- Women should be screened for a possible depressive disorder using the Edinburgh Postnatal Depression Scale (EPDS), using a score of 13 or more as an indicator for further assessment (EBR).
- In the postnatal period this should be completed between six and 12 weeks and again in the first year postnatal (CBR) or any time it is clinically indicated (p. 7).
- The language and cultural appropriateness of the tool must be considered, in particular for use with Aboriginal and Torres Strait Islander women (CBR).
- Any woman with a positive score on Question 10 of the EPDS must have the risk managed through further assessment and consideration given for support and treatment options (CBR).

It is recommended that readers access the full guidelines, which are available from: https://www.cope.org.au/wp-content/uploads/2018/05/COPE-Perinatal-MH-Guideline_Final-2018.pdf.

Prevention

Protective factors against development of PND identified in the NICE guidelines (2015) are gentle exercise, rest, getting help with baby care, talking to someone about their feelings and accessing social support networks. Possible other protective factors are optimism and self-esteem, having a good relationship and adequate preparation for physical and psychosocial changes of parenthood (Pope, 2000). Discussion and use of these strategies should be considered and included in routine postnatal care provided by midwives.

Management

The main psychosocial support and psychological approaches include education, social support groups and individual structured psychological interventions such as cognitive behavioural therapy or interpersonal psychotherapy (EBR). The education includes advising women of the symptoms of depression and the possible benefits of directed counselling (CBR).

Treatment options may include complementary therapies such as omega-3 fatty acid supplementation, however the evidence is lacking for the effectiveness (Austin et al., 2017). Antidepressants are recommended only if the woman declines counselling, if psychological interventions are ineffective, or if the woman has a history of

Box 41.9 Factors influencing treatment choice for postnatal mental illness

- Choose medications with lower risk profiles for the mother and infant
- Start at a low dose, and slowly increase to the lowest effective dose—this is particularly important where the risks may be dose related
- Use monotherapy in preference to combined treatment
- Consider additional precautions for pre-term, low-birth-weight or sick infants

(Source: NICE, 2015)

severe depression. Serotonin reuptake inhibitors (SSRIs) are recommended for the first line pharmacological treatment, however this is conditional on a woman's history and the age of the infant and breastfeeding status (EBR). When prescribing medication the health professional should take into consideration the factors outlined in Boxes 41.9 and 41.10. It is recommended that the reader access the Mental Health in the Perinatal period guideline for recommended treatment and doses (Austin et al., 2017). An important practice point is to be aware that women should be advised not to discontinue the medication without consulting with their medical practitioner as withdrawal symptoms or relapse into depression may occur.

Maternal mortality and suicide

Perinatal mental health disorders are increasingly resulting in deaths from suicide with Australia reporting 23 deaths in the period 2009 to 2018 (AIHW, 2020), and 30 women dying by suicide in New Zealand between 2006 and 2018 with an over-representation of Māori women in this number (PMMRC, 2018). This trend is reported worldwide, however due to the differences in reporting across countries the prevalence is difficult to compare (Humphrey, 2016). The risk of suicide is increased 'drastically' in women with severe or moderate mental illness compared to women with no psychiatric history (Howard & Khalifeh, 2020). Additionally, women with mental health disorders are reported to experience more complications in pregnancy including acute renal failure, cardiac arrest, cardiac failure or infarction and obstetric embolism (Easter, 2021) possibly due to misattribution of physical symptoms to anxiety or schizophrenia (Howard & Khalifeh, 2020). Assessment of risk of suicide involves asking about the extent of suicidal thoughts and planning, specifically asking about how frequent and persistent suicidal thoughts are, if the woman has a plan, if the planned method is lethal and does the woman have the means to carry out the method (Austin et al., 2017). The safety of the infant also needs consideration at this point. A safety plan should be developed with the woman and revisited and modified as needed (Austin et al., 2017). As this is outside of the midwifery scope of practice it would be important for the midwife to refer the woman for mental health assessment (ACM, 2014).

Post-traumatic stress and childbirth

Post-traumatic stress disorder (PTSD) is characterised by persistent re-experiencing of the traumatic event, persistent avoidance of stimuli associated with the event, numbing of general responsiveness, and symptoms of increased arousal (American Psychiatric Association (APA), 2012). These symptoms or reactions can develop after either experiencing or witnessing a traumatic event (COPE, 2021), so may apply to a woman, her partner or support people or staff involved in care. Although most childbirth is not traumatic, global studies report that approximately three percent of women experience PTSD in the postpartum period (Ayers et al., 2016). A longitudinal study conducted in Sweden reported that 65% of women with PTSD also experienced depression at 11 months postpartum (Söderquist et al., 2006).

Some women are more vulnerable to PTSD such as those with anxiety or previous psychological problems, or a history of trauma or sexual abuse (Ayers et al., 2016). Primiparity and birth risk factors such as poor support, negative emotions, perceived threat through operative birth and dissociation further compound this (Ayers et al., 2016). The role of support during labour and birth appears to be important for prevention of PTSD, however Ayers et al. (2016) suggest that this may also be the case for postpartum support and care, but more research is needed in this area.

COPE (2021) advise that treatment for PTSD may include psychological treatment such as trauma-focused cognitive behavioural therapy (CBT) or eye movement desensitisation and reprocessing (EMDR) and medications such as SSRIs. Support groups and resources for women and their families are listed in Box 41.11.

Consequences of poor mental health outcomes for women, children and families

Postnatal distress is associated with adverse psychosocial consequences such as relationship difficulties, poor family functioning and impaired parenting. Children of women who suffer mood disorders can have short- and long-term disturbances to their emotional, behavioural and cognitive development (Moehler et al., 2006). Ongoing and debilitating anxiety and panic attacks, depression and suicidal thoughts, feelings of rage, marital and family breakdown, sexual dysfunction and emotional detachment from their babies and other children may be experienced (Murray, 2006). Obsession with seeking answers about the traumatic episode, dissociation, terrifying

Box 41.10 Race-related mental health issues

The incidence of mental health issues is thought to be similar in different cultural groups, but may be underreported in different groups due to the stigma of mental illness. Both Australia and New Zealand have culturally diverse populations including Indigenous people and immigrant people—both by choice and because of being forced to flee the country of origin. In order for all women to receive the best care possible it is important that healthcare providers, in particular midwives, recognise the significant challenges to mental health in the perinatal period. Perinatal Clinical Practice Guidelines developed by COPE (Austin et al., 2017) provide a comprehensive resource for psychosocial assessment, treatment and care for all women and more resources are available via their website (https://www.cope.org.au/wp-content/uploads/2018/05/COPE-Perinatal-MH-Guideline_Final-2018.pdf), specifically for Aboriginal and Torres Strait Islander women and women from culturally and linguistically diverse (CALD) backgrounds. Similarly in New Zealand the Mental Health Foundation provides resources for postnatal and perinatal mental health via its website (http://www.mentalhealth.org.nz).

Aboriginal and Torres Strait Islander women

Studies regarding Aboriginal and Torres Strait Islander women's reproductive health are highly sensitive owing to tradition, culture and women's business. Currently there is a lack of data specifically about the incidence of postnatal depression for Aboriginal and Torres Strait Islander women; however, the data that are available suggest that the problems faced by these women are at least as prevalent as for non-Aboriginal women, possibly more so owing to their history of loss, their ongoing disadvantage within our communities and the barriers to their accessing help (Austin et al., 2017). In traditional Aboriginal cultures, birth is intrinsically linked to the land and plants, making these factors vital to the wellbeing of the mother, infant and families. Aboriginal women have been pushed towards institutions to give birth in a medicalised environment without appropriate recognition of the importance of tradition and culture to their birth experience (Hancock, 2006). This action disrupts their families as they leave their land to give birth among strangers, which may contribute to mental health issues. Other factors that contribute to mental health of Aboriginal and Torres Strait Islander women include a lack of basic resources and facilities such as poor literacy, family violence, and risk-associated behaviours such as smoking and alcohol use in pregnancy (Hancock, 2006). Postnatal depression and other mental health disorders may present themselves spiritually and culturally so the use of mainstream diagnostic criteria and treatment for mental illness in Aboriginal and Torres Strait islander women has been questioned. There is a need for a culturally sensitive approach to assessment and management of perinatal depression for women from Aboriginal and Torres Strait heritage, which would ideally include Aboriginal Health Workers who are recognised as being experts in community relevant knowledge (Ferguson-Hill, 2010).

Māori and Pacific Island families

A New Zealand study of the prevalence of postnatal depression using postal surveys (including the EPDS) in 2015 concluded that rates of postnatal depression in urban New Zealand were slightly higher than the worldwide average and largely go untreated, with only 13% of women with an EPDS of 13 or more seeking treatment (Deverick & Guiney, 2016). A sub study within the Growing Up in New Zealand study cohort reported that Pacific or Asian women accounted for 26% of the sample, but 37.7% of the women who had depression symptoms at antenatal interview or when surveyed nine months after birth using the EPDS (Underwood et al., 2016).

Māori and Pacific Island people's model of wellbeing see the individual as being part of the wider community, or inseparable from the family and those around them (New Zealand Guidelines Group, 2008). Culturally competent care needs to address the following issues:

- acknowledgement of the role of the broader whānau (extended family) and other environmental factors
- awareness of Māori belief systems and lifestyles
- knowledge of existing support systems such as kaiatawhai (Māori health workers), whānau, kaumātua (tribal elders), consumer advisors and other specialist service providers.

(Source: New Zealand Guidelines Group, 2008)

flashbacks and nightmares, hypervigilance with regard to their baby and isolation from other mothers are consistently reported by women who experienced distressing births (Nerum et al., 2006). Women also report fear of becoming pregnant again, which contributes to a lack of intimacy and conflict with partners, avoidance of pregnant women and voluntary infertility (Nerum et al., 2006). Women who do become pregnant again report sleep difficulties, depression, suicidal thoughts and panic attacks, particularly when attending maternity appointments, but conversely also report that developing coping strategies such as proactive planning, use of a birth plan, and seeking supportive and empathetic care providers helps them to regain a sense of control.

A recent systematic review regarding the impact of mental health on partners reported that mental health issues resulted in conflict, relationship breakdown and domestic violence (Atkinson et al., 2021). This review revealed that partners lacked knowledge of postnatal depression and found themselves looking for the cause of the change in

Box 41.11 Support groups and resources for women and their families

Australia

- beyondblue—https://www.beyondblue.org.au/. There are a number of telephone helplines and physical resources available for Australian women expressing depression in pregnancy and after birth. beyondblue is a national, independent, not-for-profit organisation working to address issues associated with depression, anxiety and related substance misuse disorders in Australia. Information provided regarding postnatal depression includes types, symptoms, treatment, helping others and self-help strategies. Resources include telephone numbers for each state and territory.
- Post and Antenatal Depression Association (PANDA)—http://www.panda.org.au. PANDA is a Victorian not-for-profit self-help organisation providing confidential information, support and referral to anyone affected by post- and antenatal mood disorders, including partners and extended family members. Information and training seminars are also provided for healthcare professionals and the wider community.

Specifically for Aboriginal and Torres Strait Islander families

- Queensland Health, Growing Deadly Families Aboriginal and Torres Strait Islander Maternity Services Strategy 2019-2025. Available from: https://www.health.qld.gov.au/atsihealth/maternity-services
- Well mob—Social, emotional and cultural wellbeing online resources for Aboriginal and Torres Strait Islander People. Available from: https://wellmob.org.au/

New Zealand

- http://www.depression.org.nz. Sponsored by the Ministry of Health, this provides information on depression and a depression helpline 0800 111 757.
- The Mental Health Foundation of New Zealand—https://www.mentalhealth.org.nz/. A charity organisation for trusted mental health information in Aotearoa, New Zealand.
- Perinatal Anxiety & Depression Aotearoa (PADA)—http://www.pada.nz/. An organisation supporting families for perinatal mental health.
- Positively Pregnant app—An app designed for women who are pregnant or planning pregnancy and who want some tools for managing stress and maintaining wellbeing during pregnancy and in the transition to parenthood—https://www.healthnavigator.org.nz/apps/p/positively-pregnant-app/.

their partner. They reported that partners felt relief when a diagnosis was made, giving them reason for hope. Partners were reluctant to disclose the illness, however those that did experienced significant relief. Further research is required for partners' mental health around screening, interventions and support (Austin et al., 2017).

Conclusion

The care of a woman and her baby in the immediate hours, days and weeks after birth can make an enormous impact on their long-term health and wellbeing, and in turn affect their family and the wellbeing of the wider society. The physical, emotional and social changes that impact on the lives of women through childbirth are often overwhelming, in particular for first-time mothers. It is important that women receive individualised care in the hours, days and weeks following birth. Many women describe ongoing health and emotional problems that occur following the birth and which have ongoing impact on their lives. Women should be encouraged to report and seek treatment for these problems. In the early postpartum period, women are at risk of postpartum haemorrhage, pregnancy-related hypertension, pulmonary embolism and endometritis. Longer-term fatigue and backache are common causes of poor health whilst, although less common, urinary and/or faecal incontinence can have a significant effect on the woman's physical and emotional recovery and longer term health. A failure to recognise postpartum complications can lead to physical discomfort, psychological distress and a poor quality of life for women. Quality and evidence-based postnatal care, including earlier identification of the problems and supportive intervention, will help the mother to achieve full recovery and restore her functional status back to her pre-pregnancy state sooner.

Review questions

1. What are some of the factors associated with poorer postpartum health?
2. List some of the barriers women face in accessing professional assistance for healthcare in the postpartum period.
3. Describe the symptoms and treatment of endometritis.
4. What assessment data would you need to determine whether a woman was experiencing a secondary postpartum haemorrhage?
5. Describe the initial treatment for a woman admitted to hospital via ambulance reporting that she is 12 days postpartum and bleeding heavily.
6. What are the factors that place women at risk of postpartum emotional distress?
7. Identify the symptoms of depression.
8. What advice would you give a woman who reported she was experiencing urinary incontinence after the birth of her child?
9. Briefly describe the effect of social support in relation to postnatal depression.
10. Describe best practice in maternity care to specifically prevent emotional distress for postpartum women.

Online resources

Australian Institute of Health and Welfare: http://www.aihw.gov.au/.
Anxiety Recovery Centre Victoria: https://www.arcvic.org.au/.
beyondblue: http://www.beyondblue.org.au/.
Centre of Perinatal Excellence: https://www.cope.org.au/.
Clinical Evidence, BMJ Publishing: http://clinicalevidence.bmj.com/ceweb/index.jsp.
Continence Foundation of Australia: http://www.continence.org.au/.
National Institute for Health and Care Excellence: http://www.nice.org.uk/.
New Zealand Ministry of Health: http://www.moh.govt.nz.

References

Abrams P, Cardozo L, Fall M, et al. The standardisation of terminology of lower urinary tract function: Report from the standardisation sub-committee of the International Continence Society. *Neurourol Urodyn*. 2002;21(2):167–178. doi:10.1002/nau.10052.

Aiken C, Mehasseb M, Prentice A. Secondary postpartum haemorrhage. *Fetal Matern Med Rev*. 2012;23(1):1–14.

Albers LL. Health problems after childbirth. *J Midwifery Womens Health*. 2000;45(1):55–57.

Alexander J, Thomas P, Sanghera A. Treatments for secondary postpartum haemorrhage. *Cochrane Database Syst Rev*. 2002;(4):CD002867.

American Psychiatric Association (APA). *Diagnostic and Statistical Manual of Mental Disorders DSM-6*. 6th ed. —text revision (DSMVI-TR). Washington, DC: American Psychiatric Publishing; 2012.

Atkinson J, Smith V, Carroll M, et al. Perspectives of partners of mothers who experience mental distress in the postnatal period: A systematic review and qualitative evidence synthesis. *Midwifery*. 2021;93:102868–102868.

Austin M-P, Highet N, and Highest the Expert Working Group. *Mental Health Care in the Perinatal Period: Australian Clinical Practice Guideline*. Melbourne: Centre of Perinatal Excellence; 2017.

Australian College of Midwives: *National Midwifery Guidelines for Consultation and Referral*. 3rd ed. Canberra: Australian College of Midwives; 2014.

Australian Institute of Health and Welfare (AIHW): *Maternal deaths in Australia*. Australian Institute of Health and Welfare; 2020.

Ayers S, Bond R, Bertullies S, et al. The aetiology of post-traumatic stress following childbirth: a meta-analysis and theoretical framework, *Psychological Medicine*. 2016;46:1121–1134.

Bastos MH, Furuta M, Small R, et al. Debriefing interventions for the prevention of psychological trauma in women following childbirth. *Cochrane Database of Syst Rev*. 2015;(4): CD007194, doi: 10.1002/14651858.CD007194.pub2.

Bastos MH, McCourt C. Morbidity during the postnatal period: impact on women and society. In: Byrom S, Edwards G, Bick D, eds. *Essential Midwifery Practice: Postnatal Care*. London: Wiley-Blackwell; 2010:113–137.

Benjamin DR, van de Water ATM, Peiris CL. Effects of exercise on diastasis of the rectus abdominis muscle in the antenatal and postnatal periods: a systematic review. *Physiotherapy*. 2013;100(1):1–8. doi:10.1016/j.physio.2013.08.005.

Benjamin DR, Frawley HC, Shields N, et al.: Relationship between diastasis of the rectus abdominis muscle (DRAM) and musculoskeletal dysfunctions, pain and quality of life: a systematic review, *Physiotherapy* 2019;105:24–34.

Bergmann R, Richter R, Bergmann KE, et al. Prevalence and risk factors for early postpartum anaemia. *Eur J Obstet Gynecol Reprod Biol*. 2010;150:126–131.

beyondblue: *Psychological treatments for anxiety*, 2021. Online: https://www.beyondblue.org.au/the-facts/anxiety/treatments-for-anxiety/psychological-treatments-for-anxiety.

Bick D, MacArthur C, Winter H. *Postnatal Care: Evidence and Guidelines for Management*. 2nd ed. Edinburgh: Churchill Livingstone; 2009.

Birch L, Doyle PM, Ellis R, et al. Risk factors for the development of postnatal anal incontinence. *Br J Midwifery*. 2006;14(5): 309–314.

Bø K, Haakstad LAH. Is pelvic floor muscle training effective when taught in a general fitness class in pregnancy? A randomised controlled trial. *Physiotherapy*. 2011;97(3):190–195. doi:10.1016/j.physio.2010.08.014.

Bø K, Mørkved S. Pelvic floor and exercise science. In: Bø K, Berghmans B, Mørkved S, et al. eds. *Evidence-Based Physical Therapy for the Pelvic Floor*. 2nd ed. Sydney: Elsevier; 2015: 111–129.

Bonet M, Brizuela V, Abalos E, et al.: *Frequency* and management of maternal infection in health facilities in 52 countries (GLOSS): a 1-week inception cohort study, *The Lancet Global Health* 8, 2020; e661–e671.

Bowyer L, Robinson HL, Barrett H, et al. SOMANZ guidelines for the investigation and management sepsis in pregnancy. *Aust N Z J Obstet Gynaecol*. 2017;57(5):540–551. doi:10.1111/ajo.12646.

Boyle R, Hay-Smith EJC, Cody JD, et al. Pelvic floor muscle training for prevention and treatment of urinary and faecal incontinence in antenatal and postnatal women. *Cochrane Database Syst Rev*. 2012;(10):CD007471, doi:10.1002/14651858.CD007471.pub2.

Brown S. *What can antenatal care do for women?* Seminar, Mother and Child Health Research, Latrobe University; 5 June 2013.

Brown S, Lumley J. Maternal health after childbirth: results of an Australian population based survey. *BJOG*. 1998;105(2): 156–161. doi:10.1111/j.1471-0528.1998.tb10045.x.

Brown S, Davey M-A, Bruinsma F. Women's views and experiences of postnatal hospital care in the Victorian Survey of Recent Mothers 2000. *Midwifery*. 2005;21(2):109–126.

Buist A, Austin M-P, Hayes B, et al. Postnatal mental health of women giving birth in Australia 2002–2004: findings from the beyondblue National Postnatal Depression Program. *Aust N Z J Psychiatry*. 2008;42(1):66–73. doi:10.1080/00048670701732749.

Burgio K, Zyczynski H, Locher JL, et al. Urinary incontinence in the 12-month postpartum period. *Obstet Gynecol*. 2003; 102(6):1291–1298.

Busowski MT, Lee M, Busowski JD, et al. Puerperal group A streptococcal infections: a case series and discussion. *Case Rep Med*. 2013;2013(3):751329. doi:10.1155/2013/751329.

Carlin E, Atkinson D, and Marley JV: 'Having a Quiet Word': Yarning with Aboriginal Women in the Pilbara Region of Western Australia about Mental Health and Mental Health Screening during the Perinatal Period, *Int J Environ Res Public Health* 2019; 16, 4253.

COAG Health Council: Woman-centred care: *Strategic directions for Australian maternity services*, Canberra, 2019, Department of Health.

Centre of Perinatal Excellence (COPE): *Postnatal anxiety*, 2021. Online: https://www.cope.org.au/new-parents/postnatal-mental-health-conditions/postnatal-anxiety/

Cox JL, Holden JM, Sagovsky R. Detection of postnatal depression; development of the 10-item Edinburgh Postnatal Depression Scale. *Br J Psychiatry*. 1987;150:782–786.

Dennis CL, Janssen P, Singer J. Identifying women at-risk for postpartum depression in the immediate postpartum period. *Acta Psychiatr Scand*. 2004;110:338–346.

Dennis CL, Falah-Hassani K, and Shiri R: Prevalence of antenatal and postnatal anxiety: Systematic review and meta-analysis. *Br J Psychiatry*. 2017;210:315–323.

Deverick Z, Guiney H. *Postnatal depression in New Zealand: Findings from the 2015 New Mothers Mental Health Survey*. Wellington: Health Promotion Agency; 2016.

Diez-Itza I, Ibañez L, Arrue M, et al. Influence of maternal weight on the new onset of stress urinary incontinence in pregnant women. *Int Urogynecol J Pelvic Floor Dysfunct*. 2009;20(10): 1259–1263.

Easter A, Sandall J, and Howard LM: Obstetric near misses among women with serious mental illness: data linkage cohort study. *The British Journal of Psychiatry*. 2021; 1–7.

Ekeroma AJ, Ikenasia-Thorpe B, Weeks S, et al. Validation of the Edinburgh Postnatal Depression Scale (EPDS) as a screening tool for postnatal depression in Samoan and Tongan women living in New Zealand. *N Z Med J*. 2012:125(1355):41–49.

Ewings P, Spencer S, Marsh H, et al. Obstetric risk factors for urinary incontinence and preventative pelvic floor exercises: Cohort study and nested randomized controlled trial. *J Obstet Gynaecol*. 2005;25(6):558–564. doi:10.1080/01443610500231435.

Ferguson-Hill S. Promoting perinatal mental health wellness in Aboriginal and Torres Strait Islander communities. In: Purdie N, Dudgeon P, Walker R, eds. *Working Together: Aboriginal and Torres Strait Islander Mental Health and Wellbeing Principles and Practice*. Barton, ACT: Commonwealth of Australia; 2010:223–242. Online. http://nceta.flinders.edu.au/files/2113/5891/4630/working_together_full_book.pdf.

Finlayson K, Crossland N, Bonet M, et al.: What matters to women in the postnatal period: A meta-synthesis of qualitative studies, *PLoS ONE*. 2020;15:e0231415.

Forster DA, McLachlan HL, Davey MA, et al. Continuity of care by a primary midwife (caseload midwifery) increases women's satisfaction with antenatal, intrapartum and postpartum care: results from the COSMOS randomised controlled trial. *BMC Pregnancy Childbirth*. 2016;16:28. doi:10.1186/s12884-016-0798-y.

Forster DA, McKay H, Powell R, et al. The structure and organisation of home-based postnatal care in public hospitals in Victoria, Australia: A cross-sectional survey. *Women Birth*. 2016;29(2): 172–179. doi:10.1016/j.wombi.2015.10.002.

Glazener C, Abdalla M, Stroud P, et al. Postnatal maternal morbidity: extent, causes, prevention and treatment. *BJOG*. 1995;102:282–287.

Hancock H. *Aboriginal Women's Perinatal Needs, Experiences and Maternity Services: A literature Review to Enable Considerations to be Made About Quality Indicators*. Alice Springs: Ngaanyatjarra Health Service; 2006. Online: http://www.lowitja.org.au/sites/default/files/docs/Ngaanyatjarra-Health-Service-Lit-Review.pdf.

Heath Quality & Safety Commission New Zealand. *Maternal Morbidity Working Group: Annual Report 1 September 2017 to 31 August 2018*. New Zealand Government; 2019.

Henderson J, Alderdice F, Redshaw M. Factors associated with maternal postpartum fatigue: an observational study. *BMJ Open* 2019: e0259. doi:10.1136/bmjopen-2018-025927.

Hollingshead JRF, Phillips RKS. Haemorrhoids: modern diagnosis and treatment. *Postgrad Med J*. 2016;92: 4–8.

Hoveyda F, MacKenzie IZ. Secondary postpartum haemorrhage: incidence, morbidity and current management. *BJOG*. 2001;108(9):927–930.

Howard LM, Khalifeh H: Perinatal mental health: a review of progress and challenges. *World Psychiatry*. 2020;19:313–327.

Howell CJ, Kidd C, Roberts W, et al. A randomised controlled trial of epidural compared with non-epidural analgesia in labour. *BJOG*. 2001;108(1):27–33. doi:10.1111/j.1471-0528.2001.00012.x.

Humphrey MD: Maternal mortality trends in Australia. *Med J Aust*. 2016;205:344–346.

Jansen AJG, Duvekot JJ, Hop WCJ, et al. New insights into fatigue and health-related quality of life after delivery. *Acta Obstet Gynecol Scand*. 2007;86(5):579–584. doi:10.1080/00016340701275424.

Khalafallah A, Dennis A, Ogden K, et al. Three-year follow-up of a randomised clinical trial of intravenous versus oral iron for anaemia in pregnancy. *BMJ Open*. 2012;2(5):e000998. doi:10.1136/bmjopen-2012-000998.

King Edward Memorial Hospital (KEMH). *Venous Thrombosis Occurring in the Present Pregnancy. Obstetric and Midwifery Clinical guidelines*. Perth, Australia: KEMH; 2016.

Koughnan BA, Carli F, Romney M, et al. Epidural analgesia and backache: a randomized controlled comparison with intramuscular meperidine for analgesia during labour. *Br J Anaesth.* 2002;89(3):466–472. doi:10.1093/bja/89.3.466.

Kristensen IH, Simonsen M, Trillingsgaard T, et al. First-time mothers' confidence mood and stress in the first months postpartum. A cohort study. *Sex Reprod Healthcare.* 2018;17:43–49.

Kurth E, Kennedy HP, Spichiger E, et al. Crying babies, tired mothers: What do we know? A systematic review. *Midwifery.* 2011;27(2):187–194. doi:10.1016/j.midw.2009.05.012.

Lemos A, de Souza A, Ferreira A, et al. Do perineal exercises during pregnancy prevent the development of urinary incontinence? A systematic review. *Int J Urol.* 2008;15:875–880.

Lim JL. Postpartum voiding dysfunction and urinary retention. *Aust N Z J Obstet Gynaecol.* 2010;50(6):502–505.

Loutzenhiser L, McAuslan P, Sharpe D. The trajectory of maternal and paternal fatigue and factors associated with fatigue across the transition to parenthood. *Australian Psychological Society Clinical Psychologist.* 2015;19:15–27.

Lumley J, Watson L, Small R, et al. PRISM (Program of Resources, Information and Support for Mothers): a community-randomised trial to reduce depression and improve women's physical health six months after birth (ISRCTN03464021). *BMC Public Health.* 2006;6:37.

MacArthur AJ, MacArthur C. Incidence, severity, and determinants of perineal pain after vaginal delivery: a prospective cohort study. *Am J Obstet Gynecol.* 2004;191(4):1199–1204. doi:10.1016/j.ajog.2004.02.064.

MacArthur C, Lewis M, Knox E. *Health After Childbirth.* London: Her Majesty's Stationery Office; 1991.

MacArthur C, Bick DE, Keighley MRB. Faecal incontinence after childbirth. *BJOG.* 1997;104(1):46–50. doi:10.1111/j.1471-0528.1997.tb10648.x.

MacArthur C, Wilson D, Herbison P, et al. Prolong study group. Urinary incontinence persisting after childbirth: extent, delivery history, and effects in a 12-year longitudinal cohort study. *BJOG.* 2016 May;123(6):1022–9. doi:10.1111/1471-0528.13395. Epub 2015 Apr 2. PMID: 25846816.

McLeish J, Redshaw M. Mothers' accounts of the impact on emotional wellbeing of organised peer support in pregnancy and early parenthood: a qualitative study. *BMC Pregnancy Childbirth.* 2017;17:28–28.

MacLennan AH, Taylor AW, Wilson DH, et al. The prevalence of pelvic floor disorders and their relationship to gender, age, parity and mode of delivery. *BJOG.* 2000;107(12):1460–1470. doi:10.1111/j.1471-0528.2000.tb11669.x.

McQueen A, Mander R. Tiredness and fatigue in the postnatal period. *J Adv Nurs.* 2003;42(5):463–469. doi:10.1046/j.1365-2648.2003.02645.x.

Marchant S, Alexander J, Garcia J, et al. A survey of women's experiences of vaginal loss from 24 hours to three months after childbirth (the BLiPP study). *Midwifery.* 1999;15(2):72–81.

Marchant S, Alexander J, Thomas P, et al. Risk factors for hospital admission related to excessive and/or prolonged postpartum vaginal blood loss after the first 24 h following childbirth. *Paediatr Perinat Epidemiol.* 2006;20(5):392–402.

Manresa M, Pereda A, Bataller E, et al. Incidence of perineal pain and dyspareunia following spontaneous vaginal birth: A systematic review and meta-analysis. *Int Urogynecol J.* 2019;30:852–868.

Mental Health Foundatin of New Zealand. *Postnatal psychosis.* 2019. Online: https://mentalhealth.org.nz/conditions/condition/postnatal-psychosis.

Ministry of Health (MOH). *Diagnosis and Treatment of Hypertension and Pre-eclampsia in Pregnancy in New Zealand. A Clinical Practice Guideline.* 2022.

Moehler E, Brunner R, Wiebel A, et al. Maternal depressive symptoms in the postnatal period are associated with long-term impairment of mother–child bonding. *Arch Womens Ment Health.* 2006;9(5):273–278.

Murray L. Socioemotional development in adolescents at risk for depression: the role of maternal depression and attachment style. *Dev Psychopathol.* 2006;18(2):489–516.

National Centre for Health and Care Excellence (NICE). *Routine Postnatal Care of Women and Their Babies*; 2015. Clinical guideline (CG37). London: NICE.

National Institute for Health and Care Excellence (NICE). *Urinary incontinence and pelvic organ prolapse in women: management. Clinical guideline (NG123).* London: NICE; 2019.

Nerum H, Halvorsen L, Sorlie T, et al. Maternal request of caesarean section due to fear of birth: can it be changed through crisis oriented counseling? *Birth.* 2006;33(3):221–228.

New South Wales (NSW) Government Health Department. *Maternal Sepsis (Puerperal Fever) due to Group A Streptococcus—Information for Clinicians fact sheet.* 2016. Online: https://www.health.nsw.gov.au/Infectious/factsheets/Pages/maternal-sepsis-info-for-HCW.aspx.

New Zealand College of Midwives (NZCOM): *Community midwives and midwifery services,* 2021. Online: https://www.midwife.org.nz/women/about-midwives/about-lead-maternity-carer-lmc-services/.

New Zealand College of Midwives (NZCOM). *Midwives Handbook for Practice.* Christchurch: New Zealand College of Midwives; 2015.

New Zealand Guidelines Group. *Identification of Common Mental Disorders and Management of Depression in Primary Care. An Evidence-based Best Practice Guideline.* Wellington: New Zealand Guidelines Group; 2008. Online: https://www.health.govt.nz/system/files/documents/publications/depression_guideline.pdf.

Nygaard I. Urinary incontinence: is cesarean delivery protective? *Semin Perinatol.* 2006;30(5):267–271. doi:10.1053/j.semperi.2006.07.007.

O'Hara MW, Wisner KL. Perinatal mental illness: definition, description and aetiology. *Best Pract Res Clin Obstet Gynaecol.* 2014;28(1):3–12. doi:10.1016/j.bpobgyn.2013.09.002.

Perinatal and Maternal Mortality Review Committee [PMMRC]: *Twelfth Annual Report of the Perinatal and Maternal Mortality Review Committee: Reporting mortality 2016.* Wellington: PMMRC; 2018.

Press J, Klein M, Kaczorowski J, et al. Does caesarean section reduce postpartum urinary incontinence? A systematic review. *Birth.* 2007;34(3):228–237.

Parera N, Liolitsa D, Iype S, et al. Phlebotoics for haemorrhoids: *Cochrane Database Syst Rev.* 2012;8 CD004322, doi:10.1002/14651858.CD004322.pub3.

Pope S. Postnatal Depression: *A Systematic Review of Published Scientific Literature to 1999: An Information Paper.* Canberra: National Health and Medical Research Council; 2000.

Poskus T, Buzinskien*fó* D, Drasutiene G, Samalavicius NE, et al. Haemorrhoids and anal fissures during pregnancy and after childbirth: a prospective cohort study. *BJOG.* 2014 Dec;121(13):1666–71. doi:10.1111/1471-0528.12838. *Epub 2014 May 9.* PMID: 24810254.

Queensland Clinical Guidelines. *VTE prophylaxis in pregnancy and the puerperium. Guideline No: MN20.9-V7-R25.* Queensland Health; 2020.

Royal Australian and New Zealand College of Obstetricians and Gynaecologists (RANZCOG). *Combined Hormonal Contraceptives*; 2016. Online: https://www.ranzcog.edu.au/.

Royal College of Obstetricians and Gynaecologists (RCOG). *The Acute Management of Thrombosis and Embolism During Pregnancy and The Puerperium. Guideline No. 37.* London: RCOG; 2010.

Russell R, Groves P, Taub N, et al. Assessing long term backache after childbirth. *BMJ.* 1993;306:1299–1303.

Russell R, Laxton C, Lucas DN, et al. Treatment of obstetric post-dural puncture headache. Part 1: conservative and pharmacological management. *Int Obstetric Anesth.* 2019;38:93–103.
Safer Care Victoria: *Postpartum haemorrhage (PPH) - prevention, assessment and management, 2019, Safer Care Victoria.* Online: https://www.bettersafercare.vic.gov.au/clinical-guidance/maternity/postpartum-haemorrhage-pph-prevention-assessment-and-management.
Sardi L, Idri A, Redman LM, et al. Mobile health applications for postnatal care: Review and analysis of functionalities and technical features, *Computer Methods and Programs in Biomedicine* 2020;184:105–114.
Schmied V, Johnson M, Naidoo N, et al. Maternal mental health in Australia and New Zealand: a review of longitudinal studies. *Women Birth.* 2013;26(3):167–178.
Schmied V, Bick D. Postnatal care-Current issues and future challenges. *Midwifery.* 2014;30: 571–574.
Schytt E, Lindmark G, Waldenström U. Physical symptoms after childbirth: prevalence and associations with self-rated health. *BJOG.* 2005;112(2):210–217.
Sheen K, Slade P. The efficacy of 'debriefing' after childbirth: Is there a case for targeted intervention? *J Reproduct Infant Psychol.* 2015;33(3):308–320. doi:10.1080/02646838.2015.1009881
Söderquist J, Wijma B, Wijma K. The longitudinal course of post-traumatic stress after childbirth. *J Psychosom Obstet Gynaecol.* 2006;27(2):113–119. doi:10.1080/01674820600712172.
Stella C, Jodicke C, How HY, et al. Postpartum headache: is your work-up complete? *Am J Obstet Gynecol.* 2007;196:318.e1–318.e7.
Taylor J, Johnson M. How women manage fatigue after childbirth. *Midwifery.* 2010;26(3):367–375. doi:10.1016/j.midw.2008.07.004.
Taylor J, Johnson M. The role of anxiety and other factors in predicting postnatal fatigue: From birth to 6 months. *Midwifery.* 2013;29(5):526–534. doi:10.1016/j.midw.2012.04.011.
Tennant E. Sepsis. *O&G Magazine.* 2013;15(1):58–59.
Thompson J, Roberts C, Currie M, et al. Prevalence and persistence of health problems after childbirth: associations with parity and method of birth. *Birth.* 2002;29(2):83–94.
Turner DP, Smitherman TA, Eisenach JC, et al. Predictors of headache before, during, and after pregnancy: a cohort study. *Headache.* 2012;52(3):348–362. doi:10.1111/j.1526-4610.2011.02066.x.
Underwood L, Underwood L, Waldie KE, et al.: A Longitudinal Study of Pre-pregnancy and Pregnancy Risk Factors Associated with Antenatal and Postnatal Symptoms of Depression: Evidence from Growing Up in New Zealand, *Matern Child Health J.* 2016;21:915–931.
United Nations (UN). *The Millennium Development Goals Report*; 2015. Online: https://sustainabledevelopment.un.org/index.php?page=view&type=400&nr=2036&menu=35.
Vanderkruik RC, Tunçalp Ö, Chou D, et al. Framing maternal morbidity: WHO scoping exercise. *BMC Pregnancy Childbirth.* 2013; 13:213. doi:10.1186/1471-2393-13-213.
Van der Woude DAA, Pijnenborg JMA, de Vries J. Health status and quality of life in postpartum women: a systematic review of associated factors. *European Journal of Obstetrics & Gynecology and Reproductive Biology.* 2015;185:45–52.
Virkus RA. Risk Factors for Venous Thromboembolism in 1.3 Million Pregnancies: A Nationwide Prospective Cohort. *PLoS ONE.* 2014;9(5):e96495.
Visness CM, Kennedy KID, Ramos RM. The duration and character of postpartum bleeding among breast-feeding women. *Obstet Gynecol.* 1997;89(2):159–163.
Waldie KE, Peterson ER, D'Souza S, et al. Depression symptoms during pregnancy: evidence from growing up in New Zealand. *Journal of Affective Disorders.* 2015;186:66–73.
Wang K, Xu X, Jia G, et al. Risk factors for postpartum stress urinary incontinence: a systematic review and meta-analysis, *Reproductive Sciences.* 2020;27:2129–2145.
Webb DA, Bloch JR, Coyne JC, et al. Postpartum physical symptoms in new mothers: their relationship to functional limitations and emotional well-being. *Birth.* 2008;35:179–187.
Wesnes SL, Lose G. Preventing urinary incontinence during pregnancy and postpartum: a review. *Int Urogynecol J Pelvic Floor Dysfunct.* 2013;24:889–899.
Wilkins C. A qualitative study exploring the support needs of first-time mothers on their journey towards intuitive parenting. *Midwifery.* 2006; 22:169–180.
Williams A, Herron-Marx S, Hicks C. The prevalence of enduring postnatal perineal morbidity and its relationship to perineal trauma. *Midwifery.* 2007;23:392–403.
Woodley SJ, Lawrenson P, Boyle R, et al. Pelvic floor muscle training for preventing and treating urinary and faecal incontinence in antenatal and postnatal women. *Cochrane Database Syst Rev.* 2020;5:CD007471.
Winter H, MacArthur C, Bick D, et al. Postnatal care and its role in maternal health and well-being. *MIDIRS Midwifery Dig.* 2001;11(1):S3–S7.
Woolhouse H, Gartland D, Perlen S, et al. Physical health after childbirth and maternal depression in the first 12 months post partum: results of an Australian nulliparous pregnancy cohort study. *Midwifery.* 2014;30(3):378–384. doi:10.1016/j.midw.2013.03.006.
World Health Organization (WHO). *Postnatal Care of the Mother and Newborn*; 2013. Online: http://apps.who.int/iris/bitstream/10665/97603/1/9789241506649_eng.pdf?ua=1.
World Health Organization (WHO). *Strategies Towards Ending Preventable Maternal Mortality (EPMM);* 2015. Online: http://who.int/reproductivehealth/topics/maternal_perinatal/epmm/en/.
Yelland J, Sutherland G, Brown SJ. Postpartum anxiety, depression and social health: findings from a population-based survey of Australian women. *BMC Public Health.* 2010;10:771.
Zaki MM, Pandit M, Jackson S. National survey for intrapartum and postpartum bladder care: assessing the need for guidelines. *BJOG.* 2004;111(8):874–876.

CHAPTER 42

The compromised neonate

Karen Walker and Jennifer Dawson

LEARNING OUTCOMES

At the completion of this chapter, the reader will have an understanding of:

1. The physiology of common birth defects that may be encountered in the neonatal period
2. The need for early identification of infants requiring resuscitation in the birthing room
3. The management of commonly occurring conditions that compromise the health of newly born infants
4. Neonatal infections that might arise in the perinatal period
5. The principles and management of supporting the mother and family of an infant who is unwell and may require transfer to a tertiary unit.

CHAPTER OVERVIEW

The aim of this chapter is to provide a brief outline of some common congenital anomalies and conditions apparent in the birthing room and early newborn period, how to recognise and resuscitate the sick infant and what to do while waiting to transfer an infant to a special or intensive care nursery. It is important to remember that infants can deteriorate very quickly and the midwife must always be prepared for the unexpected. It is not within the scope of this chapter to discuss all the neonatal disorders in detail as these can be found in neonatal textbooks such as *Neonatal Nursing in Australia and New Zealand: Principles for Practice* (Kain & Mannix, 2018).

KEY TERMS

abdominal wall defects
congenital anomaly
congenital heart disease
fetal alcohol spectrum disorder
meconium aspiration syndrome
necrotising enterocolitis
neonatal infection
neonatal resuscitation
neonatal transfer
respiratory distress syndrome

INTRODUCTION

In Australia each state and territory collects and publishes data on perinatal and maternal morbidity and mortality. Although there are some statistical differences between and within states, the data are similar. The most striking differences in outcomes are between women and babies living in rural / remote regions and those from metropolitan areas, with morbidity and mortality rates higher in babies born in rural, remote and very remote Australia (Australian Institute of Health and Welfare (AIHW), 2021). An increasing number of women choose to give birth at home and this means that sometimes mothers and babies require transfer to a tertiary facility. The majority of Australian women give birth in a hospital setting; for example, in New South Wales (NSW) 99% of mothers chose this option. The number of reported planned home births in NSW increased from 258 in 214 to 301 in 2018, with 235 women actually having a home birth in 2018 (Centre for Epidemiology and Evidence, 2019). In New Zealand in 2014, 96.4% of women gave birth at a tertiary or secondary facility, with 3.6% born at home (MOH, 2018). In New Zealand, there is a robust data collection system and process for perinatal and maternal mortality information. The Perinatal and Maternal Mortality Review Committee's report from the year 2019 shows a continuing reduction in stillbirths, although the rates of stillbirth remain significantly lower for those for NZ European mothers compared with the rates for Indian and Pacific mothers (PMMRC, 2021).

The incidence of infants with congenital anomalies from the most current Australia and New Zealand Neonatal Network report was 12.8% (Chow et al., 2019). The majority of infants with congenital anomalies are born at term, with 51.1% in Australia and New Zealand diagnosed antenatally (Chow et al., 2019).

CARE OF THE BABY WITH A CONGENITAL ABNORMALITY

If a fetus is diagnosed with a severe **congenital anomaly**, the safest place for the mother to give birth is a tertiary perinatal centre co-located with a surgical unit. In New Zealand, babies in utero diagnosed with severe congenital anomalies are generally born in tertiary maternity facilities with access to neonatal intensive care units (NICUs). However, this is not always possible because the diagnosis is made only after birth in about 50% of cases, thus the midwife should always anticipate the possibility of complications. Anticipation and preparation are particularly important because many Australian women live in rural and remote regions and maternity centres lack the facilities required to care for critically ill neonates. Irrespective of the location of an infant's birth, the midwife's first priority is always reviewing the safety of the environment and ensuring that the appropriate equipment is available and ready for the birth.

NEONATAL RESUSCITATION

Every health professional is required to be competent in basic adult and **neonatal resuscitation**. The following section provides some guidelines, but clinicians are expected to attend professional development courses in resuscitation annually.

The vast majority of newborns manage the transition from fetus to neonate without assistance Continuous positive airways pressure is the most common active resuscitation method used with only a small proportion of babies requiring intermittent positive-pressure ventilation. Less than 1% of newborn babies require cardiac massage (AIHW, 2021). Although the need for resuscitation can often be anticipated, on many occasions it is unexpected. A variety of maternal, fetal and intrapartum circumstances can increase the risk of the newborn needing resuscitation at birth, and these are listed in Box 42.1. The midwife should call for assistance from neonatologists and specialist midwives when the risk factors listed in this box are identified. In many rural, remote or community settings it is important to ask for help as early as possible and plan for transfer by the quickest route to the appropriate setting.

Since it is not always possible to predict which infants might require resuscitation it is vital that there is at least one person at every birth capable of providing assistance to infants who are not breathing. There is a multitude of different resuscitation equipment available and it is the individual midwife's responsibility to be familiar and expert in the use of equipment available in her / his work setting (Box 42.2). Prior to every birth, resuscitation equipment should be checked to ensure that it is available and functioning correctly. A plan (that works) to obtain assistance should be well established. In New Zealand and Australia most babies are born in a hospital, but a considerable number are born at home or in rural and remote settings where the most up-to-date equipment (e.g. radiant warmers, T-piece resuscitation devices) may be unavailable. Therefore, every midwife should be skilled in providing positive-pressure ventilation (PPV) with a self-inflating bag and mask. If a T-piece is available, midwives should also be competent with its use. For babies born at term a 240 mL self-inflating bag is the most appropriate size. If PPV is given it should begin with air (i.e. 21% oxygen). An air / oxygen blender should be used if available. Only if the infant does not respond after 30 seconds of effective PPV does the midwife need to give supplemental oxygen.

Transition from fetus to newborn

(See also Ch. 31.)

The transition from fetus to newborn is a normal physiological and developmental process; most infants make the transition with very little assistance. However, the first breaths are characterised by a rapid transition from liquid- to air-filled lungs with corresponding changes in pulmonary circulation.

Box 42.1 Risk factors: anticipating the need for resuscitation

Maternal
- Prolonged rupture of membranes (greater than 18 hours)
- Bleeding in second or third trimester
- Pregnancy-induced hypertension
- Chronic hypertension
- Substance abuse
- Drug therapy (e.g. lithium, magnesium, adrenergic-blocking agents, narcotics)
- Diabetes mellitus
- Chronic illness (e.g. anaemia, cyanotic congenital heart disease)
- Maternal pyrexia
- Maternal infection
- Chorioamnionitis
- Heavy sedation
- Previous fetal or neonatal death
- No prenatal care

Fetal
- Multiple gestation (e.g. twins, triplets)
- Pre-term gestation (especially less than 35 weeks)
- Post-term gestation (greater than 41 weeks)
- Large for dates
- Fetal growth restriction
- Alloimmune haemolytic disease (e.g. anti-D, anti-Kell, especially if fetal anaemia or hydrops fetalis present)
- Polyhydramnios and oligohydramnios
- Reduced fetal movement before onset of labour
- Congenital abnormalities which may affect breathing, cardiovascular function or other aspects of perinatal transition
- Intrauterine infection

Intrapartum
- Non-reassuring fetal heart rate patterns on cardiotocograph (CTG)
- Abnormal presentation
- Prolapsed cord
- Prolonged labour (or prolonged second stage of labour)
- Precipitate labour
- Antepartum haemorrhage (e.g. abruption, placenta praevia, vasa praevia)
- Meconium in the amniotic fluid
- Narcotic administration to mother within 4 hours of birth
- Forceps birth
- Vacuum-assisted (ventouse) birth
- Maternal general anaesthesia

(Source: Australian and New Zealand Resuscitation Councils (ARC/NZRC), 2021. ANZCOR Guideline 13.2—Planning for neonatal resuscitation and identification of the newborn at risk)

Umbilical cord management and placental transfusion

When to clamp the umbilical cord after birth has received much attention in recent years. Deferred cord clamping (DCC) to promote placental perfusion has been shown to reduce neonatal morbidity and mortality, especially among preterm infants (Liyanage et al., 2020). Benefits of deferring cord clamping for preterm infants includes reduced transfusions for anaemia, reduction in intraventricular haemorrhage and rate of necrotising enterocolitis. Term infants benefit from a placental transfusion with higher HCT. Hb and ferritin stores at 6 weeks of age are improved in infants following DCC. This may be especially important in low-resource settings. In preterm infants, however, cord milking is not recommended as a placental transfusion strategy (Balasubramanian et al., 2020).

The role of placental transfusion when neonatal resuscitation is required is less clear. Evidence from animal models (Polglase et al., 2015) and human studies (Katheria et al., 2016) suggest that for preterm neonates, including those who need active resuscitation, deferring clamping of the umbilical cord until ventilation is established may assist the fetal cardiorespiratory system to transition more quickly to the 'normal' postnatal circulation.

ANZCOR recommends a delay of a minimum of one minute, OR until the cord stops pulsating, prior to clamping the umbilical cord (ANZCOR, 2016). If the neonate appears to have acute, profound hypoxia (as demonstrated by a HR of less than 60 beats per minute (b.p.m.) and poor muscle tone) or if meconium is present and the neonate is apnoeic, the umbilical cord should be clamped and cut and the neonate immediately transferred to the resuscitation cot.

The need for resuscitation should be determined within 30 seconds after birth (Box 42.3). Most infants born at term will transit from fetal to extrauterine life and should remain with their mother to receive routine care. Indications for further assessment and intervention by the midwife include: apnoea (absence of spontaneous breathing), grunting or irregular respirations, heart rate <100 beats per minute (b.p.m.), poor tone and reflexes, meconium in the amniotic fluid or on the skin, and conditions such as pre-term birth or congenital anomalies such as a diaphragmatic hernia or exomphalos.

Following the initial (30-second) assessment, all subsequent assessments are based on breathing, heart rate (HR) and muscle tone. Regular respirations are adequate

Box 42.2 Equipment required for neonatal resuscitation

General equipment

- Firm, padded resuscitation surface
- Overhead warmer
- Light for the area
- Clock with timer in seconds
- Warmed towels or similar covering
- Polyethylene bag or sheet, big enough for an infant <1500 g birth weight
- Stethoscope, neonatal or paediatric sized
- Pulse oximeter with neonatal probe/sensor

Equipment for airway management

- Suction apparatus and catheters (6F, 8F, 10F or 12F)
- Oropharyngeal airways (sizes 0 and 00)
- Intubation equipment
- Laryngoscopes with infant blades (00, 0, 1)
- Spare bulbs and batteries
- Endotracheal tubes (2.5, 3, 3.5, 4 mm uncuffed)
- Endotracheal stylet or introducer
- Supplies for fixing endotracheal tubes (scissors/tape)
- End-tidal carbon dioxide detector (to confirm intubation)
- Meconium suction device (to apply suction directly to endotracheal tube)
- Magill forceps, neonatal size (optional)
- Laryngeal mask airway, size 1

Equipment for supporting breathing

- Soft, round face-masks (range of sizes suitable for premature and term infants)
- Positive-pressure ventilation device, either:
  - T-piece device, *or*
  - flow-inflating bag with a pressure safety valve and manometer, *or*
  - self-inflating bag (approximately 240 mL) with a removable oxygen reservoir
- Medical gases
  - source of medical oxygen with flow meter, tubing
  - source of medical air plus air/oxygen blender
- Feeding tubes for gastric decompression (e.g. size 6 and 8F)

Equipment for supporting circulation

- Umbilical venous catheter (UVC) kit (including UVC size 5F)
- Peripheral intravenous cannulation kit
- Skin preparation solution suitable for newborn skin
- Tapes/devices to secure UVC/IV cannula
- Syringes and needles (assorted sizes)

Drugs and fluids

- Adrenaline: 1:10,000 concentration (0.1 mg/mL)
- Volume expanders:
  - normal saline
  - blood suitable for emergency neonatal transfusion needs to be readily available for a profoundly anaemic baby

Documentation

- Resuscitation record sheet

(Source: Australian and New Zealand Resuscitation Councils (ARC/NZRC), 2021. ANZCOR Guideline 13.1—Introduction to resuscitation of the newborn infant)

if they maintain an infant's HR at >100 b.p.m. Gasping and apnoea generally indicate the need for additional interventions. Generally auscultation is the most accurate method to measure a newly born infant's heart rate (Dawson et al., 2018) with the infant under a radiant warmer. Palpation of the umbilical cord to estimate the HR is helpful if a stethoscope is not available. The HR should be >100 b.p.m. in the uncompromised newborn. A newborn's colour is unreliable for determining the need for supplemental oxygen and is no longer part of the immediate assessment to determine whether the infant requires oxygen or active resuscitation. In normal healthy infants it takes several minutes for infants to reach an oxygen saturation (S_pO_2) of 90% (Dawson et al., 2010) (Table 42.1). If an infant requires positive-pressure ventilation, or there are concerns about the infant's transition, then a pulse oximeter can be a useful addition to monitoring an infant's HR and S_pO_2. The sensor should be applied to the infant's right hand/wrist to provide preductal measurements.

CLINICAL POINT

The Apgar score is not an effective indicator of the need for active resuscitation.

Active resuscitation

Active resuscitation of a newly born infant follows the ABC algorithm (see Fig. 42.2). The midwife's first priority is to ensure adequate inflation of the lungs. Even if the infant is not breathing at birth, drying and stimulating the infant are often enough to encourage the infant to take the first breaths. If positive-pressure ventilation is required the lungs are ventilated at 40–60 inflations per minute. If bag and mask ventilation is effective, the chest will rise with each inflation and the infant should respond with an increased heart rate >100 b.p.m. A cold-stressed baby will not respond to resuscitation and so it is very important to keep the baby warm using a radiant warmer or skin-to-skin contact with the mother.

Box 42.3 Rapid evaluation of the newborn (within first 30 seconds of birth)

- Assess: breathing, heart rate, tone, reflexes
- Stimulate—dry with warm towel (discard wet towel)
- Pre-term infants (<28/40) are placed in a polyethylene bag up to neck without drying (to prevent heat loss)
- Start clock/timer
- Ensure airway open and clear mucus if it is obstructing the airway
- Keep the baby warm and place under radiant warmer if required
- Consider the need for help and if necessary begin the 'transfer' process

Table 42.1 Preductal oxygen saturation (S_pO_2) targets for the first 10 minutes after birth[a]

Time (min)	S_pO_2 (%)
1	60–70
2	65–85
3	70–90
4	75–90
5	80–90
10	85–90

[a]Using pulse oximeter sensor on infant's right hand or wrist and Fig. 42.2.

If the infant has not responded to stimulation then active resuscitation commences. The umbilical cord is clamped and cut and the baby moved to the Resuscitaire. Warming can be done by placing the infant under a radiant warmer, quickly drying the skin, removing wet linens and wrapping the baby in prewarmed blankets. The airway is cleared first by positioning the infant supine or lying on his/her side with the head in a slightly extended position known as the 'sniffing position' to maintain an open airway (Fig. 42.1). If secretions are blocking the airway, the infant can be gently suctioned—mouth first, then nose—with a suction catheter. However, aspiration of the nasopharynx is not part of routine care and is rarely necessary. These initial steps should be performed during the first 30 seconds after birth and the infant should then be re-evaluated for breathing, HR, reflexes and muscle tone (Fig. 42.2) (Australian and New Zealand Resuscitation Councils (ARC/NZRC), 2021). Warming the infant immediately after birth will decrease cold stress and oxygen consumption. Drying and stimulation *are both assessment and resuscitative interventions.*

Airway

The first priority at any birth is to ensure the patency of the airway and to ensure adequate lung inflation. The optimal position is to place the neonate supine with the head in a neutral or slightly extended (sniffing position) (see Fig. 42.1). Other methods to improve patency of the airways include 'support of the lower jaw, opening the mouth, or in some cases upper airway suction' (ARC/NZRC, 2021, Guideline 13.4). Suction should be used *only* when airway obstruction is evident.

Ventilation

If the infant continues to be apnoeic, is gasping and/or has a HR <100 b.p.m. then positive-pressure inflations with a bag and mask, or T-piece device, should be commenced (Box 42.4). Adequate ventilation is the most important and most effective step in cardiopulmonary resuscitation of the compromised newborn infant. Bag and mask ventilation is the mainstay of initial resuscitation. Before commencing positive-pressure inflations, the proper size mask must be selected, the airway must be clear, and the baby's head should be positioned in the 'sniffing position'. The mask should cover both nose and mouth to achieve a tight seal with the face. Noticeable chest wall rise, bilateral breath sounds and improved S_pO_2 and HR are indications that ventilation is effective. Inflations should be given at a rate of 40–60 per minute.

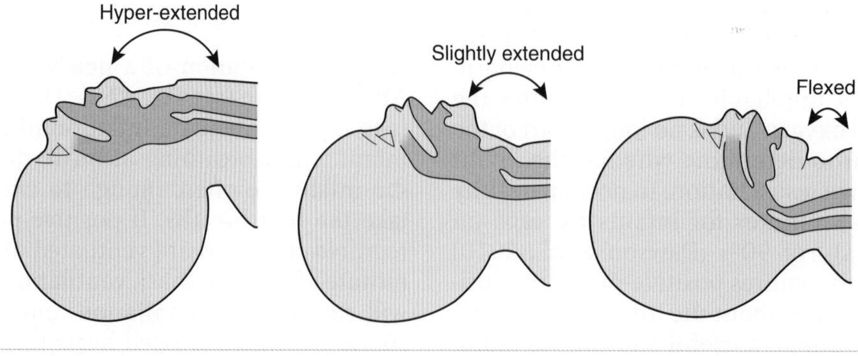

FIGURE 42.1 Position of the neonate head—the slightly extended or 'sniffing position' of the baby illustrated in the middle panel results in optimal airway patency for resuscitation
(Source: adapted from the Australian and New Zealand Resuscitation Councils (ARC/NZRC), 2021)

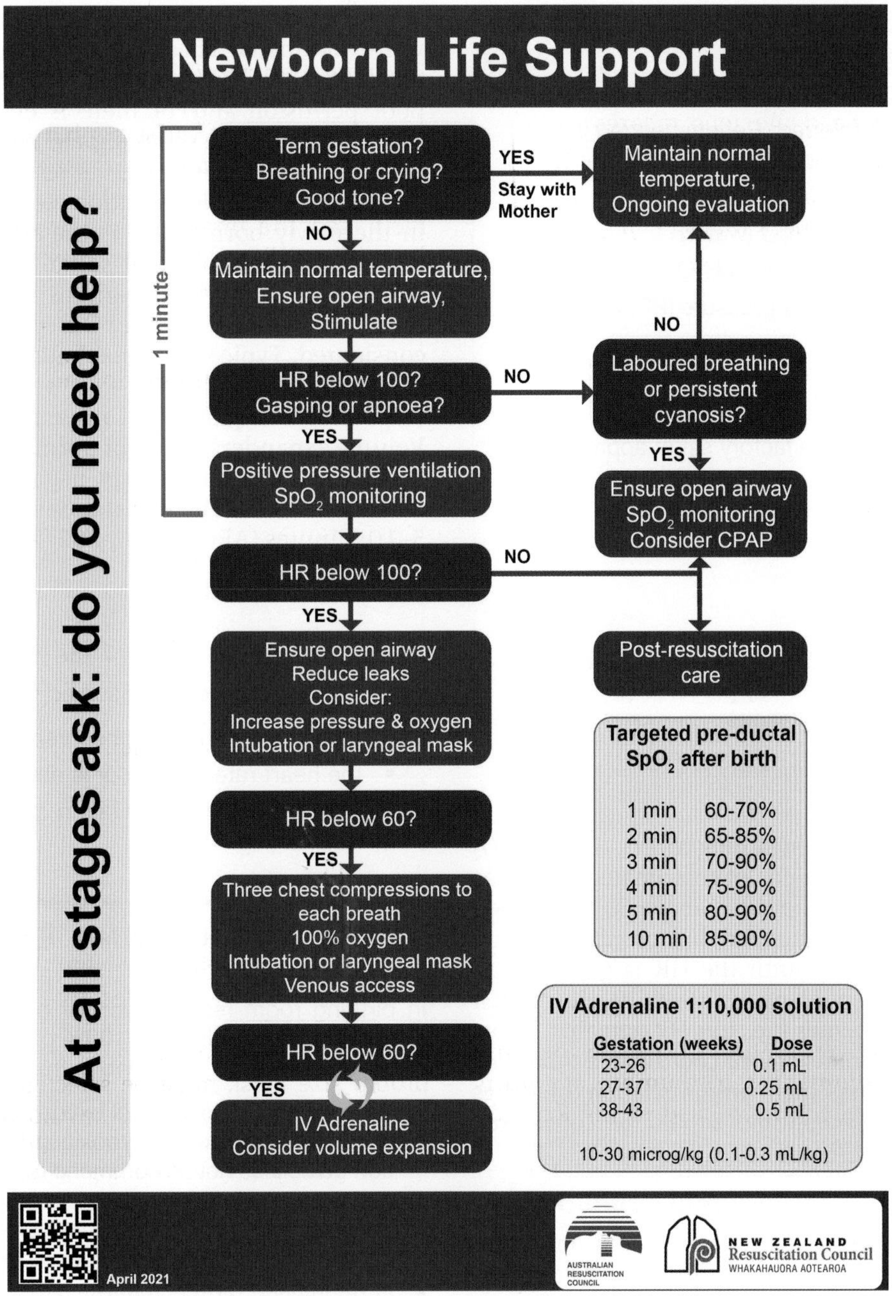

FIGURE 42.2 Newborn life support
(Source: Australian and New Zealand Resuscitation Councils (ARC/NZRC) Neonatal Guidelines 2021a; copied with permission https://resus.org.au/guidelines/flowcharts-3/)

After 30 seconds of ventilation, breathing and HR should be re-evaluated. If the baby is breathing spontaneously and the HR is greater than 100 b.p.m. then positive-pressure inflations can be stopped. However, if the infant's HR is greater than 60, but less than 100 b.p.m., then positive-pressure inflations should continue (ARC/NZRC, 2021).

Cardiac compression

If the infant's HR is less than 60 b.p.m. following initial positive-pressure inflations, it is likely that blood oxygen levels are low and myocardial contractility (and cardiac output) is poor. Chest compressions should be started and positive-pressure inflations continued until the HR improves (ARC/NZRC, 2021). Two people are needed if chest compressions are required: one to administer compressions (using the two-thumb approach) and one to continue inflations.

To perform chest compressions, enough pressure is applied to the lower third of the sternum to depress the sternum to a depth of approximately one-third of the anterior–posterior diameter of the chest, and then released to allow the heart to refill. Three compressions should be administered for every one inflation so that 120 events are given each minute (i.e. 90 compressions plus 30 inflations).

Box 42.4 Devices for providing positive-pressure ventilation (PPV)

- T-piece device is preferred. Recommended initial pressures are:
  - peak inspiratory pressure (PIP)
  - term newborn 30 cmH_2O (water)
  - pre-term newborn 20–25 cmH_2O
  - positive end-expiratory pressure (PEEP): 5–8 cmH_2O
  - maximum pressure relief valve: 50 cmH_2O
- Self-inflating bag
  - pressure release valve factory set at approximately 40 cmH_2O
- Flow-inflating (or anaesthetic) bag
- Face masks should be:
  - the appropriate size
  - cushioned
  - self-inflating bags cannot effectively deliver continuous positive airway pressure (CPAP), PEEP or sustained inflations

Re-evaluation of the infant's breathing efforts, HR and S_pO_2 should be done after 30 seconds of coordinated inflations and chest compressions. If the HR is above 60 b.p.m. then chest compressions can be stopped, but positive-pressure inflations should continue until the HR is greater than 100 b.p.m. and there is spontaneous breathing. However, if the infant is not improving (i.e. the HR remains below 60 b.p.m. despite 30 seconds of well-coordinated inflations and chest compressions) then administration of drugs such as adrenaline (epinephrine) should be considered (ARC/NZRC, 2021).

Drugs used during neonatal resuscitation

Administration of drugs is rarely needed and only with critically depressed infants. Adrenaline is a cardiac stimulant that increases contractility and HR while causing peripheral vasoconstriction (alpha-adrenergic effect). It is indicated if the neonate's heart rate remains <60 b.p.m. despite at least 30 seconds of effective ventilations and cardiac compressions. The recommended dose of adrenaline is 10–30 μg/kg (0.1–0.3 mL/kg of a 1:10,000 solution). It can be administered through an endotracheal tube for absorption by the lungs via the pulmonary veins, which drain directly into the heart. Alternatively, and preferably, adrenaline is given via an umbilical venous catheter (UVC) placed in the umbilical vein (ARC/NZRC, 2021). This route is likely to deliver more effective blood levels of the drug, but additional time is required to insert the catheter. After 30 seconds following administration, an increase in HR rate to more than 60 b.p.m. should be observed. If the HR remains depressed (<60 b.p.m.) then repeat doses of adrenaline may be given. In the meantime, good chest movement, equal bilateral breath sounds and well-coordinated chest compressions to an appropriate depth must all be continued. If the infant displays pallor, poor perfusion and/or there is evidence of blood loss then hypovolaemic shock should be considered in the infant who has not responded to resuscitative efforts.

The recommended solution for treating hypovolaemia in the newly born infant is the administration of 0.9% sodium chloride (normal saline). If there is suspected or proven blood loss, perhaps after an antepartum/intrapartum haemorrhage, O-negative blood should be considered. Typically the neonate appears to be in shock (e.g. pale, poor perfusion and weak pulse) and has not responded adequately to other resuscitative measures. Volume expanders, blood or normal saline, must be given very carefully intravenously, usually through an umbilical vein catheter. The initial dose is 10 mL/kg given over 5–10 minutes (ARC/NZRC, 2021).

CLINICAL POINT

Signs of effective ventilation

Effective ventilation is observed when:

- a rise in the chest is observed with each inflation
- the heart rate rises to or is above 100 b.p.m.

If signs of effective ventilation are not present consider MR SOPA (Fig. 42.3):

CRITICAL THINKING EXERCISE

In birthing room resuscitation of newly born infants when should you use medical air, 100% oxygen or a concentration of oxygen between these two extremes?

- When giving supplemental oxygen to newly born infants it is important to prevent hypoxia and hyperoxia. Resuscitation guidelines now recommend S_pO_2 targets when giving oxygen in the birthing room. The percentage of oxygen administered is adjusted to keep preductal oxygen saturations within the specified target range (see Fig. 42.2).
- In depressed term newborns, HR <100 b.p.m. initial resuscitation should be with air (21% oxygen). If preductal S_pO_2 is below the recommended target then oxygen should be introduced.
- In infants born pre-term <32 weeks, gestation initial resuscitation should be with air or a low percentage of oxygen (30%–50%). If preductal S_pO_2 is below recommended targets then blended oxygen should be introduced (see Fig. 42.2).
- If oxygen or a blender is not available a self-inflating bag can be used to give positive pressure.
- Local strategies for managing oxygen therapy in the delivery room will be influenced by the available equipment, the experience of the staff attending deliveries and the patient mix at the individual institution.

(Source: ARC/NZRC, 2021)

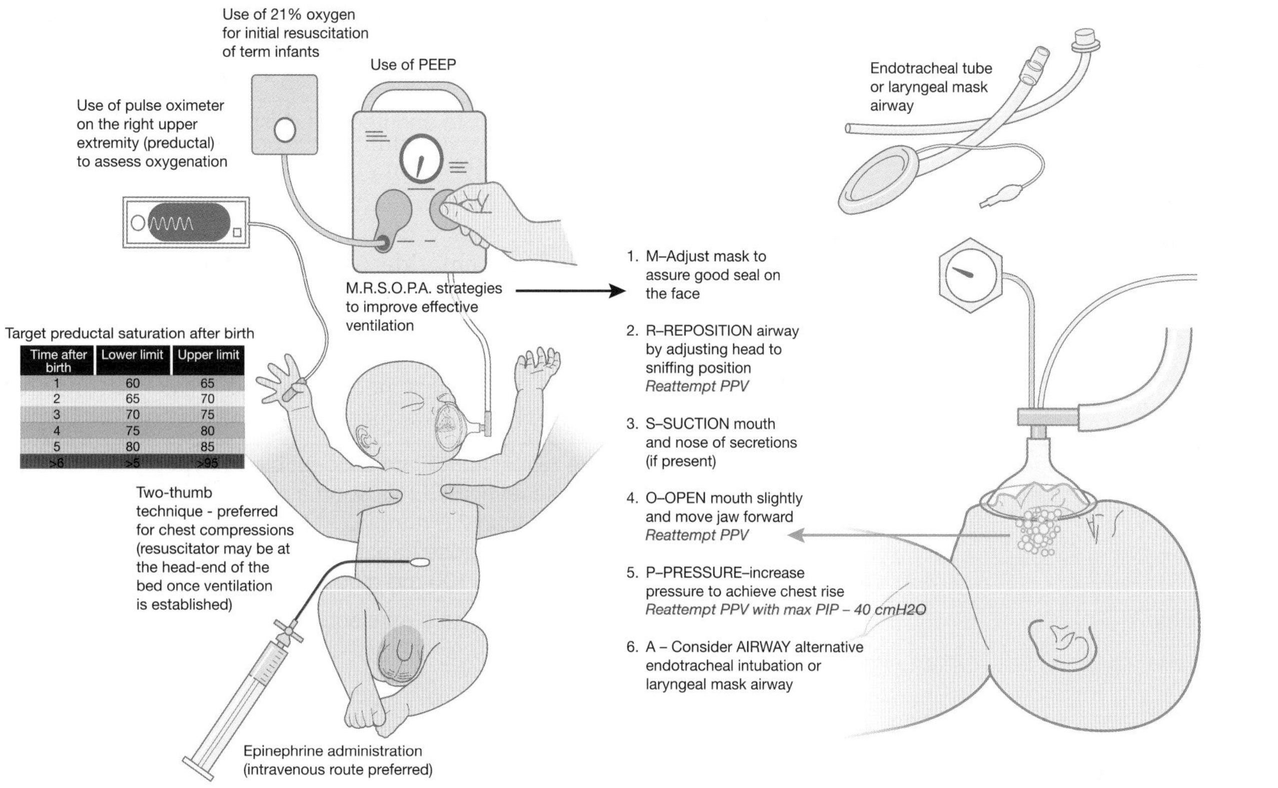

FIGURE 42.3 MR SOPA
(Source: Vali P, Mathew B, Lakshminrusimha S. Neonatal resuscitation: evolving strategies. Matern Health Neonatol Perinatol. 2015;1(1):1–4.)

CLINICAL POINT

It is important to check that the laryngoscope bulb is connected securely and that the light is bright.

CARE OF THE NEONATE AFTER RESUSCITATION

The neonate who has required active resuscitation remains at risk and requires ongoing assessment and care. It is important that the parents are included in all phases and decisions about their infant. Table 42.2 provides guidelines for ongoing care of the neonate who has required active resuscitation. These may vary according to guidelines at each institution (see also Chs 31 and 41).

COMMON CONDITIONS THAT AFFECT THE NEWLY BORN INFANT'S AIRWAY

The most common conditions that affect the airway are described in the following section. Babies born with these complications require immediate transfer to a tertiary level NICU.

Choanal atresia

Choanal atresia is a congenital anomaly of the nasal cavity in which there is narrowing of one or both nasal passages. As newborn babies breathe through their nose, in bilateral choanal atresia there is immediate obstructive breathing that is relieved only when the baby cries. Intubation will be necessary in this instance to secure the airway.

Micrognathia—Pierre Robin sequence

Pierre Robin sequence (PRS) is not a syndrome but rather a triad of features that cause respiratory compromise. These include micrognathia (small jaw), glossoptosis (large tongue) and cleft palate. At birth, infants present with airway obstruction related to the small jaw and large tongue. Placing the infant prone can frequently relieve the obstruction. Intubation should be undertaken only by experienced personnel.

Breathing

Many very pre-term infants cry and breathe after birth and therefore will require stabilisation rather than resuscitation

Table 42.2 Continuing care of the neonate after resuscitation

Care	Practice points
Location	• Assess the need for admission to an intensive or special care nursery.
Monitoring	• Monitoring required may include: • oxygen saturation • heart rate • respiratory rate and pattern • blood glucose measurement • blood gas analysis • fluid balance and nutrition • blood pressure • temperature • neurological state.
Blood glucose management	• Neonates who require resuscitation are susceptible to hypoglycaemia. • Check the blood glucose level (BGL) as soon as possible after resuscitation. • Maintain the BGL greater than 2.5 mmol/L. • Avoid large bolus doses of glucose (greater than 100–200 mg/kg): • 1 mL 10% glucose contains 100 mg glucose.
Antibiotics	• The need for resuscitation can be a consequence of sepsis. Soon after resuscitation consider: • relevant investigations • the need for antibiotics.
Induced hypothermia for hypoxic–ischaemic encephalopathy	• There is now level 1 evidence that inducing hypothermia in term and near-term infants who have moderate or severe encephalopathy following peripartum asphyxia can reduce the degree of brain injury and long-term neurodevelopmental sequelae: • Discuss any neonate with hypoxic–ischaemic encephalopathy (HIE) who is considered for induced hypothermia early with a neonatologist. • Suitable plans should be made for transfer (if required) and admission to a neonatal intensive care unit.
Inter-hospital transfer	• If the birth facility is unable to provide an appropriate level of post resuscitation monitoring and support, transfer the neonate to an appropriate higher-level facility. • To discuss the decision to transfer and to arrange transfer of the neonate to a higher-level facility, contact the appropriate provider, i.e. RFDS, NETS, etc.
Continuing care of the family	• Parent(s) find witnessing the resuscitation of their baby distressing regardless of outcome. Whenever possible: • Prepare parents for resuscitation if it is anticipated. • Keep parent(s) informed during and after resuscitation. Ideally information should be provided by a senior clinician. • Facilitate early parental contact with their baby.

NETS=Newborn and Paediatric Emergency Transport Service; RFDS=Royal Flying Doctor Service.
(Adapted from ARC/NZRC, 2021)

with respiratory support (Centre for Epidemiology and Evidence, 2019). The majority of babies who require respiratory support now receive continuous positive airway pressure (CPAP) instead of endotracheal intubation. Neonatal endotracheal intubation should be attempted only by clinicians with appropriate training and experience in the procedure. If there is no one skilled and intubation is required, the midwife continues to give positive-pressure ventilation (PPV) via a face mask or more rarely a laryngeal mask (LM). One reason to intubate a pre-term infant is to give surfactant, however there is a growing body of evidence that a more selective approach to intubation and greater use of non-invasive respiratory support with early intervention with surfactant is equally effective in preventing hyaline membrane disease (HMD) compared with birthing room intubation (Sweet et al., 2019). A small number of infants born at term (7%) will have some respiratory distress, the risk at 37 weeks gestation being three times greater than at 39–40 weeks (Edwards et al., 2013).

Common causes for breathing difficulties in pre-term and term infants

Respiratory distress syndrome and hyaline membrane disease

Respiratory distress syndrome (RDS) is caused by inadequate production of surfactant in the lungs. Surfactant is normally produced by type II pneumocytes and has the property of lowering surface tension. Most alveolar surfactant is produced after 30 weeks of gestation. Inadequate surfactant production causes air sacs to collapse on expiration and greatly increases the energy required for breathing. The development of interstitial oedema makes the lung even less compliant. This leads to hypoxia and retention of carbon dioxide. Right-to-left shunting may be severe and occurs through collapsed lung (intrapulmonary) or, if pulmonary hypertension is severe, across the ductus arteriosus and the foramen ovale (extrapulmonary).

Affected infants are usually pre-term, with RDS presenting very soon after birth with signs of respiratory distress: tachypnoea (respiratory rate over 60 per minute), expiratory grunting, subcostal and intercostal retractions, diminished breath sounds, cyanosis and nasal flaring. Many rapidly develop fatigue, apnoea and hypoxia as they struggle to breathe. These babies need to be transferred to a NICU.

CLINICAL POINT

The signs of respiratory distress can include rapid breathing >60 breaths per minute, nasal flaring, expiratory grunting, sternal recession, intercostal recession, cyanosis and low oxygen saturation.

Transient tachypnoea of the newborn

Transient tachypnoea of the newborn (TTN) is a respiratory problem that can be seen in infants soon after birth. It is the most common cause of respiratory distress in infants born >35 weeks gestation and is sometimes referred to as 'wet lung'. It is thought to be related to retained fetal lung fluid and can be complicated by a mild surfactant deficiency. It is more common in infants born by caesarean without labour (see also Ch. 41). Affected infants usually present with very rapid breathing up to 120 breaths per minute (higher than the normal range of 40–60 times per minute). They may also demonstrate nasal flaring, sternal recession, expiratory grunting and cyanosis. Usually, this condition resolves over 24–48 hours. Treatment is supportive and may include supplemental oxygen and antibiotics (Sweet et al., 2019).

Meconium aspiration syndrome

Meconium aspiration syndrome (MAS) is a serious condition in which a newborn infant breathes a mixture of meconium and amniotic fluid into the lungs around the time of birth. MAS may develop in term or post-term infants; it occurs rarely in infants born at less than 36 weeks gestation. In approximately 10%–15% of labours there is meconium-stained amniotic fluid (MSAF). The majority of infants born through MSAF will experience only mild respiratory distress that resolves over 24–48 hours. In a small number of infants (3–12%) this develops into a severe disorder (Vain & Batton, 2017).

It was once thought that oronasopharyngeal (ONP) suctioning of an infant born through MSAF would prevent or reduce aspiration of meconium-stained fluid. However, research has shown that ONP suctioning of an infant born through MSAF before the chest is delivered does not prevent MAS and may cause harm (ARC / NZRC 2021).

Immediately after birth in the presence of thick meconium, if the clinician is deemed competent, direct laryngoscopy and suctioning of residual meconium from the pharynx in infants who are not vigorous (absent or depressed respirations and decreased muscle tone) may help to prevent MAS (ARC / NZRC, 2021) (Box 42.5). There is no benefit in endotracheal intubation for suctioning of vigorous infants born through MSAF (ARC / NZRC, 2021). There is little evidence to show that endotracheal intubation for suctioning in depressed infants born through MSAF reduces the incidence of MAS (ARC / NZRC, 2021).

CLINICAL POINT

Prevention of aspiration of meconium previously involved routine suctioning of the oropharynx and nasopharynx before birth of the infant's shoulders. The seminal large multicentre trial in 2004 demonstrated that this practice does not reduce the incidence of MAS and has changed clinical practice (Vain et al., 2004).

Chronic lung disease

Bronchopulmonary dysplasia (BPD), the chronic lung disease (CLD), remains a major cause of neonatal morbidity and mortality. CLD is defined as a need for either

Box 42.5 Principles of care of a baby born into meconium

- Suctioning mouth, nose, hypopharynx before the shoulders are born is no longer recommended
- *Vigorous infant*—tracheal suction not indicated
- *Infant with absent or depressed respirations*, heart rate <100 b.p.m., or poor tone:
  - Do not stimulate infant
  - Prompt intubation to clear meconium from below the cords, if competent to do so
  - Do not delay resuscitation

mechanical ventilation or CPAP and / or receiving supplemental oxygen at a corrected gestational age of 36 weeks or beyond the 28th day of life. It is a multifactorial condition. Risk factors thought to predispose infants to CLD include lung injury from mechanical ventilation, prematurity, severity of respiratory distress syndrome, oxygen toxicity, patent ductus arteriosus, inflammatory changes in the lung and duration of mechanical ventilation. The risk for developing CLD increases with decreasing gestational age. The aim of management of CLD is supportive and may include respiratory support (mechanical ventilation, CPAP, high-flow or low-flow subnasal oxygen) and medications such as:

- bronchodilators (to help open the airways)
- steroids (to help reduce inflammation)
- diuretics (to help reduce excess fluid in the lungs)
- antibiotics (to fight infection).

Some infants will continue to require oxygen when they go home from hospital, but most of this group of infants can be weaned from oxygen by the end of their first year. Babies with CLD are at increased risk of respiratory infection, which may require hospitalisation.

Air leak syndrome

Pneumothorax is a lung disorder in which air in the lungs leaks out through holes in the lung tissue into the spaces outside the lung airways. Pneumothorax is one type of air leak. Types of air leak include the following:

- *pneumothorax*—air leaks into the space between the chest wall and the outer tissues of the lungs
- *pneumomediastinum*—air leaks into the mediastinum (the space in the thoracic cavity behind the sternum and between the two pleural sacs containing the lungs)
- *pneumopericardium*—air leaks into the sac surrounding the heart
- *pulmonary interstitial emphysema (PIE)*—air leaks and becomes trapped between the alveoli, the tiny air sacs of the lungs.

Infants most at risk for pneumothorax include those:

- with other lung diseases such as RDS or HMD
- receiving mechanical ventilation
- born pre-term
- with meconium aspiration syndrome.

Air leaks may occur suddenly or develop gradually. The degree of respiratory distress depends on the location of the leak and the amount of air involved. Affected infants may present with increasing respiratory distress, including tachypnoea, expiratory grunting, nasal flaring and chest wall retractions. It may be difficult to hear breath sounds on the affected side when listening with a stethoscope. Depending on the size of the air leak, there may be a change in the location of heart or lung sounds when these organs are moved sideways by the presence of air.

Management of air leaks will depend on the size of the leak and severity of signs. Some spontaneous air leaks that do not cause respiratory distress may resolve without treatment. As the leak seals over, air is absorbed into the body.

Congenital diaphragmatic hernia

Congenital diaphragmatic hernia (CDH) is a defect in the diaphragm muscle with herniation of the abdominal contents into the thorax through the defect. It occurs in approximately 1 : 2200–4000 live births. Mortality and morbidity are related to the degree of pulmonary hypoplasia (PH), the response to artificial ventilation and the presence of therapy-resistant pulmonary hypertension. Left-sided diaphragmatic hernias are more common, with right-sided hernias associated with increased risk of mortality. Rare occurrences of bilateral CDH are usually fatal. Increasing survival to more than 90% has been reported in some surgical units, with evidence of long-term nutritional and respiratory morbidity confirming the need for long-term multidisciplinary follow-up (Hollinger & Buchmiller, 2020; Kirby & Keijzer, 2020).

Priorities of resuscitation in the birthing room are based on the avoidance of high airway pressures and the establishment of a satisfactory (>85%) preductal S_pO_2. These infants will require intubation as the use of ventilation with a bag and mask should be avoided so as to prevent gut distension and will require a nasogastric tube inserted to vent the stomach. Infants will require transfer to a surgical centre, where surgical repair will be required when the infant is in a stable condition.

Oesophageal atresia

Oesophageal atresia (OA) is a congenital anomaly in which the oesophagus ends in a blind pouch. It has an incidence of approximately 1 : 2500–4500 live births, with an increased incidence in twins. OA may be isolated; however, in approximately 85% of cases it is associated with a fistula (connection) between the trachea and the oesophagus (tracheo-oesophageal fistula, or TOF). Midwives should have a high level of suspicion regarding OA / TOF when an infant is born following maternal polyhydramnios. Associated anomalies, including chromosomal anomalies, are found in 50% of infants with OA / TOF and it is also included as part of the VACTERL association (**V**ertebral anomalies, **A**norectal, **C**ardiac defects, **T**racheo-**E**sophageal, **R**enal and **L**imb anomalies). Infants should be screened for co-existing anomalies (van Lennep et al., 2019).

Initial management consists of nursing the baby supine in a 'head-up' position and frequent gentle suctioning to remove any secretions. The infant is kept 'nil by mouth'; intravenous fluids are commenced to maintain hydration. Transfer to a surgical centre for repair is required, with excellent survival rates reported from most centres. It is recommended that children with OA should be enrolled in long-term follow-up programs (Dingemann et al., 2020).

Pneumonia

Pneumonia is most likely to occur in the first week after birth. Prelabour rupture of membranes, maternal fever

>38°C before or during birth and clinical chorioamnionitis are significant risk factors for the development of neonatal infections including pneumonia (Coetzee et al., 2017). There is an increased risk of neonatal pneumonia to infants born to women whose labour does not start spontaneously after rupture of the membranes (Coetzee et al., 2017; see also Chs 38 and 40).

Routes of transmission and the most common types of organisms responsible for neonatal pneumonia include:

- transplacental—cytomegalovirus (CMV), tuberculosis (TB), rubella virus, *Treponema pallidum*, herpes simplex virus (HSV), varicella zoster virus (VZV)
- perinatal—anaerobic bacteria, *Chlamydia*, enteric bacteria, group B *Streptococcus* (GBS), *Haemophilus influenzae*, herpes simplex virus, *Listeria monocytogenes*, *Mycoplasma*
- postnatal—adenovirus, *Candida* spp., coagulase-negative *Staphylococcus*, CMV, Echo virus, enteric bacteria, influenza viruses A and B, parainfluenza, *Pseudomonas*, respiratory syncytial virus (RSV), *Staphylococcus aureus*.

Group B *Streptococcus* is the most common cause of neonatal pneumonia (see also Ch. 39). Early signs of pneumonia can be very non-specific and include poor feeding, lethargy, irritability, cyanosis and temperature instability (Coetzee et al., 2017). Respiratory signs include grunting, tachypnoea, retractions, nasal flaring, apnoea, lung crackles heard on auscultation, and cyanosis with increasing oxygen requirements. The respiratory distress can quickly progress to severe respiratory failure requiring endotracheal intubation and mechanical ventilation.

Management of pneumonia includes supporting the respiratory system according to the severity of clinical signs, chest X-ray, full blood count, blood cultures and arterial blood gases. For early onset infections within the first week after birth, intravenous antibiotics are required. The profile of antibiotics prescribed will depend on the type of suspected or proven disease and is likely to include: ampicillin or penicillin G + aminoglycosides (gentamicin) or cefotaxime. Antibiotics prescribed might also depend on the profile of organisms presenting within a neonatal unit.

Apnoea

Apnoea is common in pre-term infants. It is defined as no respiratory effort for greater than 20 seconds. No respiratory effort for shorter periods of time may also be classified as apnoea if accompanied by cyanosis or bradycardia (HR <100 b.p.m.). It is uncommon in term infants and is likely to have a pathological cause. In preterm infants of <34 weeks gestation, management includes administration of a methylxanthine (caffeine citrate or aminophylline). The drug can be given orally or intravenously and is usually routinely given to infants of <34 weeks gestation. It acts as a smooth muscle relaxant and a cardiac muscle and central nervous system stimulant.

CIRCULATION

The colour of the infant in the presence of a patent airway and adequate ventilation is useful in assisting with diagnosis. Many infants are pink at birth; others present as cyanotic (blue), which may indicate cyanotic congenital heart disease, with pallor, which may indicate shock and haemorrhage, and yellow, which may indicate a severe ABO incompatibility.

The healthy newborn has a HR >100 b.p.m., which should be established shortly after birth. If the HR is <60 b.p.m. despite satisfactory ventilation, with evident chest wall movement, then chest compressions should be commenced (ARC/NZRC, 2021).

Congenital heart disease

There are many conditions that affect the newborn circulation, one of the most common being **congenital heart disease** (CHD). The prevalence of CHD ranges from approximately 7–9 per 1000 of all live births. At birth, it will be obvious that an infant has a cyanotic congenital heart defect; however, acyanotic defects are less obvious. The American Academy of Pediatrics (AAP) and the American Heart Association (AHA) endorsed a recommendation in 2011 that screening for congenital heart disease using pulse oximetry should be part of routine newborn care as a useful tool in identifying infants with CHD in hospital and in the home-birth setting, and in 2018, recommended that there must be an oxygen saturation level of at least 95% in both the upper and lower limbs to pass (Martin et al., 2020). However, clinical examination of the newly born infant for cyanosis, respiratory distress and heart failure remains an important skill to alert midwives to the possibility of congenital heart disease.

Transposition of the great arteries

Transposition of the great arteries (TGA), one of the most common cyanotic heart defects, accounts for approximately 5% of all CHD cases (Galvis et al., 2021).

In TGA there are two separate circulations: the pulmonary artery arising from the left ventricle and the aorta from the right ventricle. There is often a concurrent atrial or ventricular septal defect, which with the ductus arteriosus allows mixing of the two circulations. The ductus is maintained with prostaglandin. Severe cyanosis is the most important clinical sign and immediate arterial oxygen saturation should be recorded. A chest X-ray can show a classic 'egg on the side' outline of the heart and echocardiography is required to confirm the diagnosis (Galvis et al., 2021).

An intact ventricular septum and no atrial communication is a cardiac emergency and the infant requires urgent transfer to a cardiac centre for a balloon atrial septostomy. Management consists of commencement of prostaglandin and stabilisation for transfer. (See section Neonatal transfer later in this chapter.) The definitive treatment for this condition is the arterial switch operation.

Tetralogy of Fallot

Tetralogy of Fallot is another common congenital heart disease and comprises a large ventricular septal defect, an overriding aorta and a right ventricular outflow obstruction and right ventricular hypertrophy. The severity of the anomalies dictates the timing of the surgical repair. Although the neonate is pink at birth, cyanosis with crying may be observed.

Left-sided heart obstruction

Causes include:
- coarctation of the aorta
- hypoplastic left heart.

Infants usually present within the first 2 weeks of life with signs of heart failure including tachypnoea, enlarged liver, decreased femoral pulses, decreased urine output and a cardiac murmur. Management consists of resuscitation and treatment of shock, commencement of prostaglandin and transfer to a tertiary cardiac centre.

Coarctation of the aorta (CoA)

Coarctation is narrowing of the aorta, which takes blood from the left ventricle of the heart to the rest of the body. It can occur anywhere in the aorta, but it is most commonly found just after the aortic arch and restricts the amount of oxygen-rich blood that travels to the lower part of the body.

The infant is pink and looks well at birth and is often discharged home, but re-presents with congestive cardiac failure and low cardiac output due to closure of the ductus arteriosus. Clinical signs include weak or absent femoral pulses, poor feeding and poor weight gain. X-rays may show cardiomegaly and pulmonary oedema with congestive cardiac failure. Conventional surgical repair is to remove the narrow segment. However, balloon dilation of the narrowed segment has also been used.

Hypoplastic left heart syndrome (HLHS)

The main features of HLHS are an underdeveloped left ventricle, atrial septal anomalies and hypoplastic ascending aorta and coronary arteries, with blood passing into the aorta through the patent ductus arteriosus. Although infants may be asymptomatic at birth, with the closure of the ductus there are increasing signs of cardiovascular collapse. The ductus must again be maintained with prostaglandin. Without surgery this is a lethal anomaly; the complex surgery, the Norwood procedure, is performed in three stages in infancy (Alphonso et al., 2020). Increasing survival has been reported over the last two decades, with data from the United Kingdom reporting survival to five years of age of 59% (Best et al., 2021). Developmental outcome is also improving for these children, and it is important that they are enrolled in follow-up clinics and continually evaluated (Sananes et al., 2021).

Patent ductus arteriosus

The ductus arteriosus is a normal fetal blood vessel that closes soon after birth. When this duct fails to close it is called a 'patent' (or 'persistent') ductus arteriosus (PDA). A PDA permits blood to flow from the aorta into the pulmonary artery, leading to an increase in blood flow in the lung circulation and congestive cardiac failure.

PDA is common in neonates with hypoxia, and has a high occurrence in children who were born prematurely. In hypoxic newborns, too little oxygen reaches the lungs to produce sufficient levels of bradykinin and subsequent closing of the ductus. Premature neonates are more likely to be hypoxic and thus have a PDA because of their underdeveloped heart and lungs.

Pallor

Haemorrhage is one cause of pallor in the newborn and can occur in utero, or during or soon after birth. Causes include trauma, for example following antepartum haemorrhage.

The procedure for treating pallor is summarised in Box 42.6.

Cephalhaematoma

Cephalhaematoma is bleeding that occurs between the periosteum and the skull bone and usually appears 12–72 hours after birth. Although of concern to parents, it does not generally require treatment (see also Chs 31 and 39).

Subgaleal haemorrhage

Subgaleal haemorrhage (SGH) is a potentially lethal condition that is a result of bleeding into the space between the epicranial aponeurosis and the periosteum. It is caused by rupture of the emissary veins (veins connecting the dural sinuses and the scalp veins), with the resulting blood loss often being life threatening. The signs of SGH are related to blood loss and include a boggy swelling of the scalp which continues to increase in size, increasing head circumference and signs of shock. The incidence is much higher in infants following a vacuum-assisted delivery. Management is focused on treating shock and controlling the haemorrhage. The mortality associated with this condition ranges from 3% to 14%, with improving survival in units with clear guidelines (Ojumah et al., 2017).

NEONATAL INFECTION

Neonatal infection is a major cause of morbidity and mortality, with over a million neonatal deaths throughout

Box 42.6 Procedure for an infant with pallor

- Check for anaemia
- Monitor/fluid resuscitation
- Ensure vitamin K (Konakion) has been given
- Cross-match blood

Box 42.7 Eye infections

Causes of eye infections include:

- *Neisseria gonorrhoeae*
- *Chlamydia trachomatis*
- *Staphylococcus aureus*
- *Pseudomonas aeruginosa*

the world attributed to infection annually (Rudd et al., 2020), thus it is a common condition encountered by midwives. The early detection of infection can be difficult; the signs are often non-specific. The midwife plays a pivotal role in prevention, early detection and prompt management of neonatal infections, and in providing support for the parents.

This section gives an overview of common bacterial infections including early and late onset sepsis (Cailes et al., 2018), congenital / perinatal infections such as eye infections (Box 42.7) and common fungal and viral infections (see also Ch. 37).

Prevention of infection

Hand washing

It is not surprising that diligent hand washing is the most effective means of decreasing nosocomial infection when dealing with neonates. Each midwifery and neonatal unit should have an evidence-based policy for hand washing, which should be adhered to by staff, parents and family members. Infection rates are monitored and quality assurance audits used to determine adherence to the hand-washing policy.

Environment and equipment

From an infection viewpoint it is of benefit at all times for infants to room in with their mothers. If this is not possible then adequate spacing between infant cots in nurseries is essential. The importance of the design and layout of neonatal units in the prevention of infection has been reported in a recent publication (O'Callaghan et al., 2019).

Common bacterial infections

Presentation

Neonatal sepsis can be classified as early onset (<48–72 hours from birth) or late onset (>48–72 hours from birth). Early-onset sepsis is acquired in the peripartum period and is most likely to be encountered by midwives. Group B *Streptococcus* (GBS) is the most common cause of early-onset sepsis (Dhudasia et al., 2021). The presence of maternal risk factors, as highlighted in Chapter 37, indicates that at-risk infants should be observed carefully in the postpartum period; however, not all infants who develop sepsis have identifiable risk factors.

Midwives in Australia are less likely to come across late-onset sepsis unless working in special care or neonatal intensive care units as these occur most commonly after the first week of life. However, this is not the case for New Zealand, as the midwifery model of care includes postnatal visits up to 4–6 weeks post birth. The most common causative agent in late-onset sepsis is usually coagulase-negative staphylococci, accounting for up to 77% of late-onset infections. Other causative agents include Gram-negative organisms such as *Klebsiella pneumoniae, Pseudomonas aeruginosa, Escherichia coli* and *Enterobacter* species (Gowda et al., 2017). Other more rare causes of late-onset sepsis can be found in neonatal textbooks.

CLINICAL POINT

Infants with suspected sepsis may present with the following non-specific signs: hypothermia or poor temperature control, pallor, mottling, hypotension, bradycardia, tachycardia, irregular respiratory rate, increased work of breathing, increased or decreased tone, poor feeding and abdominal distension.

Group B haemolytic *Streptococcus*

Group B haemolytic streptococci are bacteria naturally found in the digestive tract and birth canal and are the most common cause of early-onset sepsis. Between 10% and 30% of women are colonised with GBS, with an infection rate in infants of <1 per 1000 live births. A majority of infants with early-onset GBS show signs of infection within the first 12 hours of birth (Coetzee et al., 2017). (See also Pneumonia section earlier in this chapter.)

GBS can also occur following birth when infants come into contact with people who carry the GBS bacteria, 'late-onset' GBS disease. GBS has a significant morbidity and mortality, with a recent European study reporting an incidence of 12 / 1000 live births for early-onset GBS and 0.36 / 1000 live births for late-onset GBS (Coetzee et al., 2017).

Common fungal infections

These are now a major cause of neonatal sepsis. The rates have increased from 0.4 to 2 cases per 1000 live births, with the incidence in very-low-birth-weight (VLBW) infants contributing over 50%. Rates of non-albicans *Candida* species have significantly increased.

Common viral infections

Common viral infections in pregnancy include VZV, influenza, vaccinia and measles, enterovirus, CMV and HSV. Consequences of maternal viral infections result in increased stillbirths and abortions, fetal defects, neonatal illnesses and illnesses in later childhood. COVID-19 infection is now also a consideration (Box 42.8).

Congenital syphilis

Congenital syphilis is rare in Australia and may be asymptomatic in approximately 67% of cases; however, it can manifest as sepsis. Suspected or confirmed infection is treated with penicillin (see Ch. 37).

TORCH infection

TORCH includes **T**oxoplasmosis, **O**ther (syphilis, VZV, parvovirus B19), **R**ubella, **C**MV and **H**erpes infections, which are some of the more common infections associated with congenital anomalies. On cranial ultrasound, TORCH infection should be suspected when there is 'microcephaly, calcifications in the periventricular region, brain atrophy, hydrocephalus, subependymal cysts and lenticulostriate vasculopathy' (Batra et al., 2020).

Microcephaly and the Zika virus

Zika virus is a mosquito-borne flavivirus that was first discovered in a monkey in 1947. Since then occasional human infections causing mild illness with fever and rash have been reported. Large outbreaks in the Pacific Islands were seen in the mid 2000s owing to spread by the mosquito *Aedes aegypti*. Zika virus is transmitted primarily by *A. aegypti* or *Aedes africanus* mosquitoes, but can also be vertically transmitted, sexually acquired or, rarely, transmitted through infected blood products or organs. The link between microcephaly and Zika virus was first suspected in 2015 when increased microcephaly cases were noted during a large Zika virus outbreak in Brazil. A causal relationship between transplacental transmission of Zika virus and fetal abnormalities has now been established. Other birth defects include gut, eye and skeletal abnormalities. Long-term outcomes of congenital infection are not fully understood. Infection with the virus usually results in a mild and self-limiting illness, with a rash, fever and arthralgia. It can also be a cause of Guillain–Barré syndrome. Increased international travel and spread of the vector, coupled with the capacity to cause birth defects, saw Zika virus declared an infection of global importance in 2016 (WHO, 2016).

Box 42.8 Management for neonates at risk for COVID-19

Current evidence suggests that SARS-CoV-2 infections in neonates are uncommon. If neonates do become infected, the majority have either asymptomatic infections or mild disease (i.e., do not require respiratory support), and they recover. Severe illness in neonates, including illness requiring mechanical ventilation, has been reported but appears to be rare. Neonates with underlying medical conditions and preterm infants (<37 weeks gestational age) may be at higher risk of severe illness from COVID-19.

Testing: The optimal timing of testing after birth is unknown. Early testing may lead to false positives (e.g., if the neonate's nares, nasopharynx and/or oropharynx are contaminated by SARS-CoV-2 RNA in maternal fluids) or false negatives (e.g., RNA may not yet be detectable immediately after exposure following birth).

Mode of birth: Rates of SARS-CoV-2 infection in neonates do not appear to be affected by mode of birth, method of infant feeding, or contact with a mother with suspected or confirmed SARS-CoV-2 infection. All neonates born to mothers with suspected or confirmed infection should be considered as having suspected SARS-CoV-2 infection when test results are not available.

Infants in NICU: Isolating infants with suspected or confirmed SARS-CoV-2 infection in a Neonatal Intensive Care Unit (NICU) should be avoided unless the neonate's clinical condition warrants NICU admission. Locating neonates with suspected or confirmed SARS-CoV-2 infection in a NICU may unnecessarily increase the risk of exposing other vulnerable infants and NICU staff to SARS-CoV-2. In some hospitals, a NICU may be the only suitable environment for appropriate care of an isolated neonate. Therefore, determination about best placement should be made at the facility level.

Contact with the mother: Early and close contact between the mother and neonate has many well-established benefits. Current evidence suggests the risk of a neonate acquiring SARS-CoV-2 from its mother is low. Further, data suggests that there is no difference in risk of SARS-CoV-2 infection to the neonate whether a neonate is cared for in a separate room or remains in the mother's room.

Risks of transmission: A potential risk of SARS-CoV-2 transmission to the neonate may occur via contact with infectious respiratory secretions from the mother, caregiver, or other person with SARS-CoV-2 infection, including just before the individual develops symptoms when viral replication may be high. As such, all caregivers should practise infection prevention and control measures (i.e., wearing a mask, practising hand hygiene) before and while caring for a neonate.

Breastfeeding: Breastfeeding reduces morbidity and mortality for both mothers and their infants. Mothers who choose to breastfeed should take measures, including wearing a mask and practising hand hygiene, to minimise the risk of virus transmission while feeding.

(Source: CDC, 2020)

JAUNDICE

Neonatal jaundice (see Ch. 31 for management of physiological jaundice) is common and is not normally a serious concern. However, in some cases jaundice can be life threatening. Jaundice occurring less than 48 hours after birth is usually due to haemolysis, the most common causes being ABO incompatibility, Rhesus immunisation or sepsis. Management is aimed at decreasing the bilirubin level; exchange transfusion may be required. Kernicterus is caused by unconjugated bilirubin and can lead to significant sequelae including developmental delay, cerebral palsy and death.

DISABILITY

Seizures

Neonatal seizures are relatively common clinical conditions found in both term and pre-term neonates. They are defined as paroxysmal alterations in neurological function and are reported to occur in 1–5 per 1000 live term births (Pisani & Spagnoli, 2016). Causes include perinatal asphyxia, metabolic disorders (hypoglycaemia, hypocalcaemia, hypomagnesaemia), central nervous system or systemic infections, intracranial haemorrhages, hypoxic ischaemia and neonatal drug withdrawal.

CLINICAL POINT

Seizures versus jitteriness

It is important to differentiate seizures from jitteriness:

Seizure	Jitteriness
Not affected by environmental stimuli	May be evoked by environmental stimuli
Not suppressed by holding the infant	Suppressed by holding the infant
Fast contraction phase, slow relaxation phase	Similar velocity in both directions
Abnormal eye movements	Normal eye movements

It is important for midwives to identify seizures as this provides the opportunity for early treatment which ultimately will improve developmental outcome. Any infant thought to be having seizures should have a neurological examination, brain monitoring and imaging, with other investigations dependent on the clinical picture. Amplitude-integrated electroencephalogram (aEEG) is used to monitor infants at risk of seizures in neonatal units, with video electroencephalogram the gold standard for diagnosis. Clinical management consists of treating reversible causes (such as hypoglycaemia), anticonvulsants and may include therapeutic hypothermia (cooling) (Box 42.9).

Box 42.9 Therapeutic hypothermia

Current evidence supports therapeutic hypothermia (cooling) to be used for the following babies:

- Greater than or equal to 35 weeks gestational age *and*
- Greater than or equal to 1800 g
- With evidence of moderate to severe encephalopathy *and*
- With evidence of intrapartum hypoxia indicated by *at least two* of the following:
    - Apgar score of less than or equal to 5 at 10 minutes
    - needing mechanical ventilation or ongoing resuscitation at 10 minutes of age
    - cord, arterial or venous blood gas with pH of less than or equal to 7.00
    - base deficit of greater than or equal to 12 mmol/L within 60 minutes of birth.

(Adapted from Queensland Maternity and Neonatal Clinical Guidelines Program. Maternity and Neonatal Clinical Guideline. Hypoxic-ischaemic encephalopathy (HIE) review draft v0.07, 2015)

Hypoxic ischaemic encephalopathy

Hypoxic ischaemic encephalopathy occurs as a result of neural tissue destruction from hypoxic and ischaemic causes, such as placental abruption and uterine rupture. Infants with this condition have a high mortality and morbidity rate, including cerebral palsy, seizures and developmental delay (Davies et al., 2019).

Therapeutic hypothermia (cooling) following a hypoxic–ischaemic insult can benefit certain babies and is now considered standard care. It must be commenced within 6 hours of birth before secondary reperfusion injury begins. Rectal temperature should be maintained at 33.0–34.0°C with the avoidance of hyperthermia. Research is under way regarding the efficacy of the addition of erythropoietin with cooling, with promising early results (Davies et al., 2019; Wassink et al., 2019).

Neural tube defects

Neural tube defects (NTD) occur early in fetal development, at about 3–4 weeks gestation when there is disruption of the central nervous system; thus they are a problem of embryology. They occur in approximately 1–7 per 1000 live births. Types of NTD include anencephaly, encephalocele and spina bifida. Animal models suggest this disruption in development as being regulated by over 200 genes; however, NTDs are also affected by environmental factors such as folic acid intake. Mandatory fortification of folic acid has been implemented in many countries including the USA and Australia, with a reported decrease in incidence compared with countries without fortification (Arth et al., 2016). Major advances in the management of

NTDs have come from genetic and environmental factors, and advances in surgical repair, with in utero repair offered in some centres.

Anencephaly is the most serious defect as it is incompatible with life. Spina bifida can occur anywhere along the spinal cord between the head and the sacrum. However, the lumbosacral region is most commonly affected. It is classified according to the degree of nervous tissue involvement. Spina bifida occulta involves a defect of the bone seen by a tuft of hair or sinus at the base of the spine. A meningocele is where there is no skin covering the spinal defect, allowing the protrusion of the meninges and the sac. It may contain cerebrospinal fluid but does not contain neural tissue. A more serious defect is a myelomeningocele as it involves the spinal cord with the inherent risk of paralysis and meningitis. Management includes covering the defect with plastic wrap, maintaining normothormia and transport to a surgical centre.

Hydrocephalus

Hydrocephalus occurs when cerebrospinal fluid (CSF) is not absorbed adequately, resulting in enlargement of the cerebral ventricles and occasionally the subarachnoid spaces. There is a reported prevalence of congenital hydrocephalus of 50/100,000 births (Isaacs et al., 2018). Causes include NTDs, infection, intraventricular haemorrhage, trauma and tumours; however, the pathophysiology is still not obvious. Defects in genes regulating brain growth have been associated with congenital hydrocephalus (Kahle et al., 2016). The infant presents at birth with an enlarged head, widened cranial sutures, dilated scalp veins and a tense anterior fontanelle. Treatment is surgical insertion of a shunt to drain the CSF from the ventricles.

Note: Undiagnosed severe congenital hydrocephalus has the potential for maternal obstructed labour.

Fetal alcohol spectrum disorder

The term '**fetal alcohol spectrum disorder (FASD)**' is not a clinical diagnosis, but is used to describe a range of effects from prenatal alcohol exposure, including fetal alcohol syndrome (FAS), partial fetal alcohol syndrome and neurodevelopmental disorders. Fetal alcohol syndrome is at the more severe end of the spectrum. Babies present with distinctive facial features including: small eye openings, a thin upper lip, a flat midface and an absent or elongated groove between the upper lip and nose. They are also generally of low birth weight and fail to thrive (see also Ch. 35).

ABDOMINAL WALL DEFECTS

Although these defects are most often detected antenatally and the infants born in a tertiary centre, some will be born in non-tertiary perinatal units; thus it is important to know the first principles of management.

Gastroschisis

Gastroschisis is the most common congenital abdominal wall defect, where the contents of the abdomen, primarily the small and large intestine, stomach, liver, spleen, bladder and uterus, protrude through a defect in the abdominal wall, lateral to and most commonly right of the umbilicus. It does not involve the umbilical cord and is not enclosed in the peritoneal sac. Over the last decade there were reports of an increasing incidence up to 6.4 per 100 live births; however, a recent US paper reports an incidence of 4.7/1000 births (Bhatt et al., 2018).

Exomphalos/omphalocele

The diagnosis of an omphalocele or exomphalos is evident at birth, as the infant presents with herniation of the abdominal viscera through the base of the umbilical cord, covered in a sac formed by the peritoneum and amniotic membrane. It has an incidence of 1–2 per 1000 births (Somme & Langer, 2019) and is associated with chromosomal anomalies, cardiac defects and Beckwith–Wiedemann syndrome. Infants with an omphalocele have a higher mortality and morbidity (Fogelstrom et al., 2021).

Management

Immediate management of abdominal wall defects is aimed at stabilising the bowel in a midline position and avoidance of twisting or constriction as this compromises blood supply to the eviscerated intestine. The bowel is wrapped in cling film to minimise heat loss and prevent hypothermia.

There may be large fluid losses; appropriate circulation monitoring and fluid resuscitation are essential. A gastric tube should be inserted to vent the stomach and the infant must remain 'nil by mouth'. The blood sugar should be checked and prophylactic intravenous antibiotics commenced following blood cultures. The infant will need to be transferred to a tertiary surgical centre for operative care.

Necrotising enterocolitis

The majority of infants with **necrotising enterocolitis** (NEC) are pre-term, with the incidence inversely proportional to birth weight. In 2019, 1.2% of babies had confirmed NEC in the Australian and New Zealand Neonatal Network, with the majority pre-term and over 50% requiring surgery (Chow et al., 2019). Signs include abdominal distension, poor tolerance of feeds, vomiting, temperature instability and lethargy.

The infant should be kept nil by mouth and a gastric tube inserted and left on free drainage. Antibiotics are commenced following blood cultures and, depending on severity and location, the infant may be transferred to a surgical unit, and in New Zealand this would include NICUs.

NEONATAL TRANSFER

While awaiting **neonatal transfer** the priority is to keep the baby stable and prevent deterioration due to secondary factors. It is important that all units that provide maternity care have guidelines in place that document step by step how to arrange the transfer of an infant to a higher level of care. It is recommended that each unit has a visible flow diagram that details current contact numbers. It is important that midwives continue to use referred technologies (e.g. phone or telehealth) to continue communication with the receiving NICU as needed to:

- relay information regarding the baby's condition, which may influence ongoing management
- receive management advice.

How to organise a neonatal transfer

New Zealand

In New Zealand, there are no stand-alone transport services for neonates or children and most areas are serviced by staff working within the neonatal units.

The main neonatal units in the North Island are in Auckland (National Women's and Middlemore), Hamilton and Wellington and they will transport infants to their centres using their own medical and nursing staff. Christchurch is the largest NICU and main centre for paediatric surgery in the South Island, with 41 beds compared to Dunedin's 16 beds. Neonatal retrievals are undertaken by registrars or nurse specialists and transport nurses who are on a retrieval roster as part of their work in the NICU. In Dunedin, medical retrievals are undertaken by a registrar if available, or by consultants on an ad hoc basis.

Australia

All states and territories in Australia have protocols and policies regarding transfer. Some examples are included in this section. The Royal Flying Doctor Service (RFDS) provides neonatal transfers in all states, with Queensland (QLD) Retrieval Services coordinating telehealth services and retrieval of neonates across QLD including supporting NETS NSW with northern NSW and the Northern Territory. Hospital-based teams as well as the RFDS teams will retrieve neonates from these locations (Box 42.10). There are also stand-alone retrieval services in NSW and Victoria, NETS (Newborn and Paediatric Emergency Transport Service) NSW and Paediatric Infant Perinatal Emergency Retrievals (PIPER) Victoria. Similar programs are available in every Australian state and territory. For example, in Western Australia (WA), NETS work in partnership with St John's Ambulance and the RFDS. The WA service manages the world's largest, though sparsely populated, geographical area (2500 km). It includes the WA NETS hotline, which offers advice to midwives and doctors in rural and remote settings (see Box 42.10).

Box 42.10 Contact details for Australian Retrieval Services

Royal Flying Doctor Service

Western operations (24-hour medical and emergency calls)	
Statewide number (All WA bases)	1800 625 800
Satellite phone calls	08 9417 6389
Central operations SA and NT (24-hour medical and emergency calls)	
Port Augusta Base	08 8648 9555
(all of SA and in NT everywhere south of Tennant Creek)	
Queensland Section (24-hour medical and emergency calls)	
Charleville Base	07 4654 1443
24-hour emergency patient transfers	
Mt Isa Base	07 4743 2802
Cairns Base	07 4040 0500
South Eastern Section VIC, NSW, TAS, WA (24-hour medical and emergency calls)	
Broken Hill Base	08 8088 1188
PIPER (VIC)	1300 13 7650
NETS (NSW)	1300 36 2500
QNETS (QLD)	1300 79 9127
NETS WA (Western Australia)	1300 63 8792

Contact details should be easily accessible and all staff should know how to arrange a retrieval from their hospital.

NSW=New South Wales; NT=Northern Territory; QLD=Queensland; SA=South Australia; TAS=Tasmania; VIC=Victoria; WA=Western Australia

Within NSW, NETS provides the numbers to call regarding how to organise retrieval of a sick newborn, and for information on non-emergency retrieval or transfer and information about the obstetric referral/transfer processes (Box 42.11). For more information see the website: https://www.nets.org.au/.

What to do while waiting for the transport team to arrive

- Maintain normothermia at 36.4–37.3°C.
- Ensure patency of airway.
- Continuous monitoring should be applied to measure respiratory rate, oxygen saturation and heart rate, for assessment of breathing, perfusion and circulation status.
- Check blood sugar level and correct if there is hypoglycaemia according to unit policies.
- Retain the placenta for histopathological examination (in a labelled plastic bag and sealed bucket).

Box 42.11 Newborn and Paediatric Emergency Transport Service (NETS) NSW

NETS expect to be called about (and possibly retrieve) newly born babies in the following categories:

- Preterm <35 weeks or <2000 g (outside the service capability of the referring hospital)
- Preterm <30 weeks or <1500 g. Such infants may be assumed to need intensive care transport
- Respiratory distress—of early onset or rapidly progressive or persistent beyond 4 hours or with accompanying apnoea or asphyxia
- Meconium aspiration demonstrated on X-ray with a need for supplemental oxygen
- Babies needing oxygen more than:
  - F_iO_2 0.6
  - F_iO_2 0.4—if regular blood gases not possible
- Cyanosis persisting despite oxygen therapy
- Unwellness, especially if infant was initially well
- Heart failure or arrhythmia
- Shock, sepsis or seizures
- Depression following perinatal asphyxia
- Apgar score persistently less than 7
- Capillary refill persistently longer than 3 seconds
- Apnoea (cessation of breathing for 20 seconds or longer)
- Bleeding
- Surgical conditions requiring acute therapy
- Airway problems interfering with gas exchange

- If intravenous access is achieved, collect blood for blood glucose level, blood gas, culture and full blood count.
- Commence antibiotics as discussed during retrieval call.
- Discuss the transport with the family.

Box 42.12 lists the equipment required for a neonatal retrieval (Browning et al., 2008).

Telemedicine

'Vision for Life' cameras are used throughout NSW. These cameras allow live video feed to the NSW NETS base to aid in triage and acute treatment of critically ill newborn infants. It is important to know how to activate the camera in an emergency. See https://www.nets.org.au/VFL.aspx.

Documentation

This is essential to maintain care between different units and may include:

- perinatal transfer form
- parent contact details; with the parents' consent a photograph is taken of the baby to give to the parents

Box 42.12 Equipment required for a neonatal retrieval

- Warm room with a Resuscitaire and the means of providing/maintaining warmth, overhead heater, cling film (e.g. Glad Wrap)
- Infant head box for providing ambient oxygen
- Neopuff Infant Resuscitator
- Newborn self-inflating bag and masks—sizes 0/0, 0/1, 2
- Sizes 6, 10, 12 suction catheters
- Oropharyngeal airways—sizes 000, 00, 0, 1
- Endotracheal tubes—internal diameter 2.5 mm, 3 mm, 4.0 mm
- Introducer, Magill's forceps, laryngoscope and size 00/0/1 neonatal blades
- CO_2 detector (e.g. Pedicap)
- Oxygen analyser
- Air and oxygen supply with blender
- Humidifier
- Oxygen saturation monitor with neonatal probe and Coban to secure
- 500 mL bags of 10% dextrose and burette
- Preferably a paediatric syringe driver or intravenous pump
- Size 24 g cannulae, umbilical catheter or size 5 Fr gauge feeding tube
- Neonatal intraosseous cannula
- Ideally, a hands-free headset telephone to enable easy communication with retrieval consultant and consultation while resuscitating
- Digital camera and access to email or communicating images and radiology when operating at a distance

(Source: Reproduced with permission from The Royal Australian College of General Practitioners from Browning Carmo K, Terrey A. Stabilising the newborn for transfer: basic principles. *Aust Fam Physician*. 2008;37(7):510–514. Available at www.racgp.org.au/afp/200807/25414)

- photocopies of relevant medical records
- X-rays
- pathology-labelled maternal blood / placenta.

Parent transfer

A parent may travel with the team whenever possible; however, this is dependent on space restrictions in the vehicles (helicopter, aeroplane or ambulance). In Australia, if the mother is travelling with the baby, she should be >24 hours following birth and discharged from postnatal care. This is not the case in New Zealand, where mothers either travel with their baby in the majority of situations, or follow closely behind. The mother is re-admitted into a postnatal ward at the tertiary facility to which her baby has been transferred. A bed should be arranged at the receiving hospital or a co-located maternity hospital if her infant is transferred to a children's hospital. In many cases of neonatal retrieval in Australia it is not possible to transfer the mother as she is peripartum and the NETS teams are neonatal specialists not maternal specialists. The father may travel with the baby. Prior to transfer it is therefore important to facilitate touch and bonding between parents and baby and provide as much information as possible about the reasons for the transfer and the proposed management plan. Photographs of their baby should be facilitated and the parent's mobile phone details should be taken by the team to enable a 'safe arrival' text message at admission to the NICU. If the parents travel to the hospital, they need to know where this is and the names and contact details of the NICU. If necessary, an interpreter should be available before and after transfer. If the mother is planning to breastfeed her baby she should be supported to initiate her lactation and express breast milk.

SUPPORTING THE MOTHER AND FAMILY WITH A SICK BABY

Having a baby should be one of the happiest experiences. However, all this changes when the infant is born prematurely or becomes sick soon after birth. In some instances the baby is then transferred to a tertiary unit and the mother remains at the birth hospital with the father commuting between the two, causing a great deal of stress for the family. The midwife is then pivotal in caring for this mother and providing empathy and support, one of the most essential components of caring being communication (Wigert et al., 2014). Much of the literature on parental stress within the neonatal intensive care environment highlights the important role of midwives and nurses at this time (Enke et al., 2017). Much of the literature on parental stress within the neonatal intensive care environment highlights the important role of midwives and nurses at this time (Williams et al., 2018). Parents dealing with the birth of a sick infant may find it helpful to talk with parents who have been through a similar experience. Some of the support groups available are listed in the Online resources section.

REFLECTIVE THINKING EXERCISE

1. Reflect on this chapter; what was the most important aspect for you?
2. What would you like to learn more about?
3. What surprised you reading this chapter?
4. What new skills do you have after reading this chapter?
5. How will you use this new knowledge?

Conclusion

This chapter has provided a brief outline of the management of common congenital anomalies and conditions that may be encountered in the birthing room and early newborn period. Much detail has been provided on the early identification of infants requiring resuscitation and efficient and evidence-based resuscitation skills that are essential to optimise outcome.

It was not within the scope of this chapter to provide comprehensive details of each condition; hence we have included some resources, e-learning and references at the end of the chapter.

Review questions

1. A baby born today at 36 weeks gestation is admitted to the ward—you notice he is grunting. What observations are important to undertake to inform the midwifery manager?
2. The baby has a temperature of 36.2°C. Why could a low temperature be associated with grunting?
3. On assessing a baby in the postnatal ward you notice that she is visibly jaundiced. The baby was born at 39 weeks and is 18 hours old. Do you need to make any referrals at this point or do you continue observing and regularly feeding? Please explain your rationale.
4. List the babies at risk of hypothermia and the consequences of a neonatal temperature of <36.0°C.
5. Discuss the clinical assessment of a jaundiced baby.
6. Discuss the 'before and after birth' factors that increase the risk of infection for the newborn.
7. Why are newborn infants more at risk of infection than full-term infants?
8. Describe some of the factors that impede a smooth transition to extrauterine life.

Online resources

Queensland Health: https://www.health.qld.gov.au/rrcsu.
Royal Flying Doctor Service: http://www.flyingdoctor.org.au/.

Neonatal transport services

NETS NSW: http://www.nets.org.au/.
PIPER (NETS) Victoria: http://www.rch.org.au/piper/.
NeoRESQ (QLD): https://metronorth.health.qld.gov.au/rbwh/healthcare-services/neonatal-retrieval-service-neoresq.
MedSTAR (SA): http://www.saambulance.com.au/Whoweare/Emergency/SAASMedSTARandSpecialOperationsTeam.aspx.
NETS (WA): https://www.cahs.health.wa.gov.au/Our-services/Neonatology/Newborn-Emergency-Transport-Service.

Neonatal units

Newborn Services, National Women's Health at Auckland City Hospital, New Zealand: https://starship.org.nz/health-professionals/#All.
Royal Prince Alfred Newborn Care Unit, Sydney, Australia: http://www.sswahs.nsw.gov.au/rpa/neonatal/.
The Royal Women's Hospital, Melbourne, Australia: https://www.thewomens.org.au/health-professionals/clinical-resources/clinical-guidelines-gps/.
Royal Children's Hospital, Melbourne, Australia: http://www.rch.org.au/clinicalguide/index.cfm.

Parent support groups

European Foundation For the Care of Newborn Infants (EFCNI): https://www.efcni.org/.
Global Alliance for Newborn Care (GLANCE): https://www.glance-network.org/.
HeartKids is a group dedicated to provide support, encouragement and hope to families of children with heart disease: http://www.heartkids.org.au/.
Life's Little Treasures is a charity specifically tailored for families of children born premature or sick: http://www.lifeslittletreasures.org.au/.
Miracle Babies Foundation supports premature and sick newborns, their families and the hospitals that care for them: http://www.miraclebabies.org.au/.
New Zealand Ministry of Health. Alcohol and Pregnancy: A Guide for Health Professionals; 2010. http://www.health.govt.nz/publication/alcohol-and-pregnancy-practical-guide-health-professionals. This describes the New Zealand Ministry of Health preferred tool for alcohol use assessment in pregnancy (AUDIT-C) and guides referral to AOD services.
The Neonatal Trust (NZ) provides support to families of premature or sick full-term babies as they make their journey through neonatal intensive care, the transition home, and onwards: https://www.neonataltrust.org.nz/.

Resuscitation councils

Australian Resuscitation Council: http://www.resus.org.au/.
New Zealand Resuscitation Council: http://www.nzrc.org.nz/.

References

Alphonso N, Angelini A, Barron DJ, et al. Guidelines for the management of neonates and infants with hypoplastic left heart syndrome: the European Association for Cardio-Thoracic Surgery (EACTS) and the Association for European Paediatric and Congenital Cardiology (AEPC) Hypoplastic Left Heart Syndrome Guidelines Task Force. *Eur J Cadriothorac Surg.* 2020;58(3):416–499.

Arth A, Kancherla V, Pachon H, et al. A 2015 global update on folic acid-preventable spina bifida and anencephaly. *Birth Defects Res Part A Clin Mol Teratol.* 2016;106(7):520–529.

Australian and New Zealand Resuscitation Councils (ARC / NZRC). *ANZCOR Guideline 13 – Introduction to Resuscitation of the Newborn Infant.* 2021. Online: https://resus.org.au/guidelines/.

Australian Institute of Health and Welfare (AIHW). *Australia's Mothers and Babies. Cat. no. PER 101.* Canberra: AIHW; 2021. Online: https://www.aihw.gov.au/reports/mothers-babies/australias-mothers-babies/contents/about.

Balasubramanian H, Ananthan A, Jain V, et al. Umbilical cord milking in preterm infants: a systematic review and meta-analysis. *Arch Dis Child Fetal Neonatal Ed.* 2020;105(6):572–80.

Batra P, Batra M, Singh S. Epidemiology of TORCH infections and understanding the serology in their diagnosis. *J Foetal Med.* 2020;7(1):25–9.

Best KE, Miller N, Draper E, et al. The improved prognosis of hypoplastic left heart: a population-based register study of 343 cases in England and Wales. *Front Pediatr.* 2021;9:554.

Bhatt P, Lekshminarayanan A, Donda K, et al. Trends in incidence and outcomes of gastroschisis in the United States: analysis of the national inpatient sample 2010–2014. *Pediatr Surg Int.* 2018;34(9):919–29.

Browning Carmo K, Terrey A. Stabilising the newborn for transfer: Basic principles. *Aust Fam Physician.* 2008;37(7):510–514.

Cailes B, Kortsalioudaki C, Buttery J, et al. Epidemiology of UK neonatal infections: the neonIN infection surveillance network. *Arch Dis Child Fetal Neonatal Ed.* 2018;103(6):F547–53.

Centers for Disease Control and Prevention (CDC). *Evaluation and Management Considerations for Neonates at Risk for COVID-19.* 29 Dec 2020. Online: https://www.cdc.gov/coronavirus/2019-ncov/hcp/caring-for-newborns.html.

Centre for Epidemiology and Evidence. *New South Wales Mothers and Babies 2018.* Sydney: NSW Ministry of Health, 2019.

Chow SSW, Creighton P, Chambers GM, et al. *Report of the Australian and New Zealand Neonatal Network.* Sydney: ANZN; 2019. Online: https://npesu.unsw.edu.au/surveillance/report-australian-and-new-zealand-neonatal-network-2017.

Coetzee M, Mbowane NT, De Witt TW. Neonatal sepsis: Highlighting the principles of diagnosis and management. *SAJCH.* 2017;11(2):99–103.

Davies A, Wassink G, Bennet L, et al. Can we further optimize therapeutic hypothermia for hypoxic-ischemic encephalopathy? *Neural Regen Res.* 2019;14(10):1678.

Dawson JA, Schmölzer GM, Wyllie J. Monitoring heart rate in the delivery room. *Semin Fetal Neonatal Med.* 2018;1(23):327–332.

Dhudasia MB, Flannery DD, Pfeifer MR, et al. Updated guidance: prevention and management of perinatal group B streptococcus infection. *Neoreviews.* 2021;22(3):e177–88.

Dingemann C, Eaton S, Aksnes G, et al. ERNICA consensus conference on the management of patients with esophageal atresia and tracheoesophageal fistula: follow-up and framework. *Eur J Pediatr Surg.* 2020;30(06):475–82.

Edwards MO, Kotecha SJ, Kotecha S. Respiratory distress of the term newborn infant. *Paediatr Respir Rev.* 2013;14:29–37.

Enke C, Hausmann AOY, Miedaner F, et al. Communicating with parents in neonatal intensive care units: the impact on parental stress. *Patient Educ Couns.* 2017;100(4):710–719.

Fogelstrom A, Caldeman C, Oddsberg J, et al. Omphalocele: national current birth prevalence and survival. *Pediatr Surg Int.* 2021;15:1–6.

Galvis MMO, Bhakta RT, Tarmahomed A et al. Cyanotic Heart Disease. In: *StatPearls* [Internet]; 2021.

Gowda H, Norton R, White A, et al. Late-onset neonatal sepsis—a 10-year review from North Queensland, Australia. *Pediatr Infect Dis J.* 2017;36(9):883–8.

Hey E, ed. *Neonatal Formulary. Drug Use in Pregnancy and the First Year of Life.* 6th ed. London: BMJ Books; 2011.

Hollinger LE, Buchmiller TL. Long term follow-up in congenital diaphragmatic hernia. *Semin Perinatol.* 2020;44(1):151171.

Isaacs AM, Riva-Cambrin J, Yavin D, et al. Age-specific global epidemiology of hydrocephalus: systematic review, metanalysis and global birth surveillance. *PloS One.* 2018;13(10):e0204926.
Kahle KT, Kulkarni AV, Limbrick DD, et al. Hydrocephalus in children. *Lancet.* 2016;387(10020):788–799.
Kain V, Mannix T. *Neonatal Nursing in Australia and New Zealand: Principles for Practice.* Sydney: Elsevier Health Sciences; 2018.
Katheria A, Poeltler D, Durham J, et al. Neonatal resuscitation with an intact cord: a randomized clinical trial. *J Pediatr.* 2016;178(1):75–80.
Kirby E, Keijzer R. Congenital diaphragmatic hernia: current management strategies from antenatal diagnosis to long-term follow-up. *Pediatr Surg Int.* 2020;36(4):415–29.
Liyanage SK, Ninan K, McDonald SD. Guidelines on deferred cord clamping and cord milking: a systematic review. *Pediatrics.* 2020;146(5).
Martin GR, Ewer AK, Gaviglio A, et al. Updated strategies for pulse oximetry screening for critical congenital heart disease. *Pediatrics.* 2020;146(1).
Ministry of Health (MOH). *Report on Maternity 2014.* Wellington: Ministry of Health; 2015.
O'Callaghan N, Dee A, Philip RK. Evidence-based design for neonatal units: a systematic review. *Matern Health Neonatol Perinatol.* 2019;5(1):1–9.
Ojumah N, Ramdhan RC, Wilson C, et al. Neurological neonatal birth injuries: a literature review. *Cureus.* 2017;9(12). Online: http://www.asid.net.au/documents/item/368.
Perinatal and Maternal Mortality Review Committee (PMMRC). *Fourteenth Annual Report of the Perinatal and Maternal Mortality Review Committee.* Wellington, NZ: Health Quality and Safety Commission, PMMRC; 2021.
Pisani F, Spagnoli C. Neonatal seizures: a review of outcomes and outcome predictors. *Neuropediatrics.* 2016;47(1):12–9.
Polglase GR, Dawson JA, Kluckow M, et al. Ventilation onset prior to umbilical cord clamping (physiological-based cord clamping) improves systemic and cerebral oxygenation in preterm lambs. *PloS One.* 2015;10(2):e0117504.
Queensland Maternity and Neonatal Clinical Guidelines Program. *Queensland Maternity and Neonatal Clinical Guideline. Hypoxic-ischaemic encephalopathy (HIE), review draft v0.07.2015.* Online: http://www.neoresus.org.au/wp-content/uploads/2015/01/Queensland-Maternity-and-Neonatal-Guideline_Hypoxic_Ischaemic_Encephalopathy_May_20101.pdf.
Rudd KE, Johnson SC, Agesa KM, et al. Global, regional, and national sepsis incidence and mortality, 1990–2017: analysis for the Global Burden of Disease Study. *Lancet.* 2020;395(10219): 200–11.
Sananes R, Goldberg CS, Newburger JW, et al. Six-year neurodevelopmental outcomes for children with single-ventricle physiology. *Pediatrics.* 2021;147(2).
Somme S, Langer JC. Omphalocele. In: Puri P, Hollwarth M, eds. *Pediatric Surgery.* Berlin, Heidelberg: Springer; 2019:153–16.
Sweet DG, Carnielli V, Greisen G, et al. European consensus guidelines on the management of respiratory distress syndrome–2019 update. *Neonatology.* 2019;115(4):432–50.
Vain NE, Batton DG. Meconium 'aspiration' (or respiratory distress associated with meconium-stained amniotic fluid?). *Semin Fetal Neonatal Med.* 2017;22(4):214–219.
van Lennep M, Singendonk MM, Dall'Oglio L, et al. Oesophageal atresia. *Nat Rev Dis Primers.* 2019;5(1):1–21.
Wassink G, Davidson JO, Dhillon SK, et al. Therapeutic hypothermia in neonatal hypoxic-ischemic encephalopathy. *Curr Neurol Neurosci Rep.* 2019;19(1):2.
Williams KG, Patel KT, Stausmire JM, et al. The neonatal intensive care unit: Environmental stressors and supports. *Int J Environ Res Public Health.* 2018;15(1):60.
World Health Organization (WHO). WHO statement on the first meeting of the International Health Regulations (2005) (IHR 2005) Emergency Committee on Zika virus and observed increase in neurological disorders and neonatal malformations. 2016. Online: https://www.who.int/news/item/01-02-2016-who-statement-on-the-first-meeting-of-the-international-health-regulations-(2005)-(ihr-2005)-emergency-committee-on-zika-virus-and-observed-increase-in-neurological-disorders-and-neonatal-malformations.

Further reading

Centre for Epidemiology and Evidence. New South Wales Mothers and Babies 2018. Sydney: NSW Ministry of Health; 2019.
Hutchinson M, Joyce A, Peirce, A. Western Australia's Mothers and Babies, 2015. 33rd Annual Report of the Western Australian Midwives' Notification System. Western Australia: Department of Health; 2019.
Galvis MM, Bhakta RT, Tarmahomed A, Mendez MD. *Cyanotic Heart Disease.* StatPearls [Internet]; 2021.
Kain V, Mannix T. *Neonatal Nursing in Australia and New Zealand: Principles for Practice.* Sydney: Elsevier Health Sciences; 2018.

CHAPTER 43

Grief and loss during childbearing—the crying times

Natasha Donnolley and Hannah G Dahlen

LEARNING OUTCOMES

Learning outcomes for this chapter are:

1. To explore some of the feelings, thoughts and behaviours that women and their family members may have after the death of a baby
2. To highlight the complexity and individuality of grief, combined with limited evidence about the effectiveness of bereavement interventions
3. To provide definitions and legislative requirements relating to fetal and infant deaths
4. To identify principles and strategies that midwives can use as part of a toolkit to work with bereaved women and their families
5. To consider the ways in which culture and belief influence how women and families experience grief and loss
6. To explore the different needs fathers, children and grandparents may have when a baby dies.

CHAPTER OVERVIEW

Today the public expectation in developed countries is that pregnancy leads to the birth of a live and healthy baby. There is also the perception that with the advances in medical technology very little should and can go wrong during the childbearing experience. The reality is that this is not always the case—miscarriage, genetic abnormalities, premature birth, stillbirth and neonatal death still occur; the reality is they probably will always occur, even in the future we can't imagine yet. In Australia, despite rapid advances in medical technology and high rates of intervention, the perinatal mortality rate has changed little in over two decades (AIHW, 2021). So, on the one hand we have a perception that perfect baby outcomes during childbirth are increasing, yet this is not the reality we see in the perinatal statistics. Each situation where a woman and her partner experience loss creates ripples that impact significantly on family, friends and community. As De Frain et al. (1991) said, 'the death of a baby is like a stone cast into the stillness of a quiet pool; the concentric ripples of despair sweep out in all directions, affecting many, many people'. As midwives we witness the despair, we wipe the tears, we hold those shaking shoulders, and we learn to walk through the fog that grief and loss creates in lives. However, knowing what to do and say, and more importantly what not to do and say, is not always so intuitive to midwives.

It is beyond the scope of this chapter to discuss all of the events where bereavement can occur during pregnancy and childbirth. We have also not reviewed the physical care associated with different experiences of loss. This can be found in other areas of this textbook. It is our intention in this chapter to take you by the hand and show you the ripples of despair that sweep out in all directions when a baby dies and how you as midwives can make such an important contribution to the journey that families who experience perinatal loss will go on.

The chapter is divided into the following sections:

- Hannah's story—a love that never ends
- Natasha's story—a fractured future
- Pulling it all together—understanding the stages of the journey
- Should we encourage parents to parent a dying or dead child?
- How do midwives walk alongside a grieving family?
- Children and grief
- Fathers and loss
- Grandparents hurt, too
- An Aotearoa New Zealand perspective on caring after perinatal loss
- The 'sorry business': caring for Aboriginal and Torres Strait Islander women
- Facts and figures you should know.

KEY TERMS

bereavement
cultural practices
grieving
infant death
miscarriage
neonatal death
perinatal death
postmortem
stillbirth
sudden unexpected death in infancy (SUDI)

INTRODUCTION

And ever has it been that love knows not its own depth until the hour of separation.

(Kahlil Gibran, 1979, p. 8)

This chapter is written by Natasha and Hannah, two women who have experienced the loss of a baby / babies. Natasha is a mother of four children (Callum, Soraya, Rohan and Keira). Natasha works as a research project manager in maternal and perinatal health research and has become a major consumer force in Australia. Natasha's baby girl Soraya was stillborn as the result of a compressed velamentous cord insertion. Hannah is a mother of four children (Lydia, Luke, Ethan and Bronte). She is a midwife who has spent much of her professional life in political activism to get midwifery recognised as the gold standard in maternity care. Hannah's sons Luke and Ethan died a year apart shortly after their birth from a rare congenital disorder. In this chapter we begin with both our journeys through perinatal loss; we also incorporate the grief and loss experiences of men, Aboriginal and Māori women, and explore how every experience of grief and loss is different but that the effects are far reaching.

HANNAH'S STORY—A LOVE THAT NEVER ENDS

'I love you so much,' my daughter says to me, throwing her arms open as wide as she can. She looks proudly at the tiny expanse created by her chubby limbs—'I love you *this* much.'

'I love you to the moon and back,' I say.

'I love you to the sun and back ... ten times.' She grins, wallowing in this game of love we play.

'Well I love you to the stars and back ... a million times,' I say.

'What's more than the stars?' she asks, growing serious, hating to be outdone.

'The outer perimeter of the universe,' I reply, 'and that is because nobody really knows where it ends, it is just so big.'

She starts to repeat these words, of which she has little understanding, but gets tongue-tied. Laughing and waving her hands about, she silences my next sentence and shouts, 'Do you know why my love is best?' I shake my head and wonder what is coming next as we have never been beyond the perimeter of the universe in this game.

The blue eyes dance with the enormity of her secret and she drops her voice to an urgent whisper, leaning towards me.

'My love is best because ... it will never end.' She sits back on her bed, cross-legged and triumphant. 'Do I win?' she asks.

Don't our children always win?

There is a love that begins before birth. There is a love that is unmarked by death. There is a love that never ends. This is the love we have for our children. It is untouched by wind, rain and sun. Age has no impact on its ferocity, and life with all its beauty and pain cannot distract us from it. We have been privileged to know this love four times. But there has been a price to pay for this love. The price has been a broken heart.

I am a mother of four beautiful children—Lydia, Luke, Ethan and Bronte. My arms, however, hold only two children. Our first son Luke died at 2 days of age in 2002, and Ethan at 11 days of age in 2003. They were both perfect and full term but had a rare genetic disorder that was discovered only after the birth of Ethan, despite an autopsy following Luke's death. It was only after Ethan was born and did not breathe, just like Luke, that investigations commenced and continued until his death 11 days later.

While my body told me again and again that things were not right, numerous ultrasounds told me I was wrong. But I was not wrong—I have learned to trust that voice now. Women must be listened to, for their knowledge is deep and real. The pain of holding two babies in your arms as they die cannot be compared. It is a place you never want to be and yet, at that moment, there is no other place you can be.

My story is not unique, however. Millions of women through history have walked this road of pain before me, and many will walk the road after me. Our midwives of life and death came on four incredible journeys with us. That journey would have been so much harder without the strength, love and continuity of midwifery care I experienced.

My firstborn daughter Lydia went through the pregnancies, births and deaths of our boys with us. She was named after my only sister whose life also ended too early, many years ago at three-and-a-half. Lydia was our shining light, our sanity, and our hope. At times I felt tied to her with a gossamer thread, but I knew this thread was reinforced with the strongest metal. I used to call her my lighthouse in the storm. Her bright light kept us away from the rocks time and again. She pressed tissues into my crying eyes and snaked little arms around my neck. She told her sobbing mother in the shower to be a butterfly, a beautiful butterfly, to lift up her arms and fly. 'It will make you happy,' she said. And when my attempt was feeble she insisted I do it properly and, strangely, I did feel better. She never saw the tubes and lines in our boys in the intensive care unit—things that I could not see past. She would say how cute her baby was and then add 'he's got poo on his foot'. How do they see so clearly? Perhaps their vision is not clouded with fear of what may come; rather they simply trust what is.

In the months leading up to the boys' births we spent days planning, swimming and loving. Lydia found the most perfect oval stone in our garden before Luke's birth and insisted that as it looked like my tummy we should paint a baby on it (Fig.43.1).

I thank her for making me overcome my fears and enabling me to find out that I, who could never paint, suddenly found a flowing hand and an artist's eye. Luke's birthstone waited in his cot for his arrival home and then

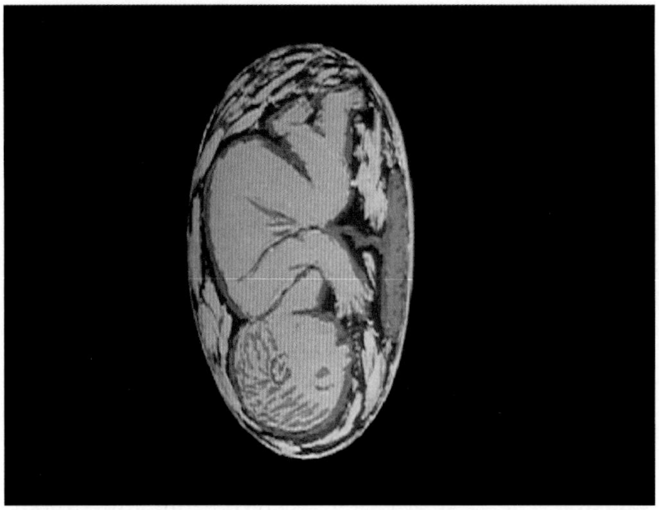

FIGURE 43.1 Luke's stone

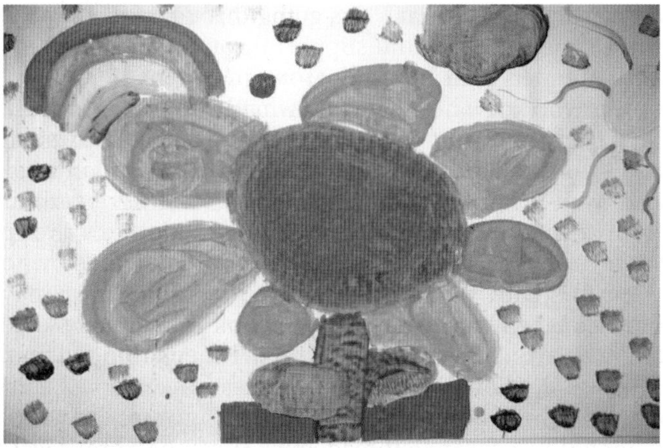

FIGURE 43.2 A rainbow of sorrow and joy

near his head in intensive care as he drifted through the short days of his life on earth. It has become so precious. I thank her mostly for understanding what we could not. I believe she was given to us first so we could bear the pain.

Just before Bronte arrived, Lydia painted the most beautiful picture for her sister. The rainbow symbolised our journey through the sorrow and tears, and the hope that we all held that we could and would smile again once more (Fig.43.2). The picture hung on Bronte's wall to remind us all of the sun that now shone through the rain.

How do you survive a broken heart? This is a question I have asked myself many times since the deaths of our two sons Luke and Ethan, only a year apart. How do you survive a heart broken, not yet healed and broken again so soon? We survive because there are others we need to survive for—our beautiful daughters, Lydia and Bronte. We survive because of what may be. We survive because as humans we are eternally hopeful in a future we cannot see. We survive because birth and death are forces that move us from the dermis of our superficial half lives into the deep life-giving marrow of our existence. We survive because that existence has meaning. We survive because not to is a worse option.

There is a love that will never end and that is the love we have for our children (Dahlen, 2009). Whether they outlive us or whether they depart this world before we do, our love for them does not end. It is this love that will make the world a better place. It is the lessons learned from the joy as well as the sorrow. This is the reason and the purpose, perhaps not *for* these tragedies, but to come *from* them.

NATASHA'S STORY—A FRACTURED FUTURE

My first child Callum was about 12 months old when we tried for our next baby. I was so in love with motherhood and my gorgeous little boy and was desperate to do it all over again. Unfortunately my next pregnancy ended in a miscarriage early in my first trimester. I thought that this was the worst thing that could ever happen to me. I sat for hours in the local hospital ED bleeding and wondering what was happening before I was told quite bluntly that my pregnancy was over and I would need a D&C. After it was over, in recovery, I lay there curled up in a ball sobbing on my own, feeling empty, betrayed and alone. The well-meaning platitudes from family and friends that it 'just wasn't meant to be' were no help at all. I never felt that I was allowed to grieve for my baby or that it was a baby at all. It seemed that miscarriage was not to be spoken about outside the confines of my home, and even then, it was in whispers. I had no idea then that there were far worse things ahead.

I was pregnant again within months and this time there was a midwife clinic up and running at my local hospital. The type of care I received from the midwives was completely different to what I had experienced with my first pregnancy under the care of one of the hospital obstetricians. They listened to my worries and never seemed to shove me out the door. I had put my miscarriage behind me and after the magic '12 weeks' felt that we were 'safe'. I had a relatively normal pregnancy and even though everything seemed to be fine, later in my pregnancy I just kept having this feeling that something was not right but was always reassured that it was normal to be 'over it' at the end.

When I was about 39½ weeks one evening I noticed a drop in my baby's movements. It was the weekend, and I didn't want to bother anyone. I figured it was probably because she did not have much room left and we were near the end and the next day the movements had increased a bit so I didn't worry too much. We were so excited when my waters broke the night before she was due and I didn't notice there were no movements. My husband and I were on top of the world, joking around about how quick this one would be after my first labour took only 4 hours.

At the hospital the midwives (who I had never met before) had trouble finding a heartbeat so put me onto a CTG. They found a heartbeat, but it was mine and not my baby's, although they did not realise it. They continued to monitor me like this for nearly 3 hours, convincing themselves and us that it was OK, turning the volume down and the monitor away from me so that I wouldn't get anxious and question them anymore. No-one ever suggested our daughter might have died. The on-call consultant finally arrived and did an ultrasound. 'No, there's no heartbeat.' That was it, just like that. Those were the words that fractured not just my future but that of my family, my friends and of course my precious baby girl, Soraya. 'Get the woman a valium.' 'You can either go home now and let labour progress there or we can give you something to speed it up.' All these words were being thrown at me with no empathy, compassion or emotion. The doctor didn't even know my name.

My daughter Soraya was born still, 40 minutes after the Syntocinon was started. Even my requests for an epidural had been denied and I birthed my beautiful baby girl through a haze of tears and Valium. She was absolutely perfect in every way but one—she did not take a breath. I was allowed home 3 hours later. The future we had planned for our family was gone with the beating of her heart. Like a shattered mirror, it lay on the floor beneath our feet in broken pieces that cut at our core. The pain in my husband's face as he rang our family, the agony in my mother's embrace as she tried to ease my own pain, the questions from my son about where his sister was, the gut-wrenching sobs as I sank to the shower floor ... I can see all of this replaying again and again when I close my eyes as if I was an observer in a macabre play. But I can no longer see our future in those broken shards.

I sought solace in my little boy and cried silently each morning in the shower so he wouldn't hear my pain. For my husband, Soraya's funeral was closure, the time for him to end his active and public grieving and to 'move on'. For me it was only the start. I had been so focused on organising her funeral and making sure she had been sent to the tertiary hospital for the autopsy that I had been on 'autopilot', being strong for everyone else and keeping it bottled up until the day of her funeral. Seeing my husband inside Soraya's grave, placing her coffin in it was my undoing. I wanted to be swallowed up in that same earth. But I had my little boy to keep me grounded. He was the reason I got up each day, tried to function as best as I could. Without that tether I don't know if I would have carried on.

It doesn't take long for the people around you to get impatient with your grief and expect that you will 'get over it'. There is no tangible outward sign that you are still missing a huge part of you. I have had two more beautiful children since Soraya died but that gaping wound in my chest is still there, I have just learned to paper over it and appreciate what I do have. I now live a new 'normal'.

PUTTING IT ALL TOGETHER—UNDERSTANDING THE STAGES OF THE JOURNEY

Our stories are very different (Hannah's and Natasha's) but both describe the importance of good midwifery care and the added trauma that comes when this is lacking. In this next section we pull together some of the important issues from our stories that midwives need to be aware of when caring for women who have experienced perinatal loss.

Everyone grieves differently, but there is comfort in the company of those who have walked in your shoes

Natasha: The best advice I received from my support group was that there was no right way to grieve, but as long as you were not hurting yourself or anyone else then it was OK. I read every book on pregnancy and child loss that I could get my hands on just trying to reach out to others that knew what I was going through and to make some sense of it. I found support through SIDS and Kids and attended their monthly group meetings to talk with others who knew how I felt and what I was going through. My family and friends meant well but they just couldn't relate to the depth of my pain and grief. The platitudes and well-meaning comments flowed fast and furious from acquaintances and friends alike. Mother's group soon dropped off as it was too awkward for those who were pregnant or had just had their babies and they didn't know what to say. I saw people I knew cross the street to avoid the small talk and the inevitable sadness. This was a relief for me as well. Some of the people I least expected became my greatest support and others who I expected more from left me feeling betrayed and alone.

Hannah: I did not attend a support group after the loss of either of my boys and this is not because I don't think it is important but because I was lucky enough to be a midwife, surrounded by wonderful midwives and they really met my needs. I found out who my friends were and this is a blessing that comes with this pain. I remember returning to work after my boys died and finding some would go out of their way to hug you and shed a tear with you while others would turn in the corridor and walk the other way. I used to think they were blaming me for what happened but now I know they were just out of their depth, not knowing what to say. Walk into women's pain, not away from it, is my advice to you. It takes a brave person to do this but midwives on the whole are incredibly brave.

Guilt

Natasha: I relived those few days before she had died and the 'what-ifs' were overwhelming. *What if* I had called the hospital when her movements had decreased, *what if* I had gotten up when her last big movement had caused me pain, *what if* I had the same carer throughout my pregnancy, *what if, what if, what if* ...

Hannah: I had chosen to have a home birth with Luke and, even though I had been transferred to hospital over 12 hours before the birth by my midwives, I felt people blamed me for my choices. After Ethan was born I realised it was not my birth choices but genetics that led to both my boys' short lives. Then I blamed myself for having a body that caused this to happen. I have learnt now to hand over those impossible feelings to the universe, as they get us nowhere. I now regret nothing, because to regret Luke is to regret Ethan and to regret Ethan is to regret Bronte and a world without Bronte is impossible to imagine. Not all women reach this place and some women reach it earlier than others. You can't hurry it up and as a midwife you need to learn to accept that grief and loss is whatever the woman and her partner say it is. Continuity of midwifery care gave me the arms to break and heal in and for that I will forever be grateful.

The stigma of losing a child

Natasha: The greatest joy I have is to hear her name said out loud—Soraya, to have her existence acknowledged, to have someone ask me about her. It is the elephant in the room that hurts the most. To be told it is better to forget and not to talk about her; to be told that I am damaging my living children by taking them to the cemetery to celebrate her life. That is what opens the wound further. Grief is not a bad thing or something that should remain hidden. Yet that is how I am often made to feel. Losing a child is one of the most painful things a parent will ever have to experience and one of the most difficult things society seems to be able to deal with. Babies aren't meant to die. Old people die, babies don't. So when it happens, people are sometimes so uncomfortable that they would rather cut all ties than have some awkward painful moments. There is nothing anyone can say to me about Soraya that would cause me pain or make me cry—her death itself did that, not talking about her.

Hannah: There is a moment whenever I am asked how many children I have that I hesitate, or when people comment on the age gap (7 years) between my two daughters that I quiver internally. There will always be four children in my life but I select whom I share that with. One of the loveliest things a midwifery colleague said to me after we had Ethan was, 'Hannah you make such good looking babies.' I needed to hear that and know that under the tubes and wires this little soul shone in all his impossible beauty to more than just his mother. Never be afraid to talk to women about their loss and comment on their baby as you would with one that is alive or will live. We are never offended if you tell us our babies are beautiful and your words honour our children.

The importance of providing options for caring for a baby once she has died

Natasha: Looking back at that time we felt so lost and had no idea that this sort of thing could happen. In our antenatal classes, the worst thing we thought we would have to deal with in labour involved a caesarean section. The only choices we thought we would have to make were about pain relief and what music to put on! We had no idea about what our options were in caring for our dead baby. We knew without a doubt that we wanted to hold her and my highest priority was ensuring she had an autopsy straight away to find out why she had died. Beyond that no one explained the other options we had regarding taking her home, bringing in our son to see his sister or even being able to bathe her. Without our knowledge the staff had at least taken some photos, a lock of her hair and hand and footprints to give us later. They never asked me if I would like to bathe her and they took her away and did this without our knowledge, returning her to us in a bright white synthetic christening-style dress an hour later. I was horrified and it no longer looked like my daughter who I had birthed just hours before. I couldn't hold her again and just wanted to get home.

The saying that 'you don't know what you don't know' was so true for our family when Soraya was stillborn. We didn't know about the options about collecting mementos, spending extended time with her, bringing others in to meet her or even being able to take her home with us. I was so focused on making sure that we got the answers to why she died and getting her off to the pathologist while she was still 'fresh' and no one caring for us told us that it wouldn't have mattered to the autopsy if we wanted to have her with us longer. No one talked to us about options. We may not have chosen to do any of those things but we never had the opportunity to make those choices. Doing those things may not be everyone's choice but they should have the opportunity to make them. It is up to the staff caring for women and their families at these times to make sure that they have all the options presented to them in a safe and appropriate way. Not everyone will want to hold their baby or spend time with them and no one should be pushed down a certain pathway, but it's about making sure that the information is there to make a choice and giving people the space to do so. It will be one of the hardest things you will have to do as a midwife but it can also have the greatest impact on the women you care for. Be open, be honest and don't be afraid to say you are sorry. They can sometimes be the kindest words you can say. An ABC National Radio Health Report I listened to recently really brought home to me what options are available now that maybe weren't available to me when Soraya died (Swan, n.d.). Sadly, they are still not available to all families after stillbirth.

Hannah: My midwives made the drab and clinical room my boys died in into a shrine fit for a goddess. They brought in flowers and candles and love and warm arms, and as I broke in those arms I also began to heal. Because every step of the way they were led by us, we live today with no regrets. We have the handprints and footprints and Lydia got to bath both her brothers and we spent precious time together. I never felt rushed or disapproved of and when we were ready we left our boys with midwives who watched over them. This is such a contrast to Natasha's story. I cannot emphasise enough how precious those memories are and that we must not rush those important hours and days after a baby dies. Some women will want to take their babies home and some women need more time than others. It is not up to us to judge what that time should be. We can guide women to collect precious memories in that time as well as give gentle suggestions along the way. I wrote once that memories are both the curse and the balm of the grieving soul. Just because creating them hurts like hell does not mean they should not be created, for later on they become the balm that makes us whole again.

Care in the postnatal period

Natasha: I didn't have the benefit of a continuity-of-carer model so I had a different midwife visit me at home each day and then nothing after a few days. I had to take myself to the GP for my 6-week check and try to track down the autopsy results and repeat my story to every new clinician I was sent to. Each time was like reliving that night over and over again.

Hannah: I remember feeling like I was leaking from both ends but bleeding from the heart. It was easy to forget my own physical needs because the emotional pain was so great. Again my story contrasts so much to Natasha's. My midwives visited me daily and weekly and then there were phone calls and I still see them and call them friends. I can't imagine having to tell a stranger about what happened and how I felt every day. They reminded me to eat, they cried with me and laughed with me and remembered with me and kept helping me and my family make memories. Lydia remembers that time as sad but also fun because she had so much love around her. Women want the best of our skills, they want the best of our knowledge and they want the best of our humanity. Without humanity the rest will soon be forgotten.

The importance of continuity of carers

Natasha: After what had happened with Soraya and the miscarriages I had before and after her, there was no joy in being pregnant and it was the thing we wanted most and feared most at the same time. When I started bleeding at 17 weeks in my next pregnancy, the staff in the labour ward couldn't understand why I was so upset at having a CTG and kept trying to explain to me that it wasn't going to be painful. How could I explain to them what it had been like 12 months before? They hadn't been there and didn't understand what we had been through when we lost Soraya. Not having the same carers meant I had to explain my story over and over again.

Hannah: Having continuity of care meant I had two amazing midwives who were like my walking medical records with warm arms. I remember meeting Natasha in 2007 at a midwives' conference where she talked about her experience of losing Soraya and I gave her a big hug and she said, as only a mother who has lost a baby could say, 'I was so jealous of your experience.' She was referring to the film 'Hannah's story' about our experiences and my amazing midwives who were there. The loss of a baby demands our greatest asset—our humanity—not our intellectual capacity. Death strips us all of pretence and soon exposes those who dare to pretend in her awesome presence. It takes a very brave and special person to walk into a mother's grief, to look into the face of a broken soul and just be there. It asks us to be blind in a seeing, doing world, to draw on senses that may have been asleep for a very long time. I was so lucky to have this for four births and two deaths.

Long-term feelings

Natasha: A new baby doesn't cancel out what had happened 12 months before. It doesn't fill the void as you hoped it would. I realised that I had been trying to replace Soraya. As hard as it was to admit, I thought that having a baby so soon after losing her would quench that pain and fill the void she had left behind. It didn't, and for a while I had resented my new baby for not being Soraya and for still feeling such acute grief. It took me many years, another miscarriage and then finally the girl I had been craving, before I realised that I could never fill that wound inside me but I could learn to live with a new version of 'normal'. You never 'get over it' or 'move on' after losing a child. When people lose a limb in an accident, there is tangible, visual evidence of what they lost. When you lose a child you don't have that. If a marathon runner lost a leg you wouldn't tell him to get over it and run another race 6 months later, but that is what happens when you lose a child.

Hannah: There is always a hole in my heart where two others should have been but that hole does not bring me to my knees any more as it once did. Having another baby did not fill this hole, and no number of children ever can, but Bronte did fill my arms and that was healing. You don't get over losing a child but you can get on with life, and life can have a richer deeper meaning. I can still be at the traffic lights and find tears welling in my eyes at the sudden thought of them and I hope that never stops.

> *The sum of the parts will never be the same as the whole. Loss never ends, it becomes a part of who we are with a potential for growth or deterioration. We [health professionals] sit at the moment when the potential sets in.*
>
> (Judith Murray, 2008 unpublished conference notes)

Subsequent pregnancies

Natasha: After Soraya, during my pregnancy with Rohan I had placenta praevia and some retroplacental clots that kept bleeding. I spent 10 weeks in hospital wondering each day if this would be the end of my baby's life yet again. It was impossible to fathom how my daughter could have died after a 40-week perfect pregnancy but that I could be bleeding for weeks and my new baby could survive. My feelings were so conflicting because all I wanted was another baby, but at the same time I couldn't accept that this baby could possibly survive under these conditions when Soraya didn't. People thought that my grieving must be over if I was having another baby. I was expected to be happy. I was wracked with guilt whenever I allowed myself a moment of happiness—did this mean I was betraying Soraya in some way? Then there was guilt when I wasn't happy about being pregnant—did this mean I wouldn't love my baby? My grief felt like my only connection to Soraya. It was only a year since she had died and now I was stuck in hospital, my husband and little boy an hour away and the uncertainty of whether I would lose another baby. Although my doctor visited every day I was forced to tell and retell my story to every new midwife who came to look after me.

Hannah: The anxiety when you get pregnant again is immense. There is a part of you that protects yourself and disconnects but of course the physical reality of pregnancy does not allow you to do this. You are more likely to want more testing and reassurance and when you have continuity of care this is easily understood. I felt so guilty wanting another baby so badly after Luke and we were pregnant within 3 months and dealing with the loss of Ethan at Luke's 1-year anniversary. I worried about how my 'selfish desire to have another baby, not to replace Luke but to fill my arms' was now going to cause added trauma to my little girl twice in a year. Guilt and worry seemed to constantly be at the forefront of my thinking and my midwives understood that and listened and walked through the fog of emotions with me.

Accepting the different journeys

Natasha: It took me several years to accept that my husband and I had such different ways of grieving for Soraya. My grief was still so raw and he seemed to move on so quickly. I used to feel so bitter about how easily he had forgotten her and how little patience he had for my continuing active grief. It is over 18 years since she died, and not once has he celebrated her birthday with me, although our surviving children do. I finally realised that, in my husband's family, death is not spoken about or dealt with in the open; what hope did I have of him openly grieving for our daughter when it was frowned upon in his family? His family has never spoken of Soraya since her funeral. We all have different ways of dealing with death; none of them are wrong but sometimes it can be hard to understand.

Hannah: Each member of the family walks their own journey and many times this journey gets more diverse as time goes on, not less, as I soon discovered. The divorce rate after the loss of a baby is around 70% and I really believe this is one of the reasons for this. We all express grief differently and yet we expect there will be a similarity in this and there is not. I remember feeling desperately caught in an eddy of grief that I could see no way out of. Carl Jung said, 'How do you find a lion that has swallowed you?' I wrote this in my diary, 'I sometimes feel my whole life has been leading up to this point. For millennia the constellations have been lining up to intersect at this one huge event. But now I am here I feel caught in a never-ending eddy that seems inescapable. Now I can see no way through or out.' Of course I did find a way out but much later than others in my family and I learnt to say that is okay, our journeys are and will be different. For me that saved my marriage, but it was hard.

Learning to trust life again

Natasha: Every morning you wake up and expect that the floor will be there where it always has been when you get up. Then one day you get up and everything you had always believed in and trusted is suddenly swept away—the floor is no longer there where it should be. How can everyone else go on like nothing happened? It takes a long time to regain that trust that the floor will be there again the next morning, and the one after that and the one after that.

Hannah: C. S. Lewis said, 'no one ever told me that grief is so like fear' (Lewis, 1961, p. 15). We are not in control of much in our lives; there's just the illusion that we are in control. The ability to sustain this illusion so effectively for the majority of our lives is perhaps the greatest kindness we have been afforded as human beings. Losing a baby smashes the illusion forever. 'Why me?' becomes 'Why not me?' 'It will never happen to me' becomes 'It did, and it could again'. Once faced with this uncertainty, life will never be the same again. The glasses we look through are no longer rose coloured; they are crystal clear. However, it is the heights of love and valleys of grief that both bring our existence into acute proximity and breathe life into the corners of worlds we rarely see or acknowledge. In the book *Tuesdays with Morrie* (Albom, 1997), Morrie says, 'once you learn how to die you learn how to live'. I have rephrased this to 'once you learn how to be with death then you truly learn how to be alive'. I came to a point when I realised that to regret is to ask the impossible; it traps you in the past. Acceptance is redemption and allows you to move on into the future. Like the rainbow that Lydia painted for Bronte when she was about to be born, beauty can come from sorrow. The tears of sorrow mingled with the sunshine of laughter form the rainbows in our lives.

CRITICAL THINKING EXERCISE

Subsequent pregnancy after loss can be traumatic and difficult for the families as well as those caring for them. There has recently been a focus on developing specific models of care for 'rainbow pregnancies' that may be higher risk both physically and psychosocially. List some of the factors that need to be considered when caring for women in a subsequent pregnancy after loss, particularly if you were developing a new model of care specifically for this.

SHOULD WE ENCOURAGE PARENTS TO PARENT A DYING OR DEAD CHILD?

When you cannot take your baby home you may not want to take them into your heart and you do this to protect you. This is the great dilemma parents may face. Holding your dying or dead baby is the last place you want to be and the only place you can be. Avoidance is simply survival and should not be judged. Sometimes parents can't see their baby but they do want to know it is being taken care of and as a midwife you can reassure them about this. You need to give some parents time to emerge from the shock into the reality. Trying to walk at their pace rather than what you think is an acceptable pace will help them avoid regret and give them time to have their baby when they are ready or for as long as they need. Rumi said, 'Don't turn away. Keep your gaze on the bandaged place. That's where the light enters you' (Barks, 2003, p. 35).

Research into perinatal loss shows the aftermath of death includes psychological and emotional disorders, PTSD, blame, guilt, hardship, avoidance of activities, feelings of isolation, relationship breakdown, chronic pain and fatigue, the desperate need to remember, the utility of autopsies and funerals, decisional conflict, the necessity for adequate support, issues surrounding surviving siblings and subsequent pregnancies, the long journey to healing, and the need to reach out and help others in distress (Burden et al., 2016). Many of these ring true for us and you will have read about some of these in what we have written about our experience. It is important though as future midwives that you base your practice not just on stories (as important as they are) but on sound scientific evidence.

The best way to care for parents and families who have lost a baby remains controversial and there are wide variations in care practices around the world (Horey et al., 2021). Over the last 40 years, recommendations and guidelines about bereavement care after stillbirth have changed significantly, swinging from recommending minimisation of contact between parents and their baby to encouraging parents to hold and get to know their stillborn baby. Studies examining the longterm effects on parents seeing and holding their stillborn baby have had conflicting results, with some showing fewer psychological complications and benefits (Cacciatore et al., 2008; Forrest et al., 1982) and others showing more severe anxiety and depression (Hughes et al., 2002). This conflicting research shows how complex an area it is and that more research is needed.

A Cochrane systematic review of support after perinatal death found no eligible trials to include in the review and concluded that more research was needed (Koopmans et al., 2013). There is clearly an ethical issue with conducting randomised controlled trials to assess the impact of holding a stillborn baby, so no trials could be included. With this in mind, Hennegan et al. incorporated more inclusive criteria in their systematic review in 2015, which included 11 studies published across 18 papers. Still, they concluded that there is no clear evidence either way regarding the impact on the mother's mental health and wellbeing after holding her stillborn baby, but that 'qualitative evidence ... suggests this contact is valued by women and that they are retrospectively satisfied with their decision' (p. 18). There is currently limited evidence available on the impact on partners following contact with their stillborn babies. In a secondary analysis from data collected through a national survey, Hennegan et al. (2018) assessed the mental health and wellbeing of partners through reports from mothers. Although their study findings suggested a negative effect from partners holding their baby, they also recommended the need for further larger and more detailed studies to properly assess the impact and acknowledged the results of other studies that consistently showed a lack of regret from parents who did hold their stillborn baby and were satisfied with their decision to do so.

Current Australian / New Zealand guidelines from the Perinatal Society of Australia and New Zealand acknowledge the conflicting evidence in this area, and recommend that clinicians assist parents in their decision making around holding their stillborn baby by giving them options and information—such as the possibility of 'cold cots' (Box 43.1)—without recommending either way (Flenady et al., 2018). Importantly, evidence from a number of studies indicates that parents should be offered the opportunity to see and hold their baby more than once (Ellis et al., 2016). There are many contributing factors that may influence a family's decision whether they should hold their stillborn baby, and also how this may impact on their mental health and wellbeing. Some of these include the condition of the baby and their gestation at birth, and how and when staff approach them with the baby (Hennegan et al., 2015). Cultural and religious practices should also be considered in this decision-making process. Although finding a lack of evidence from randomised trials, Koopmans et al. (2013) identified three themes from their review that should be considered when providing care to families following a perinatal death: 'firstly a deep respect for the individuality and diversity of grief, respect for the deceased child, and recognition of the healing power and resilience of the human spirit' (p. 9).

> *Her absence is like the sky, spread over everything.*
>
> (C. S. Lewis, 1961, p. 11)

Updated guidance from the Perinatal Society of Australia and New Zealand, developed in partnership with the NHMRC Centre of Research Excellence in Stillbirth provides a framework for respectful and supportive perinatal bereavement care based around the four pillars of good communication, shared decision making, recognition of parenthood, and effective support (Flenady et al., 2018). These guidelines are also aligned with the *Principles of Bereavement Care* developed by Sands Australia (Sands Australia, 2018). Both of these resources should be utilised to guide your practice in supportive and respectful bereavement care after perinatal loss.

HOW DO MIDWIVES WALK ALONGSIDE A GRIEVING FAMILY?

Midwives have a truly privileged role when they are part of this incredibly sad time and, as Judith Murray says, 'We

Box 43.1 Jo Hunter—a midwife's perspective on cold cots

There is plenty of research, and certainly anecdotal evidence, which suggests that parents who have physical contact with their stillborn baby find the experience positive and an important part of the grieving process. Cold cots, or 'Cuddle Cots', are now in some hospitals in Australia. Instead of needing to retrieve their baby from the morgue to have some time with their baby after it has died, Cuddle Cots give parents the opportunity to have their baby with them, for several days if they wish. It is a discrete cooling system designed to fit within a small cot and slows down the natural processes that occur after death. It offers the option for babies who have passed away to remain with their families for longer periods. A Cuddle Cot can also assist bereaved families to reconcile their loss, giving them an opportunity to say hello to their baby, before having to say goodbye.

I was midwife to a couple who were having twins, who were born via planned caesarean section and the second twin was born severely compromised and placed on life support. Eventually after running lots of tests, withdrawal of care was recommended. This couple desperately wanted to take their baby home to die and have some time with her in their own environment, away from the machines and monitors, tubes and wires and the sterile medical environment of the hospital. The hospital did have a Cuddle Cot; however, the couple were not able to take it home, seeing 'as it is an expensive piece of equipment'.

A local woman in the community fundraised and purchased a Cuddle Cot to have in the community to be used by this family but also others who may wish to do the same thing in the future. For this family, taking their baby home to die and having time with her at home after she died allowed them to be more present and aware, and it gave them the freedom and opportunity to grieve and experience their baby more deeply than they may have in the hospital setting. They hand selected the people they wanted present to support them. They were free to do whatever they wished, without inhibition and without feeling as though they had to gain permission, and they left no stone unturned.

In the future we must work to allow bereaved families to take a Cuddle Cot home with them, subsequently giving them more time with their baby.

[health professionals] sit at the moment when the potential sets in'. It is an awesome responsibility and you will never be forgotten when you are part of parents' lives at this vulnerable time. Lundqvist and colleagues found in their study that a sense of empowerment emerged when health professionals 'saw through the mother's eyes' and 'felt with the mother's feelings' (Lundqvist et al., 2002, p. 198). Women felt empowered when they experienced a sense of nearness, a sense of encouragement and a sense of empathy. They felt powerless when there was a sense of distance, a sense of violation and a sense of disconnection. Midwives can never hope to become an expert when it comes to death, but you can learn to become comfortable with being in its presence:

When birth and death meet we mix two of life's most powerful emotions. Our job is to protect the natural process, to 'midwife' the grief and not to attempt to cure it. We have the choice to be an outsider or insider in grief. Women will know which choice you have made.

Continuity of midwifery care is the best way to provide quality perinatal loss care because it facilitates the relationship between mother / family and midwife (Box 43.2). Fenwick et al. (2007) reported that midwives found the most satisfying aspect of midwifery when dealing with loss was connecting with families and providing what was seen as the 'very best' care. This was seen to include sensitive supportive care, being flexible and responding to individual needs, facilitating understanding, creating special memories (Box 43.3), listening to and sharing grief, making a positive difference and creating a supportive environment; the least satisfying was the personally challenging experiences, being emotionally overwhelmed, feeling unsure and feeling unsupported (Fenwick et al., 2007).

CRITICAL THINKING EXERCISE

Most women and families who lose their baby will not know what their options are for spending time with their baby or creating memories. They may need to have ideas provided to them and their options presented multiple times to consider. Prepare a list of suggestions for ways families can spend time with their baby and ways they can create their own special memories (keeping in mind available services at your hospital). Locate resources or services in your area that you could recommend if the situation arose for a woman for whom you were caring.

CHILDREN AND GRIEF

As caregivers we need to remember to include and respect the grief of others. This includes partners, siblings, grandparents and other relatives and friends. Parents can assist children to become familiar with birth and death as part of life. Hiding death from children does not make it easier for them to cope because they see a changed parent and are left wondering why. Involving children in the experience of loss is a way for them to understand why you are sad and to make sense of the emotions around them. Children understand much more than we give them credit for. Children can also be an enormous comfort

Box 43.2 Do's and don'ts for midwives

- Make sure you have the time.
- Sit down at the couple's level and use their names.
- Don't be defensive.
- Watch your body language.
- Find out the baby's name first and use it.
- It's okay to cry and touch women as your tears honour the baby, your touch connects you to another and soothes, and your comments reinforce and establish the baby's existence.
- Watch out for technical language.
- Use diagrams.
- Don't hide behind social workers; you are important.
- Don't avoid women as they will think they have done something or that you are trying to hide something, or that nobody cares and this breeds distrust.
- Parents want privacy, not abandonment.
- Try and get one person to give the information and make it consistent.
- Don't be positive if you're not and don't be devastating.
- Take your time and don't rush the process.
- It is okay to say 'we don't know'. In the long run this will be respected more than answers forced into the yawning gaps in order to make it better.
- Allow parents the opportunity to think about what you have said and offer a contact number or time for a further visit.
- Always ask and don't make decisions on their behalf.
- Support parents to express their concerns.

when a baby dies. As you will have read in our stories, Hannah involved Lydia in everything whereas Natasha did not do this with Callum. The type of care and gentle suggestions along the way can determine whether or not this happens. In the end the parents are the best people to judge whether this will be okay for their children.

FATHERS AND LOSS

Gary Sillett

Losing a child at birth (or at any time) is one of the most painful and devastating experiences that someone can go through. Sadly, so many men, once excited at the prospect of being a dad (many for the first time), never get to experience a 'normal' childbirth. Some also never get to experience a 'normal' fatherhood at all. These men are part of a club that swells by over 3000 new members each year through stillbirth or neonatal or infant loss alone.

Modern society has conditioned men to conceal their emotions as a sign of strength, but a grieving father feels the loss of a child just as keenly as the mother. Although men don't express themselves as women do, it does not mean that we grieve any less. Whilst the grieving process may be different for men and women the grieving process is often based on individuality rather than gender. However, there is a significant feeling that fathers are often forgotten in the grieving process.

During the pregnancy and birth of a child a father's role is predominantly to support his partner emotionally and physically. A father is expected to be the pillar of support (strength) for the mother, extended family and friends. He is also the communication channel to the outside world and on many occasions, if he has other children, he becomes their chief caretaker while his partner recovers from surgery and the birth. Although of course he did not carry the child, there is still a deep bond that reaches a whole new dimension once the child is outside the womb.

During the period immediately after loss there is little time for dads to do something for themselves or get support. They feel the need to provide it to everyone else (particularly their partners) to ensure that everything continues in some sense of 'normality'. Many men take on the protector role in the family, supporting their wives or partners and not allowing time for their own grief. Even in today's society, some men find it difficult to express their emotions and feelings can get locked up. Many men need time and space to grieve and this may happen many weeks, months or even years later.

For some fathers sadly our role is to support our child's memory rather than supporting them through life. I am a bereaved dad. My son was born 14 weeks prematurely, and passed away after 2 days in the NICU at RNS hospital in December 2010. My son's passing changed my world forever. However, fatherhood, once reached, is timeless.

Coping with the loss of your child at any time is both emotionally heartbreaking and physically devastating. It is a pain that endures. You never know the moment when your next 'down day' will come, no matter how long ago you lost your child.

Being in this situation you will find that friends and family always offer support or to do something for you, but there really isn't anything they can do to help you with your grief and the guilt of not being able to do anything to fix things. Fathers tend to take on the practicalities and keep themselves busy. Men also often find that other people ask about how their partner is coping without seeming to realise that they are grieving too. Men may feel helpless when they see their partner so distressed. However, it is important to recognise that although men may not show symptoms of grief they are grieving and need support too.

The important thing is to respect and support each family member when they are dealing with their loss. Acknowledge the father and ask how he is doing—although it may seem small it will go a long way. Acknowledge him and acknowledge their child and recognise their loss, no matter when it occurred. It's a loss that never goes away. Affirm his role as dad.

Box 43.3 Helping to make memories

To avoid prescribing the parents' grief, use the concept of 'guided participation' (Kobler et al., 2007) to quietly do or suggest activities the couple might want to consider which other grieving parents have found helpful:

- Hold the baby's hand. We suggest the midwife consciously behave *as though the baby were alive* (Culling, 2005), gently and courteously taking the baby's hand or holding the baby herself. Seeing this can give the parents confidence and offers a chance to say 'hello' before saying 'goodbye'.
- Hold the baby; lie down with the baby.
- Bathe and dress the baby.
- Take photographs.
- Arrange to take the baby to a place that is special to the family.
- If a cold cot or 'Cuddle Cot' is available, offer parents the opportunity to take their baby home or to stay longer with them in the hospital.

Remember, whatever you suggest may be declined, and it can be useful to say to parents that they can slow down, and that in time they may wish to do something they previously felt uncomfortable about doing (Kobler et al., 2007).

Photographs:

- Seek consent before taking any photographs.
- Take lots of photographs with different combinations of family members, e.g. parents and baby; parents, siblings and baby, etc.
- Digital images have now largely replaced the instant Polaroid photos that fade over time.
- Consider what the baby wears, e.g. make sure the clothes fit or, in the case of a second trimester miscarriage, use a piece of soft material as a wrap.
- Be aware that the skin of babies less than around 24 weeks is translucent (the veins are visible because there is little subcutaneous tissue), red and sticky, so handle the baby carefully.
- Think about where the baby is photographed, e.g. inside a room, outside in the garden, in a Moses basket of a suitable size, lying or propped on a pillow, holding a toy/stuffed animal.
- Avoid having too much white in photographs—it can emphasise the pallor or redness of their skin, e.g. white sheets and a flash-lit exposure can create a stark photograph.
- Think about having a professional photographer in the way they might to celebrate the arrival of a live baby.

GRANDPARENTS HURT, TOO

The death of a much planned and loved baby affects many people close to the parents. Often forgotten are the grandparents, who are also robbed of the future they had imagined with their grandchild. Their grief is complicated by the dual experience of losing a grandchild and watching their own child suffer indescribable pain. Feelings of helplessness, disbelief and anguish are often described by the grandparents. In some cases the death may trigger memories of their own child loss previously kept secret. There has been little in the way of research specifically about the effects of perinatal loss on grandparents, with Murphy and Jones (2014) describing it as 'by the way knowledge' gathered incidentally through other research. Lockton et al. (2020) studied the effects of perinatal loss on grandmothers, finding it was a devastating experience, and a grief like no other, compounded by the 'ambiguity' of pregnancy loss. Participants in the study described feelings of disbelief, isolation, a loss of hope and powerlessness. The same study also reported grandmothers valued being given the opportunity to create mementoes of the baby and spending time with their grandchild, including holding them. The participants acknowledged that while they wanted to hide their grief from their children to avoid adding to their burden, sharing their grief with others and not internalising it was important. Encourage them to talk about their loss if they wish and provide them with resources for grandparents' grief.

A GRANDMOTHER'S STORY

Tania (Natasha's mother)

I can still see your smile as you left your house to go to the hospital. You were so happy to finally have your baby. Then came the phone call—I heard your scream and 'the baby's dead'. I could not comprehend what was happening—it can't be true. I can't remember how we got to the hospital, but I do remember thinking that this is a nightmare and we will all wake up. The baby was born and I kept thinking that she would be all right, that you would be spared the pain you were going through. But it was not to be—I could not share your pain with you because I had never lost a baby. All I could see was my child in such pain, the pain I could not comprehend. I kept wanting to turn the clock back and start again, this time with a happy ending. You put on her plaque 'like a butterfly on delicate petals, you touched our lives'; to me it was always a sledgehammer. I dread the anniversary of Soraya's death because I know that you go through such pain, pain I cannot share with you, nor prevent.

AN AOTEAROA NEW ZEALAND PERSPECTIVE ON CARING AFTER PERINATAL LOSS

Vicki Culling

Health and caring professionals can make an incredible difference to the experience of parents facing perhaps one of the most heart-wrenching moments of their lives. What was joyous and full of wonder—the impending arrival of a beautiful, much loved baby—is now heavy with sadness, grief and shattered hopes.

Parents will look to those around them, those 'in charge', for some indication of what they can and cannot do, what they should and should not do. The information you give, the advice you impart and the approach you take might just make all the difference to their experience of perinatal or infant loss. And it may be something small, and seemingly unimportant, that makes all the difference—just one word, one gesture or one suggestion—that impacts how they meet and say farewell to their precious baby.

Practices around the death of a baby have changed throughout the Western world. Whereas it was once believed that best practice was the removal of the baby as promptly as possible, and without the mother seeing or holding her baby at all, we now embrace the notion that seeing, holding, spending time with the baby and making memories is a positive and healing practice.

New Zealand's perinatal death practices have followed suit, but one of the major influences on our death and funeral customs in general is our indigenous Māori population and their approach to death. Despite the effects of colonisation, population decline, detrimental government policies and a subsequent revival of Māori language and culture, the one tradition that has remained unchanged is the tangihanga or death ritual / funeral.

Māori death rituals ensure that the deceased person is never left alone and is cared for by the extended family. Family and mourners stay with the deceased at a marae (a communal and / or sacred place that serves social and religious purposes), usually for three days with burial on the third day. New Zealand's mainstream culture has adopted aspects of Māori death practices, with many families of all ethnicities bringing their deceased loved ones home for a short time prior to a farewell service or funeral.

In New Zealand, parents are routinely asked in hospital whether they wish to take their deceased baby home and, whilst there are no statistics collected on the practice, anecdotal evidence suggests over 50% of bereaved families do take their baby home.

Babies are taken home for a matter of hours through to a number of days. This depends on funeral arrangements and the parents' desire for time with their baby. Siblings may wish to meet their little brother or sister and this may be the only time they get to be together as a family. Funeral directors are often involved and advise on care of the body. Taking care of the deceased baby is relatively straightforward; because there is little need for a baby to be embalmed, they simply need to be kept cool with a cooling device or ice / chiller pads. Babies are taken home prior to or following a postmortem; this does not obstruct the parents' opportunity to be with their baby.

For many parents bringing their deceased baby home is a natural and normal thing to do. Despite their grief and sadness, the act of taking their baby home is part of their parenting that baby and is a further way of creating precious memories.

One of the best things you can do as a health professional is to gather together a range of information and options for bereaved parents, such as taking their baby home, and let them know not only what they can do but also why they might want to do it. Your knowledge, your approach, your kindness—that may be the one small thing that makes all the difference to the next family you support through a perinatal loss.

THE 'SORRY BUSINESS': CARING FOR ABORIGINAL AND TORRES STRAIT ISLANDER WOMEN

Tanya Martin

Aboriginal people are the original inhabitants of the Australian continent and they are one of the best-known and least-understood people in the world, in regards to their traditional heritage and culture. Many Aboriginal childbearing women in Australia have had to contend with many traumatic dispiriting situations within their lives and family situations. The women's continued strength, devotion and commitment to family and domestic responsibilities are evident by a strong kinship structure that is central to cultural practices and their connection to their spiritual country still practised today. Therefore, when traditional woman's business such as 'Sorry Business' associated with perinatal loss is being discussed it must be treated with the utmost respect. Cultural safety must be acknowledged at all times and integrated within maternal health services in a manner that acknowledges cultural beliefs and is respectful of Aboriginal culture. This empowers Aboriginal woman to make informed decisions that impact on their social and emotional wellbeing during their childbearing experiences within mainstream health services.

The significance of Aboriginal women's spiritual connection of giving birth on country is linked spiritually with the Dreaming and is paramount. Perinatal loss and bereavement is to be approached and understood with this in mind. Dreaming is a way of doing and being in the world; it is not abstract or external to the individual. It is also an instrument in maintaining and strengthening cultural belief and cultural identity.

Babies, irrespective of gestation at the time of loss, should be returned to country. Midwives need to understand the significance of human spirit conceived from the land and returned upon death. Child spirit is to return to the mother's country so that the spirit can freely roam with the spiritual ancestors. The woman should be supported by a family member, owing to the importance of kinship structure. If she is on her own, all attempts must be made to contact the family and if this is not possible then a health worker with understanding of cultural safety and sensitivity should be sought. The right of all women is to be treated respectfully especially at such a vulnerable time; however, it should be highlighted that Anglo-Saxon constructs of the afterlife such as heaven and angels are not appropriate and not particularly helpful for the Aboriginal mother in her grief.

Women who lose a baby that is under 20 weeks gestation are often restricted in having their and their baby's cultural needs met. Currently in Australia, legislation is based on a biomedical model and restricts the transport of these babies outside of the health system. As a result, babies under the age of 20 weeks are often unable to be returned to their mother's country and this breaks with traditional protocol. In some towns, cremation services are offered to enable the baby to be taken home, returned to country and final ceremony. Consideration should be given to developing local relationships with Aboriginal medical services and funeral directors to facilitate this.

Mothers of stillborn babies are to be offered the opportunity to hold and nurture their babies. Family members are invited in to say goodbye and the baby will be washed, dressed and named. Many women will opt for mainstream services and ceremonies on their own country; however, the babies may be buried in mainstream cemeteries or the baby cremated with the mother keeping her baby's ashes. The family will have a traditional tribute to the child with the family gathering at a significant place. There will be a smoking ceremony that heals, purifies, strengthens and protects the baby's soul. Every year the mother and her family will go out to the site to honour the child.

To date very little research has been done on Aboriginal women's perinatal 'Sorry Business'. The knowledge around this is sacred and should be respected as such.

FACTS AND FIGURES YOU SHOULD KNOW

Definitions—mortality

- *Miscarriage*—baby born with no signs of life before 20 weeks of pregnancy, or weighing <400 g. (Regardless of gestational age or weight, if there are signs of life, such as breathing, beating of the heart, pulsation of the umbilical cord, or definite movement of voluntary muscles, then this is termed a live birth—even if prior to 20 weeks.)
- *Therapeutic termination of pregnancy (TOP)*—pregnancy medically terminated for reasons as decreed by a country's legal system, e.g. fetal abnormality incompatible with viability / reasonable quality of life, maternal mental health significantly threatened. Fetus dies during process or shortly after, usually.
- *Stillbirth*—baby born after 20 completed weeks gestation, or birth weight ≥400 g, who shows no sign of life at birth; it is also termed 'fetal death'.
- *Neonatal death*—the death of a baby that occurs during the first 28 days of life. This may be subdivided into early neonatal deaths, occurring during the first 7 days of life, and late neonatal deaths, occurring after the seventh day but before 28 completed days of life.
- *Sudden unexpected death in infancy (SUDI), previously sudden infant death syndrome (SIDS)*—death of a neonate or an infant where the postmortem fails to diagnose cause of death. Some of these can occur in the first 6 weeks after birth.
- *Infant mortality rate*—rate per 1000 live births, of deaths of babies from birth to 1 year of age.
- Perinatal mortality rates (Table 43.1):
  - in Australia, measured as rate of babies who die from age 20 weeks gestation up to 28 days after birth, out of 1000 live and stillborn babies, per year
  - in New Zealand, the rate of babies who die from age 20 weeks gestation (or 400 g birth weight) to 168 completed hours (7 days) after birth (early neonatal deaths), out of 1000 live and stillborn babies, per year.
  - in New Zealand, the *perinatal related mortality rate* is the rate of babies who die from age 20 weeks gestation (or 400 g birth weight) up to 28 days after birth (early and late neonatal deaths), out of 1000 live and stillborn.

The legislative requirements for Australian and New Zealand midwives involved with the death of a baby are given in Tables 43.2 and 43.3 respectively.

Another area about which midwives are required to be well informed and prepared is postmortems (Box 43.4).

CRITICAL THINKING EXERCISE

You are caring for family members who experience the unexpected stillbirth of their baby at term. Their religious beliefs prevent them from consenting to a full postmortem for their baby. What alternatives can you suggest to the family that would honour their wishes but might also assist in finding the cause of death of their baby? Locate information and resources about these alternatives so that you are fully aware of what they involve.

Table 43.1 Mortality rates (per year) in Australia and New Zealand

	Australia	New Zealand
Miscarriage	Varies. Best estimate is 15–25% of all pregnancies	
Therapeutic termination of pregnancy (TOP)	General rate per 1000 women of childbearing age 15–44 years[a]:	
	2004: 19.3	2015: 14.2 2016: 13.5 2017: 13.7
Stillbirth	Number of fetal deaths × 1000 divided by total births (live and fetal deaths):	
	2016: 6.7 2017: 7.1 2018: 7.0	2016: 7.6 2017: 7.0 2018: 7.6
Infant mortality rate	Per 1000 live births, of deaths of babies from birth to 1 year of age:	
	2016: 3.1 2017: 3.3 2018: 3.1	2015: 4.3 2016: 4.2 2017: 4.7
SUDI/SIDS[b]	Per 1000 live births, of deaths of babies from birth to 1 year of age[c]:	
	2016: 0.3 2017: 0.3 2018: 0.3	2015: 0.4 2016: 0.4 2017: 0.5
Perinatal mortality rate[d]	Rate of babies who die from age 20 weeks gestation to 28 days after birth, per 1000 live and stillborn babies	Rate of babies who die from age 20 weeks gestation (or 400 g birth weight) to 28 days after birth (early and late neonatal deaths), per 1000 live and stillborn babies
	2016: 9.1 2017: 9.7 2018: 9.4	2016: 10.1 2017: 9.8 2018: 10.2

[a]Estimate only for Australia.
[b]SIDS = sudden infant death syndrome; SUDI = sudden unexpected death in infancy.
[c]In NZ SIDS rate includes deaths where either the underlying or contributing cause of death was SIDS. In Australia it includes underlying cause of death only.
[d]In NZ this is known as perinatal-related mortality to include neonatal deaths < 28 days.
(Sources: Stillbirths and neonatal deaths in Australia, 2017 and 2018 (AIHW, 2021); Stillbirths and neonatal deaths in Australia, 2015 and 2016 (AIHW, 2019); PMMRC 14th Annual Report (Perinatal and Maternal Mortality Review Committee, 2021); Births and Deaths: Year Ended December 2015 (Statistics New Zealand, 2016); Abortion Statistics: Year Ended December 2017 (Statistics New Zealand, 2018); Causes of Death, Australia 2016 (Australian Bureau of Statistics, 2017); Causes of Death, Australia 2017 (Australian Bureau of Statistics, 2018); Causes of Death, Australia 2018 (Australian Bureau of Statistics, 2019); NZ Ministry of Health Fetal and Infant Deaths 2016 (Ministry of Health, 2019); NZ Ministry of Health Fetal and Infant Deaths web tool (Ministry of Health, 2020))

REFLECTIVE THINKING EXERCISE

Midwives need to be aware of their own views about bereavement, death and grieving. Take the time to work through these reflective exercises. Choose *when* and *how* you do this work. You might:

- return to it over several weeks at quiet times
- record your thoughts in your journal
- talk about some aspects with a friend, colleague or professional supervisor.

1. Think about a situation where you 'lost' something. It does not need to be a person; it might just be a set of keys or your wallet.
   a. What were your feelings?
   b. What did you think about?
   c. What did you do?
   d. To whom did you turn for help?
2. What are your thoughts about your own death?
   a. If you could choose, how old would you like to be when you die?
   b. If you could choose, how would you like to die?
   c. How would you like your funeral to be?
   d. Have you made a will?
3. How has the death of a family member or a friend affected you? What is the story that you would tell about this death and the effect it has had for you in terms of feelings, how you coped, who helped you?
4. What are the practices/rituals that you have taken part in, after the death of a person?

Table 43.2 Legislative requirements of Australian midwives involved with the death of a baby

Miscarriage	The birth does not need to be registered. The legal role of the midwife varies from state to state. Example: Western Australia (WA) has a multidisciplinary approach. Midwives are part of a team that includes an obstetrician, GP, social worker and chaplain. Consent is required for funeral arrangements such as cremation at the hospital and return of ashes, or interment in a memorial garden; there is an option for families to take the baby home and bury, whereby a disclaimer is required.
Therapeutic termination	After 20 weeks gestation, the birth needs to be registered and a Medical Certificate of Cause of Death needs to be completed. If the baby is born alive at any gestation, including termination, even if the only sign of life is a pulsing cord, a Notification of Birth for Registration must be completed by the parents.
Stillbirth	If a Medical Certificate of Cause of Death has been issued and if the coroner is *not* involved then a Notification of Birth for Registration, which includes acknowledgement of the baby's death (stillbirth), is completed by the parents. The certificate must be completed by a medical officer, or coroner if it is a coronial case.
Neonatal death	The birth must be registered, as must the death. If the coroner is *not* involved then a Medical Certificate of Cause of Death must be completed by a medical officer. A Notification of Death for Registration is completed by the parents or their representative, e.g. funeral director, within 3 working days after disposal of the body.

(Sources: Births, Deaths and Marriages Registration Act [NZ] 1995; Births, Deaths, Marriages and Relationships Registration Amendment Act [NZ] 2008; Burial and Cremation Act [NZ] 1964)

Table 43.3 Legislative requirements of New Zealand midwives involved with the death of a baby

Miscarriage	Neither a birth nor a death needs to be registered. The midwife advises the family that the baby may be cremated or buried, or disposed of by the hospital (may be incinerated or cremated). If the baby is being buried at a cemetery or being cremated, the midwife writes a letter for the family confirming that the baby's death was defined as miscarriage.
Therapeutic termination	After 20 weeks gestation, the birth needs to be registered and a Medical Certificate of Cause of Death needs to be completed. If the baby is born alive at any gestation, including termination, even if the only sign of life is a pulsing cord, a Notification of Birth for Registration (BDM27) must be completed by the parents.
Stillbirth	Either the 'occupier' of the hospital or the midwife must notify Births, Deaths & Marriages (BD&M) of the stillbirth, within 5 working days. A Medical Certificate of Cause of Fetal and Neonatal Death (HP4721) must be completed by the midwife or doctor, *or* a Coroner's Order must be issued.
	If a Medical Certificate of Cause of Death has been issued, i.e. if the Coroner is *not* involved, then a Notification of Birth for Registration (BDM27), which includes acknowledgement of the baby's death (stillbirth), is completed by the parents.
Neonatal death	The midwife must notify BD&M of the birth. If the baby subsequently dies at any age, and the Coroner is *not* involved, i.e. Medical Certificate of Cause of Death has been completed, a Notification of Death for Registration (BDM28) is completed by the parents or their representative, e.g. midwife or funeral director, within 3 working days after disposal of the body.

(Sources: Births, Deaths and Marriages Registration Act [NZ] 1995; Births, Deaths, Marriages and Relationships Registration Amendment Act [NZ] 2008; Burial and Cremation Act [NZ] 1964)

Box 43.4 Postmortems

The issue of postmortem will arise for most parents of stillborn babies and all those who are bereaved following sudden unexpected death in infancy (SUDI). Postmortems are a legal requirement when requested by the coroner because a medical practitioner cannot certify the cause of death.

Families need to have an explanation of what is involved and the opportunity to ask questions of a healthcare professional who is experienced and familiar with postmortems. This person must also know how to work with the particular cultural and spiritual preferences of families (e.g. a paediatric or perinatal pathologist, or an obstetrician/paediatrician). This is particularly important to address any concerns families may have about having body organs and tissues being retained by the pathologist for research or future investigation. It is also important to explain to families that, if they are concerned about a full autopsy, there are alternatives such as a limited autopsy, a step-wise examination or an external examination only. An experienced perinatal pathologist can assist parents by explaining the different approaches. Consent must always be given for such procedures.

Generally, a preliminary report is sent to the treating doctor within a few weeks of the autopsy. It may take several months for the final report to be ready, at which time the family should be offered the opportunity to meet or talk with a doctor to discuss the findings. The coroners' websites in New Zealand and in Australia provide clear information about postmortems, and information for both clinicians and families is available from the Stillbirth CRE website (https://stillbirthcre.org.au/). Sometimes there may be significant delays in receiving the postmortem results, which may result in additional stress for the family, particularly if they are concerned about future pregnancies.

There are two questions that most families ask:

1. *Why do a postmortem?* Answer: because it can provide information about the cause of death which may also be relevant for future pregnancies. The results of a postmortem could also help other families in the future.
2. *What happens in a postmortem?* Answer: it is a respectful operation undertaken by a skilled doctor over a period of several hours. It involves incisions to the chest (partial postmortem) and/or back of the head (full postmortem). Tissues are examined, samples may be sent for analysis if families give consent, and organs are examined and weighed. The organs are replaced unless consent has been given for them to be examined further; the incisions are then sutured and covered with a dressing. There are other options for partial or step-wise postmortem examinations that are available.

If at all possible, when English is the family's second language use an interpreter.

Be evidently knowledgeable—speak confidently and honestly about the legalities, physiology and pathology. If you cannot supply an explanation, then tell them this and find the appropriate resource or person to clarify it for them. Good resources for clinicians are the PSANZ *Clinical Practice Guideline for Care Around Stillbirth and Neonatal Death*, which can be obtained from the Centre of Research Excellence in Stillbirth website (see Online resources).

(Source: Perinatal Society of Australia and New Zealand, https://stillbirthcre.org.au/researchers-clinicians/download-resources/clinical-practice-guidelines-and-position-statements/)

Conclusion

Grief and grieving is experienced and expressed differently by individuals, cultures, religions and genders. There is no right or wrong way to grieve and as midwives your role is to walk the journey with women and their families as they make a life-changing transition. Although it is not your journey to make, you can guide the women and families under your care to ensure they have a safe and respectful space and support them to make memories of their baby by providing them with information, choices and support. We hope this little walk in our shoes will provide you with some tools as you care for women and their families following the death of a baby. Don't try to understand it as you never will. Learn to be there and to accept that whatever the person says the experience is for them, that is how it is. Don't try to rush them through grief or decisions and most importantly don't ever think parents and families get over it; we know, however, that with good care, time and understanding most people can have wonderfully meaningful lives following the death of a baby.

The reality is that you will grieve forever. You will not 'get over' the loss of a loved one; you will learn to live with it. You will heal and you will rebuild yourself around the loss you have suffered. You will be whole again but you will never be the same. Nor should you be the same, nor would you want to.

Elisabeth Kübler-Ross

Review questions

1. What, if any, differences do you think that differing countries of origin for sample groups might have on research findings about bereavement stages and phases?
2. Looking at the different experiences of Hannah and Natasha, what difference do you think continuity of carer made to Hannah's experience?
3. We can't always work in a continuity-of-carer model. What sorts of things could you do if you were caring for a woman you hadn't previously met who had a stillborn baby? If you had been caring for Natasha and her family, what could you have done to make their experience better?

Acknowledgements

About our contributors:

Vicki Culling PhD is the principal trainer for Vicki Culling Associates, a NZ company that specialises in perinatal and infant loss training for health and caring professionals.

Gary Sillett is a director of Pillars of Strength and a bereaved dad.

Tanya Martin is the Clinical Rural and Remote Coordinator-Poche Centre for Indigenous Health RN/RM and Associate Lecturer in Nursing and Midwifery at the University of Sydney.

Jo Hunter is a midwife working in private practice in the Blue Mountains area of Sydney. Prior to becoming a midwife, Jo worked as a mothercraft nurse in the UK, then as a birth and postnatal doula and childbirth educator.

Hannah discuses being a midwife and a mother who lost two babies on the following podcast:

http://circleofbirth.com/e30-mother-midwife-professor-hannah-dahlen-shares-stories-midwifery-birth-loss/.

Online resources

Asia Pacific Coroners Society: http://www.asiapacificcoroners.org/links/.

Australian Government mothers and babies statistics: https:// www.aihw.gov.au/reports-statistics/population-groups/mothers-babies/overview.

New Zealand Coroners: https://coronialservices.justice.govt.nz/.

New Zealand Ministry of Health fetal death statistics: http://www.health.govt.nz/nz-health-statistics/health-statistics-and-datasets/fetal-and-infant-death-data-and-stats.

New Zealand Perinatal and Maternal Mortality Review Committee: http://www.hqsc.govt.nz/our-programmes/mrc/pmmrc/.

PSANZ *Clinical Practice Guideline for Care Around Stillbirth and Neonatal Death*: https://stillbirthcre.org.au/researchers-clinicians/download-resources/clinical-practice-guidelines-and-position-statements/.

Vicki Culling Associates—online resources and training for health professionals and parents around perinatal and infant loss: http://vca.co.nz/.

Information, contacts, forums about specific situations of loss

Bears of Hope: http://www.bearsofhope.org.au.

Centering Corporation provides education on grief and loss for professionals: http://www.centering.org/.

Heartfelt volunteer photographers: www.heartfelt.org.au.

Support and information about death of a twin / triplet: https://www.miraclebabies.org.au/content/loss-of-your-twin-triplet-or-higher-multiple-babies/gjssmw.

The Lost Ones: http://www.thelostones.co.nz.

Support and information for families after stillbirth, newborn and infant death in NZ and Australia:

Australian Centre for Grief and Bereavement: http://www.grief.org.au.

National Association for Loss and Grief (NALAG): http://www.nalag.org.au/.

Red Nose (AU): https://rednose.com.au/.

SIDS and Kids (NZ): http://www.sidsandkids.org.nz.

Stillbirth and Newborn Death Support (AU): http://www.sands.org.au.

Stillbirth and Newborn Death Support (NZ): http://www.sands.org.nz.

Stillbirth Centre of Research Excellence: https://stillbirthcre.org.au/parents/care-after-loss/.

References

Albom M. *Tuesdays with Morrie: An Old Man, a Young Man and Life's Greatest Lesson*. New York: Doubleday; 1997:24.

Australian *Bureau of Statistics. Causes of Death 2016—3303.0.* Canberra: ABS; 2017.

Australian *Bureau of Statistics. Causes of Death 2017—3303.0.* Canberra: ABS; 2018.

Australian *Bureau of Statistics. Causes of Death 2018—3303.0.* Canberra: ABS; 2019.

Australian Institute of Health and Welfare (AIHW). *Stillbirths and neonatal deaths in Australia 2015 and 2016. Perinatal statistics series no. 36. Cat. no. PER 102*. Canberra: AIHW; 2019.

Australian Institute of Health and Welfare (AIHW). *Stillbirths and neonatal deaths in Australia 2017 and 2018. Perinatal statistics series no. 38. Cat. no. PER 115*. Canberra: AIHW; 2021.

Barks C. *Rumi: The Book of Love: Poems of Ecstasy and Longing*. New York: Harper Collins Publishers; 2003:35.

Births, Deaths and Marriages Registration Act [NZ]. Wellington: New Zealand Government; 1995.

Births, Deaths, Marriages and Relationships Registration Amendment Act [NZ]. Wellington: New Zealand Government; 2008.

Burden C, Bradley S, Storey C, et al. From grief, guilt pain and stigma to hope and pride – a systematic review and meta-analysis of mixed-method research of the psychosocial impact of stillbirth. *BMC Pregnancy Childbirth*. 2016;16(1):9–9.

Burial and Cremation Act [NZ]. Wellington: New Zealand Government; 1964.

Cacciatore J, Radestad I, Froen F. Effects of contact with stillborn babies on maternal anxiety and depression. *Birth*. 2008;35(4):313–320.

Culling V. What Can Midwives Learn From Bereaved Parents? A presentation for SANDS Fifth National Conference, October 2005, Wellington: SANDS; unpublished. 2005.

Dahlen H. A love that never ends. *Birth Matters*. 2009;13(1).

De Frain JD, Jakub DK, Mendoza BL. The psychological effects of sudden infant death on grandmothers and grandfathers. *Omega (Westport)*. 1991;24(3):165–182.
Ellis A, Chebsey C, Storey C, et al. Systematic review to understand and improve care after stillbirth: a review of parents' and healthcare professionals' experiences. *BMC Pregnancy Childbirth*. 2016;16:16.
Fenwick J, Jennings B, Downie J, et al. Providing perinatal loss care: satisfying and dissatisfying aspects for midwives. *Women Birth*. 2007;20:153–160.
Flenady V, Oats J, Gardener G, et al. for the PSANZ Care Around the Time of Stillbirth and Neonatal Death Guidelines group. *Clinical Practice Guideline for Care Around Stillbirth and Neonatal Death. Version 3*. Brisbane, Australia: NHMRC Centre of Research Excellence in Stillbirth; 2018. Online: https://stillbirthcre.org.au/researchers-clinicians/download-resources/clinical-practice-guidelines-and-position-statements/.
Forrest GC, Standish E, Baum JD. Support after perinatal death: a study of support and counselling after perinatal bereavement. *BMJ*. 1982;285:1475–1479.
Gibran K. *The Prophet*. London: Heinemann; 1979. (Originally published 1923 in New York by Alfred A. Knopf.)
Hennegan JM, Henderson J, Redshaw M. Contact with the baby following stillbirth and parental mental health and well-being: a systematic review. *BMJ Open*. 2015;5:e008616.
Hennegan JM, Henderson J, Redshaw M. Is partners' mental health and well-being affected by holding the baby after stillbirth? Mothers' accounts from a national survey. *J Reprod Infant Psychol*. 2018;36(2):120–31.
Horey D, Boyle F, Cassidy J, et al. Parents' experiences of care offered after stillbirth: An international online survey of high and middle-income countries. *Birth*. 2021;00;1–9.
Hughes P, Turton P, Hopper E, et al. Assessment of guidelines for good practice in psychosocial care of mothers after stillbirth: a cohort study. *Lancet*. 2002;360:114–118.
Kobler K, Limbo R, Kavanaugh K. Meaningful moments: the use of ritual in perinatal and pediatric death. *Am J Matern Child Nurs*. 2007;32(5):289–295.
Koopmans L, Wilson T, Cacciatore J, et al. Support for mothers, fathers and families after perinatal death. *Cochrane Database Syst Rev*. 2013;(6):CD000452. doi:10.1002/14651858.CD000452.pub3.
Lewis CS. *A Grief Observed*. New York: HarperCollins; 1961:11–15.
Lockton J, Due C, Oxlad M. Love, Listen and Learn: Grandmothers' Experiences of Grief Following Their Child's Pregnancy Loss. *Women Birth*. 2020;33(4):401–7.
Lundqvist A, Nilstun T, Dykes AK. Both empowered and powerless: mothers' experiences of professional care when their newborn dies. *Birth*. 2002;29(3):192–199.
Ministry of Health (MOH). *Fetal and Infant Deaths 2016*. Wellington: Ministry of Health; 2019.
Ministry of Health (MOH). *Fetal and Infant Deaths web tool*. 2020. Online: https://minhealthnz.shinyapps.io/fetal-and-infant-deaths-web-tool/.
Murphy S, Jones KS. By the way knowledge: Grandparents, stillbirth and neonatal death. *Hum Fertil (Camb)*. 2014;17(3):210–3.
Perinatal and Maternal Mortality Review Committee (PMMRC). Fourteenth Annual Report of the Perinatal and Maternal Mortality Review Committee. Reporting Mortality and morbidity 2018. Wellington: Health Quality & Safety Commission Perinatal and Maternal Mortality Review Committee; 2021.
Sands Australia. *Sands Australian Principles of Bereavement Care—Miscarriage, Stillbirth and Newborn Death*; 2018.
Statistics New Zealand. *Births and Deaths: Year Ended December 2015*. 2016. Online: http://www.stats.govt.nz/browse_for_stats/population/births/BirthsAndDeaths_HOTPYeDec15.aspx.
Statistics New Zealand. *Abortion Statistics: Year Ended December 2017*. 2018. Online: https://www.stats.govt.nz/information-releases/abortion-statistics-year-ended-december-2017.
Swan N. *A Stillborn Inequity. Health report*. N.d. Online: http://www.abc.net.au/radionational/programs/healthreport/a-stillborn-inequity/7835698.

Further reading

Miscarriage and perinatal death specifically
Clendon-Miller N. *Life After Baby Loss: A Guide to Pregnancy and Infant Loss and Subsequent Pregnancy in New Zealand*. Auckland: Tandem Press; 2003.
Faldet R, Fitton K, eds. *Our Stories of Miscarriage*. Minneapolis: Fairview Press; 1997.
Hindmarch C. *On the Death of a Child*. 2nd ed. Oxford: Radcliffe Medical Press; 2000.
Kohner N, Henley A. *When a Baby Dies: The Experience of Late Miscarriage, Stillbirth and Neonatal Death*. New York: Routledge; 2001.
Moulder C. *Miscarriage: Women's Experiences and Needs*. 3rd ed. London: Routledge; 2001.
Radestad I. *When a Meeting is Also Farewell*. Cheshire, UK. Hale: Books for Midwives; 2000.
Spence A (compiler). *Our Babies Have Died: Stories of Miscarriage, Stillbirth and Neonatal Death*. South Yarra: Michelle Anderson Publishing; 2008.

Death of a baby, including neonatal death and SUDI
Fleming P, Sidebotham P. *Unexpected Death in Childhood: a Handbook for Practitioners*. Chichester: Wiley; 2008.
Hindmarch C. *On the Death of a Child*. 2nd ed. Oxford: Radcliffe Medical Press; 2000.
Nicol M. *Loss of a Baby. Death of a Dream*. Sydney: HarperCollins; 1997.
Warland J. *The Midwife and the Bereaved Family*. Melbourne: Ausmed; 2000.

For grandparents
Cerza Kolf J. *Grandma's Tears*. Grand Rapids, MI: Baker Books; 1995.
Gerner M. *For Bereaved Grandparents*. Omaha, NE: Centering Corporation; 2008.
Leininger L, Ilse S. *Grieving Grandparents*. Wayzata, MN: Pregnancy and Infant Loss Center; 1985.
Schwiebert P. *A Grandparent's Sorrow*. Omaha, NE: Centering Corporation; 2008.

For siblings
Gryte M. *No New Baby*. Omaha, NE: Centering Corporation; 2008.
Johnson M, Johnson J. *Where's Jess?* Omaha, NE: Centering Corporation; 2008.
Lamb J, Dodge N. *Sharing with Thumpy: My Story of Love and Grief*. Omaha, NE: Centering Corporation; 2008.
There are many journal and blog sites for children and teenagers, e.g. 'Fire in my heart', on the Centering Corporation website: http://www.centering.org/.

About some rituals and beliefs
Field D, Hockey J, Small N, eds. *Death, Gender and Ethnicity*. London: Routledge; 1997.
Ho S, Brotherson SE. Cultural influences on parental bereavement in Chinese families. *Omega (Westport)*. 2007;55(1):1–25.
Hockey J, Katz J, Small N, eds. *Grief, Mourning and Death Ritual*. Buckingham: Open University Press; 2001:185–211.
Parkes CM, Laungani P, Young B, eds. *Death and Bereavement Across Cultures*. London: Routledge; 1997.

Statutes
Births, Deaths, and Marriages Registration Act 1995 [NZ].
Births, Deaths, Marriages and Relationships Registration Amendment Act [NZ].
Burial and Cremation Act 1964 [NZ].

Films
Hannah's Story by Shea Caplice
Men and Grief by Shea Caplice

Photo credits

p. 37 Fig 2.12 'The mother of all marches'—home-birth protest, Canberra, 7 September 2009 (Photo: Sue Kruske)

p. 129 Fig 7.2 Auscultation of baby's heart with Pinard stethoscope (Reproduced with the permission of the New Zealand College of Midwives)

p. 131 Fig 7.3 Range of body postures to be supported (Source: Bianca Lepori, 1994, Freedom of movement in birth places)

p. 134 Fig 7.4 Courtyard garden at the Helensville Birth Centre, NZ, providing a private, calming, natural environment. (Source: Helensville Birthing Centre. Helensville Birthing Centre. http://www.helensvillebc.co.nz/)

p. 134 Fig 7.5 Comparing a space for observation and intervention (top) with a space for private birth (below) (Sources: (above) iStockphoto/baranozdemir; (below) iStockphoto/thelinke)

p. 361 Fig 17.1 Example of text message received by a midwife (Image courtesy the author (SM))

p. 381 Fig 17.7 Tūranga Kaupapa poster (© Ngā Maia)

p. 513 Fig 23.1 Antenatal visit (Reproduced with the permission of the New Zealand College of Midwives)

p. 529 Fig 23.2 A midwife taking an antenatal blood pressure recording (Reproduced with the permission of the New Zealand College of Midwives)

p. 532 Fig 23.3 Abdominal palpation (Reproduced with the permission of the New Zealand College of Midwives)

p. 539 Fig 23.14 An antenatal Doppler assessment (Reproduced with the permission of the New Zealand College of Midwives)

p. 622 Fig 27.1 The growing popularity of water birth is largely due to the women who have experienced its benefits (Photograph copyright David Hancock.)

p. 624 Fig 27.2 The relaxing effect of water immersion during labour (Photograph copyright David Hancock.)

p. 632 Fig 27.3 Partner support during a water birth (Photograph copyright David Hancock.)

p. 684 Fig 30.1 Maternal transitions

p. 731 Fig 31.4 Calibrated mat for measuring crown–heel length

p. 732 Fig 31.5 Posture: (a) term posture (flexed); (b) pre-term posture (extended) (Source: Thureen et al., 2005)

p. 732 Fig 31.6 Scarf sign: (a) full-term infant; (b) pre-term infant (Source: Thureen et al., 2005)

p. 737 Fig 31.9 Port wine stain (Source: Callen et al., 2000)

p. 738 Fig 31.10 Strawberry naevus: (a) 4 days after birth; (b) 6 weeks after birth (Source: Thureen et al., 2005)

p. 738 Fig 31.11 Skin variations: (a) vernix caseosa; (b) and (c) erythema toxicum; (d) *Candida* dermatitis; (e) hyperpigmented macules; (f) harlequin sign; (g) 'stork bites' (Source: Thureen et al., 2005; photograph (g) Eichenfield LF 2015)

p. 740 Fig 31.12 Abdominal palpation: liver (Source: Davies L, McDonald S. *Examination of the Newborn and Neonatal Health.* 2nd ed. 2020. London: Elsevier; 2021: p. 26)

p. 740 Fig 31.13 Abdominal palpation: spleen (Source: Davies L, McDonald S. *Examination of the Newborn and Neonatal Health.* 2nd ed. 2020. London: Elsevier; 2021: p. 27)

p. 741 Fig 31.14 Abdominal palpation: kidneys (Source: Davies L, McDonald S. *Examination of the Newborn and Neonatal Health.* 2nd ed. 2020. London: Elsevier; 2021: p. 27)

p. 741 Fig 31.15 Femoral pulses (Source: Davies L, McDonald S. *Examination of the Newborn and Neonatal Health.* 2nd ed. 2020. London: Elsevier; 2021: p. 27)

p. 742 Fig 31.16 Ventral suspension (Source: Fraser & Cooper, 2009)

p. 743 Fig 31.17 Traction response (Source: Fraser & Cooper, 2009)

p. 743 Fig 31.19 Moro reflex (Source: Davies L, McDonald S. *Examination of the Newborn and Neonatal Health.* 2nd ed. 2020. London: Elsevier; 2021: p. 34)

p. 744 Fig 31.20 Ortolani's test (Source: Davies L, McDonald S. *Examination of the Newborn and Neonatal Health.* 2nd ed. 2020. London: Elsevier; 2021: p. 33)

p. 744 Fig 31.21 Barlow's test (Source: Davies L, McDonald S. *Examination of the Newborn and Neonatal Health.* 2nd ed. 2020. London: Elsevier; 2021: p. 33)

p. 767 Fig 32.5 The nine newborn instinctual behavioural phases (Dr Kajsa Brimdyr, Healthy Children Project)

p. 769 Fig 32.6 Mother–infant positioning (Copyright: Charly Rose Photography)

p. 769 Fig 32.7 Wide-open mouth, head slightly extended, chin touching the breast (Copyright: Charly Rose Photography)

p. 769 Fig 32.8 Anchoring bottom lip onto the areola (Copyright: Charly Rose Photography)

p. 769 Fig 32.9 Infant–breast latching—nose free, chin touching breast (Copyright: Charly Rose Photography)

p. 827 Fig 34.2 Female condom (Femidom) (Source: Guillebaud, 2009)

p. 827 Fig 34.3 The CAYA (Source: Terri Foran)

p. 828 Fig 34.4 Intrauterine contraceptive devices: (a) Copper-T 380; (b) Multiload Cu 375; (c) Mirena (Source: Contraceptive Flipchart—SHine SA; (c) SHINE SA)

p. 830 Fig 34.5 Contraceptive implant (Implanon) (Source: Shutterstock/Akkalak Aiempradit)

p. 834 Fig 34.6 Hormonal vaginal contraceptive ring (NuvaRing) (Source: WikimediaCommons/Sakky)

p. 873 Fig 36.2 Anteroposterior diameters of a newborn head: for occiput anterior delivery, the suboccipitobregmatic diameter (green) typically passes through the outlet and over the perineal body. For occiput posterior deliveries, the larger occipitofrontal (yellow) or occipitomental (red) diameters typically pass through the outlet as a result of extension of the fetal head. (Source: Barth, 2015)

p. 888 Fig 36.9 The art of vaginal breech: (a) 7.45 a.m.: the mother-to-be is on all fours talking to her husband while the attending midwife (vB-S) calmly awaits further events. (b) The hips progressively descend with the sacrum in the anterior position. (c) The lower part of the body in the frank breech position progressively distends the perineum. The mother is encouraged to continue to push. (d) Watchful waiting. At this stage of birth, the hands of the attending midwife do not touch the lower part of the body of the baby. (e) The left leg of the baby has now been born spontaneously, while the right leg remains in flexion, with extension at the knee. The cord is clearly visible. (f) The attending midwife applies both hands at the trunk and both legs of the baby while the mother is encouraged to push. (g) Following the spontaneous release of both arms, the midwife ushers the body of the baby with gentle anterior and downward traction. (h) The body continues to descend until the head becomes visible. (i) 8.04 a.m.: the baby is born. (j) The first gasps of the baby while she is shown to her parents (Reproduced from Wildschut HIJ, van Belzen-Slappendel H, Jans S. The art of vaginal breech birth at term on all fours. *Clin Case Rep*. 2017;5(2):182–186, with permission of Hinke van Belzen-Slappendel, Midwife, Independent Midwifery Practice)

p. 1012 Fig 39.11 Baby with a chignon (Source: Henderson & Macdonald, 2004)

p. 1079 Fig 40.16 Starting chest compressions and pulling the gravid uterus laterally (Source: Saksena & Camm, 2012. Figure 73-8B. *Electrophysiological Disorders of the Heart*. 2nd ed. ©2005, 2012 by Saunders, an imprint of Elsevier Inc.)

p. 1098 Fig 41.1 The woman sits on an armrest with legs apart, feet on the floor, flexed hips and straight back with the perineum resting on the armrest. The instruction is to squeeze around the pelvic openings and lift the skin away from the armrest without rising up or putting any pressure on the feet (Source: Bø K & Mørkved S, 2015)

Index

Page numbers followed by "*f*" indicate figures, "*t*" indicate tables, and "*b*" indicate boxes.

C